Implantable Cardioverter-Defibrillator

Edited by

Igor Singer, MBBS,
FRACP, FACP, FACC, FACA

Associate Professor of Medicine
Chief, Arrhythmia Service
Director of Electrophysiology and Pacing
University of Louisville
Louisville, Kentucky

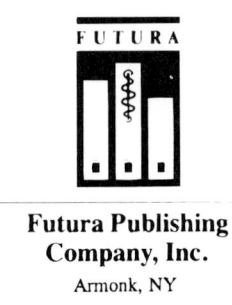

Futura Publishing Company, Inc.
Armonk, NY

Library of Congress Cataloging-in-Publication Data

Implantable cardioverter defibrillator / edited by Igor Singer.
    p.   cm.
   Includes bibliographical references and index.
   ISBN 0-87993-593-6
   1. Implantable cardioverter-defibrillators.   I. Singer, Igor.
   [DNLM: 1. Defibrillators, Implantable.   2. Arrhythmia—therapy.
   3. Death, Sudden, Cardiac—prevention & control. WG 330 I341 1994]
   RC684.E4I465   1994
   617.4′120645—dc20
   DNLM/DLC
   for Library of Congress   94-14074
                                                                    CIP

Copyright © 1994

Published by
Futura Publishing Company, Inc.
135 Bedford Road
Armonk, New York 10504

LC #: 94-14074
ISBN #: 0-87993-593-6

Every effort has been made to ensure that the information in this book is as up to date and accurate as possible at the time of publication. However, due to the constant developments in medicine, neither the author, nor the editor, nor the publisher can accept any legal or any other responsibility for any errors or omissions that may occur.

All rights reserved.

No part of this book may be translated or reproduced in any form without written permission of the publisher.

Printed in the United States of America.

Printed on acid-free paper.

Special thanks for typing and secretarial support to Nancy Mattingly and to Sherry Roark for artwork.

To my wife Sylvia, my children Justin, Jessica, Chrissy and my parents, Dr. D. Singer and Ivan Singer

Contributors

Peter R. Accorti, Jr., MS, BME
Senior Research Engineer,
Telectronics Pacing Systems, Miami,
Florida

John Adams
Vice President of Engineering,
InControl Inc., Redmond, Washington

Lesa Adams, RN, BSN
Cardiovascular Associates, Louisville,
Kentucky

Stuart W. Adler, MD
Cardiovascular Division University of
Minnesota, Minneapolis

Clif A. Alferness, BSEE
InControl Inc., Redmond, Washington

Mark H. Anderson, BSc, MBBS, MRCP
Department of Cardiological Sciences,
St. Georges's Medical School, London,
United Kingdom

Erle Austin, MD, FACS
Professor of Cardiothoracic Surgery,
University of Louisville, Louisville,
Kentucky

Gregory M. Ayers, MD, PhD
InControl Inc., Redmond, Washington

Gust H. Bardy, MD, FACC
Associate Professor of Medicine,
Division of Cardiology, University of
Washington School of Medicine,
Seattle, Washington

S. Serge Barold, MBBS, FRACP, FACP, FACC, FESC
Professor of Medicine, The Genesee
Hospital, University of Rochester,
School of Medicine and Dentistry,
Rochester, New York

David Benditt, MD, FACC
Professor of Medicine, Director of
Cardiac Arrhythmia Service,
University of Minnesota Medical
School, Minneapolis, Minnesota

J. Thomas Bigger, Jr., MD, FACC
Professor of Medicine and
Pharmacology, College of
Physicians & Surgeons of Columbia
University, New York, New York

Susan M. Blanchard, PhD
Assistant Research Professor,
Department of Biomedical
Engineering Duke University,
Durham, North Carolina

Michael Block, MD
Hospital of the Westfälische
Wilhelms-University of Münster,
Department of Cardiology/Angiology
and Institute for Research in
Arteriosclerosis, Münster, Germany

Günter Breithardt, MD, FESC, FACC
Hospital of the Westfälische
Wilhelms-University of Münster,
Department of Cardiology/Angiology
and Institute for Research in
Arteriosclerosis, Münster, Germany

A. John Camm, MD, FACC, FRCP, FESC
Professor of Clinical Cardiology, and
Chairman of Medicine, Department of
Cardiological Sciences, St. George's
Hospital Medical School, London,
United Kingdom

Eric Dolla, MD
Clinical Assistant Professor,
University of Marseille, Marseille,
France

Edwin G. Duffin
Bakken Fellow, Medtronic, Inc., Minneapolis, Minnesota

Andrew E. Epstein, MD, FACC
Professor of Medicine, Division of Cardiovascular Disease, University of Alabama at Birmingham, Birmingham, Alabama

Richard Fogoros, MD, FACC
Director, Clinical Electrophysiology, Allegheny General Hospital, Associate Professor of Medicine, Medical College of Pennsylvania, Pittsburgh, Pennsylvania

Jerry C. Griffin, MD, FACC
Vice President, Medical Affairs, InControl Inc., Redmond, Washington

Gerard Guiraudon, MD, FRCS(C), FACC
Professor of Surgery, University of Western Ontario, London, Ontario, Canada

Raymond E. Ideker, MD, PhD
Professor, Department of Pathology, Professor, Department of Biomedical Engineering, Associate Professor, Department of Medicine, Duke University, Durham, North Carolina

Ross Infinger
InControl Inc., Redmond, Washington

Werner Irnich, PhD
Professor of Biomedical Electronics, Chief, Department of Medical Engineering of the Justus-Liebeg-University Hospital Giessen, Germany

Greg K. Jones, MD
Division of Cardiology, University of Washington School of Medicine, Seattle, Washington

Janice L. Jones, PhD
Chief, Cardiac Research, Georgetown University and Department of Veterans Affairs Medical Center, Washington, D.C.

Werner Jung, MD
Department of Medicine and Cardiology, University of Bonn, Bonn, Germany

G. Neal Kay, MD, FACC
Professor of Medicine, Division of Cardiovascular Disease, University of Alabama at Birmingham, Birmingham, Alabama

Bruce H. KenKnight, MS
Cardiac Pacemakers, Inc., Therapy Research Department, St. Paul, Minnesota

George J. Klein, MD, FRCP(C), FACC
Director of Arrhythmia Service, Professor of Medicine, University of Western Ontario, Ontario, Canada

Helmut Klein, MD, FACC, FESC
Professor of Medicine, Chief, Department of Medicine, Otto-Von-Guericke-University, University Hospital, Magdeburg, Germany

Lawrence S. Klein, MD, FACC
Krannert Institute of Cardiology, Indiana University School of Medicine and the Richard E. Roudebush Veterans's Administration Hospital, Indianapolis, Indiana

Stephen B. Knisley, PhD
Assistant Research Professor, Department of Biomedical Engineering, Duke University, Durham, North Carolina

Theofilos M. Kolettis, MD, PhD
Clinical Research Associate, Arrhythmia and Pacemaker Service, Eastern Heart Institute, and Division of Cardiology, UMDNJ, New Jersey Medical School, Passaic, New Jersey

Douglas J. Lang, PhD
Cardiac Pacemakers, Inc., Therapy Research Department, St. Paul, Minnesota

Keith G. Laurie, MD
Cardiovascular Division, Department of Medicine, University of Minnesota, Minneapolis, Minnesota

Samuel Lévy, MD, FACC, FESC
Professor of Medicine, Chief, Division of Cardiology, University of Marseille, Marseille, France

Berndt Lüderitz, MD, FESC, FACC
Professor of Medicine, Head, Department of Medicine and Cardiology, University of Bonn, Bonn, Germany

Matthias Manz, MD
Associate Professor of Medicine, Director of Cardiac Electrophysiology and Pacing, Department of Medicine and Cardiology, University of Bonn, Bonn, Germany

William M. Miles, MD
Associate Professor of Medicine, Krannert Institute of Cardiology, Indiana University School of Medicine and the Richard E. Roudebush Veteran's Administration Hospital, Indianapolis, Indiana

L. Brent Mitchell, MD, FRCP(C)
Professor and Head, Director of Clinical Electrophysiology, Foothill Hospital, University of Calgary, Canada

Morton Mower, MD, FACP, FACC, FCCP
Visiting Associate Professor of Medicine, The Johns Hopkins University School of Medicine, Baltimore, Maryland, and Vice President of Medical Sciences, Cardiac Pacemakers, Inc., St. Paul, Minnesota

Tibor Nappholz
Vice President, Strategic Research and Development, Telectronics Pacing Systems, Inc., Englewood, Colorado

Seah Nisam
Director, Medical Sciences, CPI Europe, Brussels, Belgium

Walter H. Olson, PhD
Senior Research Fellow, Tachyarrhythmia Research, Medtronic, Inc., Minneapolis, Minnesota

Eliot L. Ostrow, BA
Clinical Research Scientist-Tachycardia Projects, Intermedics, Inc., A company of SULZERmedica, Angleton, Texas

Merritt H. Raitt, MD
Division of Cardiology, University of Washington School of Medicine, Seattle, Washington

Stephen C. Remole, MD
Cardiovascular Division, Department of Medicine, University of Minnesota, Minneapolis, Minnesota

Philippe Ricard, MD
Assistant Professor, University of Marseille, Marseille, France

Scott Sakaguchi, MD
Cardiovascular Division, University of Minnesota, Minneapolis, Minnesota

Sanjeev Saksena, MD, FACC, FCCP
Director, Arrhythmia and Pacemaker Service, Eastern Heart Institute, Passaic, and Clinical Associate Professor of Medicine and Pediatrics, Divisions of Cardiology, UMDNJ-New Jersey Medical School and Children's Hospital of New Jersey, Newark, New Jersey

Gena Sears, RN, BSN
InControl Inc., Redmond, Washington

Igor Singer, MBBS, FRACP, FACP, FACC, FACA
Associate Professor of Medicine, Chief, Arrhythmia Service, Director of Electrophysiology and Pacing, University of Louisville, Louisville, Kentucky

David A. Slater, MD, FACS
Associate Professor of Cardiothoracic Surgery, University of Louisville, Louisville, Kentucky

R. K. Thakur, MD
Department of Surgery and Cardiology, University of Western Ontario, Ontario, Canada

Hans-Joachim Trappe, MD
Department of Cardiology, University Hospital, Hannover, Hannover, Germany

Gregory P. Walcott, MD
Research Associate, Department of Pathology, Duke University, Durham, North Carolina

Kurt Wheeler
InControl Inc., Redmond, Washington

Raymond Yee, MD, FRCP(C), FACC
Director, Arrhythmia Monitoring Unit, University Hospital, London, Ontario, Canada

Preface

Great advances in science are rarely if ever accomplished by the efforts of groups or collective thinkers. Usually, these advances result from the inspiration of a single individual mind and unbending perseverance in the face of myriad obstacles. The birth of the implantable cardioverter-defibrillator (ICD) is no exception. A single individual should be credited not only with the very concept, but with the implementation of a working model of an implantable device to treat ventricular tachycardia and ventricular fibrillation. This individual is the late Dr. Michel Mirowski who labored from the early 1970s through the 1980s until his premature death to bring to fruition perhaps one of the greatest advances in the management of sudden cardiac death. At first, this logical and unique concept had many detractors and some determined enemies, and it still continues to engender emotional and sometimes even illogical opposition in some very knowledgeable circles. This sometimes visceral response is not unique to this invention and usually accompanies any great leap in scientific thinking.

Dr. Mirowski's idea evolved with help and contributions from many scientists, engineers, physicians, surgeons, and many nonmedical experts into a breathtaking array of sophisticated devices capable of multitiered therapies and bradycardia pacing. The methods for implantation of ICDs have evolved from the surgical approaches requiring thoracotomy to transvenous implantation techniques, which offer relative simplicity comparable to pacemaker implantation techniques. With these technological breakthroughs we are at the threshold of new applications for primary prophylaxis of sudden cardiac death, an idea that intrigued Dr. Mirowski at the inception of his original scientific work.

The progress in ICD technology is in fact so rapid that any textbook dealing with the subject risks obsolescence by the time that it is actually published. With this in mind, I have set out to write and compile this textbook *Implantable Cardioverter-Defibrillator* so that it would be generic enough, yet sufficiently specific to be of actual use to physicians, engineers, implanters, cardiology trainees, and practicing electrophysiologists for some time to come.

The textbook is organized in five sections:

The first section provides the basic background and foundation to comprehend the context of the historical development and pathophysiological mechanisms underlying ventricular tachycardia and ventricular fibrillation.

The second section provides the engineering background, and deals with the essential components of ICD therapy, including detection, logic, data processing, defibrillation waveforms, tiered therapy and antitachycardia pacing algorithms, lead design and technology, and also reviews fundamental theories of defibrillation.

The third section describes the current clinical practice of implantable defibrillators, including patient selection, preoperative, operative and postoperative management of ICD therapy; available implantation techniques and patient follow-up are described; and clincial results with thoracotomy and nonthoracotomy lead systems are reviewed. A special chapter deals with controlled clinical trials with ICD therapy, as well as ongoing clinical trials evaluating prophylactic ICD applications. Economic ramifications of ICD therapy are carefully analyzed in light of the currently available information.

The fourth section of the book discusses some available alternatives to ICD management of ventricular dysrrhythmias including pharmacological therapy, surgical, and catheter ablation techniques.

The final section of the book is devoted to future technologies not yet clinically available, but that could, in the next decade, become the next frontier in ICD development. These include implantable atrial defibrillators, dual-chamber defibrillators, and combined infusion pump-ICDs (ICDIs). Some or all of these concepts may come to fruition. Future development is dictated by the perceived needs and available technologies on one hand and the economic realities and constraints on the other.

I am indebted to my many contributors and scientific experts for their excellent contributions. Without their talents this textbook would not be possible.

It is our hope that this textbook will provide a unique resource for the experts, engineers, and clinicians, and all others who care for patients with life-threatening arrhythmias and require use of ICD therapy.

Above all, I remain indebted to Dr. Michel Mirowski whose perseverance, inspiration, and hard work enriched the science and the art of caring for patients at risk for sudden cardiac death. I have personally been extremely fortunate to have been associated with this extraordinary individual whose humanistic qualities were only surpassed by his scientific genius.

Igor Singer

Contents

Contributors vii

Preface xi

Part 1. Basic Concepts

Chapter 1.   Clinical and Historical Perspective
Morton M. Mower 3

Chapter 2.   Ventricular Tachycardia
Igor Singer 13

Chapter 3.   Ventricular Fibrillation
Janice L. Jones 43

Part 2. Engineering Aspects

Chapter 4.   Tachyarrhythmia Sensing and Detection
Walter H. Olson 71

Chapter 5.   Tachyarrhythmia Termination: Lead Systems and Hardware Design
Rahul Mehra and Zach Cybulski 109

Chapter 6.   Defibrillation Theory and its Clinical Impact
Werner Irnich 135

Chapter 7.   Defibrillation Waveforms
Susan M. Blanchard, Stephen B. Knisley, Gregory P. Walcott, and Raymond E. Ideker 153

Chapter 8.   Leads Technology
Peter R. Accorti, Jr. 179

Chapter 9.   A Logical Approach to Tiered-Therapy Implantable Cardioverter-Defibrillator Design
Eliot L. Ostrow 207

Chapter 10. Implant Support Devices
Douglas J. Lang and Bruce H. KenKnight 223

Chapter 11. Device Telemetry
Igor Singer 253

Chapter 12. Antitachycardia Pacing
Berndt Lüderitz, Werner Jung, and Matthias Manz 271

Part 3. Clinical Aspects of Implantable Cardioverter-Defibrillator Therapy

Chapter 13. Indications for Implantable Cardioverter-Defibrillator Therapy
Theofilos M. Kolettis and Sanjeev Saksena 303

Chapter 14. Evaluation of a Prospective Patient for Implantable Cardioverter-Defibrillator Therapy
Michael Block and Günter Breithardt 315

Chapter 15. Operative Techniques for Implantation and Testing of Implantable Cardioverter-Defibrillators
Erle Austin and Igor Singer 327

Chapter 16. Implantation of Cardioverter-Defibrillators in the Electrophysiology Laboratory
Andrew E. Epstein and G. Neal Kay 357

Chapter 17. Unipolar Defibrillation Systems
Gust H. Bardy, Merritt H. Raitt, and Greg K. Jones 365

Chapter 18. Interactions of Implantable Cardioverter-Defibrillators With Antiarrhythmic Drugs and Pacemakers
Igor Singer and David A. Slater 377

Chapter 19. Postoperative Care and Follow-up of Implantable Cardioverter-Defibrillator Patients
Igor Singer and Lesa Adams 389

Chapter 20. Complications of Implantable Cardioverter-Defibrillator Surgery: Diagnosis and Management
Igor Singer 415

Chapter 21. Troubleshooting of Patients With Implantable Cardioverter-Defibrillators
Seah Nisam and Richard N. Fogoros 433

Chapter 22. Programming of Implantable Cardioverter-Defibrillators
Seah Nisam and Richard N. Fogoros 457

Chapter 23. Clinical Results With Implantable Cardioverter-Defibrillator Therapy: An Overview
Igor Singer 471

Chapter 24. Clinical Results With Implantable Cardioverter-Defibrillator Therapy
Hans-Joachim Trappe and Helmut Klein 487

Chapter 25. Clinical Results With Nonthoracotomy Lead Systems and Implications for Implantable Cardioverter-Defibrillator Practice: The European Experience
Samuel Lévy, Philippe Ricard, and Eric Dolla 507

Chapter 26. Primary Prevention of Sudden Cardiac Death Using Implantable Cardioverter-Defibrillators
J. Thomas Bigger, Jr. 515

Chapter 27. The Implantable Cardioverter-Defibrillator: Economic Issues
Mark H. Anderson and A. John Camm 547

Part 4. Alternative Approaches to Implantable Cardioverter-Defibrillator Therapy

Chapter 28. Pharmacological Therapy
L. Brent Mitchell 577

Chapter 29. Surgical Treatment of Ventricular Tachycardia Associated With Coronary Artery Disease
Gerard M. Guiraudon, George J. Klein, Raymond Yee, and R. K. Thakur 615

Chapter 30. Catheter Ablation for Ventricular Tachycardia
William M. Miles and Lawrence S. Klein 633

Part 5. Future Perspectives

Chapter 31. Antitachycardia Pacing and Implantable Cardioverter-Defibrillators for Treatment of Supraventricular Tachyarrhythmias
David G. Benditt, Stuart W. Adler, Stephen C. Remole, Scott Sakaguchi, and Keith G. Lurie 651

Chapter 32. Rationale for an Implantable Atrial Defibrillator
Jerry C. Griffin, Gena Sears, Gregory M. Ayers, John Adams, Clif A. Alferness, Ross Infinger, and Kurt Wheeler 675

Chapter 33. Automated Rhythm Systems
Mark H. Anderson and A. John Camm 687

Chapter 34. Dual Chamber Defibrillator: From Theoretical Concepts to Implementation
Tibor Nappholz 711

Chapter 35. Combination of Drug Delivery Systems and Implantable Cardioverter-Defibrillators: Is There a Possible Future Marriage?
Tibor Nappholz 731

Chapter 36. Implantable Cardioverter-Defibrillators: An Overview and Future Directions
Edwin G. Duffin and S. Serge Barold 751

Index 769

Part 1
Basic Concepts

Chapter 1

Clinical and Historical Perspective

Morton M. Mower

The history of the implantable cardioverter-defibrillator (ICD) is really quite straightforward, spanning almost a quarter of a century.[1,2] It is perhaps no longer apropos to continue to refer to it as being in its "infancy" or that its technology is "immature" as it has progressed quite a long way. It is perhaps because of this very position that some conceptual problems related to the therapy have arisen, which are just now being addressed.

Over the course of the development of the ICD a large number of different individuals became involved in different timeframes and at different places, all of whom were crucial for its ultimate success (Figure 1). The initial development was pioneered in the late 1960s by Dr. Michel Mirowski, who was deeply affected by the death of Dr. Harry Heller, his Chief of Medicine, his mentor, and close personal friend. Dr. Heller had been hospitalized with a short history of recurrent episodes of ventricular arrhythmia. Knowing that any of Dr. Heller's episodes could potentially be life-threatening, and frustrated by the lack of a means for continuous therapeutic intervention, Dr. Mirowski conceived of miniaturizing a defibrillator to a size that could be implanted, similar to a pacemaker, and deliver defibrillating shocks to the heart when required through a transvenous catheter. At this time, external cardiac defibrillation in the coronary care unit and elective cardioversion were becoming known as effective treatments for ventricular fibrillation and atrial fibrillation and flutter, respectively.

A number of observations validated the need for an implantable device. In the United States alone, approximately 450,000 people were thought to be dying of sudden cardiac death each year. Most of these deaths were suspected to be due to ventricular fibrillation. Although mobile advanced life support rescue units had potential, it was acknowledged that most victims of sudden cardiac death outside the hospital could not be reached in time to implement effective external defibrillation therapy.

In 1969, Sinai Hospital of Baltimore was constructing a new Coronary Care Unit and Dr. Mirowski was recruited from Israel to be its first director, a post in which he was to be given considerable time for research. I had received virtually all my postgraduate training at Sinai Hospital, and was a very visible figure in the research laboratories. It was only natural that our Chief of Medicine, Dr. Albert Mendeloff would bring the two of us together to collaborate on the new project. Dr. Mirowski brought with him and presented his idea of an automatic implantable defibrillator. Working in the hospital's clinical engineering and animal research facilities, we designed, constructed, and successfully tested a prototype automatic defi-

---

From Singer I, (ed.) Implantable Cardioverter-Defibrillator. Armonk, NY: Futura Publishing Company, Inc.; © 1994.

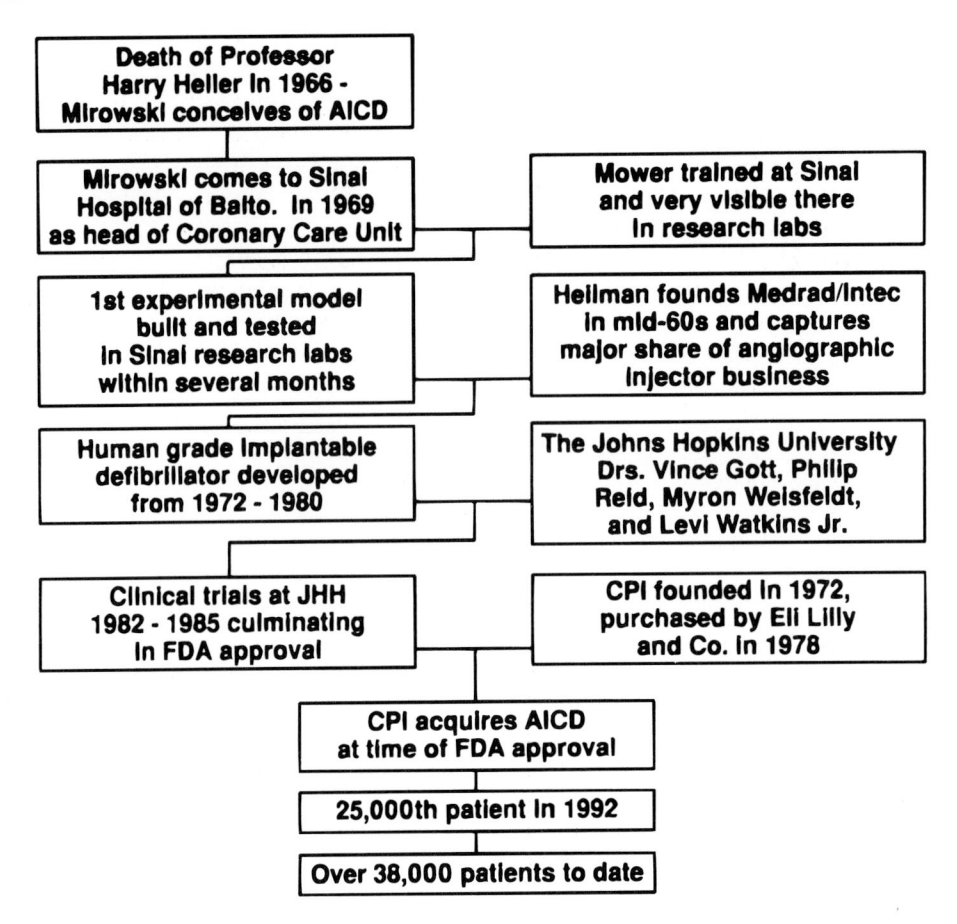

```
┌─────────────────────────┐
│   Death of Professor    │
│  Harry Heller in 1966 - │
│ Mirowski conceives of AICD │
└─────────────────────────┘
         │
┌─────────────────────────┐      ┌─────────────────────────┐
│ Mirowski comes to Sinai │      │  Mower trained at Sinai │
│  Hospital of Balto. In 1969 │──│   and very visible there │
│ as head of Coronary Care Unit │ │    in research labs     │
└─────────────────────────┘      └─────────────────────────┘
         │
┌─────────────────────────┐      ┌─────────────────────────┐
│   1st experimental model │      │ Heilman founds Medrad/Intec │
│      built and tested    │──────│  in mid-60s and captures │
│   in Sinai research labs │      │  major share of angiographic │
│   within several months  │      │    injector business    │
└─────────────────────────┘      └─────────────────────────┘
         │
┌─────────────────────────┐      ┌─────────────────────────┐
│ Human grade implantable │      │ The Johns Hopkins University │
│  defibrillator developed │──────│  Drs. Vince Gott, Philip │
│      from 1972 - 1980    │      │   Reid, Myron Weisfeldt, │
└─────────────────────────┘      │   and Levi Watkins Jr.  │
         │                       └─────────────────────────┘
┌─────────────────────────┐      ┌─────────────────────────┐
│   Clinical trials at JHH │      │   CPI founded in 1972,  │
│  1982 - 1985 culminating │──────│   purchased by Eli Lilly │
│      in FDA approval     │      │     and Co. in 1978     │
└─────────────────────────┘      └─────────────────────────┘
                    │                    │
              ┌─────────────────────────┐
              │   CPI acquires AICD     │
              │  at time of FDA approval │
              └─────────────────────────┘
                        │
              ┌─────────────────────────┐
              │ 25,000th patient in 1992 │
              └─────────────────────────┘
                        │
              ┌─────────────────────────┐
              │ Over 38,000 patients to date │
              └─────────────────────────┘
```

Figure 1. Block diagram indicating how various groups interacted at critical times after the original conception to finally achieve a widely available implantable cardioverter-defibrillator (ICD) device. Note the early training in research of Mower at Sinai Hospital, the founding of a medical device company by Heilman, the development of the cardiovascular division at The Johns Hopkins University, and the development of Eli Lilly and Co.'s interest in cardiovascular devices.

brillator in dogs.[3] This was achieved in less than 3 months, and without any institutional or outside financial support.

During that same time period, a discussion was underway in the medical literature concerning issues of device safety. We were impressed with a published definition that said "a device is safe, when its use is safer for the patient than the prognosis of his disease, and is the best available." Aside from our small group of investigators, the project did not find sympathetic ears in those early days. There were some in the medical and engineering communities who doubted that a workable device would be possible. Even the very concept and possible clinical usefulness were challenged editorially in prominent medical and engineering journals by eminently qualified experts in the fields of cardiology and medical instrumentation. However the disease chosen for attack was a highly lethal one, and there did not appear to be any suitable alternative therapeutic intervention to compete with our approach.

The prototype performed quite reliably in the animal experiments. It was larger than what we would have considered desirable for implantation and the current drain was higher than wanted for long battery life. However, we made no special effort to enhance these features in our original prototype. The goal was simply to demonstrate that such a device could be reasonably designed and constructed to perform the task of automatic defibrillation. The experimental model clearly demonstrated the practicality of the concept.

An investigation to determine human defibrillation requirements was then performed during bypass surgery operations at The Johns Hopkins Hospital, using a catheter electrode in the right ventricular apex and a platinum electrode incorporated onto one of the bypass cannulae in the superior vena cava so as to simulate a single transvenous catheter system (Figure 2). Defibrillation was accomplished using energies of 5–15 J with truncated pulses through this system.[4] Although these experiments validated the effectiveness of low-energy defibrillation shocks through a transvenous catheter system, there were some practical negative aspects of this approach that precluded its use in the initial clinical models. These included the sensitive dependence of the catheter's positioning within the right ventricle for proper functioning, and the possibility of dislodgement of the electrode from the apex. There was also the theoretical possibility of myocardial damage from high-current density through a relatively small electrode surface area.

In 1972 we began collaboration with Medrad Inc. (later Intec Systems was a wholly-owned subsidiary) of Pittsburgh, Pennsylvania that eventually resulted in the development of the clinical model of the automatic implantable defibrillator (Figure 3). One of the initial priorities of this phase of the work was to explore alternatives to the single intravascular catheter system. The experiments clearly indicated that by far the lowest, most consistent, and most stable energy requirements for successful defibrillation were achieved with insulated patch electrodes placed directly on the heart. Truncated exponential waveforms were adopted because they required low peak voltage and current for effective defibrillation and the circuits required to generate them were simple. Initial shocks were delivered at 25 J approximately 15 seconds after detection of ventricular fibrillation.

During the period from 1972–1976, considerable effort was made to optimize

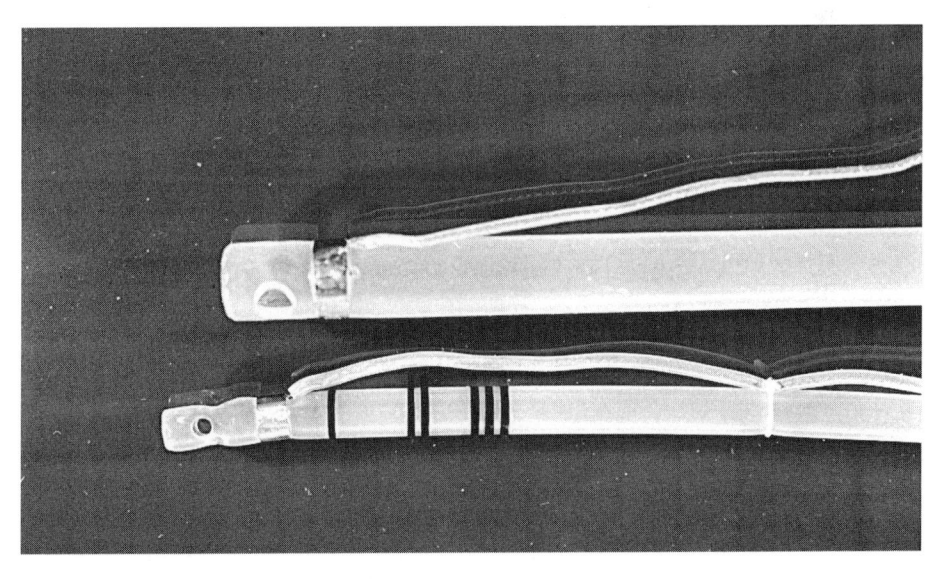

Figure 2. Some of the superior vena cava cannulae incorporating platinum defibrillating electrodes used to simulate a single intravascular defibrillating catheter. The system was used during bypass operations in order to determine energy requirements in human.

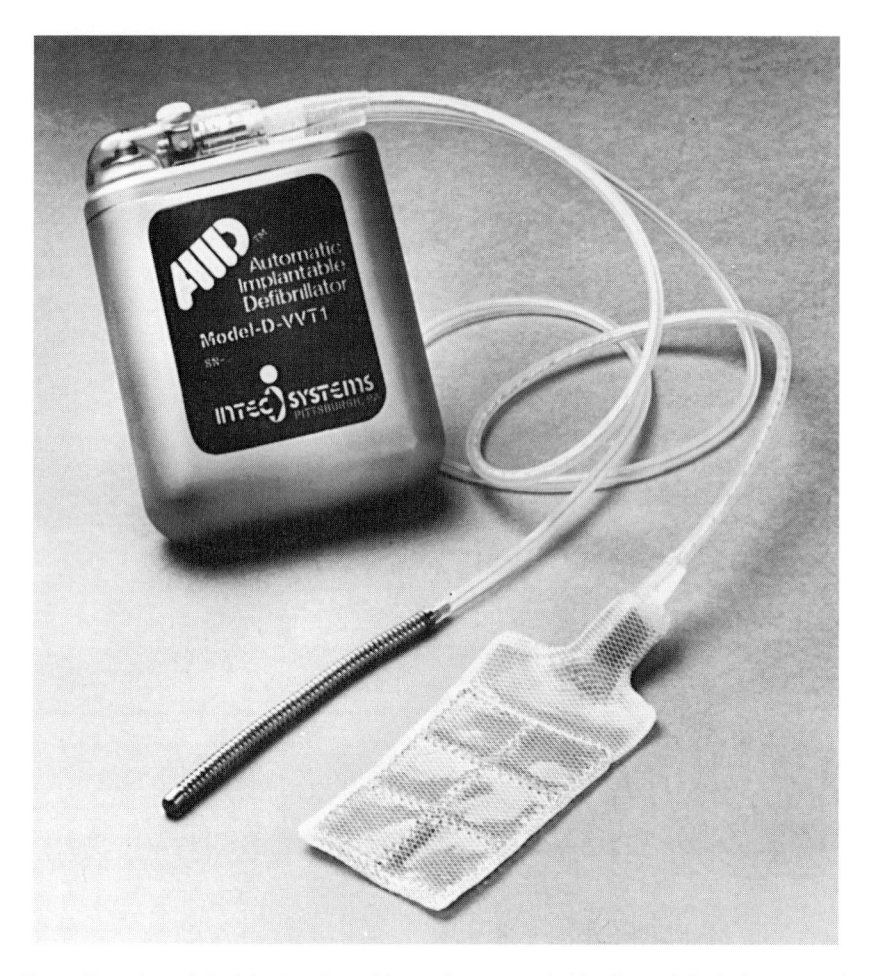

Figure 3. First clinical model of the implantable cardioverter-defibrillator (ICD) shown with superior vena cava catheter and patch electrode.

the design of the defibrillator so that it would eventually be suitable for implantation in humans. Reliability and safety were paramount in the design objectives. A very conscious decision was made to make the device as sensitive as possible, so as never to miss an episode of malignant arrhythmia, even at the cost of delivering some shocks into more normal rhythms.

The clinical device was ready for the first long-term implants in animals in 1976. In order to demonstrate that the device could perform as intended, it was necessary to be able to repeatedly induce ventricular fibrillation on demand in active, conscious animals. An implantable "fibrillator" was designed for this purpose. This unit delivered a fibrillating current of approximately 50 mA directly to the heart of the animal through a right ventricular catheter electrode. This provided a convenient and reliable experimental model of sudden arrhythmic death in active animals. One very important milestone was a motion picture showing the induction and automatic termination of episodes of ventricular fibrillation in such an animal. When this film was shown, a colleague jokingly suggested we had used Pavlovian conditioning to teach the animal to perform such wonderful tricks. We returned to the laboratory to film additional sequences, this time with simul-

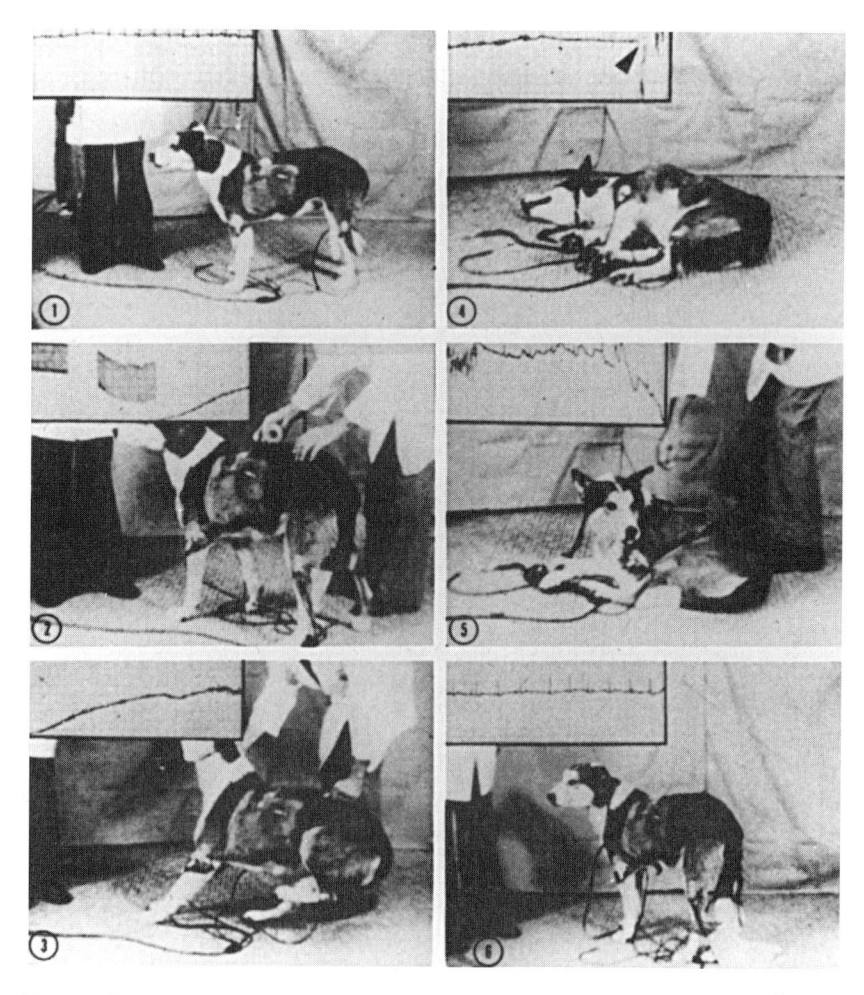

Figure 4. Frames from a motion picture showing induction and automatic reversion of ventricular fibrillation in a conscious animal. Note the superimposed electrocardiogram (ECG) strips in the upper left corner of each frame. Fibrillation and resultant syncope are depicted in frames 2 and 3, the moment of the defibrillating shock in frame 4, frame 5 is immediately after defibrillation, and frame 6 is 15 seconds after defibrillation.

taneous electrocardiogram (ECG) tracings superimposed (Figure 4). Little did we realize that in the very near future, similar fibrillation-defibrillation sequences were to become routine events during clinical electrophysiologic studies.

The first implantation of an ICD device in a human took place on February 4, 1980 at the Johns Hopkins Hospital. This model was eventually implanted in 37 patients and then a second-generation unit incorporating cardioversion was phased into the study. The units appeared to be highly successful in detecting and terminating ventricular fibrillation. Even in those early days, our initial findings were considered striking, and far from what the literature would have predicted the prognosis for repeated cardiac arrest patients to have been and what we inferred the sudden death rate would have been based on an analysis of the symptomatic device firing rate (Figure 5). The original clinical trials lasted from February, 1980 through October, 1985. At that time the ICD received approval from the United States Food and Drug Administration (FDA) for

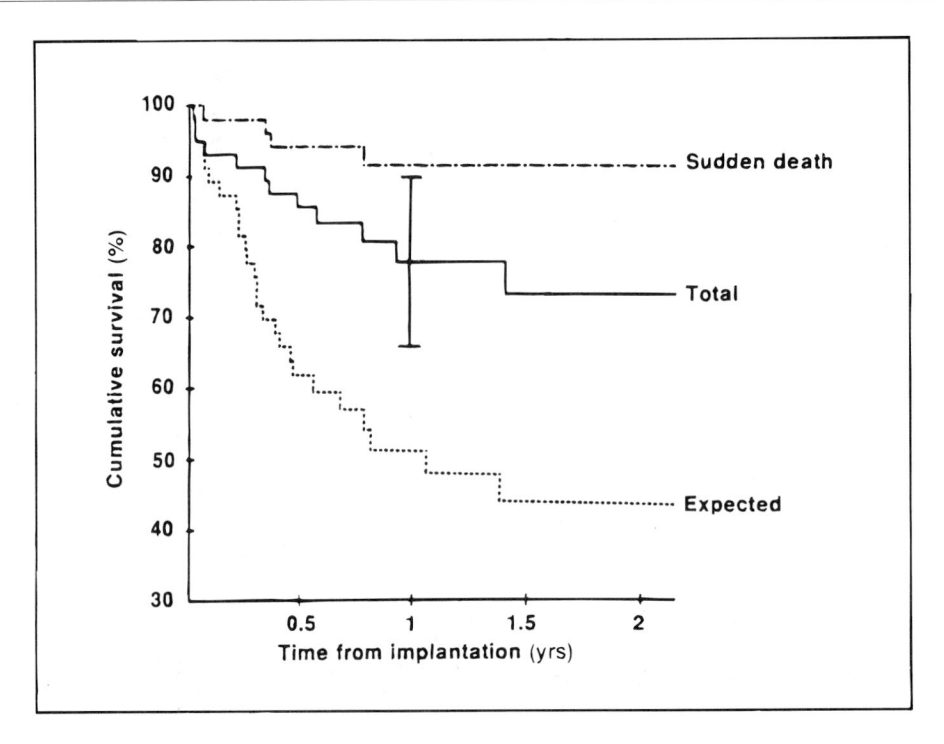

Figure 5. Initial survival curves in the first 52 patients. The upper two curves depict actual sudden and total mortality, respectively, and the lower curve indicates what we inferred the total mortality would have been based on the numbers of symptomatic firings of the devices.

market release. Intec was acquired by Cardiac Pacemakers Incorporated (CPI) and its parent company, Eli Lilly and Company in May, 1985.

The first nonthoracotomy system was implanted in late 1986. It consisted of a transvenous defibrillating lead called the Endotak™ (CPI, St. Paul, MN), designed to be implanted in a manner similar to conventional pacemaker leads, and a subcutaneous patch that can optionally be added to control or steer the direction of the shock pulses given through the lead system. The optimal positioning appears to be with a pronounced S curve and with the body of the catheter lying against the septum. The lead incorporates tines for good fixation in the apex, and is rather sturdy, further guarding against displacement from the intended positioning. The system was market released by the FDA in 1993 (Figure 6).

In 1989 other manufacturers introduced devices (Ventritex Cadence™ [Ventritex, Sunnyvale, CA] and Medtronic PCD™ [Medtronic, Minneapolis, MN) into clinical trials and these were finally market released in 1993. Telectronics (Engelwood, CO) and Intermedics (Angleton, TX) have also begun clinical trials, and CPI has entered a number of new and improved devices into clinical trials, including the PRxI and II, and P2.

Since the widespread availability of the device after market release by the FDA in 1985, at least two major trends have evolved. One of these was the rapid adoption of the therapy by the medical community (Figure 7). In 1992 alone, over 9,000 ICDs were implanted, and to date, some 38,000 devices have been implanted worldwide in over 32,000 patients.[2] This high acceptance rate occurred because of the apparent high degree of effectiveness of the therapy against sudden arrhythmic death. The other development, somewhat opposite in direction, was the mounting of a consid-

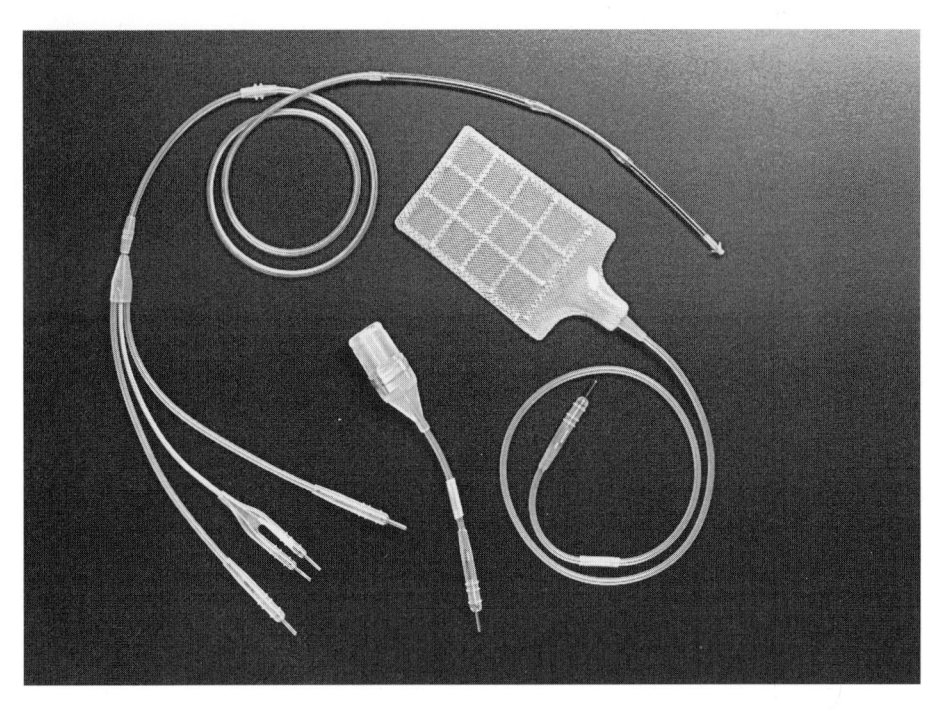

Figure 6. Endotak™ (CPI, St. Paul, MN) defibrillating lead with subcutaneous patch and Y-adapter used to connect the electrodes in various ways.

WORLDWIDE GROWTH IN CPI AICD PATIENTS AND TECHNOLOGICAL MILESTONES

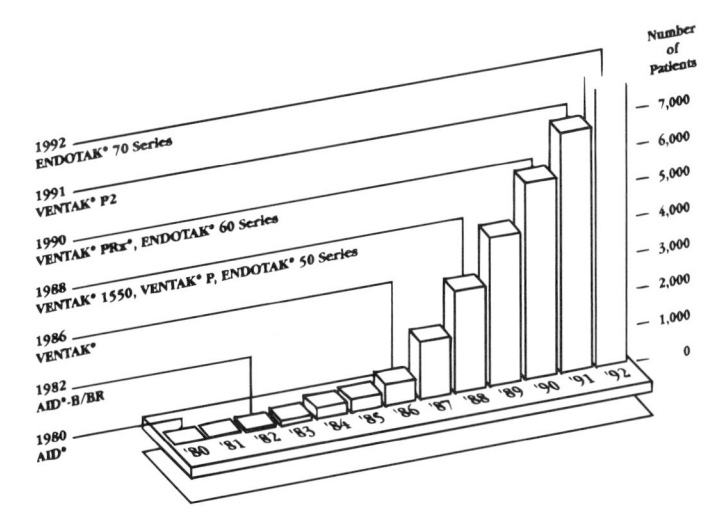

Figure 7. Bar graph of number of new implantable cardioverter-defibrillator (ICD) implantees per year on the x axis versus the year on the y axis from 1980–1992. Also indicated are the times of significant hardware and regulatory developments.

erable number of major large-scale studies involving ICDs in response to questions that had been raised concerning the expense of the therapy and scientific proof of its efficacy.

Early in the development of the ICD, attempts to interest investigator groups in randomized trials in patients resuscitated from previous cardiac arrest proved fruitless. Most physicians felt unable to ethically enter high-risk subjects into a randomization schema, obliging some to receive conventional treatments many believed ineffective. Some compelling, but in retrospect, circumstantial evidence of ICD effectiveness became apparent. Many large series have indicated sudden cardiac death rates with the ICD of less than 2% and 5% at 1 and 3 years, respectively, even under conditions of severe myocardial disease.[5-9] In comparison, drug trials such as CASCADE with amiodarone have shown 17% 1-year and 35% 3-year incidences of recurrent cardiac arrests,[10] and recently even the moricizine arm of CAST has shown excess mortality in the drug-treated population.[11] Although uncontrolled case studies, and historical control group comparisons have been considered valid to assess clinical utility in many other therapeutic areas, some have vigorously asserted that the favorable ICD literature should not be relied on because a proper randomized trial was never done.[12] This has recently given rise to some degree of backlash against the treatment.[13]

Several variations on this theme have also appeared. Because in many series the reduction in total mortality is significantly less than that of sudden death, what is suggested to be happening is the shifting of mortality to myocardial failure a short time later, and thus, not really benefitting the patients. Another assertion is that, even if the device works, its cost is so high that it cannot be cost effective. Or, more to the point, that society simply cannot afford expensive therapies.[14] Even so, the most basic of the criticisms is that the available efficacy data is suspect.

Partly in an effort to address these issues, CPI has helped in the development and funding of trials in selected high-risk patients who have no previous history of episodes of serious ventricular arrhythmias or cardiac arrests, ie, prophylactic ICD uses. We believe it will be quite reasonable to analogize the data so obtained to the cardiac arrest group for whom it would at least be very difficult to randomize. The prospective risk factors being looked at are similar to those thought important in the postcardiac arrest groups, namely reduced left ventricular function, nonsustained ventricular tachycardia, positive signal-averaged ECG, and electrophysiologic inducibility and nonsuppressibility. As an additional motivation, most patients who die suddenly do so without warning, and it is clear that in order to validate prophylactic indications, clear and convincing scientific bases have to be prepared.

The studies presently ongoing include "CABG Patch" (coronary artery disease patients scheduled for elective coronary artery bypass graft [CABG] surgery, with ejection fractions less than 0.36 and positive signal-averaged ECG); "MADIT" (coronary artery disease patients not suitable for, or having had bypass surgery, with ejection fractions less than 0.36 and nonsustained ventricular tachycardia, inducible and unresponsive to procainamide); and "MUSTT" (asymptomatic nonsustained ventricular tachycardia with ejection fractions less than 0.41 and positive electrophysiological inducibility). Four other trials supported by CPI are in the planning stage. To a large extent, they all depend on the availability of a transvenous lead system to make the trials feasible, since by and large they deal with patient groups somewhat more ill than those studied so far. These studies are "Bridge to Transplant," "DEFIBRILAT" (Defibrillator as a Bridge to Later Transplant), "EDIT" (Early Defibrillator Implantation Trial), and "DCM" (Dilated CardioMyopathy) and deal with severe heart failure, early (subacute) myocardial infarctions, and dilated cardiomyopathy patient groups. While these do not exhaust the total possible range of study groups that may be envisioned, there is a wide range of substrate in terms of coronary artery disease versus cardiomyopathy, congestive heart failure, and acute as well as old myocardial infarction encompassed by this program.

Following the efforts that led to the development of the above studies, some movement toward the development of randomized trials in conventional cardiac arrest groups finally occurred. The Canadian Implantable Defibrillator Study (CIDS)[15] has begun and is attempting to randomize a variety of manufacturer's defibrillator models against amiodarone therapy. The trial started over a year ago, and recruitment, although initially slow, is believed to be increasing gradually.

Under the direction of Dr. Karl-Heinz Kuck, CASH (The Cardiac Arrest Study Hamburg), also began several years ago in Germany, evaluating ICD versus amiodarone, propafenone, and metoprolol in a four-armed, randomized trial. Recruitment is about two thirds complete. The propafenone arm was stopped in mid-1992 by the Data and Safety Monitoring Committee due to clearly less effectiveness compared to the other arms.[16] The other arms are continuing, but no data is available at this time.

Another interesting study is the Netherlands Cost-Effectiveness Study under the direction of Dr. Richard Hauer of Utrecht.[17] This is purely an examination of the cost of various strategies of therapy, and not an effectiveness trial per se, but it appears that a substantial cross-over is occurring from the drug limb to ICD implantation. Recruitment is complete and the data is shortly to be formally reported.

Finally, the NIH has recently started a randomized defibrillator clinical trial to be called AVID (Amiodarone Versus Implantable Defibrillators) in cardiac arrest and serious ventricular arrhythmia patients.[18] The trial design is presently problematical, and only time will tell whether or not it will be possible to enroll patients in such a study.

Thus, the ICD effectiveness database is now being well addressed, and even if not all the above referenced studies are carried to satisfactory conclusions, the next few years should certainly see a plethora of critically useful clinical data being generated from them.

References

1. Mirowski M, Mower MM, Staewen WS, et al: Standby automatic defibrillator: an approach to prevention of sudden coronary death. *Arch Intern Med* 126:158, 1970.
2. Mirowski M, Mower MM, Staewen WS, et al: The development of the transvenous automatic defibrillator. *Arch Intern Med* 129:773, 1972.
3. Mirowski M, Mower M, Staewen WS, et al: Ventricular defibrillation through a single intravascular catheter electrode system. *Clin Res* 19:328, 1971.
4. Mirowski M, Mower MM, Gott VL, et al: Feasibility and effectiveness of low energy catheter defibrillation in man. *Circulation* 47:79, 1973.
5. Winkle RA, Mead RH, Ruder MA, et al: Long-term outcome with the automatic implantable cardioverter-defibrillator. *J Am Coll Cardiol* 13:1353, 1989.
6. Levine JH, Mellits ED, Baumgardner RA, et al: Predictors of first discharge and subsequent survival in patients with automatic implantable cardioverter-defibrillators. *Circulation* 84:558, 1991.
7. Fogoros RN, Elson JJ, Bonnet CA, et al: Efficacy of the automatic implantable cardioverter-defibrillator in prolonging survival in patients with severe underlying cardiac disease. *J Am Coll Cardiol* 16:381, 1990.
8. Akhtar M, Jazayeri M, Sra J, et al: Implantable cardioverter defibrillator for prevention of sudden cardiac death in patients with ventricular tachycardia and ventricular fibrillation: ICD therapy in sudden cardiac death. *PACE* 16:511, 1993.
9. Nisam S, Mower M, Moser S: ICD clinical update: first decade, initial 10,000 patients. *PACE* 14:255, 1991.
10. Greene HL, CASCADE Investigators: Cardiac arrest in Seattle: conventional versus amiodarone drug evaluation. The CASCADE Study. *Am J Cardiol* 67:578, 1991.
11. Cardiac Arrhythmia Suppression Trial In-

vestigators: Effect of the antiarrhythmic agent moricizine on survival after myocardial infarction. *N Engl J Med* 327:227, 1992.
12. Furman S: Implantable cardioverter defibrillator statistics. *PACE* 13:1, 1990.
13. Kim SG: Implantable defibrillator therapy: does it really prolong life? How can we prove it? *Am J Cardiol* 71:1213, 1993.
14. Campbell RFW: Life at a price: the implantable defibrillator. *Br Med J* 64:171, 1990.
15. Connolly, Dr. Stuart J: Personal communication, 1992.
16. Siebels J, Cappato R, Rüppel R, et al: ICD versus drugs in cardiac arrest survivors: preliminary results of the Cardiac Arrest Study Hamburg. *PACE* 16:552, 1993.
17. Hauer RNW, Wever EFD, Crijns JGM: Automatic implantable cardioverter defibrillator: cost effectiveness. *PACE* 16:559, 1993.
18. Greene, Dr. Leon: Personal communication, 1993.

Chapter 2

Ventricular Tachycardia

Igor Singer

Ventricular tachyarrhythmias are a significant cause of morbidity and mortality in patients with organic heart disease. Reentry and abnormal impulse generation are the two main mechanisms implicated in the genesis of arrhythmias.

Mechanisms

Reentry

The available clinical and experimental evidence suggests that reentry is the mechanism of most clinically observed ventricular arrhythmias.[1-3] The evidence supporting this conclusion is derived from electrophysiologic studies, intracardiac activation mapping studies, and response of ventricular tachycardia to antiarrhythmic drugs.

Reentry requires two physiologically distinct conduction pathways with differing electrophysiologic properties (Figure 1). The reentry pathway may be either anatomically or functionally determined. Figure 1 illustrates the model of reentry with two functionally dissimilar pathways. Pathway I and pathway II are connected proximally and distally. Pathway I has a shorter refractory period, but slower conduction velocity than pathway II, enabling the impulse to conduct slowly in antegrade direction in pathway I. Pathway II has substantially longer refractory period than pathway I, but faster conduction velocity. As the impulse enters both pathways proximally, it is blocked antegradely in pathway II but is conducted slowly in pathway I. By the time the impulse returns, pathway II has recovered sufficiently to conduct the impulse in retrograde direction and reentry tachycardia may be initiated, if pathway I is sufficiently recovered to be able to conduct the impulse antegradely. For reentry to perpetuate, the impulse must always find excitable tissue in the direction in which it propagates, ie, the wavelength of the circulating impulse (conduction velocity × refractory period) must be less than the length of the circuit. Presence of slow conduction has been demonstrated clinically. During sinus rhythm mapping, low-amplitude fractionated potentials have been demonstrated in patients with recurrent ventricular tachycardia, suggesting presence of slow conduction.[4-6] Activation mapping frequently localizes the origin of ventricular tachycardia to the region from which these fractionated electrical potentials can be recorded.[7-9]

Further evidence for existence of slow conduction is derived from pace mapping of the endocardium close to the site of the

---

From Singer I, (ed.) Implantable Cardioverter-Defibrillator. Armonk, NY: Futura Publishing Company, Inc.; © 1994.

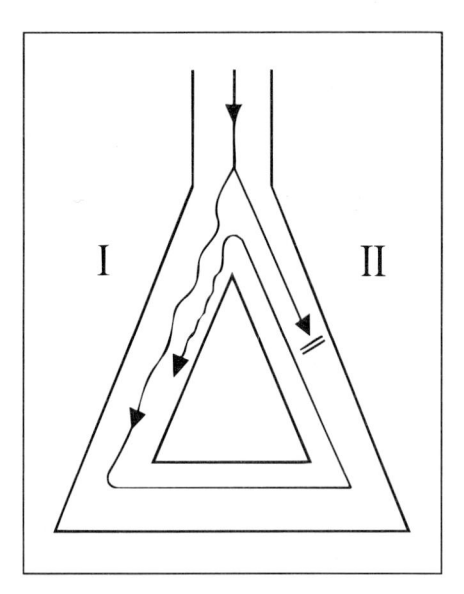

Figure 1. A schematic representation of a reentry loop. The prerequisites for reentry are two anatomically and/or physiologically separate conduction pathways connected proximally and distally. Pathway I has a shorter refractory period, but slower conduction velocity than pathway II, enabling the impulse to conduct slowly in antegrade direction in pathway I. Pathway II has a substantially longer refractory period than pathway I, but faster conduction velocity. As the impulse enters both pathways, it is blocked antegradely in pathway II, but is conducted slowly in pathway I. By the time the impulse returns, pathway II has recovered sufficiently to conduct the impulse in retrograde direction and reentry tachycardia may be initiated (see text). (Adapted with permission from Fogoros RN: *Electrophysiologic Testing*. Blackwell Scientific Publications; 1990.)

may or may not affect the site of origin of ventricular tachycardia.[15,16]

If extrastimuli interact with the tachycardia circuit, a noncompensatory pause may follow. When a noncompensatory pause is observed, the tachycardia is said to reset. Most ventricular tachycardia may be reset by one or more extrastimuli. However, the ability to demonstrate resetting of an arrhythmia does not support a specific mechanism of the tachycardia. Triggered activity may also be reset by premature extrastimuli, but unlike reentry, automatic rhythms cannot be reliably initiated or terminated by programmed stimulation.

Several responses may be observed as a result of programmed stimulation. It is characteristic of reentry that an inverse relationship usually exists between the coupling interval of the premature impulse to the last impulse of the basic cycle drive and the first impulse of the tachycardia.[17] In contradistinction, a direct relationship usually exists in triggered rhythms, ie, the shorter the coupling interval, between the paced drive and the extrastimulus, the shorter the interval between the premature stimulus and the first beat to the tachycardia.[17] A flat response, ie, a fixed first postpacing interval in response to a decrement in the extrastimulus coupling interval, may be observed due to triggered or reentry mechanisms.

Presence of fusion strongly supports reentry as the mechanism of tachycardia.

presumed origin of ventricular tachycardia. Pacing close to the site results in a long stimulus—QRS interval consistent with presence of slow conduction.[10-14]

Response of Ventricular Tachycardia to Programmed Extrastimulation

Supporting evidence for reentry mechanism may be derived from the ability to initiate and terminate ventricular tachycardia by programmed stimulation. Extrastimuli delivered during ventricular tachycardia

Table 1 Criteria for Entrainment
1) Constant fusion during rapid pacing except for the last beat (which demonstrates the morphology of spontaneous tachycardia)
2) Demonstration of progressive fusion
3) Evidence of a localized conduction block
4) Demonstration of electrogram equivalent of progressive fusion

* Adapted from Waldo et al. Transient entrainment: concepts and applications. In Rosen MR, Janse MJ, Wit AL (eds.) *Cardiac Electrophysiology: A Textbook*. Futura Publishing Company Inc, 1990:627, with permission.

Fusion requires that two wave fronts of activation coexist within the same tissue at the same time. Conditions required for fusion during resetting or entrainment include separate entrance and exit points and a region of slow conduction. Waldo et al.[18] proposed a set of criteria that define entrainment based on the presence of fusion (Table 1). Fulfillment of these criteria strongly supports reentry as the mechanism of ventricular tachycardia.

Finally, destruction of a part of the reentrant circuit by surgical means or by catheter techniques should stop the tachycardia, if the destroyed tissue is an integral part of the reentry circuit.

Triggered Activity

Triggered activity has been implicated as a less frequent cause of ventricular tachycardia. Triggered activity results from oscillations in membrane potentials known as afterdepolarizations.[19] If afterdepolarizations reach a threshold an action potential may result. If this action potential results in further afterdepolarizations, sustained arrhythmia may follow.

Two types of afterdepolarization have been described: 1) early and 2) late afterdepolarizations. Early afterdepolarizations (Figure 2) occur before complete repolarization of the action potential has occurred. These have been observed under different conditions, including hypoxia, acidosis, hypokalemia, exposure of cells to cesium, and a variety of antiarrhythmic drugs.[20,21] Early afterdepolarization may be the underlying mechanism of polymorphic ventricular tachycardia associated with the acquired long QT syndrome (bradycardia-dependent) and the congenital long QT syndromes.[22]

Delayed afterdepolarizations are the result of membrane oscillations that occur after repolarization of the action potential has occurred (Figure 3). It is currently believed that afterdepolarizations are the result of calcium loading within the cell, which is followed by an increase in sodium conductance.

Triggered rhythms secondary to delayed afterdepolarizations can also be initiated and terminated by programmed stimulation. However, rapid pacing is usually the most efficacious method for initiation of

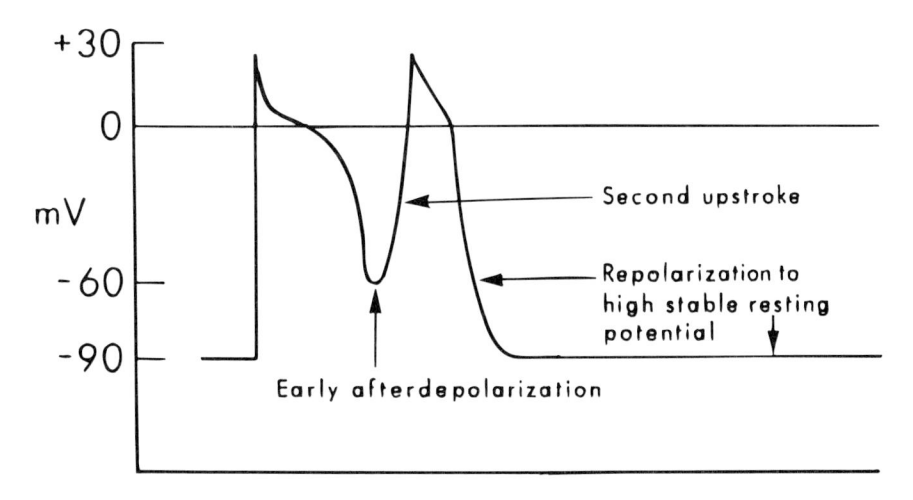

Figure 2. Diagram of an action potential in which repolarization is interrupted by an early afterdepolarization from which a second, nondriven upstroke arises. The second upstroke is followed by repolarization to the high stable level of resting potential (-90 mV). (Reproduced with permission from Cranefield PF, Aronson RS: *Cardiac Arrhythmias: The Role of Triggered Activity and Other Mechanisms*. Futura Publishing Company; 1988.)

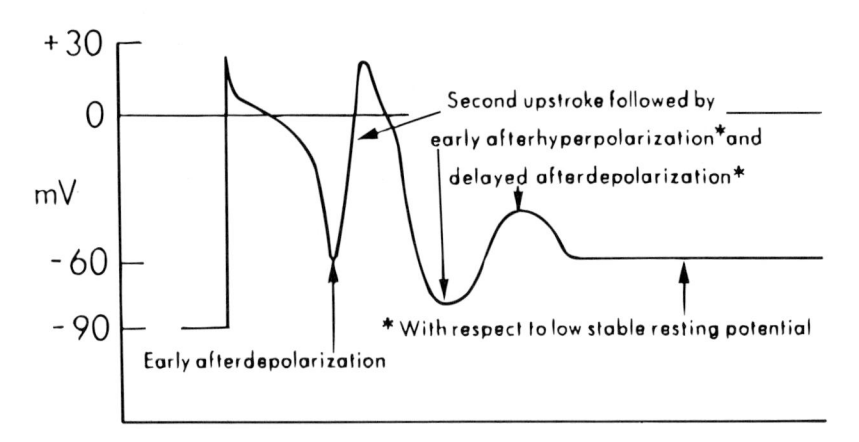

Figure 3. Diagram showing an early afterdepolarization and a delayed afterdepolarization defined with reference to the low level of diastolic potential (−60 mV). The repolarization of the first driven potential is interrupted by an early afterdepolarization which is followed by a second, nondriven upstroke. Repolarization of the nondriven action potential is interrupted by an early afterdepolarization which is followed by a second, nondriven upstroke. Repolarization of the nondriven action potential is followed by an early hyperpolarization and a delayed afterdepolarization, both of which are defined as hyperpolarizing or depolarizing with respect to the low stable level of the resting potential. (Reproduced with permission from Cranefield PF, Aronson RS: *Cardiac Arrhythmias: The Role of Triggered Activity and Other Mechanisms.* Futura Publishing Company; 1988.)

triggered arrhythmias. Extrastimuli are much less efficacious in initiating sustained triggered activity. Triggered rhythms frequently exhibit gradual acceleration or a "warm up" phenomenon at onset, and a gradual deceleration prior to termination.

Limitation of Programmed Stimulation in Identifying the Mechanism of Ventricular Tachycardia

Characteristic responses to programmed electrical stimulation are summarized in Table 2. Although response to programmed electrical stimulation is helpful in suggesting the presumptive mechanism of ventricular tachycardia, it is not specific enough to reliably differentiate reentry from triggered activity. Limitations of programmed electrical stimulation can be summarized as follows: 1) reentry or triggered activity can be initiated and terminated by single or multiple extrastimuli; 2) more than one mechanism may be operative in initiation and perpetuation of arrhythmia; and 3) the technique of programmed electrical stimulation involves application of extrastimuli and trains of stimuli at short coupling intervals, shorter than the spontaneous sinus cycle length or rate set by pacing. Therefore, this technique is not helpful in eliciting bradycardia-induced arrhythmias.

Although programmed stimulation has clear limitations, it is the only readily available method clinically for determination of the presumed mechanism of ventricular tachycardia, other than the analysis of the surface electrocardiogram (ECG). Response to programmed stimulation is not specific enough to allow one to distinguish always whether triggered activity or reentry is the primary mechanism.[23–26]

Detection of fragmented and continuous diastolic electrical activity in association with ventricular arrhythmias has been taken as evidence supporting reentry. However, fragmentation and continuous electrical activity may also be caused by mechanisms other than reentry. One such cause may be continuous diastolic electrical activity, which may be due to oscillatory afterpo-

Table 2
Characteristic Responses to Programmed Electrical Stimulation

Criteria	Response		
	REENTRY	DADs[1]	EADs[2]
Single extrastimulus			
induction	yes	yes	yes
termination	yes	yes	yes
resetting	yes	yes	yes
Multiple extrastimuli			
induction	yes	yes*	no
termination	yes	yes	yes
resetting	yes	yes	unknown
Relationship of S_1S_2[3] and first beat of tachycardia			
direct	occasionally	yes	unknown
inverse	yes	occasionally	unknown
Response to rapid pacing or spontaneous rate	rarely	characteristic	no
Favored by slow pacing or bradycardia	unknown	no	yes*
Response to decreased cycle length of stimulation by increasing number of responses and the number of induced beats	unknown	characteristic	no
"Warm Up" phenomenon (acceleration to a stable rate) initiation depends on number of preceding extrastimuli	occasional / occasional	characteristic / characteristic	unknown / no
Entrainment or capture	occasional	occasional	no

Adapted from Cranefield PF, Aronson RS (eds.) *Cardiac Arrhythmias: The Role of Triggered Activity and Other Mechanisms*. Futura Publishing Company Inc, 1988:507, with permission.

1. DADs: delayed afterdepolarizations
2. EADs: early afterdepolarizations
3. S_1S_2: last beat of drive (S_1) and first coupled extrastimulus (S_2)
* Higher characteristic response

tentials that are out of phase, but associated with triggered activity. Therefore, presence of continuous diastolic activity cannot exclude triggered activity as a possible mechanism.

To summarize, it is sometimes difficult or impossible to distinguish clinical arrhythmias due to triggered activity from those due to reentry, using programmed electrical stimulation techniques.

Cellular Mechanisms Causing Reentry in the Setting of Ischemia and Infarction

Myocardial ischemia or infarction can give rise to slow conduction and unidirectional block, the two preconditions necessary for reentry to occur.[27] Slow conduction and block depend on the alteration in the action potentials (APs). The velocity of impulse propagation in the ventricular muscle mainly depends on the inward, fast Na^+ current during the upstroke of the AP. A reduction in the rate or amplitude of the AP may result in either slowing of conduction, or in a unidirectional block.

The fraction of Na^+ channels available for opening is determined by the level of the resting potential. A decrease in the resting membrane potential inactivates some of the resting channels, decreases inward Na^+ current and causes slowing in conduction. Fast Na^+ channel is inactivated completely when the resting potential is depolarized to approximately -50 mV. However, the slow, Ca^{2+} channel is not inactivated. The slow current may give rise to an AP, though conduction velocity due to the slow Ca^{2+} channel activity is sluggish, and a unidirectional block may occur. Dispersion of conduction due to either depressed fast or slow responses may result in reentry.

Electrophysiologic Effects Due to Acute Ischemia

Although most sustained ventricular tachycardias encountered clinically are seen in relation to a remote infarction in the setting of coronary artery disease, sustained ventricular tachycardia is also encountered in the setting of acute myocardial infarction. Ischemia is characterized by oxygen and substrate deprivation and accumulation of ions and products of anaerobic metabolism in the extracellular space. Ischemia leads to K^+ loss by cells and extracellular K^+ accumulation. This may be due to partial depression of Na^+/K^+ pump, K^+ efflux coupled to cellular anion loss, and increased K^+ conductance due to adenosine triphosphate (ATP) depletion,[28] resulting in a decrease in the resting membrane potential. Other factors may contribute, eg, intracellular Ca^{2+} overload or lipid metabolites accumulation. A decrease in pH, decrease in Po_2, and catecholamine excess may also contribute to arrhythmogenesis.[29,30]

Changes in conduction velocity occur rapidly in the ischemic myocardium (within 5 minutes) due to a decrease in amplitude and upstroke velocity of APs and increase in intracellular and extracellular resistance. After 4–5 minutes of ischemia, conduction block occurs.

Ischemic cells exhibit postrepolarization refractoriness.[31] The inhomogeneity of recovery in excitability may give rise to unidirectional block, and a decrease in conduction velocity may provide an area of slow conduction, thus setting up conditions for reentry to occur.

Abnormal automaticity may occur in the surviving subendocardial Purkinje fibers, giving rise to triggered activity. Abnormal automaticity, triggered activity, and reentry may contribute to the arrhythmogenesis following an acute myocardial infarction.

The distinction between myocardial ischemia and infarction is clinically important. Myocardial infarction results in irreversible tissue necrosis. This is followed by a period of healing with tissue remodeling and scar formation. The acute period of infarction extends up to 72 hours and is subsequently followed by healing, which takes 6–8 weeks. The remodeling process and scarring causes tissue inhomogeneity and potentially results in an unstable milieu, which may be arrhythmogenic.

It has been observed that in the border zone between the healed myocardial infarction and the surrounding normal tissue, clusters of cells exist with reduced resting potentials, upstroke amplitudes, velocities, and shortened AP durations.[32] Border cells with reduced transmembrane resting potentials are found to have significant reduction in intracellular K^+ and a corresponding increase in intracellular Na^{2+}.[33] These data suggest that there may be a decreased K^+ and/or increased Na^+ conductance during depolarization of the border cells. Observed abnormalities may be due to intracellular Ca^{2+} accumulation, increased background K^+ currents, or accumulation of cytosolic Ca^{2+} due to cellular uncoupling.[34]

Regional variability in responsiveness to autonomic stimulation may also exist in the border zone. Tissue in the border zone can be stimulated to give rise to afterdepolarizations and triggered activity in response to α- and β-adrenergic agonists, which may be blocked by specific receptor blockers.[35-37] Regional abnormalities may provide the substrate for electrical instability, resulting in arrhythmogenesis.

Clinical Features of Ventricular Tachycardia

Morphological Characteristics

Ventricular tachycardias have been characterized on morphological grounds as monomorphic (having a stable QRS morphology) and polymorphic (without a constant morphology). Polymorphic ventricular tachycardia may occur in the setting of normal QT interval or it may be associated with congenital or acquired long QT interval syndromes.

Further distinction is made between sustained ventricular tachycardia (tachycardia that lasts > 30 seconds or requires intervention for termination, eg, antitachycardia pacing or cardioversion due to hemodynamic collapse) and nonsustained ventricular tachycardia (> five complexes induced during programmed electrical stimulation not due to bundle branch reentry and > 100 beats per minute). Nonsustained ventricular tachycardia is defined by continuous electrocardiogram (ECG) recording (eg, 24-hour Holter monitoring) as three or more consecutive ventricular beats > 100 beats per minute.

Based on the 12-lead ECG appearance, ventricular tachycardia may be further described as having either a left or a right bundle branch block appearance in the precordial leads, and a superior, inferior, or indeterminate axis in the frontal leads.

Diagnostic Features of Ventricular Tachycardia

Twelve-Lead ECG

Several features of the 12-lead ECG are helpful in diagnosing ventricular tachycardia. These include: 1) QRS duration > 0.14 seconds in the absence of antiarrhythmic drugs; 2) presence of atrioventricular (AV) dissociation; 3) presence of fusion complexes; 4) superior and rightward frontal QRS axis; 5) precordial concordance; 6) left bundle branch block pattern; and 7) monophasic or biphasic QRS complex in V_1.[38,39]

Although these features are helpful, none are specific enough to diagnose ventricular tachycardia without the use of intracardiac recordings with the exception of fusion complexes.

Use of Intracardiac Recordings to Diagnose Ventricular Tachycardia

Intracardiac recordings have simplified diagnosis of ventricular tachycardia. During normal conduction His activation precedes the ventricular depolarization with H-V interval of 35–55 msec. During ventricular tachycardia, however, no con-

be used to determine the origin, the presumptive mechanism, and to differentiate ventricular from AV reciprocating and supraventricular tachycardias with aberrant conduction. Using programmed electrical stimulation, reentrant arrhythmias can be readily initiated and terminated when reentry is the underlying mechanism.

Electrophysiologic study is recommended to clarify the diagnosis in a patient with symptomatic or recurrent wide QRS tachycardia.

Aborted Sudden Cardiac Death

Patients who are resuscitated from cardiac arrest and have no evidence of a new myocardial infarction are at significant risk of subsequent recurrence of sudden death posthospital discharge if left untreated. In this high-risk population the 1-year and 2-year recurrence rates of cardiac arrest is reported to be 30% and 45%, respectively.[76]

Ventricular tachycardia or fibrillation may be initiated during electrophysiologic studies in 70% to 80% of patients resuscitated from cardiac arrest. In the majority, monomorphic ventricular tachycardia is inducible. In others, polymorphic ventricular tachycardia, nonsustained ventricular tachycardia, or ventricular fibrillation are inducible.[77–81]

Effective drug therapy may be identified in up to 80% of survivors.[77–82] However, patients who remain inducible on antiarrhythmic drug therapy remain at a significantly higher risk for sudden cardiac arrest (estimated risk of 23% at 1 year and 30% at 3 years).[82,83] Conversely, in patients in whom arrhythmias have been successfully suppressed by antiarrhythmic drugs or surgery or a combination of therapies, have a reduced risk of recurrent cardiac arrest (6% at 1 year and 15% at 3 years).[82] Cardiac arrest survivors who remain inducible on electrophysiological testing should be considered for nonpharmacological therapies, including coronary artery revascularization, subendocardial resection, and/or implantable cardioverter-defibrillator (ICD) therapy.

Another important question is what to do with patients who are noninducible at electrophysiological study. Postcardiac arrest due to ventricular fibrillation or ventricular tachycardia, noninducibility at electrophysiologic study does not necessarily signify good prognosis in a patient with significant LV dysfunction (ejection fraction < 40%). These patients remain at a significant risk of cardiac arrest or nonfatal recurrent ventricular tachycardia. Therefore, ICD therapy should be considered in such patients in absence of clearly identifiable ischemia.[82–84]

In summary then, all patients resuscitated from cardiac arrest who do not have evidence of an acute myocardial infarction or clearly identifiable underlying cause (eg, ischemia, aortic stenosis, proarrhythmia, or severe electrolyte abnormality) should undergo electrophysiologic evaluation. Presence of advanced multisystem or terminal disease, or inability of patients to cooperate may preclude electrophysiologic studies in specific circumstances.

Patients With Established Diagnosis of Ventricular Tachycardia Where Electrophysiologic Studies Are Used for Management

Available data suggest that electrophysiologic studies are the method of choice to assess antiarrhythmic drug efficacy in patients with sustained inducible ventricular tachycardia, but insufficient spontaneous ventricular ectopy to allow assessment by serial long-term ECG recordings.[85,86]

All patients who are considered candidates for device therapy (ICDs) must undergo electrophysiologic studies prior to device implantation. The goal of electrophysiologic studies in these patients is to: 1) identify features of ventricular tachycardia, eg, rate, morphology; 2) demonstrate pace terminability and identify the most effective antitachycardia pacing sequence to terminate ventricular tachycardia; 3) document hemodynamic stability or instability; and 4) ascertain effectiveness of ICD or antitachycardia pacing.

Similarly, all patients considered to be candidates for ventricular tachycardia surgery (eg, subendocardial resection, aneurysmectomy) require preoperative electrophysiologic studies to localize the tachycardia circuit because intraoperative mapping may not be possible in some patients (due to the effect of anesthesia on inducibility of ventricular tachycardia in the operating room).[87,88] Electrophysiologic studies may be used postoperatively to assess the results of operative intervention.

Electrophysiologic Techniques Used to Diagnose and Treat Ventricular Tachycardia

Programmed Stimulation in the Electrophysiology Laboratory

Programmed electrical stimulation is commonly used to study ventricular tachycardia. The ability to initiate and terminate arrhythmias by programmed electrical stimulation has been considered to be characteristic of reentrant arrhythmias. However, as previously discussed, arrhythmias due to triggered activity may also be started, stopped, or modified by programmed stimulation.

Techniques used to initiate triggered activity and their characteristics differ from those used to initiate reentrant arrhythmias (Table 2). The data available in the literature support the value of programmed electrical stimulation for diagnosis and therapy of sustained monomorphic ventricular tachycardia.

Factors that influence ability to initiate ventricular tachycardia include: 1) number of extrastimuli; 2) paced cycle length; 3) site of stimulation; 4) voltage; and 5) pulse width used for stimulation.

Number of Extrastimuli

The sensitivity of programmed stimulation for induction of sustained monomorphic ventricular tachycardia increases with the number of extrastimuli used. Beyond three extrastimuli, however, the sensitivity increases only slightly at a cost of a significant decrease in specificity and a possibility of induction of nonspecific polymorphic ventricular tachycardia or ventricular fibrillation.[89-93]

In patients with normal ventricular function or in patients with clinically manifest monomorphic ventricular tachycardia, induction of polymorphous ventricular tachycardia or ventricular fibrillation may be a nonspecific finding and should not be used as an end point for therapeutic decisions. This is particularly true if more than three extrastimuli or very short coupling intervals are used (< 180 msec). Conversely, induction of polymorphous ventricular tachycardia or fibrillation during electrophysiologic studies may be a significant finding, which may have serious prognostic implications.[77-82]

In most electrophysiology laboratories (including our own) up to three extrastimuli are considered optimal. This finding is supported by several studies that suggest that the relationship of the sensitivity and specificity is most optimal using this approach.[89-93]

Drive Cycle Length

Most studies support the use of at least two—a long and a short—drive cycle lengths.[94-96] In our laboratory we typically use drive cycle lengths of 600 and 400 msec. Abrupt changes in cycle lengths may facilitate ventricular tachycardia induction.[97]

Some investigators advocate the use of ventricular extrastimuli in normal sinus rhythm. In our experience, most ventricular tachycardias that are inducible by this method are also inducible by ventricular pacing and extrastimulus techniques.

Therefore, we do not routinely use programmed electrical stimulation during spontaneous rhythm because it prolongs the study without conferring a significant additional diagnostic benefit.

Multiple cycle lengths used for ventricular drive increase sensitivity for inducing ventricular tachycardia by altering the prematurity with which extrastimuli are delivered.[96-98] Additional cycle lengths may be used if ventricular tachycardia cannot be initiated by this protocol.

Sites of Stimulation

Previous studies support the use of at least two sites for programmed stimulation. For example, in one study[99] monomorphic ventricular tachycardia was induced from right ventricular outflow tract in 58% of patients in whom triple extrastimuli at two drive cycle lengths were unsuccessful from the right ventricular apex.

In select patients in whom stimulation from the right ventricular apex and outflow tracts fails to induce ventricular tachycardia, LV programmed electrical stimulation may be used. Although the additional yield is relatively small (up to 10%), if a specific ventricular tachycardia can be induced by this technique, this information may be useful to guide therapeutic decisions.

Use of Isoproterenol

The use of isoproterenol for facilitation of induction of ventricular tachycardia has been suggested.[100,101] Isoproterenol may be particularly useful for initiating ventricular tachycardia in exercise-induced ventricular tachycardia or ventricular tachycardia originating in the right ventricular outflow tract. These arrhythmias are thought to be caused by triggered activity, which may be potentiated by a β-agonist drug.

Current Strength

Increasing current strengths from 5 to 20 mA minimally increases the sensitivity, but decreases the specificity of programmed electrical stimulation for inducing ventricular tachycardia with increased frequency of induction of polymorphous ventricular tachycardia or ventricular fibrillation. The increased yield of induction is thus far outweighed by the loss of specificity.[102] Therefore, we and others recommend that programmed electrical stimulation be conducted at currents twice the diastolic threshold (but < 5 mA) and at the pulse widths of 1 or 2 msec.

Technique of Programmed Electrical Stimulation for Induction of Ventricular Tachycardia

The technique for induction of ventricular tachycardia using programmed electrical stimulation is described in detail elsewhere.[103] Briefly, single, double, and triple extrastimuli are used consecutively from at least two right ventricular sites at two cycle drives for ventricular tachycardia induction. Diastole is scanned by a single extrastimulus to ventricular refractoriness. If ventricular tachycardia is not induced, second, then third extrastimuli are added. Isoproterenol infusion and/or programmed LV stimulation are used in specific circumstances, as discussed. The end point of programmed electrical stimulation is induction of sustained monomorphic ventricular tachycardia or noninducibility. In survivors of cardiac arrest, polymorphous ventricular tachycardia or fibrillation may be accepted as the end points of programmed electrical stimulation, although the caveats discussed should be kept in mind when interpreting the results.[104-107]

Polymorphous ventricular tachycardia, which has the potential to degenerate to ventricular fibrillation, may also occur in patients with normal repolarization (normal QT interval) or in patients with long QT intervals. In patients with normal QT intervals, the most common substrate is coronary artery disease. Patients with long QT syndrome may have either congenital or acquired abnormalities of repolarization. In the acquired form, bradycardia often precipitates torsade de pointes and follows a short-long-short sequence of spontaneous or induced extrastimuli.[108–110] Certain drugs have been associated with prolonged QT interval, including antiarrhythmic drugs, tricyclic antidepressants, and phenothiazines. Repolarization abnormalities have also been associated with electrolyte abnormalities (hypokalemia or hypomagnesemia) and nutritional imbalance (especially liquid protein diet).[111–113]

Because bradycardia facilitates torsade de pointes, measures that shorten repolarization, eg, administration of catecholamine agonists or pacing are often effective in suppressing torsade de pointes. In contrast, in congenital long QT syndrome, polymorphic ventricular tachycardia is usually not pause- or bradycardia-dependent. Adrenergic stimulation or emotional stress often precipitate onset of polymorphic ventricular tachycardia.[114,115] Programmed electrical stimulation is rarely useful in provoking ventricular tachycardia in patients with congenital long QT syndrome and should not be used for diagnosis, or to guide therapy in such patients.[103]

In patients with normal QT interval associated with coronary artery disease, with clinically manifest polymorphous ventricular tachycardia or ventricular fibrillation, these arrhythmias may be inducible in up to 85% of patients.[104–107] Because polymorphic ventricular tachycardia and ventricular fibrillation may also be induced in normal patients if aggressive protocols for stimulation are used, the results of programmed electrical stimulation must be interpreted with caution, and particular attention must be paid to the clinical history and presentation. For example, patients with a history of prior myocardial infarction, previous history of cardiac arrest or syncope, or clinically documented polymorphous ventricular tachycardia in whom a signal-averaged ECG is positive for late potentials, induced ventricular fibrillation during programmed electrical stimulation must be regarded as relevant, and should be evaluated and treated aggressively.

Use of Programmed Stimulation During Sustained Monomorphic Ventricular Tachycardia

Programmed stimulation may be used during sustained monomorphic ventricular tachycardia to study mechanisms or to evaluate antitachycardia pacing techniques for ventricular tachycardia termination. Programmed extrastimuli may be used to study the mechanism of the tachycardia. One of several outcomes are possible in response to premature extrastimuli during ventricular tachycardia: 1) no effect; 2) resetting (entrainment); 3) overdrive suppression (without termination); 4) acceleration; and 5) ventricular tachycardia termination.

To study the effects of programmed electrical stimulation, the tachycardia must be well tolerated hemodynamically and have a stable cycle length. Presence of rapid or hemodynamically destabilizing tachycardia precludes a systematic study and requires prompt termination by overdrive burst pacing or cardioversion.

Initially, single ventricular extrastimuli are introduced, which are delivered at a coupling interval slightly shorter than the ventricular tachycardia cycle length. It is subsequently decreased, typically by 10-msec decrements, until refractoriness is reached. If resetting or termination is not achieved, double, triple, or multiple extrastimuli are introduced (Figure 5).

Synchronized rapid pacing may be effective when multiple extrastimuli are ineffective in terminating ventricular tachycardia, or when hemodynamic compromise ensues. A series of paced beats delivered at cycle lengths shorter than the tachycardia cycle length should be assessed. With faster tachycardias, usually cycle lengths of < 300 msec, pacing may be ineffective and cardioversion may be required for ventricular tachycardia termination. For faster ventricular tachycardias, overdrive pacing is more

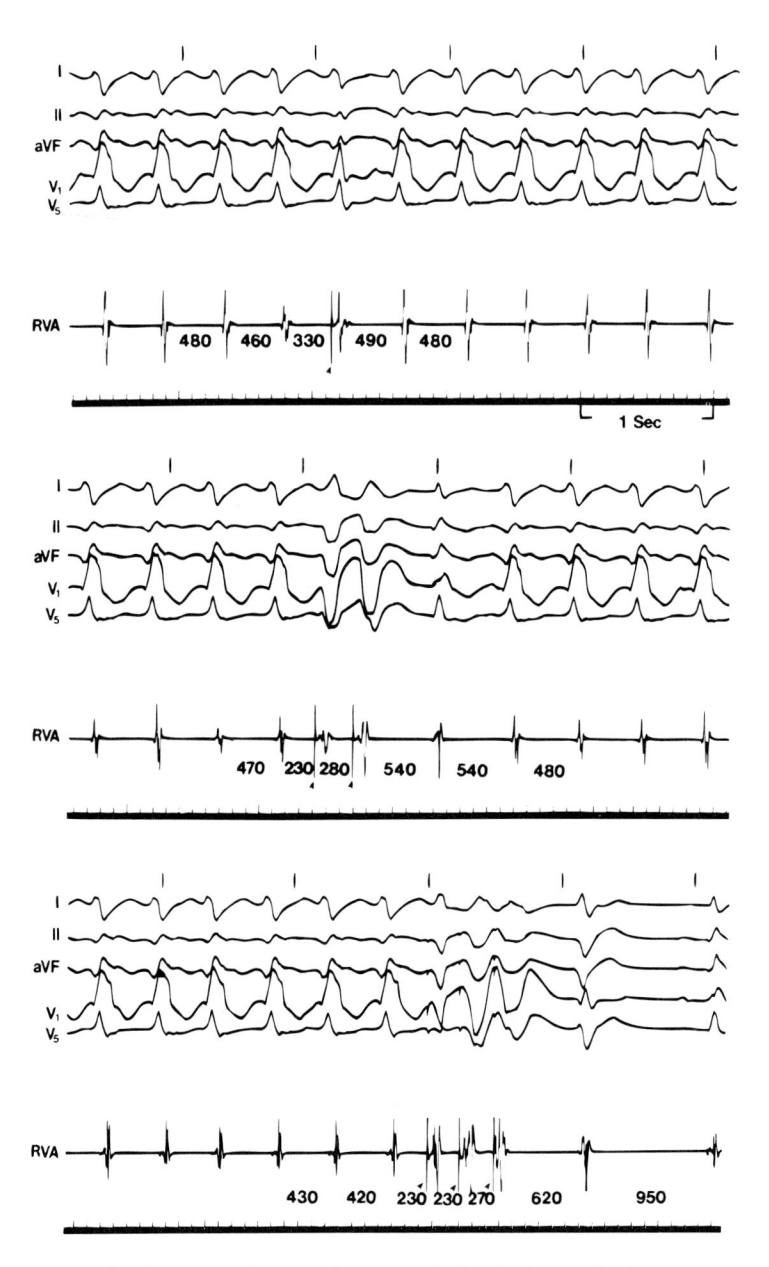

Figure 5. Programmed extrastimulation during ventricular tachycardia. From top to bottom each panel is labeled identically: Surface leads I, II, aVF, V$_1$, and V$_5$, and right ventricular electrogram (RVA). Single (upper panel), double (middle panel) and triple extrastimuli (bottom panel) are introduced in an attempt to terminate ventricular tachycardia (VT). Arrowheads mark extrastimuli. Note that single and double extrastimuli fail to terminate VT, but triple extrastimuli are effective in terminating VT. (Reproduced with permission from Reference 103.)

likely to lead to ventricular tachycardia acceleration. The ability to influence ventricular tachycardia by timed extrastimuli (single or multiple) depends on the tachycardia cycle length, the duration of the excitable gap of the tachycardia, refractoriness at the stimulation site, and conduction time from the stimulation site to the tachycardia circuit.[116,117]

Termination of Ventricular Tachycardia

Cycle length of ventricular tachycardia influences the ability of programmed electrical stimulation to terminate it. Most tachycardias that can be terminated by single extrastimuli are relatively slow (> 400 msec). The faster the tachycardia, the less likely it is that it can be terminated by single extrastimuli. Rapid or burst ventricular pacing is the most effective way to terminate ventricular tachycardia, regardless of the tachycardia cycle length. Rapid pacing may also accelerate the tachycardia.[116]

Acceleration of ventricular tachycardia rarely occurs with single or double extrastimuli, but occurs in up to 35% of cases with rapid ventricular pacing.[118] Change in morphology of ventricular tachycardia may also result during acceleration. Accelerated ventricular tachycardia may be terminated by even faster pacing in roughly half the cases, but it may require cardioversion in the rest. Hence, when antitachycardia pacing techniques are used in the ventricle back-up cardioversion and defibrillation is mandatory.

Factors that influence the ability of pacing to terminate ventricular tachycardia include: 1) refractoriness at the site of stimulation; 2) distance from the site of stimulation; 3) tachycardia cycle length; and 4) duration of the excitable gap. Thus, one may be able to modify the ability to terminate ventricular tachycardia by one of the following techniques: 1) multiple extrastimuli to decrease refractoriness at the stimulation site; 2) increase in current to decrease local refractoriness; 3) change in the site of stimulation; 4) increase in the ventricular tachycardia cycle length by antiarrhythmic drugs, thereby increasing the excitable gap, prolonging conduction and preventing perpetuation of reentry.

Localization of Ventricular Tachycardia

Localization of the site of origin of ventricular tachycardia during electrophysiologic study is essential if surgical or catheter ablation are contemplated. The technique of endocardial mapping requires that ventricular tachycardia is easily and predictably initiated, that it is hemodynamically stable and that access to the left ventricle is possible by endocardial catheter (absence of significant peripheral vascular disease precluding advancement of the catheter to the left ventricle, or a mechanical prosthetic aortic valve). Antiarrhythmic drugs may be used to slow ventricular tachycardia and to facilitate endocardial mapping.

Mapping schema has previously been described by Horowitz et al.[119] and is shown in Table 3. Endocardial mapping requires the use of multiple catheters. Catheters are typically positioned at the right ventricular

Table 3
Mapping Sites for Ventricular Tachycardia

Left Ventricle	Right Ventricle
Apex	His (A-V junction)
Septum	Apex
High	
Middle	Outflow tract
Low	Anterior
Anterior	
Lateral	
Low	
High	

A-V = atrioventricular.
Reproduced from Singer I: *Ventricular tachycardia*. Singer I, Kupersmith J (eds.) *Clinical Manual of Electrophysiology*. Williams and Wilkins Medical Publishers, 1993:113, with permission.

apex, right ventricular outflow tract, coronary sinus (optional, to identify the base of the heart), and left ventricle for mapping. Fluoroscopic visualization in multiple views is required to ascertain the anatomical position of the catheters, and cine is used to record and store the fluoroscopic information for later review. If the left ventricle is catheterized, it is essential to administer a full dose of heparin to the patient (100 U/kg body weight bolus, and 1,000 U/h infusion).

For LV mapping, we usually use a steerable LV catheter with 5-mm interelectrode distance. Bipolar electrograms from the distal electrode pair of electrodes are recorded with filter gain settings of 30 and 500 Hz. The site of origin of ventricular tachycardia is determined by the earliest recorded electrogram. This electrogram is commonly fractionated and may display continuous electrical activity. The earliest presystolic electrogram closest to mid-diastole is defined as the site of origin (Figure 6). The earliest site should be at least 50 msec before the inscription of the QRS complex.

Continuous electrical activity may occasionally be recorded in patients with ventricular tachycardia associated with coronary disease. These sites may represent the localized sites of reentry. To prove that the continuous activity is related to reentry tachycardia, one must demonstrate that its presence is required to maintain ventricular tachycardia and that the fractionated electrograms bears a fixed relationship to the surface QRS.[119,120] Intraoperative mapping has provided further corroborative evidence that most sustained monomorphic ventricular tachycardias arise from a circumscribed area.[120]

Mapping During Sinus Rhythm

Occasionally, when ventricular tachycardia mapping is not possible, the ventricle

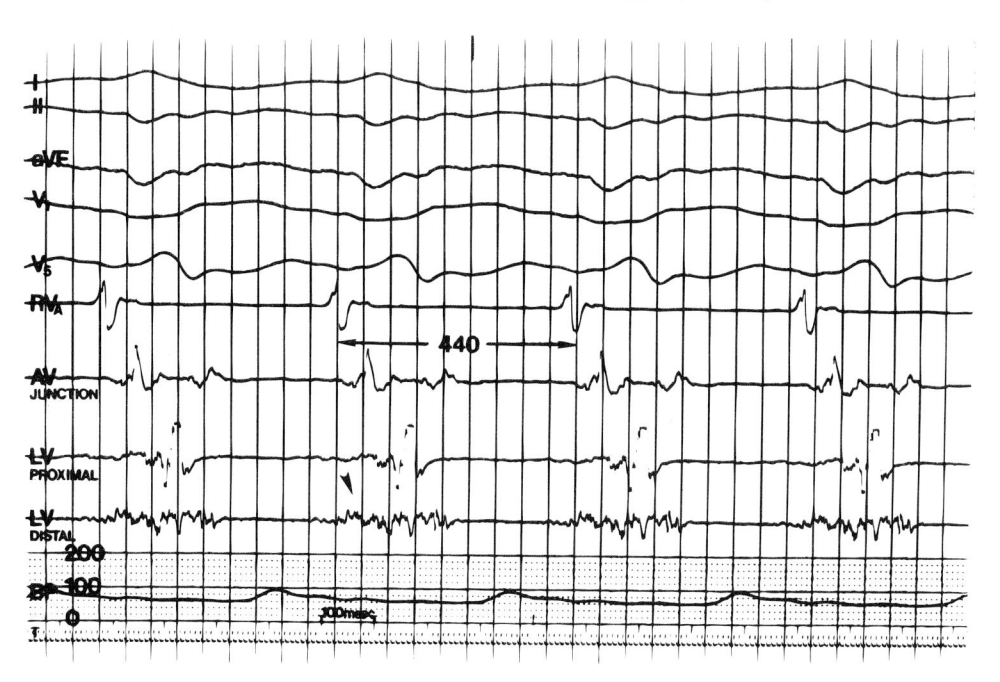

Figure 6. Endocardial mapping during ventricular tachycardia. The earliest site of ventricular activation (arrowhead) was localized to the basal septum. Note that the left ventricle distal electrogram precedes the surface QRS activation by 60 msec. From top to bottom: surface leads I, II, aVF, V$_1$, and V$_5$, intracardiac electrograms from right ventricular apex RVA, atrioventricular junction (AV junction), proximal bipolar part of a quadripolar ventricle (LV proximal), and a distal bipolar pair of electrodes (LV distal). (Reproduced with permission from Reference 103.)

may be mapped during normal sinus rhythm. Abnormal or late electrograms may be identified that may be associated with the arrhythmogenic focus.[121,122] Unfortunately fractionated or late electrograms are not specific or sufficiently precise to identify the site of origin of ventricular tachycardia and may occur throughout the infarcted myocardial tissues. Furthermore, approximately 15% of ventricular tachycardias may arise at sites that appear normal during sinus rhythm mapping.[121]

Nevertheless, when mapping during ventricular tachycardia is not possible, mapping during sinus rhythm may provide useful clues about the site of origin of ventricular tachycardia.

Usefulness of Twelve-Lead ECG to Localize Ventricular Tachycardia

Twelve-lead ECG may be used for approximate localization of ventricular tachycardia. Josephson et al.[123] have demonstrated that Q waves are present in leads I, V_1, V_2, and V_6 when ventricular tachycardia originates near the LV apex, regardless of the bundle branch block morphology. Conversely, the presence of R waves in leads I, V_1, V_2, and V_6 was demonstrated to be specific for posterior sites of origin, irrespective of the bundle branch block pattern. Presence of Q waves in leads I and V_6, associated with left bundle branch block, was localized to septo-apical location, but the presence of R waves in the same leads identified an inferobasal and septal origin of ventricular tachycardia. Although the 12-lead ECG lacks precision, it helps focus attention to a specific area, permitting more elaborate endocardial mapping at that site.

Pace Mapping

Pace mapping may be used as an adjunctive technique to confirm the suspected site of origin of ventricular tachycardia. Theoretically, pacing close to the site should reproduce ventricular tachycardia morphology similar to tachycardia that which is observed clinically. There are some limitations, however. These include: 1) adequate contact of the pacing electrode with the endocardium and 2) relative lack of precision due to a relatively large area of myocardium that may be involved in reentry, even when the catheter is close to the presumed site of origin of ventricular tachycardia. Thus, pace mapping is most useful as a confirmatory technique when a presumptive site has already been localized by endocardial mapping techniques during tachycardia.

Operative Techniques for the Treatment of Ventricular Tachycardia

Direct cardiac mapping has been shown to increase the effectiveness of surgery for recurrent ventricular tachycardia. Preoperative and intraoperative mapping must be performed to guide surgical ablation.[124-129] Because it is often difficult to sustain ventricular tachycardia in the operating room multichannel data acquisition systems have been developed for experimental and clinical use.[130-132] Many types of sensing electrodes have been designed and developed for experimental and clinical mapping, including plunge electrodes,[133] electrodes embedded in socks or plaques,[134] intracavitary probes, and balloons.[135]

Multiple signal acquisition and display of isopotential maps enables the electrophysiologist and the surgeon to construct an instantaneous activation map that can be used to locate and guide surgical therapy. Epicardial mapping is generally performed first and provides some useful information. However, the site of the arrhythmia epicardial breakthrough may be removed from the endocardial site. Therefore, this technique is generally complemented by endocardial mapping using an endocardial balloon with multiple electrodes with a computerized acquisition system, or by using a single probe mapping after a ventriculotomy is made. Detailed discussion of the surgical techniques for ventricular tachycardia ablation is beyond the scope of this chapter and is discussed in Chapter 29 of this book.

Treatment of Ventricular Tachycardia

Although therapy for ventricular tachycardia by ICDs is the subject of this textbook, alternative methods for the therapy of ventricular tachycardia and ventricular fibrillation are also discussed in this volume (see Chapters 28–30). Therefore, only a brief reference will be made to each one of these possible therapeutic approaches here.

Therapy of ventricular tachycardia may be pharmacological, ablative (surgical and nonsurgical), or electrical (ICD). It should be emphasized, however, that these therapeutic approaches are not mutually exclusive. Frequently, a combination of these techniques is used.

The first decision is to identify which patients to treat. Some clinical features may be helpful in this regard. Patients with depressed LV function (LV ejection fraction < 40%), multiple documented ventricular tachycardia episodes, or patients who present with aborted sudden cardiac death should be vigorously treated, because prognosis is generally poor without therapy.[136-139] Patients with normal ventricular function and nonsustained ventricular tachycardia, however, generally have a good prognosis and may not require therapy.

Antiarrhythmic Drug Therapy

Antiarrhythmic drugs may be used as the initial therapeutic modality for patients with sustained ventricular tachycardia. Drug therapy guided by programmed electrical stimulation is currently preferred by most electrophysiologists. This is especially true for patients who present with life-threatening symptoms, because recurrence of arrhythmias may be fatal in these patients.[84,139] The likelihood that these patients will require ablative or device therapy is relatively high. The use of noninvasive testing to guide drug therapy should be reserved only for patients who have sustained ventricular tachycardia without life-threatening symptoms or as an adjunct to the electrophysiologic assessment.[140]

Baseline electrophysiologic study is generally performed after discontinuation of all antiarrhythmic drugs for a period of > 5½ half-lives. An antiarrhythmic agent is then administered either intravenously or orally and the patient restudied when steady-state levels of antiarrhythmic drugs are achieved. Because procainamide and quinidine are both available in intravenous and oral form, these drugs are commonly tested first in the electrophysiology laboratory. For more extensive discussion of antiarrhythmic drug therapy for ventricular tachycardia see Chapter 28.

Antiarrhythmic drug serum levels must be correlated with drug efficacy. Serum levels should always be obtained prior to the electrophysiologic study to confirm therapeutic level of the drug, and during or after the induction protocol. Patients who do not respond to antiarrhythmic drugs (ie, in whom induction of ventricular tachycardia cannot be suppressed) should be considered for device or ablative therapy. Factors that predict poor outcome to antiarrhythmic drugs include the following: 1) lack of significant slowing of ventricular tachycardia after drug administration; 2) hemodynamic collapse requiring cardioversion; 3) repeated induction of ventricular fibrillation or rapid and polymorphic ventricular tachycardia on drug therapy.[141]

Induction of a well-tolerated ventricular tachycardia during treatment is associated with lower risk (4% to 6% at 1 to 2 years) for sudden cardiac death, but not for arrhythmia recurrence.[141-143] However, in patients who present with poorly tolerated ventricular tachycardias, slowing of the tachycardia during electrophysiologic study does not necessarily predict favorable outcome.[144] Therefore, in the author's opinion, ICDs should be considered for therapy of ventricular tachycardia in addition to, or instead of antiarrhythmic therapy in these patients.

Ablative Therapy

Surgical

Some patients have ventricular tachycardias that are refractory to antiarrhythmic drug therapy. Ablative therapy is considered the preferred therapeutic alternative in patients with frequent episodes of ventricular tachycardia despite drug therapy, particularly in patients who present with a single morphology tachycardia and a discrete resectable LV aneurysm. The aim of ablative therapy is to destroy the critical part of the reentrant circuit of the ventricular tachycardia.

Successful ablation is critically dependent on the ability to localize the involved myocardium necessary to initiate and perpetuate the ventricular tachycardia.[145] Diagnostic techniques used to localize the reentry circuit include analysis of the 12-lead ECG, catheter mapping during ventricular tachycardia, and pace mapping. Once the site of origin of ventricular tachycardia is localized, ablative procedures (surgical or catheter directed) can be performed. The techniques used for surgical and catheter ablation are discussed in more detail in Chapters 29 and 30.

The largest surgical experience to date has been with localized subendocardial resection guided by preoperative and intraoperative endocardial mapping.[146,147] Cryoablation or laser ablation may be combined with subendocardial resection or used instead of subendocardial resection to destroy the reentrant tissues. These techniques are particularly useful in the region of the mitral valve and papillary muscles.[148]

The operative mortality of electrophysiologically guided subendocardial resection has been reported to be between 5% and 15% in experienced clinical centers.[147] Because of significant immediate operative risk, subendocardial resection should be considered in drug-refractory ventricular tachycardia or in patients with discrete resectable LV aneurysm. Predictors of poor outcome (perioperative heart failure or death) are LV ejection fraction of $< 20\%$, history of prior cardiac surgery, and evidence of prior anterior and inferior myocardial infarctions.[149] In experienced centers, cure rates have been reported to be as high as 90%.[148,149]

Catheter Ablation

Catheter ablation theoretically offers an attractive alternative for ventricular tachycardia ablation. However, a number of technical problems limit the usefulness of this technique at the present time. These include, but are not limited to the following: 1) ability to localize the site of origin precisely by a single catheter technique; 2) inability to fixate the catheter to the ablation site; and 3) limited size of lesions generated by radiofrequency current, and to a lesser extent, DC shock. In addition, significant morbidity and mortality may be associated with the procedure (particularly with DC ablation), which limits the usefulness of this technique at present.

Results of catheter ablation are difficult to evaluate and to compare among different investigators and clinical investigative sites since the technique is not standardized. Therefore, it is not possible to provide precise data on the success of this procedure. Response rates have been variously reported to be between 25% and 50% (defined as noninducibility of ventricular tachycardia postablation).[150,151] Unfortunately, long-term results are difficult to evaluate because no true control group exists and many patients remain on antiarrhythmic drugs after catheter ablation.

We find this technique particularly useful for incessant ventricular tachycardia in patients who are not surgical candidates and who are unresponsive to antiarrhythmic drug therapy. In these patients, termination of ventricular tachycardia can be lifesaving, and is therefore justified, because all other attempts at ventricular tachycardia termination have already failed. Catheter ablation of right ventricular outflow ventricular tachycardia and bundle branch block reentry tachycardia is highly effective and represents aspecial subset of tachyarrhythmias. It is likely that further improvements in catheter mapping techniques, particularly the use of multiple electrode catheters or probes with computer-assisted maps in the electrophysiology laboratory, with improved energy sources (eg, radiofrequency current, microwave) may improve the outlook for catheter ablative therapy of ventricular tachycardias. A detailed description of catheter ablation techniques can be found in Chapter 30.

Device Therapy

Implantable cardioverter-defibrillators have revolutionized therapy for patients with sustained ventricular tachycardias. Electrical therapy is designed to terminate ventricular tachycardia by creating a block in the reentrant circuit (antitachycardia pacing) or uniformly depolarizing the tissue involved in the tachycardia circuit (cardioversion/defibrillation). Implantable cardioverter-defibrillators have provided a significant therapeutic advance for patients who present with aborted sudden cardiac death or with hemodynamically unstable ventricular tachycardias. Implantable cardioverter-defibrillator therapy is the treatment of choice for patients who have poorly tolerated ventricular tachycardia, who remain inducible on antiarrhythmic therapy, and patients who are not candidates for surgical ablative therapy.

Antitachycardia pacing techniques and cardioversion/defibrillation are now available in the third-generation devices. Further advancements of this technology, particularly the development of transvenous, nonthoracotomy lead systems have simplified the implantation techniques and will result in more widespread application of this therapeutic approach and acceptance, including the prophylactic ICD use for the high-risk group of patients.

Ventricular Tachycardia Not Associated with Coronary Artery Disease

Ventricular tachycardia may occur in structurally normal hearts, or in association with other pathological entities. Other causes of ventricular tachycardia include arrhythmogenic right ventricular dysplasia, dilated cardiomyopathy, hypertrophic cardiomyopathy, and mitral valve prolapse. These pathological entities are discussed.

Ventricular Tachycardia in a Structurally Normal Heart

Some patients have ventricular tachycardia without identifiable structural abnormalities. Sudden cardiac death has been reported rarely in association with ventricular tachycardia in these patients. The hallmark of this type of ventricular tachycardia is absence of slow conduction, with a generally normal signal-averaged ECG, noninducibility by programmed electrical stimulation, and inducibility by atrial or ventricular pacing, exercise testing, and β stimulation.[70,71]

Tachycardias originating in the left ventricle have a right bundle branch block QRS morphology and a superior frontal plane axis.[152,153] These tachycardias are usually responsive to verapamil and occasionally to β-blockade.

Another type of tachycardia can be localized to the right ventricular outflow tract.[71] This tachycardia typically has a left bundle branch block QRS morphology and an inferior frontal plane axis. Repetitive salvos or monomorphic ventricular tachycardia are noted. This ventricular tachycardia is critically dependent on the heart rate and is often initiated by exercise or exertion.[152,153] It usually cannot be initiated by programmed ventricular stimulation,[71] although it can be initiated by atrial and ventricular pacing, or with isoproterenol infusion.[154] If it can be terminated with adenosine, a cAMP-mediated triggered activity is suggested as the underlying mechanism.[155] Localization of the arrhythmia to the right ventricular outflow makes this ventricular tachycardia amenable to the catheter ablation or surgical ablation.

Arrhythmogenic Right Ventricular Dysplasia

Arrhythmogenic right ventricular dysplasia is a rare disorder caused by infiltration of the right ventricle with fatty tissue and fibrosis. This abnormality tends to occur in young adults, but can be found at in patients of any age and is more common in males. This disorder is characterized by right ventricular dilatation and diffuse or localized disease. Histopathology demonstrates fatty tissue with strands of surviving or partially degenerating myofibrillar fascicles. Pseudodiverticula or aneurysmal appearance may be observed grossly with focal ventricular thinning. Signal-averaged ECG is usually positive, and the patient is frequently inducible by programmed ventricular stimulation, suggesting reentry as the underlying mechanism.[156] Ventricular tachycardia usually has a left bundle branch block QRS morphology. This particular ventricular tachycardia is amenable to antiarrhythmic drug therapy. Alternatively, ablative approaches are available, including surgical resection or isolation procedures[157] or catheter directed ablation.[158]

Dilated Cardiomyopathy

Sustained ventricular tachycardia is uncommon in dilated cardiomyopathies. However, nonsustained ventricular tachycardias, frequent ventricular ectopic beats, and sudden cardiac death are relatively frequent occurrences in patients with dilated cardiomyopathies.[159] The signal-averaged ECG is usually positive, and in most patients ventricular tachycardia is inducible with programmed electrical stimulation. Frequently, multiple ventricular tachycardia morphologies are elicited during ventricular programmed stimulation. Because antiarrhythmic drugs are frequently ineffective in preventing inducibility of ventricular tachycardia, ICD therapy should be considered early in this group of patients.

Most patients have severe LV dysfunction. When LV dysfunction is marked and heart failure symptoms predominate, cardiac transplantation should be considered as a therapeutic alternative.

Hypertrophic Cardiomyopathy

Hypertrophic cardiomyopathy is a relatively infrequent disorder that usually presents in young adults and may cause sudden cardiac death.[160] The mechanism of sudden death in this cardiac disorder is complex and may be related to a number of factors including myocardial ischemia due to impaired coronary artery reserve, conduction abnormalities, or ventricular tachycardia related to reentry. Although β-blocker and calcium channel blocker therapy usually relieves the hemodynamic abnormalities they do not prevent ventricular tachycardia or ventricular fibrillation.[161-163]

Electrophysiologic studies are useful for guiding antiarrhythmic drug therapy. Polymorphic ventricular tachycardia is usually induced during electrophysiologic study.[163-166] In patients at risk of sudden cardiac death (patients who present with near syncope or syncope) ICD therapy should be considered early.

Mitral Valve Prolapse

Mitral valve prolapse (MVP) is generally a benign disease of young adults, predominately females. Palpitations and frequent premature beats are a common occurrence, although syncope and cardiac arrest have been reported rarely.[73,167-169] The precise mechanisms of ventricular tachycardia in this patient population is not established, but triggered activity[170] and adrenergic heart hyperresponsiveness have been suggested as possible mechanisms.[171] Reentry has also been suggested as a possible mechanism. Therefore, β blockers and electrophysiologically guided antiarrhythmic drug therapy have been suggested in the inducible patients. Patients who present with aborted sudden cardiac death should be considered candidates for ICD implantation.

Conclusion

Ventricular tachycardia is a serious and often lethal arrhythmia. It is most commonly associated with coronary artery disease and prior myocardial infarction. Ventricular tachycardia may also occur in association with other cardiac pathological entities, or occasionally it may occur in a structurally normal heart. Evaluation of the high-risk patients is recommended, because successful therapy of ventricular tachyarrhythmias markedly improves prognosis.

The advent of implantable cardioverter-defibrillators has revolutionized the approach to therapy of ventricular tachycardia and ventricular fibrillation.

References

1. Josepheson ME, Almendral JM, Buxton AE, et al: Mechanisms of ventricular tachycardia. *Circulation* 75:41, 1987.
2. Miller JM, Harken AH, Hargrove WC, et al: Patterns of endocardial activation during sustained ventricular tachycardia. *J Am Coll Cardiol* 6:1280, 1985.
3. Mason JW, Stinson EB, Winkle RA, et al: Mechanisms of ventricular tachycardia: wide complex ignorance. *Am Heart J* 102:1083, 1981.
4. Klein H, Karp RB, Kouchoukos NT, et al: Intraoperative electrophysiologic mapping of the ventricles during sinus rhythm in patients with a previous myocardial infarction. *Circulation* 66:847, 1982.
5. Cassidy DM, Vassallo JA, Marchlinski FE, et al: Sinus rhythm endocardial mapping in humans with normal left ventricles: activation patterns and electrogram characteristics. *Circulation* 70:37, 1984.
6. Cassidy DM, Vassallo JA, Buxton AE, et al: The value of sinus rhythm catheter mapping to localize ventricular tachycardia site of origin. *Circulation* 69:1103, 1984.
7. Vassallo JA, Cassidy DM, Kindwall KE, et al: Nonuniform recovery of excitability in the left ventricle. *Circulation* 78:1365, 1988.
8. Wellens HJJ, Lie KI, Durrer D: Further observation on ventricular tachycardia as studied by electrical stimulation of the heart. *Circulation* 39:647, 1994.
9. Josephson ME, Horowitz LN, Farshidi A, et al: Recurrent sustained ventricular tachycardia. 1. Mechanisms. *Circulation* 57:431, 1978.
10. Josephson ME, Horowitz LN, Farshidi A, et al: Recurrent sustained ventricular tachycardia, 2. Endocardial mapping. *Circulation* 57:440, 1978.
11. deBakker KMT, Janse MK, van Capelle FJL, et al: Endocardial mapping by simultaneous recording of endocardial electrograms during cardiac surgery for ventricular tachycardia. *J Am Coll Cardiol* 2:947, 1983.
12. Miller JM, Harken AH, Hargrove WC, et al: Patterns of activation during sustained ventricular tachycardia. *J Am Coll Cardiol* 5:1280, 1985.
13. Morady F, Frank R, Kou WH, et al: Identification and catheter ablation of a zone of slow conduction in the reentrant circuit of ventricular tachycardia in humans. *J Am Coll Cardiol* 11:775, 1988.
14. Gough WB, Mehra R, Restivo M, et al: Reentrant ventricular arrhythmias in the late MI period in the dog: correlation of activation and refractory maps. *Circ Res* 57:422, 1985.
15. Almendral JM, Stamato NJ, Rosenthal ME, et al: Resetting response patterns during sustained ventricular tachycardia: relationship to the excitable gap. *Circulation* 74:722, 1986.
16. Almendral JM, Rosenthal ME, Stamato NJ, et al: Analysis of resetting phenomenon in sustained uniform ventricular tachycardia: incidence and relation to termination. *J Am Coll Cardiol* 8:294, 1986.
17. Josephson ME, Marchlinski FE, Buxton AE, et al: Electrophysiologic basis for sustained ventricular tachycardia-role of reentry. In:

Tachycardias: Mechanisms, Diagnosis, Treatment. Edited by ME Josephson, HJJ Wellens. Philadelphia, PA: Lea and Febiger; 1984, p. 305.
18. Waldo AL, Henthorn RW, Plumb VJ, et al: Demonstration of the mechanism of transient entertainment and interruption of ventricular tachycardia with rapid atrial pacing. *J Am Coll Cardiol* 3:422, 1984.
19. Sano T, Sawanobori T: Abnormal automaticity in canine Purkinje fibers focally subjected to low external concentrations of calcium. *Circ Res* 31:158, 1972.
20. Strauss HC, Bigger JT, Hoffman BF: Electrophysiological and beta-receptor blocking effects of MI 1999 on dog and rabbit cardiac tissue. *Circ Res* 26:661, 1970.
21. Damiano BP, Rosen MR: Effects of pacing on triggered activity induced by early afterdepolarizations. *Circulation* 69:1013, 1984.
22. Jackman WM, Friday KL, Alderson JL, et al: The long QT syndromes: a critical review, new clinical observations and unifying hypothesis. *Prog Cardiovasc Dis* 31:115, 1988.
23. Johnson N, Danilo P, Wit AL, et al: Characteristics of initiation of catecholamine-induced triggered activity in atrial fibers of the coronary sinus. *Circulation* 74:1168, 1986.
24. Brugada P, Green M, Abdollah H, et al: Significance of ventricular arrhythmias initiated by programmed stimulation: the importance of type of ventricular arrhythmia induced and number of premature stimuli required. *Circulation* 69:87, 1984.
25. Morady F, DiCarlo L, Winston S, et al: A prospective comparison of triple extrastimuli and left ventricular stimulation in studies of ventricular tachycardia induction. *Circulation* 70:52, 1984.
26. Moak JP, Rosen MR: Induction and termination of triggered activity by pacing in isolated canine Purkinje fibers. *Circulation* 69:149, 1984.
27. Hoffman BF, Rosen MR: Cellular mechanisms for cardiac arrhythmias. *Circ Res* 49:1, 1984.
28. Kléber AG: Extracellular potassium accumulation in acute myocardial ischemia. *J Mol Cell Cardiol* 16:380, 1984.
29. Clusin WT, Buchbinder M, Harrison DC: Calcium overload, "injury current" and early ischemic cardiac arrhythmias—a direct connection. *Lancet* I:272, 1983.
30. Corr PB, Gross RW, Sobel BE: Arrhythmogenic amphiphilic lipids and the myocardial cell membrane. *J Mol Cell Cardiol* 14:619, 1982.
31. Downar E, Janse MJ, Durrer D: The effect of acute coronary artery occlusion on subepicardial transmembrane potentials in the intact porcine heart. *Circulation* 546:217, 1977.
32. Wong SS, Basset AL, Cameron JS, et al: Dissimilarities in the electrophysiological abnormalities of lateral border and center infarction zone cells after healing of myocardial infarction in cats. *Circ Res* 51:486, 1982.
33. Kimura S, Basset AL, Gaide MS, et al: Regional changes in intracellular potassium and sodium activity after healing of experimental myocardial infarction in cats. *Circ Res* 58:202, 1986.
34. Kimura S, Bassett AL, Kolya et al: Automaticity, triggered activity, and responses to adrenergic stimulation in cat subendocardial Purkinje fibers after healing of myocardial infarction. *Circulation* 75:651, 1987.
35. Kammerling JJ, Green FJ, Watanabe AM, et al: Denervation suprasensitivity of refractoriness in non-infarcted areas apical to transmural myocardial infarction. *Circulation* 756:383, 1987.
36. Kozlovaskis PL, Smeets MJD, Bassett AL, et al: Regional beta adrenergic receptors and adrenergic cyclase activity after healing of myocardial infarction in cats (abstract). *J Am Coll Cardiol* (Suppl A):252A, 1988.
37. Kozlovakis PL, Fieber LA, Bassett AL, et al: Regional reduction in ventricular norepinephrine after healing of experimental myocardial infarction in cats. *J Mol Cell Cardiol* 18(4):413, 1986.
38. Wellens HJJ, Bar FWHM, Lie KI: The value of electrocardiogram in the differential diagnosis of a tachycardia with a widened QRS complex. *Am J Med* 64:27, 1987.
39. Kindwall KE, Brown J, Josephson ME: Electrocardiographic criteria for ventricular tachycardia in wide complex left bundle branch block morphology tachycardias. *Am J Cardiol* 61:1279, 1988.
40. Akhtar M, Denker S, Lehman MH, et al: Macroreentry within the His-Purkinje system. *PACE* 6:1010, 1983.
41. Casceres J, Jazayeri M, McKinnie J, et al: Sustained bundle branch reentry as a mechanism of clinical tachycardia. *Circulation* 79:256, 1989.
42. Kuchar DL, Thornburn CL, Sammel WL: Prediction of serious arrhythmic events after myocardial infarction: signal-averaged electrogram, Holter monitoring, and radionuclide ventriculography. *J Am Coll Cardiol* 9:531, 1987.
43. Gomes JA, Winters JL, Stewart D, et al: A new noninvasive index to predict sustained ventricular tachycardia and sudden death in the first year after myocardial infarction:

based on signal-averaged electrocardiogram, radionuclide ejection fraction and Holter monitoring. *J Am Coll Cardiol* 10:349, 1987.
44. Breithardt G, Borggrefe M, Haerten K: Role of programmed ventricular stimulation and noninvasive recording of ventricular late potentials for the identification of patients at risk of ventricular tachyarrhythmias after acute myocardial infarction. In: *Cardiac Electrophysiology and Arrhythmias*. Edited by DP Zipes, J Jalife. Orlando, FL: Grune & Stratton; 1985, p. 553.
45. Dennis AR, Ross DL, Richards DA, et al: Differences between patients with ventricular tachycardia and ventricular fibrillation as assessed by signal-averaged electrocardiogram, radionuclide ventriculography and cardiac mapping. *J Am Coll Cardiol* 11:276, 1988.
46. Stevenson WG, Brugada P, Waldecker B, et al: Clinical, angiographic and electrophysiologic findings in patients with aborted sudden death as compared with patients with sustained ventricular tachycardia after myocardial infarction. *Circulation* 71:1146, 1985.
47. Freedman RA, Gillis A, Keren A, et al: Signal-averaged electrocardiographic late potentials in patients with ventricular fibrillation or ventricular tachycardia: correlation with clinical arrhythmia and electrophysiologic study. *Am J Cardiol* 55:1350, 1985.
48. Simson MB: Use of signals in the terminal QRS complex to identify patients with ventricular tachycardia after myocardial infarction. *Circulation* 64:235, 1981.
49. Denniss AR, Richards DA, Cody DV, et al: Prognostic significance of ventricular tachycardia and fibrillation induced at programmed stimulation and delayed potentials detected on the signal-averaged electrocardiograms of survivors of acute myocardial infarction. *Circulation* 74:731, 1986.
50. Marchlinski FE, Waxman HL, Buxton AE, et al: Sustained ventricular arrhythmias during the early postinfarction period: electrophysiologic findings and prognosis for survival. *J Am Coll Cardiol* 2:240, 1983.
51. Poll DS, Marchlinski FE, Buxton AE, et al: Sustained ventricular tachycardia in patients with idiopathic dilated cardiomyopathy: electrophysiologic testing and lack of response to antiarrhythmic drug therapy. *Circulation* 70:451, 1984.
52. Poll DS, Marchlinski FE, Falcone RA, et al: Abnormal signal-averaged electrocardiogram in nonischemic congestive cardiomyopathy; relationship to sustained ventricular arrhythmias. *Circulation* 72:1308, 1985.
53. Poll DS, Marchlinski FE, Buxton AE, et al: Usefulness of programmed stimulation in idiopathic dilated cardiomyopathy. *Am J Cardiol* 58:992, 1986.
54. Marcus F, Fontaine GH, Guiraudon G, et al: Right ventricular dysplasia: a report of 24 adult cases. *Circulation* 65:384, 1982.
55. Horowitz LN, Vetter VL, Harken AH, et al: Electrophysiologic characteristics of sustained ventricular tachycardia occurring after repair of tetralogy of Fallot. *Am J Cardiol* 46:446, 1980.
56. Kugler JD, Pinsky WW, Cheatham JP, et al: Sustained ventricular tachycardia after repair of tetralogy of Fallot: new electrophysiologic findings. *Am J Cardiol* 51:1137, 1983.
57. Garson A Jr, Porter CJ, Gillett PC, et al: Induction of ventricular tachycardia during electrophysiologic study after repair of tetralogy of Fallot. *J Am Coll Cardiol* 1:1494, 1983.
58. McKenna WJ, Harris L, Percy G, et al: Arrhythmia in hypertrophic cardiomyopathy. II. Comparison of amiodarone and verapamil in treatment of arrhythmias. *Am Heart J* 46:173, 1981.
59. McKenna WJ, Chetty S, Oakley CM, et al: Arrhythmia in hypertrophic cardiomyopathy: exercise and 48 hour ambulatory electrocardiographic treatment with and without beta adrenergic blocking therapy. *Am J Cardiol* 45:1, 1980.
60. Nocid P, Polikar R, Peterson KL: Hypertrophic cardiomyopathy and death. *N Engl J Med* 318:1255, 1988.
61. Anderson KP, Stinson EB, Derby G, et al: Vulnerability of patients with obstructive hypertrophic cardiomyopathy to ventricular arrhythmia induction in the operating room. *Am J Cardiol* 51:811, 1983.
62. Schiavone WA, Maloney JD, Lever HM, et al: Electrophysiologic studies of patients with hypertrophic cardiomyopathy presenting with syncope of undetermined etiology. *PACE* 9:476, 1986.
63. Watson RM, Schwartz JL, Maron BJ, et al: Inducible polymorphic ventricular tachycardia and ventricular fibrillation in a subgroup of patients with hypertrophic cardiomyopathy at high risk for sudden death. *J Am Coll Cardiol* 10:761, 1987.
64. Morady F, Shen E, Bhandari A, et al: Programmed ventricular stimulation in mitral valve prolapse: analysis of 36 patients. *Am J Cardiol* 53:135, 1984.
65. Rosenthal ME, Hamer A, Gang ES, et al: The yield of programmed ventricular stimulation in mitral valve prolapse patients

with ventricular arrhythmias. *Am Heart J* 110:970, 1985.
66. Durer DR, Becker AE, Dunning AJ: Long term follow up of identifying mitral valve prolapse in 300 patients: a prospective study. *J Am Coll Cardiol* 11:42, 1988.
67. Wit AL, Fenoglio JJ, Hordof AJ, et al: Ultrastructure and transmembrane potentials of cardiac muscle in the human anterior mitral valve leaflet. *Circulation* 59:1284, 1979.
68. Boudoulas H, Wooley CF: Mitral valve prolapse syndrome. Evidence of hyperadrenergic state. *Postgrad Med* 152, 1988.
69. Buxton AE, Waxman HL, Marchlinski FE, et al: Right ventricular tachycardia: clinical and electrophysiologic characteristics. *Circulation* 68:917, 1983.
70. Ohe T, Shimomura K, Aihara N, et al: Idiopathic sustained left ventricular tachycardia: clinical and electrophysiologic characteristics. *Circulation* 77:560, 1988.
71. Palileo EV, Ashley WW, Swiryn S, et al: Exercise provocable right ventricular outflow tract tachycardia. *Am Heart J* 104:185, 1982.
72. Moss AJ, Davis HT, DeCamilla J, et al: Ventricular ectopic beats and their relation to sudden and nonsudden cardiac death after myocardial infarction. *Circulation* 60:998, 1979.
73. Ruberman W, Weinblatt E, Goldberg JD, et al: Ventricular premature complexes and sudden death after MI. *Circulation* 64:297, 1981.
74. Bigger JT Jr, Webb FM, Rolnitzky LM: Prevalence, characteristics and significance of ventricular tachycardia (three or more complexes) detected with ambulatory ECG recording in the late hospital phase of acute MI. *Am J Cardiol* 48:815, 1981.
75. Cardiac Arrhythmia Suppression Trial Investigators: Preliminary report: effect of encainide and flecainide on mortality in a randomized trial of arrhythmia suppression after myocardial infarction. *N Engl J Med* 321:406, 1989.
76. Baum RS, Alvarez H III, Cobb LA: Survival after resuscitation from out-of-hospital ventricular fibrillation. *Circulation* 50:1231, 1974.
77. Ruskin JN, DiMarco JP, Garan H: Out-of-hospital cardiac arrest. Electrophysiologic observations and selection of long-term antiarrhythmic therapy. *N Engl J Med* 303:607, 1980.
78. Morady F, Scheinman MM, Hess DS, et al: Electrophysiologic testing in the management of survivors of out-of-hospital cardiac arrest. *Am J Cardiol* 51:85, 1983.
79. Roy D, Waxman HL, Kienzle MG, et al: Clinical characteristics and long-term follow up in 119 survivors of cardiac arrest: relation to inducibility at electrophysiologic testing. *Am J Cardiol* 52:969, 1983.
80. Benditt DG, Benson DW Jr, Klein GJ, et al: Prevention of recurrent sudden cardiac arrest: role of provocative electropharmacologic testing. *J Am Coll Cardiol* 2:418, 1983.
81. Skale BT, Miles WM, Heger JJ, et al: Survivors of cardiac arrest: prevention of recurrence by drug therapy as predicted by electrophysiologic testing or ECG monitoring. *Am J Cardiol* 57:113, 1986.
82. Wilber DJ, Garan H, Kelly E, et al: Out-of-hospital cardiac arrest: role of electrophysiologic testing in prediction of long term outcome. *N Engl J Med* 318:19, 1988.
83. Weaver WD, Lorch GS, Alvarez HA, et al: Angiographic findings and prognostic indicators in patients resuscitated from sudden cardiac death. *Circulation* 54:895, 1976.
84. Wilber DJ, Kelly E, Garan H, et al: Determinants of inducible ventricular arrhythmias in survivors of out-of-hospital cardiac arrest (abstract). *Circulation* 72(Suppl III):III-45, 1985.
85. Wellens HJJ: Value and limitations of programmed electrical stimulation in ventricular tachycardia. *Circulation* 57:845, 1978.
86. Buxton AE, Marchlinski FE, Flores BT, et al: Nonsustained ventricular tachycardia in patients with coronary artery disease: role of electrophysiologic study. *Circulation* 75:1178, 1987.
87. Gallagher JJ, Kassell JH, Cox JL, et al: Techniques of intraoperative mapping. *Am J Cardiol* 49:221, 1982.
88. Miller JM, Marchlinski FE, Harken AH, et al: Subendocardial resection for sustained ventricular tachycardia in the early period after acute MI. *Am J Cardiol* 55:980, 1985.
89. Buxton AE, Waxman HL, Marchlinski FE, et al: Role of triple extrastimuli during electrophysiologic study of patients with documented sustained ventricular tachyarrhythmias. *Circulation* 69:532, 1984.
90. Brugada P, Abdollah H, Heddle B, et al: Results of ventricular stimulation protocol using a maximum of 4 premature stimuli in patients without documented or suspected ventricular arrhythmias. *Am J Cardiol* 52:1214, 1983.
91. Morady F, DiCarlo L, Winston S, et al: A prospective comparison of triple extrastimuli and left ventricular stimulation in studies of ventricular tachycardia induction. *Circulation* 70:52, 1984.
92. DiCarlo LA Jr, Morady F, Schwartz AB, et al: Clinical significance of ventricular fibrillation-flutter induced by ventricular pro-

grammed stimulation. *Am Heart J* 10:959, 1985.
93. Brugada P, Green M, Abdollah H, et al: Significance of ventricular arrhythmias initiated by programmed ventricular stimulation: the importance of the type of ventricular arrhythmia induced and the number of premature stimuli required. *Circulation* 69:87, 1984.
94. Estes NAM III, Garan H, McGovern B, et al: Influence of drive cycle length during programmed stimulation on induction of ventricular arrhythmias: analysis of 403 patients. *Am J Cardiol* 57:108, 1986.
95. Gillis AM, Winkle RA, Echt DS: Role of extrastimulus prematurity and intraventricular conduction time in inducing ventricular tachycardia or ventricular fibrillation secondary to coronary artery disease. *Am J Cardiol* 60:590, 1987.
96. Vassallo JA, Marchlinski FE, Casidy DM, et al: Shortening of ventricular refractoriness with extrastimuli: role of the degree of prematurity and number of extrastimuli. *J Electrophysiol* 2:227, 1988.
97. Denker S, Lehmann M, Mahmud R, et al: Facilitation of ventricular tachycardia induction with abrupt changes in ventricular cycle length. *Am J Cardiol* 53:508, 1984.
98. Cain ME, Martin TC, Marchlinski FE, et al: Changes in ventricular refractoriness after an extrastimulus: effects of prematurity, cycle length and procainamide. *Am J Cardiol* 52:996, 1983.
99. Doherty JU, Kienzle MG, Waxman HL, et al: Programmed ventricular stimulation at a second right ventricular site: An analysis of 200 patients, with special reference to sensitivity, specificity and characteristics of patients with induced ventricular tachycardia. *Am J Cardiol* 52:1184, 1983.
100. Freedman RA, Swerdlow CD, Echt DS, et al: Facilitation of ventricular tachyarrhythmia induction by isoproterenol. *Am J Cardiol* 54:765, 1984.
101. Reddy CP, Gettes LS: Use of isoproterenol as an aid to electric induction of chronic recurrent ventricular tachycardia. *Am J Cardiol* 44:705, 1979.
102. Morady F, DiCarlo LA Jr, Liem LB, et al: Effects of high stimulation current on the induction of ventricular tachycardia. *Am J Cardiol* 56:73, 1985.
103. Singer I: Ventricular tachycardia. In: *Clinical Manual of Electrophysiology*. Edited by I Singer, J Kupersmith. Williams and Wilkins Medical Publishers; 1993, p. 107.
104. Josephson ME, Horowitz LN, Spielman SR, et al: Electrophysiologic, and hemodynamic studies in patients resuscitated from cardiac arrest. *Am J Cardiol* 49:948, 1980.
105. Spielman SR, Farshidi A, Horowitz LN, et al: Ventricular fibrillation during programmed ventricular stimulation: incidence and clinical implications. *Am J Cardiol* 42:913, 1987.
106. Freedman RA, Swerdlow CD, Soderholm-Difatte V, et al: Prognostic significance of arrhythmias induced at electrophysiologic study in cardiac arrest survivors. *Circulation* 72(Suppl III):III-45, 1985.
107. Swerdlow CD, Bardy GH, McAnulty J, et al: Determinants of induced sustained arrhythmias in survivors of out-of-hospital ventricular fibrillation. *Circulation* 76:1053, 1987.
108. Jackman WM, Friday KJ, Anderson JL, et al: The long QT syndromes: a critical review, new clinical observation and a unifying hypothesis. *Prog Cardiovasc Dis* 31:115, 1988.
109. Jackman WM, Clark M, Friday KJ, et al: Ventricular tachyarrhythmias in the long QT syndromes. *Med Clin North Am* 68:1079, 1984.
110. Kay GN, Plumb VJ, Arciniegas JG, et al: Torsade de pointes: the short-long-short initiating sequence and other clinical features. Observations in 32 patients. *J Am Coll Cardiol* 2:806, 1983.
111. Keren A, Tzivoni D, Gavish D, et al: Etiology, warning signs and therapy of torsade de pointes. *Circulation* 64:1167, 1981.
112. Bauman JL, Baurenfiend RA, Hoff JV, et al: Quinidine syncope: torsades de pointes due to quinidine. Observations in 31 patients. *Am Heart J* 107:425, 1984.
113. Bhandari AK, Scheinman M: The long QT syndrome. *Mod Concepts Cardiovasc Dis* 54:45, 1985.
114. Coumel P, Fidelle J, Lucet V, et al: Catecholamine-induced severe ventricular arrhythmias with Adams-Stokes syndrome in children: report of four cases. *Br Heart J* 40(Suppl):28, 1987.
115. Coumel LP, Laclercq JF, Lucet V, et al: Possible mechanisms of the arrhythmias in the long QT syndrome. *Eur Heart J* 6(Suppl D):115, 1985.
116. Roy D, Waxman HL, Buxton AE, et al: Termination of ventricular tachycardia: role of tachycardia cycle length. *Am J Cardiol* 50:1346, 1982.
117. Almendral JM, Rosenthal ME, Stamato NJ, et al: Analysis of the resetting phenomenon in sustained uniform ventricular tachycardia: incidence and relation to termination. *J Am Coll Cardiol* 8:294, 1986.
118. Almendral JM, Gottlieb CD, Rosenthal

ME, et al: Entrainment of ventricular tachycardia: explanation for surface electrocardiographic phenomena by analysis of electrograms recorded within the tachycardia circuit. *Circulation* 77:569, 1988.
119. Horowitz LN, Josephson ME, Harken AH: Epicardial and endocardial activation during sustained ventricular tachycardia in man. *Circulation* 61:1227, 1980.
120. Josephson ME, Horowitz LN, Spielman SR, et al: Comparison of endocardial catheter mapping with intraoperative mapping of ventricular tachycardia. *Circulation* 61:395, 1980.
121. Cassidy DM, Vassallo JA, Buxton AE, et al: The value of catheter mapping during sinus rhythm to localize site of origin of ventricular tachycardia. *Circulation* 69:1103, 1984.
122. Cassidy DM, Vassalo JA, Miller JM, et al: Endocardial catheter mapping in patients in sinus rhythm: relationship to underlying heart disease and ventricular arrhythmias. *Circulation* 73:645, 1986.
123. Josephson ME, Horowitz LN, Waxman HL, et al: Sustained ventricular tachycardia: role of the 12-lead electrocardiogram in localizing site of origin. *Circulation* 64:257, 1981.
124. Mason JW, Stinson EB, Winkle RA, et al: Surgery for ventricular tachycardia: efficacy of left ventricular aneurysm resection compared with operation guided by electrical activation mapping. *Circulation* 65:1148, 1982.
125. Josephson ME, Horowitz LN, Spielman SR, et al: The role of catheter mapping in the preoperative evaluation of ventricular tachycardia. *Am J Cardiol* 49:207, 1982.
126. Hauer RNW, deZwart MT, deBakker JMT, et al: Endocardial catheter mapping: wire skeleton technique for representation of computed arrhythmogenic sites compared to intraoperative mapping. *Circulation* 74:1346, 1986.
127. Waspe LE, Brodman R, Kim SG, et al: Activation mapping in patients with coronary artery disease with multiple ventricular tachycardia configurations: occurrence and therapeutic implications of widely separate apparent sites of origin. *J Am Coll Cardiol* 5:1075, 1985.
128. Saksena S, Hussain SM, Gieldinsky I, et al: Intraoperative mapping guided Argon laser ablation of malignant ventricular tachycardia. *J Am Coll Cardiol* 59:78, 1987.
129. Caceres J, Werner P, Jazayeri M, et al: Efficacy of cryosurgery alone for refractory monomorphic sustained ventricular tachycardia due to inferior wall infarction. *J Am Coll Cardiol* 11:1254, 1988.
130. deBakker JMT, Janse MJ, van Capelle FJL, et al: Endocardial mapping by simultaneous recording of endocardial electrograms during cardiac surgery for ventricular aneurysm. *J Am Coll Cardiol* 2:947, 1983.
131. Downar E, Harris L, Mickleborough LL, et al: Endocardial mapping of ventricular tachycardia in the intact human ventricle: evidence for reentrant mechanisms. *J Am Coll Cardiol* 11:783, 1988.
132. Harris L, Downar E, Mickleborough LL, et al: Activation sequence of ventricular tachycardia: endocardial and epicardial mapping studies in the human ventricle. *J Am Coll Cardiol* 10:1040, 1987.
133. Kassell J, Gallagher JJ: Construction of multipolar needle electrode for activation study of the heart. *Am J Physiol* 233:H312, 1977.
134. Wit AL, Allessie MA, Bonke FIM, et al: Electrophysiologic mapping to determine the mechanisms of experimental ventricular tachycardia initiated by premature impulses: experimental approach and initial results demonstrating reentrant excitation. *Am J Cardiol* 49:166, 1982.
135. Taccardi B, Arisi G, Macchi E, et al: A new intracavitary probe for detecting the site of origin of ventricular ectopic beats during one cardiac cycle. *Circulation* 75:272, 1987.
136. Lampert S, Lown B, Graboys TB, et al: Determinants of survival in patients with malignant ventricular arrhythmia associated with coronary artery disease. *Am J Cardiol* 61:791, 1988.
137. Swerdlow CD, Winkle RA, Mason JW: Determinants of survival in patients with ventricular arrhythmias. *N Engl J Med* 308:1436, 1983.
138. DiCarlo LA, Morady F, Suavae MJ, et al: Cardiac arrest and sudden death in patients treated with amiodarone for sustained ventricular tachycardia or ventricular fibrillation: risk stratification based on clinical variables. *Am J Cardiol* 55:372, 1985.
139. Schoenfeld MH, McGovern B, Garan M, et al: Determinants of outcome of electrophysiologic study in patients with ventricular tachyarrhythmias. *J Am Coll Cardiol* 6:298, 1985.
140. Graboys T: Long-term survival of patients with malignant ventricular arrhythmia treated with antiarrhythmic drugs. *Am J Cardiol* 50:437, 1982.
141. Waller TJ, Kay HR, Spielman SR, et al: Reduction in sudden death and total mortality by antiarrhythmic therapy evaluated by electrophysiologic drug testing: criteria of efficacy in patients with sustained ventricular tachyarrhythmia. *J Am Coll Cardiol* 10:1083, 1987.
142. Horowitz LN, Greenspan AM, Spielman

SR, et al: Usefulness of electrophysiologic testing in evaluation of amiodarone therapy for sustained ventricular tachyarrhythmias associated with coronary heart disease. *Am J Cardiol* 35:367, 1985.
143. Kadish AH, Buxton AE, Waxman HL, et al: Usefulness of electrophysiologic study to determine the clinical tolerance of arrhythmia recurrences during amiodarone therapy. *J Am Coll Cardiol* 10:90, 1987.
144. Gottlieb CD, Berger MD, Miller JM, et al: What is an acceptable risk for cardiac arrest patients treated with amiodarone? *Circulation* 78(II):500, 1988.
145. Marchlinski FE, Josephson ME: Appropriate diagnostic studies for arrhythmia surgery. *PACE* 7:902, 1984.
146. Josephson ME, Harken AH, Horowitz LN: Endocardial excision: a new surgical technique for the treatment of recurrent ventricular tachycardia. *Circulation* 76:332, 1987.
147. Haines DE, Lerman BB, Kron IL, et al: Surgical ablation of ventricular tachycardia with sequential map-guided subendocardial resection: electrophysiologic, assessment and long term follow up. *Circulation* 7:131, 1988.
148. Caceres J, Werner P, Jazayeri M, et al: Efficacy of cryosurgery alone for refractory monomorphic sustained ventricular tachycardia due to inferior wall infarction. *J Am Coll Cardiol* 11:1254, 1988.
149. Miller JM, Gottlieb CD, Hargrove WC, et al: Factors influencing operative mortality in surgery for ventricular tachycardia. *Circulation* 78:II-44, 1988.
150. Morady F, Scheinman MM, DiCarlo LA, et al: Catheter ablation of ventricular tachycardia with intracardiac shocks: results in 33 patients. *Circulation* 75:1037, 1987.
151. Fontaine G, Frank R, Tonet J, et al: Fulguration of chronic ventricular tachycardia: results of forty-seven consecutive cases with follow-up ranging from 11 to 65 months. In: *Cardiac Electrophysiology: From Cell to Bedside*. Edited by DP Zipes, J Jalife. Philadelphia: W.B.Saunders; 1990, p. 978.
152. German LD, Packer DL, Bardy GH, et al: Ventricular tachycardia induced by atrial stimulation in patients without symptomatic cardiac disease. *Am J Cardiol* 52:1202, 1983.
153. Lin FC, Finley CD, Rahimtoola SH, et al: Idiopathic paroxysmal ventricular tachycardia with a QRS pattern of right bundle branch block and left axis deviation: a unique clinical entity with specific properties. *Am J Cardiol* 52:95, 1983.
154. Sung RJ, Keung EC, Nguyen NX, et al: Effects of beta-adrenergic blockade on verapamil-responsive and verapamil-irresponsive sustained ventricular tachycardias. *J Clin Invest* 81:688, 1988.
155. Lerman BB, Belardinelle L, West GA, et al: Adenosine-sensitive ventricular tachycardia: evidence suggesting cyclic AMP-mediated triggered activity. *Circulation* 74:270, 1986.
156. Belhassen B, Caspi A, Miller H, et al: Extensive endocardial mapping during sinus rhythm and ventricular free wall: surgical treatment of right ventricular tachycardia associated with right ventricular dysplasia. *J Am Coll Cardiol* 4:1302, 1984.
157. Guiraudon GM, Klein GJ, Gulamhusein SS, et al: Total disconnection of the right ventricular free wall: surgical treatment of right ventricular tachycardia associated with right ventricular dysplasia. *Circulation* 67:463, 1983.
158. Leclerq JF, Chouty F, Cauchemez B, et al: Results of electrical fulguration in arrhythmogenic right ventricular disease. *Am J Cardiol* 62:220, 1988.
159. Poll DS, Marchlinski FE, Buxton AE, et al: Sustained ventricular tachycardia in patients with idiopathic dilated cardiomyopathy: electrophysiologic testing and lack of response to antiarrhythmic drug therapy. *Circulation* 70:451, 1984.
160. Maron BJ, Savage DD, Wolfson JK, et al: Prognostic significance of 24 hour ambulatory electrocardiographic monitoring in patients with hypertrophic cardiomyopathy: a prospective study. *Am J Cardiol* 48:252, 1987.
161. Mc Kenna WJ, Harris L, Percy G, et al: Arrhythmia in hypertrophic cardiomyopathy. II. Comparison of amiodarone and verapamil in treatment. *Am Heart J* 46:173, 1981.
162. McKenna WJ, Chetty S, Oakley CM, et al: Arrhythmia in hypertrophic cardiomyopathy: exercise and 48 hour ambulatory electrocardiographic treatment with and without beta adrenergic blocking therapy. *Am J Cardiol* 45:1, 1980.
163. Nicod P, Polikar R, Peterson KL: Hypertrophic cardiomyopathy and death. *N Engl J Med* 318:1255, 1988.
164. Anderson KP, Stinson EB, Deraby G, et al: Vulnerability of patients with obstructive hypertrophic cardiomyopathy to ventricular arrhythmia induction in the operating room. *Am J Cardiol* 51:811, 1983.
165. Schiavone WA, Maloney JD, Lever HM, et al: Electrophysiologic studies of patients with hypertrophic cardiomyopathy presenting with syncope of undetermined etiology. *PACE* 9:476, 1986.
166. Watson RM, Schwartz JL, Maron BJ, et al: Inducible polymorphic ventricular tachycardia and ventricular fibrillation in a

subgroup of patients with hypertrophic cardiomyopathy at high risk for sudden death. *J Am Coll Cardiol* 10:761, 1987.
167. Morady F, Shen E, Bhandari A, et al: Programmed ventricular stimulation in mitral valve prolapse: analysis of 36 patients. *Am J Cardiol* 53:135, 1984.
168. Rosenthal ME, Hamer A, Gang ES, et al: The yield of programmed ventricular stimulation in mitral valve prolapse patients with ventricular arrhythmias. *Am Heart J* 110:970, 1985.
169. Duren DR, Becker AE, Dunning AJ: Long term follow up of identifying mitral valve prolapse in 300 patients: a prospective study. *J Am Coll Cardiol* 11:42, 1988.
170. Wit AL, Fenoglio JJ, Hordof AJ, et al: Ultrastructure and transmembrane potentials of cardiac muscle in the human anterior mitral valve leaflet. *Circulation* 59:1284, 1979.
171. Boudoulas H, Wooley CF: Mitral valve prolapse syndrome. Evidence of hyperadrenergic state. *Postgrad Med* 152, 1988.

Chapter 3

Ventricular Fibrillation

Janice L. Jones

Initialization and Stabilization

Ventricular fibrillation (VF) was defined by Zipes[1] in 1975 as a "chaotic, random, asynchronous electrical activity of the ventricles due to repetitive re-entrant excitation and/or rapid focal discharge." The resulting uncoordinated excitation and contraction of the ventricles is incapable of pumping blood. Therefore, blood pressure drops rapidly and approaches the mean circulatory pressure within approximately 4–10 seconds. This lethal arrhythmia is a leading cause of death[2-4] that kills over 400,000 persons per year in the United States alone.[5] A fundamental understanding of the relationship between cardiac arrhythmias and syncope first developed early in the 19th century.[6] In spite of continuing research since that time, the mechanisms underlying the initiation and maintenance of fibrillation have yet to be completely determined. Yet, an understanding of these mechanisms is very important, not only to the research scientist, but also to the practicing clinician because the defibrillation threshold (DFT) in an individual patient depends on the characteristics of the arrhythmia to be terminated.

Ventricular fibrillation occurs primarily in the presence of a transient or permanent conduction block. Under normal conditions, the excitation wave causing ventricular contraction passes across the ventricle before cells become reexcitable. Therefore, the wave of excitation dies out and the ventricle remains quiescent until the next impulse arrives through the conduction system. However, as originally shown by Mines[7] and Garrey,[8] if a conduction slowing or block occurs so that cells that have previously been stimulated recover excitability before the excitation wave reaches the area, then reentry can occur. A schematic drawing of their original experiments is shown in Figure 1. This figure represents a ring of cardiac tissue. The white areas represent excitable tissue. After each section of tissue is excited, it becomes completely refractory as shown by the black areas. If the ring is excited so that propagation is rapid and is allowed in only one direction, propagation passes around the ring and arrives back at the starting point while the tissue is still in the absolute refractory period. Therefore, the impulse dies out as shown in the upper panel. However, if propagation is slow, as shown in the lower panel of Figure 1, then the impulse travels slowly, so that by the time it reaches the first areas that were stimulated, these regions are no longer completely refractory. Therefore, they will be reexcited and reentry will have begun. The ability of the ring to sustain continual reen-

---

From Singer I, (ed.) Implantable Cardioverter-Defibrillator. Armonk, NY: Futura Publishing Company, Inc.; © 1994.

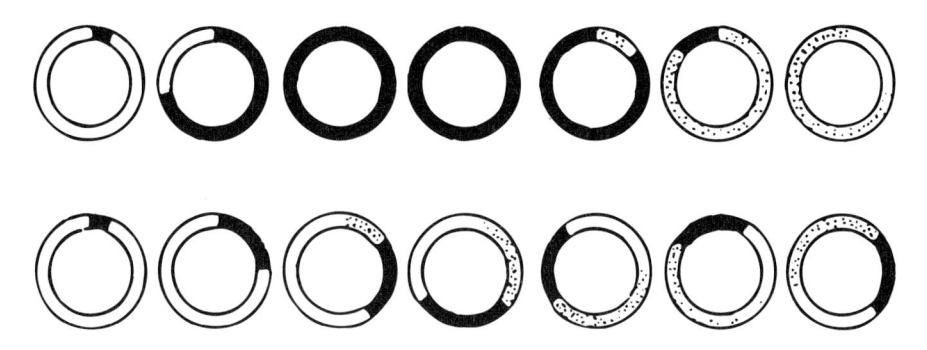

Figure 1. Schematic drawing showing conduction in a ring of cardiac tissue. The white regions represent excitable tissue. The black regions represent tissue in the absolute refractory period. The speckled regions represent tissue in the relative refractory period. The upper panel shows rapid conduction leading to extinction of the excitation wave. The lower panel shows slow conduction leading to reentry. (Modified with permission from Reference 7.)

try depends on the conduction velocity and the duration of the refractory period. Therefore, either shortening the refractory period or slowing conduction (or both) will facilitate reentry.

Ventricular fibrillation occurs under a variety of conditions. These include: 1) electrical induction with a single, low-intensity stimulus delivered during the "vulnerable period" when the ventricles are repolarizing; 2) electrical induction with a burst, usually 1 second in duration, of 60 Hz AC current; 3) spontaneous fibrillation during conditions such as ischemia that lead to conduction block; 4) reperfusion-induced fibrillation; and 5) fibrillation following high-intensity electric shocks.

Electrically Induced Vulnerable Period Fibrillation

When the heart is excited during the T wave of the electrocardiogram (the vulnerable period), either by a naturally occurring extrastimulus or by an external electrical stimulus, it is likely to fibrillate. The mechanism underlying vulnerable period fibrillation is shown in Figure 2.[9] This schematic diagram shows simultaneous action potentials from fibers in three regions of the heart (upper panels) and the corresponding electrocardiogram (lower panel). During a normal heartbeat the wave of excitation spreads throughout the ventricle from the septum in a general pattern of apex to base, and endocardium to epicardium. Because epicardial cells have shorter action potentials than endocardial cells, repolarization proceeds in a direction that is generally the opposite from excitation. During the repolarization phase, cells may be found in many different stages of repolarization at the same time. Therefore, a premature stimulus delivered during the repolarization phase will interact with cells in all stages of repolarization.

In Figure 2, a premature stimulus is given to the heart at the time of the arrow. Note that at this time some regions of the heart (eg, Fiber 1) have recovered excitability while other regions (eg, Fiber 3) are completely refractory. Different regions (eg, Fiber 2) are in the relative refractory period. These regions do not produce a normal action potential, but rather a small slowly rising response that propagates slowly and exhibits characteristics of decremental conduction. This provides the substrate for reentrant arrhythmias. When the premature stimulus is delivered, it produces an almost normal action potential in Fiber 1. The impulse can travel to Fiber 2, where it is delayed because that fiber is still partially re-

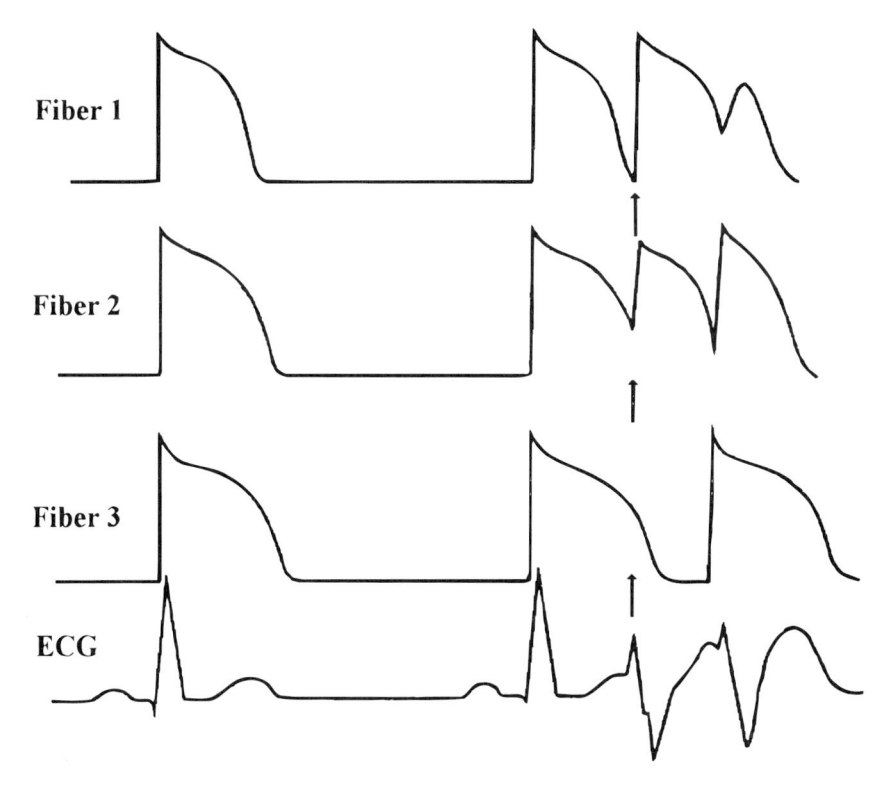

Figure 2. Schematic drawing showing the development of fibrillation. The upper three panels show action potentials from different regions of the ventricle. The lower panel shows the corresponding electrocardiogram (ECG). The arrows indicate the time of delivery of a premature stimulus. (Modified with permission from Reference 9.)

fractory. The impulse is completely blocked when it reaches Fiber 3. The slowly propagating response then cycles around to reexcite each fiber. However, the new impulse again finds fibers in different stages of refractoriness. The resultant combination of conduction slowing and block in nonexcitable regions leads to increased probability of reentry with each succeeding action potential and finally to fibrillation. This mechanism was described for atrial fibrillation by Moe and Abildskov[10] as a "multiple wavelet" hypothesis. They stated that as fibrillation develops, the " . . . grossly irregular wavefront becomes fractionated as it divides about islets or strands of refractory tissue, and each of the daughter wavelets may now be considered as independent offspring. Such a wavelet may accelerate or decelerate as it encounters tissue in a more or less advanced state of recovery. It may become extinguished as it encounters refractory tissue; it may divide again or combine with a neighbor; it may be expected to fluctuate in size and change in direction. Its course, though determined by the excitability or refractoriness of surrounding tissue, would appear as random as Brownian motion. Fully developed fibrillation would then be a state in which many such randomly wandering wavelets coexist."[10] Although more recent experiments have refined our understanding of activation patterns during fibrillation,[11-13] Moe and Abildskov's description remains accurate.

Vulnerable period fibrillation occurs in humans, as well as in experimental models such as canines, pigs, and isolated rabbit

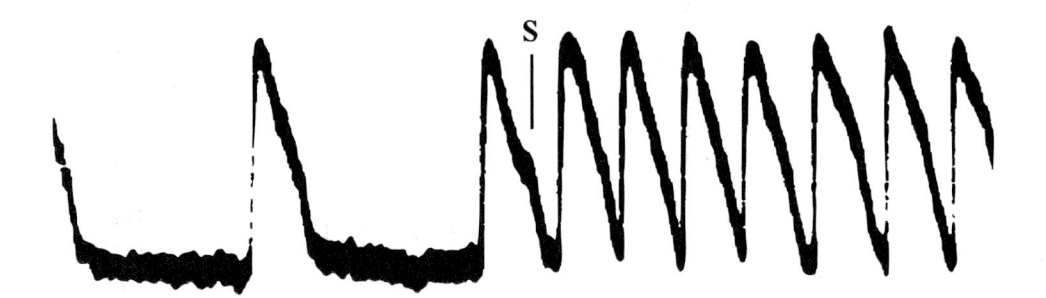

Figure 3. Monophasic action potentials recorded from the epicardium during induction of vulnerable period fibrillation in the isolated rabbit heart. "S" indicates the time of delivery of a premature stimulus leading to fibrillation.

hearts. Figure 3 shows monophasic action potentials recorded during induction of fibrillation by a single extrastimulus in the isolated rabbit heart (J. Jones, unpublished data). Note that the region of the heart from which the recording is taken is in the process of repolarizing at the time when the stimulus is delivered. Vulnerable period fibrillation can only be induced by stimulation at specific coupling intervals during the T wave and only by stimuli of specific intensity. The lowest level of stimulus that can induce fibrillation is defined as the lower limit of vulnerability. This is the lowest stimulus intensity that can stimulate partially refractory cells. Stimuli of very high intensity can no longer cause the heart to fibrillate. The highest intensity stimulus that will induce fibrillation is defined as the upper limit of vulnerability (ULV).

Determining the ULV and the mechanisms underlying it has become an important area of investigation because, under some conditions, it predicts DFT.[14,15] Therefore, shocks delivered during the vulnerable period are frequently used to induce fibrillation during internal defibrillator testing. However, the relationship varies depending on experimental conditions, such as drugs and defibrillator waveform. For example, lidocaine increased the ULV from 5.3 J–13.1 J, whereas it only increased DFT from 4.4 J–8.7 J.[16] With biphasic waveforms, the ULV and DFT also differed significantly. In one study, the ULV$_{50}$ was 250 J while the DFT$_{50}$ was 332 J.[17] Therefore, this technique cannot be routinely applied without further investigation at the research level to determine differences between mechanisms underlying fibrillation induction with a premature stimulus and defibrillation.

Electrically Induced Fibrillation Using Burst Stimuli

Delivery of an approximately 1- to 2-second pulse of 60-Hz stimuli is another technique commonly used for induction during internal defibrillator testing. This is also the method that induces fibrillation when a person contacts normal AC power. The mechanism by which these rapid stimuli induce fibrillation is illustrated in Figure 4. This figure shows optical recordings of transmembrane potential from a group of cells during application of rapid stimuli.[18] Because the stimuli are applied very rapidly at intervals that are shorter than the normal action potential, each cell responds to a stimulus very early in its relative refractory period. The resulting reentry leads to fibrillation by mechanisms similar to those described above. However, with burst stimuli, the timing of the burst to the cardiac cycle is not important because some stimuli within the 1-second burst will fall in the vulnerable period.

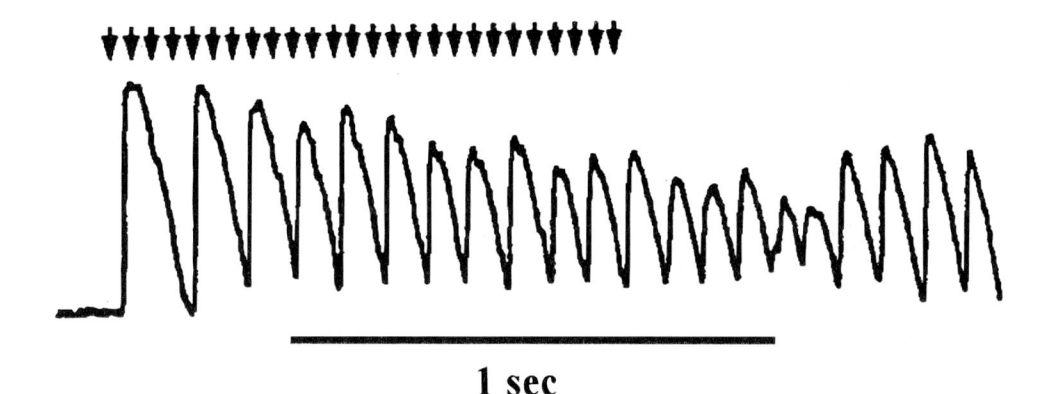

Figure 4. Optically recorded action potentials from the isolated rabbit heart recorded during induction of fibrillation using rapidly delivered stimuli. The arrows indicate the time of delivery of each stimulus. (Modified with permission from Reference 18.)

Ischemia-Induced Fibrillation

Fibrillation commonly occurs during early ischemia due to reentry caused by functional block. For example, in one study cats subjected to proximal left anterior descending coronary artery occlusion developed fibrillation in approximately 25% of animals within 1–5 minutes.[19] The tachyarrhythmia leading to fibrillation was maintained primarily by intramural reentry involving multiple activation sites in and around the border zone of the ischemic area, although nonreentrant mechanisms also contributed. The transition to fibrillation was characterized by intramural reentry and rapid, inhomogeneous recovery of excitability, which led to increased conduction delay, and development of multiple reentrant circuits.

Inhomogeneities between effects of developing ischemia and reperfusion on action potentials in different regions of the heart are partially responsible for inducing fibrillation. For example, transmembrane potentials recorded from cat endocardium and epicardium during ischemia and reperfusion, as shown in Figure 5,[20] show that while action potential morphology and conduction time deteriorated rapidly in both regions, the magnitude was greater in epicardial cells than in endocardial cells. The action potential duration of endocardial cells progressively decreased during 30 minutes of ischemia, and the refractory period paralleled the action potential duration during the entire 30 minutes. In contrast, the action potential duration of epicardial cells decreased maximally at 10 minutes, then began to return toward normal. However, in epicardial cells, the refractory period duration paralleled the action potential duration only during the first 10 minutes. Refractory period then began to increase due to postrepolarization refractoriness. The resulting dispersion of refractoriness contributes to ischemia-induced fibrillation.

In general, there are several conditions that contribute to the development of fibrillation, and that tend to develop almost simultaneously. First, inhomogeneous repolarization, which is accentuated by ischemia, allows creation of a unidirectional conduction block and allows some depolarization waves to travel throughout the ventricle without being extinguished. Second, the resulting rapid stimulation of ventricular cells causes a decrease in conduction velocity and shortening of the refractory period that enhances the probability of reentry into the region. Third, the impulses divide around refractory tissue so that a single excitation wave degenerates into multiple wavelets. This produces longer pathways

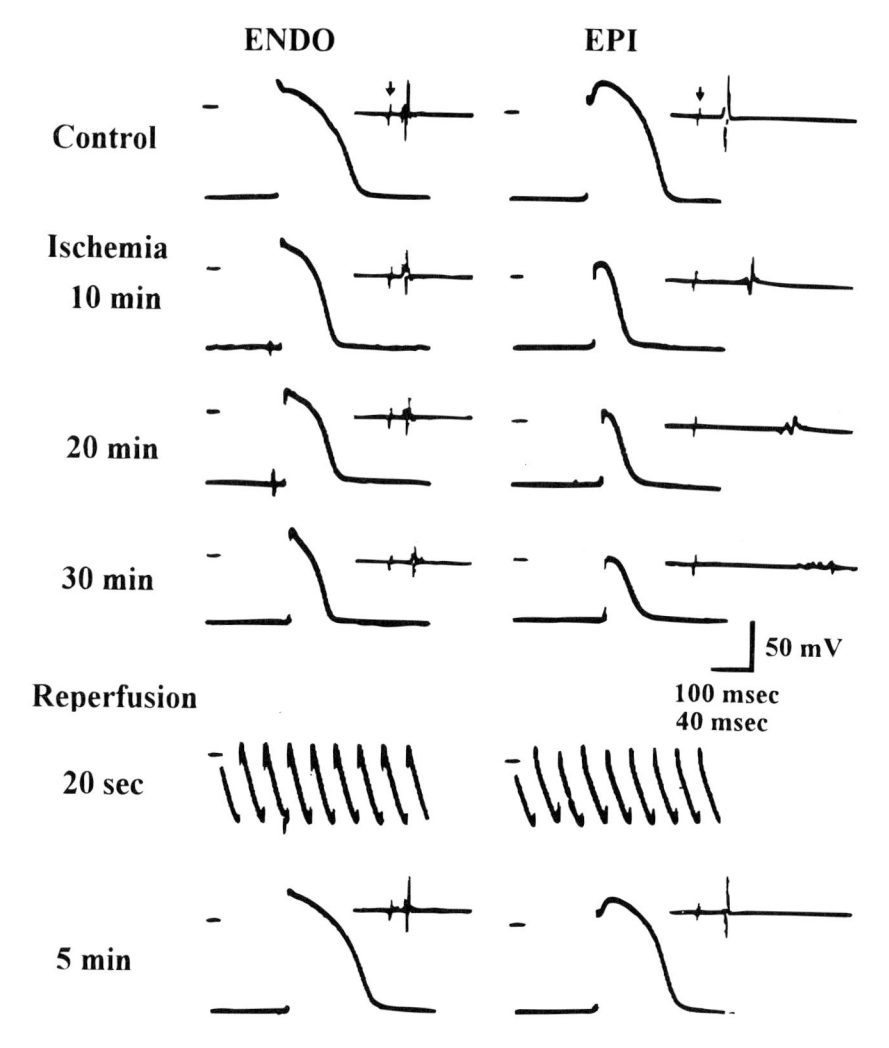

Figure 5. Transmembrane action potentials and bipolar electrograms recorded from the endo- and epicardium of the isolated cat ventricle during ischemia.[20]

for each wave front, and patchy areas of refractory tissue. Finally, the tissue reaches a stable condition in which, as each area leaves the refractory period, an excitation wave front is nearby, ready to reexcite the regions. At this point, fibrillation is stabilized.

Role of the Autonomic Nervous System in Initiating Fibrillation

There is growing evidence that an imbalance in sympathetic tone may be an important element leading to sudden cardiac death.[21,22] Myocardial ischemia resulting from coronary artery occlusion increases cardiac sympathetic tone and reduces parasympathetic tone. These changes are more pronounced in animals that are susceptible to VF than in animals that are resistant.[23] Ohyanagi et al.[24] also showed that increased localized β adrenergic activity during ischemia sensitized the heart to VF. In their study, 15 minutes of ischemia increased sarcolemmal β adrenergic receptors and cyclic adenosine monophosphate (cAMP) levels in the ischemic area of animals that developed spontaneous VF. β Blockers suppressed development of fibrillation. Similar results were obtained by Skinner,[25] who found autonomic transmitter imbalances in regions distal to a transmural infarction.

When catecholamine concentrations vary in different regions of the heart, they produce variable effects on action potential duration. Similar epinephrine concentrations also produce different effects on action potential duration in epicardial, endocardial, and midmyocardial tissue.[26] Therefore, action potential durations may vary greatly in different regions of the ventricle with strong adrenergic stimulation. Ventricular fibrillation occurs predominantly in the setting of coronary disease. It may be caused by interaction between selective ischemia (spasm or infarct with dying tissue) with imbalance of sympathetics to the heart leading to dispersion of repolarization. During ischemia, metabolite and ionic imbalances may also play an important role in producing ventricular arrhythmias.[27-29]

Even in the absence of ischemia, stimulation of cardiac sympathetic nerves increases vulnerability to VF.[30] Although vagal stimulation alone had no effect on fibrillation inducibility, vagal stimulation in the presence of sympathetic stimulation attenuated the increased vulnerability produced by sympathetic stimulation. Behavioral stress causes similar increased vulnerability.[31]

Although the normal sympathetic transmitter in the heart is norepinephrine (primarily an α agonist), under conditions of stress,[31] the large catecholamine release is primarily epinephrine (a mixed α/β agonist). Epinephrine may not only convert tachyarrhythmias to fibrillation by shortening action potential duration,[32,33] but may also stabilize fibrillation by altering cellular coupling.[34] Epinephrine also reduces fibrillation threshold (defined as 80% probability of inducing fibrillation from a curve of fibrillation success versus stimulus intensity) from 23 ± 4 V to 5 ± 1 V.[33]

Because catecholamines are implicated in arrhythmias leading to sudden cardiac death, β blockers are commonly given after myocardial infarction to help prevent these arrhythmias.[35-38]

Reperfusion-Induced Fibrillation

Reperfusion of ischemic tissue can also lead to VF. Although the mortality due to fibrillation in dogs is similar after occlusion and during reperfusion, the mechanism underlying reperfusion-induced fibrillation differs from that by which fibrillation is induced during early ischemia.[39-41] In an early study, Penkoske et al.[39] showed that the arrhythmia is initiated by rapidly repeating sequences originating from the reperfused area. More recently, Pogwizd and Corr[42] showed that in cats in which 10 minutes of regional ischemia was followed by reperfusion, reperfusion was followed by tachyarrhythmia that degenerated into fibrillation in 50% of the animals. The ventricular tachycardia (VT) originated in the subepicardium at the border of the reperfused area by nonreentrant mechanisms, and was maintained by both nonreentrant and reentrant mechanisms. During the transition to fibrillation, the nonreentrant mechanisms led to rapid acceleration and fibrillation. Another study of activation patterns during the transition to fibrillation after reperfusion in dogs also showed a period of organized epicardial activation.[43]

The incidence of reperfusion-induced fibrillation in dogs is increased in the presence of ventricular hypertrophy and is independent of hypertension. Taylor et al.[41] showed that following reperfusion after 15 minutes of coronary artery occlusion, 7 of 17 dogs with ventricular hypertrophy fibrillated. In contrast, fibrillation occurred in only 1 of 18 control dogs. In hypertrophied hearts, mechanisms initiating reperfusion-induced fibrillation appear similar to those in control hearts.

Fibrillation Induced with High-Intensity Electric Stimuli

A high-intensity electric shock that is significantly above the ULV can also induce fibrillation in normal myocardium. Transthoracic stimulation of increasing intensity, beginning at about 20 times excitation threshold, produces "minor arrhythmias such as several extrasystoles, temporary tachycardia or bradycardia; moderate but fully reversible arrhythmias involving longer lasting changes of rhythm including VT and ventricular extrasystoles; severe changes such as marked electrocardiographic deformations and ventricular rhythm changes lasting up to several minutes; and severe arrhythmias changing into VF which could not be corrected by a second shock."[44] Saumont et al.[45] also described a similar pattern of arrhythmias ranging from tachycardia to irreversible fibrillation. The fibrillation observed by both groups following high-voltage stimulation is very different in nature from fibrillation that occurs after low-voltage stimulation during the vulnerable period because it cannot be corrected by a second shock and has a characteristic electrocardiographic appearance. Shock intensities required to produce irreversible fibrillation with poor defibrillator waveforms having low safety factors (ratio of shock intensity required to produce dysfunction to intensities required to defibrillate) were not much higher than those required to defibrillate.[46,47] Similar arrhythmia patterns are produced in cultured myocardial cells by similar intensity shocks.[47-49] The mechanism underlying production of irreversible fibrillation appears to be calcium overload.[50] After high-intensity shock, intracellular calcium increases due to the formation of transient sarcolemmal microlesions during the shock.[51] The high intracellular calcium causes erratic, calcium-induced, calcium release from the sarcoplasmic reticulum. This leads to erratic contraction of individual myofibrils within the cardiac cell. The gross manifestation of this cellular fibrillation[52] is an unusual type of VF that cannot be corrected by a defibrillating shock. Because cardiac glycosides can dramatically increase the probability of postshock arrhythmias,[53] including irreversible fibrillation after electric countershock (unmasking of "digitalis toxicity"), some investigators recommend withdrawing cardiac glycosides 1–3 days prior to elective cardioversion.[54-56] However, serum digoxin levels alone cannot predict the probability of such arrhythmias.[57,58]

Control of Human Fibrillation Cycle Length by Refractory Period

Fibrillation Cycle Length

The ECG, as usually recorded, shows voltage as a function of time. However, much useful information can be obtained about mean heart rate and heart rate variability both during normal sinus rhythm and during fibrillation by displaying the power of the ECG signal as a function of frequency using a fast Fourier transform as shown in Figure 6.[59,60] During early fibrillation, much of the power is contained in a sharp, low-frequency band. Allen et al.[61] found that in humans with primary VF, the peak of this band in the lead II ECG was at 5.18 ± 0.3 Hz (corresponding to a cycle length of 193 msec). Similar results have been obtained in several other studies.[62,63]

Role of Refractory Period in Controlling Fibrillation Cycle Length

The cellular mechanisms that underlie fibrillation are only poorly understood. Yet these mechanisms play an important role in understanding defibrillation mechanisms. For example, if there is an excitable gap during VF, as there is in atrial fibrillation,[64] then cells could be stimulated in diastole and a pacing level regimen could be used to defibrillate. Conversely, if cells are restimulated by new fibrillation wave fronts immediately after termination of their refractory period, then refractory period stimulation is important for defibrillation.[65,66]

Studies by Allessie et al.[67-69] in isolated sheets of rabbit atrium suggested that the

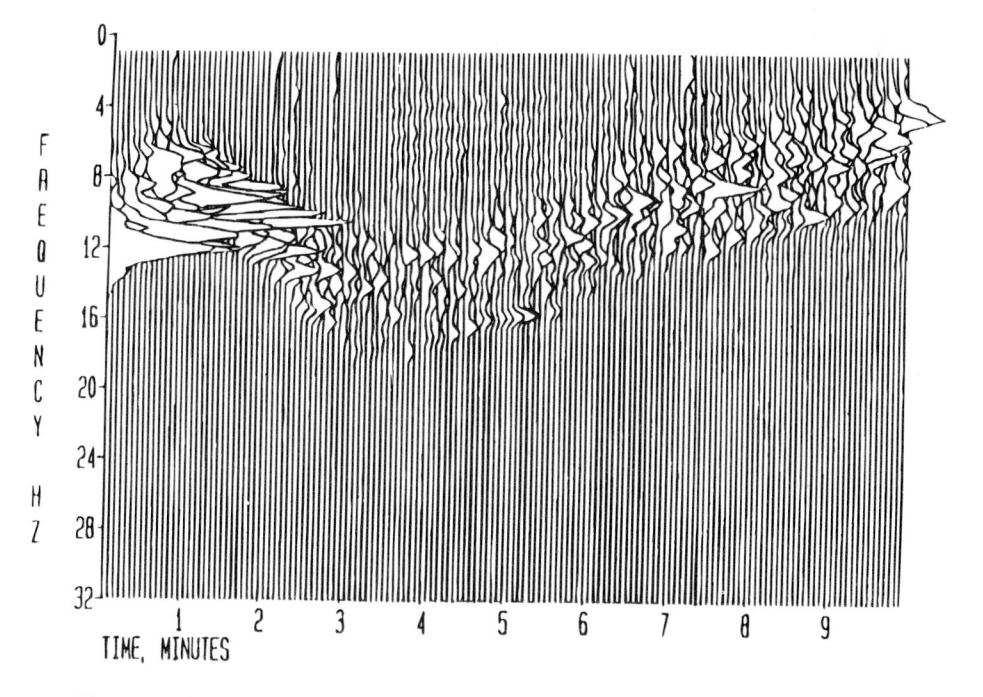

Figure 6. Electrocardiogram (ECG) power spectrum recorded during fibrillation in the swine. The x axis represents fibrillation duration (downtime) in minutes; the y axis represents frequency; and the z axis the power amplitude. (Reproduced with permission from Reference 96.)

cycle length of fibrillation in each region of the ventricle is controlled by the cellular refractory period in that region. They mapped the spread of excitation with multiple electrodes during the initiation of reentry and found that the impulse circulated in the smallest possible pathway for which the tissue just ahead was in the relative refractory period. They designated this small pathway as a leading circle for which the head of the circulating wave front was continuously "biting" its own tail of relative refractoriness. These functional circuits were small, very rapid, and very unstable. These findings in rabbit tissue suggested that the local cycle length during fibrillation is determined by the cellular refractory period (or action potential duration in the absence of postrepolarization refractoriness). These findings also suggested a critical criterion for defibrillation, that defibrillation involved stimulation of partially refractory tissue and that the local defibrillating stimulus must be stronger than that provided by the local reentrant excitation. It is this finding that has provided the impetus for the many recent studies of defibrillation mechanisms that are based on the hypothesis that defibrillation involves stimulation of refractory tissue.[65,70,71]

Monophasic Action Potentials During Fibrillation

In order to determine whether fibrillation cycle length in humans is controlled primarily by the cellular refractory period as predicted by Allessie, or whether it is determined by timing of arrival of a fibrillation wave front to the region so that a diastolic interval occurs between action potentials, Swartz et al.[72] recorded right ventricular endocardial monophasic action potentials during routine nonthoracotomy internal defibrillator implants. Tachyarrhythmia episodes that resulted in loss of blood pressure were classified as VF/poly-

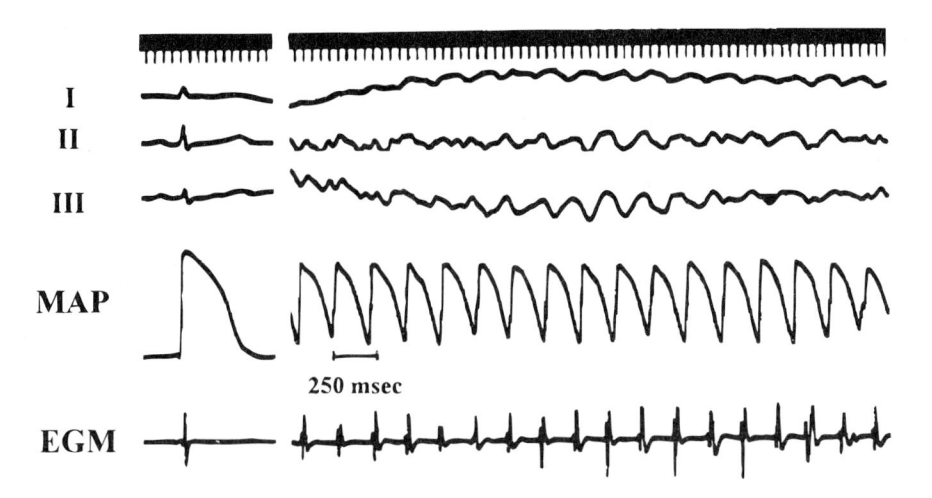

Figure 7. Recordings taken during ventricular fibrillation (VF) in a human. Leads I, II, and III are body surface electrocardiograms (ECGs). MAP: right ventricular monophasic action potentials. EGM: local bipolar electrogram. Note that there is no period of diastole between action potentials. (Modified with permission from Reference 72.)

morphic VT if they had irregular limb lead I morphology. Typical recordings during fibrillation are shown in Figure 7. In this figure, leads I, II, and III of the ECG confirm fibrillation (as opposed to another tachyarrhythmia). The monophasic action potential is identified as MAP and the output of the defibrillator's sensing lead is labeled as EGM. The left panel shows recordings during normal sinus rhythm; the right panel shows recordings during fibrillation. The figure shows clearly that fibrillation action potentials usually occur immediately following partial repolarization from each previous action potential so that there is no period of diastole. Mean cycle length recorded in humans during the first 15 seconds of fibrillation was 213 ± 27 msec. Episodes

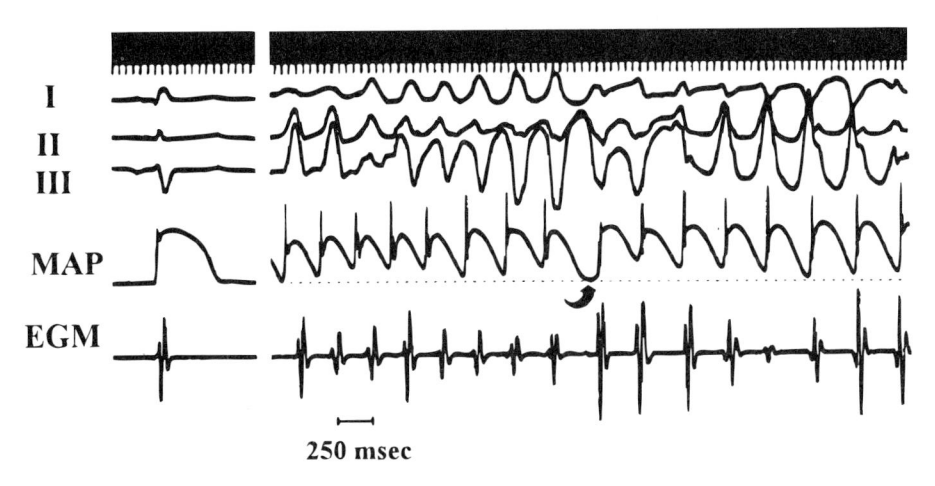

Figure 8. Recordings taken during polymorphic ventricular tachycardia in the human. Leads I, II, and III are body surface electrocardiograms (ECGs). MAP: right ventricular monophasic action potentials. EGM: local bipolar electrogram. Note that there are occasional periods of diastole between action potentials. (Modified with permission from Reference 72.)

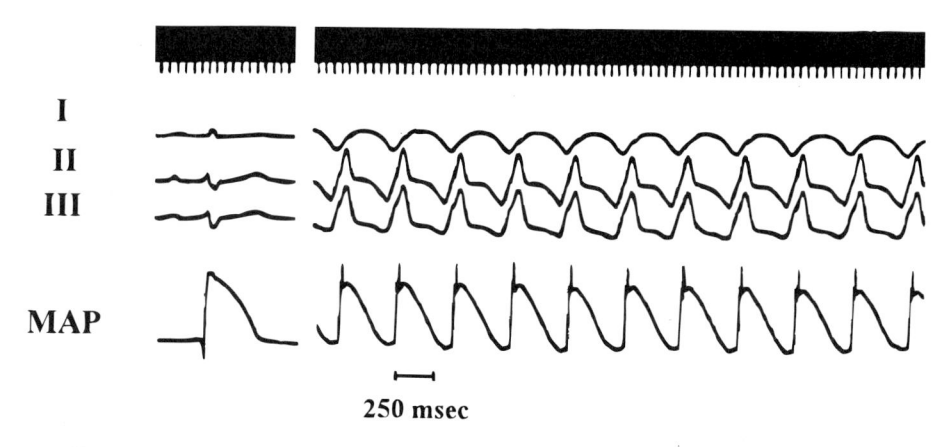

Figure 9. Recordings taken during "slow" monomorphic ventricular tachycardia in the human. Leads I, II, and III are body surface electrocardiograms (ECGs). MAP: right ventricular monophasic action potentials. EGM: local bipolar electrogram. Note that there are well-defined periods of diastole between action potentials. (Modified with permission from Reference 72.)

characterized as polymorphic VT, which occurred primarily in patients on amiodarone therapy, had a slower mean cycle length of 257 ± 22 msec and had occasional MAP diastole as shown by the curved arrow in Figure 8. In contrast, episodes of slow monomorphic tachycardia with for example, cycle length of 360 msec, were always characterized by diastolic intervals as shown in Figure 9. The cycle lengths recorded using monophasic action potentials during fibrillation are in close agreement with those found by direct measurement with bipolar sensing electrodes during internal defibrillator testing and with those found using power spectrum analysis of the external ECG.[61]

Importance of Arrhythmia Morphology and Cycle Length for Successful Conversion

The finding that there is no diastolic interval during VF is important in understanding the high shock intensity required to defibrillate in contrast to that required for pacing or antitachycardia devices. For example, Kerber et al.[73] tested the hypothesis that current requirements for transthoracic termination of tachyarrhythmia depend on morphology as determined from the surface ECG. They compared shock intensities required for conversion of different tachyarrhythmias in 203 patients who received a total of 569 shocks. They defined monomorphic VT by uniform QRS morphology with rate greater than 100 beats per minute (cycle length < 600 msec), polymorphic VT by nonuniform QRS morphology and heart rate ≤ 300 beats per minute (cycle length > 200 msec), and VF by nonuniform QRS morphology with rate > 300 beats per minute (cycle length < 200 msec). The results in Figure 10 show that low-intensity shocks of 18 and 25 amps have a high probability of converting monomorphic VT, but only a low probability of converting polymorphic VT or VF. Low-intensity shocks (18 and 25 amps) had a higher probability of success for slow monomorphic VT (89%) than for fast VT (72%, $P < 0.01$).

The findings of Kerber et al. findings support the conclusion that the morphology and rate of the arrhythmia are important determinants of the electric shock energy required to terminate it. Because the shock intensity which is required to convert the arrhythmia depends on its type, it is important during defibrillator testing to ensure that the patient is actually in fibrillation, rather than in another tachyarrhythmia.

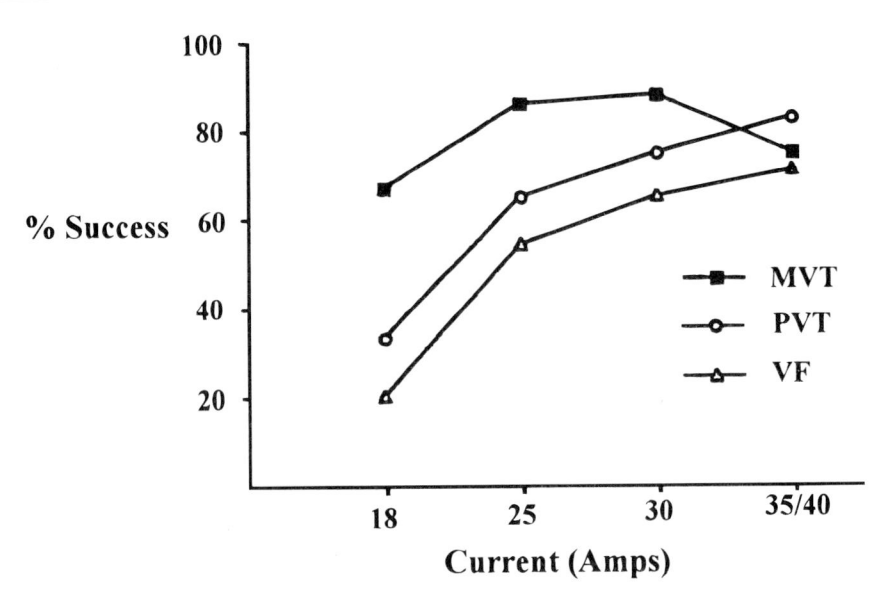

Figure 10. Probability of successful conversion in humans of monomorphic ventricular tachycardia (MVT), polymorphic ventricular tachycardia (PVT), and ventricular fibrillation (VF) as a function of electrode current using transthoracic electrodes. (Modified with permission from Reference 73.)

Kerber et al.'s results can be explained by the monophasic action potentials recorded by Swartz et al.[65] during fibrillation. Monomorphic VT, for which there is usually a diastolic interval, could be successfully terminated by a low-intensity shock in most cases. In contrast, polymorphic VT and VF, which were usually characterized by a lack of diastolic interval, required a much higher current intensity to successfully convert. In agreement with the occurrence of a greater number of short diastolic intervals with polymorphic VT than with VF, the probability of conversion with low-intensity shocks was slightly greater.

Because cells during fibrillation or fast polymorphic VT are seldom found in diastole, conversion of VF requires interaction of the electric field primarily with refractory tissue.[65,66,74] During defibrillation, the shock acts on the cell during its action potential to prolong the refractory period. This prevents fibrillation wave fronts from entering the area and causes fibrillation to cease.[65,70,75] However, the shock intensity required to produce refractory period extension with monophasic defibrillator waveforms is approximately 3–4 times that required for excitation during diastole.[74] Also, this high-current intensity must be produced throughout all or a critical mass of the ventricle. Because local shock intensity varies by a factor of approximately 20 in different regions of the heart for epicardial electrode placements,[76] and by an even larger ratio with nonthoracotomy electrode placements, a very large shock is required for defibrillation compared to that required for pacing.

The requirement for refractory period stimulation to convert fibrillation also has a major impact on the choice of defibrillator waveform. Recent research has shown that biphasic waveforms in which the polarity is reversed partway through the pulse can lower defibrillation energy threshold to approximately one half that required for similarly shaped monophasic waveforms.[77] During fibrillation, cells seldom repolarize fully. Therefore, sodium channels, which are inactivated following the upstroke of the action potential, are not fully recovered at the time of the shock, and a high shock intensity is required to produce a well-

Monophasic

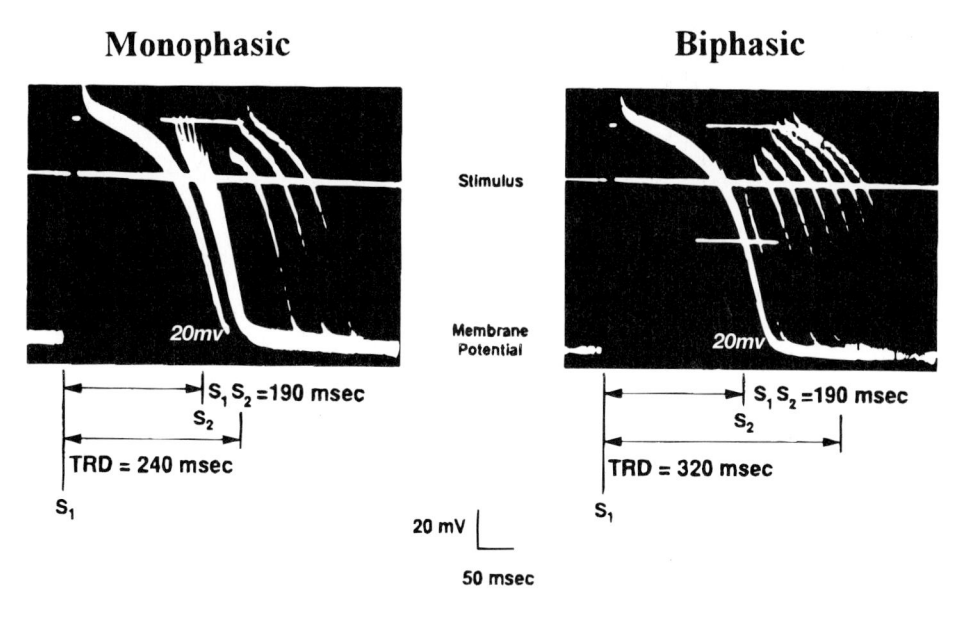

Biphasic

Figure 11. Transmembrane potentials recorded from myocardial cell aggregates during refractory period stimulation using intracellular current injection with depolarizing monophasic and hyperpolarizing/depolarizing biphasic stimuli. Each panel shows 10 superimposed action potential responses produced by stimuli of 1.5 times the monophasic waveform diastolic threshold at different coupling intervals. The biphasic stimulus produces better formed responses at short coupling intervals. (Modified with permission from Reference 65.)

formed graded response. One mechanism by which biphasic waveforms reduce threshold is by accelerating repolarization during the first phase, thereby shortening the cellular refractory period, and allowing sodium channel recovery. Therefore, the tissue is able to produce a longer, better formed graded response at short coupling intervals as shown in Figure 11.[65,66,78] The longer response prolongs the total response duration (TRD in Figure 11) and total refractory period. Therefore, the tissue is refractory during arrival of fibrillation wave fronts, and fibrillation ceases.

Species Differences in Ventricular Fibrillation

In situ animal and isolated tissue models are commonly used to study fibrillation-defibrillation mechanism and also to determine optimal electrical waveshapes and electrode configurations for defibrillation. Although these models are very useful and allow experiments that could not ethically be performed on humans, it is important to note differences between these models and humans and to interpret data acquired in such model systems with caution. Fibrillation cycle length varies widely among species. In humans, it is approximately 200 msec. In dogs, the mean peak frequency of the power spectrum is at 9.9 ± 0.7 Hz, which corresponds to a mean cycle length of 101 msec. This value is similar to the value found by Worley et al. with direct activation mapping during the first 15 seconds of fibrillation. In pigs, another model that is commonly used for defibrillation studies, fibrillation cycle length is approximately 95 msec (frequency of 10.4 Hz at 30 seconds fibrillation).[59] In sheep, cycle length is approximately 110 msec (C. Alferness, unpublished data). In isolated rabbit hearts, cycle length is approximately 100 msec, similar to that found in dogs.[33] It is possible that these differences may reflect differences in the underlying electrophysiology between these species. This may have an impact on choosing an animal model in which to develop new drugs or defibrillator waveforms to improve defibrillation efficacy in humans.

Relation Between Duration of Fibrillation and Defibrillation Success

Short Fibrillation Durations

Internal defibrillators are designed so that the first defibrillating shock is delivered within 10–20 seconds after the initiation of fibrillation. During the implantation procedure, several test shocks must be delivered to ensure that the device will function properly. For this testing, fibrillation duration prior to delivering the test shocks is usually set at 10 or 15 seconds. This short time minimizes the ischemia to which the patient is subjected. However, during actual use in the field, the duration of fibrillation may be longer especially if the first shock fails and the unit must deliver a second shock. The effects of fibrillation duration on DFT remain uncertain.

In the biventricular working rabbit heart model,[79] defibrillation voltage threshold for single pulses using monophasic waveforms increases with fibrillation duration from 5–30 seconds as shown in Figure 12. This corresponds to an increase from 0.18 J at 5 seconds to 0.33 J at 30 seconds, a 1.8 times increase in energy threshold. Similar results have been obtained in other experimental models. In dogs, energy threshold increased from 19 J at 5 seconds to 29 J at 30 seconds, so that threshold was increased by 1.5 times during that period.[80]

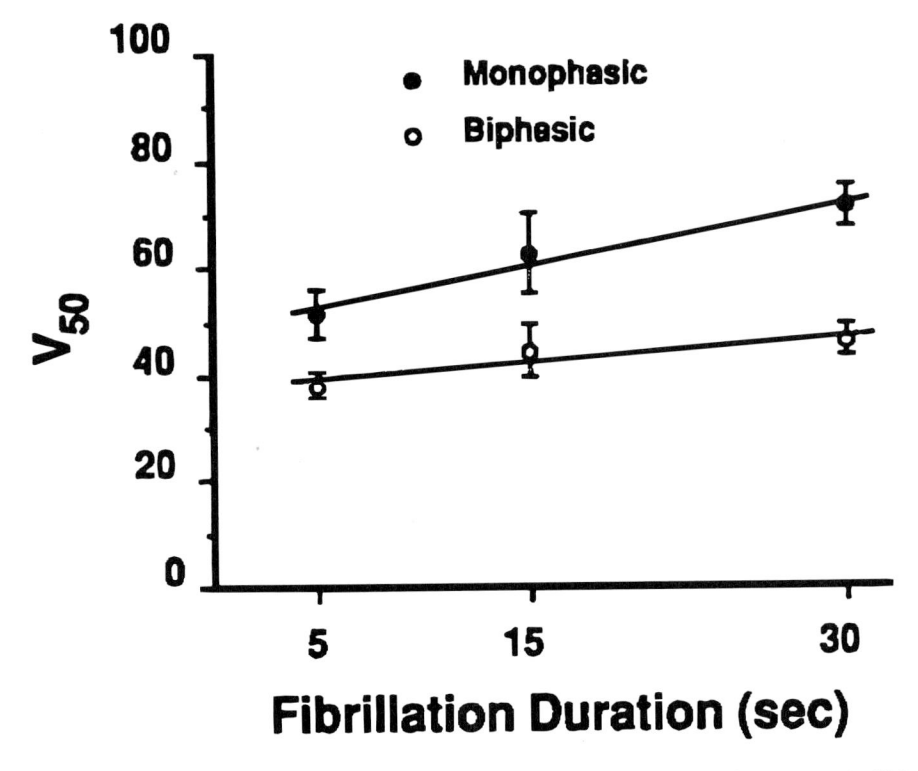

Figure 12. Defibrillation threshold for 5-msec monophasic (closed circles) and asymmetrical biphasic (open circles) waveforms as a function of fibrillation duration. (Reproduced with permission from Reference 79.)

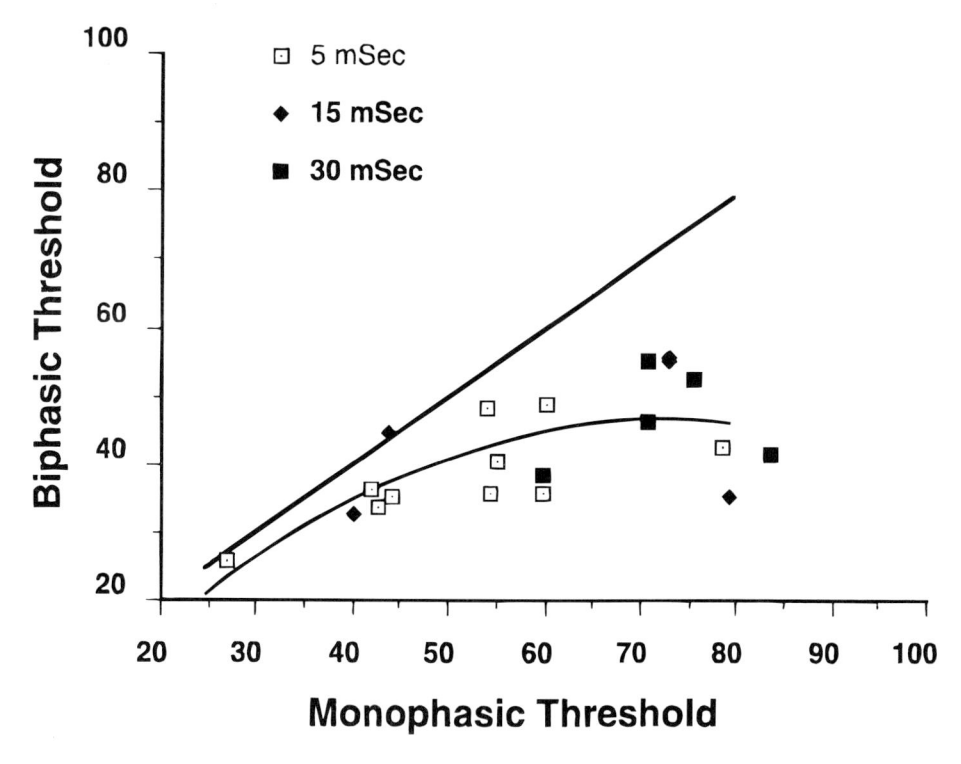

Figure 13. Defibrillation threshold for biphasic waveform as a function of monophasic waveform threshold. (Reproduced with permission from Reference 79.)

With the sequential pulse technique, Fujimura et al.[81] found a smaller threshold increase of 1.4 times between 10- and 40-seconds fibrillation in the open chest pig.

Human studies have produced varying results. One study failed to show an increase between 10- and 20-seconds fibrillation in 10 patients during defibrillator implantation.[82] However, another study in 14 patients showed an increase from 10.9 J at 12 seconds to 17.6 J at 28 seconds.[83] This corresponds to an increase of approximately 1.6 times.

The increase in DFT with fibrillation duration, which occurs for monophasic defibrillator waveforms, does not appear to occur with biphasic waveforms as shown in Figure 12. Figure 13 shows DFT for the biphasic waveform as a function of monophasic waveform threshold (note clustering of filled squares, representing 30-seconds fibrillation at the higher monophasic thresholds). Biphasic waveforms (5-msec duration, 50% undershoot) reduce DFT at all fibrillation durations. However, the relative efficacy of the biphasic waveform increases at long fibrillation durations because as monophasic waveform threshold increases, biphasic waveform threshold remains relatively stable. A possible mechanism for the increased monophasic waveform threshold with increasing fibrillation duration and its stabilization with biphasic waveforms may be the physiological changes in the cellular milieu, such as increased extracellular potassium and acidosis, which develop as fibrillation continues.

Prolonged Fibrillation

The probability of survival decreases significantly with prolonged fibrillation duration as shown in Figure 14.[84–86] After approximately 7 minutes, only 60% of fibrillation episodes are converted to any other

% surviving VF

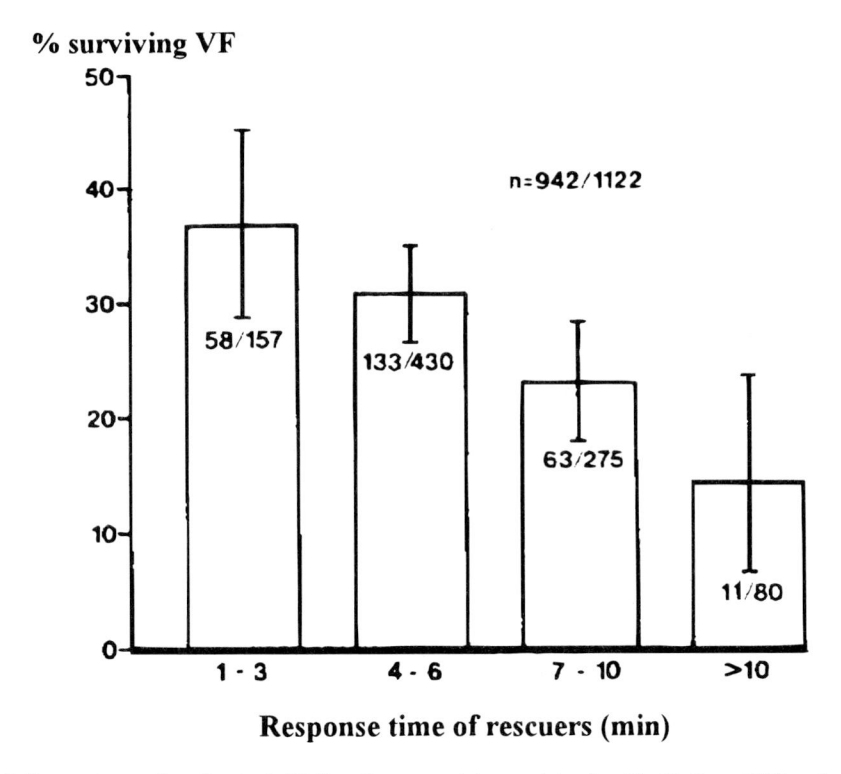

Figure 14. Percentage of patients, initially discovered in ventricular fibrillation (VF), who survive to hospital discharge as a function of response time of rescuers trained to defibrillate. (Modified with permission from Reference 85.)

rhythm. Since half of these conversions are to ventricular standstill, only 30% of patients are converted to a perfusing rhythm resulting in survival.[85] These results are far better than those obtained in most geographic locations. For example, a very recent study showed that in Chicago, only about 3% of out-of-hospital resuscitations are successful.[87] Yet it is known from animal experiments that myocardial tissue can withstand at least 15 minutes of total ischemia before irreversible injury takes place. If fibrillation could be successfully converted to normal sinus rhythm in these patients, new developments in treating ischemia-induced dysfunction could allow these patients to return to a productive lifestyle. Factors producing the lack of success for defibrillation between 1 and 10 minutes fibrillation are largely unknown. However, especially after longer fibrillation durations, the defibrillating shock appears to convert fibrillation to cardiac standstill rather than to a perfusing rhythm due, in part, to potentiation of dysfunction caused by the shock itself[47,51] by the preexisting ischemia. The resulting ionic imbalances lead to increased ventricular standstill. A second mechanism by which biphasic waveforms may improve defibrillation success is by reducing the severity of these postshock arrhythmias and allowing improved postshock cardiac function.[88,89]

Cellular Electrophysiology of Fibrillation

Ionic Channel Alterations During Short Duration Fibrillation

During normal sinus rhythm, the action potential upstroke is caused by a large and fast sodium current that can be blocked by tetrodotoxin. These channels are inactivated during depolarization. During repolarization, recovery of the channels that carry this current is time and voltage dependent. The end of the cellular refractory period is usually characterized by the recovery of these channels to the resting state. Because during fibrillation new action potentials are formed immediately after repolarization from the previous action potential as shown in Figures 3, 4, and 7, it is possible that the fast sodium current is not yet completely available. In one study using the open chest dog model, intracellular microelectrodes were used to examine action potential morphology during early vulnerable period induced fibrillation. This study showed that a small, but variable sodium channel activity remains during the first 20 seconds of fibrillation.[90] In contrast, Akiyama[91] showed that during the first minute of reperfusion-induced fibrillation, action potentials arose from a depolarized membrane as shown in the upper panel of Figure 15. They had a slow upstroke and lack of tetrodotoxin sensitivity that suggested primarily slow calcium channel dependence. Therefore, the role of the fast sodium channel in maintaining fibrillation may vary depending on its initiating cause. However, because with either type of induction, new fibrillation action potentials arise as soon as a cell leaves its refractory period, the defibrillating shock is delivered during the refractory period when little sodium channel activity is available. Therefore, monophasic waveforms may directly activate slow channels, whereas biphasic waveforms may

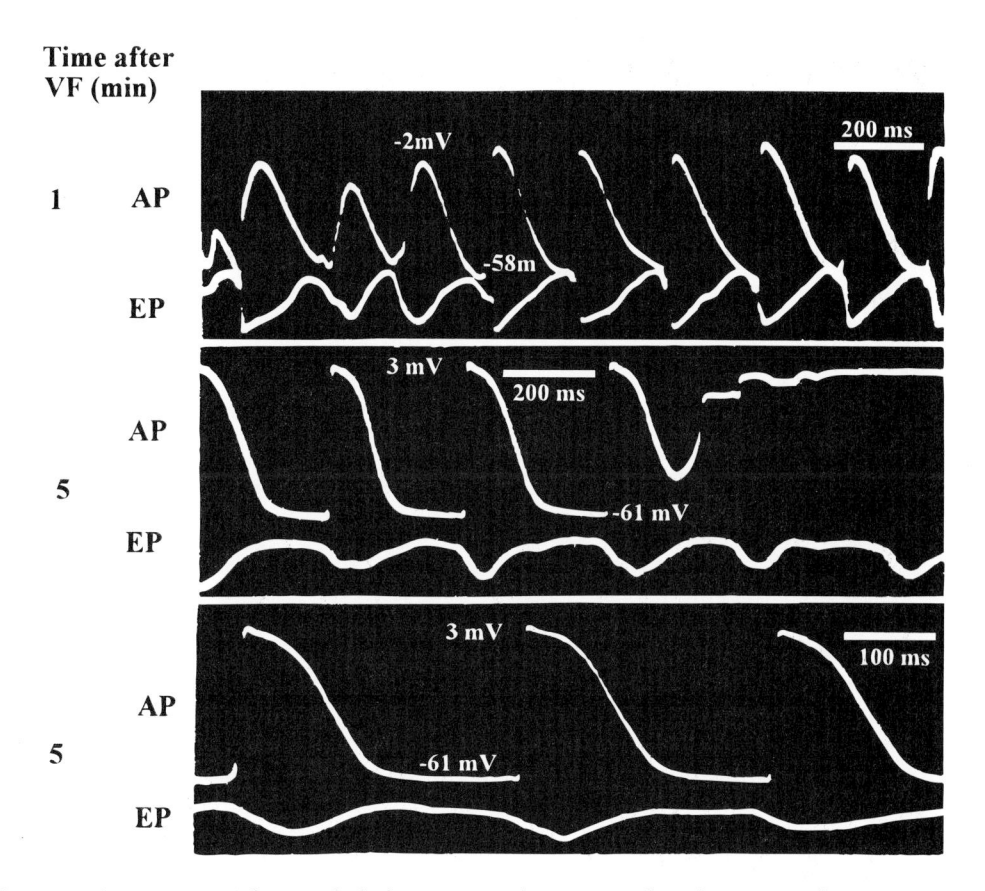

Figure 15. Action potentials recorded after 1 minute (upper panel) and 5 minutes (lower two panels) of reperfusion-induced fibrillation in the dog. (Modified with permission from Reference 91.)

lower threshold by causing early sodium channel recovery as discussed earlier.

Electrophysiology of Prolonged Fibrillation

In agreement with the decreasing probability of successful defibrillation with increasing fibrillation duration shown in Figure 14, it appears that electrophysiologic characteristics of the heart change after 1–10 minutes of fibrillation. After short fibrillation durations, cells are restimulated before complete repolarization from their previous action potential. After long fibrillation durations, ventricular cells in the epicardium are found in diastole but are depolarized as shown in the lower panels of Figure 15. Therefore, fibrillation cycle length of epicardial cells becomes longer between 1 and 5 minutes fibrillation. A similar epicardial cycle length slowing is shown by Worley et al.[92] who examined activation rates throughout the myocardium as a function of fibrillation duration. Figure 16 shows activation patterns in the endocardium, midmyocardium, and epicardium during 20 minutes of fibrillation. During the first minute of fibrillation, rapid activations appear in all locations. After the first minute, endocardial activation rate slows, but remains regular; midmyocardial and epicardial activations occur only infrequently. The regular activations observed at the endocardium may be produced by Purkinje fibers near the blood pool.

Similar results were found by Carlisle et al.[93] who found that the dominant frequency at the body surface in dogs decreased from 12 Hz (cycle length = 83 msec for fibrillation induced by occlusion of the left descending coronary artery) to 5–6 Hz (cycle length = 200 msec) after 120 seconds of fibrillation. There was no corresponding decrease in frequency of endocardial recordings. The slowing of fibrillation with duration as shown by the decrease in me-

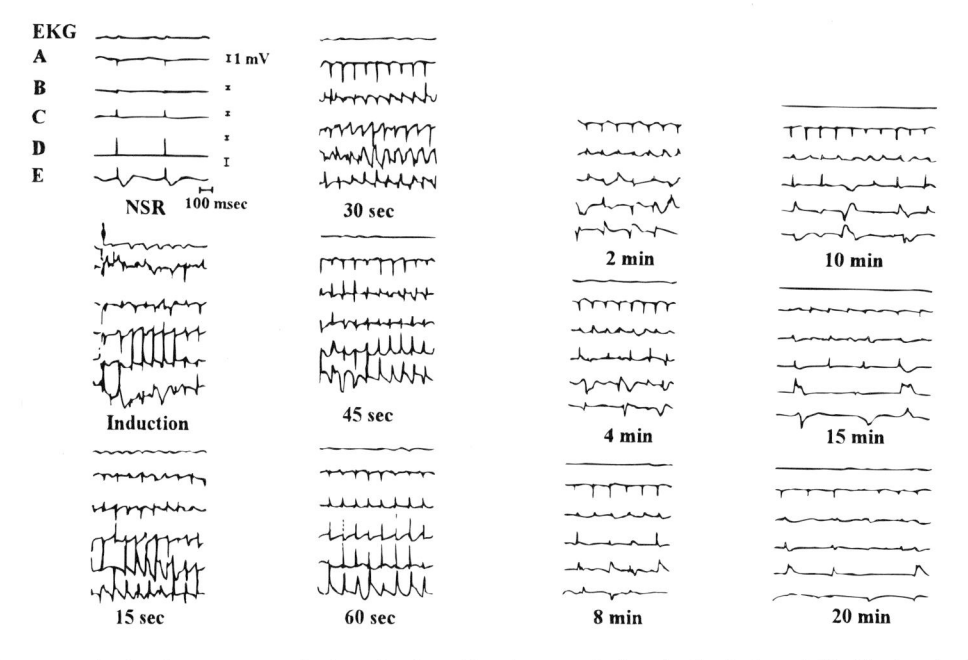

Figure 16. Activation patterns during the first 20 minutes of electrically induced fibrillation in the dog. The upper tracing in each panel is the body surface electrocardiogram (EKG). Tracings A–E are bipolar recordings from plunge electrodes. A is near the endocardium; E is near the epicardium. (Modified with permission from Reference 92.)

dian frequency of the power spectrum also correlates well with fibrillation duration in pigs.[94] This study suggested that the power spectrum of the body surface ECG could be used to predict fibrillation duration during out-of-hospital resuscitation.

The slowing of excitation rate and appearance of diastole as fibrillation duration increases suggests that the fundamental electrophysiology of fibrillation, and perhaps the mechanism underlying defibrillation changes with fibrillation duration. During early fibrillation, cells in the ventricle are contracting asynchronously and cells are found in all phases of their refractory period. However, as fibrillation duration increases, as can be seen in Figure 15, new action potentials no longer occur immediately following the previous action potential as was the case during early fibrillation.

During the global ischemia that occurs during prolonged fibrillation, greater epicardial action potential morphology deterioration and postrepolarization refractoriness occurs compared to endocardial action potentials as shown in Figure 5.[20] This difference may be responsible for the differing endocardial versus epicardial activation patterns observed by Worley et al.,[92] as well as the appearance of diastole in epicardial cells that was observed by Akiyama.[91] It may also be responsible for changes in the primary frequency of the body surface ECG power spectrum morphology that occur with increasing fibrillation duration and that have been used to predict the duration of fibrillation in out-of-hospital patients.[62,63,95,96] The increased epicardial cycle length as fibrillation duration increases past 1 minute, may be due to postrepolarization refractoriness[97] during the developing ischemia. Similar postrepolarization refractoriness is also observed in isolated cells after 1 minute of rapid stimulation (200-msec cycle length) in 10 mM K_o.[78] An additional cause may be cellular uncoupling[98] caused by increased cytosolic calcium[50] during ischemia. As cells become less coupled, the effective space constant in the direction of the electric field decreases and the electric field intensity required to excite the cell increases. This would increase DFT.

Secondary Fibrillation

The relationship described between fibrillation cycle length and fibrillation duration is valid only for primary fibrillation that is induced by an electrical or naturally occurring extrastimulus or conduction block. It does not hold for secondary fibrillation that is induced metabolically or by other chemical changes. In this case, cycle length alone cannot predict fibrillation duration. For example, fibrillation cycle length, measured using fast Fourier transform, differs even in the same species depending on the method by which fibrillation is induced. Several studies have found a power spectrum peak during early electrically induced fibrillation in dogs to be between 9 and 12 Hz (cycle length = 83–111 msec).[60,99] However, Allen et al.[61] showed that while the mean cycle length of fibrillation in dogs was 9.9 ± 0.7 Hz (cycle length = 101 msec) with electrical induction, it was reduced to 7.1 ± 1.1 Hz (cycle length = 141) when fibrillation was induced with ouabain infusion. Ouabain would be expected to produce ventricular depolarization leading to fibrillation due to inhibition of the Na^+/K^+-ATPase. When fibrillation was induced with potassium infusion that produced direct ventricular depolarization, the mean peak frequency was reduced to 4.8 ± 0.8 Hz (cycle length = 208 msec). Under both of these conditions, hearts were very difficult to defibrillate.

A reduction of cycle length as predicted by ECG power spectrum frequency was also observed in humans with secondary fibrillation. In this case the mean peak frequency was 3.95 ± 0.3 Hz (cycle length = 253 msec) and only 7.7% of patients could be successfully defibrillated. In contrast, with primary fibrillation having a higher frequency of 5.18 ± 0.3 Hz (cycle length = 193 msec), 95% of patients could be defibrillated.

These findings suggest that the fibrillation cycle length as predicted by the power spectrum cannot be used alone to determine electrophysiologic characteristics of fibrillation and the potential ease of defibrillation. For example, with potassium or ouabain infusion, the mean peak frequency decreased and hearts became difficult to defibrillate. However, in the presence of Class III antiarrhythmics, which prolong the action potential, a similar slowing of cycle length occurs,[72] but hearts do not become more difficult to defibrillate. The mechanism underlying slowing of the fibrillation cycle length is probably very different in these two cases. With the Class III antiarrhythmics, the fibrillation cycle length is still controlled primarily by the cellular refractory period[72] and defibrillation involves a similar stimulation of partially refractory tissue that is necessary in untreated hearts. However, when fibrillation is induced with ouabain or potassium infusion, the fibrillation cycle length may no longer be controlled by cellular refractory period, but rather by fibrillation wave front arrival to tissue that is capable of being stimulated, as shown in the lower panel of Figure 15. Fibrillation cycle length may be controlled by late wave front arrival due to slow conduction perhaps caused by cellular uncoupling. Also, because cells are depolarized and may exhibit postrepolarization refractoriness, they would be difficult to stimulate. Therefore, defibrillation would be more difficult than in untreated hearts.

In summary, slow cycle length indicates either prolonged or secondary fibrillation and can be used to predict difficulty of defibrillation. However, this relationship holds only in the absence of drug treatment with Class III antiarrhythmics that also slow cycle length, but decrease DFT. A complete differentiation between these two types of fibrillation is only possible with monophasic action potential recordings which show both depolarization and repolarization characteristics of tissue during fibrillation.

Spontaneous Defibrillation

Occurrence of Spontaneous Defibrillation in Humans and Experimental Models

It is widely believed that once initiated, VF cannot spontaneously convert. However, now that internal defibrillators are frequently implanted in patients subject to risk of sudden cardiac death, spontaneous conversion is being observed more frequently than expected. There are numerous verbal anecdotal accounts of spontaneous conversion among cardiologists who induce fibrillation during defibrillator testing. During testing at the VA Medical Center in Washington, DC, spontaneous defibrillation in episodes that are clearly identified as true fibrillation by surface ECGs is not uncommon. Figure 17 shows an example of spontaneous conversion episode in a typical patient (J. Swartz, unpublished data). Spontaneous defibrillation has also been reported during programmed ventricular stimulation in the catheterization laboratory in 4 of 10 patients in whom fibrillation was induced using a double ventricular extrastimuli protocol.[100] Therefore, it is important clinically to look for episodes of spontaneous conversion during defibrillator implant testing because they may occur during the time while the defibrillator is charging and discharging. If spontaneous conversion were to occur prior to the shock, it would of course invalidate the results from that episode.

Mechanisms Underlying Stabilization of Fibrillation by Epinephrine

Mechanisms underlying spontaneous defibrillation are unknown. However, because spontaneous conversion also frequently occurs in the isolated rabbit heart model, it provides an excellent model for studying this phenomenon. The electrophysiologic patterns preceding spontaneous defibrillation in both humans and in the isolated rabbit heart model are similar. These similarities suggest that fibrillation

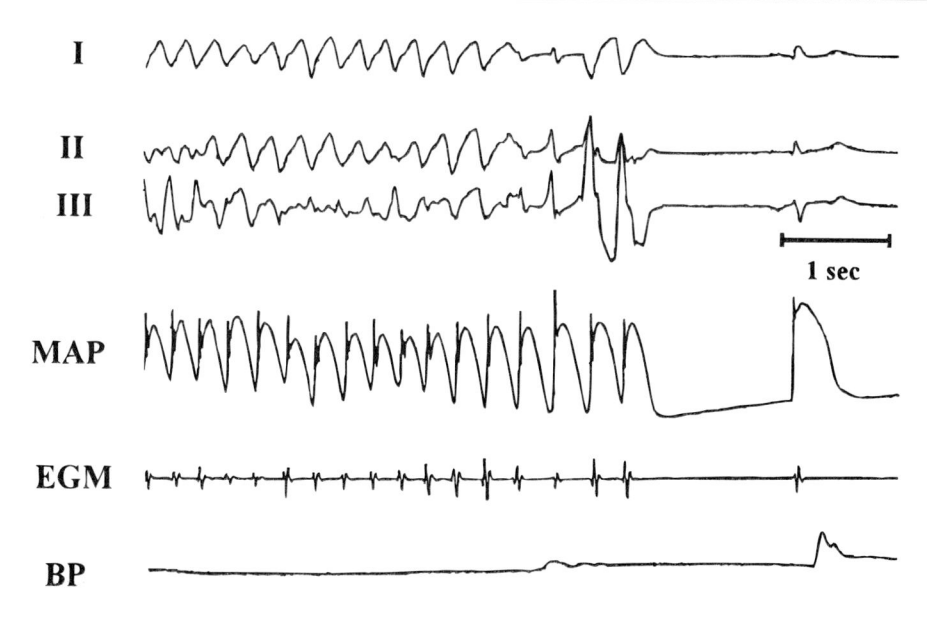

Figure 17. Spontaneous defibrillation observed during a clinical internal defibrillator implant. Leads I, II, and III are body surface electrocardiograms (ECGs). MAP: right ventricular monophasic action potentials; EGM: bipolar electrograms; BP: blood pressure.

develops and spontaneously converts through a tachyarrhythmic phase.[33,101] Spontaneous defibrillation may occur because fibrillation wave fronts occasionally become blocked because cells in a region have not yet repolarized. This leads to late arrival of excitation in other regions that allows improved repolarization and increased duration of the subsequent action potential. This produces a transitional tachyarrhythmic phase. If another wave front becomes blocked during this phase, the tachyarrhythmia converts to normal rhythm; otherwise, it degenerates back into fibrillation.

When fibrillation is induced electrically, there is no preceding catecholamine imbalance before the fibrillating stimulus. In contrast, when fibrillation occurs in the setting of myocardial ischemia (eg, infarction), it may be induced by catecholamine imbalance so that large concentrations of epinephrine are present as fibrillation begins. Epinephrine stabilizes fibrillation in the isolated rabbit heart[33] so that the incidence of spontaneous defibrillation is reduced from 29% under control conditions to only 8% of episodes in the presence of epinephrine. Cycle length measured with monophasic action potentials during the first 5 seconds of fibrillation also decreased from 108 ± 3 msec to 75 ± 3 msec in the presence of epinephrine. Because new action potentials occurred immediately after repolarization both with and without epinephrine, the shorter cycle length was associated with a shorter fibrillation action potential duration. Similar action potential duration shortening by epinephrine also occurred in isolated cells and was especially evident at the short cycle lengths associated with fibrillation.[32] Because the refractory period is shorter in the presence of epinephrine, fibrillation waves encounter less refractory tissue. Therefore, a greater number of fibrillation wave fronts can be simultaneously present on the ventricle and fibrillation is stabilized.

It is not yet known whether epinephrine stabilizes fibrillation in humans by producing a similar shortening of action potential duration at short cycle length characteristic of fibrillation. It is also unknown whether spontaneous defibrillation occurs in humans in a setting of high catecholamine concentration or if it only occurs after electrical induction such as that used for internal defibrillator testing.

References

1. Zipes DP: Electrophysiological mechanisms involved in ventricular fibrillation. *Circulation* 51(Suppl III):III-120, 1975.
2. Gillum RF: Sudden coronary death in the United States: 1980–1985. *Circulation* 79: 756, 1989.
3. Luna AB, Coumel P, Leclercq JF: Ambulatory sudden cardiac death: mechanisms of production of fatal arrhythmia on the basis of data from 157 cases. *Am Heart J* 117:151, 1989.
4. Cobb LA, Wener JA, Trobaugh GB: Sudden cardiac death I. A decade's experience with out-of-hospital resuscitation. *Mod Concepts Cardiovasc Dis* 49:31, 1980.
5. Lown B: Sudden cardiac death: the major challenge confronting contemporary cardiology. *Am J Cardiol* 43:313, 1979.
6. Fye WB: Ventricular fibrillation and defibrillation: historical perspectives with emphasis on the contributions of John MacWilliam, Carl Wiggers, and William Kouwenhoven. *Circulation* 71:858, 1985.
7. Mines GR: On dynamic equilibrium in the heart. *J Physiol* 46:349, 1913.
8. Garrey WE: The nature of fibrillary contraction of the heart. Its relation to tissue mass and form. *Am J Physiol* 33:397, 1914.
9. Watanabe Y, Dreifus LS: *Cardiac Arrhythmias—Electrophysiologic Basis for Clinical Interpretation*. Grune & Stratton, Inc., 1977.
10. Moe GK, Abildskov JA: Atrial fibrillation as a self-sustaining arrhythmia independent of focal discharge. *Am Heart J* 58:59, 1959.
11. Witkowski FX, Penkoske PA: Activation patterns during ventricular fibrillation. *Ann NY Acad Sci* (June 8):219, 1990.
12. Johnson EE, Ideker RE: Ventricular fibrillation: update. In: *Current Topics in Cardiology*. New York: Elsevier Science Publishing Co, Inc.; 1991, p. 121.
13. Damle RS, Kanaan NM, Robinson NS, et al: Spatial and temporal linking of epicardial activation directions during ventricular fibrillation in dogs. Evidence for underlying organization. *Circulation* 86:1547, 1992.
14. Chen PS, Shibata N, Dixon EG, et al: Comparison of the DFT and the upper limit of ventricular vulnerablility. *Circulation* 73: 1022, 1986.
15. Chen PS, Feld GK, Mower MM, et al: Effects of pacing rate and timing of defibrillation shock on the relation between the defibrillation threshold and the upper limit of vulnerability in open chest dogs. *J Am Coll Cardiol* 18:1555, 1991.
16. Topham SL, Cha YM, Peters BB, et al: Effects of lidocaine on relation between defibrillation threshold and upper limit of vulnerability in open-chest dogs. *Circulation* 85:1146, 1992.
17. Souza JJ, Malkin RA, Smith WM, et al: Relationship between upper limit of vulnerability and defibrillation threshold in a nonthoracotomy pig model. *PACE* 16:156, 1993.
18. Dillon SM: Synchronized repolarization after defibrillation shocks. A possible component of the defibrillation process demonstrated by optical recordings in rabbit heart. *Circulation* 85:1865, 1992.
19. Pogwizd SM, Corr PB: Mechanisms underlying the development of ventricular fibrillation during early myocardial ischemia. *Circ Res* 66:672, 1990.
20. Kimura S, Bassett AL, Kohya T, et al: Simultaneous recording of action potentials from endocardium and epicardium during ischemia in the isolated cat ventricle: relation of temporal electrophysiologic heterogeneities to arrhythmias. *Circulation* 74:401, 1986.
21. Vanoli E, DeFerrari GM, Stramba-Badiale M, et al: Vagal stimulation and prevention of sudden death in conscious dogs with a healed myocardial infarction. *Circ Res* 68: 1471, 1991.
22. Zipes DP, Levy MN, Cobb LA, et al: Task Force 2: sudden cardiac death. Neural-cardiac interactions. *Circulation* 76:I202, 1987.
23. Collins MN, Billman GE: Autonomic response to coronary occlusion in animals susceptible to ventricular fibrillation. *Am J Physiol* 257:H1886, 1989.
24. Ohyanagi M, Matsumori Y, Iwasaki T: β-Adrenergic receptors in ischemic and nonischemic canine myocardium: relation to ventricular fibrillation and effects of pretreatment with propranolol and hexamethonium. *J Cardiovasc Pharmacol* 11:107, 1988.
25. Skinner JE: Regulation of cardiac vulnerability by the cerebral defense system. *J Am Coll Cardiol* 5:88, 1985.
26. Taggert P, Sutton P, Lab M, et al: Interplay between adrenaline and interbeat interval on ventricular repolarization in intact heart in vivo. *Cardiovasc Res* 24:884, 1990.

27. Corr PB, Gross RW, Sobel BE: Amphipathic metabolites and membrane dysfunction in ischemic myocardium. *Circ Res* 55:135, 1984.
28. Corr PB, Pitt B, Natelson BH, et al: Task Force 3: sudden cardiac death. Neural-chemical interactions. *Circulation* 76(1 Pt 2):I208, 1987.
29. Gross RW, Sobel BE: Lysophosphatidylcholine metabolism in the rabbit heart. *J Biol Chem* 257:6702, 1982.
30. Kolman BS, Verrier RL, Lown B: The effect of vagus nerve stimulation upon vulnerability of the canine ventricle. *Circulation* 52:578, 1975.
31. Verrier RL, Lown B: Behavioral stress and cardiac arrhythmias. *Ann Rev Physiol* 46:155, 1984.
32. Tovar OH, Milne KB, Bransford PP, et al: Epinephrine facilitates fibrillation by shortening action potential duration and refractory period at VT/fibrillation cycle lengths (abstract). *J Soc Pacing Electrophysiol* 16:68, 1993.
33. Bransford PP, Varghese PJ, Tovar OH, et al: Epinephrine reduces ventricular fibrillation threshold and stabilizes fibrillation by reducing cellular refractory period during fibrillation (abstract). *J Soc Pacing Electrophysiol* 16:67, 1993.
34. Manoach M, Basat MB: The structural-functional basis of spontaneous ventricular defibrillation. *Int J Cardiol* 26:129, 1990.
35. Yusuf S, Sleight P, Rossi P, et al: Reduction in infarct size, arrhythmias and chest pain by early intravenous beta blockade in suspected acute myocardial infarction. *Circulation* 67:I-32, 1983.
36. Lichstein E, Morganroth J, Harrist R, et al: Effect of propranolol on ventricular arrhythmia. The beta-blocker heart attack trial experience. *Circulation* 67:I-5, 1983.
37. Woosley RL, Kornhauser D, Smith R, et al: Suppression of chronic ventricular arrhythmias with propranolol. *Circulation* 60:819, 1979.
38. Gillis AM, Clusin WT: The role of β-adrenergic receptor antagonists in the prevention of sudden cardiac death. *Comp Ther* 10:60, 1984.
39. Penkoske PA, Sobel BE, Corr PB: Disparate electrophysiological alterations accompanying dysrhythmia due to coronary occlusion and reperfusion in the cat. *Circulation* 58:1023, 1978.
40. Kimura S, Bassett AL, Saoudi NC, et al: Cellular electrophysiologic changes and "arrhythmias" during experimental ischemia and reperfusion in isolated cat ventricular myocardium. *J Am Coll Cardiol* 7:833, 1986.
41. Taylor AL, Winter R, Thandroyen F, et al: Potentiation of reperfusion-associated ventricular fibrillation by left ventricular hypertrophy. *Circ Res* 67:501, 1990.
42. Pogwizd SM, Corr PB: Electrophysiologic mechanisms underlying arrhythmias due to reperfusion of ischemic myocardium. *Circulation* 76:404, 1987.
43. Ideker RE, Klein GJ, Harrison L, et al: The transition to ventricular fibrillation induced by repolarization following acute ischemia in the dog: a period of organized epicardial activation. *Circulation* 63:1371, 1981.
44. Peleska B: Cardiac arrhythmias following condenser discharges and their dependence upon strength of current and phase of cardiac cycle. *Circ Res* 13:21, 1963.
45. Saumont R, Brunet JP, Fabiato A, et al: Exploration of the cardiac cycle with timed electric shocks. *Arch Mal Coeur* 58:246, 1965.
46. Lepeschkin E, Jones JL, Rush S, et al: Local potential gradients as a unifying measure for thresholds of stimulation, standstill, tachyarrhythmia and fibrillation appearing after strong capacitor discharges. *Adv Cardiol* 21:268, 1977.
47. Jones JL, Jones RE: Post-shock arrhythmias—a possible cause of unsuccessful defibrillation. *Crit Care Med* 8:167, 1980.
48. Jones JL, Lepeschkin E, Jones RE, et al: Response of cultured myocardial cells to countershock-type electric field stimulation. *Am J Physiol* 235:H214, 1978.
49. Jones JL, Jones RE: Determination of safety factor for defibrillator waveforms in cultured heart cells. *Am J Physiol* 242:H662, 1982.
50. Jones J, Jones R, Balasky G, et al: Defibrillator induced dysfunction and calcium overload. *Fed Proc* 46:409, 1987.
51. Jones JL, Jones RE, Balasky G: Microlesion formation in myocardial cells by high-intensity electric field stimulation. *Am J Physiol* 253:H480, 1987.
52. Jones JL, Lepeschkin E, Jones R, et al: Cellular fibrillation appearing in cultured myocardial cells after application of strong capacitor discharges. *Am J Cardiol* 39:273, 1977.
53. Jones JL, Jones RE: Postcountershock fibrillation in digitalized myocardial cells in vitro. *Crit Care Med* 8:172, 1980.
54. Chung EK: Digitalis and ventricular arrhythmias after cardioversion. *Heart Lung* 5:147, 1976.
55. Lown B, Wittenberg S: Cardioversion and digitalis. III. Effect of change in serum potassium. *Am J Cardiol* 21:513, 1968.
56. Reneskov L: Drug therapy before and after

the electroversion of cardiac dysrhythmias. *Prog Cardiovasc Dis* 16:531, 1974.
57. Lown B: Cardioversion and the digitalized patient (editorial comment). *J Am Coll Cardiol* 5:889, 1985.
58. Mann DL, Maisel AS, Atwood JE, et al: Absence of cardioversion-induced ventricular arrhythmias in patients with therapeutic digoxin levels. *J Am Coll Cardiol* 5:882, 1985.
59. Martin DR, Brown CG, Dzwonczyk R: Frequency analysis of the human and swine electrocardiogram during ventricular fibrillation. *Resuscitation* 22:85, 1991.
60. Herbschleb JN, Heethaar RM, Tweed L, et al: Frequency analysis of the ECG before and during ventricular fibrillation. *IEEE Comput Cardiol* 365, 1980.
61. Allen JD, Stewart AJ, Carlisle EJF, et al: Fibrillation frequency and ventricular defibrillation. *Proc IEEE Eng Med Biol Soc* 655, 1992.
62. Stewart AJ, Allen JD, Adgey AAJ: Frequency analysis of ventricular fibrillation and resuscitation success. *Q J Med* 85:307, 1992.
63. Brown CG, Dzwonczyk R, Martin DR: Physiologic measurement of the ventricular fibrillation ECG signal: estimating the duration of ventricular fibrillation. *Ann Emerg Med* 22:70, 1993.
64. Allessie M, Kirchhof C, Scheffer GJ, et al: Regional control of atrial fibrillation by rapid pacing in conscious dogs. *Circulation* 84:1689, 1991.
65. Swartz JF, Jones JL, Jones RE, et al: The conditioning prepulse of biphasic defibrillator waveforms enhances refractoriness to fibrillation wavefronts. *Circ Res* 68:438, 1991.
66. Jones JL, Jones RE, Milne KB: Refractory period prolongation by biphasic defibrillator waveforms is associated with enhanced sodium current in computer models of the ventricular action potential. *IEEE Trans Biomed Eng* 41:60, 1994.
67. Allessie MA, Bonke FIM, Schopman FJG: Circus movement of rabbit atrial muscle as a mechanism of tachycardia. *Circ Res* 32:54, 1973.
68. Allessie MA, Bonke FIM, Schopman FJG: Circus movement in rabbit atrial muscle as a mechanism of tachycardia. II. The role of nonuniform recovery of excitability in the occurrence of unidirectional block as studied with multiple microelectrodes. *Circ Res* 39:168, 1976.
69. Allessie MA, Bonke FIM, Schopman FJG: Circus movement in rabbit atrial muscle as a mechanism of tachycardia. III. The "leading circle" concept: a new model of circus movement in cardiac tissue without the involvement of an anatomic obstacle. *Circ Res* 41:9, 1977.
70. Sweeney RJ, Gill RM, Steinberg MI, et al: Ventricular refractory period extension caused by defibrillation shocks. *Circulation* 82:965, 1990.
71. Dillon SM: Optical recordings in the rabbit heart show that defibrillation strength shocks prolong the duration of depolarization and the refractory period. *Circ Res* 69:842, 1991.
72. Swartz JF, Jones JL, Fletcher RD: Characterization of ventricular fibrillation based on monophasic action potential morphology in the human heart. *Circulation* 87:1907, 1993.
73. Kerber RE, Kienzle MG, Olshansky B, et al: Ventricular tachycardia rate and morphology determine energy and current requirements for transthoracic cardioversion. *Circulation* 85:158, 1992.
74. Jones JL, Jones RE: Effects of monophasic defibrillator waveform intensity on graded response duration in a computer simulation of the ventricular action potential. *Proc IEEE Eng Med Biol Soc* 13:598, 1991.
75. Witkowski FX, Penkoske PA: Refractoriness prolongation by defibrillation shocks. *Circulation* 82:1064, 1990.
76. Chen P, Wolf PD, Claydon FJ, et al: The potential gradient field created by epicardial defibrillation electrodes in dogs. *Circulation* 74:626, 1986.
77. Dixon EG, Tang ASL, Wolf PD, et al: Improved defibrillation thresholds with large contoured epicardial electrodes and biphasic waveforms. *Circulation* 76:1176, 1987.
78. Jones JL, Jones RE, Balasky G: Improved cardiac cell excitation with symmetrical biphasic defibrillator waveforms. *Am J Physiol* 253:H1418, 1987.
79. Jones JL, Swartz JF, Jones RE, et al: Increasing fibrillation duration enhances relative asymmetrical biphasic versus monophasic defibrillator waveform efficacy. *Circ Res* 67:376, 1990.
80. Echt DS, Barbey JT, Black JN: Influence of ventricular fibrillation duration on defibrillation energy in dogs using bidirectional pulse discharges. *PACE* 11:1315, 1988.
81. Fujimura O, Jones DL, Klein GJ: Effects of time to defibrillation and subthreshold preshocks on defibrillation success in pigs. *J Soc Pacing Electrophysiol* 12:358, 1989.
82. Bardy GH, Ivey TD, Allen M, et al: A prospective randomized evaluation of effect of ventricular fibrillation duration on defibrillation thresholds in humans. *J Am Coll Cardiol* 13:1362, 1989.
83. Bardy GH, Ivey TD, Johnson G, et al: Pro-

spective evaluation of initially ineffective defibrillation pulses on subsequent defibrillation success during ventricular fibrillation in survivors of cardiac arrest. *Am J Cardiol* 62:718, 1988.
84. Yakaitis RW, Ewy A, Otto CW, et al: Influence of time and therapy on ventricular defibrillation in dogs. *Crit Care Med* 8:157, 1980.
85. Weaver WD, Cobb LA, Hallstrom AP, et al: Factors influencing survival after out-of-hospital cardiac arrest. *J Am Coll Cardiol* 7:752, 1986.
86. Dalzell GWN, Adgey AAJ: Determinants of successful transthoracic defibrillation and outcome in ventricular fibrillation. *Br Heart J* 65:311, 1991.
87. Becker LB, Han BH, Meyer PM, et al: Racial differences in the incidence of cardiac arrest and subsequent survival. *N Engl J Med* 329:600, 1993.
88. Jones JL, Jones RE: Improved defibrillator waveform safety factor with biphasic waveforms. *Am J Physiol* 245:H60, 1983.
89. Jones JL, Jones RE: Decreased defibrillator-induced dysfunction with biphasic rectangular waveforms. *Am J Physiol* 247:H792, 1984.
90. Zhou X, Guse P, Wolf PD, et al: Existence of both fast and slow channel activity during the early stages of ventricular fibrillation. *Circ Res* 70:773, 1992.
91. Akiyama T: Intracellular recording of in situ ventricular cells during ventricular fibrillation. *Am J Physiol* 240:H465, 1981.
92. Worley SJ, Swain JL, Colavita PG, et al: Development of an endocardial-epicardial gradient of activation rate during electrically induced, sustained ventricular fibrillation in the dog. *Am J Cardiol* 55:813, 1985.
93. Carlisle EJF, Allen JD, Kernohan WG, et al: Fourier analysis of ventricular fibrillation of varied aetiology. *Eur Heart J* 11:173, 1990.
94. Dzwonczyk R, Brown CG, Werman HA: The median frequency of the ECG during ventricular fibrillation: its use in an algorithm for estimating the duration of cardiac arrest. *IEEE Trans Biomed Eng* 37:640, 1990.
95. Brown CG, Griffith RF, Ligten PV, et al: Median frequency—a new parameter for predicting defibrillation success rate. *Ann Emerg Med* 20:787, 1991.
96. Brown CG, Dzwonczyk R, Werman HA, et al: Estimating the duration of ventricular fibrillation. *Ann Emerg Med* 18:1181, 1989.
97. Rozanski GJ, Jaliffe J, Moe GK: Determinants of post repolarization refractoriness in depressed mammalian ventricular muscle. *Circ Res* 55:486, 1984.
98. Jones RE, Jones JL: Cell-to-cell uncoupling under "fibrillation conditions" in myocardial cell aggregates (abstract). *J Mol Cell Cardiol* 20:13, 1988.
99. Carlisle EJF, Allen JD, Bailey A, et al: Fourier analysis of ventricular fibrillation and synchronization of DC countershocks in defibrillation. *J Electrocardiol* 21:337, 1988.
100. Spielman SR, Farshidi A, Horowitz LN, et al: Ventricular fibrillation during programmed ventricular stimulation: incidence and clinical implications. *J Am Coll Cardiol* 42:913, 1978.
101. Varghese PJ, Bransford PP, Tovar OH, et al: Mechanisms of spontaneous defibrillation in the rabbit heart (abstract). *J Am Coll Cardiol* 21:306, 1993.

Chapter 4

Tachyarrhythmia Sensing and Detection

Walter H. Olson

Introduction

Sensing of electrogram signals and the detection algorithms for ventricular fibrillation (VF) and ventricular tachycardia (VT) in implantable cardioverter-defibrillators (ICDs) use high-gain amplifier systems and only the analysis of time intervals between ventricular depolarizations. The design philosophy has been to assure high sensitivity for detection of VF despite slight undersensing during VF and to accept decreases in detection specificity for some supraventricular rhythms. The rationale is that the negative consequences of underdetection of VF and VT outweigh the risks of some inappropriate therapy. The challenge for the design of future ICDs is to increase detection specificity by analyzing electrogram waveshapes, atrial and ventricular electrograms, and perhaps hemodynamic sensors without sacrificing prompt high-sensitivity detection of VT and VF.

The first step in tachyarrhythmia recognition is sensing of the electrogram signal from two implanted cardiac electrodes. Sensing systems attempt to find only the time of occurrence for each R wave generated by ventricular depolarization. The time interval between the latest sensed R wave and the previous one determines the cardiac cycle length. The primary challenge for sensing is to avoid missing too many of the low-amplitude fragmented R waves that occur during VF. At the same time, the high sensitivity must not cause double counting of the R waves or oversensing of the T waves, P waves, myopotentials, or electromagnetic interference.

Detection is the process of analyzing the recent cycle lengths between sensed R waves with an algorithm to identify a sustained tachyarrhythmia that should be treated with antitachycardia pacing (ATP) or shocks. The detection algorithm should discriminate between VF and VT using ventricular rate and other criteria because different electrical therapies are usually prescribed. Detection should be prompt so that therapy is given before a patient develops syncope, before electrogram amplitude and slew rate deteriorate, and before defibrillation thresholds rise. However, detection should not occur too quickly because some tachyarrhythmias are nonsustained and should not be treated.

Spontaneous ventricular tachyarrhythmia episodes have a distinct beginning and end, are usually infrequent, occur in a variety of circumstances, may be sustained, hemodynamically stable or unstable, and tend to be grouped in time.[1,2] Implantable cardioverter-defibrillators should respond to these episodes with a series of detection and therapy processes until the termination of

From Singer I, (ed.) Implantable Cardioverter-Defibrillator. Armonk, NY: Futura Publishing Company, Inc.; © 1994.

the episode is detected or all the prescribed therapies have been delivered. After unsuccessful therapies, redetection is required prior to each additional therapy in the progression of prescribed therapies. After a successful therapy, the ICD must detect a nontachycardia rhythm to conclude its recognition of the episode, complete data storage, and reset therapy sequences.

The types of detection processes include initial detection that initiates an ICD episode and initiates the first automatic therapy, confirmation of the detected tachyarrhythmia during and/or upon completion of capacitor charging to determine if the tachyarrhythmia is sustained, synchronization to assure delivery of a shock during a ventricular depolarization, redetection of the same or possibly a different tachyarrhythmia in an episode after a therapy, and detection of episode termination when the tachyarrhythmia has stopped.

Figure 1 shows an example of an induced VF episode with the duration of each process shown by a horizontal bracket. Each detection process is composed of individual cardiac events, such as sensed R waves, that occur at some point in time. Each event is classified according to the time interval between successive events and each event is marked as paced, normal sense, VT, or VF. Recent strings of these events are analyzed by the detection algorithms. The first event in Figure 1 was a normal sense during sinus rhythm. Then pacing and a T shock were used to induce VF, which was detected after sensing 18 VF events. The capacitors were charged, the tachyarrhythmia was confirmed, and a synchronized 10-J shock was not successful. Ventricular fibrillation was

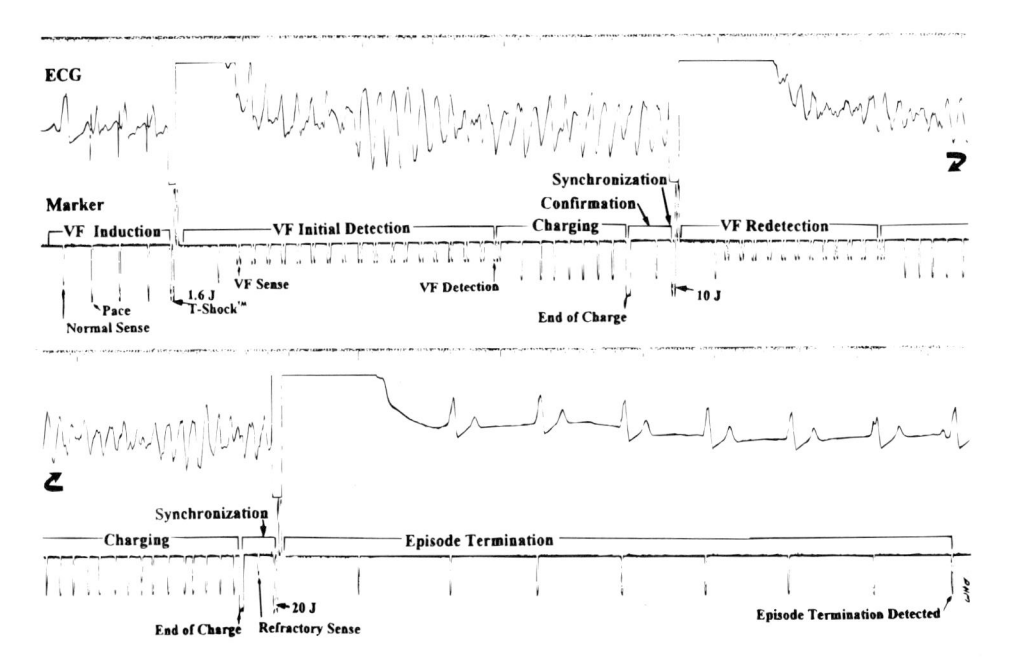

Figure 1. The components of an induced tachyarrhythmia episode are shown with the surface electrocardiogram (ECG) and marker in this continuous recording. Ventricular fibrillation (VF) induction by pacing and a T-shock™ converts sinus rhythm to VF; VF initial detection for 18 VF sensed events; charging; confirmation, synchronization and delivery of a 10-J shock; VF redetection for 12 VF sensed events; charging again; synchronization and delivery of a 20-J committed shock; and detection of episode termination requiring eight consecutive long intervals. Each type of event marker is labeled below the marker symbol. This example of an episode was recorded for the PCD Jewel™ Model 7219D (Medtronic, Inc., Minneapolis, MN) ICD.

redetected after sensing 12 VF events, charging was longer, and a synchronized 20-J shock terminated the VF. After 8 normal sensed events the device detected episode termination.

The variety of arrhythmias that may be presented to a detection process is large, and methods for the analysis and evaluation of detection algorithms with real tachyarrhythmia databases and simulators are not well established. The criteria for physician diagnoses of rhythms may not be the same as the detection criteria for automatic control of electrical therapy. For example, fast VT (FVT) may not be terminated by ATP therapy and may need to be detected and treated as VF by an ICD. The discrimination of VF from polymorphic nonsustained VT with short cycle lengths can be extremely difficult and yet shock therapy is needed if polymorphic rapid VT persists. A confounding distinction exists between short runs of VT separated by sinus beats and true VT with some sinus capture beats that conduct to the ventricle. Similarly, supraventricular tachyarrhythmias with aberrant ventricular conduction can be very difficult to distinguish from VT with 1:1 retrograde conduction. The success of current ICDs, that rely only on ventricular rate for detection with high sensitivity, is tempered by a less than perfect detection specificity with inappropriate detections that occur in 10% to 40% of patients. Patients with ICDs have a reduced risk of sudden cardiac death.

Properties of Electrograms from Sensing Leads

Endocardial or epicardial electrograms used by ICDs differ from the surface electrocardiograms (ECGs) used by physicians to diagnose cardiac arrhythmias in several important ways. When at least one of the two electrodes in contact with the myocardium has a surface area less than about 50 mm^2, the amplitude of the R wave in the electrogram is 5–10 times the size of a normal 1 mV QRS in the surface ECG. Also, the frequency content of electrograms is higher than that of ECGs, and discrete ventricular depolarization durations are shorter for all ventricular rhythms including VF. The direction of local wave front propagation with respect to the electrode geometry affects the electrogram amplitude and shape. The electrogram wave shape may be the same for arrhythmias that have different surface QRS morphologies. The volume of cardiac tissue that contributes to the bipolar electrogram is usually quite small and decreases as electrode separation and surface area decrease, whereas the entire myocardium contributes to the surface ECG.

Early automatic implantable defibrillators developed for Mirowski used the loss of right ventricular (RV) pressure waveform as the means of detecting VF. This concept was abandoned in favor of electrical sensing of high ventricular rate using a superior vena cava spring electrode on a catheter and a flexible conical apex patch electrode that were optimized for defibrillation.[3] This classic paper by Langer et al.[3] also describes the probability density function (PDF) that detects VF based on the fraction of time the signal spends between positive and negative amplitude thresholds that are close to the baseline. Rate detection was later added because fast nonsinusoidal VT was not detected reliably by PDF alone. Unfortunately, the large surface area electrodes permitted double counting due to large amplitude T waves, P waves, and postshock ST-T waves caused many inappropriate detections. The reliability of VF and VT sensing was greatly improved when local ventricular bipolar electrograms from two closely spaced small surface area epicardial screw-in electrodes were used with a high-sensitivity automatic gain control amplifier.[4] For 25 episodes of induced VT, the mean unfiltered local bipolar screw-in electrograms were 9.9 mV compared to 5.2 mV for the spring-patch electrodes. Electrogram amplitudes in sinus rhythm were also greater (10.4 mV) for local bipolar sensing than for large surface area spring-patch electrodes (4.1 mV).

A. Bipolar Epicardial Sensing

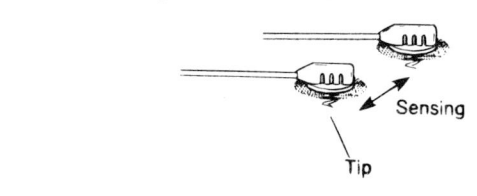

B. Standard Bipolar Endocardial Sensing

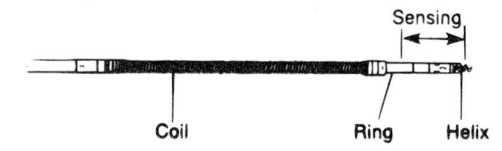

C. Integrated Bipolar Endocardial Sensing

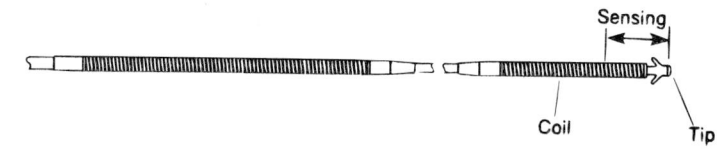

Figure 2. Most epicardial implantable cardioverter (ICD) lead systems have used two myocardial screw-in leads, shown in panel **A**, placed 1 cm apart for bipolar sensing from two small surface area electrodes. In problem cases, bipolar endocardial pacemaker leads have been used with epicardial patch defibrillation electrodes. Transvenous ICD leads have used either standard bipolar sensing between the tip and a separate ring electrode, as shown for the Transvene™ (Medtronic, Inc., Minneapolis, MN) lead in panel **B**, or integrated bipolar sensing between the tip and the right ventricular shocking coil, as shown for the Endotak™ (CPI, St. Paul, MN) lead in panel **C**.

Typical sensing electrodes for endocardial or epicardial leads used with ICDs are shown in Figure 2. Small separation (approximately 1 cm) of the two epicardial screw-in electrodes as shown in Figure 2A is important to prevent inappropriate sensing of atrial activity, myopotentials, and external electromagnetic interference. Bipolar endocardial pacemaker leads have been used to sense electrograms for ICDs that use epicardial patch defibrillation leads. Transvenous endocardial defibrillation leads have either standard bipolar sensing from a distal tip electrode to a small sensing ring as shown in Figure 2B (Transvene, Medtronic, Inc., Minneapolis, MN, 12-mm spacing) or integrated bipolar sensing from a distal tip electrode to a large RV shocking coil as shown in Figure 2C (Endotak™ 60 series, 6-mm spacing; or Endotak™ 70 series, 12-mm spacing, CPI, St. Paul, MN), and the Cadence TVL Lead System™ (11-mm spacing, Ventritex, Inc., Sunnyvale, CA).

Bipolar ventricular electrograms during VF have discrete depolarizations with variable amplitudes and 100–300-msec cycle lengths. Filtered electrogram amplitudes during induced tachyarrhythmias from 63 patients undergoing ICD implantation averaged 8–9 mV during VF.[5] However, 11 of 69 VF episodes (16%) had minimum amplitudes of 1 mV or less. Electrograms from endocardial bipolar leads were slightly larger than epicardial bipolar electrograms but not significantly different. In 60% of VF episodes there was at least a 50% change in electrogram amplitude during 10 seconds. In half the patients, at least a 5-mV change in amplitude was seen between different episodes of VF.

The correlation between sinus rhythm electrogram amplitudes and VF electrogram amplitudes was poor ($r = 0.19$) in one study.[5] Although a stronger correlation was found ($r = 0.70$) in another study,[6] the 95% confidence intervals were very large and the ratio of sinus to VF electrogram amplitudes ranged from 0.29–1.05 with a mean of 0.55 ± 0.20. The large interpatient variation of this ratio makes it impractical to estimate VF electrogram amplitude with any precision from sinus electrograms in individual patients. Nevertheless, electrogram amplitudes in sinus rhythm of at least 5 mV measured when the leads are implanted have proven adequate in several large ICD clinical studies.

Little information is available on chronic electrograms, particularly for VF, and little is known about the differences between induced and spontaneous tachyarrhythmias. The long-term reliability of epicardial leads that are properly implanted and tested is similar to endocardial pacing leads.[7] The mean and minimum chronic amplitudes of telemetered electrograms for induced VF in 10 patients followed for 1 year increased slightly, but not significantly (unpublished data). Differences between induced and spontaneous tachyarrhythmia cycle lengths are minimal with some indication that spontaneous rhythms have slightly longer cycle lengths.

Electrogram Sensing and Interval Classification

The primary functional operations within the sensing system of an ICD are

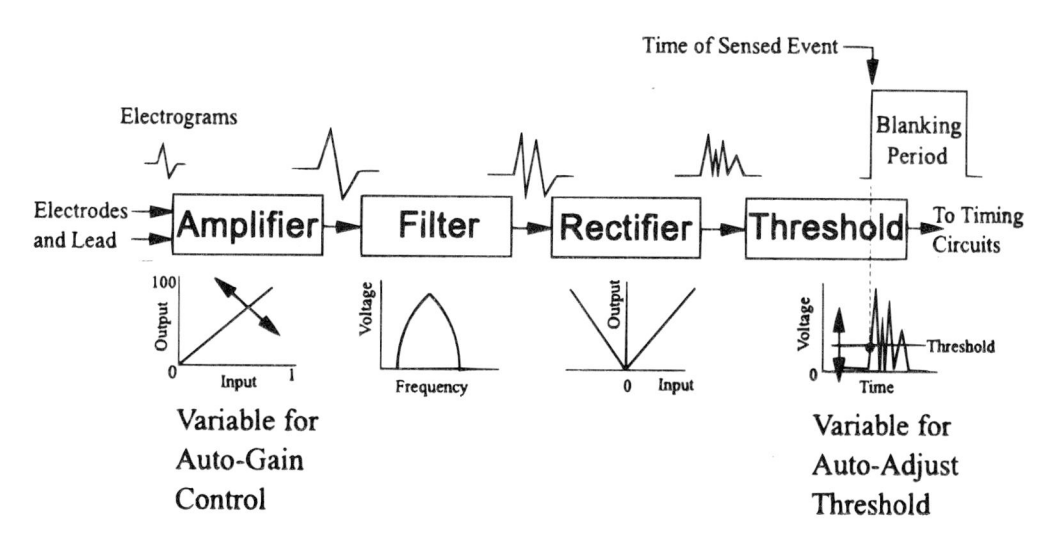

Figure 3. A functional block diagram for an implantable cardioverter-defibrillator (ICD) sense amplifier consists of an amplifier that may be fixed or have automatic gain control, a bandpass filter to reject low-frequency T waves and high-frequency noise, a rectifier to eliminate polarity dependency, and a threshold detector that may be fixed or autoadjusting. The net result is a single pulse for each sensed event that is used by timing circuits to determine a series of cycle lengths. The effects of each block on a biphasic electrogram are shown above the blocks and each functional operation is shown below each block. In actual circuits, some functions such as amplification and filtering may be integrated.

shown in Figure 3. The raw signal coming from the leads, connector and hermetic feedthroughs encounters protection circuitry, such as zener diodes, before reaching the amplifier. Sensing systems use either automatic gain control or autoadjusting threshold to dynamically adjust the sensitivity for reliable sensing of VF without oversensing T waves in sinus rhythm or other inappropriate signals. Automatic gain control is a feedback system that attempts to keep the amplifier output signal amplitude constant for any input signal and then uses a fixed threshold to sense the R waves. Auto-adjusting threshold uses constant amplification and the peak amplitude of the R waves provides the feedback for adjusting the starting amplitude of a time decaying threshold. Both systems have an "attack" time that determines how rapidly the gain or threshold can increase as well as a "decay" time for gain or threshold decreases. Practical amplifiers have a limited dynamic range so the electrogram is saturated or clipped when it exceeds a maximum value. Amplifiers must recover quickly after pacing pulses and defibrillation shocks, reject large DC offsets due to electrode polarization, and reject common mode noise applied to both inputs. They also must have high signal-to-noise ratios while using only a few microamperes of battery current.

The bandpass filter is designed to accept the electrogram ventricular depolarization signal for all rhythms while rejecting lower frequency signals such as the T waves and higher frequency signals, such as myopotentials and most electromagnetic interference. In the actual circuits, the filter is usually incorporated into the several stages of amplification. The filter bandpass shape is designed to match the frequency spectrum of the ventricular electrograms with particular attention to VF signals before and after shocks. The filter typically rejects signals with frequencies less than about 10 Hz and greater than about 60 Hz. The filtered electrogram signal intentionally distorts the electrogram waveshapes to optimize the signal for the subsequent sensing threshold.

Telemetered and stored electrograms typically use 0.5–200 Hz-filters that do not distort the electrogram signal waveshapes.

A full wave rectifier circuit is usually used to flip any negative signal deflection upward so that sensing threshold is not affected by the polarity of the R wave that may vary for different rhythms. The polarity of the sensing electrodes are sometimes labeled by the pacing function they usually share.

The threshold circuit compares the amplified-filtered-rectified signal amplitude to a threshold voltage and senses an R wave when the signal exceeds the threshold. This comparator circuit sends out a pulse when an event is sensed. The beginning of this pulse is used by the timing circuits as the time of the sensed event.

The sensing blanking period is an artificial absolute refractory period as it prevents further sensing for an interval of time following every sensed event. The primary purpose of blanking is to sense each ventricular depolarization only once regardless of the number of times the filtered-rectified R wave crosses the sensing threshold. The blanking period cannot be used to prevent T wave oversensing in an ICD as the typical RT interval is longer than the smallest RR intervals observed during VF. The minimal programmable interval for VF rate detection should be at least twice the blanking period so that alternate ventricular depolarizations cannot hide in the blanking period and cause failure to detect VF. However, if minimal VF cycle lengths are less than the blanking period, the sum of two such VF intervals should be less than the minimal cycle length that can be classified as VF. The blanking period after sensing is 120 msec in Medtronic ICDs; 135–140 msec for various Cardiac Pacemaker, Inc. ICDs; 135 msec in Ventritex ICDs; 70–100 msec for various Telectronic ICDs; and 135–165 msec for Intermedics ICDs. Electronic refractory periods that frequently follow blanking periods for sensed events in bradycardia pacemakers are not usually used in ICDs because of the need to sense the very short cycle lengths of VF.

For the automatic gain control method, the amplifier gain that is the slope of the line relating the amplifier input and output, shown on the left of Figure 3, varies (double arrow) according to the signal amplitude while the threshold voltage is fixed. For auto-adjusting threshold, the amplifier gain is fixed and the horizontal line representing the threshold voltage, shown on the right of Figure 3, varies (double arrow) according to peak signal amplitude and the time since an R wave was last sensed.

Figure 4 illustrates the differences between automatic gain control and automatic adjusting thresholds. Both systems may undersense a few cycles during VF when R wave amplitudes change abruptly or signal amplitude becomes extremely small. For automatic gain control, the amplifier increases the gain when the amplitudes of several R waves decrease from large values in sinus rhythm to smaller amplitudes during VF. The amplifier tries to maintain a constant peak amplitude at the output as shown in Figure 4B. The first few beats of VF may be missed at the onset of spontaneous VF depending on how quickly the gain is increased. When the R waves increase in amplitude during VF or after spontaneous termination of nonsustained rhythms, oversensing of T waves may occur until the gain automatically decreases.

For autoadjusting threshold, Figure 4C shows that the threshold for sensing an-

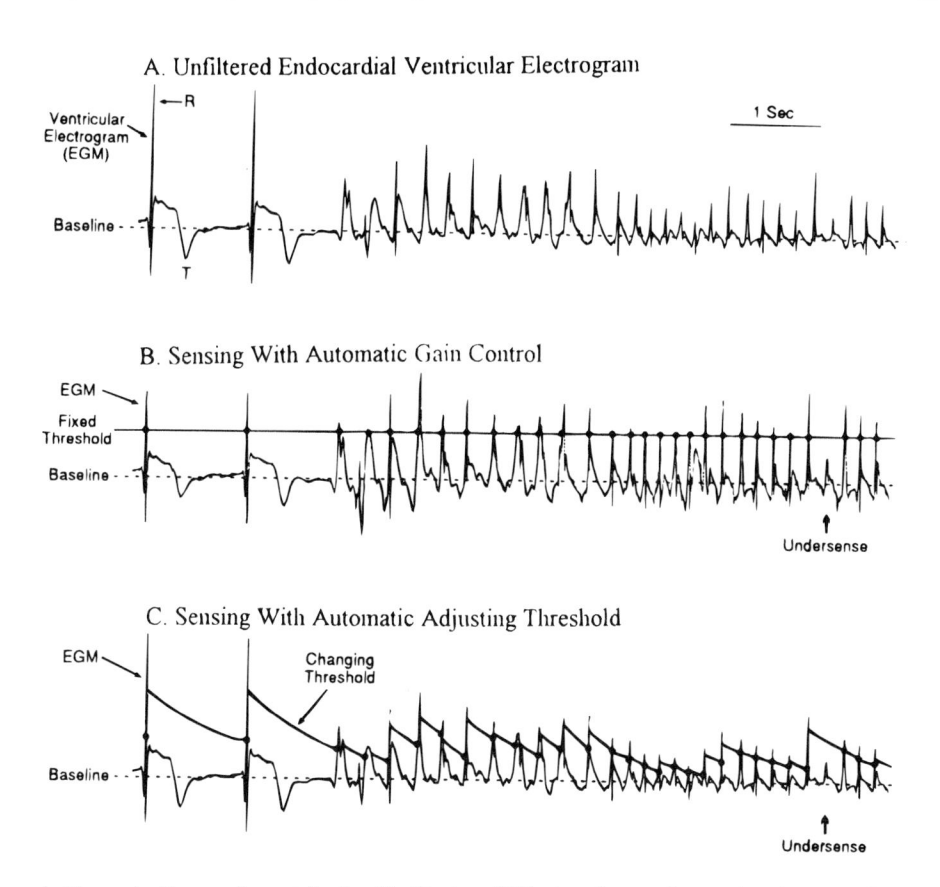

Figure 4. Sinus rhythm and ventricular fibrillation (VF) signals are shown for the raw electrogram in panel **A**, for automatic gain control in panel **B**, and automatic adjusting threshold in panel **C**. For panel B, the small electrograms are amplified compared to panel A and the sensing is shown by the dots where the signal crosses the fixed threshold. For panel C, the electrograms are the same as in panel A, and the threshold varies according to the amplitude of the electrogram, and sensing is again shown by the dots where the signal crosses the variable threshold.

other R wave is increased for each beat to a fraction of the peak R wave amplitude or a multiple of the programmed sensitivity, whichever is less. This is equivalent to a very rapid gain increase for an automatic gain control amplifier. The threshold for sensing another R wave then decreases exponentially until it reaches the programmed sensitivity. T waves are rejected well because the threshold increases more for a large R wave amplitude that will usually have a larger T wave. The threshold decay time is similar to the decay time of the amplification for an automatic gain control amplifier.

Sensing Performance and Problems

Sensing of a low-amplitude VF by autoadjusting threshold with various programmed values of sensitivity is shown in Figure 5. Manual estimates of ideal sensing times for this low-amplitude VF signal (black dots on the local bipolar electrogram [EGM] waveform) can be compared to sensing times shown by the rising edge of each 120-msec pulse that also illustrates the blanking period. The undersensing of VF increases as the programmed sensitivity values increase (maximum amplifier gain decreases). This figure shows why high sensitivity should be used whenever possible to minimize VF undersensing. While slight undersensing of VF for some episodes cannot be eliminated with either autogain or autothreshold methods, underdetection of VF by the detection counting algorithms is exceedingly rare.

A histogram of manually measured VF cycle lengths has a peak at about 200 msec and a range from 130 msec to 300 msec for

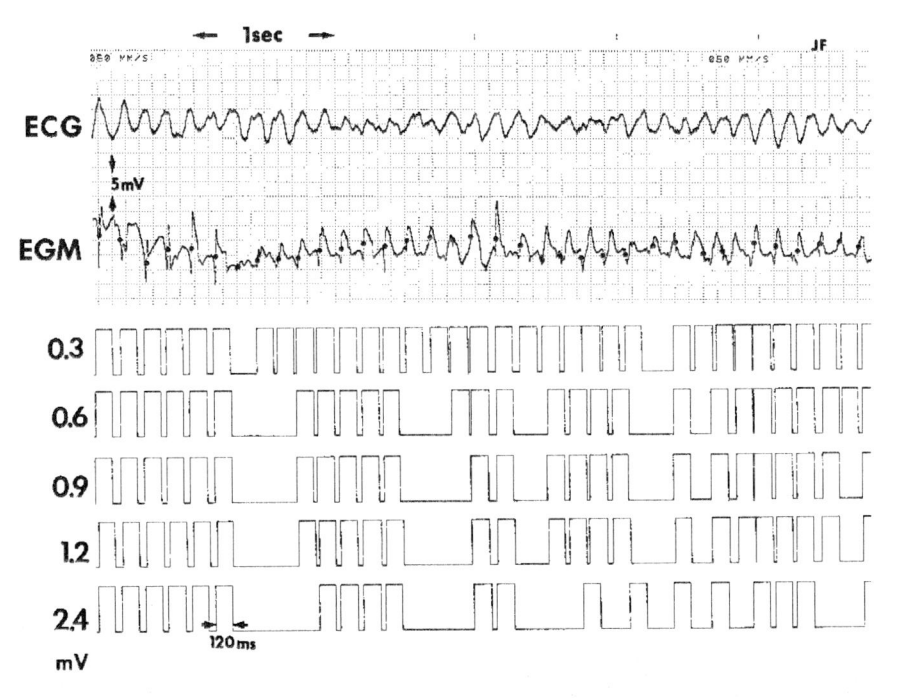

Figure 5. Sensing for automatic adjusting threshold is illustrated for various minimum thresholds from 0.3 to 2.4 mV sensitivity. On the electrogram, the black dots indicate where ideal sensing would occur. The rising edge of each pulse is the time of sensing and the pulse duration of 120 msec represents the blanking period. Note that undersensing of this difficult ventricular fibrillation (VF) increases as the programmed sensitivity rises from 0.3 to 2.4 mV. Sensing of 0.3 mV is the recommended setting. The 5-mV calibration shown applies only to the local bipolar electrogram (EGM) signal.

patients who are not taking antiarrhythmic drugs. Occasional VF oversensing and variability of the cycle lengths due to sensing different parts of the electrogram waveshapes is common. Cycle lengths > 300 msec usually represent occasional brief undersensing during VF.

Rare cases of VF underdetection for induced VF have been observed for extremely disorganized and low-amplitude VF. Ventricular fibrillation underdetection has been seen due to reduced amplitude electrograms following an apical infarction at the site of the endocardial sensing electrodes that required repositioning of the lead.[8] Ventricular fibrillation underdetection was reported when large R-to-R wave electrogram amplitude variability could not be followed by the automatic gain control.[9] This case of VF underdetection was resolved by repositioning the epicardial sensing lead during implantation to obtain a more uniform, although smaller amplitude, VF electrogram. Automatic gain control or autoadjusting thresholds may undersense some R waves during VF if large decreases in R-to-R wave electrogram amplitude occurs as shown on the right side of Figure 4. These extremely variable VF signals may arise from heterogeneous diseased tissue with irregular conduction of the wave fronts during VF. Such irregular electrograms need to be identified at the time the leads are implanted, when lead repositioning is most feasible. Other cases reported have attributed underdetection of VF and VT to ventricular hypertrophy[10] or immature leads.[11] Oversensing of T waves and ST segments have been reported.[12,13] Inappropriate sensing, detection, and shocks have been reported following telemetry[14] and magnet tests.[15]

Sensing systems with inadequate constant sensitivity may underdetect VF. Constant sensing in Telectronic ICDs has resulted in VF underdetection for 10% of patients[16] that could be corrected in all but two patients by reprogramming and lead repositioning.[17] A maximum sensitivity of 0.7 mV may not be adequate to detect some VFs, yet T wave oversensing in sinus rhythm also occurred. For the Guardian 4210™ ICD, 12.9% of patients required reoperation due to oversensing and other sensing/pacing lead complications[18] and VF undersensing at 1-mV maximum sensitivity has been reported.[19] The Guardian ATP II 4211™ ICD has an automatic sensitivity tracking (AST) system that uses the autoadjusting threshold concept with a maximum sensitivity of 0.375 mV.

Sinus rhythm sensing errors in ICDs with automatic gain control and autoadjusting threshold have been observed.[20-22] Sinus rhythm R wave amplitude spontaneously varied by 24%[20] and short runs of VT have caused changes in automatic gain that caused undersensing of subsequent sinus rhythm and inappropriate bradycardia pacing that induced VT in two patients with the Ventritex ICDs.[21] This occurred because the automatic gain control abruptly increased (150%) or decreased (67%) the gain after a fixed number of different beats or passage of a fixed time. Sinus rhythm amplitude changes of 39% following premature beats,[20] that did not cause automatic gain changes, also led to undersensed sinus beats and bradycardia pacing that induced VT in 3 patients.[22] Medtronic ICDs have oversensed T waves after paced beats[22] that will reduce the effective bradycardia pacing rate and may inhibit ATP, but will not cause inappropriate detection. T wave oversensing can also cause inappropriate confirmation or synchronization of shocks. The Cardiac Pacemakers, Inc. and Telectronic ICDs have also been observed to oversense T waves. Medtronic ICDs do not increase the autoadjusting threshold after a pacing pulse, whereas the Ventritex ICDs switch to maximal sensitivity after three consecutive paced beats. This assures that bradycardia pacing due to VF undersensing does not contribute to additional VF undersensing. Automatic gain control and autoadjusting threshold can cause changes in the exact time of sensing during an R wave that can affect cycle lengths or cause intermittent double counting.

Postshock sensing is critical to redetection after unsuccessful tachyarrhythmia treatments and proper detection of tachyarrhythmia termination. Considerable postshock signal distortion and ST segment changes on spring-patch shocking electrodes was described by Winkle et al.[4] They found minimal postshock distortion on separate standard bipolar electrodes used only for sensing. Another study[23] also found no significant postshock changes in R wave amplitudes on standard bipolar epicardial sensing electrodes. For two large surface area (125 mm^2) endocardial catheter shocking electrodes separated by 5 mm, substantial postshock decreases in R wave amplitudes and increases in pacing thresholds were seen that persisted for up to 10 minutes.[24,25] Recordings from separate sensing electrodes during transthoracic shocks showed that these effects were localized to electrodes that were used for both shocking and sensing. Studies with transvenous Endotak 60™ series leads showed failure to sense VF after shocks and decreases in sinus rhythm electrograms from 10.5 mV preshock to 1.9 mV postshock, which is well below the 5-mV implant criterion.[26] The electrograms did not fully recover for up to 2 minutes after the shock. This lead uses integrated bipolar sensing between the pacing tip electrode and the RV shocking coil, which are separated by 6 mm. A subsequent report[27] showed smaller decreases in electrogram amplitude for Endotak 70 series leads with 12-mm spacing between the electrodes. Electroporation, which creates microscopic holes in the cardiac cell membranes near the shocking electrode, has been proposed as the mechanism for these postshock phenomena.[28] During the postoperative period (8–24 hours) after multiple VF inductions during ICD implantation, there were no significant changes in electrogram amplitude, slew rate, or resistance.[29] Also, serial serum creatine kinase and MB isoenzymes showed no evidence of myocardial necrosis.

Rate Detection Algorithms

The ventricular rate is defined by algorithms that use the recent series of cycle lengths between sensed ventricular depolarizations. The early automatic implantable cardiac defibrillator devices used analog circuits to apply a small charge that was inversely proportional to the cycle length to a capacitor and resistor that had a fixed decay constant. Detection occurred when the accumulated charge caused the voltage on the capacitor to reach a threshold value. This decaying average of the recent cycle lengths can approach the threshold for detection even if none of the cycle lengths quite reach the threshold. A short run of small cycle lengths may not generate enough charge to reach the threshold. Thus, the time to detection decreased as the rate and its rate of change increased.

All modern ICDs use digital circuits and microprocessors to classify each cycle length into a distinct range of cycle lengths called a zone. Then, detection algorithms analyze recent series of cycle lengths with concurrent and serial calculations, logic, and counting. Implantable cardioverter-defibrillator detection algorithms for VF are designed to have very high sensitivity despite reduced specificity, because the consequences of underdetecting VF are so grave. This basic philosophy pervades all aspects of detection processes from initial detection through episode termination. For VT, more specificity is needed and can be obtained by the method of counting VT events and the use of optional algorithms such as stability.

Implantable cardioverter-defibrillators from different manufacturers use quite different initial detection algorithms. Confirmation, synchronization, redetection, detection of episode termination, and optional detection features such as onset, stability, and PDF will be described later.

The Medtronic, Inc. PCD™ ICDs use up to three rate detection zones for VF, FVT, or VT and two types of counting to detect tachyarrhythmias.[30–33] The latest cycle length preceding each sensed event is classi-

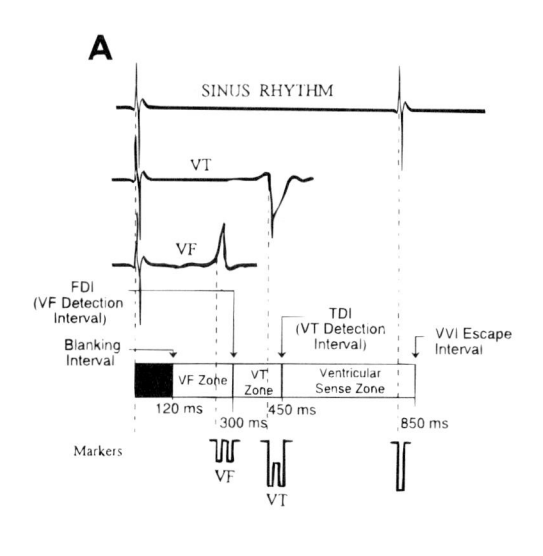

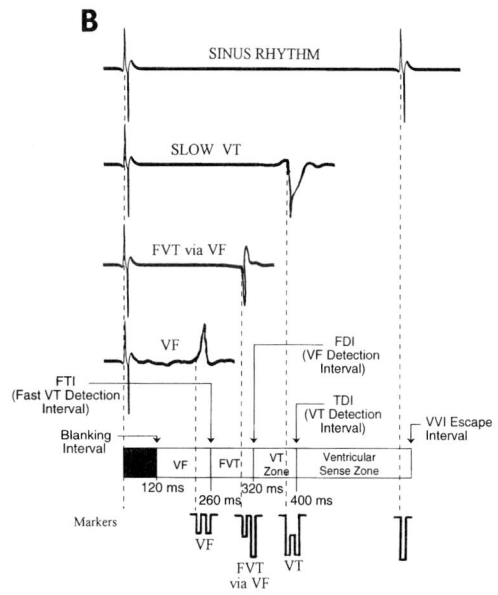

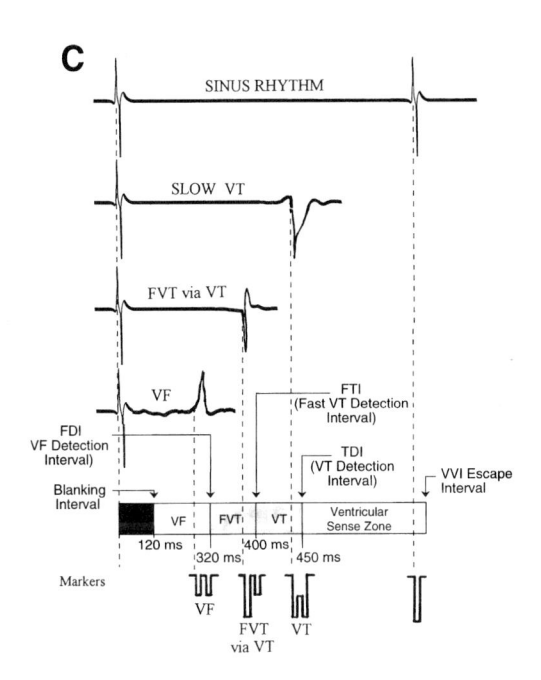

Figure 6. The classification of each sensed cycle length by the PCD™ device (Medtronic, Inc., Minneapolis, MN) is shown for ventricular fibrillation (VF) and ventricular tachycardia (VT) zones in panel **A**. Sensed events between 120 msec and the fibrillation detection interval (FDI) are classified as VF and marked by a short double marker as shown in Figure 1. Longer sensed intervals between the FDI and the tachycardia detection interval (TDI) are classified as VT cycle lengths marked by tall double markers. Still longer cycle lengths greater than the TDI are classified as normal sensed events such as sinus rhythm. In panel **B**, the VF zone is divided into a VF zone and a fast VT zone by the fast tachy interval (FTI) denoted by a short-long marker. In panel **C**, the VT zone is divided into a fast VT zone and a slow VT zone by the FTI, and a fast VT cycle length is denoted by a long-short marker.

fied into the detection zones shown in Figure 6. A sensed event (vertical dashed line) is classified in the VF zone if its cycle length is greater than blanking (120 msec) and less than the programmable fibrillation detection interval (FDI) (Figure 6A). A sensed event is classified in the VT zone if its cycle length is greater than or equal to the FDI and less than the tachycardia detection interval (TDI). A cycle length greater than or equal to the TDI is considered a normal sensed event and does not count toward detection. Ventricular fibrillation events are counted with an X-of-Y sliding window counter (VFCNT). Ventricular fibrillation detection requires a percentage of the prior events to be classified in the VF zone. This type of counter can increase, decrease or neither for each event. Ventricular fibrillation is detected when the VF counter reaches the programmable number of intervals for detection (VFNID, nominally 18 of the last 24). For VT detection in the PCD device, an independent VT counter (VTCNT) increments for VT events, is reset to zero by a single normal sensed event and is not affected by VF events. Ventricular tachycardia is detected when the VTCNT reaches the number of intervals for detection (VTNID; nominally 16). This consecutive type of counter has considerable specificity for rejecting atrial fibrillation that conducts rapidly and irregularly to the ventricle. Highly variable VT that usually does not respond well to ATP therapy may be underdetected. To avoid detection delay due to counter competition, VF is detected if the sum of the VT and VF counters reaches 7/6 of the VFNID (nominally 21) with at least 6 VF events, unless all of the last 8 events are VT, in which case VT is detected.

If a third intermediate zone between the VF and VT zones is desired, then a FVT zone can be added that shares either the VF-type of counting or the VT-type of counting. If the fast tachy interval (FTI) is programmed to be less than the FDI, then the VF-type counter (VFCNT) increments for events that are in either the VF zone or the FVT zone (shaded in Figure 6B). A flowchart for a three-zone detection algorithm with FVT via VF is shown in Figure 7A, using nominal programmable parameter values. If the VF counter reaches the VFNID (nominally 18 of 24), and all of the last eight cycle lengths are longer than the FTI, then FVT is detected. If one or more of the last eight cycle lengths are in the VF zone, then VF is detected. This FVT via VF type of detection is recommended when a patient has a fast pace-terminable VT with cycle lengths in the range 240–320 msec that may overlap with some of the cycle lengths during VF.

When the FTI is programmed greater than the FDI, the VT-type counting (VTCNT) is used for the FVT zone and the slow VT zone (shaded in Figure 6C). All events in the shaded FVT and VT zones increment a single VT-type counter. When this VT counter reaches the VTNID (nominally 16), and all of the last 8 events are greater than the FTI, then slow VT is detected. If one or more of the last eight events are less than the FTI, then the FVT is detected. This FVT-via-VT-type of detection is recommended when a patient has both a slow hemodynamically stable VT and another faster VT with cycle lengths greater than about 320 msec that requires a more aggressive set of therapies.

The Cadence ICD initial detection algorithm can have up to three distinct tachyarrhythmia RD zones for fibrillation, Tach B and Tach A with separate counters and independently programmable criteria.[34,35] A simplified flowchart of this device's detection algorithm is shown in Figure 7B. For fibrillation detection, a minimum number of intervals, nominally 12, must be classified and counted (VFCNT) in the VF zone, which is less than the programmable FDI. Similarly, the minimum number of intervals required for detection of Tach B in its zone and counter (BCNT) or Tach A in its zone and counter (ACNT) are independently programmable with nominal values of 8.

The classification of a sensed event into a tachycardia zone depends not only on the latest interval, but also on the average of the current interval with the previous three intervals (CLAVE). If both the latest interval and the average interval are in one of the three tachycardia zones, then the counter for that zone is incremented by 1. If the latest interval and the average interval are in different tachycardia zones, then the latest sensed event is always classified in the zone with the shorter cycle length. For example, if the latest interval is classified as Tach A and the average interval is fibrillation, then the latest event is counted toward fibrillation detection. If only the latest interval or the average interval is longer than the slowest tachyarrhythmia interval, then the latest interval is thrown out and not counted toward detection of either tachyarrhythmia or sinus rhythm. If both the latest interval and

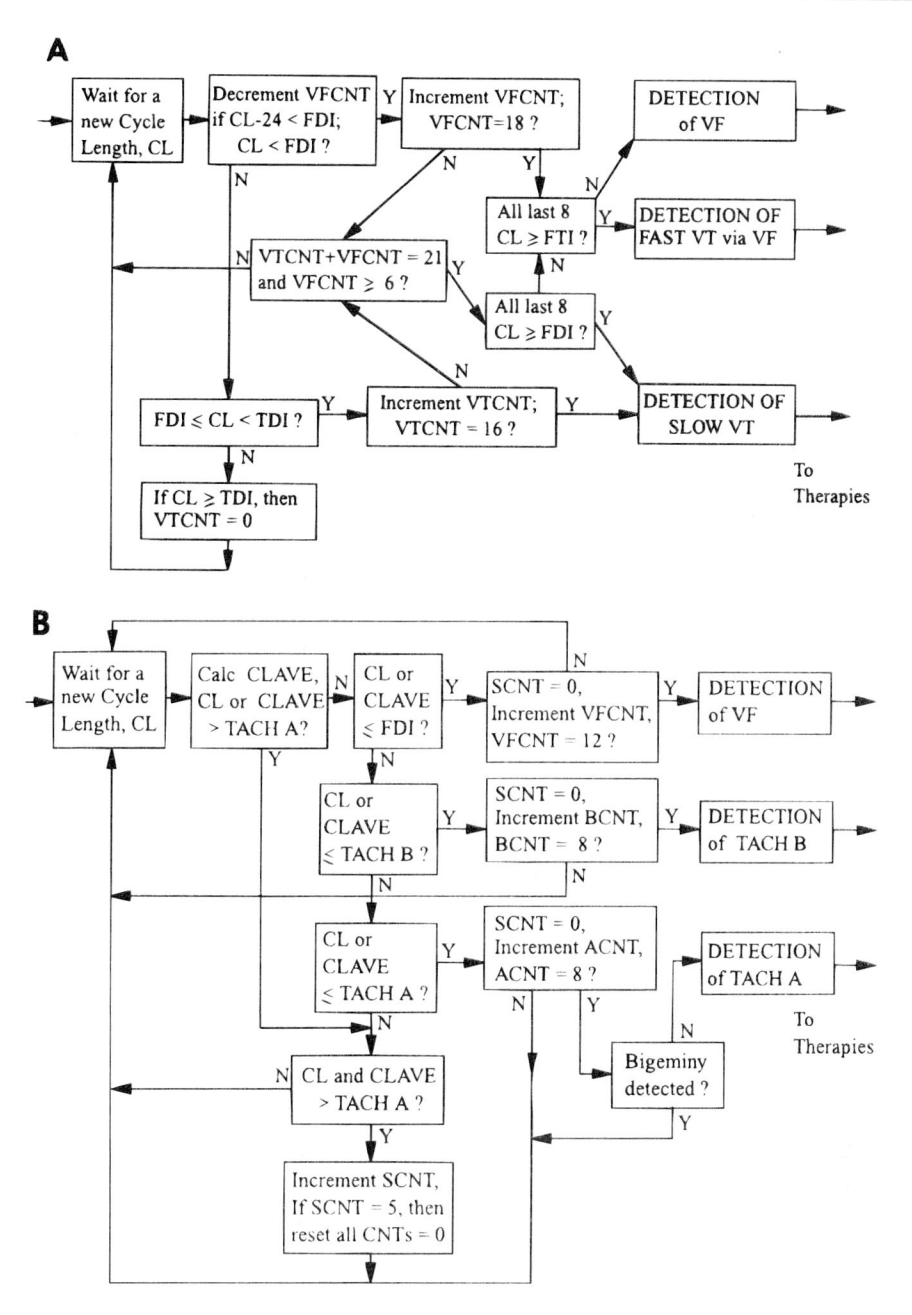

Figure 7. Simplified detection algorithm flowcharts. **Panel A**: Medtronic, Inc. PCD Jewel™ 7219 (Medtronic, Inc., Minneapolis, MN); **Panel B**: Ventritex, Inc. Cadence V-100™ (Ventritex, Inc., Sunnyvale, CA).

the average interval are longer than the slowest tachyarrhythmia interval, then the latest interval is classified as "sinus" and a sinus counter (SCNT) is incremented. This sinus rhythm counter is reset to zero whenever any interval is classified as Fib, Tach B, or Tach A. Sinus rhythm will be detected, causing all counters to be reset to zero, when the sinus counter reaches a programmable number (5 if nominal, 3 if "fast", 7 if "slow"). In order to avoid detecting bigeminal rhythms with an average interval in the

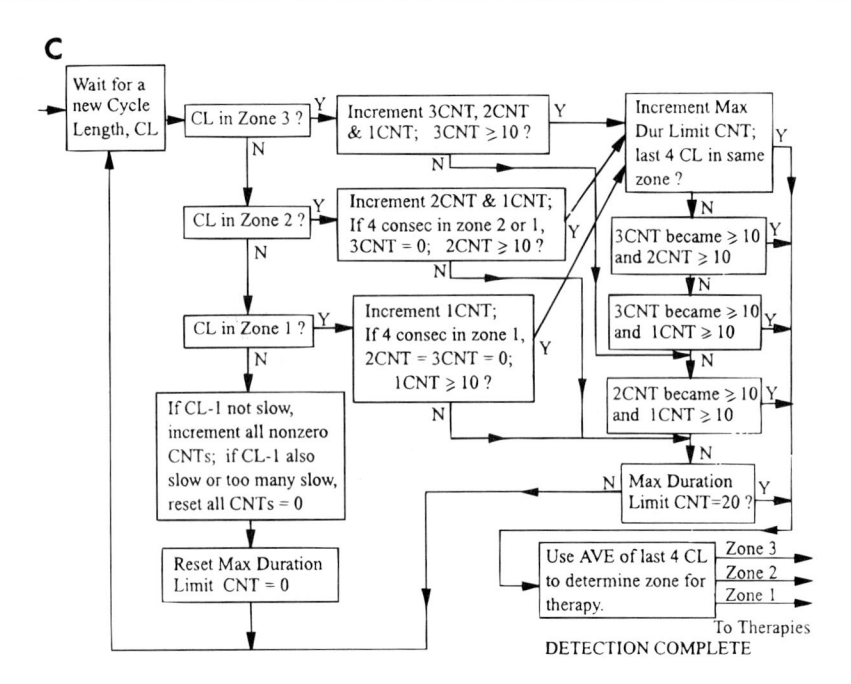

Figure 7. *(continued)* **Panel C:** Cardiac Pacemakers, Inc. Ventak PRx 1700™ (Cardiac Pacemakers, Inc., St. Paul, MN). Each flowchart takes in new cycle lengths (CL) on the left and may detect a tachyarrhythmia in one of three zones labeled as VF, fast VT, or VT for the PCD; VF, Tach B, or Tach A for the Cadence; and Zone 3, Zone 2, or Zone 1 for the PRx. Integer event counters with various prefixes are labeled *CNT. Programmable integers for the duration of sustained tachyarrhythmias are shown as integer constants with nominal values. "Increment" means to increase an integer counter by 1 and "decrement" means to decrease a counter by 1. CLAVE is the average of the last 4 CLs. CL-24 means the 24th previous CL, and CL-1 means the previous CL. For each new CL, each algorithm is processed, and if a tachyarrhythmia is not detected on that CL, the algorithm returns to get another CL, and the process repeats. Nominal values were assumed when possible and various optional algorithms such as Stability, Onset, Extended High Rate, etc. were not included for the sake of simplicity.

tachycardia zone, the device uses an additional bigeminy detection algorithm that requires more tachyarrhythmia than sinus intervals. If a bigeminal pattern is detected, tachycardia therapy is withheld.

The Cadence ICD also has a concurrent extended high rate (EHR) detection algorithm that limits the duration of redetections and low-energy therapies to a programmable time period. The EHR timer starts when the average cycle length is less than or equal to a separate programmable EHR detection interval that is nominally equal to the Tach A interval. If the programmable timer expires (10 seconds to 5 minutes) and the tachycardia persists, the low-energy tachycardia therapies are abandoned and defibrillation therapy is initiated. The EHR timer is reset by delivery of defibrillation therapy via the regular detection algorithm or detection of sinus rhythm.

The Ventak PRx™ (CPI, St. Paul, MN) ICD can have up to three separate tachyarrhythmia zones with increasing rate limits labeled 1, 2, and 3 with separate, programmable counters and therapy regimens for each zone.[36,37] A simplified flowchart for this detection algorithm is shown in Figure 7C. Each tachycardia interval increments the counter for the zone it falls into and also increments the counters for any lower rate zones. The count for a zone is reset to zero when four consecutive intervals fall in slower zones. A single nontachycardia interval increments all nonzero counters to compensate for occasional undersensing during VF. If the number of these nontachycardia intervals exceeds 30% of the programmed duration value (PDV, nominally 10) for the counter in the zone of the most recent tachy interval, then all zone counters are reset to zero. The counter also resets to zero if two consecutive nontachycardia intervals occur. When the counter for any zone reaches its PDV, therapy is delivered provided that the last four intervals are all in the same zone. Otherwise, detection continues and therapy is delivered when either: 1) four consecutive intervals occur in a zone with PDV satisfied; or 2) PDVs in any two zones are satisfied; or 3) the maximum duration limit counter is reached. When initial detection is complete, the four most recent intervals are averaged to determine the detection zone for therapy delivery.

The Guardian ATP II 4211 device has two tachyarrhythmia detection zones for initial detection.[38] The high rate detection (HRD) algorithm is used for tachyarrhythmias such as VF that require immediate high-energy defibrillation. This HRD algorithm uses a programmable high rate interval (HRI) (160–600 msec) and a fixed 8 of 10 counter. The RD algorithm for VT uses a programmable rate detect interval (RDI) (160–600 msec) and a programmable rate detect criterion with an X-of-Y counter that is programmable from 8 of 10 to 48 of 60. All therapies are available to treat tachyarrhythmias detected using RD.

The Res-Q ACD™ (Arrhythmia Control Device) (Intermedics, Inc., Angleton, TX) has fibrillation detection and tachycardia detection that can be subdivided into up to three zones labeled TACH-1, TACH-2, and TACH-3 (shortest interval).[39] The FIB detection simultaneously uses two criteria, counting of consecutive intervals in the FIB zone that may detect sooner than the X-of-Y-type counter (nominally 12 of 16). The number of consecutive intervals, the X, and the Y can be independently programmed with the number of consecutive intervals no greater than X-1 and the ratio X/Y must be greater than 0.5 for X and Y ranging from 5 to 31. The tachycardia detection relies primarily on high rate and uses a consecutive interval counter that resets to 0 for a single long interval. If this tachycardia region is subdivided into two or three zones, then the rate of 2 of the last 3 intervals determines the type of therapy delivered. In addition to high rate, sudden onset, rate stability and sustained high rate can be combined using "and" and "or" logic into 10 specific algorithms for use in the tachycardia zones.

Stability is an optional detection feature available in the PCD, Ventak PRx, and Res-Q devices that limits counting of events in the VT detection zone when cycle length variability occurs. The main objective of these algorithm enhancements is to reject atrial fibrillation that conducts rapidly to the ventricle. Other rhythms such as polymorphic nonsustained VT and complex ectopy that usually do not respond well to ATP therapy may also be rejected. Unstable sustained VT should not be rejected. Studies of VT variability show mean cycle length differences of 7%,[40] decreasing variability over time,[41] more variability for slower VTs, and 45% of VTs stabilized within the first 15 beats.[42] The PCD stability operates when the VT count reaches four by comparing the latest interval with each of the three previous intervals. If the absolute value of any of these interval differences is greater than the programmed stability interval in milliseconds, then the VT counter is reset to zero. This resetting of the VT counter must occur often enough to avoid inappropriate detection. Testing of this algorithm with spontaneous VT[42] showed good separation of VT from spontaneous atrial fibrillation.[30,43] A detailed clinical evaluation with stability of 40 msec showed a 95% decrease of inappropriate detection of induced atrial fibrillation without significant impairment of VT detection.[44]

The Ventak PRx stability algorithm compares the latest interval to the average of the current interval with three previous intervals. The rhythm is judged unstable if over 20% of the intervals in the programmed duration period for the slowest zone differ from the average by more than the programmed stability value in milliseconds.[36] The Res-Q device stability algorithm requires a programmable number of intervals to not vary from each other by more than twice the programmed stability delta in milliseconds. The Cadence and Guardian ICDs do not have a stability algorithm.

Onset is an optional detection feature available in the PCD, Cadence, Ventak PRx, Guardian, and Res-Q devices. Onset attempts to discriminates sinus tachycardia, which accelerates slowly, from VT, which begins abruptly.[43-47] When onset is "on," VT detection will not occur unless the onset algorithm is satisfied. A major weakness of all onset algorithms is that VT that begins during sinus tachycardia may not be detected. The PCD Jewel device compares the average of the latest four events to the average of the four previous events and uses a percent change threshold.[33] Earlier PCD devices compared the latest interval to the average of the four previous intervals.[31] The Cadence device compares the average interval to previous averages, and the difference must exceed the programmable sudden onset delta of 50 to 500 msec. The Ventak PRx onset algorithm finds the maximum difference between adjacent intervals for the five intervals on each side of the lowest rate boundary. If this maximum difference exceeds the programmable onset parameter of 9% to 34%, the algorithm selects the shorter of these two intervals as the pivot interval. Then, the difference between the average of the four intervals before the pivot interval and three of the four intervals starting with the pivot interval must also be greater than the programmable 9% to 34% to satisfy the onset criterion. The Guardian 4211 ICD uses a separate onset detection interval (ODI) and a calculated sinus average to find a decrease in cycle length of at least onset delta (50–250 msec) for the next two intervals. Then, an X-of-Y counter must find that all Y intervals remain less than the sinus average by the onset and X of the Y intervals must be less than the ODI. The Res-Q ICD uses a programmable sudden onset δ in milliseconds that must exist between the first two consecutive HRI and the two preceding intervals. This difference must be found in order to count the subsequent intervals in the tachycardia zone toward the number of intervals for detection.

A cycle length median filtering method using five consecutive cycle lengths performed better than onset algorithms that compare single intervals to medians and comparisons of median percent changes.[48]

Various signal processing methods have been used to improve the discrimination between VF, VT, and supraventricular tachycardia (SVT). The PDF and its digital counterpart, the turning point morphology (TPM) algorithm, use the concept that VF has less isoelectric line than other rhythms.[3,49] The Ventak PRx morphology algorithm, (TPM), provides more aggressive therapy if the electrogram has less isoelectric time than a threshold percentage designed to avoid noise. Clinical experience with the PDF concept has shown that it may reduce sensitivity and delay detection of fast monomorphic VTs (cycle length < 250 msec) that have isoelectric segments but need to be shocked.[4,49-53] The PDF uses the entire cardiac cycle, so it increases even when only cardiac rate increases. It is also susceptible to large T waves and ST segments. Another published technique uses threshold crossings to create a binary sequence and a probability distribution to perform sequential hypothesis testing that trades off detection accuracy for time-to-detection.[54,55]

Some proposed rhythm discrimination techniques use simultaneous electrogram signals from two sites in the ventricle, which has obvious practical limitations. For eight patients, the time intervals between the intrinsic deflections in two ventricular electrograms allowed patient-specific separation of sinus and VT rhythms.[56] A least-mean-square algorithm was used to implement a form of coherence analysis for two ventricular electrogram signals to distinguish between SVT, VT, and VF.[57] The magnitude-squared coherence compares two signals in the frequency domain. It has been shown to differentiate monomorphic VT from polymorphic VT and VF for 45 episodes in 15 patients, whereas rate alone was less able to distinguish, and beat-to-beat irregularity could not discriminate.[58,59] Rank ordered differences of wave front arrival times for two unipolar electrograms for 11 cardiac cycles was able to separate VT from VF in 8 of 9 patients.[60]

Confirmation, Synchronization, Redetection, Episode Termination

Confirmation may occur during or after capacitor charging to verify that a detected tachyarrhythmia has not spontaneously terminated. If VF is undersensed during the confirmation period, failure to confirm would inappropriately abort a necessary shock. A synchronization process may require sensing of several events to assure that the shock is delivered into the early part of the R wave and not into late activity or even an oversensed T wave. For defibrillation, an asynchronous shock may be delivered at the end of an escape interval if no R waves are sensed during the synchronization process.

The PCD Jewel device confirms prior to the first VF shock and will abort the shock if four consecutive sinus rhythm events are sensed (the older PCD 7217B is always committed for VF). All PCD devices confirm as a part of the synchronization sequence prior to delivery of a cardioversion shock for VT. The Cadence device is noncommitted for rhythms detected as VT or VF. During the charging and synchronization process, continuing presence of the tachyarrhythmia requires that six tachyarrhythmia intervals with tachyarrhythmia average intervals be counted before therapy is delivered. When charging is complete, and the tachyarrhythmia intervals have been counted, the Cadence ICD will deliver the shock synchronously with the next sensed event having an interval and an average interval that are tachyrhythmic. The Ventak PRx device can be programmed as committed or noncommitted. If committed, the shock is delivered at the first sensed event after a 200-msec postcharge blanking period and no later than the interval for the slowest rate zone. The Guardian 4211 ICD always confirms the presence of a tachyarrhythmia before delivery of ATP therapy or cardioversion/defibrillation, unless committed therapy is selected. All confirmations use a TCI, which is usually equal to the RDI, and a 6 of 10 counting algorithm. If the onset detection algorithm is used, then the TCI is calculated dynamically to be related to the average interval before onset. Therapy will be aborted if the 6 of 10 confirmation is not met.

After automatic therapy, redetection of tachyarrhythmias during an episode is needed to determine whether the rhythm accelerated or continued unchanged so that additional therapy can be promptly delivered. Most algorithms simplify the initial detection criteria and allow reduction of the number of intervals for redetection to keep the overall duration of episodes to a minimum. After ATP therapies or shocks, tachyarrhythmias sometimes terminate spontaneously after a few rapid polymorphic beats. Thus, redetection that is too quick may interfere by applying more therapy too soon after a previous therapy. During redetection, a rhythm may accelerate or decelerate within a zone, or change to a different zone.

PCD Jewel device redetection uses the same initial detection counting algorithms, except for a separately programmable number of intervals for detection. PCD devices detect acceleration within a zone if the average of the last four intervals of redetection decreases by 60 msec or more from the average for initial detection (7217B) or a previous (re)detection (7219). Detection of such an acceleration causes skipping of any remaining ATP sequences in the VT therapy and a more aggressive therapy is given. When the PCD algorithm redetects in a slower zone, the therapy for that zone is given. After defibrillation shocks, the PCD device suspends VT detection for 16 events (64 in the 7217B) to allow nonsustained rhythms to self-terminate. For redetection, the Cadence ICD uses the same initial detection algorithm except that the minimum required number of intervals is fixed at six for all tachyarrhythmia zones. The device also has a separate programmable postshock detection interval that allows continuation of a therapy sequence if the tachyarrhythmia is redetected in a slower tachyarrhythmia zone. The Cadence ICD never allows the use of less aggressive therapy within an episode. The Ventak PRx device posttherapy monitoring counts intervals in all zones with a single counter. Redetection is completed at 6 to 10 intervals after an ATP therapy, and at 6–105 intervals after a shock, depending on the zone programmable postshock delay of 5–100 intervals. The optional Ventak PRx acceleration function provides a full-energy shock as the next therapy if the latest therapy resulted in a rate increase that is greater than a programmed percentage (9% to 50%). The Guardian 4211 ICD uses a 6 of 10 redetection algorithm between therapies using the TCI. This TCI is equal to the TDI unless the onset detection algorithm is being used, whereupon the TCI adapts to the sinus rate. The Res-Q ICD uses the same fibrillation algorithm to redetect VF and tachycardia redetection uses only the high-rate and the stability algorithms. The number of intervals for tachycardia redetection can be independently programmed to a smaller value than for initial detection.

Episode termination is a process that determines when an ongoing tachyarrhythmia episode is concluded, therapy sequences are reset to initial values, and initial tachyarrhythmia detection algorithms resume. The episode termination algorithm is processed concurrently with redetection after each therapy. If an ICD detects episode termination before actual termination of the tachyarrhythmia, then the therapy sequence is reset inappropriately and previously unsuccessful therapies will be repeated. If, on the other hand, episode termination is too difficult to satisfy, then recurring spontaneous episodes may be inappropriately detected as one long episode, and the ICD may inappropriately run out of therapies.

The PCD device requires eight consecutive intervals that are longer than the TDI (or FDI) to detect episode termination. The Cadence device detects episode termination when sinus rhythm is detected, which requires a programmable number (nominally five) of sinus intervals since the last tachyarrhythmia interval. In the Ventak PRx device, posttherapy monitoring nominally analyzes 10 events after ATP or 15 events after a shock. The episode is terminated if 3 or 4 of the last 4 events are nontachy or if 2 of the 4 events are nontachy and the average of the 4 events is nontachy. For the Guardian 4211 device an episode is considered terminated after ATP if the arrhythmia is not immediately confirmed using the 6 of 10 counter. After shock therapy, episode termination occurs if 6 of 10 intervals less than TCI are not found during a fixed 5-second time-out after the 6 of 10 confirmation period. The Res-Q ICD uses an X-of-Y criterion to detect sinus rhythm and conclude an episode.

Electrogram Morphology

Wave shape analysis of the QRS complexes in the surface ECG has been used for several decades in Holter monitor scanners and intensive care monitoring units. Correlation waveform analysis (CWA), various template matching techniques, and heuristic feature extraction have been used to classify many ectopic and normal QRS morphologies. Of course, supraventricular rhythms with bundle branch block may cause inappropriate detection, but at least this errs in the direction of false-positive detections. The surface ECG integrates the electrophysiology of the entire heart, whereas electrogram signals record primarily local activation, and therefore, do not contain the same types of morphological information. Intracardiac bipolar or far-field R wave electrograms may be useful for discriminating VT from SVT. Most electrogram morphology research has been conducted on the bipolar electrograms that are used for rate sensing. Unipolar and bipolar electrograms were comparable for CWA,[61] although results varied with electrode position.[62,63] Patch-patch electrodes and intracardiac shocking coils with larger surface areas appear to provide more morphology information and may be better suited to morphology analysis.[64,65] Appropriate filtering of electrograms prior to any waveform analysis is clearly important.[66] Finally, sympathetic tone,[67] exercise,[68] heart rate,[69] lead maturation, and other sources of variability[70] are known to alter the amplitude and shape of intracardiac electrograms.

The CWA method[71,72] has been widely used to distinguish supraventricular rhythms from VT. Although computationally demanding, CWA is amplitude and baseline invariant and is often used as a basis for evaluating other methods. Down sampling of 250 samples per second digitized data by 5:1 with preservation of extrema prior to CWA had negligible effects on the results.[73] Several computationally simpler methods called bin area method, normalized area of difference, and the derivative area method have been shown to be comparable to CWA.[74] Further reductions in computation were achieved with signature analysis (SIG) that finds the fraction of samples that are outside template window boundaries.[75,76] Another method, called gradient pattern detection (GPD), approximates the wave shape with a series of signed straight lines with quantized lengths.[77,78] A similar method, named temporal electrogram analysis (TEA) uses the sequence and duration of signal excursions above or below positive or negative thresholds.[79] A time sequenced adaptive algorithm uses linear prediction of electrogram morphology for the entire cycle to find a relative increase in an error function at the onset of VT followed by a decrease in the error function by the 20th beat of VT.[80] A step function model for the pulse shape near the peak of the R wave in the electrogram has been proposed to classify electrogram morphologies.[81] Standard linear and quadratic statistical discrimination methods were used and data from only three patients showed that increasing the number of pulse parameters improved performance.

An area of difference method that is illustrated in Figure 8 superimposes an unknown waveform over a stored template waveform and sums the area between the two curves.[82] With a limited number of acute bipolar electrograms, this method gave patient specific separation of SVT and VT. A study comparing coherence, area of difference with 6 features, a histogram with 10 features, moment of inertia, correlation coefficient, and PDF showed that coherence may be useful; however, little additional discriminating power is available in single lead electrograms.[83] The integrated electrogram evoked response, called the paced depolarization integral (PDI), showed promise for discriminating between SVT and VT.[84] An artificial neural network with a multilayer feed forward architecture used waveform morphology and heart rate to classify electrogram morphology[85] without patient-specific decision thresholds and templates.

Many practical issues may limit the usefulness of these wave shape measurements when used to supplement RD algorithms, however, additional electrodes are not required. Clearly bundle branch block or any type of aberrant conduction may confound these measurements and some method of dealing with multiple VT morphologies is needed. Electrogram amplitudes and morphologies undergo considerable change during the first few months after implantation due to growth of a fibrotic capsule over the electrodes and lead. As implantable device technology allows more advanced signal processing in implanted devices, some of these electrogram

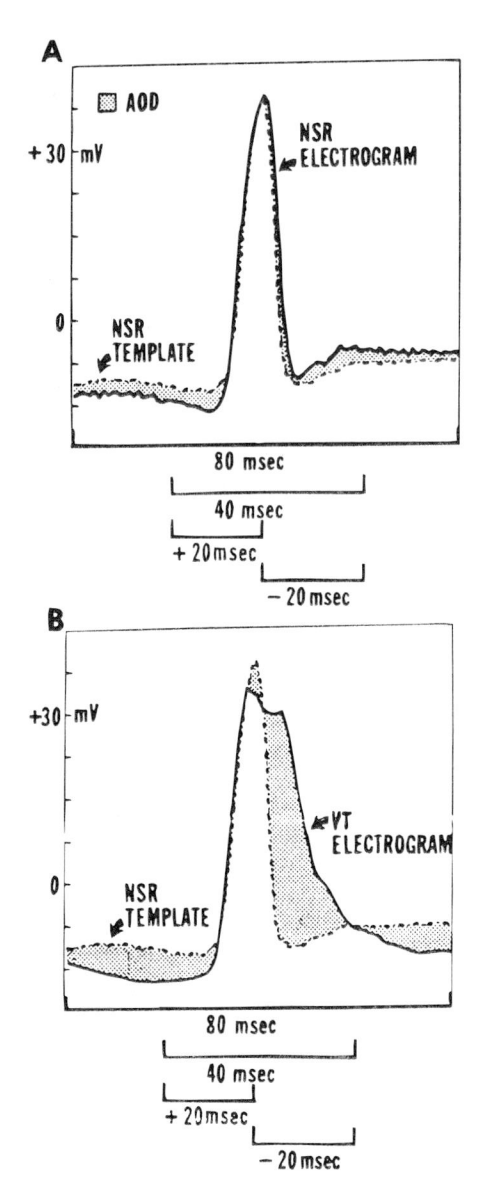

Figure 8. Electrogram template matching by the "area of difference" (AOD) method is illustrated by aligning waveform peaks of a normal sinus rhythm (NSR) template with the unknown waveform morphology. Panel **A** shows the NSR template superimposed on a slightly different NSR waveform, and the AOD is small as depicted by the shading that is accumulated for the 80-msec window. Panel **B** shows a similar result when the NSR template is compared to the depolarization for a VT electrogram. Note the AOD is much larger for VT than for NSR. (Reproduced with permission from Reference 82.)

morphology measurements will be investigated during chronic human clinical trials.

Dual Chamber Interval Analysis

Dual chamber ICDs that sense and pace in both the atrium and the ventricle are being developed to improve tachyarrhythmia detection accuracy and to improve cardiac output with dual chamber pacing. There are many practical difficulties that make a dual chamber ICD complex. If accurate atrial and ventricular sensing is assumed, then a simple comparison of the number of atrial and ventricular events, as shown in Figure 9, can discriminate most tachyarrhythmias.[86,87] The AA, AV, VA, and VV intervals were analyzed to confirm the diagnosis and refine the classification of the SVTs. This algorithm misclassified only 1 of 22 rhythms tested because a VT had retrograde conduction for 7 of 8 beats. In another study, 29 of 30 episodes (97%) of induced monomorphic VT would have been correctly detected by ventricular cycle lengths that were less than atrial cycle lengths and by AV interval tracking.[88]

Atrial sensing for a dual chamber ICD is challenging because atrial electrograms are typically less than one third the size of ventricular electrograms for all rhythms, and particularly for atrial fibrillation, which must be sensed well for accurate dual chamber arrhythmia analysis. Sinus rhythm and induced atrial fibrillation electrograms from chronic canine bipolar atrial leads could be discriminated using an automatic threshold atrial rate detector or amplitude histograms.[89] Acute induced atrial fibrillation recorded from 17 patients was reliably sensed by a 0.15-mV autoadjusting threshold sense amplifier, and no oversensing was seen in sinus rhythm.[90] Electrograms from patients with persistent chronic atrial fibrillation may have no discrete deflections on their atrial electrograms. Studies using amplitude distribution analysis and power spectral analysis of electrograms showed

TACHYCARDIA ANALYSIS

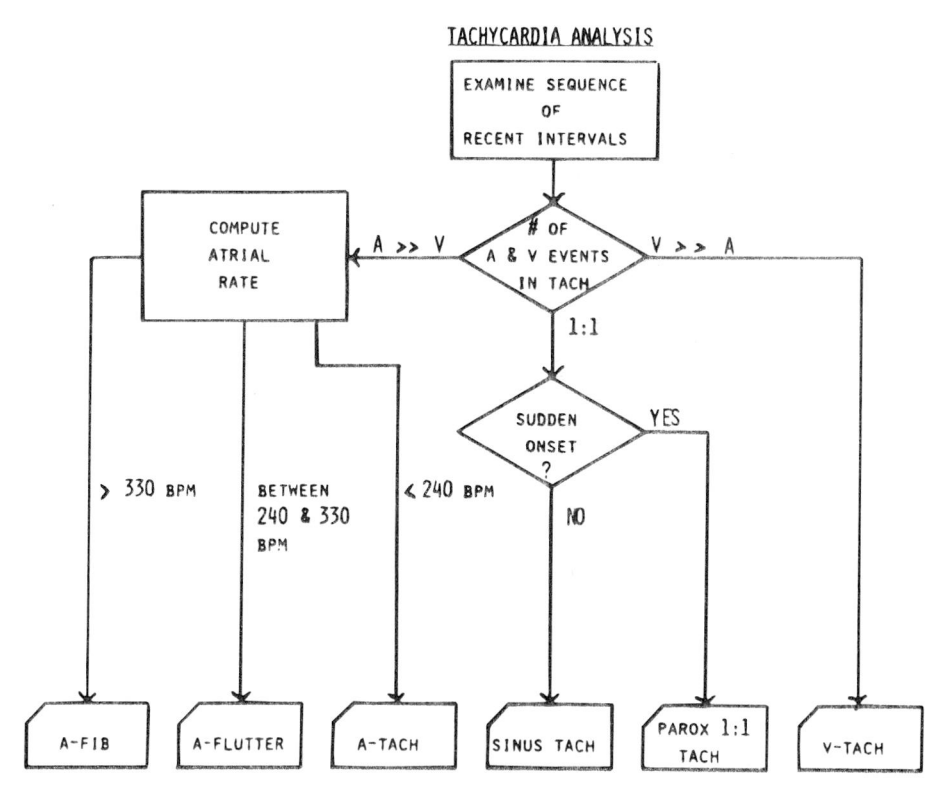

Figure 9. Dual chamber detection algorithm flowchart for 36 recent atrial (A) events and ventricular (V) events with AA and VA or VV and AV intervals, respectively. The difference between the number of A events and the number of V events and the atrial rate are used to diagnose all but the 1:1 tachyarrhythmias for which sudden onset was required. (Reproduced with permission from Reference 87.)

that over time and after treatment with propranolol and lidocaine, discrimination of sinus and atrial fibrillatory rhythms decreased.[91] For 11 episodes of atrial fibrillation in 8 patients, procainamide significantly reduced the accuracy of atrial fibrillation detection using rate, median frequency and amplitude PDF.[92]

Proposed methods for discriminating between the 1:1 tachycardias include onset criteria at the start of the tachyarrhythmia, electrogram morphology analysis, and use of the response to a premature atrial stimulus. At the start of spontaneous VT, an intrinsic atrial event usually will not occur between the last sinus ventricular event and the first ectopic ventricular event, whereas for the onset of sinus tachycardia there will be consistently one atrial event before every ventricular event. An algorithm based on this principle would be quite vulnerable to inappropriate detection due to atrial undersensing. CWA has been used to discriminate successfully between antegrade and retrograde atrial depolarization wave shapes for 19 patient-specific thresholds at a sampling rate of at least 1,000 Hz.[93] An orthogonal atrial catheter was able to discriminate antegrade from retrograde atrial conduction in all 18 patients studied.[94] The chronic performance of orthogonal electrograms in canines was poor (unpublished data). When tachycardia with a 1:1 atrioventricular (AV) relationship is detected, a single late diastolic atrial extrastimulus can be given and the timing of the next ventricular event examined.[95,96] For sinus tachycardia in 14 of 15 patients, stimuli that were 80–100 msec premature made the next ventricular event premature by 30–50 msec;

whereas, 13 patients with 1:1 paroxysmal tachycardia had 80–120 msec atrial prematature extrastimuli that failed to make the next beat premature by more than 10 msec. This method may fail because the antegrade conduction for the premature atrial stimulus may block during tachycardia. Also, the atrial extrastimulus might induce ventricular arrhythmias in some ICD patients. The incidence of VA conduction in ICD patients tested for retrograde conduction was only 23% of patients, and the shortest cycle length with 1:1 VA conduction was 496 ± 100 msec (mean ± standard deviation) and ranged from 280 to 600 msec.[97] None of these patients had 1:1 VA conduction during induced VT. Another study[88] found up to 48% 1:1 retrograde conduction for ventricular pacing intervals as short as 300 msec.

Dual chamber detection algorithms using both timing and morphology information in both chambers have been described. A cycle-by-cycle coding scheme that classifies morphology as normal or abnormal and AA, AV, VV timing intervals as short, normal, or long has been combined with a prioritized contextual analysis to detect 34 of 36 episodes accurately.[98] Errors were caused by incorrect associations between atrial and subsequent ventricular events. A similar algorithm was tested on 28 episodes of SVT and VT with 99.5% accuracy for 641 cardiac cycles.[99] A different dual chamber morphology and timing intracardiac classifier (MATIC)[100] used a neural network morphology classifier and a decision tree for timing analysis. The MATIC achieved 99.6% accuracy on a database of 12,483 R waves from 67 patients compared to 75.9% accuracy for the Guardian ATP 4210® device on the same database. A dual chamber detection algorithm that uses only atrial and ventricular event timing was described that uses an AV interval ratio and AV delay creep.[101] Another dual chamber timing algorithm that used only timing information and the atrial extrastimulus concept detected 66 episodes correctly, but erred for three slow and regular atrial fibrillation rhythms that were diagnosed as atrial flutter.[102]

Hemodynamic Sensors

The direct measurement of hemodynamic collapse with implantable sensors has been appealing since the beginning of ICD therapy. The sensing system of the first experimental prototype automatic implantable defibrillator championed by Mirowski et al.[103] monitored pulsatile RV pressure. Practical technological limitations led to electrical sensing instead. Detection of VT and VF by the absence of hemodynamic parameters poses the added difficulty that inappropriate detection may occur if the sensor or its lead fails.

For 180 ICD patients, only 15% reported syncope associated with their shocks, and this did not depend on previous history of syncope.[104] In a different group of 184 patients only 21% had syncope during their shock episode.[105] The short detection times and high success rates of ATP in tiered therapy ICDs has probably reduced syncope further. Many VTs are hemodynamically stable so electrical criteria would still be required. Also, stable VT is often unstable for the initial 10–15 seconds of a spontaneous tachyarrhythmia until cardiovascular reflexes can increase peripheral resistance. Therefore, the clinical utility of a hemodynamic sensor to control the aggressiveness of therapy may be limited to a small number of episodes. In addition to RV pressure, the following physiological signals have been proposed for ICDs: RV and peripheral arterial impedance plethysmography, RV mixed venous oxygen saturation, coronary sinus blood temperature, and dissociated atrial heart rate.

In a group of 40 patients with VT, Figure 10 shows that half these supine patients became syncopal when the mean arterial pressure fell below 50 mm Hg.[106] The left ventricular ejection fraction did not predict syncope. In these supine patients syncope did not occur in < 10 seconds, and the time to syncope was typically 20 seconds. All of the patients with VT rates below 200 beats per minute were awake; all with rates above 230 beats per minute were syncopal. How-

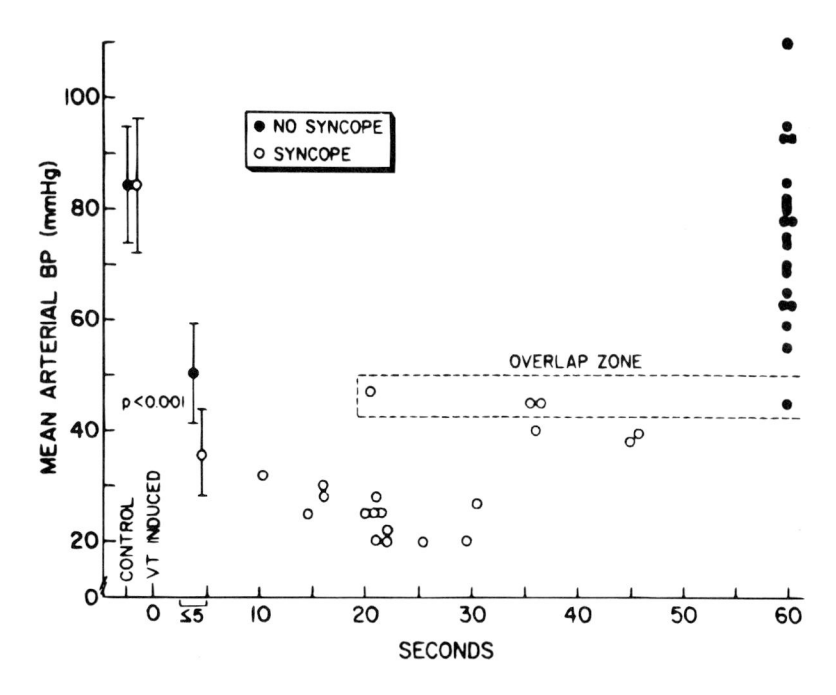

Figure 10. The mean arterial blood pressure is plotted versus time after induction of ventricular tachycardia (VT) in 20 patients with syncope and 20 patients without syncope. Within 5 seconds, a statistically significant difference in mean arterial pressure was observed for patients who went on to syncope versus those who did not. None of these supine patients with syncope was able to generate a mean pressure > 50 mm Hg. All but one of the nonsyncopal patients had mean pressures that recovered to values > 50 mm Hg within 60 seconds. (Reproduced with permission from Reference 106.)

ever, 40% of the patients were in the 200–230 beats per minute overlap region.

Left ventricular peak systolic pressure decreased from 123 mm Hg in sinus rhythm to 77 mm Hg during induced VT in 20 supine patients[107] and correlated with the VT cycle length. Right ventricular systolic pressure and dP/dt declined during the first five beats of the VT. A 25% sustained decline criteria for identifying syncopal VT was sensitive for all patients,[108] but the specificity is unknown. Right ventricular pulse pressure during hemodynamically unstable episodes decreased from 46 to 13 mm Hg[109] and overlapped with the stable VT group, but only stable episodes showed recovery of the RV pulse pressure during the episode so that after 30 seconds there was no overlap between stable and unstable VT patients. For VF, 1 second after the induction, the RV pulse pressure decreased from 25 to 6 mm Hg and recovered immediately upon defibrillation.

Figure 11 shows the results from another study[110] with 27 supine patients where unstable VT, shown in the lower panel, had a 22% decrease in RV pulse pressure. In contrast, the upper panel shows the stable VT group had RV pulse pressure decreases of only 12%. The percent decrease in RV pulse pressure correlated well with decreases in mean arterial pressure. Another smaller human study with only five patients found the normalized RV pulse pressure was a good indicator of unstable VT while VT cycle length, RV maximum negative and maximum positive dP/dt were poor discriminators.[111] Measurement of right atrial and RV pulse pressure combined with a high-ventricular rate has been proposed for use in an algorithm to increase the specificity of rate-only detection while maintaining 100% specificity.[112] Characteristic changes in the right atrial pressure signal during induced VT have been described.[113] Chronic implantation of an RV

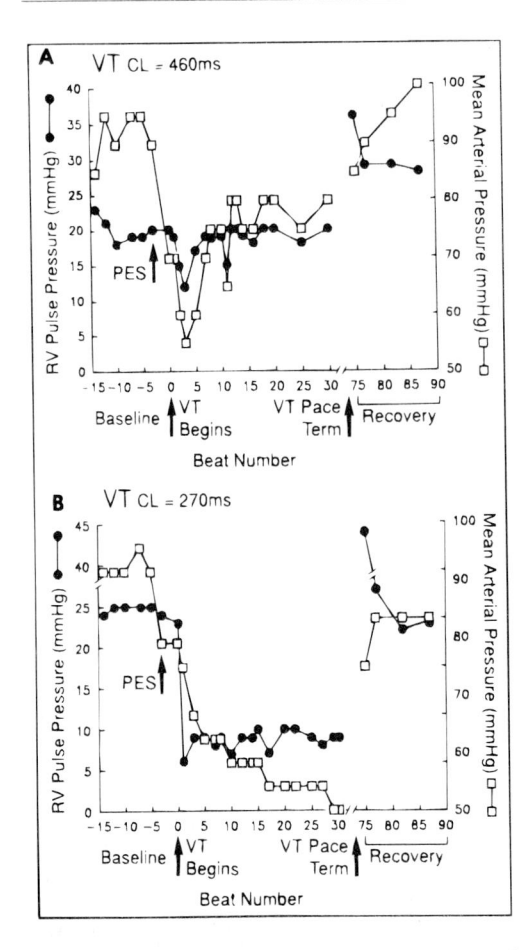

Figure 11. Right ventricular pulse pressure and mean arterial pressure are compared versus time during induced episodes of stable ventricular tachycardia (VT) (cycle length = 460 msec) in panel **A** and for unstable VT (cycle length = 270 msec) in panel **B**. In 27 supine patients, there were 47 stable VTs and 23 unstable VTs. (Reproduced with permission from Reference 110.)

pulse pressure sensor in canines is feasible and this study showed pulse pressure decreased by 82% during VF.[114] Such a sensor must be able to withstand defibrillation shocks, remain hermetically sealed, and not complicate the implant procedure.

Right ventricular impedance plethysmography uses subthreshold high frequency applied constant amplitude currents and measures the resulting voltage on electrodes that is demodulated to assess chamber volume changes. This technique has great practical appeal as no special sensor is required. A detection algorithm for using RV impedance to confirm RD was described[115]; optimal electrode spacing was determined[116]; and chronic canine results showed a 90% decrease in RV impedance for induced VF.[117] Two human studies of RV impedance showed significant decreases in signal amplitude for VF and FVT.[118,119] However, the impedance signals remained high at sinus rhythm levels for several episodes of ventricular flutter that clearly required defibrillation. Inconsistent results were also reported from another group of investigators.[120] Other groups have reported good statistical correlations between impedance amplitudes and arterial pressure changes although standard deviations were large.[121-124] Some of the conflicting results may be due to the number of electrodes used to measure intracardiac impedance. An implantable systemic arterial pulse sensor using impedance measurements has been reported for detection of VF.[125] Practical concerns for this concept include the complex surgical procedure and the possibility of erosion and rupture of the artery.

Mixed venous oxygen saturation has been proposed for sensing unstable tachyarrhythmias.[126-129] While the oxygen saturation decreases for stable VT, it changes little or not at all for unstable VT and VF because reduced blood transport does not return the desaturated blood to the sensor in the right ventricle. A detection algorithm for coping with this lack of decline has been proposed when the tachyarrhythmia cycle lengths are < 230 msec.[127]

Pulsatile changes in the temperature of the coronary sinus blood measured with a rapid response thermistor-tipped catheter have been studied during various rhythms including asystole, sinus, VT, and VF.[130] The small oscillations that are typically 40 m°C in amplitude also contain a respiratory component. The amplitude of the cardiac signal decreases during bradycardia or tachycardia and nearly disappears during asystole or VF.

Usually there is AV dissociation during VT and the atrial rate could be monitored during VT. The atrial rate increases during the first 10 seconds of VT and continues increasing for hemodynamically stable VT. However, the atrial rate decreases after 10 seconds of unstable VT.[131] This difference may be caused by imbalances in the autonomic reflexes. The different time courses of the changes in the atrial rate during stable and unstable VT might be used to control therapy in a dual chamber ICD.

Interference

Because ICD sense amplifiers are almost 10 times as sensitive as bradycardia pacemaker amplifiers, susceptibility of ICDs to electromagnetic interference is increased and inappropriate shocks may result. The larger size of the ICD metal case can also affect the coupling of external energy to the device. Although many types of external energy may adversely affect ICDs and pacemakers, clinically important interactions are very rare for modern devices. Patients are exposed to external energy sources in the home, workplace, public places and medical facilities. The effects could include overdetection and inappropriate shocks, inadvertent temporary suspension of detection, disabling of detection, erroneous end-of-battery-life indications, reset to power-up conditions, permanent damage to circuitry, and physical damage to the leads. Important factors include the type and level of energy, timing and the duration of the exposure, and particularly the spatial orientation and proximity to the source and the device.[132] Energy forms include, but are not limited to: radiated electromagnetic fields, directly conducted galvanic currents, DC magnetic fields, ionizing radiation, acoustic radiation, thermal heating, external pressure, mechanical trauma, and twiddling.

Exclusive use of bipolar sensing with closely spaced electrodes in ICDs reduces the spatial field for coupling of electrical interference to the sense amplifier. However, ICDs have very high sensitivities (up to 0.15 mV) that increase their susceptibility to interference. When using two epicardial electrodes for sensing, it is important to position them as close together as possible, typically 1 cm apart, and to keep the lead bodies together to minimize the area for magnetic induction. Endocardial sensing leads have fixed spacing that is usually small and both wires are in the same lead that minimizes magnetic induction. Leads that use integrated bipolar sensing between a small tip electrode and the long RV shocking coil such as the Endotak lead, are more susceptible to interference than standard bipolar sensing between a small tip electrode that is close to a small ring electrode such as the Transvene lead. P wave oversensing has been reported to cause inappropriate shocks for integrated bipolar sensing in small hearts when the proximal end of the RV coil gets close to atrial tissue. Undesired interactions with bradycardia pacemakers is much less for standard bipolar sensing.

There have been very few incidents of inappropriate ICD shocks due to electromagnetic interference. In one case, an inappropriate shock occurred while the patient was operating a radial arm saw in a wet environment. The probable cause was inappropriate detection via conducted leakage current. In another anecdotal ICD case, a patient received a shock while operating a large orbital electric sander that was pressed against his abdomen directly over the ICD.[133] The presumed mechanism in this case was electromagnetic induction into the sensing system from electromagnetic fields generated by the electric motor that was very close to the ICD and its leads. Careful testing of an arc welder with an implanted ICD that used standard bipolar sensing electrodes resulted in no disturbance of the sensing function and the patient was able to return to work.[134]

Interference or damage to the ICD from other medical devices and instruments is probably the greatest risk to patients. External transthoracic defibrillator paddles can apply several thousand volts and tens of amperes of current to implanted ICDs and their leads. External defibrillator paddles should be placed so that current will flow around epicardial patch electrodes. Implantable cardioverter-defibrillators have high-voltage protection circuits but may have the memory reset by large shocks. Electrosurgical electrodes should be kept at least 6 inches away from ICD devices and leads. Implantable cardioverter-defibrillators should be deactivated during these procedures. The effects of radiofrequency ablation on pacemakers in canines showed inhibition, high-rate pacing and resetting of parameters.[135] An in vitro study of magnetic resonance imagers (MRI) on ICDs[136] showed enough voltage amplitude and frequency to induce VF on the leads alone and when connected to an ICD. Extracorporeal shock wave lithotripsy used to dissolve renal or uretheral calculi can damage internal ICD components and should be kept away from ICDs. There is one successful case report of lithotripsy on the right side while an ICD was implanted an unknown distance away on the left side.[137] Therapeutic ionizing radiation including x-rays, gamma rays, electrons, protons, neutrons, and cosmic particles including cobalt radiators, linear accelerators, and betatrons can damage the thin oxide layers on CMOS integrated circuits in ICDs. The effects are cumulative and as little as 14 Gy have caused permanent damage to pacemakers.[138] Medical diathermy, TENS, cardiomyoplasty stimulators, hyperbaric chambers and various medical devices can interact with ICDs. Interactions between ICDs and cardiac pacemakers are described in Chapter 18.

Sensing and Detection Analysis and Evaluation

Clinical performance of the AICD device manufactured by Cardiac Pacemaker

Rhythm at the time of unnecessary ICD shock

- NSVT: 4 Pts (6 shocks)
- ATP: AF/SVT > ATP > VT, 5 Pts (9 shocks)
- NSR: 10 Pts (19 shocks)
- SVT: 11 Pts (16 shocks)
- AF: 30 Pts (82 shocks)

Number of Pts

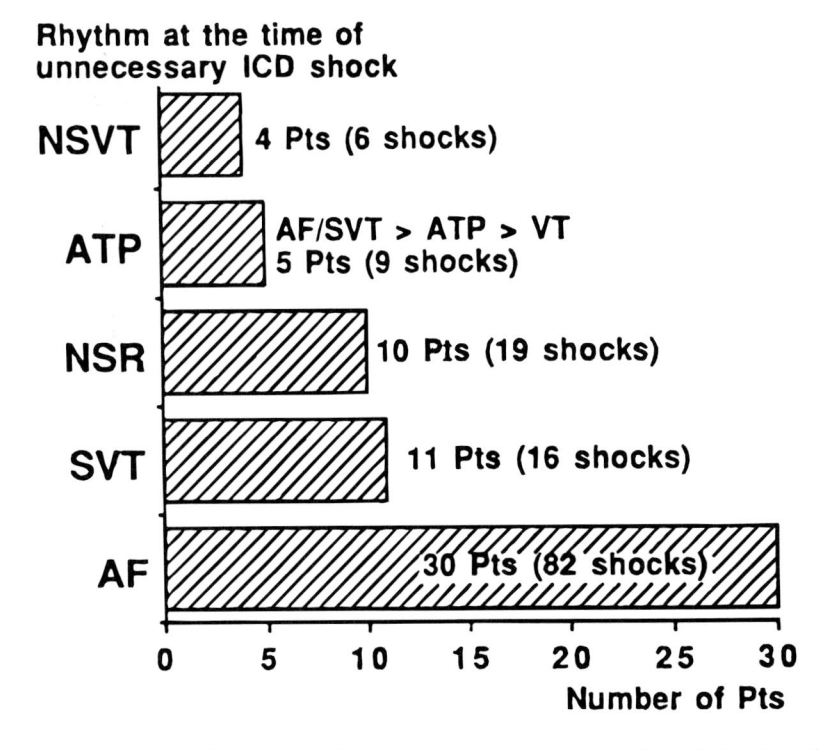

Figure 12. The incidence and cause of 132 spontaneous unnecessary automatic implantable cardiac defibrillator shocks with electrogram (EGM) documentation in 54 of 241 patients (22%) are plotted versus the number of patients. By far the most common cause was atrial fibrillation (AF), followed by regular supraventricular tachycardia (SVT), baseline rhythm (NSR), antitachycardia pacing (ATP), and nonsustained ventricular tachycardia (NSVT). (Reproduced with permission from Reference 145.)

Inc. for 101 spontaneous discharges that were documented with Holter monitors[139] in 23 patients showed that 8 shocks were for only 5 episodes of true VF, 68 shocks were for 63 episodes of sustained VT, 20 were for nonsustained VT that terminated before the shock was delivered, 3 were for SVT, and 2 were spurious in sinus rhythm. Patients were symptomatic prior to all VF episodes, about half the VT episodes and two thirds of the nonsustained VT episodes. In other studies of the AICD device with less documentation, 27%, 41%, 46%, and 20%[140–143] of patients had inappropriate shocks due primarily to atrial fibrillation, sinus tachycardia, nonsustained VT, pacemaker stimuli, or magnet testing. In these studies individual patients also received inappropriate shocks associated with shivering, arm movement, device malfunction, or sensing lead fracture. Atrial fibrillation with a rapid ventricular response has been inappropriately detected and shocks induced VT or VF that was not terminated by the device so an external rescue shock was required.[144] Reliability problems with epicardial sensing and pacing leads led to the addition of an endocardial bipolar pacing lead in approximately one third of the patients.[142]

For newer tiered therapy devices, 54 of 241 patients (22%) received 132 unnecessary shocks that were documented with Holter, telemetry monitoring, or electrograms stored in the ICD.[145] Figure 12 shows the rhythm preceding the shock was nonsustained VT in 4 patients, atrial fibrillation or SVT that initiated inappropriate ATP therapy that induced VT in 5 patients, sinus rhythm or pacemaker rhythm in 10 patients, sinus tachycardia or SVT in 11 patients, and atrial fibrillation in 30 patients. Figure 13 shows an example of a stored electrogram for inappropriate detection of atrial fibrillation that was rapidly conducted to the ventricle. Other major studies have similar findings and rate stability or sudden onset algorithms were used in selected patients to eliminate inappropriate therapies.[44,146–148]

The incidence of atrial fibrillation in-

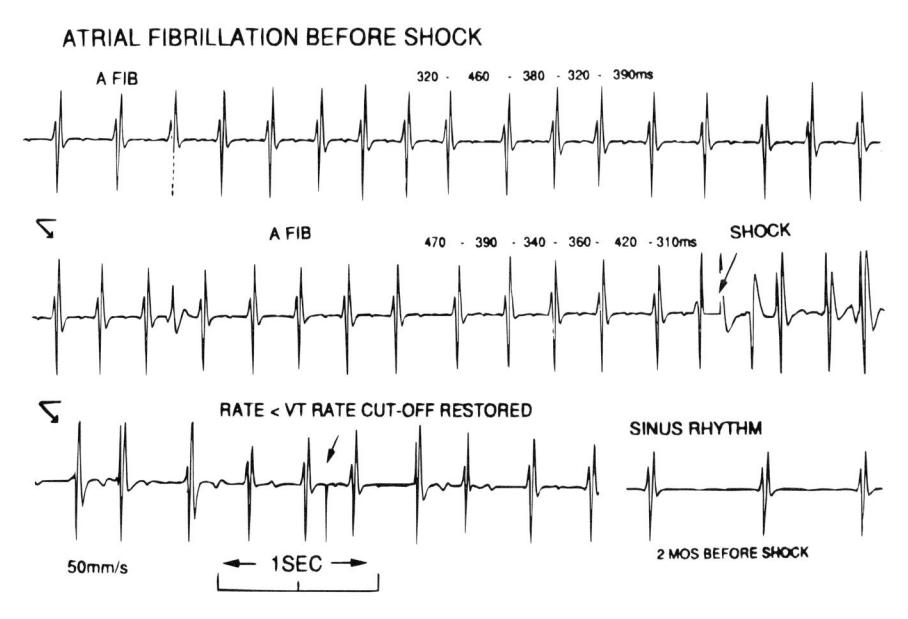

Figure 13. Stored bipolar ventricular electrogram from the Cadence V-100® (Ventritex, Inc., Sunnyvale, CA) ICD showing inappropriate detection of nonsymptomatic atrial fibrillation, shock delivery, and detection of a rate less than the ventricular tachycardia (VT) rate limit. The diagnosis was "made with certainty based on the electrogram morphology and the stability of the ventricular rate."[156]

duction by intracardiac ventricular defibrillation shocks ranged from 14% to 29% of patients.[149,150] Inappropriate detection and therapy can occasionally induce arrhythmias.[151,152] Confirmation of tachyarrhythmias was used to abort shocks for nonsustained arrhythmias in 37% of patients.[153] However, underdetection of VT also resulted,[154] and the time to defibrillation has been shown to affect shock efficacy[155] for lower energy shocks. Implantable cardioverter-defibrillator data storage,[156] and particularly stored electrograms[157] have been shown to reduce uncertainty of the cause for the shocks. Other techniques such as transtelephonic recordings,[158] phonograms recorded from the AICD,[159] and Holter monitors modified to continuously record telemetered marker signals[160,161] are useful troubleshooting aids.

Quantitative testing and evaluation of the accuracy of tachyarrhythmia sensing and detection has been studied by ICD manufacturers using their own proprietary databases. Methods for conducting the tests probably differ although sensitivity and specificity are usually used and few results have been published. The problems with algorithm evaluation are similar to the testing of arrhythmia detectors for surface ECG intensive care monitors and Holter recording systems. Databases of surface ECG recordings for testing ECG algorithms have been distributed,[162-164] and methods for evaluating performance have been developed[162-168] and standardized.[169] Each beat in these databases was annotated by cardiologists, and the emphasis was on PVC detection. These complete databases and particular recordings have achieved qualitative reputations among algorithm designers for their degree of difficulty. A critical issue throughout this long process was the need to keep algorithm development databases separate from algorithm evaluation databases so that algorithm designers could not "tune" their algorithm to perform well on distributed databases. The use of separate secure databases that are reserved exclusively for evaluation has not been successful.

The compilation of substantial databases of human arrhythmia recordings with intracardiac electrograms from the various epicardial and endocardial lead systems for induced and spontaneous rhythms requires substantial effort, and three large databases have been described.[170-172] Smaller databases have been developed for testing various algorithms.[64,77,83,85] There are very few published comparisons of full tachyarrhythmia detection algorithms. Rate alone, rate irregularity, and amplitude distribution algorithms were compared for 35 episodes of SVT, VT, and VF that were matched with 35 sinus rhythm episodes.[173] Each algorithm could separate the tachyarrhythmias from sinus rhythm for various sets of algorithm parameters. Rate alone could separate SVT from VF, but not SVT from VT. Rate and rate irregularity used together could discriminate VT from VF, but not SVT from VT. The amplitude distribution algorithm gave the best separation of SVT from VT (82% sensitivity and specificity). The rate and amplitude distribution provided little advantage over rate alone. Three X-of-Y RD algorithms were compared[174] for rejection of 1,126 spontaneous atrial fibrillation episodes and a 12 of 12 consecutive counting algorithm was best as shown in Figure 14. Several studies[74,83,175] compared various electrogram morphology algorithms, and no optimal algorithm was identified. Specificity for discrimination of VT and VF for 118 episodes was improved about 20% when an FVT RD zone was added, while maintaining 100% sensitivity for detection of VF.[32] The performance of several onset and stability algorithms have been compared.[43,44]

The use of statistical models as an adjunct to databases of actual arrhythmias can be helpful to increase basic understanding of algorithm behavior, but cannot be used to evaluate performance. Autoregressive moving average models have been used to synthesize VF electrograms with similar root mean square amplitudes, number of

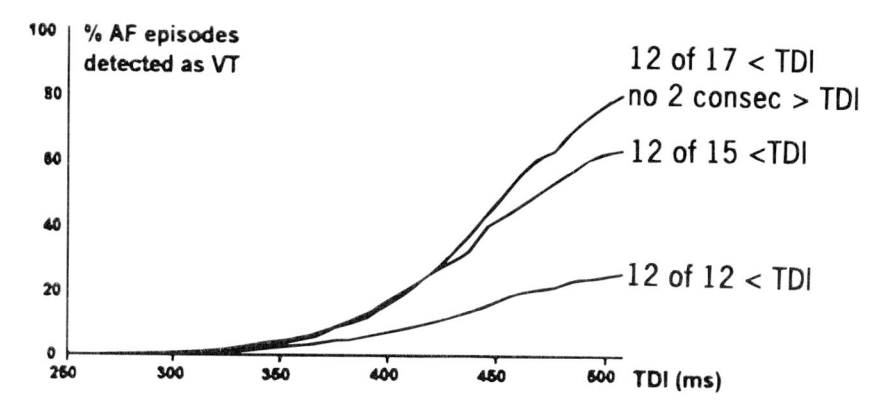

Figure 14. Percent of 1,126 episodes of atrial fibrillation (AF) that were misdiagnosed as ventricular tachycardia by 3 implantable cardioverter-defibrillator (ICD) detection algorithms plotted versus the programmable tachycardia detection interval (TDI). For all values of TDI, the algorithm that requires a consecutive number of intervals to be < the TDI (12 of 12 < TDI) was less likely to inappropriately detect spontaneous AF. (Reproduced with permission from Reference 174.)

crossings per second, amplitude distributions, rates and percent variations of rate when compared to true VF signals.[176] Thousands of 50-interval series of cycle lengths with Gaussian distributions have been synthesized with means and standard deviations that are themselves uniformly distributed on a graph of standard deviation versus mean cycle length.[32] Figure 15 shows an example for the PCD detection algorithm programmed to have a VF zone, a fast VT via VF zone, and a slow VT zone. Each symbol on the graph represents the type of detection that occurred when one of the 50-interval strings of random cycle lengths was applied to the algorithm. Refer to the figure legend for symbol definitions. As the variability represented by the standard deviation increases, "episodes" with means slightly greater than the FTI are detected as VF. Also, note that variable "rhythms" with mean cycle lengths less than the TDI are not detected. Actual rhythms in this region are predominately atrial fibrillation. Slow VT detection intended primarily for ATP therapy does not occur for highly variable rhythms. The borders between the zones become less distinct as the cycle length variability increases. Real tachyarrhythmias probably do not obey Gaussian statistics and the incidence of real tachyarrhythmias are not distributed uniformly on this graph as shown in this simulation. This type of graph is not a substitute for testing with real tachyarrhythmia data. These random interval string simulations show properties of a detection algorithm for an unlimited large number of "episodes" that challenge an algorithm with a very wide range of interval patterns.

Conclusions

Previous reviews of tachyarrhythmia sensing and detection have focused on VT detection,[177] rate and morphology detection,[178,179] or all aspects of the subject.[37,180–182]

Electrograms with amplitudes from 20 mV to a few tenths of a millivolt must be reliably sensed for all cardiac rhythms including VF. Sensing electrode systems in ICDs must be bipolar to reject myopotentials and other interference that can cause inappropriate shocks. The sensing of ventricular electrograms must use very high-gain amplifiers that have either automatic gain control or autoadjusting thresholds to reliably sense VF without oversensing T waves in sinus rhythm.

Ventricular tachyarrhythmia rates from 100 beats per minute to over 500 beats

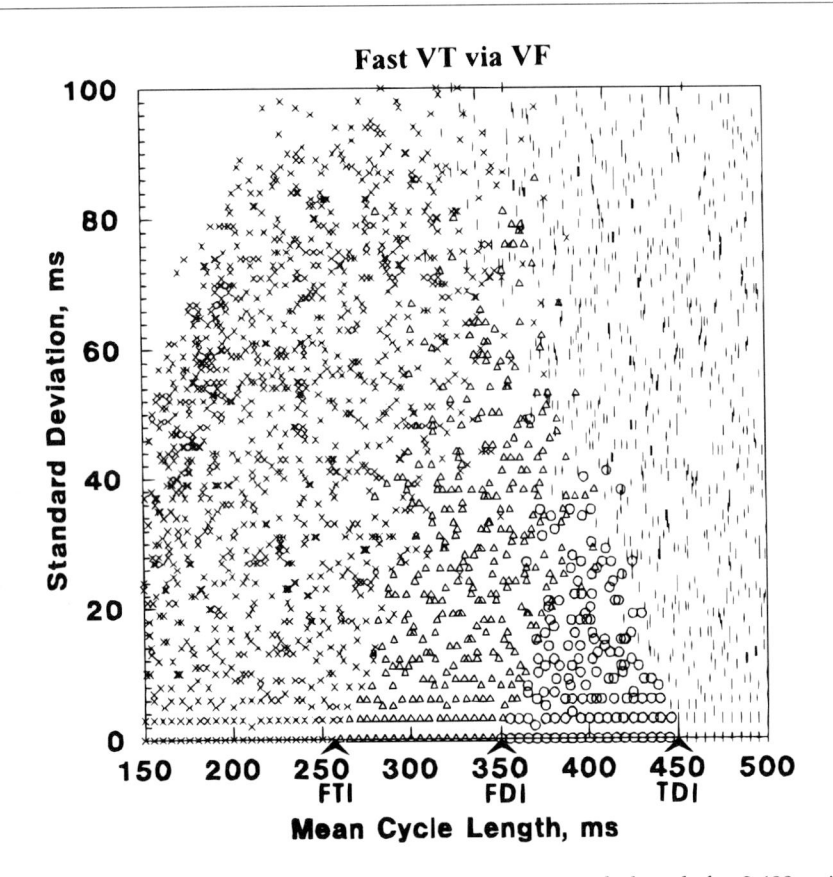

Figure 15. Cycle length variability is plotted versus the mean cycle length for 2,400 strings each with 50 cycle lengths that had Gaussian statistics with means and standard deviations that were uniformly distributed on the graph. Each symbol shows the type of detection that occurred for one interval string that represents one tachyarrhythmia episode. Detection of ventricular fibrillation (X), fast ventricular tachycardia via ventricular fibrillation (△), slow ventricular tachycardia (○), and no detection (|) for the PCD Jewel 7219™ (Medtronic, Inc., Minneapolis, MN) detection algorithm are shown. (Reproduced with permission from Reference 32.)

per minute, that are sustained and are not due to confounding supraventricular tachyarrhythmias, must be detected despite their extremely low incidence. High ventricular rate is sensitive for detection of ventricular tachyarrhythmias unless changes in drug therapy have altered the cycle lengths or an unknown slower VT occurs. The specificity of rate-only detection algorithms depends on the design of the algorithm, its programming, and whether optional stability and onset algorithms are used. Rejection of atrial fibrillation with a rapid ventricular response and sinus tachycardia are particularly important. Electrogram morphology and atrial sensing should increase algorithm specificity, although decreases in the sensitivity of VT and VF detection must be negligible. Hemodynamic sensors may be used to confirm detection and control the type and timing of therapy for tachyarrhythmias; however, simplicity and reliability of lead systems are also important.

Improved methods and databases for evaluating the performance of both sensing systems and detection algorithms are important to assure that new sensing techniques and detection algorithms maintain the high sensitivity of simple rate-only systems while reducing the number of inappropriate detections and therapies.

Acknowledgments: I appreciate reviews of the commercial ICD descriptions for technical accuracy by Stanley Bach from Intermedics; Eric Fain from Ventritex; Douglas Lang from CPI; and Maria Poczobutt-Johanos from Telectronics. I am grateful for critical reviews of the manuscript by Larry DiCarlo, MD, Chuck Swerdlow, MD, Ed Duffin, PhD, Jeff Gillberg, Bruce Gunderson, Bill Kaemmerer, PhD, Jack Keimel, Ann Pearson, Dave Peterson, PhD, Linda Ruetz, Lyn Stepaniak, and Li Wang, PhD. Thanks also go to the Information Resource Center at Medtronic, Inc. for, "if they cannot find it, it was never published!"

References

1. Bardy GH, Olson WH: Clinical characteristics of spontaneous-onset sustained ventricular tachycardia and ventricular fibrillation in survivors of cardiac arrest. In: *Cardiac Electrophysiology: From Cell to Bedside*. Edited by DP Zipes DP, J Jalife. Philadelphia, PA: W.B. Saunders Co.; 1990, p. 778.
2. Wood MA, Simpson PM, Farina DR, et al: The time intervals between episodes of ventricular tachyarrhythmias in patients with implantable defibrillators are nonrandomly distributed. *Circulation* 88(4 Pt 2):I-156, 1993.
3. Langer A, Heilman MS, Mower MM, et al: Considerations in the development of the automatic implantable defibrillator. *Med Instrum* 10:163, 1976.
4. Winkle RA, Bach SM, Echt DS, et al: The automatic implantable defibrillator: local ventricular bipolar sensing to detect ventricular tachycardia and fibrillation. *Am J Cardiol* 52:265, 1983.
5. Ellenbogen KA, Wood MA, Stambler BS, et al: Measurement of ventricular electrogram amplitude during intraoperative induction of ventricular tachyarrhythmias. *Am J Cardiol* 70:1017, 1992.
6. Leitch JW, Yee R, Klein GJ, et al: Correlation between the ventricular electrogram amplitude in sinus rhythm and in ventricular fibrillation. *PACE* 13:1105, 1990.
7. Helguera ME, Maloney JD, Woscoboinik JR, et al: Long-term performance of epimyocardial pacing leads in adults: comparison with endocardial leads. *PACE* 16:412, 1993.
8. Stanton MS: Personal communication. 1992.
9. Bardy GH, Ivey TD, Stewart R, et al: Failure of the automatic implantable defibrillator to detect ventricular fibrillation. *Am J Cardiol* 58:1107, 1986.
10. Grubb BP, Durzinsky D, Temesy-Armos P, et al: Tachycardia sensing failure of an implantable cardioverter defibrillator in a patient with hypertrophic cardiomyopathy. *PACE* 15:845, 1992.
11. Glicksman FL, Zaman L, Huikuri HV, et al: Reversible failure to sense ventricular tachycardia early after surgical implantation of the automatic implantable cardioverter-defibrillator. *Am J Cardiol* 62:833, 1988.
12. Singer I, DeBorde R, Veltri EP, et al: The automatic implantable cardioverter defibrillator: T wave sensing in the newest generation. *PACE* 11(Pt 1):1584, 1988.
13. Vlay SC, Moser SA, Seifert F: Sensing aberration by the automatic implantable cardioverter defibrillator during intraoperative testing. *PACE* 11:331, 1988.
14. Gottlieb C, Miller JM, Rosenthal ME, et al: Automatic implantable defibrillator discharge resulting from routine pacemaker programming. *PACE* 11:336, 1988.
15. Kim SG, Furman S, Matos JA, et al: Automatic implantable cardioverter/defibrillator: inadvertent discharges during permanent pacemaker magnet tests. *PACE* 11:579, 1987.
16. Sperry RE, Ellenbogen KA, Wood MA, et al: Failure of a second and third generation implantable cardioverter defibrillator to sense ventricular tachycardia: implications for fixed-gain sensing devices. *PACE* 15:749, 1992.
17. Wilber DJ, Poczobutt-Johanos M: Time dependent sensing alterations in implantable defibrillators: lessons from the Telectronics Guardian 4202/4203. *PACE* 14(4 Part II):624, 1991.
18. Stambler BS, Wood MA, Damiano RJ, et al: Sensing/pacing lead complications with a newer generation implantable cardioverter-defibrillator: worldwide experience from the Guardian ATP 4210 clinical trial. *J Am Coll Cardiol* 23:123, 1994.
19. Singer I, Adams L, Austin E: Potential hazards of fixed gain sensing and arrhythmia reconfirmation for implantable cardioverter defibrillators. *PACE* 16(5 Part I):1070, 1993.
20. Callans DJ, Hook BG, Marchlinski FE: Effect of rate and coupling interval on endocardial R wave amplitude variability in permanent ventricular sensing lead systems. *J Am Coll Cardiol* 22:746, 1993.
21. Callans DJ, Hook BG, Marchlinski FE: Paced beats following single nonsensed complexes in a "codependent" cardioverter defibrillator and bradycardia pacing sys-

tem: potential for ventricular tachycardia induction. *PACE* 14:1281, 1991.
22. Callans DJ, Hook BG, Kleiman RB, et al: Unique sensing errors in third-generation implantable cardioverter-defibrillators. *J Am Coll Cardiol* 22:1135, 1993.
23. Bardy GH, Olson WH, Ivey TD, et al: Does unsuccessful defibrillation adversely affect subsequent AICD sensing of ventricular fibrillation? *PACE* 11:485, 1988.
24. Yee R, Jones DL, Jarvis E, et al: Changes in pacing threshold and R wave amplitude after transvenous catheter countershock. *J Am Coll Cardiol* 4:543, 1984.
25. Yee R, Jones DL, Klein GJ: Pacing threshold changes after transvenous catheter countershock. *Am J Cardiol* 53:503, 1984.
26. Jung W, Manz M, Moosdorf R, et al: Failure of an implantable cardioverter-defibrillator to redetect ventricular fibrillation in patients with a nonthoracotomy lead system. *Circulation* 86:1217, 1992.
27. Jung W, Manz M, Pfeiffer D, et al: Change in the amplitude of endocardial electrograms following defibrillator discharge: comparison of two lead systems. *J Am Coll Cardiol* 21:128A, 1993.
28. Bardy GH: Ensuring automatic detection of ventricular fibrillation. *Circulation* 86:1634, 1992.
29. Grubb BP, Durzinsky D, Mancini MC, et al: Serum creatine kinase activity and sensing characteristics after intraoperative arrhythmia induction using implantable defibrillator rate sensing leads. *PACE* 15:9, 1992.
30. Olson WH, Bardy GH, Mehra R, et al: Onset and stability for ventricular tachyarrhythmia detection in an implantable pacer-cardioverter-defibrillator. *Computers in Cardiology 1986*. IEEE Computer Society Press.; 1987; p. 167.
31. *PCD Model 7217B Technical Manual*. Minneapolis, MN: Medtronic, Inc.; December 1992.
32. Olson WH, Peterson DK, Ruetz LL, et al: Discrimination of fast ventricular tachycardia from ventricular fibrillation and slow ventricular tachycardia for an implantable pacer-cardioverter-defibrillator. *Computers in Cardiology 1993*. IEEE Computer Society Press.; 1993; p. 835.
33. *PCD Jewel Model 7219 Technical Manual*. Minneapolis, MN: Medtronic, Inc.; June 1993.
34. *Cadence Model V-100 Technical Manual*. Sunnyvale, CA: Ventritex, Inc.; January 1993.
35. Fain ES, Winkle RA: Implantable cardioverter defibrillator: Ventritex Cadence. *J Cardiovasc Electrophysiol* 4(2):211, 1993.
36. *Ventak PRx Model 1700 Physician's Manual*. St. Paul, MN: Cardiac Pacemakers, Inc.; September 1992.
37. Bach SM, Hsung JC: Implantable device algorithms for detection and discrimination of tachyarrhythmia. In: *The Implantable Cardioverter/Defibrillator*. Edited by E Alt, H Klein, JC Griffin. Berlin: Springer-Verlag; 1992, p. 67.
38. *Guardian ATP II Model 4211 Physician's Manual*. Lane Cove, Australia: Telectronics Pacing Systems; September 1992.
39. *Res-Q ACD (Arrhythmia Control Device) Model 101–01 Physicians Manual*. Angleton, TX: Intermedics, Inc.; October 1993.
40. Geibel A, Zehender M, Brugada P, et al: Changes in cycle length at the onset of sustained tachycardias—importance for antitachycardiac pacing. *Am Heart J* 115:588, 1988.
41. Volosin KJ, Beauregard LM, Fabiszewski R, et al: Spontaneous changes in ventricular tachycardia cycle length. *J Am Coll Cardiol* 17:409, 1991.
42. Olson WH, Bardy GH: Cycle length and morphology patterns at the onset of spontaneous ventricular tachycardia and fibrillation. *PACE* 9(2):284, 1986.
43. Olson WH, Bardy GH, Mehra R, et al: Comparison of different onset and stability algorithms for detection of spontaneous ventricular arrhythmias. *PACE* 10:439, 1987.
44. Swerdlow CD, Chen PS, Kass RM, et al: Discrimination of ventricular tachycardia from sinus tachycardia and atrial fibrillation in a tiered-therapy cardioverter-defibrillator. *J Am Coll Cardiol* 23:1342, 1994.
45. Fisher JD, Goldstein M, Ostrow E, et al: Maximal rate of tachycardia development: sinus tachycardia with sudden exercise vs. spontaneous ventricular tachycardia. *PACE* 6(2 Part 1):221, 1983.
46. Mercando AD, Gableman G, Fisher JD, et al: Comparison of the rate of tachycardia development in patients: pathologic vs sinus tachycardias. *PACE* 11(4):516, 1988.
47. Brown JP, Gillette PC, Goh TH, et al: Discrimination of tachycardia by rate of onset. *Computer Interpretation of the ECG XI, Engineering Foundation* 98–101, 1986.
48. Chiang CJ, Jenkins JM, Silka MJ: Median filtering as a sudden onset criterion to separate sinus tachycardia from ventricular tachycardia. *Computers in Cardiology 1992*. IEEE Computer Society Press; 1992; p. 227.
49. Routh AG, Larnard DJ: The probability density function as an arrhythmia discriminator in cardiac electrogram analysis. *Miami Technicon International Conference IEEE TH0206*. p. 19, 1987.
50. Gamache C, Redd RM, Janosik DI, et al:

Analysis of probability density function by programmed electrical stimulation. *J Am Coll Cardiol* 15(2):200A, 1990.
51. Tomaselli GF, DeBorde R, Griffith LSC, et al: The role of AICD probability density function in tachycardia discrimination. An in vivo study. Cardiostim 1990 Abstract 465, RBM 12(3):125, 1990.
52. Hemmer W, Weismuller P, Lass M, et al: Morphology sensing for tachycardia detection—reliability of PDF in the Ventak P AICD. *Herz Schrittmacher* 10(4):187, 1990.
53. Toivonen L, Viitasalo M, Jarvinen A, et al: The performance of the probability density function in differentiating supraventricular from ventricular rhythms. *PACE* 15(5):726, 1992.
54. Thakor NV, Zhu YS, Pan KY, et al: Ventricular tachycardia and fibrillation detection by a sequential hypothesis testing algorithm. *IEEE Trans Biomed Eng* 37(9):837, 1990.
55. Thakor NV, Natarajan A, Tomaselli GF: Multiway tachyarrhythmia detection algorithm. *Computers in Cardiology 1992*. IEEE Computer Society Press; 1992; p. 227.
56. Mercando AD, Furman S: Measurement of differences in timing and sequence between two ventricular electrodes as a means of tachycardia differentiation. *PACE* 9(6 Part II):1069, 1986.
57. DuFault RA, Wilcox AC: Dual lead fibrillation detection for implantable defibrillators via LMS algorithm. *Computers in Cardiology 1986*. IEEE Computer Society Press.; 1987, p. 163.
58. Ropella KM, Sahakian AV, Baerman JM, et al: The coherence spectrum: a quantitative discriminator of fibrillatory and nonfibrillatory cardiac rhythms. *Circulation* 80(1):112, 1989.
59. Ropella KM, Baerman JM, Sahakian AV, et al: Differentiation of ventricular tachyarrhythmias. *Circulation* 82(6):2035, 1990.
60. Bardy GH, Olson WH, Taepke B, et al: A detection algorithm for the automatic discrimination of ventricular tachycardia from ventricular fibrillation. *J Am Coll Cardiol* 19(3):287A, 1992.
61. Greenhut SE, DiCarlo LA, Jenkins JM, et al: Identification of ventricular tachycardia using intracardiac electrograms: a comparison of unipolar versus bipolar waveform analysis. *PACE* 14(3):427, 1991.
62. DiCarlo LA, Jenkins JM, Chiang CJ, et al: Ventricular tachycardia detection using bipolar electrogram analysis is site specific. *PACE* 15(11 Part II):2154, 1992.
63. Jenkins JM, DiCarlo LA, Chiang CJ, et al: Impact of electrode placement and configuration on performance of morphological measures of intraventricular electrograms. *Computers in Cardiology 1991*. IEEE Computer Society Press.; 1991, p. 367.
64. Callans DJ, Hook BG, Marchlinski FE: Use of bipolar recordings from patch-patch and rate sensing leads to distinguish ventricular tachycardia from supraventricular rhythms in patients with implantable cardioverter defibrillators. *PACE* 14(11 Part II):1917, 1991.
65. Block M, Neuzner J, Bocker D, et al: Initial clinical experience with a new multiprogrammable implantable cardioverter-defibrillator. *PACE* 16(9):1913, 1993.
66. Jenkins JM, DiCarlo LA, Chiang CJ, et al: Impact of filtering upon ventricular tachycardia identification by correlation waveform analysis. *PACE* 14(11 Part II):1809, 1991.
67. Finelli CJ, DiCarlo LA, Jenkins JM, et al: Effects of increased heart rate and sympathetic tone on intraventricular electrogram morphology. *Am J Cardiol* 68:1321, 1991.
68. Ross BA, Zinner A, Ziegler V, et al: The effect of exercise on the atrial electrogram in humans. *J Am Coll Cardiol* 9(2):32A, 1987.
69. Paul VE, Bashir Y, Murphy T, et al: Variability of the intracardiac electrogram: effect on specificity of tachycardia detection. *PACE* 13(12 Part II):1925, 1990.
70. Rosenheck S, Schmaltz S, Kadish AH, et al: Effect of rate augmentation and isoproterenol on the amplitude of atrial and ventricular electrograms. *Am J Cardiol* 66:101, 1990.
71. Collins SM, Arzbaecher RC: An efficient algorithm for waveform analysis using the correlation coefficient. *Comput Biomed Res* 14:381, 1981.
72. DiCarlo LA, Jenkins JM, Kreigler C: Discrimination of ventricular tachycardia from ventricular fibrillation by morphologic analysis of electrograms. *Computers in Cardiology 1991*. IEEE Computer Society Press.; 1992, p. 201.
73. Steinhaus BM, Wells RT, Greenhut SE, et al: Detection of ventricular tachycardia using scanning correlation analysis. *PACE* 13(12 Part II):1930, 1990.
74. Throne RD, Jenkins JM, DiCarlo LA: A comparison of four new time-domain techniques for discriminating monomorphic ventricular tachycardia from sinus rhythm using ventricular waveform morphology. *IEEE Trans Biomed Eng* 38(6):561, 1991.
75. Greenhut SE, Steinhaus BM, Murphy AJ: Comparison of a new template matching algorithm, correlation, and area of difference methods for detection of ventricular tachycardia. *Computers in Cardiology 1991*. IEEE Computer Society Press.; 1992, p. 371.

76. Greenhut SE, Deering TF, Steinhaus BM, et al: Separation of ventricular tachycardia from sinus rhythm using a practical, real-time template matching computer system. *PACE* 15(11 Part II):2146, 1992.
77. Davies DW, Wainwright RJ, Tooley MA, et al: Detection of pathological tachycardia by analysis of electrogram morphology. *PACE* 9(2):200, 1986.
78. Tooley MA, Davies DW, Nathan AW, et al: Recognition of multiple tachyarrhythmias by rate-independent means using a small microcomputer. *PACE* 14(2 Part II):337, 1991.
79. Paul VE, O'Nunain S, Malik M, et al: Temporal electrogram analysis: algorithm development. *PACE* 13(12 Part II):1943, 1990.
80. Finelli CJ, Li PC, Jenkins JM, et al: The time-sequenced adaptive algorithm: application to morphological adaptation and arrhythmia onset detection. *Computers in Cardiology 1991.* IEEE Computer Society Press.; 1992, p. 205.
81. Turner TR, Thomson PJ, Cameron MA: Statistical discriminant analysis of arrhythmias using intracardial electrograms. *IEEE Trans Biomed Eng* 40(11):1189, 1993.
82. Langberg JJ, Gibb WJ, Auslander DM, et al: Identification of ventricular tachycardia with use of the morphology of the endocardial electrogram. *Circulation* 77(6):1363, 1988.
83. Gibb WJ, Auslander DM, Griffin JC: Selection of myocardial electrogram features for use by implantable devices. *IEEE Trans Biomed Eng* 40(8):727, 1993.
84. Belz MK, Ellenbogen KA, Camm AJ, et al: Differentiation between monomorphic ventricular tachycardia and sinus tachycardia based on the right ventricular evoked potential. *PACE* 15(11 Part I):1661, 1992.
85. Farrugia S, Yee H, Nickolls P: Implantable cardioverter defibrillator electrogram recognition with a multilayer perceptron. *PACE* 16(1 Part II):228, 1993.
86. Jenkins J, Bump T, Glick K, et al: Automated recognition of tachycardias from electrograms: decision rules for diagnosis. *Computers in Cardiology 1983.* IEEE Computer Society Press; 1983, p. 93.
87. Arzbaecher R, Bump T, Jenkins J, et al: Automatic tachycardia recognition. *PACE* 7(3 Part II):541, 1984.
88. Schuger CD, Jackson K, Steinman RT, et al: Atrial sensing to augment ventricular tachycardia detection by the automatic implantable cardioverter defibrillator: a utility study. *PACE* 11(10):1456, 1988.
89. Jenkins J, Noh KH, Guezennec A, et al: Diagnosis of atrial fibrillation using electrograms from chronic leads: evaluation of computer algorithms. *PACE* 11(5):622, 1988.
90. Ruetz L, Yee R, Bardy G, et al: Reliable sensing of human atrial fibrillation. *PACE* 16(4 Part II):902, 1993.
91. Bump TE, Ripley KL, Guezennec A, et al: The effect of drugs and lead maturation on atrial electrograms during sinus rhythm and atrial fibrillation. *Am Heart J* 117(3):577, 1989.
92. Ropella KM, Sahakian AV, Baerman JM, et al: Effects of procainamide on intra-atrial electrograms during atrial fibrillation: implication for detection algorithms. *Circulation* 77(5):1047, 1988.
93. Throne RD, Jenkins JM, Winston SA, et al: Discrimination of retrograde from anterograde atrial activation using intracardiac electrogram waveform analysis. *PACE* 12(10):1622, 1989.
94. Gerstenfeld EP, Sahakian AV, Baerman JM, et al: Detection of changes in atrial endocardial activation with use of an orthogonal catheter. *J Am Coll Cardiol* 18(4):1034, 1991.
95. Munkenbeck FC, Bump TE, Arzbaecher RC: Differentiation of sinus tachycardia from paroxysmal 1:1 tachycardias using single late diastolic atrial extrastimuli. *PACE* 9(1 Part I):53, 1986.
96. Jenkins J, Noh KH, Bump T, et al: A single atrial extrastimulus can distinguish sinus tachycardia from 1:1 paroxysmal tachycardia. *PACE* 9(6 Part II):1063, 1986.
97. Li HG, Zardini M, Thakur RK, et al: Ventriculo-atrial conduction in patients with implantable cardioverter-defibrillators: implication for tachycardia discrimination by dual chamber sensing. *Circulation* 88(4 Part 2):I-54, 1993.
98. Chiang CJ, Jenkins, JM, DiCarlo LA, et al: Real-time arrhythmia identification from automated analysis of intraatrial and intraventricular electrograms. *PACE* 16(1 Part II):223, 1993.
99. DiCarlo LA, Lin D, Jenkins JM: Automated interpretation of cardiac arrhythmias: design and evaluation of a computerized model. *J Electrocardiol* 26(1):53, 1993.
100. Leong PHW, Jabri MA: MATIC—An intracardiac tachycardia classification system. *PACE* 15(9):1317, 1992.
101. Murphy AJ, Mason D, Bassin D: Dual-chamber rhythm classifier for implantable cardioverter defibrillators. *PACE* 16(4 Part II):928, 1993.
102. Arzbaecher R, Polikaitis A: Dual chamber tachycardia identification. *PACE* 16(5 Part II):1110, 1993.
103. Mirowski M, Mower MM, Staewen WS, et al: Standby automatic defibrillator: an ap-

proach to prevention of sudden coronary death. *Arch Intern Med* 126:158, 1970.
104. Kou WH, Calkins H, Lewis RR, et al: Incidence of loss of consciousness during implantable cardioverter-defibrillator shocks. *Ann Intern Med* 115(12):942, 1991.
105. Axtell KA, Akhtar M: Incidence of syncope prior to implantable cardioverter defibrillator discharges. *Circulation* 82(4):III-211, 1990.
106. Hamer AWF, Rubin SA, Peter T, et al: Factors that predict syncope during ventricular tachycardia in patients. *Am Heart J* 107(5): 997, 1984.
107. Saksena S, Ciccone JM, Craelius W, et al: Studies on left ventricular function during sustained ventricular tachycardia. *J Am Coll Cardiol* 4(3):501, 1984.
108. Wasty N, Pantopoulos D, Rothbart ST, et al: Detection of sustained ventricular tachyarrhythmias using right ventricular hemodynamic parameters: a prospective study. *J Am Coll Cardiol* 9(2):141A, 1987.
109. Sharma AD, Bennett TD, Erickson M, et al: Right ventricular pressure during ventricular arrhythmias in humans: potential implications for implantable antitachycardia devices. *J Am Coll Cardiol* 15(3):648, 1990.
110. Ellenbogen KA, Lu B, Kapadia K, et al: Usefulness of right ventricular pulse pressure as a potential sensor for hemodynamically unstable ventricular tachycardia. *Am J Cardiol* 65(16):1105, 1990.
111. Jadvar H, Bump T, Arzbaecher R: Computer analysis of right ventricular pressure for improved discrimination of ventricular tachyarrhythmias. *Computers in Cardiology 1990*. IEEE Computer Society Press.; 1991, p. 35.
112. Cohen TJ, Liem LB: A hemodynamically responsive antitachycardia system: development and basis for design in humans. *Circulation* 82(2):394, 1990.
113. Kaye GC, Astridge P, Perrins J, et al: Tachycardia recognition and diagnosis from changes in right atrial pressure waveform—a feasibility study. *PACE* 14(9):1384, 1991.
114. Olson WH, Bennett TD, Huberty KP, et al: Automatic detection of ventricular fibrillation with chronically implanted pressure sensors. *J Am Coll Cardiol* 7(2):182A, 1986.
115. Bourland JD, Terry RS, Geddes LA: Automatic detection of ventricular fibrillation using the ECG and intraventricular electrical impedance changes. *Med Instrum* 12(1): 52, 1978.
116. Tacker WA, Bourland JD, Thacker JR, et al: Optimal spacing of right ventricular bipolar catheter electrodes for detecting cardiac pumping by an automatic implantable defibrillator. *Med Instrum* 14(1):27, 1980.
117. Wibel FH, Kallok MJ, Schollmeyer MP, et al: Impedance mechanogram and electrogram for detection of ventricular fibrillation in dogs. *Med Instrum* 15(5):328, 1981.
118. Olson WH, Miles WM, Zipes DP, et al: Intracardiac electrical impedance during ventricular tachycardia and ventricular fibrillation in man. *J Am Coll Cardiol* 5(2):506, 1985.
119. Bardy GH, Olson WH, Fishbein DP, et al: Transvenous right ventricular impedance during spontaneous ventricular arrhythmias in man. *Circulation* 72(Suppl III):474, 1985.
120. Shapland JE, Bach SM, Baumann L, et al: New approaches for tachyarrhythmia discrimination. *PACE* 11(6 Part II):821, 1988.
121. Woodard JC, Bertram CD, Gow BS, et al: Right ventricular volumetry by catheter measurement of conductance. *PACE* 10(4 Part I):862, 1987.
122. Khoury D, McAlister H, Wilkoff B, et al: Continuous right ventricular volume assessment by catheter measurement of impedance for antitachycardia system control. *PACE* 12(12):1918, 1989.
123. Wood MA, Ellenbogen KA, Kapadia K, et al: Comparison of right ventricular impedance, pulse pressure and maximal dP/dt for determination of hemodynamic stability of ventricular arrhythmias associated with coronary artery disease. *Am J Cardiol* 66:575, 1990.
124. Voelz MB, Wessale JL, Geddes LA, et al: Detection of ventricular fibrillation with a ventricular monopolar catheter electrode. *Biomed Instrum Tech* 25:387, 1991.
125. Konrad PE, Tacker WA, Bourland JD, et al: A new implantable arterial pulse sensor for detection of ventricular fibrillation. *Med Instrum* 22(6):304, 1988.
126. Van Riper DF, Horrow JC, Kutalek SP, et al: Mixed venous oximetry during automatic implantable cardioverter-defibrillator placement. *J Cardiothorac Anesth* 4(4): 453, 1990.
127. Cohen TJ, Liem LB: Mixed venous oxygen saturation for differentiating stable from unstable tachycardias. *Am Heart J* 122(3): 733, 1991.
128. Erickson MK, Cheng F, Bennett TD, et al: Behavior of mixed venous oxygen saturation during ventricular fibrillation in dogs. *PACE* 14(4 Part II):708, 1991.
129. Venditti FJ, Qiang ZZ, Grubelich F, et al: Hemodynamic stability of tachyarrhythmia as determined by use of pulmonary artery

O₂ saturation monitoring. *PACE* 14(4 Part II):708, 1991.
130. Hiles MC, Bourland JD, Wessale JL, et al: Detection of ventricular tachycardia and fibrillation using coronary sinus blood temperature: a feasibility study. *PACE* 16(12): 2266, 1993.
131. Huikuri HV, Zaman L, Castellanos A, et al: Changes in spontaneous sinus node rate as an estimate of cardiac autonomic tone during stable and unstable ventricular tachycardia. *J Am Coll Cardiol* 13(3):646, 1989.
132. Olson WH: The effects of external interference on ICDs and PMs. In: *Implantable Cardioverter-Defibrillators: A Comprehensive Text*. Edited by PJ Wang, NAM Estes, AS Manolis. New York: Marcel Dekker; 1994; p. 139.
133. Herre JM: Personal communication. February 28, 1993.
134. Embil JM, Geddes JS, Foster D, et al: Return to arc welding following defibrillator implantation. *PACE* 16(12):2313, 1993.
135. Chin MC, Rosenqvist M, Lee MA: The effect of radio-frequency catheter ablation on permanent pacemakers: an experimental study. *PACE* 13(1):23, 1990.
136. Stanton MS, Stahl W, Gray JE: Interaction between magnetic resonance imaging and implantable defibrillators. *J Am Coll Cardiol* 19(3):243A, 1992.
137. Long AL, Venditti FJ: Lithotripsy in a patient with an automatic implantable cardioverter defibrillator. *Anesthesiology* 74(5):937, 1991.
138. Rodriguez F, Filimonov A, Henning A, et al: Radiation-induced effects in multiprogrammable pacemakers and implantable defibrillators. *PACE* 14(12):2143, 1991.
139. Maloney J, Masterson M, Khoury D, et al: Clinical performance of the implantable cardioverter defibrillator: electrocardiographic documentation of 101 spontaneous discharges. *PACE* 14(2 Part II):280, 1991.
140. Marchlinski FE, Flores BT, Buxton AE, et al: The automatic implantable cardioverter-defibrillator: efficacy, complications, and device failures. *Ann Intern Med* 104(4):481, 1986.
141. Gabry MD, Brodman R, Johnston D, et al: Automatic implantable cardioverter-defibrillator: patient survival, battery longevity and shock delivery analysis. *J Am Coll Cardiol* 9(6):1349, 1987.
142. Kelly PA, Cannom DS, Garan H, et al: The automatic implantable cardioverter-defibrillator: efficacy, complications and survival in patients with malignant ventricular arrhythmias. *J Am Coll Cardiol* 11(6):1278, 1988.
143. Winkle RA, Mead RH, Ruder MA, et al: Long-term outcome with the automatic implantable cardioverter-defibrillator. *J Am Coll Cardiol* 13(6):1353, 1989.
144. Manz M, Gerckens U, Luderitz B: Erroneous discharge from an implanted automatic defibrillator during supraventricular tachycardia induced ventricular fibrillation. *Am J Cardiol* 57(4):343, 1986.
145. Grimm W, Flores BF, Marchlinski FE: Electrocardiographically documented unnecessary, spontaneous shocks in 241 patients with implantable cardioverter defibrillators. *PACE* 15(11 Part I):1667, 1992.
146. Wietholt D, Block M, Isbruch F, et al: Clinical experience with antitachycardia pacing and improved detection algorithms in a new implantable cardioverter-defibrillator. *J Am Coll Cardiol* 21(4):885, 1993.
147. Bardy GH, Hofer B, Johnson G, et al: Implantable transvenous cardioverter-defibrillators. *Circulation* 87(4):1152, 1993.
148. Brachmann J, Sterns LD, Hilbel T, et al: Regularity of spontaneously occurring ventricular tachycardias and its influence on stability criteria for detection. *Circulation* 88(4 Part 2):I-353, 1993.
149. Jones GK, Johnson G, Troutman C, et al: Incidence of atrial fibrillation following ventricular defibrillation with transvenous lead systems in man. *J Cardiovasc Electrophysiol* 3(5):411, 1992.
150. Jung W, Mletzko R, Hügl B, et al: Incidence of atrial tachyarrhythmias following shock delivery of implantable cardioverter/defibrillator. *Eur Heart J* 12(Suppl):364, 1991.
151. Johnson NJ, Marchlinski FE: Arrhythmias induced by device antitachycardia therapy due to diagnostic nonspecificity. *J Am Coll Cardiol* 18(5):1418, 1991.
152. Birgersdotter-Green U, Rosenqvist M, Lindemans FW, et al: Holter documented sudden death in a patient with an implanted defibrillator. *PACE* 15(7):1008, 1992.
153. Hurwitz JL, Hook BG, Flores BT, et al: Importance of abortive shock capability with electrogram storage in cardioverter-defibrillator devices. *J Am Coll Cardiol* 21(4):895, 1993.
154. Swerdlow C, Hwang C, Ahern T, et al: Incidence and significance of underdetection of ventricular tachycardia by algorithms to enhance specificity in an advanced antiarrhythmic device. *Circulation* 88(4 Part 2): I-156, 1993.
155. Winkle RA, Mead RH, Ruder MA, et al: Effect of duration of ventricular fibrillation on defibrillation efficacy in humans. *Circulation* 81(5):1477, 1990.
156. Marchlinski FE, Gottlieb CD, Sarter B, et al:

ICD data storage: value in arrhythmia management. *PACE* 16(3 Part II):527, 1993.
157. Hook BG, Marchlinski FE: Value of ventricular electrogram recordings in the diagnosis of arrhythmias precipitating electrical device shock therapy. *J Am Coll Cardiol* 17(4):985, 1991.
158. Steinberg JS, Sugalski JS: Cardiac rhythm precipitating automatic implantable cardioverter-defibrillator discharge in outpatients as detected from transtelephonic electrocardiographic recordings. *Am J Cardiol* 67(1):95, 1991.
159. Chapman PD, Troup P: The automatic implantable cardioverter-defibrillator: evaluating suspected inappropriate shocks. *J Am Coll Cardiol* 7(5):1075, 1986.
160. Feldman CL, Olson WH, Hubelbank M, et al: Holter monitoring continuous telemetry from an ICD for troubleshooting and improved programming. *Computers in Cardiology 1992*. IEEE Computer Society Press.; 1992, p. 387.
161. Feldman CL, Olson WH, Hubelbank M, et al: Identification of an implantable defibrillator lead fracture with a new Holter system. *PACE* 16(6):1342, 1993.
162. Ripley KL, Oliver GC: Development of an ECG database for arrhythmia detector evaluation. *Computers in Cardiology 1977*. IEEE Computer Society Press.; 1977, p. 203.
163. Moody GB, Mark RG: The MIT-BIH arrhythmia database on CD-ROM and software for use with it. *Computers in Cardiology 1990*. IEEE Computer Society Press.; 1991, p. 185.
164. Taddei A, Biagini A, Distante G, et al: The European ST-T database: development, distribution and use. *Computers in Cardiology 1990*. IEEE Computer Society Press.; 1991, p. 177.
165. Hermes RE, Cox JR: A methodology for performance evaluation of ventricular arrhythmia detectors. *Computers in Cardiology 1980*. IEEE Computer Society Press.; 1981, p. 3.
166. Schluter P, Mark R, Moody G, et al: Performance measures for arrhythmia detectors. *Computers in Cardiology 1980*. IEEE Computer Society Press.; 1981, p. 267.
167. Cox JR, Hermes RE, Ripley KL: Evaluation of performance. In: *Ambulatory Electrocardiographic Recording*. Edited by NK Wenger, MB Mock, I Ringqvist. Chicago: Yearbook Medical Publishers; 1981, p. 183.
168. Greenwald SD, Albrecht P, Moody GB, et al: Estimating confidence limits for arrhythmia detector performance. *Computers in Cardiology 1985*. IEEE Computer Society Press.; 1985, p. 383.
169. Mark R, Wallen R: Testing and reporting performance results of ventricular arrhythmia detection algorithms. *AAMI ECAR Recommended Practice* 1–16, 1987.
170. Igel DA, Rashidi R, Bassin D, et al: Ventricular fibrillation library testing of implantable defibrillators. *Circulation* 84(4):II-607, 1991.
171. Jenkins JM: Ann Arbor Electrogram Libraries. 13 Eastbury Court, Ann Arbor, MI.
172. Developing and verifying an ICD detection system. *Tachyarrhythmia Technical Concept Paper* 1(6):1–5, (UC9202328EN), Medtronic Inc. 1993.
173. Ripley KL, Bump TE, Arzbaecher RC: Evaluation techniques for recognition of ventricular arrhythmias by implanted devices. *IEEE Trans Biomed Eng* 36(6):618, 1989.
174. Anderson MH, Murgatroyd FD, Hnatkova K, et al: Computer modelling of misdiagnosis of atrial fibrillation as ventricular tachycardia by algorithms used in the implantable defibrillator. *Computers in Cardiology 1993*. IEEE Computer Society Press.; 1993, p. 847.
175. Paul V, Farrell T, Saumarez R, et al: Comparative sensitivity of tachycardia detection algorithms. *J Am Coll Cardiol* 17(2):85A, 1991.
176. Throne R, Wilber D, Olshansky B, et al: Autoregressive modeling of epicardial electrograms during ventricular fibrillation. *IEEE Trans Biomed Eng* 40(4):379, 1993.
177. Furman S, Fisher JD, Pannizzo F: Necessity of signal processing in tachycardia detection. In: *The Third Decade of Cardiac Pacing*. Edited by SS Barold, J Mugica. Mount Kisco NY: Futura Publishing Company, Inc.; 1982, p. 265.
178. Camm AJ, Davies DW, Ward DE: Tachycardia recognition by implantable electronic devices. *PACE* 10(5):1175, 1987.
179. Pannizzo F, Mercando AD, Fisher JD, et al: Automatic methods for detection of tachyarrhythmias by antitachycardia devices. *J Am Coll Cardiol* 11(2):308, 1988.
180. Khoury DS, Wilkoff BL: Tachycardia recognition algorithms for implantable systems. *IEEE Eng Med Biol Magazine* 9(2):40, 1990.
181. Camm AJ, Paul V, Ward DE: Recognition of tachyarrhythmias by implantable devices. In: *Electrical Therapy for Cardiac Arrhythmias*. Edited by S Saksena, N Goldschlager. Philadelphia: WB Saunders, Co; 1990, p. 589.
182. *Practical Aspects of Staged Therapy Defibrillators*. Edited by LJ Kappenberger, FW Lindemans. Mount Kisco, NY; Futura Publishing Company, Inc.; 1992.

Chapter 5

Tachyarrhythmia Termination: Lead Systems and Hardware Design

Rahul Mehra and Zach Cybulski

Effective defibrillation depends on efficient delivery of current density or voltage gradient in a critical myocardial volume. To achieve this essential result, optimal lead design, electrode configuration and adequate power delivery are essential. These issues will be described here in some detail. This chapter, therefore, discusses currently available lead configurations and power sources, capacitors and switching circuits required to optimize defibrillation.

Lead Systems

One of the primary technological requirements of implantable defibrillators is that the devices be efficacious and small so that they can be easily implanted in appropriate patients. Because size of these devices is directly related to their maximum energy output, in order to reduce their size, the energy required for ventricular defibrillation must be reduced. The lead systems in conjunction with the shock waveform play an important role in reducing defibrillation threshold (DFT). Presently, most devices deliver 30–40 J and their relatively large size requires implantation in the abdomen. Smaller devices that can be implanted in the subpectoral region have only recently been developed.

In order to design optimal electrode systems, it is first necessary to define the primary requirements for defibrillation. Even though the mechanism of defibrillation is controversial, most experimental work indicates that defibrillation can be achieved by developing adequate current density or voltage gradient in a critical volume of the myocardium in order to excite the tissue and interrupt the multiple wavelets that sustain fibrillation[1-4] (see Appendix A for description of current density and voltage gradient). Based on this, the ideal electrode system is one that sets up this minimum current density in most of the ventricular mass. Because most defibrillation electrodes are placed relatively close to the myocardium, they create a nonuniform current density distribution. Due to this nonuniformity, certain regions of the heart are exposed to relatively high-current density that can result in tissue damage or be proarrhythmic by setting up focal activity. This nonuniformity creates a second requirement for defibrillation electrodes, ie, that the volume of tissue that is exposed to high fields be kept to a minimum. Apart from these requirements, the electrodes should be easy to implant, safe, and facilitate pacing and sensing.

Initially, defibrillator implants were

From Singer I, (ed.) Implantable Cardioverter-Defibrillator. Armonk, NY: Futura Publishing Company, Inc.; © 1994.

primarily done with epicardial electrodes. Recent studies have shown that the perioperative mortality and morbidity associated with epicardial electrodes is higher than with endocardial systems.[5] Due to this finding, the use of endocardial electrode systems has increased significantly. There are certain basic electrode configurations that are applicable to both epicardial and transvenous systems and these will be discussed first.

Electrode Configurations

Defibrillation can be performed with two or more electrodes (Figure 1). When two electrodes are used, single or multiple shocks can be delivered through a pathway. When two shocks are delivered, they can be opposite in polarity (biphasic shocks) or be of the same polarity. The latter pulsing configuration has been called dual pulse defibrillation.

When three or more electrodes are used for defibrillation they can be connected to deliver Simultaneous or Sequential shocks. With Simultaneous defibrillation, there is only one pulse and the current is distributed across multiple pathways. For example, in a three-electrode system, two of the electrodes are connected and the shock is delivered across this electrode pair and the third electrode (Figure 1). The defibrillation current is distributed between the two pathways. With Sequential pulse defibrillation, the shocks are temporally separated and delivered across different pathways. For a three-electrode Sequential pulse defibrillation, the first shock is across two of the electrodes and the second shock across the third electrode and one of the electrodes used for the first shock (Figure 1). If four electrodes were used, then the second shock would be across a completely separate pair of electrodes.

Single, Simultaneous or Sequential pulsing configurations can be used with epicardial or transvenous electrode systems. There are certain advantages and shortcomings of each method and these are discussed.

DEFIBRILLATION PULSING METHODS

1. SINGLE PULSE

2. DUAL PULSE

3. SEQUENTIAL PULSE

4. SIMULTANEOUS PULSE

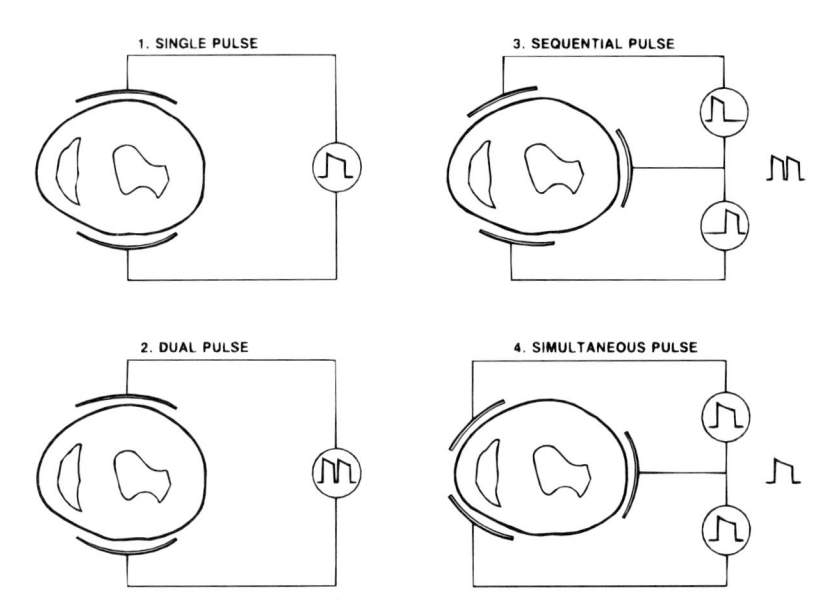

Figure 1. Various pulsing methods that can be used with two electrodes (single and dual pulse) and three-electrode systems (Sequential and Simultaneous pulse). Although the figure depicts them for epicardial defibrillation, they are similarly applicable for transvenous defibrillation.

Epicardial Lead Systems

Two-Electrode Defibrillation

The two-electrode system is most commonly used with implantable defibrillators. There are several variables that effect DFT with two electrodes. Apart from defibrillation pulse waveform, it is well appreciated that electrode size and placement are important variables. Most animal and clinical studies indicate that epicardial patches must be positioned appropriately and that DFT decreases as the patch electrode area increases.[6]

In an attempt to understand the fundamental basis of this observation, we developed a finite element model of a dog's heart. This computer model allows the current density distributions created by any electrode system to be plotted, and based on certain assumptions regarding the basic requirements for defibrillation, compute the DFT for those electrodes. We assumed that for successful defibrillation, the current density in 90% to 95% of the ventricular mass must be above a certain threshold value. In order to create this three-dimensional model, a dog's heart was fixed in formalin, sliced into 15 sections, and each slice digitized. These digitized sections were used for creating a 57,000-tetrahedral element, isotropic, linear model of the heart using the Ansys® (Swanson Analysis Systems, Houston, PA) 4.0 Software (Figure 2).

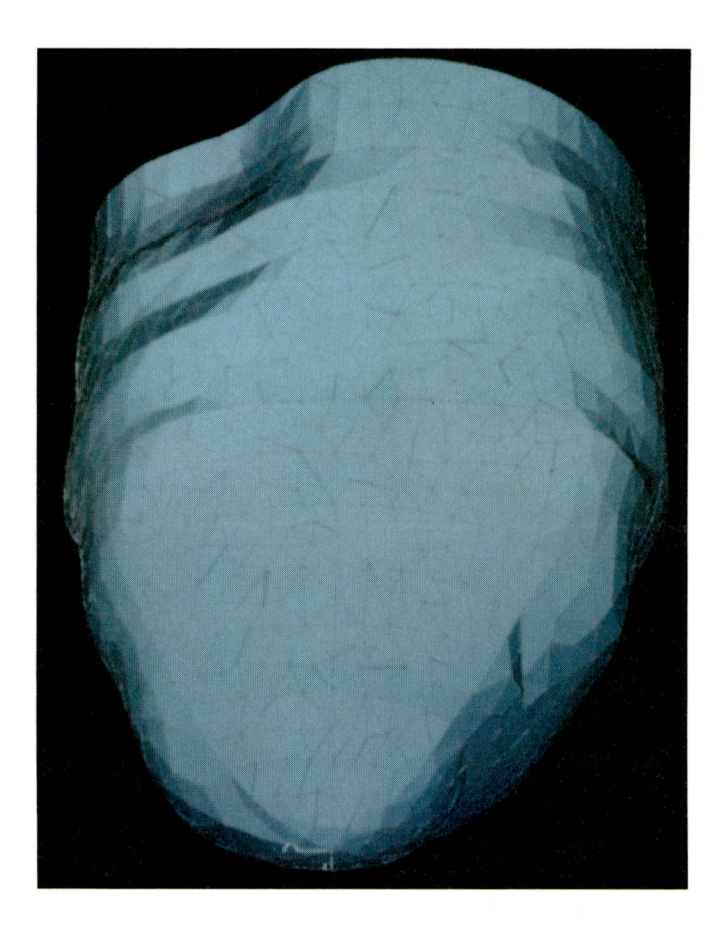

Figure 2. An epicardial view of the finite element model of the heart. The computer model has 57,000 tetrahedral elements.

In order to collect experimental data so that the computer model could be eventually validated, the heart was isolated and set up in a Langendorff preparation prior to sectioning. An epicardial sock electrode with 61 unipolar electrodes was slipped on the epicardium and two epicardial defibrillation patches were sutured. One hundred-volt shocks were delivered across the two epicardial patches during diastole and the voltages at each of the 61 sites measured. Before sectioning the heart, the sites of the 61 epicardial potential measurements were delineated by inserting needle electrodes at those locations.

Once the computer model was complete, epicardial patches of the same dimensions and at the same location as in the experimental preparation were simulated and the epicardial voltages at each of the 61 sites computed. The resistivity values used for cardiac muscle and blood were 400 and 150 Ω cm. The correlation between the experimental and the computed potentials was 0.97 ($P < 0.01$), confirming that the computer model was a reasonable simulation. It should be noted that there are two primary limitations of this model. First, cardiac tissue is assumed to be isotropic and linear, and second, the thoracic cavity is not included in the model.

Effect of Electrode Area

In this heart model, the effect of size of epicardial patches was analyzed. Two epicardial patches each with a surface area of 9 cm², 15 cm², 30 cm², 46 cm², 56 cm², and 66 cm² were placed on the heart, and the DFT and the impedance were computed in each case. For the 46-cm², 56-cm², and 66-cm² electrodes, the distance between adjacent edges of the two patch electrodes was at 3, 2, and 1 cm, respectively. These six sizes of electrodes covered 12% to 87% of

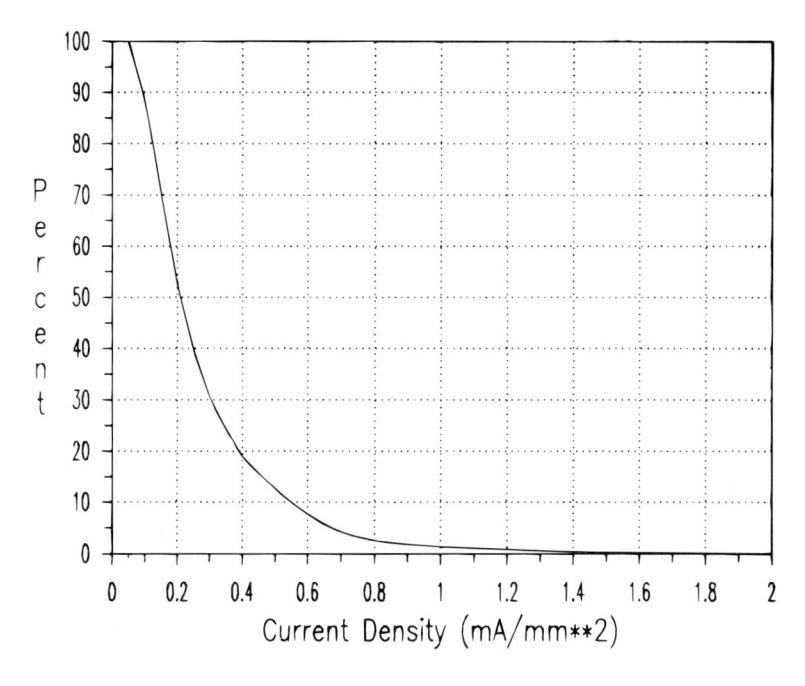

Figure 3. A graph of the percentage of the ventricular myocardium that has current density greater than the values depicted in the abscissa when a 100-V shock is delivered across two patches. For example, about 55% of the myocardium has current density greater than 0.2 mA/mm².

the epicardial surface of this heart, whose total epicardial surface area was 152 cm².

Defibrillation threshold was computed based on the hypothesis that defibrillation occurs when 95% of the myocardium has a current density of at least 0.3 mA/cm². This corresponds to a voltage gradient of 12 V/cm (This value may be larger than reported by other investigators. The thresholds can be scaled for other values of critical voltage gradient.) and a resistivity of 400 Ω cm (12/400 = 0.03 amps/cm² = 0.3 mA/mm²). The DFT is determined from a graph of current density versus percentage of myocardial volume that has a current density greater than that value as computed for a 100-V shock (Figure 3). The current density in 95% of the volume is read from that graph. In order that the current density be at least equal to 0.3 mA/cm², this 100-V value is appropriately scaled to determine the DFT. For example, in this figure, 95% of the myocardium has a current density greater than 0.05 mA/mm² for a 100-V shock. For 95%

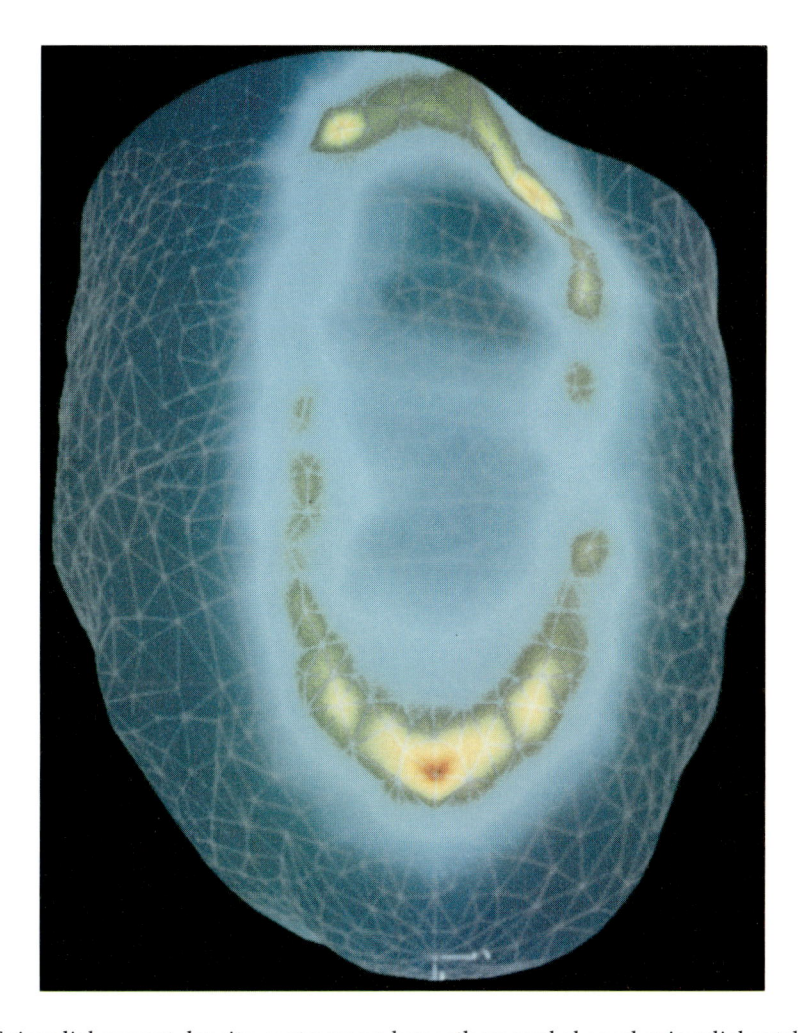

Figure 4. Epicardial current density contours underneath an oval-shaped epicardial patch electrode. The red and yellow regions have very high-current density. The light blue regions have lower current density and the dark blue region is the lowest. Note the region of low density in the central region of the patch and high density at the circumference.

of the muscle to have current density greater than 0.3 mA/mm² so that defibrillation can occur, the voltage required would be 600 V.

Figure 4 shows the pattern of epicardial current density with large patches. The current density at the circumference of the patch is much higher than at the central part even though the same potential is applied across the complete patch. This occurs because most of the current flows from the outer edge. This high-current density area can damage the tissue. Preliminary studies indicate that current densities > 100 V/cm can cause irreversible damage. With epicardial patches this damaged tissue can be visualized as a silhouette of the patch electrode and typically can constitute < 1.6% of the myocardium based on histopathological studies conducted in our laboratory.[7] Lower voltage gradients between 60 and 70 V/cm can cause reversible modification of electrophysiologic properties such as excitability and conduction.[8]

The effect of increasing surface area on DFT and impedance is shown in Figures 5 and 6. The results indicate that increasing the area up to 46 cm² (61% of epicardial coverage) causes a reduction in DFTs, but the thresholds plateau as the area is further increased. This occurs in spite of a decrease in impedance and is due to a degradation of the field distribution caused by the shunting of current between the closely spaced largest electrodes. This is indicated by the current thresholds that tend to go up when the electrode area is relatively large. These conclusions are not altered even if the threshold current density is altered between 0.2 and 0.4 mA/cm² or the critical mass of the myocardium is varied between 75% and 95% (Figures 7 and 8). The impedance values of 39 Ω with 35-cm² electrodes observed in the model are comparable to 43 Ω observed experimentally.[9,10] These results indicate that increasing electrode area reduces thresholds, but using extremely large electrodes are not necessarily advantageous for

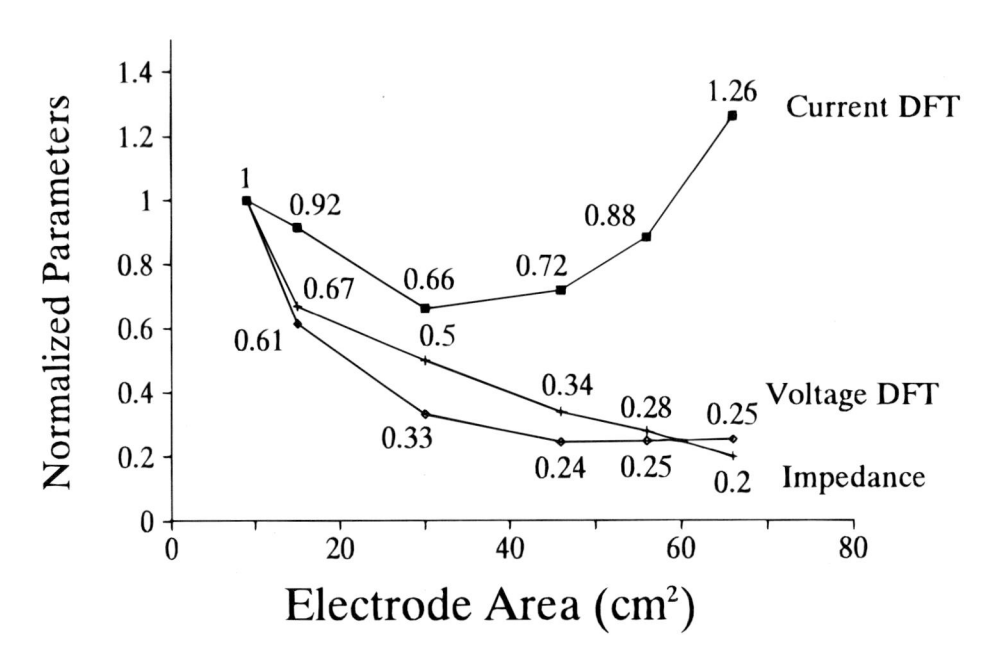

Figure 5. Effect of increasing electrode area on current and voltage defibrillation thresholds as well as interelectrode impedance determined from the computer model. The parameters are normalized to unity for two 9-cm² electrodes. The voltage defibrillation thresholds (DFTs) impedance generally decrease with increasing area whereas the current thresholds reach a minimum and then increase.

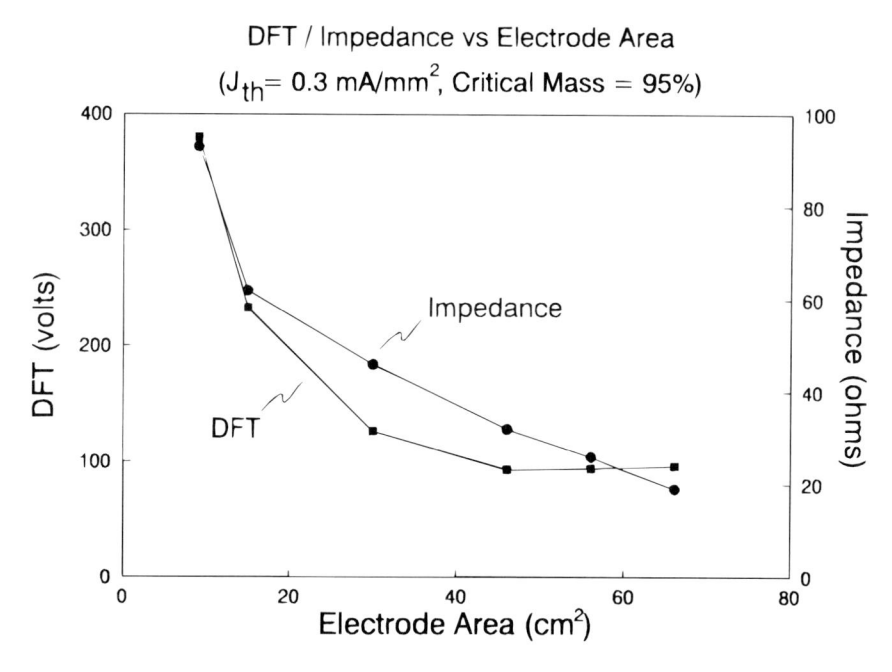

Figure 6. Absolute values of impedance and voltage defibrillation thresholds as a function of patch electrode area computed from the heart model. The threshold current density is assumed to be 0.3 mA/cm² and the critical mass is 95%.

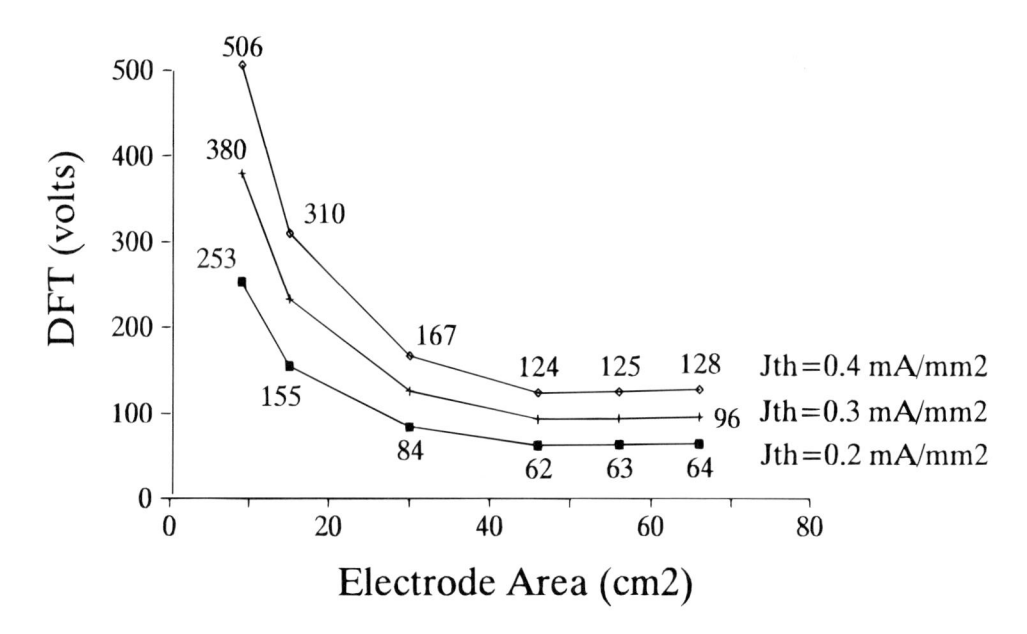

Figure 7. Voltage defibrillation threshold as a function of electrode area as computed at various threshold current densities. In each case, the critical mass is 95%.

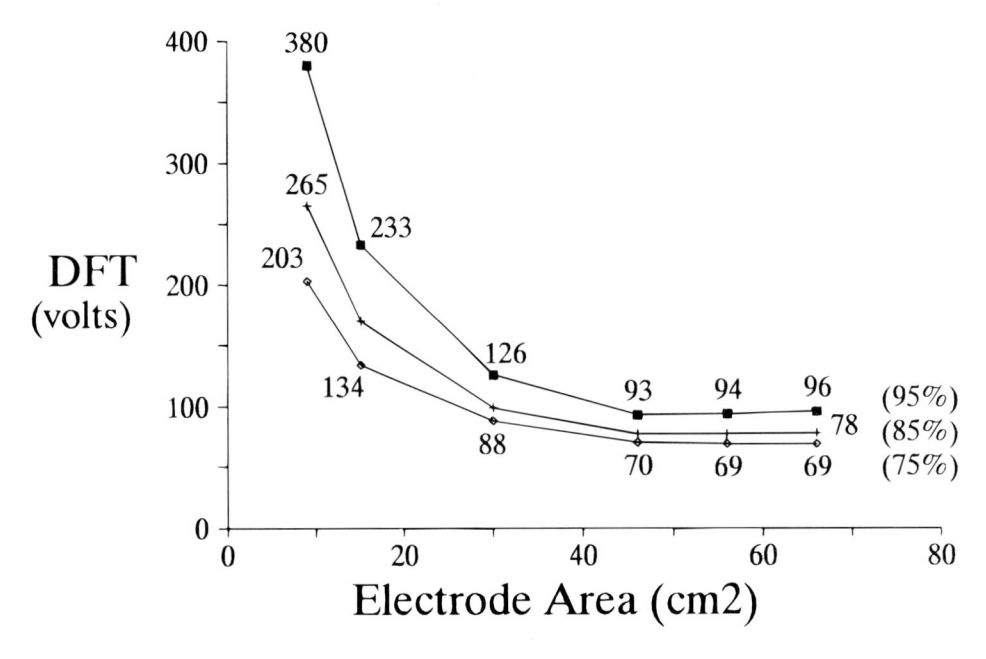

Figure 8. Voltage defibrillation threshold as a function of electrode area computed at a critical mass of 95%, 85%, and 75%. In each case, the threshold current density is 0.3 mA/mm².

defibrillation. Another reason for limiting the patch area is that large insulative patches increase the transthoracic DFTs because they impede current flow across the myocardium.[11] Large patches can also impair ventricular filling chronically. This can be potentially minimized by positioning the patches on the pericardium. The inverse relationship between electrode area and DFTs has also been observed in clinical and animal studies.[6] Most clinicians appreciate that if the DFTs are high in a patient, using a larger area patch will frequently lower the threshold.

Effect of Electrode Location

The effect of electrode location placement of a patch electrode on clinical defibrillation efficacy have not been investigated systematically. The placement is primarily based on surgical ease and attempt is made to position the patches opposite each other. However, if adequate defibrillation efficacy cannot be established, moving the patches can frequently help. In our computer model, we analyzed the effect of patch position on DFTs. Two small oval-shaped patches (each 9 cm²; 12% of epicardial coverage) were used for the simulation. Keeping the posterior patch stationary and moving the anterior patch from an apical to a midventricular and a basal position altered the thresholds from 412 to 350 and 307 V respectively when a threshold current density of 0.3 mA/cm² and a critical mass of 95% was used for the computation. This reduction in DFT of about 25% from apical to the basal position occurred in spite of an increase in impedance from 89 to 98 Ω. This difference in DFTs might have been less if larger size patches were used. There are other variables that can also effect DFT such as positioning the patches on compromised versus healthy myocardium. These variables have not been investigated in experimental preparations.

Effect of Patch Design

One of the problems that has been encountered in the design of patch electrodes is related to the use of a screen mesh as the defibrillation electrode. Since the epicardial patch electrode must be flexible to conform to the ventricles, rigid plates cannot be used and the flexible screen mesh was a reasonable alternative. However, long-term testing and chronic clinical studies indicate that the wires of the mesh can sometimes fray due to repeated flexing. One of the alternative designs is the use of multiple concentric coils that can withstand flexing to a much greater degree. We analyzed the difference in epicardial impedance and DFT between an oval plate and a three coil oval patch electrode: both of the same shadow area (area enclosed within outermost circumference) of 30 cm^2. The impedance of the plate and multiple coil electrodes were 45.8 and 48.4 Ω and the DFT 126 and 136 V, respectively. This difference is relatively small to be of clinical significance. It is important to note that the exposed metallic electrode area of the coil patch electrode is significantly less than of a plate electrode and yet the impedances were within 6% of each other. This is because the shadow area of both the electrodes was equal. The shadow area rather than the exposed electrode area is the critical variable. These results indicate that the multiple coil design is a reasonable alternative to a continuous patch electrode and it provides a significant advantage in flex life.

Another variable that lends itself to computer simulations is the effect of shape. Commercial epicardial electrodes vary from being oval to rectangular and circular. Computer modeling could also help us determine the optimal shape of these electrodes.

Three-Electrode Defibrillation

The initial rationale for using three electrodes for defibrillation was to reduce the threshold. As mentioned previously, this can be done by using sequential or simultaneous pulse defibrillation. There is conflicting data in the literature regarding the difference between these methods and single pulse defibrillation.[12,13] In order to understand the fundamental aspects of these configurations, they were also simulated using the finite element method.

For Sequential pulse defibrillation, three oval epicardial patches (each 9 cm^2) were placed equilaterally (at 120° angle) around the ventricles midway between the apex and the base of the heart. The DFT for the Sequential pulse was computed by taking the maximum of the current densities produced at each node by either of the two pulses and developing a current density versus percent myocardial volume curve equivalent to the one shown in Figure 3. With three electrodes, either one of them can be the common electrode. With the lateral, anterior or the posterior patch as the common electrode, the DFTs varied only between 225 and 231 V; an insignificant difference (threshold current density: 0.3 mA/cm^2; critical volume: 95%). However when the three electrodes were pulsed in a Simultaneous mode with equilateral patch placement and the lateral electrode as the common, the DFT increased to 312 V. Analysis of the field distributions in the individual cardiac sections indicated that this was a result of the low-current density between the two electrodes at the same potential (Figure 9). This was because the anterior and posterior electrodes were at the same potential and due to the low voltage difference in the myocardium between the electrodes, there was insignificant current flow there, resulting in a high DFT. The volume of tissue between the anterior and posterior electrodes with low-current density could be minimized by moving them closer to each other. When these electrodes were placed at 95°, the Simultaneous pulse threshold reduced to 266 V and at an angular separation of 70°, it was further reduced to 239 V. At each of these separations, the sequential pulse thresholds remained relatively stable at 221 and 226 V, respectively. Figure 9 illustrates the simultaneous and Sequential pulse current density distributions from one of the cardiac sections with angular placement of electrodes at 120° and 70°. The figure shows that as the angle between the anodes de-

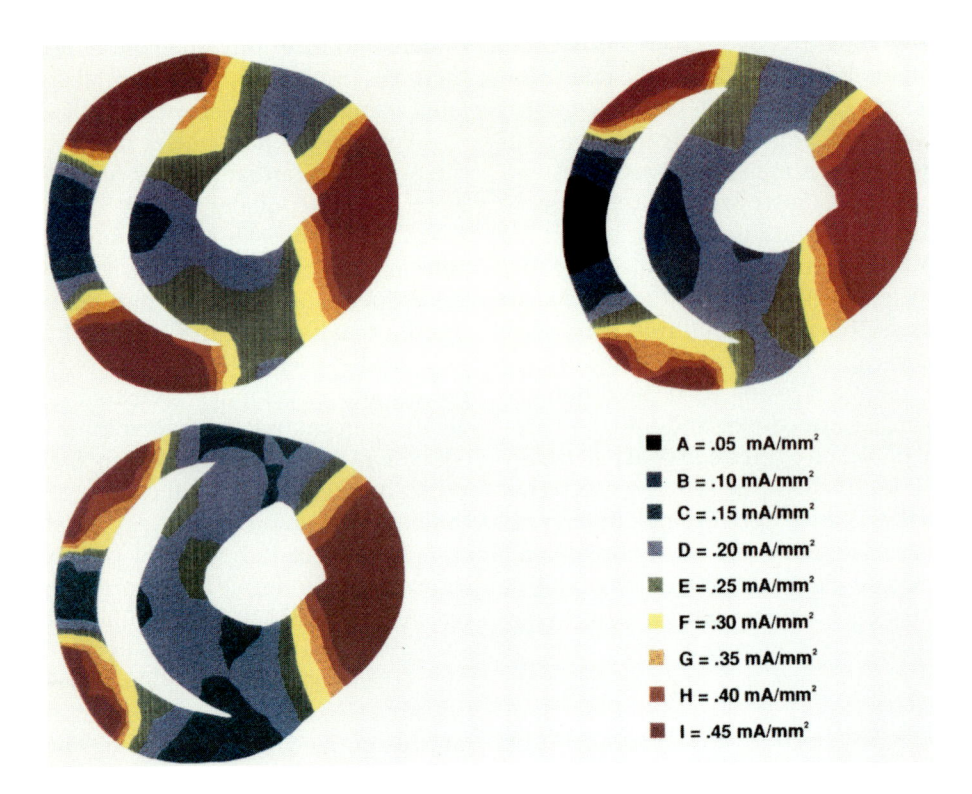

Figure 9. Isocurrent density plots across one cardiac section when a 100-V shock is delivered through epicardial patches. **Top left:** Current density plots with sequential shocks when the three epicardial electrodes were 120° apart. The patch on the left ventricular free wall was the common electrode. **Top right:** Plots during Simultaneous pulse defibrillation with the same electrodes. Note the large low-density black region between the two isopotential electrodes on the right ventricle. **Bottom:** For Simultaneous pulse defibrillation, the two right ventricular electrodes are now closer and 70° apart. This shrinks the low-current density region substantially, thus reducing the computed defibrillation threshold (DFT).

creased the volume of myocardium exposed to the low-current density decreased for Simultaneous pulse defibrillation, resulting in an improvement of DFT. There are two primary conclusions that can be drawn from this analysis. First, to optimize simultaneous pulse DFTs, the electrodes should not be placed equilaterally around the ventricles. The two anodes should be close to each other. Second, the Simultaneous and Sequential pulse DFTs are almost equal provided the patch placement is optimized for each method (Figure 10). One advantage of epicardial Sequential pulse method is that its threshold is less sensitive to electrode placement. The disadvantage of Sequential pulse defibrillation is that is requires additional hardware switches and tends to increase the size of the device slightly.

Animal studies have also validated these concepts.[14] In one study, with equidistant placement of three 10-cm² epicardial electrodes, the Sequential pulse DFTs were 255 ± 52 V. When the same three electrodes were connected for Simultaneous pulses, the threshold increased to 555 ± 149 V. However moving the two anodes together so that they were separated by 3.5 cm reduced the Simultaneous threshold to 269 ± 46 V, a result which is compatible with the general conclusions of the finite element modeling.

Comparison of DFTs between two- and

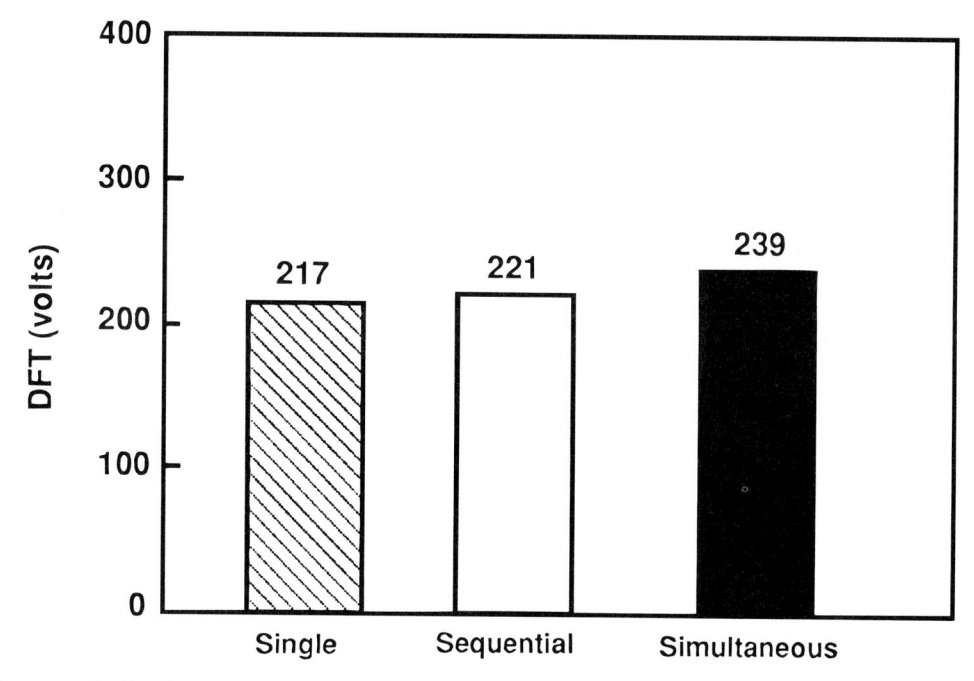

Figure 10. Defibrillation thresholds computed with sequential, simultaneous, and single pulse shocks when the total patch area in each case is 27 cm² and the electrode location is optimized for each method.

three-electrode systems was also investigated with this model. In our previous analysis with three 9-cm² electrodes, the Sequential pulse thresholds were about 221 V. This is much lower than the 307-V threshold measured with two 9-cm² patches. It should be noted that the total electrode area of the three electrodes is about 27 cm² as compared to 18 cm² with the two electrodes. If the area of the two epicardial electrodes is made approximately equal to 27 cm², then the DFT with the two-electrode system is computed to be 217 V; a value not significantly higher than the three-electrode threshold of 225 V (Figure 10).

Transvenous Lead Systems

Analysis of the transvenous defibrillation electrode systems requires a finite element model of the complete human thorax. This is because some of the electrodes used in the transvenous system are located outside the heart; such as the electrodes in the superior vena cava or the subcutaneous electrodes. Since our human thorax model is in the process of being completed, we cannot as yet present theoretical results regarding computer simulation of transvenous electrodes. Therefore, all the data presented here will be the animal and clinical results with transvenous electrodes.

It is generally observed that the DFTs with epicardial systems tend to be lower than with transvenous electrodes. For example in 51 implants with epicardial electrodes with the Medtronic PCD System[005] (Medtronic, Inc., Minneapolis, MN) using a monophasic pulse, the mean DFT was 10.6 ± 5.1 J.[15] This threshold is significantly lower than that observed with the transvenous electrode system.[10,16,17] As with epicardial systems, two or three electrodes can be used for transvenous defibrillation.

Two-Electrode Systems

The goal of the transvenous system is to provide adequate current density in most of the myocardium. The location of the transvenous leads is limited by the anatomical constraints and due to the fact that electrodes on the arterial side are not used because of the concerns of arterial thrombi. If one were not restricted by the latter constraint, canine studies comparing various lead configurations indicate that the lowest thresholds are obtained with a transvenous electrode in the left ventricle and four subcutaneous electrodes are located around the thorax. The threshold with biphasic shocks was 158 ± 32 V as compared to 235 ± 51 V when the left ventricular catheter was replaced with one in the right ventricle (RV).[18] The threshold with the left ventricular lead was only slightly greater than the 100–120 V threshold obtained with large epicardial patches in canine studies.[19]

In the clinical studies, electrodes for transvenous defibrillation have been located in the RV, superior vena cava (SVC)/right atrium (RA), coronary sinus (CS), and subcutaneous or cutaneous electrodes on the thoracic cavity. With RV-cutaneous/subcutaneous, RV-SVC, and RV-CS electrode configurations, the DFTs have been measured using biphasic shocks and are shown in Table 1. All these measurements were made using a one capacitor biphasic waveform in which the tilt of the positive and negative phases was set at 65% and the output capacitance was 120 microfarads.

(Tilt is defined as the difference between the leading and the trailing voltage divided by the leading voltage of the pulse.) These results indicate that the lowest voltage or energy thresholds are obtained with RV to subcutaneous or cutaneous electrodes. The lowest thresholds of 9.3 ± 4.6 J were obtained in a 25 patient study by Bardy et al.,[20,21] when biphasic shocks were delivered between the RV electrode and a Can electrode in the pectoral location (Figure 11). This data has also been reproduced by other investigators.[22,23] Another important observation is that the location on the thoracic cavity of the cutaneous or the subcutaneous electrode has a significant influence on the optimization of the field configuration and therefore the DFT. In general there are two factors one must analyze to appreciate the differences between the various methods. First, since defibrillation is dependent on obtaining adequate current density, the current threshold is a good indicator of the efficiency of the fields created by the electrode system, ie, how evenly are the fields distributed across the ventricular muscle. Second, the voltage or energy thresholds are also dependent on the impedance of the electrode system, ie, the higher the impedance the greater will be the voltage and energy threshold. For example, the biphasic current threshold with subcutaneous/cutaneous electrodes in the pec-

Table 1

Reference	Config	N	EF (%)	DFT (volts)	DFT (joules)	DFT (Amps)	Resistance (ohms)	Patch Position
Bardy[10]	CP-RV	15	45 ± 20	608 ± 148	23.4 ± 11.1	8.9 ± 4.0	74 ± 17	Anterolateral
	RV-CS	16	41 ± 20	495 ± 124	15.6 ± 7.2	8.5 ± 2.8	60 ± 8	
	Epi	20	39 ± 18	262 ± 107	4.8 ± 4.1	6.9 ± 3.8	41 ± 10	
Wyse[17]	CP-RV	12	34 ± 17	407 ± 101	12.3 ± 5.3	5.5 ± 1.5		High midaxillary line
Bardy[9]	RV-CS	12	41 ± 21	504 ± 155	18.6 ± 11.6	9.1 ± 3.6	57 ± 6	
Bardy[20]	RV-Can	40	39 ± 16	376 ± 119	9.3 ± 6.0		58 ± 7	
Zardini[22]	Can-RV	9	42 ± 15	348 ± 63	9.6 ± 4.2	6.8 ± 1.9	53 ± 9	
	SVC-RV	9	42 ± 15	399 ± 60	12.7 ± 3.7		52 ± 8	
Adler[23]	Can-RV	9	36 ± 16	368 ± 62	8.0 ± 2.7	7.1 ± 1.6	52 ± 6	
Desai[24]	CP-RV	14	38 ± 14		15.1 ± 5.6	7.1 ± 1.6	71 ± 8	Left axilla
		14	38 ± 14		12.8 ± 5.7	5.6 ± 1.4	81 ± 12	Left pectoral
		14	38 ± 14		9.8 ± 4.2	6.2 ± 1.4	65 ± 9	Interscapular

CP: chest patch; Can: infraclavicular Can in subcutaneous tissue; Epi: epicardial patches.

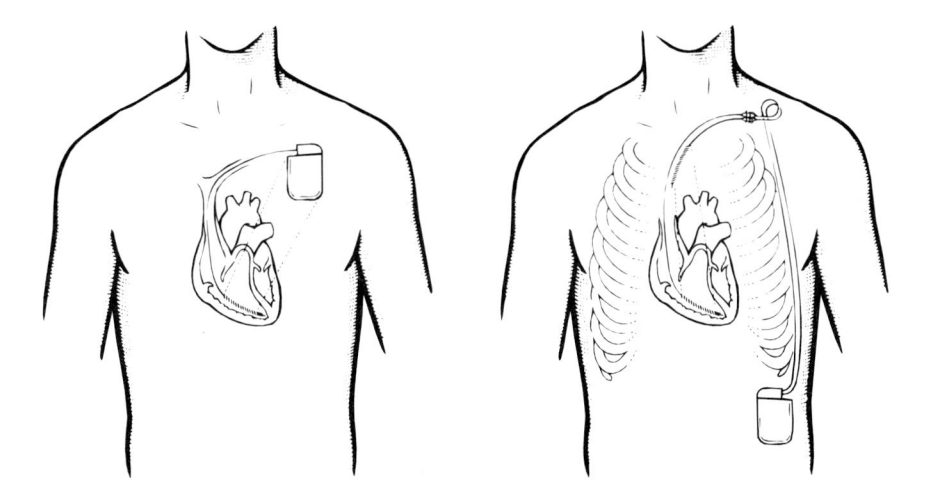

Figure 11. The figure on the left shows a transvenous two-electrode system utilizing an electrode in the right ventricular (RV) and a subpectoral Can electrode. The figure on the right illustrates the RV-SVC defibrillation electrode system with the device implanted in the abdomen.

toral location[20] are significantly lower than with those located at the anterior axillary line[10] indicating that the former has a more optimal field distribution. The study by Wyse et al.[17] indicates that the current thresholds are also low with a high placement of the patch in the midaxillary line. Studies with a posterior (subscapular) placement of the patch are presently in progress. Preliminary results indicate that the current thresholds are the same as with a subpectoral patch placement.[24] The subpectoral placement of the electrode is attractive not only from its ability to yield low thresholds, but also because it facilitates implantation of a unipolar system with one surgical incision and the use of the subpectoral can as the active defibrillation electrode. The use of the active Can electrode as opposed to a subcutaneous patch has also resulted in lower energy thresholds because the impedance of the system tends to be lower. The mean impedance of RV-CAN was 53 Ω[20,22] versus between 65 and 73 Ω with RV-subcutaneous patch.[10,16,17] Recent studies indicate that if a subcutaneous electrode is made of three coils that are about 12 cm long and connected at a yoke thus creating a large shadow area, low DFTs are also obtained.[25] This is partially due to the low impedance of such electrodes. The primary concern with this electrode system is the surgical complexity for its placement.

It is interesting to note that RV-Can biphasic thresholds are lower than when two intraventricular electrodes in the RV and the CS are utilized.[9,10] The impedance between the RV-CS and RV-Can systems are not significantly different and therefore the difference in their DFTs is due to the field configurations of these two systems. Based on this and without computer modeling results, one can only speculate that the RV-CS thresholds are higher because the CS electrode is typically located in the proximal CS, causing shunting of current across the posterior regions of the RV and CS electrodes. Also, the CS electrode typically resides posteriorly and the anterior as well as the apical aspect of the left ventricle may not have adequate current density. With the RV to pectoral Can configuration, the anterior aspect of the left ventricle probably has a higher current density distribution. The mean DFTs with RV-Can are also lower than those observed with electrodes in the RV and the SVC.[22] This study showed that the biphasic shock thresholds were 9.6 ± 4.2 J with the RV-subpectoral Can configuration and lower than 12.7 ± 3.7 J with the RV-SVC system ($P < 0.05$). Since the impedance with the two configurations were equal, this difference can only be attributed to an improved field distribution with the Can electrode. Experimental animal studies have been conducted to investigate the field distributions with RV-SVC configuration.[26] The results indicate that the regions of low gradient or current density tend to be in the left ventricular free wall and the apex of the heart and the current density is highest at the lateral and posterior RV. The current density decreased rapidly with distance away from the catheter electrode. This configuration also has the limitation that it requires the use of a large diameter lead with RV and SVC electrodes or two separate leads; one in the RV and the other in the SVC. It is likely that due to all these factors, the use of the Can electrode would become much more prevalent when the technology allows development of smaller devices that can be readily implanted in the pectoral region.

The biphasic current thresholds with two epicardial patches of 6.9 amps[10] is not significantly different from 6.6 amps obtained in the RV-subpectoral Can configuration. This indicates that the lower epicardial thresholds of 4.8 J are primarily based on lower impedance associated with epicardial patches.

Three-Electrode Systems

The primary motivation for using three-electrode systems has been to lower DFTs. In the earlier implantable cardioverter-defibrillators (ICDs) that did not have biphasic defibrillation and the maximum output of the devices was between 30 and 35 J, two-electrode systems were not able to meet the implantation criteria with an adequate safety margin in some patients. The use of three electrodes with Sequential and/or Simultaneous pulse defibrillation generally lowered the thresholds and the devices could be implanted in a greater percentage of the patients. There are, however, few scientific studies that have systematically compared clinical thresholds with various configurations prospectively. Some of these studies are listed in Table 2. We will discuss these results in two sections: systems using RV-SVC with thoracic electrodes and those with the CS electrode (Figure 12).

RV, SVC, and Thoracic Electrode Systems

This configuration with the RV electrode as the common cathode and the SVC and the thoracic electrode as the two anodes has been most frequently used in ICD implants.[27,28] This simultaneous pulse configuration has two arms; the RV-SVC and the RV-patch pathway. The former thresholds tend to be much higher. There are no paired studies with the RV-patch configuration. These results can be explained based on the voltage gradient measurements

Table 2

Reference	Config	M/B	N	EF (%)	DFT (volts)	DFT (joules)	Patch Position
Saksena[32]	(SVC + CP)-RV	B	12		473 ± 97	14.3 ± 5.3	Infraclavicular
		B	12		405 ± 80	10.2 ± 3.8	Infraaxillary
		B	12		479 ± 84	14.4 ± 4.8	Apical
Bardy[34]	(SVC + Can)-RV	B	9		325 ± 100	6.9 ± 4.1	
	Can-RV	B	9		319 ± 102	6.7 ± 4.4	
Bardy[35]	CV + CS-Can	B	10		408 ± 115	10.8 ± 5.4	
	RV-Can	B	10		451 ± 104	12.9 ± 5.7	
Bardy[9]	RV-CS	B	12	41 ± 21	504 ± 155	18.6 ± 11.6	
	RV-CS, CP-CS	M	12	41 ± 21	469 ± 180	14.8 ± 12.9	Ant. axillary line
	(RV + CP)-CS	M	12	41 ± 21	515 ± 178	18.0 ± 10.8	Ant. axillary line
Yee[37]	SVC-RV, CS-RV	M	7	32 ± 14		15.6 ± 2.9	

CP: chest patch; Can: Infraclavicular Can in subcutaneous tissue.

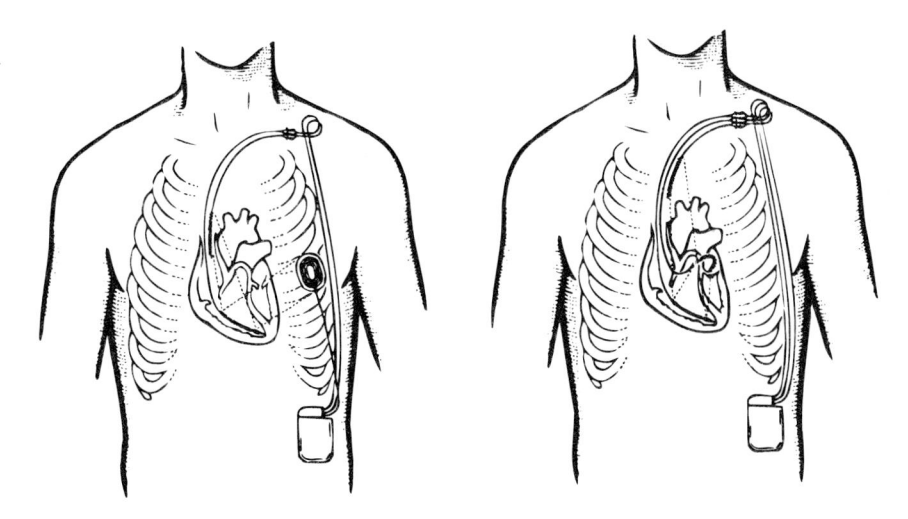

Figure 12. Three-electrode defibrillation systems utilizing RV-SVC and subcutaneous patch electrodes (left) and with RV, SVC, and coronary sinus electrodes (right).

made in dogs with RV-SVC, RV-chest patch, RV-SVC + chest patch configurations.[26] Simultaneous (SVC + patch) combination had the highest gradient present in more than 90% of the myocardium and would therefore have the lowest thresholds. Also, this configuration is not affected by the low gradient between the two anodes as observed in epicardial defibrillation (Figure 9) because this low-gradient region is in extracardiac structures. Another advantage of this method is that the peak current around the RV is increased because the total system impedance is reduced (see Appendix B). All these reasons explain the higher effectiveness of this configuration. In that study Simultaneous and Sequential pulse defibrillation methods were not directly compared. In order to compute the gradients with sequential shocks, the higher of the gradients produced by each shock would be assigned at each location and the volume/gradient graphs determined. This assumes that there is no electrophysiologic interaction between the two shocks that are temporally separated. There are various clinical studies that have attempted to compare the clinical effectiveness of Sequential and Simultaneous shocks.[29–31] The results have been conflicting. When we analyzed the Medtronic PCD™ (Medtronic, Minneapolis, MN) database we found that there was no significant difference in their efficacy to defibrillate at 18 J with monophasic shocks. However, there were many patients in whom one configuration satisfied the implant criteria and the other failed. Statistical analysis showed this incremental benefit was greater than what would be expected based on greater number of attempted configurations.[30] Therefore, having the option of Sequential and Simultaneous pulse defibrillation allowed ICD implantation in a larger patient group.

The defibrillation efficacy of this configuration is also influenced by the position of the subcutaneous patch.[32] Clinical data indicate the lowest Simultaneous monophasic pulse DFTs (current or stored energy) are observed when the patch is located laterally in the midaxillary line than at the infraclavicular location or on the apex beat of the heart. It is also possible that the optimal patch position for Simultaneous pulse defibrillation may be different than for Sequential shocks.

Defibrillation implants have also been attempted with the RV + SVC to patch combination with marginal success.[33] This is consistent with the gradient maps that indicate the voltage gradient in > 90% of the myocardium to be the same as with RV-SVC configuration.[26] There is one other permutation with this three-electrode system, ie, the use of the SVC as the common electrode. For Simultaneous pulse defibrillation, this is a very poor theoretical combination because one of the pathways is extracardiac (SVC to chest patch) and the region of low-current density between the two anodes would be in the left ventricle.

Addition of a third electrode to the RV-subpectoral Can system has also been attempted to lower the thresholds even further. Unfortunately, recent reports indicate that if an SVC electrode is added, the simultaneous pulse thresholds with biphasic shocks are not lower than observed with RV-Can system even though the system impedance is reduced significantly.[34] This indicates that the field is compromised and significant shunting probably occurs across the RV-SVC pathway. Similar results were obtained when an attempt was made to increase defibrillation efficacy by improving the field across the posterior left ventricle with a CS electrode.[35] The DFTs with RV-subpectoral Can and RV+CS-subpectoral Can configurations were 12.9 ± 5.7 and 10.8 ± 5.4 J, respectively, and not significantly different.

Three-Electrode Systems Using the Coronary Sinus Electrode

The initial impetus to use the CS electrode arose primarily because it was felt that it would increase the current density in the left ventricle and provide the opportunity to develop a totally transvenous three-electrode system. This concept provided certain challenges such as fixation of the CS lead, the concern about CS obstruction, and the its response to a defibrillation shock. There were reports in the literature that showed that with high-energy DC ablation shocks delivered through small surface area electrodes, the wall of CS could be torn. However, with our animal studies using long coil electrodes we found that not only was the damage insignificant, there was no obstruction to the CS with long-term implants lasting 3 months. Long-term evaluation revealed that a thin fibrous capsule was formed over the lead and the lead typically sat at the floor of the sinus. The distal end of the deep cardiac vein was typically thrombosed but there was adequate collateralization. Similar observations have been made clinically in hearts that have undergone autopsy.[36]

Evaluation of DFT in the clinical setting has occurred with two types of lead systems using three electrodes. They are the RV,SVC,CS and the RV,SVC thoracic patch combination. The former is the completely transvenous three-electrode system, and in a series of seven ICD patients Yee et al.[37] reported that the monophasic pulse thresholds were 15.6 ± 2.9 J when Sequential pulse defibrillation was conducted with the RV as the common cathode. There are no clinical results with Simultaneous shocks. In a prospective study on 12 patients, Bardy et al.[9] observed that the sequential or the simultaneous energy thresholds with RV/CS and patch electrode (CS as common) were not statistically lower than with the two-electrode RV/CS system.

These data do not show that across a patient population, a three-electrode CS system lowers thresholds below those obtained with other systems. However, further analysis has shown that it does provide versatility and patients who cannot meet implant criteria without a CS lead frequently do so when it is used.[30,38] Well-controlled prospective studies need to be done to quantitate this difference.

Conclusions

It is clear that due to their low morbidity and mortality, implantable defibrillators are primarily going to be used with transvenous leads. The initial phase of transvenous defibrillation has gone through various permutations of lead systems and pulsing configurations. Recent studies indicate that a unipolar defibrillation system using a single

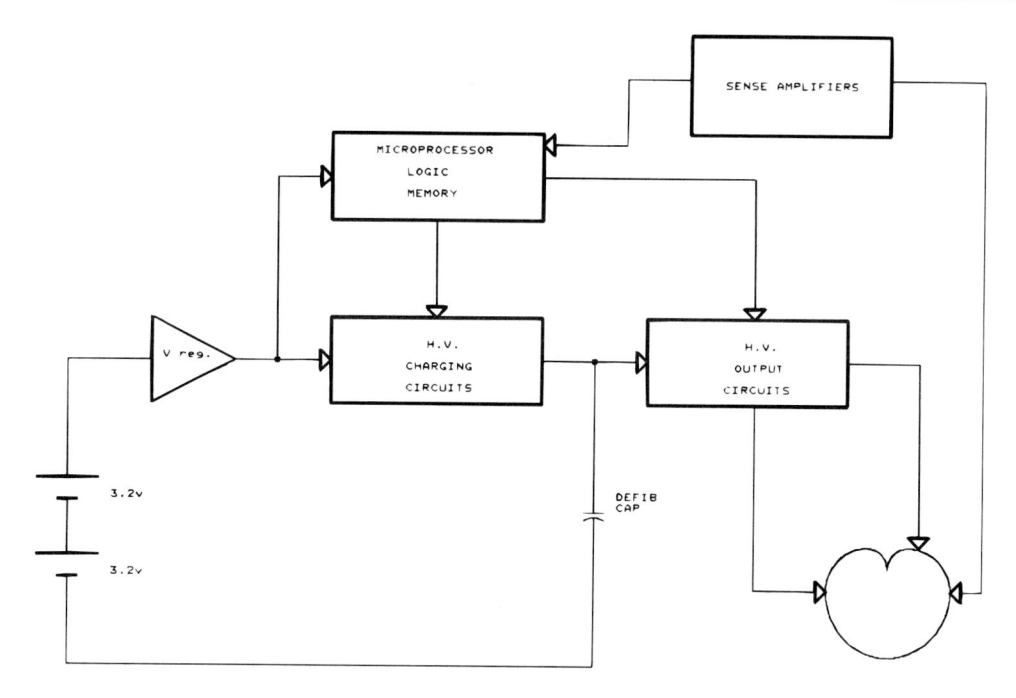

Figure 13. Defibrillator system block diagram.

defibrillation lead in conjunction with the Can as the other high-voltage electrode and a biphasic shock will become the method of choice because of the simplicity in implanting such a system and because the DFTs are as low as those observed with any technique. Computer models are being developed to explain these low thresholds.[39] These models will help in developing new electrode designs and shock waveforms to lower thresholds even further and consequently reduce the size of these devices. Our past experience with the use of finite element models to explain epicardial defibrillation systems has been very encouraging. The correlation between the clinical and modeling results has helped us understand the effect of electrode variables and pulsing methods on defibrillation efficacy. It is important that we continue in this direction and develop a strong scientific discipline in this field.

Hardware Design

The ICD has six basic components: a battery; sense amplifier; control circuits comprised of the microprocessor, logic and memory; high-voltage charging circuits that consists of a DC-DC converter and control circuitry; a defibrillation energy storage capacitor; and a high-voltage output switching circuit. The battery, defibrillation energy storage capacitor, and the electronic circuitry consume roughly one third of the volume of the device. The low voltage stored by the battery is converted to a high voltage by the DC-DC converter that is stored on the high-voltage defibrillation capacitor and then discharged across the heart through the high-voltage output circuitry. A voltage regulator (V reg) is used typically to supply stable power for the control circuits. Other designs may include microprocessor, logic, memory, and bradycardia sense and pacing circuits to implement more complex systems than the basic defibrillator. The block diagram of a defibrillator is shown in Figure 13.

The defibrillator must be capable of monitoring the electrical status of the heart through the sense amplifier, analyzing the waveforms for abnormal conditions and delivering therapy when appropriate to restore normal cardiac electrical function. The device must have a high degree of reliability and a clinically significant lifetime before battery depletion. This section focuses on the delivery of the therapy from the time of detection of a ventricular tachycardia or ventricular fibrillation.

Table 3
Battery Parameters

Lithium Silver Vanadium Oxide Battery

Voltage @ Beginning of Life	3.2 V/Cell
Energy Density	1800 J/CC
Maximum Current Rating	3.0 Amps typical
Series Resistance	<1 Ohm typical

Power Requirements

Power requirements of implantable electronic defibrillators present many engineering challenges. In most devices DC voltages of about 750 V across a capacitor are required to perform the defibrillation function of the device. This high voltage is generated from either a single battery of 3.2 V or two cells connected in series giving 6.4 V. The requirements of the device demand that the battery be capable of supplying high peak currents to ensure rapid charging of the defibrillation capacitors. The same battery must also supply a stable noise-free power for the low-voltage sense amplifiers, microprocessor, logic, and memory circuits inside the device. The higher the voltage of the battery, the easier the problem of charging to high voltage becomes. At the same time, the other circuitry in the device for power consumption require a lower voltage. For defibrillator systems where two cells are connected in series, the 6.4 V is typically regulated down for the sense amplifier, microprocessor, logic, and memory. Using only one of the two cells for this would result in unequal depletion of the two cells, reducing overall device life.

All currently available defibrillators at present use a lithium silver vanadium oxide (Li/SVO) battery. This chemistry is the only one available that meets the requirements for implantable defibrillators due to the high-peak currents required. Other chemistries used for pacemakers cannot supply the high-peak currents required for defibrillators, which may be up to 3 amps. The anode of the battery is lithium with a silver vanadium oxide cathode and a liquid organic electrolyte. An ideal defibrillator battery would have high stored energy per cubic centimeter of battery volume resulting in a small size, zero internal DC resistance, and completely predictable and reproducible end-of-life characteristics. Battery parameters of design and device importance are listed in Table 3 for typical batteries used in current devices.

A typical 10-cc defibrillator battery can store 18,000 J of electrical energy. This is roughly 500 34-J shocks. This shock capacity is reduced by the additional overhead currents associated with powering the device circuitry and energy conversion losses. A significant energy consumption is associated with a bradycardia pacing function. For 100% pacing a significant reduction in device lifetime can be expected. The lifetime of a device varies with the number of shocks and the relative percentages of times spent monitoring and pacing along with the beginning battery capacity. Manufacturers typically express lifetime in terms of combinations of these parameters. Device size is strongly influenced by the size of the battery required. A design trade off must be made between device size and battery capacity/device life. Overhead currents can be minimized with the careful design of circuits and other nondefibrillation functions.

Important parameters of the battery are its voltage during the charging of the defibrillator capacitor, battery end-of-life voltage, and the battery voltage at which the device loses function. The Li/SVO battery has two voltage plateaus as shown in Figure 14. The upper curve is the voltage under low current drain, when the battery is powering only the control circuits and the sense

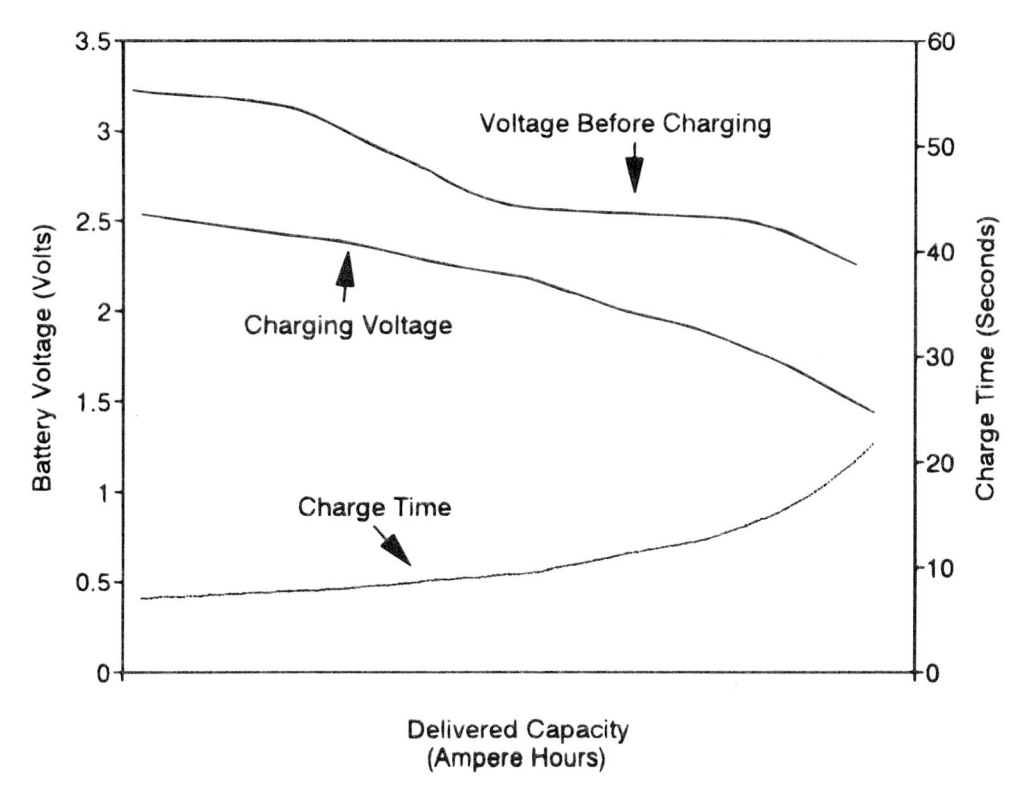

Figure 14. LI/SVO battery characteristics for a typical 3.2-V battery.

amplifiers. The current drawn from the battery is in the order of microamps. The lower voltage curve (charging voltage) represents the battery voltage during the high-voltage charging cycle. The voltage is lowered because the internal voltage drop in the battery increases with increased current demand. When high-voltage capacitor charging is active, amps of current are drawn from the battery. As the battery approaches end-of-life, it rapidly becomes more resistive and the difference between the two curves widens. This is undesirable because at worst the battery voltage during charging could drop below the point at which the device resets to the end of life parameters resulting in premature replacement. As the charging voltage decreases, the time required for charging also rapidly increases, as seen in Figure 14. These battery characteristics, along with the device design and usage practices must be considered when selecting the elective replacement voltage and the end-of-life voltage for a particular design.

Lithium silver vanadium oxide batteries may swell as they approach end-of-life. When the battery reaches approximately 2 V, an electrochemical reaction with one of the components of the electrolyte begins to occur. One of the products of this reaction is a gas, propylene. The gas pressure causes the battery to swell. The extent of the swelling depends on how much the battery is discharged beyond the point where gas production begins and the ease with which the case of the battery deforms.

Defibrillation Capacitor

The energy standard for today's defibrillators is about 34 J. To achieve this energy, the battery voltage of 3.2 or 6.4 V must be transformed to a DC voltage 100–300 times the battery voltage available. There are two electronic components capable of storing energy: inductors and capacitors. The inductor stores energy in the magnetic field created by passage of current through its windings. In the capacitor, energy is stored in the electric field created by an accumulation of charge in the capacitor. It is easier to store energy in a defibrillator on a capacitor.

The stored energy in a capacitor is given by the following formula:

$$E = \frac{1}{2} CV^2$$

where C is capacitance and V is voltage. Depending on the capacitance for a particular design, the required voltage to achieve 34 J varies as shown in Table 4.

The volume of capacitors is nearly linear with respect to stored energy. There is a fixed volume component associated with the capacitor packaging and electrical connections. An ideal 34-J 90-μF capacitor is nearly the same size as a 34-J 120-μF capacitor. The capacitors are only available in given maximum voltage ratings, eg, 360 V. Therefore, achieving 34 J with 90 μF of capacitance (1,065 V) will require three 270-μF capacitors rated at 360 V connected in series. Similarly, achieving 34 J with 150 μF of capacitance (673 V) only requires two 300-μF capacitors rated at 360 V connected in series. The second approach requires fewer capacitors and is more space efficient because interconnecting two capacitors requires less space than interconnecting three. However, the second approach has excess capacity. The capacitors are capable of 720 V, but are only being charged to 673 V. This excess capacity also uses up volume in the device. The selection of capacitance is a trade-off between maximizing defibrillation efficacy and packaging efficiency and minimizing excess storage capacity.

The high-voltage created by the DC-DC converter is stored on the defibrillation capacitor. Aluminum electrolytic capacitors are used in all current defibrillator designs. The defibrillator aluminum electrolytic capacitor is essentially the same as those used in photographic flash units. Typical capacitance values range from 60 to 240 μF for existing designs. These capacitors have a rating of 360-V working voltage. The peak current rating typically is 80 amps and the equivalent series resistance is typically 1.5 Ω. The energy storage density of the aluminum electrolytic capacitor is approximately 1.5 J/cc. An undesirable characteristic of this technology is that when voltage is removed, the dielectric slowly deteriorates. The dielectric of the capacitor needs to be reformed periodically by charging the capacitor. It is for this reason that the current generation of implantable defibrillation capacitors must be charged periodically to ensure proper operation of the device. Today aluminum electrolytic capacitors offer the highest energy storage density available for a high-voltage capacitor.

Many manufacturers are exploring alternative capacitor technologies seeking to increase energy density and achieve size reduction and eliminate the capacitor forming problem. Alternative technologies include ceramic, thin film, and double-layer technology. Their energy density ranges from 4 to 5 J/cc and do not require capacitor reforming. Problems such as weight, capacitance variation with applied voltage, reliability and manufacturability have precluded their implementation into a design. As the technical and economic issues are resolved one or more of the alternative technologies will migrate into implantable defibrillator designs. This could result in significant size reduction given the amount of

Table 4
Relationship of Capacitance and Voltage

Energy	Capacitance	Voltage
34 J	60 μF	1,065
34 J	90 μF	869
34 J	120 μF	753
24 J	150 μF	673

space consumed in current designs and eliminate capacitor reformation.

DC-DC Converters

A DC-DC converter is required to transform the battery voltage to the high-voltage energy needed for defibrillation. Unlike AC voltage where passive transformers are available to step up AC voltage, none are available for DC. The transformation of DC voltages requires the use of active components such as transistors along with inductors, transformers, and capacitors.

Ideally, the DC-DC converter would be 100% efficient, not create electromagnetic interference (EMI) or electrical noise, and be capable of charging the defibrillation capacitor instantly. Practical design of DC-DC converters require that these parameters must be traded off if the smallest device is to be achieved.

To step a voltage up or down, energy must be switched between the inductors and capacitors in a design. To do this, switches are implemented with diodes and transistors. Because the switches have a finite DC resistance, energy losses occur. An ideal inductor and capacitor would have zero resistance and energy would be stored with no losses. This is not realistic and energy loss occurs in both components when current flows. Practical conversion efficiencies of current converters are typically < 80% with size the main design trade-off.

The basic DC-DC converter used in defibrillators is a variation of the circuit shown in Figure 15. This implementation is referred to as a "flyback" converter.[40] The transformer T1 provides isolation and reduces the voltage seen by the transistor S1 depending on the turns ratio. In this design, transistor S1 and diode D1 are used as switches. When S1 is closed, current builds up in Lp, the inductance of the primary. The energy stored by the inductance of Lp is proportional to the inductance and the square of the current passing through. When S1 opens, the energy stored in the primary of the transformer is transferred to the secondary, charging the capacitor C2. Diode D1 prevents the capacitor C2 from discharging back through the secondary side of the transformer. This cycle is repeated by switching S1 on and off until the desired voltage on C2 is reached.

An actual DC-DC converter is more complicated than the basic "flyback" shown in Figure 15. Circuitry to sense the level of the output voltage and feedback control to the primary side of the converter is needed. Additional circuits are needed to sense and control charging currents and filter EMI.

Defibrillator Output Switching Circuits

The defibrillation energy stored on the capacitor must now be steered to the various electrodes on or in the heart. A generalized switching system is shown in Figure 16.

With various combinations of switches, S1–S4 monophasic and biphasic waveforms may be realized. Switch S5 is not used for the biphasic pulse. To create a biphasic

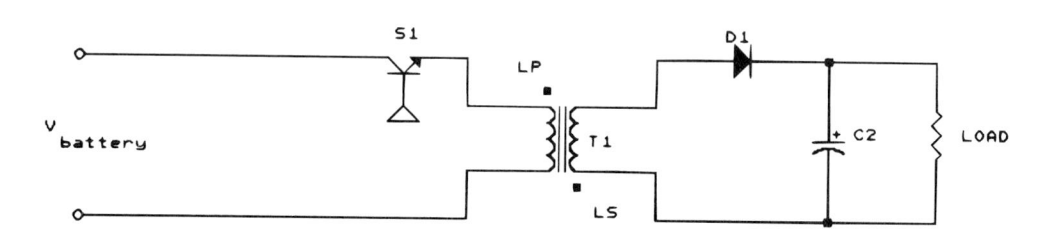

Figure 15. A basic flyback DC-DC converter schematic.

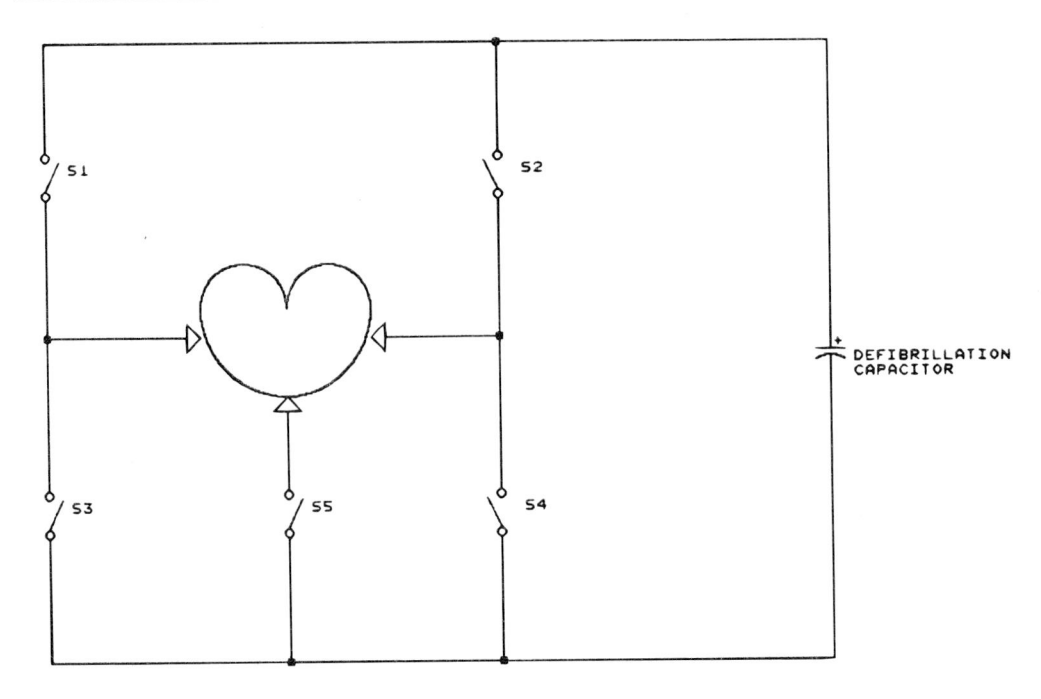

Figure 16. A general defibrillation capacitor switching matrix.

waveform, first S1 and S4 would be closed with S2 and S3 open. In this configuration current would flow from the positive capacitor terminal through S1, the heart, S4, and back to the negative terminal of the capacitor. At the end of phase one, S1 and S4 are opened and S2 and S3 are closed. In this configuration the direction of current flow is reversed through the heart. This sequence of switching can also be reversed to create the biphasic waveform of the opposite polarity. The monophasic waveform is created by only executing the first half of the previously described switching sequence. To implement sequential pulsing a third electrode and another switch S5 is added to this configuration. For the first pulse, S1 and S5 would be closed with S2, S3, and S4 open. S1 then would be opened and S2 closed for the second pulse. Simultaneous pulsing is achieved by closing S1, S2, and S5. The ability to alter the timing of switch closure allows control of the capacitor voltage at the termination of the pulse or pulse width. The voltage on the capacitor during discharge is described by the equation:

$$V = V_{initial} e^{-(T/RC)}$$

where V is the voltage on the capacitor and $V_{initial}$ is the voltage on the capacitor prior to the start of the discharge. T is the time the capacitor C has discharged through R. R is comprised of the switch and heart resistance. For $T/RC = 1$ the voltage remaining on the capacitor is 37% of its initial value. This would correspond to a 63% tilt waveform. Tilt control is implemented by monitoring the voltage on the capacitor and terminating the pulse when the desired voltage of discharge is achieved. In an actual circuit the switches are implemented with silicon controlled rectifiers (SCRs), TRIACs (bidirectional SCRs), power metal oxide semiconductor field effect transistors (MOSFETs), gate turn-off thyristors (GTOs), or insulated gate bipolar transistors (IGBTs). In a real output switching matrix design, additional circuitry would be needed to control tilt and provide transthoracic shock protection, which is extremely important when an exposed electrode may be close to the skin. Tolerance of voltages

> 1,200 V may be required. Other circuits are needed to implement voltage and current clamps, drive the gates of the power switches, and control the sequencing and timing of the switches. The H bridge configuration illustrated in Figure 16 is a more general implementation than is required in most designs.

Appendix A

Current density (J) is defined as current per unit area and voltage gradient (G) as voltage difference per unit length. The two parameters are proportional to each other.

$$G = JP$$

Where P is the resistivity of the tissue. G has units of V/cm; J has units of amps/cm^2, and P has units of Ω cm. For example, if a 1-cm radius spherical electrode is in blood pool and 10 amps of current flows through it, then the current density at the surface of the electrode is $10/4\pi = 0.8$ amps/cm^2. Since the resistivity of blood is 150 Ω cm, the voltage gradient at the surface of the sphere would be $0.8 \times 150 = 120$ V/cm.

Appendix B

A three-electrode defibrillation system can be simulated as a "Y" network (Figure 17). The resistance R1 represents the electrode tissue impedance and the bulk tissue impedance under electrode 1. R2 and R3 are for the other two electrodes. Electrode 3 is the common electrode for Sequential or Simultaneous pulse defibrillation. During Sequential pulse defibrillation, the current in pathway 1 during the first shock is V/(R1 + R3) and in pathway 2 during the second shock it is V/(R2 + R3). During Simultaneous pulse defibrillation, electrodes 1 and 3 are interconnected and the same voltage shock is delivered simultaneously across the two pathways. In this situation, the total impedance of the system is R3 + (R1*R2)/(R1 + R2) and the current in electrode 3 is V divided by this impedance. Note that this current is greater than with sequential pulse defibrillation. This current however is split between electrode 1 [V/{R1 + R3 + (R1*R3/R2)}] and electrode 2 [V/{R2 + R3 + (R2*R3/R1)}] and

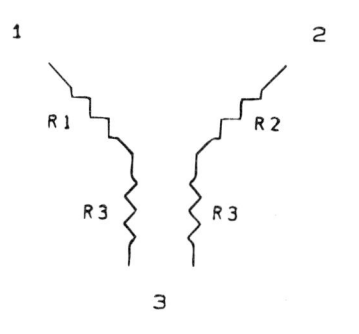

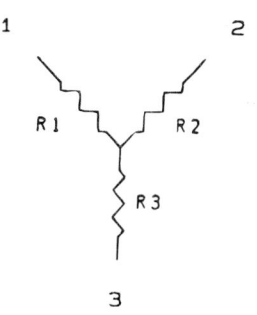

Figure 17. Circuit diagram for sequential and simultaneous pulse defibrillation.

is lower in each arm than with Sequential pulse defibrillation. Therefore, Simultaneous pulse defibrillation tends to increase the current through the common electrode and decrease it in the two other electrodes.

References

1. Wiggers CJ: The physiologic basis for cardiac resuscitation from ventricular fibrillation: method for serial defibrillation. *Am Heart J* 20:413, 1940.
2. Zipes DP, Fischer J, King RM, et al: Termination of ventricular fibrillation in dogs by depolarizing a critical amount of myocardium. *Am J Cardiol* 36:37, 1975.
3. Chen PS, Shibata N, Dixon EG, et al: Comparison of the defibrillation threshold and the upper limit of ventricular vulnerability. *Circulation* 73:1022, 1986.
4. Jones JL, Lepeschkin E, Jones RE, et al: Response of cultured myocardial cells to countershock-type electric field stimulation. *Am J Physiol* 235:H214, 1978.
5. Saksena S: Defibrillation thresholds and perioperative mortality associated with endocardial and epicardial defibrillation lead systems. *PACE* 16(1 Pt 2):202, 1993.
6. Troup PJ, Chapman PD, Olinger GN, et al: The implanted defibrillator: relation of defibrillation lead configuration and clinical variables to defibrillation threshold. *J Am Coll Cardiol* 6(6):1315, 1985.
7. Medtronic PMA Application for Model 7216A and 7217IB devices and Epicardial Patch Leads. September 1990.
8. Yabe S, Smith WM, Daubert JP, et al: Conduction disturbances caused by high current density electric fields. *Circ Res* 66:1190, 1990.
9. Bardy GH, Allen MD, Mehra R, et al: An effective and adaptable transvenous defibrillation system using the coronary sinus in humans. *J Am Coll Cardiol* 16:887, 1990.
10. Bardy GH, Troutman C, Johnson G, et al: Electrode system influence on biphasic waveforms defibrillation efficacy in humans. *Circulation* 84:665, 1991.
11. Walls JT, Schuder JC, Curtis JJ, et al: Adverse effect of permanent cardiac internal defibrillator patches on external defibrillation. *J Am Coll Cardiol* 64:1144, 1989.
12. Jones DL, Klein GJ, Guiraudon GM, et al: Sequential pulse defibrillation in humans: orthogonal sequential pulse defibrillation with epicardial electrodes. *J Am Coll Cardiol* 11(3):590, 1988.
13. Bardy GH, Ivey TD, Allen MD, et al: Prospective comparison of sequential pulse and single pulse defibrillation with use of two different clinically available systems. *J Am Coll Cardiol* 14:165, 1989.
14. Mehra R, Norenberg MS, DeGroot P: Comparison of defibrillation thresholds with pulsing techniques requiring three epicardial electrodes. *PACE* 11:527, 1988.
15. Fromer M, Brachmann J, Block M, et al: Efficacy of automatic multimodal device therapy for ventricular tachyarrhythmias as delivered by a new implantable pacing cardioverter-defibrillator: results of a European Multicenter Study of 102 implants. *Circulation* 86:363, 1992.
16. Bardy GH, Allen MD, Mehra R, et al: Transvenous defibrillation in humans via the coronary sinus. *Circulation* 81:1252, 1990.
17. Wyse DG, Kavanagh KM, Gillis AM, et al: Comparison of biphasic and monophasic shocks for defibrillation using a nonthoracotomy system. *Am J Cardiol* 71:197, 1993.
18. Guse PA, Kavanagh KM, Alferness CA, et al: Defibrillation with low voltage using a left ventricular catheter and four cutaneous patch electrodes in dogs. *PACE* 14:443, 1991.
19. Dixon EG, Tang AS, Wolf PD, et al: Improved defibrillation thresholds with large contoured epicardial electrodes and biphasic waveforms. *Circulation* 76:176, 1987.
20. Bardy GH, Johnson G, Poole JE, et al: A simplified, single lead unipolar transvenous cardioverter-defibrillator system. *Circulation* 88:543, 1993.
21. Bardy GH, Johnson G, Poole JE, et al: Simplicity and efficacy of a single incision pectoral implant unipolar defibrillation system. *J Am Coll Cardiol* 21:66A, 1993.
22. Zardini M, Yee R, Mehra R, et al: Improved defibrillation efficacy with a simple non-thoracotomy lead configuration. *J Am Coll Cardiol* 21:66A, 1993.
23. Adler SW, Remole SC, Lurie KG, et al: Prepectoral anode electrode position optimizes defibrillation efficacy for a "unipolar" transvenous implantable defibrillator. *PACE* 16:853, 1993.
24. Desai P, DeGroot P, Casavant D, et al: Is patch position critical for successful nonthoracotomy (NTL) ICD implant with biphasic shocks? *Circulation* 88:I-215, 1993.

25. Jordaens L, Vertongen P, Bellegham YV: A subcutaneous lead array for implantable cardioverter defibrillators. *PACE* 16:1429, 1993.
26. Tang A, Wolf P, Afework Y, et al: Three-dimensional potential gradient fields generated by intracardiac catheter and cutaneous patch electrodes. *Circulation* 85:1857, 1992.
27. Block M, Hammel D, Isbruch F, et al: Results and realistic expectations with transvenous lead systems. *PACE* 15:665, 1992.
28. Saksena S, The PCD Investigators and Participating Institutions: Defibrillation thresholds and perioperative mortality associated with endocardial and epicardial defibrillation lead systems. *PACE* 16:202, 1993.
29. Saksena S, An H, Mehra R, et al: Prospective comparison of biphasic and monophasic shocks for implantable cardioverter- defibrillators using endocardial leads. *Am J Cardiol* 70:304, 1992.
30. Mehra R, Norenberg MS, DeGroot PD, et al: Multicenter clinical results with an implantable defibrillator utilizing transvenous leads. *PACE* 15:566, 1993.
31. Mehra R, Norenberg M, DeGroot P, et al: Comparison of initial clinical results with transvenous and epicardial defibrillation systems. In: *Pacemaker Leads*. Edited by GE Antonioli, AE Aubert, M Ector. New York, NY: Elsevier Science Publishers; 1991, p. 375.
32. Saksena S, Krol RB, John T, et al: Optimal thoracic electrode or device location for cardioverter-defibrillators with endocardial defibrillation leads. *Circulation* 86:I-443, 1992.
33. Bhandari AK, and the USA Endotak Investigators Group: Intraoperative defibrillation efficacy of endocardial subcutaneous lead configurations. *Circulation* 86:790, 1992.
34. Bardy GH, Johnson G, Poole J, et al: Simplicity and efficacy of a single incision pectoral implant unipolar defibrillation system. *J Am Coll Cardiol* 21:66A, 1993.
35. Bardy GH, Kundenchuck PJ, Dolack GL, et al: A prospective randomized comparison in humans of the unipolar pectoral defibrillation system within one incorporating an additional electrode in the coronary sinus. *Circulation* 88:I217, 1993.
36. Bardy GH, Swerdlow C, Reichenbach D, et al: Anatomic findings in patients having had a coronary sinus defibrillation lead. *PACE* 16:903, 1993.
37. Yee R, Klein G, Leitch J, et al: A permanent transvenous lead system for an implantable maker cardioverter-defibrillator: nonthoracotomy approach to implantation. *Circulation* 85:196, 1992.
38. Bardy G, Hofer B, Johnson G, et al: Implantable transvenous cardioverter-defibrillators. *Circulation* 85:196, 1992.
39. Mehra R, DeGroot P, Norenberg S: Three dimensional finite element model of the heart for analysis of epicardial defibrillation: effect of patch surface area. *PACE* 12:652A, 1989.
40. Slobodan C, Middlebrook RD: Advances in switched-mode power conversion. Part I. In: *Advances in Switched Mode-Power Conversion*. Edited by RD Middlebrook, C Slobodan. Pasadena, CA: TESLAco; 1983, p. 520.

Chapter 6

Defibrillation Theory and its Clinical Impact

Werner Irnich

Introduction

The optimum defibrillation pulse is that which can defibrillate with the lowest energy. As pulses are physically characterized by amplitude, shape, pulse duration, and direction of current (monophasic, biphasic, ambiphasic), it seems that researchers are faced with a difficult if not hopeless search for the proverbial needle in the haystack. Therefore, we believe that a theory that can serve as a guide is of inestimable value, especially in defibrillation research where experiments are difficult, time consuming, and occasionally difficult to produce.

The principles on which the design of defibrillators are based and that are electrophysiologically justified may be outlined as follows: 1) an electric pulse of sufficient intensity is capable of interrupting fibrillation[1]; 2) the electric pulse must be truncated, otherwise the defibrillation success rate is reduced by refibrillation[2]; 3) monophasic pulses are less efficient than biphasic pulses[3]; 4) the energy is the physical parameter responsible for defibrillation dose; and 5) the optimum tilt of capacitor discharge for defibrillation is 60% to 75%.[4,5]

Although alternative principles or hypotheses may exist, it is somewhat surprising how little theoretical electrophysiologic knowledge has entered defibrillation technology to date. Moreover, some of the outlined hypotheses conflict with theory and practical findings on defibrillation. The constant energy dose concept is especially problematic because it contradicts the existence of the rheobase. *Constant energy concept* means that every defibrillation pulse, regardless of pulse shape or duration will have the same effect if its energy is the same. Incidentally, the hypothetical defibrillation probability curves, if assumed sigmoidal in shape, similarly contradict the rheobase concept, which postulates an intersection of the curve with the dose axis, below which the probability is zero.

Other questions remain that are not only of theoretical but clinical importance: 1) If the constant energy concept is questionable, what is a suitable alternative? 2) What are the consequences that follow from this concept with respect to programming? 3) Assuming that capacitor discharge for defibrillation should be truncated to avoid refibrillation, what degree of truncation is necessary? 4) Is "tilt" independent of pulse duration? 5) If the pulse duration and the energy are programmable, which combination is optimal? and 6) Are monophasic pulses, if optimally truncated, inferior to biphasic pulses? This chapter introduces one aspect of a defibrillation theory and attempts to provide answers to these questions.

From Singer I, (ed.) Implantable Cardioverter-Defibrillator. Armonk, NY: Futura Publishing Company, Inc.; © 1994.

Defibrillation Theory

Termination of cardiac fibrillation can be caused by a condenser discharge,[1] a method that was developed between 1938–1939. Gurvich and Yuniev[1] found that the amplitude of the voltage to which a capacitor had to be charged was a declining curve with increasing capacitance. The similarity of their findings to that of Hoorweg in 1892[6] with respect to stimulation is remarkable. Koning et al.[7] later demonstrated that defibrillation can be described by similar functions to those that are known for stimulation. Geddes and Tacker[8] found curves for defibrillation energy, peak current, and charge for capacitor discharge, which seem to deviate from the well-known strength duration curves in that energy, peak current, and charge are higher than anticipated if a time constant of more than 5 msec was reached or exceeded. Tacker and Geddes[9] adopted the suggestion of Schuder et al.[2] "that, if very long duration pulses are used for defibrillation with capacitor discharge, the long, exponentially decaying tail refibrillates the ventricles." Although their investigations were carried out with external defibrillators, there is no reason to assume that implantable defibrillators obey different rules.

How is Defibrillation Acting on the Cellular Level?

Fibrillation is explained either by ectopic foci or by circus movements.[10] Whether one or the other theory or both are valid, fibrillation requires that: 1) the dominance of the sinus node is lost; 2) ventricular excitation along predetermined paths and with uniform and fast velocity is abolished; and 3) the duration of refractoriness is converted from long to short duration, thus permitting early preexcitation.

An electric pulse of sufficient intensity, applied for defibrillation, can act in that it: 1) depolarizes excitable cells, outside refractory period (400–600 V/m is necessary); 2) prolongs refractory period of excited cells (600–900 V/m); and 3) damages cells with subsequent inhibition of up to 4 seconds (above 8,000 V/m?).

Common to all three effects is that something happens within the membrane. Either pores are opened to allow sodium influx or small holes are created causing loss of potassium or other elements causing inactivity of the cell.[11] In all these cases, a model of influencing the membrane can be assumed, with the aid of which we have explained electrostimulation physically.[12]

Opening of pores or producing holes always requires a mechanical force acting on the membrane, whether in moving obstacles at or within the pores, or in puncturing it. As there are ionized or polarized particles at or within the membrane, the force is due to attraction or repulsion of charged particles within an electric field. If the force is acting for a short period of time, the (physical) impulse is relevant for this effect and the exogenic force must, in any case, be stronger than that fixing the obstacle at or within the membrane. An example for the latter requirement can be illustrated by a magnetic latch of a cupboard. To open the door, the force applied must be greater than the magnetic force holding the door closed. Physical impulse is defined as the product of force × exposition duration. If the force is not steady with time, the product must be replaced by the time integral over the force.

Thus, this idea can be formulated mathematically:

$$\int^{\tau} (F_{exog} - F_{stat}) \, dt \geq I_{Pmin} \qquad (1)$$

with:
τ = exposition duration called pulse duration; F_{exog} = exogenic force acting on the obstacles; F_{stat} = static force fixing the obstacle at or within the membrane; and I_{Pmin} = minimum mechanical impulse required to move the obstacles.

As we assumed the obstacles to not be neutral electrically, we can substitute the exogenic force, by an exogenic electric field using the familiar relation:

$$F_{exog} = q * E_{exog} \qquad (2)$$

with q = charge of the obstacle; and E_{exog} = exogenic electrical field strength.

Inserting Equation 2 into Equation 1, we get Equation 3:

$$\int^{\tau} (F_{exog} - E_{stat})\, dt \geq I_{Pmin}/q \quad (3)$$

By rearranging and dividing both sides of Equation 3 by the pulse duration τ, we get Equation 4, the interpretation of which reads: The mean value of the exogenic electric field applied to a membrane during the pulse duration τ must be equal to or larger than a minimum field strength, termed "rheobase field strength," $\times$ a hyperbolic expression of the duration τ to reach opening of the pores or the holes:

$$\frac{1}{\tau}\int^{\tau} E_{exog}\, dt \geq \frac{I_{Pmin}}{q * \tau} + E_{stat}$$
$$= E_{rheo}(1 + t_{chr}/\tau) \quad (4)$$

with E_{rheo} = identical with the electric field; E_{stat} = fixing the obstacle; and t_{chr} = chronaxie calculated from:

$$t_{chron} = \frac{I_{Pmin}}{q * E_{stat}} \quad (5)$$

Multiplying Equation 4 by τ yields a similarly structured equation as the linear "formula fondamentale" found by Weiss[13] for electrostimulation:

$$\int^{\tau} E_{exog}\, dt \geq E_{rheo}(\tau * t_{chr}) \quad (6)$$

Equations 4 and 6 are identical, if and only if the amplitude of the electric field in Equation 4 is given as a mean value.

Under the assumption of "removing obstacles by an electric field" or of "punching holes into the membrane by excessive electric fields," we get a physical Equation 4 that is formally identical for stimulation, defibrillation, and mechanical damage of the cell. The differences are:

1. In electrostimulation of the heart, a small critical mass in the immediate vicinity must be excited from which an excitation wave spreads to the whole heart. Preferably fibers are stimulated whose long-axis orientation are in parallel to the field orientation. One can simply estimate[12] that fibers perpendicular to the field orientation need a four to six times higher field strength to be excited (ratio: fiber length to fiber diameter). Opening of the sodium channels initiates excitation, which can be accomplished with a rheobase field strength of about 60 V/m.[14]

2. In defibrillation, a large critical mass must be influenced including longitudinally and transversely orientated fibers. Efficiency of defibrillation is determined in the areas farthest from the electrodes. Whereas a smaller percentage of cells are to be excited by opening the sodium channels, the majority of cells are refractory, and a proportion of which is in relative refractoriness. The latter part must be influenced for prolonging the refractory period by reopening sodium channels.[15] As reopening needs about 1.5 times higher field strengths and influencing of transversal fibers require a four- to sixfold higher one, defibrillation rheobase field strength must be assumed between 350 and 440 V/m. There is no indication why opening of the sodium channels and its reopening should yield another chronaxie time.

For damaging the cell membrane, the electric field strengths must be essentially at least 10 times stronger than in the case of defibrillation. Most probably the chronaxie of the damaging strength duration curve is greater than for stimulation, as the mass of the particles torn out of the membrane are larger and with it the necessary minimum impulse (see Equation 5).

If the circumstance can be assumed to be ohmic, as is the case in defibrillation, the mean value of the electric field in Equation 4 is proportional to the mean value of the applied voltage of a defibrillator and proportional to the mean value of the current flowing.

Which Experimental Results Support the Correctness of This Theory?

Several, investigators claim that stimulation and defibrillation is best described by the electric field or its synonym, by the potential gradient.[15-18] The derivation of the stimulation/defibrillation law (Equations 4 and 6) can be interpreted as the combination of very old knowledge[13,19] with recent findings, yielding probably the best method to describe stimulation and defibrillation.

Keeping the proportionality of electric field and current in mind, the findings of Bourland et al.[20] and that of Walker et al.[21] are in agreement with this theory, that it is the mean value of current, voltage, or field that is responsible for electrophysiologic effects. We must, however, add that this is only valid as long as the pulse intensity is above the rheobase. Exponential decaying or slowly increasing or decreasing ramp functions must be excluded from this rule.

There are at least three studies[7,20,22] proving that energy, current, and charge as a function of pulse duration have features, given by the hyperbolic so-called strength duration curve. Important in this context is that the defibrillation energy must have a minimum when chronaxie is reached.

The estimated electric field strength necessary for defibrillation is with 350–440 V/m (rheobase) very close to what has been measured so far (Ideker et al.[15] 600 V/m, 14 msec, Kavanagh et al.,[23] 400–900 V/m). If Equations 4 or 6 are regarded as being the fundamental law of defibrillation, what are the consequences for implantable cardioverter-defibrillator (ICD) practice?

Theory of Truncation

The following theory is based upon the hypothesis that defibrillation obeys the Fundamental Law of Electrostimulation[12]

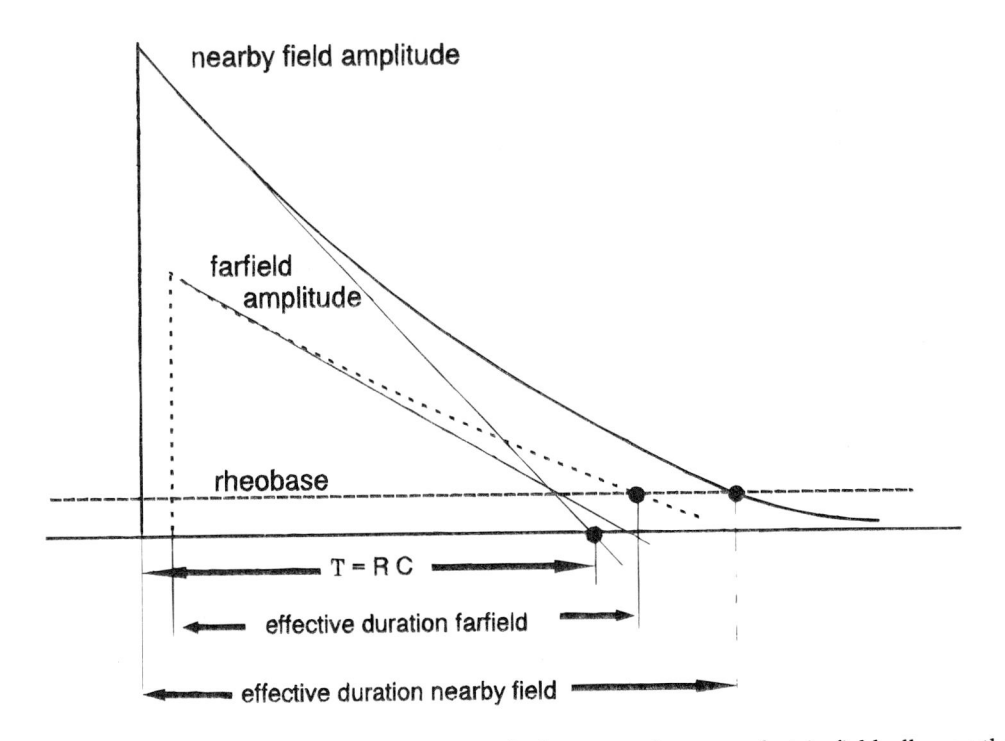

Figure 1. An exponential decay of a capacitor discharge produces an electric field all over the heart that is similar in shape, but different in amplitude decreasing with increasing distance from the electrode(s). Therefore, the far-field intersects rheobase (which is equal all over the heart) much earlier than the nearby field.

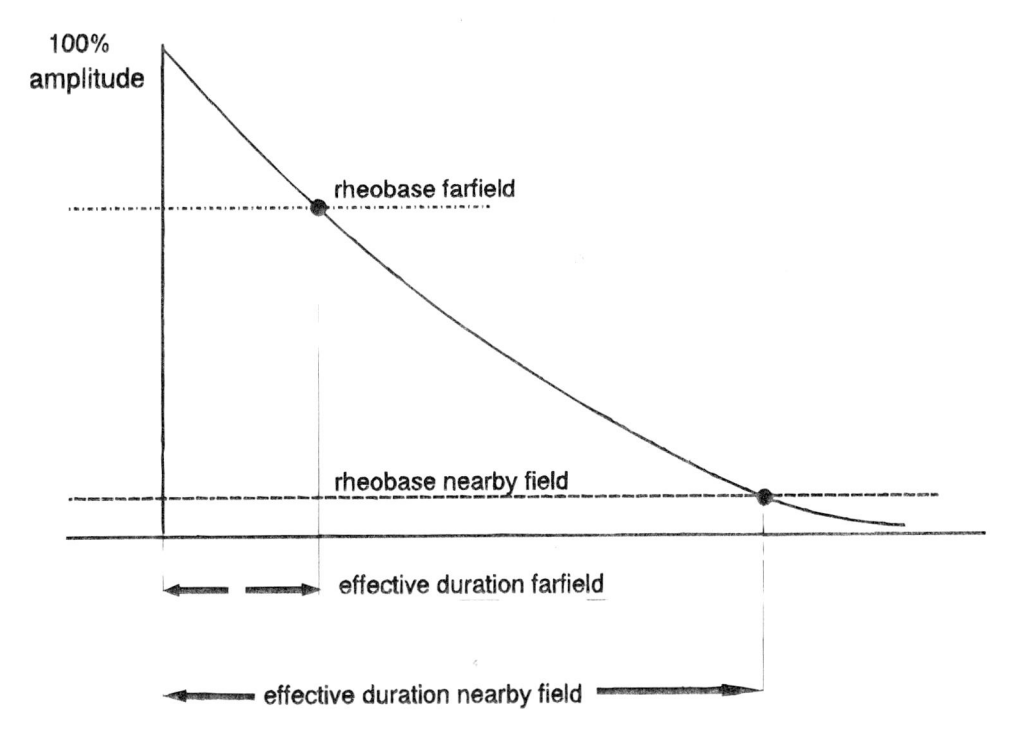

Figure 2. It can be derived from Figure 1A that the ratio of rheobase field related to maximum amplitude is the higher, the more distant from the electrodes cardiac tissue is. The higher the ratio, the smaller the effective duration. Prolongation of the pulse duration beyond effective duration of the far-field is not useful, as there is no benefit for the far-field below rheobase but possibly refibrillation due to longer and more intensive stimulation field strengths in the regions close to the electrodes. Thus, temporal and regional irregularities are created which may form the basis on which circus movements are reinitiated.

that is presented by a hyperbola and is characterized by Lapicque's terms of rheobase and chronaxie.[19] The essential message of the rheobase is that any intensity below a threshold value, called rheobase no longer has a stimulating effect. Applied to defibrillation the rheobase is modified in that an electric field spread all over the heart is no longer capable of defibrillating all sites simultaneously. This means that for exponentially decaying capacitor discharges, if the electric field is below rheobase, the most distant regions of the heart are no longer electrically affected, while in contrast, the closest regions may be stimulated much longer (Figures 1 and 2). This regional and temporal irregularity forms the basis upon which renewed fibrillation by circus movements can be reinitiated.

Assuming that the above hypothesis is true, the problem of correct truncation of a defibrillation pulse can be treated mathematically by the application of the Weiss "formule fondamentale" (Equation 6) to an exponentially decaying pulse, combined with the boundary condition that the intensity at the end of the pulse is equal to rheobase (Figure 3), thus:

$$\int^{\tau} E(t)\, dt = E_0 \int^{\tau} e^{-t/RC}\, dt$$
$$= RCE_0(1 - e^{-\tau/RC}) \qquad (7)$$
$$\geq E_{rheo}(t_c + \tau)$$

with E = electrical field strength; τ = pulse duration; E_0 = initial field strength due to the capacitor discharge; RC = product of lead resistance and discharge capacitor;

$$U_{exp}(t) = U_i \cdot e^{-t/T}$$

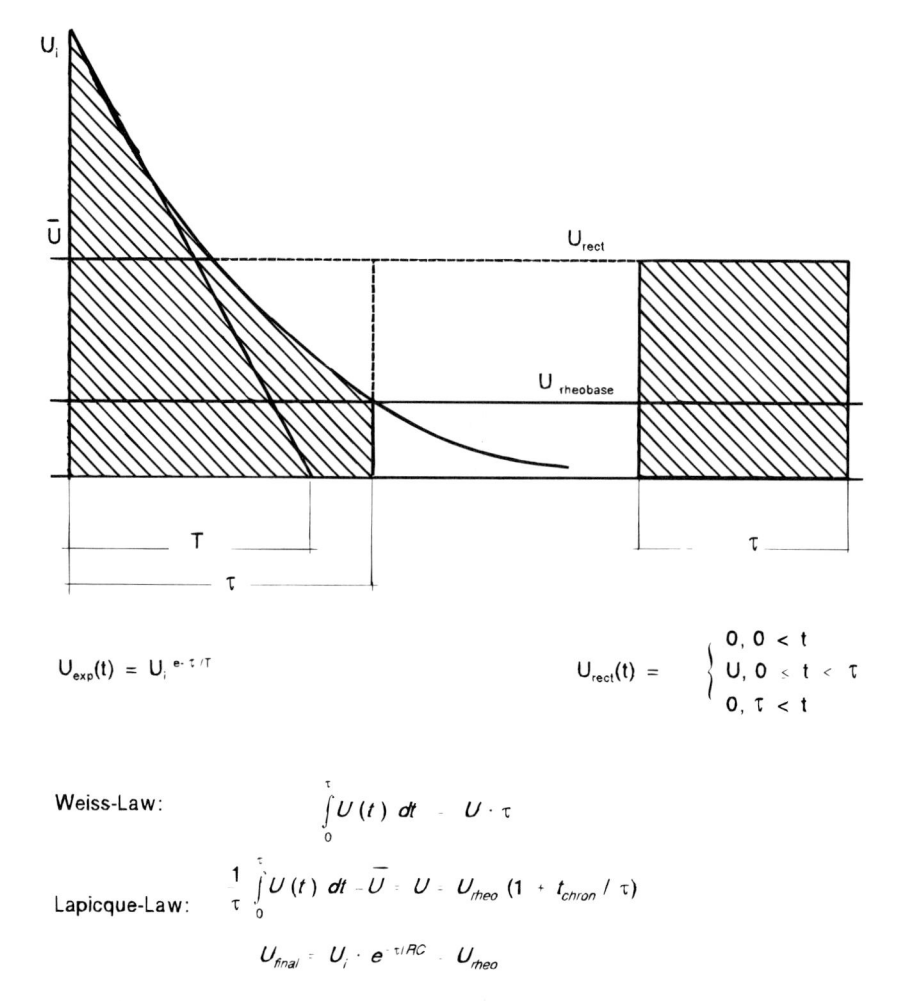

$$U_{rect}(t) = \begin{cases} 0, & 0 < t \\ U, & 0 \leq t < \tau \\ 0, & \tau < t \end{cases}$$

Weiss-Law: $\quad \int_0^\tau U(t)\, dt = U \cdot \tau$

Lapicque-Law: $\quad \dfrac{1}{\tau}\int_0^\tau U(t)\, dt = \bar{U} = U = U_{rheo}(1 + t_{chron}/\tau)$

$$U_{final} = U_i \cdot e^{-t/RC} = U_{rheo}$$

Figure 3. Equivalence of rectangular and exponential decaying pulses: By two or more threshold measurements the rheobase voltage is calculated. Introducing rheobase into the exponentially decaying voltage, the intersection with rheobase yields the effective pulse duration τ. If the mean voltage of the exponential pulse U is equal to the threshold voltage Ū of the rectangular pulse, then both are equally effective and, thus, equivalent according to Weiss' Law.

E_{rheo} = rheobase field strength; t_c = chronaxie time.

Introducing the boundary condition that requires:

$$E_0 \cdot e^{-\tau/RC} = E_{rheo}, \quad (8)$$

Equation (7) can be rearranged to:

$$E_{rheo} \cdot RC(e^{\tau/RC} - 1) \geq E_{rheo}(t_c + \tau) \quad (9)$$

The solution of Equation 9 is independent of the rheobase field strength and can be formulated simply by normalizing pulse duration τ and RC to chronaxie t_c:

$$e^{X/V} - 1 \geq 1/V + X/V \quad (10)$$

with: $X = \tau/t_c$ and $V = RC/t_c$.

Equation 10 represents a transcendental function that can be solved by a simple iteration method. The solution is depicted in Figure 4. The highly nonlinear correlation can be approximated by functions entered in Figure 4. Their accuracy is better than 1.5%.

Similarly, the energy needed for defibrillation can be expressed in a normalized form:

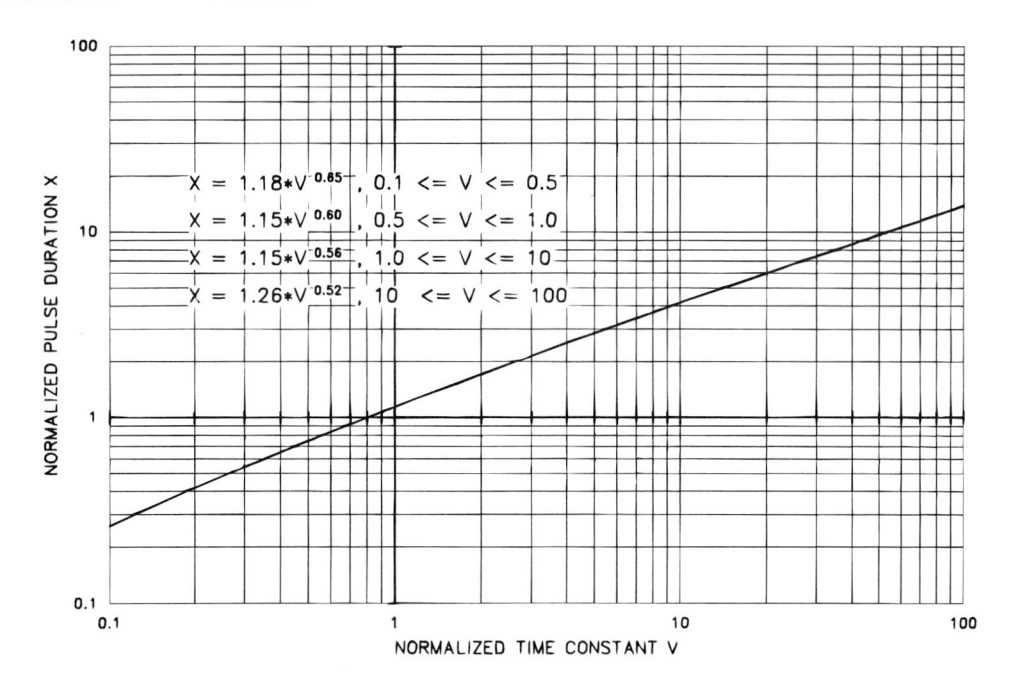

Figure 4. Equivalent normalized pulse duration X of a capacitor discharge with normalized time constant V: X = t/t$_{chron}$; t = pulse duration; t$_{chron}$ = chronaxie; V = RC/t$_{chron}$; R · C = resistance-time-product of the discharge circuit. Depending on V, the function can be approximated as indicated.

$$\frac{E(V)}{E_{min}} = 0.1018 \cdot V \cdot e^{2X/V} \quad (11)$$

with: E(V) = the stored capacitor energy, E$_{min}$ = minimum energy. The solution of Equation 11 is depicted in Figure 5.

The curve in Figure 5 or Equation 11 was calculated under the assumption that the stored energy of the output capacitor should be minimized. This is based on the philosophy that the rest energy, stored at the end of the pulse duration, is lost energy if the defibrillation attempt is successful. A curve comparable to Figure 5 for delivered energy is similar, but shifted to the right. The optimal pulse duration or the minimal energy in this case is given for V = 1.46 or X = 1.46 or τ = 1.42t$_{ch}$. If comparisons between different results are made, one should keep in mind that there are differences between stored and delivered energy with respect to threshold results.

To determine whether and where there is a minimum, the calculation yields: The energy is minimal if the time constant and the pulse duration is:

$$RC = 0.8t_c \quad \text{and} \quad \tau = t_c \quad (12)$$

Equation 11 and Figure 5 are the strongest argument against the constant energy concept. If we assume the chronaxie to be 2 msec, the energy minimum is located where τ/t$_s$ = X = 1 or, the pulse duration is equal to chronaxie = 2 msec.

If we compare the minimum energy with those of 10-msec or 20-msec duration, the energy for the same defibrillation effect is 2.92 or 7.9 higher if optimal truncation, according to Equation 10 or Figure 4 is carried out. If this is not the case, the elevation factor can be even higher. One could state this fact in colloquial language by saying that there are "good Joules" and "bad Joules" in the defibrillation art. If the normalized energy is plotted versus the normalized time constant (Figure 6) the region

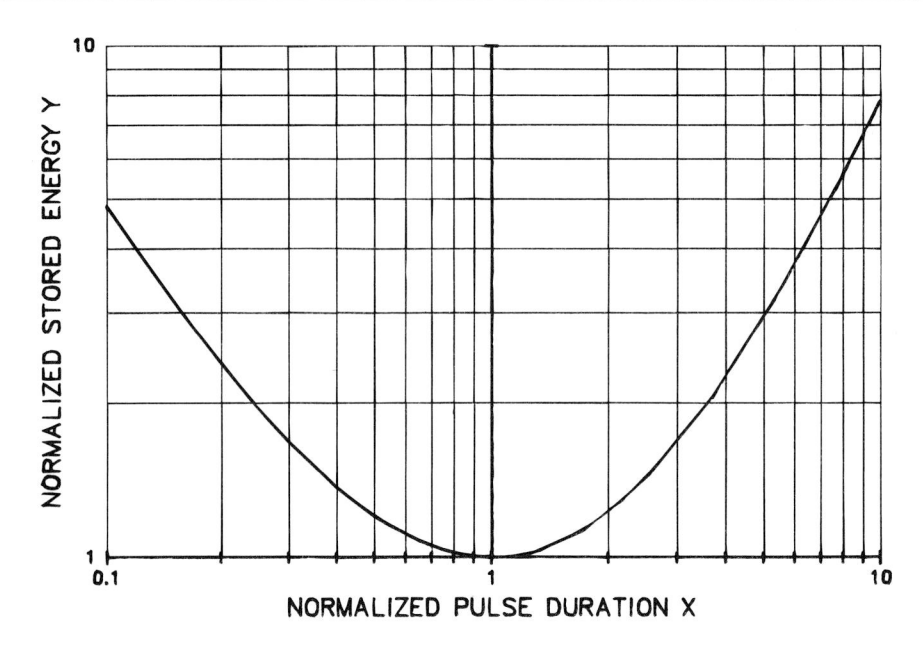

Figure 5. Normalized threshold energy Y as a function of normalized pulse duration X. Y = ratio of energy with duration X related to minimum energy with X = 1.

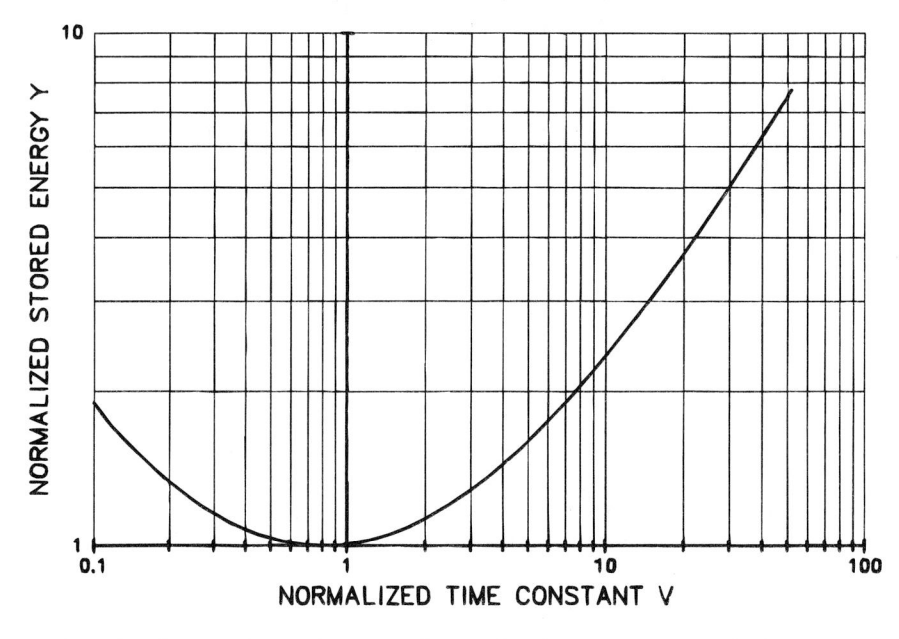

Figure 6. Normalized energy Y as a function of normalized time constant V. Today's time constants may go up to V = 15. Between $0.3 \leq V \leq 2.5$ the energy needed for defibrillation can be assumed to be constant ($1 \leq Y \leq 1.2$) or this is the range of V for optimum performance.

of practical interest is between 0.4 and 15 demonstrating that even with optimized pulse duration the energy needed may be up to 2.3 times higher than the minimum located at 0.8.

In contrast to the constant energy concept the following is valid:

1. Pulse duration: With a given RC-time constant the energy needed for defibrillation is the lowest, if optimal truncation according to Figure 4 is carried out. A shorter pulse duration than given with Figure 4 needs higher energies, as the initial voltage to which the capacitor is charged must be higher. The energy of the capacitor at the end of the pulse duration then is unnecessarily high as the decay was stopped above rheobase. A longer pulse duration than calculated implies possible refibrillation.
2. Pulse shape: A shorter RC-time constant is more favorable as it is closer to the optimal working point $V = RC/t_c = 0.8$ according to Equation 12. The higher efficiency of shorter time constants has the electrophysiologic advantage that the energy needed is lowest around chronaxie. Moreover, voltages, to which the capacitor must be charged are higher as the time constants are reduced. The remaining rest energy at the end of the pulse duration is relatively unimportant.
3. The tilt (T): T is the decrease in capacitor voltage ΔU related to initial voltage U_i and can be expressed similarly by the normalized values X and V yielding:

$$T = 1 - e^{-X/V} \quad (13)$$

Equation 13 can be evaluated by looking for the corresponding pairs of values X, V, or by calculation with the approximation formula in Figure 4 and inserting them into Equation 13. The solution is depicted in Figure 7.

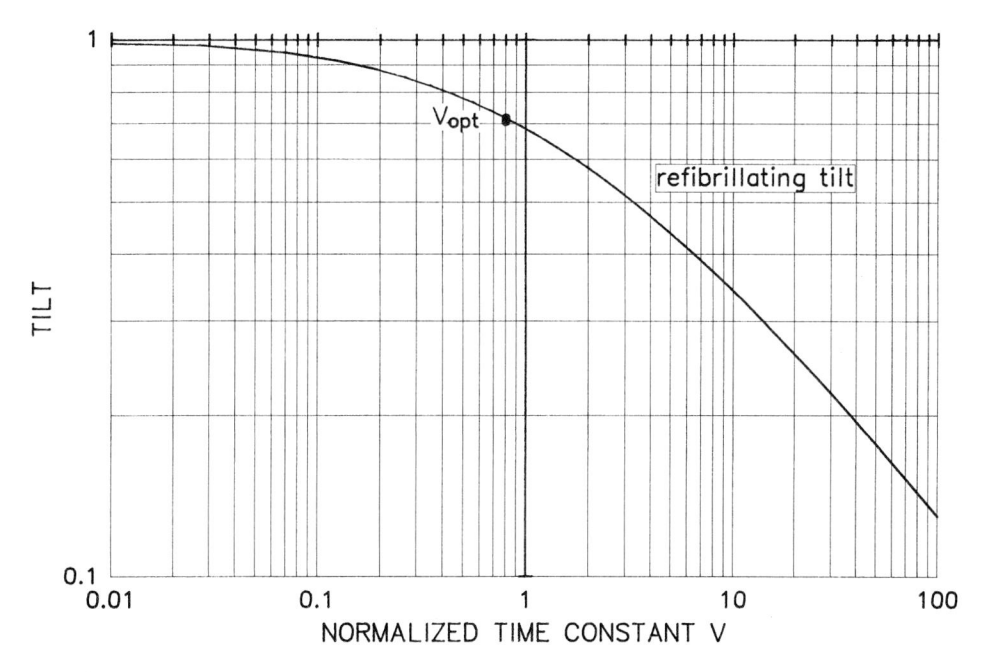

Figure 7. Tilt (change in capacitor voltage ΔU related to initial voltage U_i) as a function of normalized time constant V. If the tilt is above curve, the pulse may have refibrillating qualities. The tilt for lowest energy at $V = 0.8$ is 71.3% (see Table 1).

According to the theory of truncation, there is a correlation between the three parameters: pulse duration, chronaxie, and RC product of the discharge circuit. For a given RC, V can be determined if the chronaxie is known. Based upon earlier calculations[12] and findings of other authors[4,21,22,24] we conclude that the chronaxie for defibrillation is close to 2 msec which is typical for stimulation with large area electrodes (such as used with external transchest stimulation). Under this assumption the curve in Figure 7 allows for determination of whether current defibrillators with monophasic pulses operate satisfactorily or not. All tilt values above the curve indicate that voltage decrease of the discharging capacitor is too great, possibly giving rise to refibrillation. For today's ICDs the capacitance of the output capacitor is between 60 and 300 μF. This, together with a lead load of 50 Ω and a V value of 1.5–7.5, requires a tilt of 61.7% to 38.7%, whereas current ICDs operate at 60% to 75%. A tilt of 75% would only be adequate if V is below 1 (RC < t_c) which means the capacitor would have 30 μF or less.

Best performance of a monophasic ICD would be reached if V is 0.8 with the parameters C = 32 μF, τ = 2 msec, and the tilt = 71%. Our calculated values are very close to what was recently found by Kroll.[4] As the minimum energy for defibrillation is about 50% or less of that of a volt with 7.5, we are of the opinion that this optimized system will operate with even lower energies than today's biphasic systems.

What Experimental Results are Supporting the Correctness of This Assumption and the Theory Based Upon It?

First, it is known that defibrillation thresholds expressed as mean current or voltage for truncated and untruncated exponential pulses are increased for long durations of more than 10 msec.[9,22,25] This is in contrast to normal stimulation strength-duration-curves in which a rheobase value exists for pulse durations reaching infinity or for infinitely long time constants for untruncated exponential decay pulses. The tail of the exponential pulse below rheobase can no longer defibrillate the most distant regions, but may introduce prolonged refractory periods in the immediate vicinity of the electrode(s). We believe that this inhomogeneity is causing refibrillation that must be overcome by higher voltages and currents and consequently higher energies.

Second, the investigations of Walker et al.[21] were tested to determine whether they are in agreement with our theory of correct truncation. They measured "strength duration curves for short time constant truncated exponential monophasic waveforms" with time constant of 4 and 7 msec in dogs weighing approximately 20 kg. They found for the 7-msec time constant, that the leading edge voltage of 422 V of the capacitor discharge remained constant for pulse durations longer than 5 msec. This means that approximately at 180 V, rheobase voltage was reached and any prolongation of pulse duration had no further defibrillation effect. Though they did not observe refibrillation by prolongation of the pulse duration, this is probably not as severe in healthy small 20-kg dogs, it must be suspected that an ineffective truncated tail below rheobase may cause refibrillation in humans with impairment of the heart. The observation of Walker and co-workers[21] confirms experimentally the assumption that a tail below rheobase no longer has a positive defibrillating effect.

Third, results based on Equation 13, which predict higher tilts for shorter time constants (Figure 7), are confirmed by the investigation of Walker et al.[21] who suggest "that truncation may not be necessary for short time constant waveforms."

Fourth, there are several investigations proving that the energy as a function of pulse duration involves a minimum[7,20,24,25] with a chronaxie of between 2 and 4 msec.

Application of the Theory to Defibrillation

If, together with Geddes et al.,[24] we postulate that defibrillation is governed by the same rules as all other stimulation phenomena, we must determine if today's defibrillation practice is in accordance with theory, and further, which improvements can be developed from it. This is especially important in a therapeutic treatment that is life-saving or, when failing, life-threatening. In contrast to pacing the heart, exact measurements of defibrillation thresholds are nearly impossible.[26] To investigate thresholds in animals, more than 30–70 defibrillation attempts are necessary, not to define a threshold, but to statistically obtain a function called "defibrillation success rate versus energy."[27–30] In contrast to cardiac stimulation, the threshold is said not to be a step function and therefore must be replaced by a "probability of success function." This starts anywhere at the lowest possible energy threshold, the rheobase energy, below which no defibrillation takes place and asymptomatically approaches the 100% line. Under these conditions it is highly desirable that a trial-and-error investigational system is replaced, at least partially, by theoretical considerations based on the fundamental law of electrostimulation. We believe that a theoretical result as complex as our derived correlation between pulse duration and time constant, depicted in Figure 4, has no chance to be detected by the trial-and-error method.

The Shape of the Defibrillation Pulse

It is already an old question, which by the way initiated the work of Weiss, as to which pulse shape is best suited to reach optimum stimulation conditions. It is not surprising that those engaged in defibrillation are similarly trying to find their own concepts. The answer was already given by Weiss in 1901.[13] With today's knowledge, taking into account the physical meaning of Equation 1 in combination with Equation 4 we can formulate that as long as the stimulation amplitude is above the rheobase value, the shape of the pulse is irrelevant. Stimulation is determined only by the time integral over the pulse duration. Weiss found that several pulses of short duration coupled immediately to a pulse train of the same duration as one pulse, have the same effect, if the time integral over the pulse duration is the same (see Equation 6). This stimulation phenomenon, formulated by Weiss in 1901, was confirmed as valid for defibrillation by Geddes et al.[24] and Bourland et al.[20] They found that it is best to use the mean current (averaged over given pulse durations) to describe the threshold, if the pulse shapes are different. Mean current, however, multiplied by the pulse duration, is identical with the threshold charge which is the determining parameter in electrostimulation, according to Weiss.[13]

One interesting aspect of the Weiss phenomenon is that a pulse with threshold intensity demands an increase in energy if the amplitude during pulse duration deviates from its mean value. The lowest possible energy is reached as the pulse approaches rectangular shape. As applied to implantable defibrillators, this means that the output capacitor should be large, to have the lowest possible decline during pulse. Conversely, practical considerations demand a compromise as the unused energy of a truncated pulse stored in the output capacitor is lost energy after successful defibrillation. This increase in energy with a pulse shape deviating from rectangular is the reason why the minimum delivered energy with truncated exponential decay is not reached at chronaxie, as is the case with rectangular pulses, but at a time 1.42 times larger (see comment to Equation 11).

The Stimulation Dose

Typically, the defibrillation dose used is the energy. This has historical reasons, as the external defibrillators could not measure voltage, current, or duration of the pulse, as is usually done in electrostimulation. The only measurable value was the voltage to which the output capacitor was charged. Using the well-known formula:

$$E_c = \frac{1}{2}CU^2 \quad (14)$$

with: E_C = charged energy; C = capacitance of the capacitor; U = voltage of the capacitor and assuming that all stored energy is delivered to the body, the manufacturers were able to specify the energy of an outgoing pulse. The load within the discharge circuit, which is mainly determined by the electrodes size and by the skin and body conductivity, determines how long the discharge will take place. In implantable defibrillators the discharge time normally is limited, yielding truncated exponential voltages and currents. In this case, the energy delivered is determined by the resistance of the leads. Only if truncation takes place at a predetermined tilt, the delivered energy is known, but with the disadvantage that the pulse duration is unknown.

Referring back to Figure 5 or 6 it is quite clear and has been known since 1892[6] that there is no general energy threshold, regardless of output capacitor and pulse duration. Schuder and co-workers[31] showed that the contour graphs for constant success rate for mono- and biphasic pulses do not follow a constant energy line, indicating that a 16-msec pulse needs double the energy than a 4-msec pulse, the same success rate assumed for both. Similarly they demonstrated that with a given energy the success rates tend to increase as the current amplitude is raised (corresponding to a decrease in pulse duration). The threshold curves expressed as energy threshold have always a defined minimum, which is determined by the chronaxie, as stated by Lapicque in 1909.[19] The concept of constant energy, introduced by Nernst in 1908[32] has its electrophysiologic shortcomings. The weakness of the energy dose may be one of the reasons why the results are so divergent. Energy, therefore, is not a good predictor of defibrillation outcome.[33,34] Conversely, the energy dose has a practical disadvantage, which physicians should be aware of: if the field strength hypothesis is accepted as true, the linear physical quantities such as voltage and current, are closer to the field strength than the energy. This means, if a given field strength has failed to stimulate or to defibrillate, the field strength must be increased by at least 10% or 20%. Projecting this to defibrillators, it is not physiological, and could be even dangerous if the programmable dose of an implantable defibrillator increases in steps from 20 to 22, 24, 27, and 30 J corresponding to an increase in voltage of 100%, 105%, 110%, 116%, and 122%. Each physician experienced in pacing would never increase an external pacemaker output with such low incremental steps. If, for technical reasons, the highest energy is limited to, for example 30 J, a downward scaling of 19, 12, 8, 5, 3.2, 1, 3, and 0.8 would correspond to a decrease in field strength in steps of 20% referring always to the last value.

We claim that a characterization of the defibrillation threshold indicating the mean output voltage and the pulse duration would drastically reduce the uncertainties of today's practice, due to the energy dose, and would probably reduce the threshold variations, which make programming the output of an ICD a problem. At least energy and pulse duration should be indicated to characterize the defibrillator's quality and not to forget, there are "good Joules" and "bad Joules" according to Figure 5.

Programming of Defibrillators

Today's defibrillators have programming features that do not always allow for optimal output characteristics. We calculated that the lowest energy stored is reached with a pulse duration equal to chronaxie and a time constant of the capacitor discharge circuit 0.8 times chronaxie (see Equation 12). To get an indication, the chronaxie could be measured by stimulation trials with the defibrillation electrode[12] as we assume stimulation chronaxie very close to defibrillation chronaxie (around 2 msec). Having found an individual chronaxie time or taking our approximation of 2 msec, we can determine the optimal output capacitor with Equation 12, if the resistance of the output circuit R is measured and known:

$$C_{opt} = \frac{0.8 t_{chron}}{R} = \frac{1.6 \text{ ms}}{R} \quad (15)$$

Let us assume the resistance R to be close to 50 Ω, Equation 15 has the solution:

$$C_{opt} = \frac{1.6 \text{ ms}}{50 \text{ Ω}} = 32 \text{ μF}$$

Charging this optimal capacitance to 790 V means an optimal energy of 10 J, which should have the same defibrillation effect as a 36-J, 10- to 12-msec pulse (this follows from Equation 11 and Figure 5). Reduction or increase in energy should be done in steps of at least 20% to 25% (10% in voltage), which would give a sequence downwards of 8, 6.5, 5, 4, 3.3, 2.5, 2.0, 1.5, 1.2, and 1 J and upwards of 12.5, 15.5., 20, 24, and 30 J.

A 30-J energy with 32 μF yields a voltage of 1,370 V, which is still a technical problem. As long as such high voltages are not tolerated by capacitors, another strategy for defibrillation could consist of having a constant voltage of, for example, 800 V and programming the output capacitors and the pulse duration accordingly. For implantable units the stored energy of 5 J would be reached at 16 μF. A pulse duration of 1.3 msec would be optimal according to Figure 4 with a resistance of 50 Ω assumed. An energy of 20 J then, is reached optimally by 64 μF and 3-msec pulse duration. Together with the energy setting 10 J and a pulse duration of 2 msec, the energy curve in Figure 5 would be used between X = 0.65 and 1.5, which guarantees a nearly flat part of the energy curve (not more than 6.2% elevation as compared to the optimum). With this strategy of programming the output capacitance around the energy minimum, it is justified in assuming the threshold to be constant in energy (Table 1).

Table 1

Capacitance/μF	16	32	64
Time constant/msec	0.8	1.6	3.2
V = R·C/t_c	0.4	0.8	1.6
X = t/t_c (Figure 3)	0.65	1.0	1.5
Pulse duration/msec	1.3	2	3
Tilt/% (Figure 6)	80.3	71.3	60.8
Energy (790V)	5.0	10.0	20.0
Normalized energy (Figure 4)	1.050	1.000	1.062
Delivered versus stored energy	96%	91%	85%
Energy (250 V)/J	0.5	1.0	2.0

Concept of variable capacitance defibrillators. Assumptions: lead resistance = 50Ω, chronaxie = 2 msec. The equations necessary for calculations are compiled in the Appendix.

If no programmable output capacitors are available, but the time constant and the chronaxie is known, then Figure 4 helps to find the best combination between output voltage and pulse duration. Let us assume the capacitor to have a capacitance of 140 μF, the resistance is 50 Ω and the chronaxie is 2 msec. The calculation should proceed with the following calculation (all equations necessary for the following calculations are compiled in the Appendix:

Step 1: R·C = 50 Ω·140 μF = 7 msec

Step 2: V = R·C/t_{chron} = 7 msec/2 msec
= 3.5 (Equation 10)

Step 3: With the aid of Figure 3 or the approximation for conversion V to X, we get:

X = 1.15·V$^{0.56}$ = 1.15·3.5$^{0.56}$ = 2.32

Step 4: Pulse duration t is given by

t = X·t_{chron} = 2.32·2 msec

= 4.6 msec

Program pulse duration to 4.6 msec. With this pulse duration, the stored energy is the most effective but still 34% higher than the minimum at chronaxie.

Step 5: Energy is given by Equation 14 that yields a voltage with 10 J assumed of

$$U = \sqrt{\frac{2E}{C}} = \sqrt{\frac{2 \cdot 10J}{140\ \mu F}} = 378\ V.$$

Program voltage to 380 V.

Step 6: If other energies are needed, step down voltages in 10%, energies in 20% decrements or increase it in 12.5% or 25% increments respectively.

The tilt T can be calculated with Equation 13 to be 48.5%. This value is remarkably lower than today's tilts of 60% to 75%, but it means that 26.6% of the stored energy is left in the output capacitor. Is this really loss in energy? It is surely not wasted energy if its release to the myocardium would yield refibrillation that can only be overcome by initially higher energies. Similar calculations for other lead resistances are summarized in Table 2, proving that neither constant tilt nor constant pulse duration satisfies electrophysiology of defibrillation.

We see no problem if this unused energy is reversed and given to the electrodes as a biphasic part of the defibrillation pulse. This energy rest, which is below rheobase for the farthest region, cannot do any harm there, but may help to avoid dysfunction of the myocardium in closest vicinity of the electrode(s) by closing pores within the membrane due to the reversion of the field direction. This is our hypothesis of how biphasic pulses could reduce refibrillation tendency.

As another practical example we assume the output capacitor to be 60 μF and we ask for the optimized pulse duration for lead resistances of 25, 50, 75, and 100 Ω. The results are summarized in Table 3 (for calculations see Appendix).

Step 1: The RCs are: 1.5 msec, 3 msec, 4.5 msec, and 6 msec.

Step 2: The ratio V = RC/t_{chron} with t_{chron} = 2 msec is:

V = 0.75, 1.5, 2.25, 3

Step 3: The pulse durations can be calculated with Equation 1 of the Appendix:

X: 0.97, 1.45, 1.81, 2.13

Step 4: The optimized pulse duration for the various resistances would be:

R = 25 Ω, t = 1.96 msec; R = 50 Ω, t = 2.89 msec;

R = 75 Ω, t = 3.62 msec; R = 100 Ω, t = 4.26 msec;

Step 5: Use the energies as needed and re-

Table 2

Lead resistance/Ω	25	50	75	100
Time constant RC/msec	3.5	7.0	10.5	14.0
V = RC/t_c	1.75	3.5	5.25	7.0
X = t/t_c (Figure 3)	1.57	2.32	2.91	3.42
Pulse duration/msec	3.14	4.64	5.82	6.84
Tilt/% (Figure 6)	59.3	48.5	42.6	38.6
Normalized energy (Figure 4)	1.08	1.34	1.62	1.89
Delivered versus stored energy	83.4%	73.4%	67.0%	62.4%

Correlations:

t/msec = 1.04 + 0.024·R/Ω

Tilt = 0.642 − 2.7·10^{-3}·R/Ω

Programming of the pulse duration with variable lead resistance and 140 μF output capacitance assumed. Assumptions: chronaxie = 2 msec. The equations necessary for calculations are compiled in the Appendix. For pulse duration t and tilt, linear regression lines are calculated to approximate others than the four values for lead resistance in the table.

Table 3

Lead resistance/Ω	25	50	75	100
Time constant RC/msec	1.5	3.0	4.5	6.0
V = RC/t_c	0.75	1.5	2.25	3.0
X = t/t_c (Figure 3)	0.97	1.44	1.81	2.13
Pulse duration/msec	1.94	2.89	3.62	4.26
Tilt/% (Figure 6)	72.5	62.0	55.3	50.8
Normalized energy (Figure 4)	1.014	1.05	1.15	1.26
Delivered versus stored energy	92%	85%	80%	76%

Correlations:

$$t/msec = 1.14 + 0.034 \cdot R/\Omega$$

$$Tilt = 0.782 - 2.9 \cdot 10^{-3} \cdot R/\Omega$$

Programming of the pulse duration with variable lead resistance and 60 µF output capacitance assumed. Assumptions: chronaxie = 2 msec. The equations necessary for calculations are compiled in the Appendix. For pulse duration t and tilt, linear regression lines are calculated to approximate others than the four values for lead resistance in the table.

---

member that longer pulse durations, than calculated with Step 4, will not increase the effectiveness of the pulse, though the delivered energy is increased slightly. This tail is below rheobase and, therefore, cannot but refibrillate.

The tilt can be calculated wth Equation 4 of the Appendix or estimated with Figure 6:

T(25 Ω) = 72.6%; T(50 Ω) = 62.0%; T(75 Ω) = 55.3%; T(100 Ω) = 50.8%.

This example demonstrates clearly that a constant tilt concept whose physiological usefulness has never been proven is not in accordance with our theory. Based on the defibrillation theory, the following conclusions may be provided to the initial rhetorical questions.

Alternatives to the Constant Energy Concept

The proposed programming procedures are examples of how the constant energy concept can be replaced by a concept based on the fundamental law of electrostimulation. To characterize the defibrillation pulse, energy, corresponding mean voltage, pulse duration, and time constant should be described to give an indication of how close or distant the defibrillation pulse is with respect to its optimum according to Figures 5 and 6.

Programming Consequences

The output capacitors must be reduced to optimally 30 µF in order to operate around the optimum. Programmable capacitance, as demonstrated above, would render the defibrillator more effective. Programmable pulse durations are obligatory to reach refibrillation-free pulses.

Degree of Truncation

The degree of truncation can be calculated with Equation 4 of the Appendix and is dependent on pulse duration, time constant, and chronaxie. The calculated values are simultaneously most effective without being refibrillating.

Tilt and Pulse Duration

For a given chronaxie but changing time constant, due to changes in lead resistance the tilt is a function of the time constant in a nonlinear way according to Figure

7. It is therefore undesirable conceptionally to have installed a fixed tilt with a variable pulse duration. The larger the pulse duration the lower the tilt should be. Today's ICD possess without exceptions refibrillating tilts.

Programming of Pulse Duration and Intensity

We have demonstrated that the optimal pulse duration is given by the time constant and the chronaxie for the calculation of which Figure 4 can be used. For this fixed pulse duration all intensities may be programmed as adequate. Prolongation of the pulse duration beyond that calculated though increasing the output energy, may reduce the defibrillation probability due to refibrillating effects of the tail below rheobase.

Monophasic Versus Biphasic Pulses

There is no proof yet that optimized monophasic pulses, operating around the ideal working point at a pulse duration equal to chronaxie and an output circuit time constant of 80% of the chronaxie are superior or equal to biphasic pulses. Besides the fact that biphasic defibrillation needs optimization too, it is difficult to perceive why a monophasic pulse should need higher energies if it does not have refibrillating qualities due to pulse optimization. To reverse the remaining capacitor energy and give it to the electrode(s), as a pulse for closing electrically opened or reopened pores within the membranes, is an additional security measure that does not need additional energy. We are awaiting anxiously further experimental results in this respect.

Summary

Is defibrillation really governed by the rules of electrostimulation? The answer is ambiguous: yes, but there are obviously additional effects that must be taken as amendments to the law: the prolongation of refractoriness and the suppression of refibrillation by reduced pulses of opposite polarity at the end of a defibrillating pulse[15,34–37] both are not present in simple electrostimulation. Additionally, the field strength must be stronger to affect cells still refractory. However, do the additional effects, such as suppression of refibrillation and prolongation of refractoriness justify the assumption that the Nernst Law of constant energy will overrule Weiss' fundamental law of electrostimulation? We are of the opinion that all of the effects result from electric fields, for which strength-duration relationship exist as they were formulated by Lapicque in 1909 with the two important parameters: rheobase and chronaxie.

Appendix

Compilation of formulae:

1) Normalized pulse duration X as a function of the normalized time constant V, both normalized to chronaxie t_c according to

$$t/t_c = X \quad RC/t_c = V$$

Correlation between X and V is given by:

$$e^{X/V} - 1 - 1/V - X/V = Z$$

with Z = zero function, ie, pair of X, V must be chosen such that $Z \rightarrow 0$

Approximation:

$$X = 1.15 V^{0.56}$$

for $0.8 \leq V \leq 15$ Error $\leq 1.5\%$

2) Charged energy normalized to minimal energy at V = 0.8 and X = 1

$$\frac{E(V)}{E_{min}} = 0.1018 \cdot V \cdot e^{2X/V}$$

Approximation:

$$\frac{E(V)}{E_{min}} = 0.1018 \cdot V \cdot e^{2.3V^{-0.44}}$$

Error ≤ 3.3%

3) Delivered energy related to stored energy

$$\frac{E_d}{E_{st}} = 1 - e^{-2X/V}$$

Approximation:

$$\frac{E_d}{E_{st}} = 1 - e^{-2.3V^{-0.44}}$$

Error ≤ 0.6%

4) Tilt = Decrease in capacitor voltage ΔU related to initial voltage U_0

$$\text{Tilt} = 1 - e^{-X/V}$$

Approximation:

$$\text{Tilt} = 1 - e^{-1.15V^{-.044}}$$

Error ≤ 0.9%

5) Mean voltage $\overline{U}$ related to initial voltage U_0

$$\frac{\overline{U}}{U_0} = \frac{V}{X}(1 - e^{-X/V})$$

Approximation

$$\frac{\overline{U}}{U_0} = 0.87 \cdot V^{0.44}(1 - e^{1.15V^{-0.44}})$$

Error ≤ 0.7%

References

1. Gurvich NL, Yuniev GS: Restoration of heart rhythm during fibrillation by a condenser discharge. *Am Rev Soviet Med* 4:252, 1947.
2. Schuder JC, Stoeckle H, West JA, et al: Transthoracic ventricular defibrillation in the dog with truncated exponential stimuli. *IEEE Trans Bio Med Eng* 18:410, 1971.
3. Schuder JC, Gold JH, Stoeckle H, et al: Defibrillation in the calf with bidirectional trapezoidal wave shocks applied via chronically implanted epicardial electrodes. *Trans Am Soc Artif Intern Organs* 27:467, 1981.
4. Kroll MW: A minimal model of the monophasic defibrillation pulse. *PACE* 16:769, 1993.
5. Bach StM, Shapland JE: Engineering aspects of implantable defibrillators. In: *Electrical Therapy of Cardiac Arrhythmias*. Edited by S Saksena, N Goldschlager. Philadelphia, PA: W.B. Saunders Co.; 1990, p. 371.
6. Hoorweg JL: Über die elektrische Nervenerregung. *Pflügers Arch* 52:87, 1892.
7. Koning G, Schneider H, Hoelen AJ, et al: Amplitude-duration relation for direct ventricular defibrillation with rectangular current pulses. *Med Biol Eng* 13:388, 1975.
8. Geddes LA, Tacker WA: Engineering and physiological consideration of direct capacitor discharge ventricular defibrillation. *Med Biol Eng* 9:185, 1971.
9. Tacker WA, Geddes LA: *Electrical Defibrillation*. Boca Raton, FL: CRC Press Inc.; 1980, p. 68.
10. Trautwein W: Erregungsphysiologie des Herzens. In: *Herz und Kreislauf*. Edited by OH Gauer, K Kramer, R Jung. München-Berlin-Wien: Urban & Schwarzenberg; 1972, p. 74.
11. Ideker RE, Frazier DW, Krassowska W, et al: Physiologic effects of electrical stimulation in cardiac muscle. In: *Electrical Therapy for Cardiac Arrhythmias*. Edited by S Saksena, N Goldschlager. Philadelphia, PA: W.B. Saunders Co.; 1990, p. 357.
12. Irnich W: The fundamental law of electrostimulation and its application to defibrillation. *PACE* 13:1433, 1990.
13. Weiss G: Sur la possibilité de rendre comparable entre eux les appareils servant a l'exitation électrique. *Arch Ital Biol* 35:413, 1901.
14. Irnich W: Electrostimulation by time-varying magnetic fields. *MAGMA* 1 (in press).
15. Ideker RE, Tang ASL, Frazier DW, et al: Basic mechanisms of ventricular defibrillation. In: *Theory of Heart*. Edited by L Glass, P Hunter, A McCulloch. New York, NY: Springer Verlag; 1991, p. 533.
16. Klee M, Plonsey R: Stimulation of spheroidal cell—the roll of cell shape. *IEEE Trans Biomed Eng* 4:347, 1976.
17. Jones JL, Lepeschkin E, Jones RE, et al: Response of cultured myocardial cells to counter-shock-type electric field stimulation. *Am J Physiol* 235:H214, 1978.
18. Reilly JP: *Electrical Stimulation and Electropathology*. Cambridge: Cambridge University Press; 1992.

19. Lapicque L: Definition expérimental de l'excitabilité. *Soc Biol* 77:280, 1909.
20. Bourland JD, Tacker WA, Geddes LA: Strength-duration curves for trapezoidal waveforms of various tilts for transchest defibrillations in animals. *Med Instrum* 12:45, 1978.
21. Walker RG, Walcott GP, Smith WM, et al: Strength duration curves for short time constant truncated exponential monophasic waveforms (abstract). *PACE* 16:915, 1993.
22. Wessale JL: *Bipolar Catheter Defibrillation in Dogs Using Trapezoidal Waveforms of Various Tilts.* West Lafayette, IN: Purdue University; 1978. Doctoral Thesis.
23. Kavanagh KM, Simpson EV, Wolf PD, et al: Minimum gradient required for biphasic defibrillation (abstract). *PACE* 16:916, 1993.
24. Geddes LA, Niebauer MJ, Babbs CF, et al: Fundamental criteria underlying the efficacy and safety of defibrillating current waveforms. *Med Biol Eng Comput* 23:122, 1985.
25. Chapman PD, Wetherbee JN, Vetter JW, et al: Strength-duration curves of fixed pulse width variable tilt truncated exponential waveforms for nonthoracotomy internal defibrillation in dogs. *PACE* 11:1045, 1988.
26. McDaniel WC, Schuder JC: The cardiac ventricular defibrillation threshold—inherent limitations in its interpretation. AAMI 20th Ann Meeting, Boston, MA, 1985.
27. Davy J-M, Fain ES, Dorian P, et al: The relationship between successful defibrillation and delivered energy in open-chest dogs: reappraisal of the "defibrillation threshold" concept. *Am Heart J* 113:77, 1987.
28. Rattes MF, Jones DL, Sharma AD, et al: Defibrillation threshold: a simple and quantitative estimate of the ability to defibrillate. *PACE* 10:70, 1987.
29. Church T, Martinson M, Kallok M, et al: A model to evaluate alternative methods of defibrillation threshold determination. *PACE* 11:2002, 1988.
30. Lehmann MH, Steinmann RT, Schuger CD, et al: Defibrillation threshold testing and other practices related to AICD implantation: do all roads lead to Rome? *PACE* 12:1530, 1989.
31. Schuder JC, Gold JH, Stoeckle H, et al: Transthoracic ventricular defibrillation in the 100 kg calf with symmetrical one-cycle bidirectional rectangular wave stimuli. *IEEE Trans Biomed Eng* 30:415, 1983.
32. Nernst W. Zur Theorie des elektrischen Reizes. *Pflügers Arch* 122:275, 1908.
33. Geddes LA, Tacker WA, Rosborough AG, et al: Electrical dose for ventricular defibrillation of large and small animals using precordial electrodes. *J Clin Invest* 53:310, 1974.
34. Chen P-S, Shibata N, Dixon EG: Activation during ventricular defibrillation in open-chest dogs. *J Clin Invest* 77:810, 1986.
35. Dillon SM, Wit AL: Action potential prolongation by shock as a possible mechanism for electrical defibrillation. *Circulation* 80:II-96, 1989.
36. Frazier DW, Wolf PD, Wharton JM, et al: Stimulus-induced critical point. *J Clin Invest* 83:1039, 1989.
37. Shibata N, Chen P-S, Dixon EG, et al: Influence of shock strength and timing on induction of ventricular arrhythmia in dogs. *Am J Physiol* 255:H891, 1988.

Chapter 7

Defibrillation Waveforms

Susan M. Blanchard, Stephen B. Knisley, Gregory P. Walcott, and Raymond E. Ideker

Patients who have implantable cardioverter-defibrillators (ICDs) receive an average of three shocks annually from their devices.[1] With more than 25,000 ICDs implanted in patients worldwide since first being introduced in 1980,[1,2] more than 100 life-saving shocks are probably delivered on any given day to prevent sudden cardiac deaths outside of hospitals. The type and duration of the shock waveforms given by these devices affect both the likelihood of successful defibrillation and the life expectancy of the ICD. To be completely successful, a defibrillation shock must stop fibrillation without reinitiating it and must not decrease cardiac function or cause myocardial necrosis.[3-6] Because there are some people for whom the shock is too weak at the highest defibrillator setting, the probability of success will increase and the likelihood of causing tissue damage or reinitiating fibrillation will lessen if the energy required for defibrillation can be reduced.[5-8] Improvements in energy requirements will lead to the development of a better ICD by: 1) allowing it to be smaller so that it can be implanted subpectorally; 2) decreasing the charge time so that the patient is hypotensive for less time before the shock is delivered; and 3) increasing the number of shocks that can be delivered before the battery is depleted. Much research is currently being done to develop more effective shock waveforms that will decrease energy requirements without reducing effectiveness.

Shape, duration, tilt, and electrical characteristics such as the leading edge voltage or current and delivered energy, are used to describe defibrillation waveforms. A monophasic truncated exponential shock waveform consists of a single pulse that decays exponentially from its initial to its final value at a rate that depends upon the capacitor in the defibrillator and the total resistance of the defibrillator-electrode-heart circuit (Figure 1, first two waveforms). In ICDs, truncated exponential waveforms were originally thought to be superior to nontruncated waveforms for defibrillation[9,10] because they avoided the refibrillatory effects of the low-voltage tail of a straight capacitor discharge.[11,12] Recent work has shown that this is true for waveforms that decay slowly, ie, those with long

---

Supported in part by the National Institutes of Health (Research Grants HL-42760, HL-44066, HL-28429, and HL-33637), the National Science Foundation Engineering (Research Center Grant CDR-86222011), the North Carolina Affiliate of the American Heart Association (Grant NC-91-G-14), the North Carolina Biotechnology Center (Grant 913-ARG-0612), and a grant from The Whitaker Foundation.

From Singer I, (ed.) Implantable Cardioverter-Defibrillator. Armonk, NY: Futura Publishing Company, Inc.; © 1994.

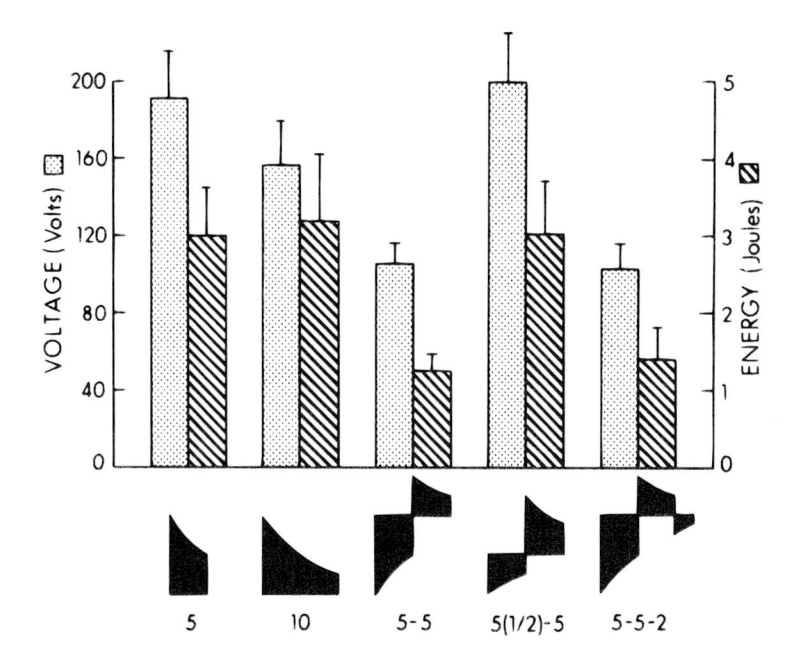

Figure 1. Defibrillation threshold (DFT) voltage and energy values for five waveforms. Shocks were delivered through large contoured patch electrodes located on the epicardial surfaces of the right ventricle (RV) and left ventricle (LV). Diagrams of the waveforms are shown at the bottom of the figure. The tops of each bar correspond to mean values with one standard deviation indicated by the lines on the top. The leading edge voltage and energy at the DFT were significantly lower for the 5-5 (both phases 5 msec in duration) biphasic and 5-5-2 (first two phases 5 msec and third phase 2 msec in duration) triphasic waveforms than for the other three waveforms. The leading edge voltage at the DFT was significantly lower for the 10-msec monophasic waveform versus the 5-msec monophasic or 5(1/2)-5 (first phase one half the leading edge voltage of the second phase) biphasic waveforms, but the energy requirements did not differ. (Reproduced and modified with permission from Reference 64.)

time constants (> 10 msec), but that waveforms with short time constants do not need to be truncated to be effective.[13] The duration of a monophasic waveform is measured as the time between the beginning and end of the pulse. Biphasic waveforms have two pulses of opposite polarity (Figure 1, third and fourth waveforms). The polarity of each phase of a waveform is determined by the defibrillator. A single capacitor can be used to create a biphasic waveform in which the trailing edge voltage of the first phase equals the leading edge voltage of the second phase (Figure 1, third waveform). Two capacitors must be used if the leading edge voltage of the second phase is equal to or larger than that of the first phase (Figure 1, fourth waveform).

Triphasic waveforms can be produced with one or more capacitors and have three pulses with the first and last pulses having the same polarity (Figure 1, last waveform). The duration of shock waveforms is expressed in terms of the duration of each phase, eg, a 3.5/2-msec (or 3.5-2) biphasic waveform has a first phase that is 3.5 msec long and a second phase that lasts for 2 msec.

Waveform tilt can be calculated by dividing the difference between the initial and final voltages of a pulse by the initial voltage value[14] and is usually expressed in terms of percent. The leading and trailing edges of low-tilt waveforms (Figure 2C) differ only slightly while high-tilt waveforms have much larger leading than trailing edge

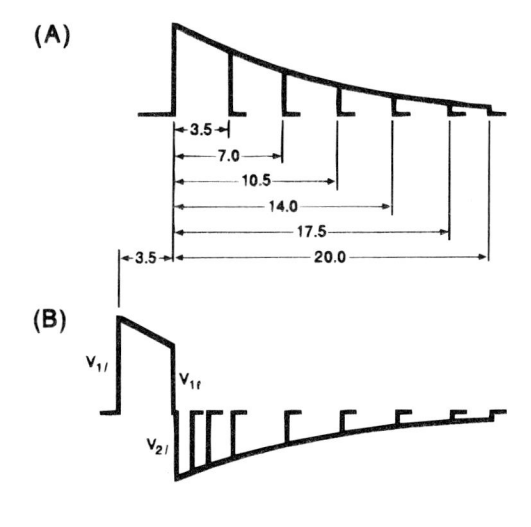

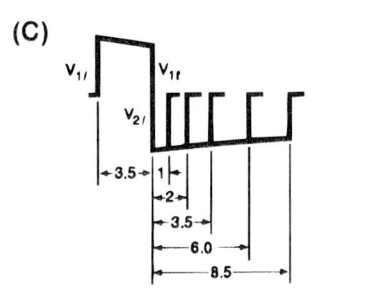

For $C = 140$ µF and $R_T = 50$ Ω, the tilt of a 3.5-msec monophasic waveform would be 39%, while the tilt of a 7-msec waveform would be 63% (Figure 2A).

The electrical properties of waveforms are described in terms of the leading edge current or voltage or the total delivered energy. Energy (E) is the integral of V∗I over the duration of the shock, where V is voltage and I is current. If the impedance (R_T) is constant then

$$E = \int \frac{V^2}{R} dt.$$

For a rectangular pulse, the delivered energy is:[14]

$$E = \left(\frac{V^2}{R_T}\right) d \text{ or } E = I^2 R_T d.$$

For a truncated monophasic waveform,

$$V = V_0 \exp\left(\frac{-d}{R_T C}\right)$$

where V_0 is the leading edge voltage.

Mechanisms of Defibrillation

New investigational tools have been responsible for much of the recent progress in understanding the basic mechanisms that describe how defibrillation works.[16,17] For example, the development of cardiac mapping systems that can record before, during, and after a defibrillation shock has allowed investigators to demonstrate that the distribution of potential gradients generated throughout the heart by a shock is an important factor for successful versus unsuccessful defibrillation attempts, and that following a shock that is slightly weaker than needed to defibrillate, the earliest postshock activations appear where the potential gradient is lowest.[18–20] Other new investigational tools that have added significantly to understanding defibrillation mechanisms are optical recording systems[21–24] and microelectrodes[25–28] that can record the action potential before and after shocks. Knowledge about the relationship between the ex-

Figure 2. Monophasic and biphasic truncated exponential waveforms. **(A)** High-tilt monophasic waveforms with durations of 3.5 to 20.0 msec. **(B)** High-tilt biphasic waveforms with a 3.5-msec first phase and second phases of 1.0–20.0 msec. **(C)** Low-tilt biphasic waveforms with a 3.5-msec first phase and 1.0- to 8.5-msec second phases. (Reproduced and modified with permission from Reference 74.)

voltages (Figure 2A and 2B). The tilt of a pulse, expressed as

$$\left[1 - \exp\left(\frac{-d}{R_T C}\right)\right] * 100\%$$

is determined by the capacitance of the defibrillator (C in mF), the total resistance (R_T in ohms), and the duration of the waveform (d in milliseconds). Due to space considerations, the capacitor in most ICDs is currently limited to 125–150 µF,[15] but a value of < 100 µF may be better for future devices.[14]

defibrillation, it is necessary to review how the potential gradient field of a shock can initiate ventricular fibrillation when it is given during the vulnerable period of normal rhythm. In a study by Frazier et al.,[40] regular pacing (S_1) was performed simultaneously from a row of eight epicardial stimulating wires located to the right of an array of 117 recording electrodes (Figure 5A). Approximately parallel activation isochrones (solid lines in Figure 5A) were created by pacing from the row of S_1 electrodes. Refractory periods to local 2-mA cathodal stimuli were similar throughout the tissue beneath the recording array (166 ± 3 msec). Therefore, isorecovery lines were also parallel (dashed lines in Figure 5A). A large premature monophasic shock (S_2), delivered from a mesh electrode spanning the bottom of the array of recording electrodes (Figure 5B), created potential gradient isolines that were perpendicular to the isorefractory lines shown in Figure 5A. S_2 shocks were given to scan the vulnerable period of the last S_1 stimulus.[41] Figure 5C shows the first activation pattern at the start of ventricular fibrillation that was initiated by giving the S_2 shock 191 msec after the last S_1 stimulus. The initial postshock activation front ended blindly in the center of the plaque at the critical point where a shock potential gradient of 5–6 V/cm intersected tissue that was just passing out of its refractory period to a 2-mA local stimulus. This front formed a functional reentrant circuit around the critical point for several cycles that then broke down into ventricular fibrillation.

Whenever a critical point is created within the myocardium, reentry will begin and either halt spontaneously after a few cycles have formed repetitive beats or lead to ventricular fibrillation.[42] This result implies there should be an ULV, ie, a shock strength above which ventricular fibrillation will not be initiated during the vulnerable period of regular rhythm because the potential gradient throughout the myocardium exceeds the critical minimum value (4–9 V/cm for a typical monophasic waveform).[18-20] The fact that this upper limit exists and that it approximately equals the defibrillation threshold (DFT) supports the ULV hypothesis as one of the mechanisms of defibrillation.[43,44]

The activation pattern by which a shock induces ventricular fibrillation during the vulnerable period of regular rhythm (Figure 5C) is similar to the activation pattern frequently observed following a failed defibrillation shock (Figure 4, E2). This similarity also supports the ULV defibrillation hypothesis. To exceed either the ULV or the DFT, the shock electric field must exceed the critical potential gradient level throughout

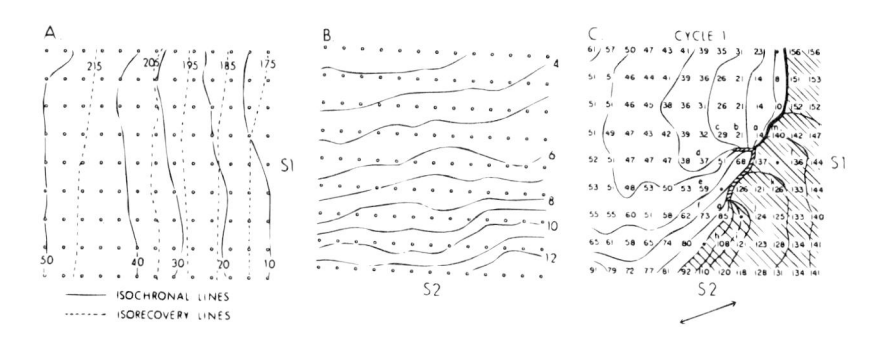

Figure 5. Initiation of reentry and ventricular fibrillation after orthogonal interaction of myocardial refractoriness and potential gradient field created by a large stimulus. **Panel A:** Distribution of activation time (solid lines) and refractoriness (dashed lines) in milliseconds during the last S_1 beat. **Panel B:** S_2 stimulus field (V/cm). **Panel C:** Initial activation pattern just after the S_2 stimulus. The hatched region is thought to be directly excited by the S_2 stimulus field. (Reproduced and modified with permission from Reference 40.)

the myocardium to ensure that no critical points are formed that can produce functional circuits which lead to ventricular fibrillation. The one or two rapid responses sometimes observed following a successful defibrillation shock may correspond to the repetitive responses observed following a shock during the vulnerable period of regular rhythm.

The effects of shocks on action potentials have been measured to determine how reentrant circuits form around a critical point.[25,26,28,45–47] In one study, the array of electrodes shown in Figure 5 was split into two pieces that were separated by a small opening. A monophasic action potential (MAP) electrode was used to record action potentials at various sites along this opening (Figure 6).[47] The shock directly excited tissue where the potential gradient was sufficiently high and the myocardium was sufficiently recovered. A strength interval curve with stimulus strength expressed in terms of potential gradient was derived from this study and was used to estimate what portion of the tissue in Figure 5C was sufficiently recovered and exposed to a sufficiently large potential gradient to be directly excited by the S_2 shock (hatched area). In the top half of Figure 5C, where the myocardium was exposed to a potential gradient that was less than the critical value of 5–6 V/cm, the more recovered tissue to the right was directly excited, while the less recovered, more highly refractory tissue to the left was not. After the shock, an activation front formed at the border of the directly excited region and propagated from right to left into the tissue that was not directly excited by the shock.

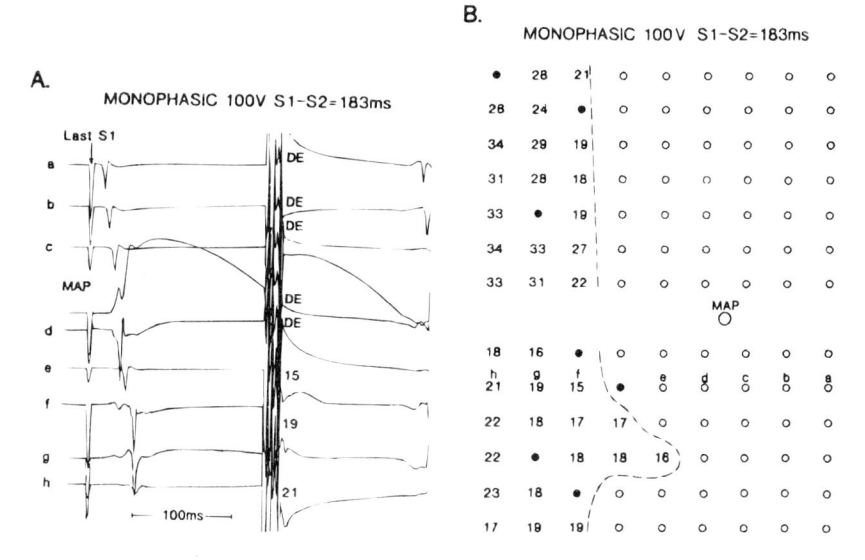

Figure 6. Panel A shows recordings from MAP electrode and 8 plaque electrodes located as shown in Panel B. S_1 and S_2 electrodes are on right side. Activations recorded after last S_1 stimulus indicate that an activation front spread away from S_1 pacing side. Gain and voltage divider circuit change artifacts appear before and after the 75-V S_2 shock. Electrodes a-e and the monophasic action potential (MAP) electrode are over tissue directly excited by the S_2 shock. An activation front spreads away from the directly excited (DE) border (between e and f) to g and h. S_2 activation times, measured in milliseconds after the S_2 stimulus, are indicated above electrograms for electrodes not DE. **Panel B** is the S_2 activation map. The 9 × 13 electrode plaque has a 15-mm gap between middle rows for the MAP electrode. Open circles: electrodes over directly excited tissue. Filled circles: bad electrodes. S_2 activation times are displayed at electrode sites for electrodes recording from tissue not DE by S_2. Dashed lines show the DE border from which an activation front propagates toward the left. (Reproduced with permission from Reference 47.)

Intriguingly, an activation front did not propagate away from the directly excited region in the lower half of Figure 5C where the potential gradient was greater than the critical value of 5–6 V/cm. The explanation for this appears to be that action potential prolongation (also known as a graded response)[48] and refractory period extension were induced by the shock field in the myocardium just to the left of the directly excited region (Figure 7) in tissue that was exposed to a shock field greater than the critical value.[28,46] Shock potential gradients greater than the critical value prolong action potential duration and hence the refractory period by an amount that increases as the potential gradient is increased and/or as the S_1-S_2 interval is increased (Figure 8A). Almost no refractory period extension is observed for potential gradients less than the critical value. At longer S_1-S_2 intervals, direct excitation takes place while at shorter

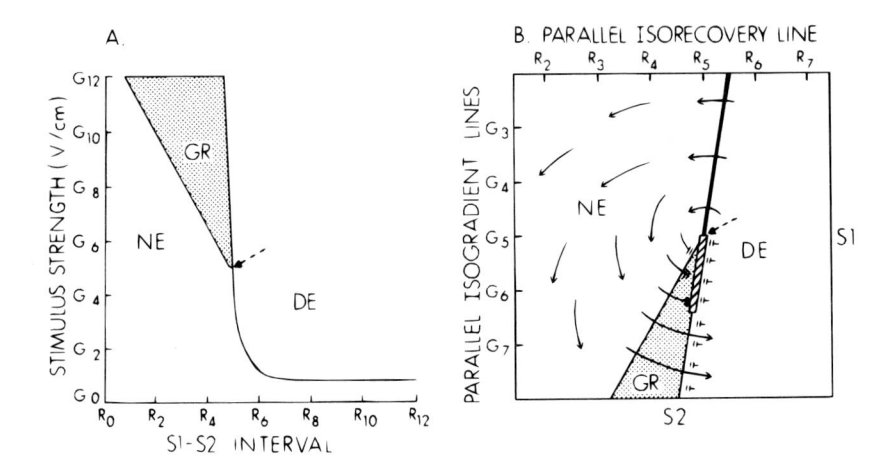

Figure 7. Graded response theory for reentry. **Panel A:** Strength interval curve. A modified strength interval curve is shown with stimulus strength in volts per centimeter on the y axis and S_1-S_2 interval, or refractoriness, on the x axis. On the y axis, G_{12} represents the largest potential gradient and G_0 the smallest. On the x axis, R_{12} represents the most recovered tissue and R_0 the most refractory. R_0 does not represent phase 0 of the action potential, but merely tissue fully refractory to a premature stimulus. Interaction of the isorecovery and isogradient lines produces either direct excitation (DE), graded response (GR), or neither effect (NE). The potential gradient at G_5 is ≈ 5 V/cm while the potential gradient at the rheobase is ≈ 0.8 V/cm.[87] The critical refractory period (for the 2 mA stimuli) equals the preshock interval at R_5. The dashed arrow represents the position of the critical point in this panel and in Panel B. **Panel B:** Perpendicular isorecovery and isogradient lines. A diagrammatic representation of the results of Figure 5C is shown, with gradient and refractory values corresponding to the diagram in A. The row of pacing wires (S_1) on the right creates parallel isorecovery lines (R_7 through R_2) with R_7 the least refractory R_2 the most refractory. The S_2 from the bottom creates parallel isogradient lines (G_7 through G_3) with G_7 the largest gradient and G_3 the weakest. The solid and hatched lines are the frame (which separates beats) and block lines, respectively. The lines with double bars at the end represent areas of temporary unidirectional conduction block. For this idealized diagram, the S_1-S_2 interval equals the recovery period (preshock interval equals the critical refractory period) at R_5, and the S_2 voltage creates a potential gradient of 5 V/cm at G_5. The S_2 shock directly excites the area near the S_1 site (DE) and produces a region of graded response (GR). Activation fronts only propagate away from part of the directly excited area. Activation fronts do not propagate away from the directly excited area abutting regions of graded response, thus forming an area of temporary unidirectional conduction block. An activation front conducting towards the S_2 site from the early sites of activation produces another region of conduction block (hatched line) when it enters tissue insufficiently repolarized from graded response or direct excitation. When the myocardium has recovered, activation can conduct through this area and form a reentrant circuit, as shown by the arrows spanning the GR zone and entering the DE zone. (Reproduced and modified with permission from Reference 40.)

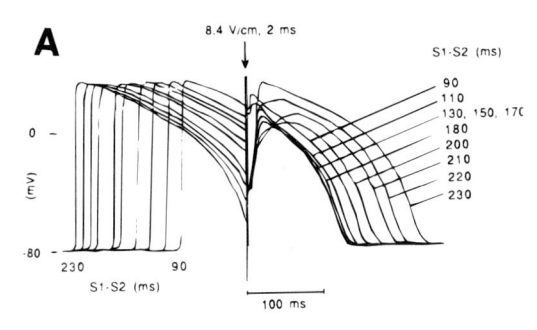

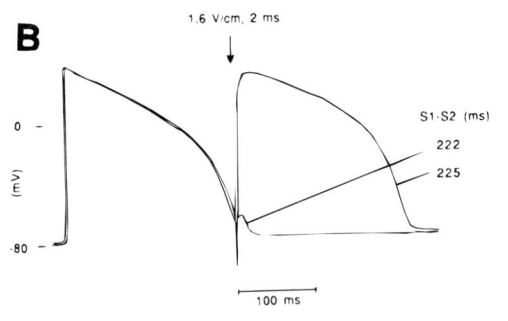

Figure 8. Panel A illustrates a range of action potential extensions produced by an S_2 stimulus having a strength of 8.4 V/cm oriented along fibers. The action potential recordings, which were obtained from one cellular impalement, are aligned with the S_2 time. An S_1 stimulus was applied 3 msec before phase zero of each recording. The longest and shortest S_1-S_2 intervals tested, 230 and 90 msec, are indicated with their respective phase zero depolarizations. The S_1-S_2 intervals for each response after S_2 are indicated to the right. Panel B shows recordings that illustrate the response to an S_2 stimulus of 1.6 V/cm oriented along the fibers. The two S_2 aligned recordings were obtained from the same cell as in panel A. The S_1-S_2 stimulus intervals for each of the responses are indicated to the right of the recordings. The responses were markedly different depending on a change in the S_2 timing of only 3 msec. An S_1-S_2 interval of 222 msec produced only a small response, whereas an S_1-S_2 interval of 225 msec produced a new action potential. (Modified and reprinted with permission from Reference 28.)

S_1-S_2 intervals no response is observed (Figure 8B). Refractory period extension is thought to affect defibrillation in two ways: 1) since new action potentials are prevented, propagating activation fronts do not form immediately following the shock[21,38,39] and/or 2) since refractory period extension is greater for those cells that are less recovered, the dispersion of refractoriness is greatly decreased by the shock making it more likely that any activation fronts present immediately after the shock will die out rather than form a new reentrant pathway.[49]

The amount of action potential prolongation for four different potential gradients generated by a monophasic shock are shown in Figure 9. The data from Figure 9 were used to estimate the distribution of intracellular potentials immediately after the shock (Figure 10) for the configuration shown in Figure 5. In the upper portion of Figure 10, where the potential gradient was less than the critical value, there was a large change in transmembrane potential at the boundary of the directly excited region with a transmembrane potential of +25 mV on the excited side of the border very close to a transmembrane potential of −64 mV on the nonexcited side of the border. Thus, intracellular current crossed from the cells that were directly excited to those cells that were not excited and initiated a propagating activation front at the border between those cells. There was no abrupt change in transmembrane potential in the region in which the electric field was greater than the critical potential gradient (Figure 5B) due to the range of prolongation of action potentials (Figure 8A). In tissue exposed to a shock field greater than the critical value there was no region where excited cells were adjacent to nonexcited cells with an abrupt change in transmembrane potential at the boundary. An activation front will not occur immediately after the shock in an area where the potential gradient produced by the S_2 is higher than the critical value. At a later time, the high-potential gradient region undergoing action potential prolongation will have recovered enough for the activation front arising in the low-potential gradient region to sweep down to excite it. When the region to the right that was directly excited by the S_2 shock has recovered (hatched in Figure 5C), the activation front can pivot into that region and eventually reach its origin at the top center (Figure 7).

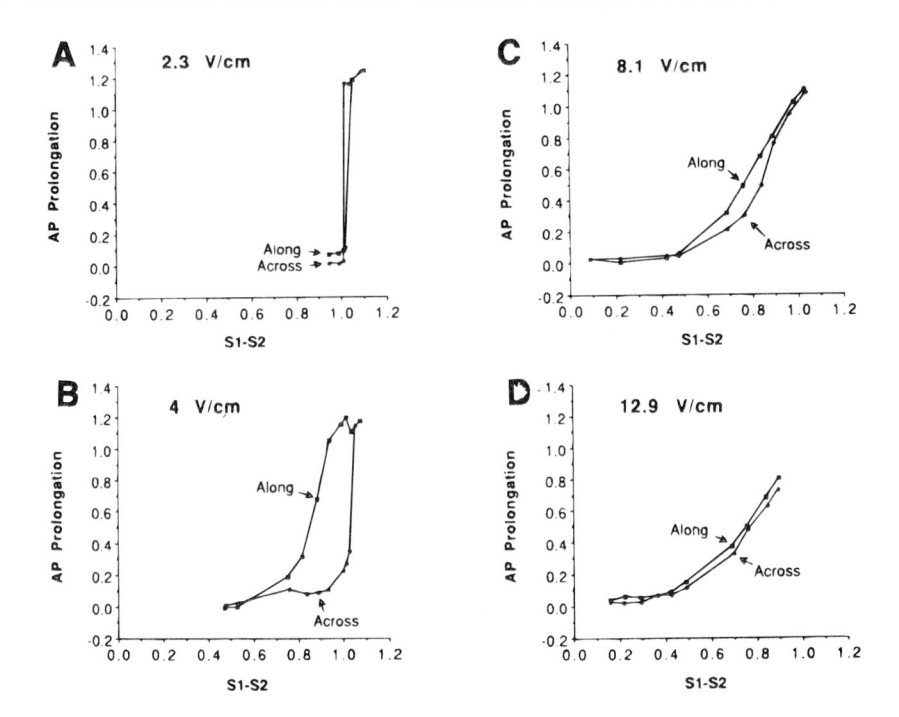

Figure 9. Action potential (AP) prolongation versus the S_1-S_2 interval for S_2 fields of 2.3, 4, 8.1, and 12.9 V/cm. Each data point represents a different trial from one cellular impalement. S_1-S_2 interval and action potential prolongation are given as fractions of control AP duration at 90% repolarization. **Panel A:** The 2.3 V/cm S_2 given as late as the time of 90% repolarization produced only a small AP prolongation. When this strength S_2 was given only 2–3 msec later, a new AP was produced. **Panel B:** The 4 V/cm S_2 produced slight action potential prolongation when given at intermediate S_1-S_2 intervals that was greater for potential gradient oriented along than across fibers. **Panel C:** The 8.1 V/cm S_2 produced a greater AP prolongation. **Panel D:** AP prolongation occurred for the 12.9 V/cm S_2 given as early as the midpoint of the AP. For this S_2 strength, AP prolongation was not markedly different for potential gradient vectors along versus across fibers. (Reprinted with permission from Reference 28.)

Thus, the activation front completes the first postshock cycle of reentry by propagating around the critical point, although reentry first occurred when the front entered the directly excited region at the bottom of the plaque. The role of action potential prolongation in reentry induction has been demonstrated in a recent study that used a voltage sensitive fluorescent dye and a laser scanner system to record 64 simultaneous transmembrane action potentials.[50] The results showed the close spatial correlation between the center of the reentrant circuit and the boundary between the region of direct excitation and the region of action potential prolongation.

A floating microelectrode method in which a glass microelectrode was attached to a flexible fine wire to record the intracellular potential in a region with known potential gradient in the in vivo dog heart, has been used to show that a 5-V/cm monophasic shock field has the same effects during ventricular fibrillation as it does during paced rhythms.[26] At longer coupling intervals, direct excitation occurs, while at very short coupling intervals no response is seen. Action potential prolongation occurs at intermediate coupling intervals. Thus, depending upon the state of the myocardium and the strength of the shock field in different parts of the heart, some portions may be directly excited while more highly refractory cells may have their action potentials

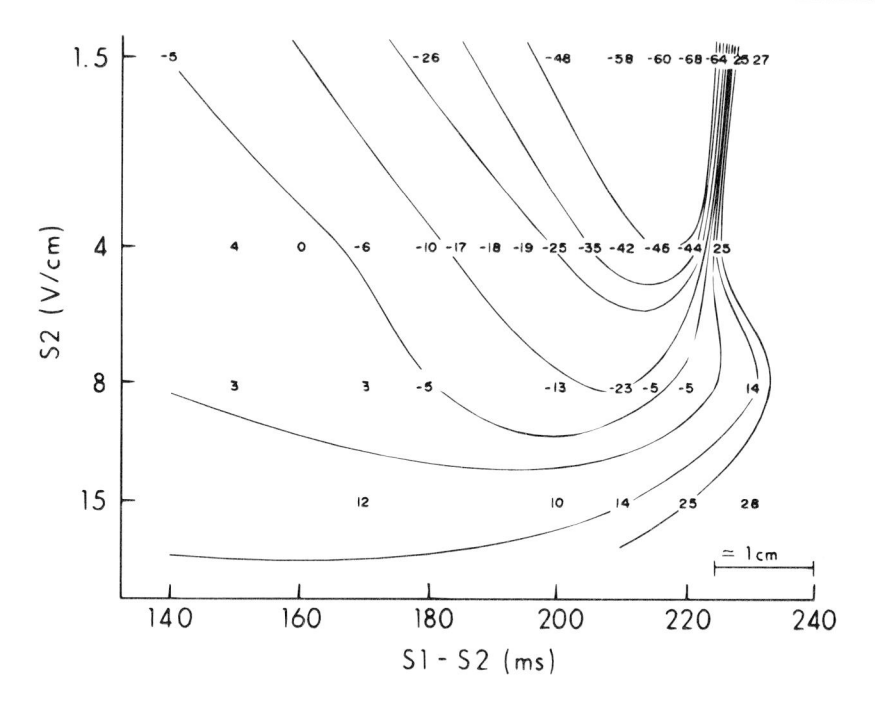

Figure 10. Intracellular potentials immediately after the S_2 stimulation shown in Figure 5 estimated from the data in Figure 9. Isopotential contours, determined by bivariate polynomial interpolation and smoothing by hand, represent intracellular potentials from -45 to 25 mV in 10-mV increments. Contours for intracellular potentials more negative than -45 mV are not shown. Where S_2 potential gradient is ≤ 4 V/cm, an abrupt boundary (upper right) occurs between tissue that is directly excited by S_2 and tissue that is not directly excited. A large intracellular potential gradient at the boundary, about 0.5 V/cm, can account for the initiation of propagation from right to left in this region in Figure 2C. The large intracellular potential gradient at the boundary is comparable to that which occurs at a propagating activation front in normal tissue. In the region having an S_2 potential gradient ≥ 8 V/cm, there is no abrupt boundary between high- and low-intracellular potentials. Instead, on the line of an S_2 potential gradient of 15 V/cm, the largest intracellular potential gradient, ignoring discontinuities of intracellular resistance, is only 0.017 V/cm. Also, intracellular potentials on the 15 V/cm line are in the range in that sodium current is inactivated. The absence of a large intracellular potential gradient and the presence of intracellular potentials that inactivate sodium current (important for propagation) may explain the absence of propagation after a shock where the electric field strength during the shock is high. (Reprinted with permission from Reference 28.)

prolonged, and some cells early in their absolute refractory period may be relatively unaffected by the shock. Depending upon the distribution of these regions of myocardium, activation fronts occurring at the border of directly excited regions may lead to resumption of ventricular fibrillation and to failure of the defibrillation shock.

Not all defibrillation failures can be explained by the ULV critical point hypothesis. In some cases after a failed defibrillation shock, earliest activation appears to arise by a focal mechanism from the region of low-potential gradient (Figure 11) rather than by conduction away from the border of a directly activated region (Figure 5C). This has been observed both in two-dimensional epicardial maps[20] as well as in three-dimensional intramural maps with 5-mm between electrodes.[51] It is not known if shock-induced triggered activity is the source of these foci. In a few cases, defibrillation may fail because of activation fronts that arise from the high-, not the low-potential gradient region. Activation fronts originating from the high-gradient region adjacent to

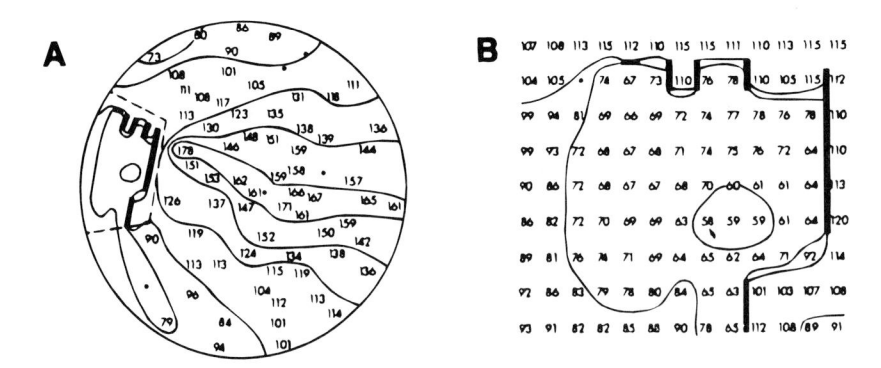

Figure 11. Isochronal maps from the sock are shown in panel A and from the plaque electrodes in panel B for the first activation after a monophasic shock that produced potential gradient of 1.6 V/cm beneath the plaque displayed in the same manner as in Figure 4E. After the shock, the activation fronts of ventricular fibrillation were halted, and new postshock fronts arose in a focal pattern, near the center of the plaque for the first three postshock cycles. (Modified and reprinted with permission from Reference 20.)

the defibrillation electrode have been mapped during ventricular tachycardia that occurred after a successful defibrillation shock (Figure 12).[19]

Monophasic Truncated Exponential Waveforms

The effectiveness of monophasic truncated exponential waveforms for defibrillation has been studied extensively (Table 1). Wessale et al.[52] demonstrated that peak current dose (peak current divided by body weight) increased with decreasing pulse duration (20 msec to 2 msec) and increasing tilt (< 5% to 80%) when shocks were given through a bipolar catheter with electrodes in the apex of the RV and superior vena cava (SVC) of dogs. In a study with a transvenous catheter in the RV to subcutaneous patch system in dogs, shorter pulse durations resulted in lower defibrillation energy requirements for monophasic truncated exponential waveforms with fixed pulse width and variable tilt.[53] Lower threshold voltages were associated with durations in the middle of the range when compared with the shortest (2.5 msec) and longest (20 msec) pulse width durations. With this

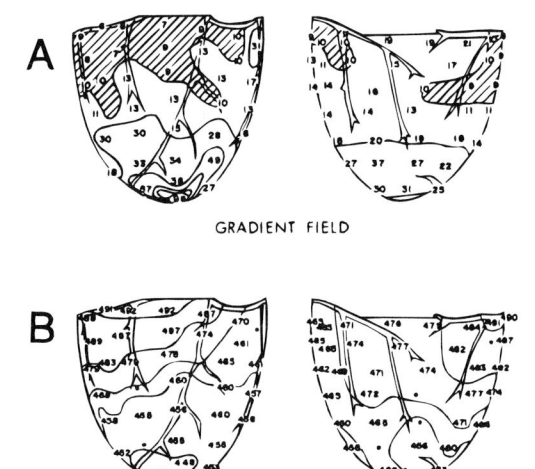

Figure 12. Panel A: Potential gradient field for a 284-V shock via a cathode on the left ventricular (LV) apex and dual anodes on the right atrium (RA) and LV base in a dog. Anterior view to left, posterior to right. Cross-hatched area indicates region with potential gradient ≤ 10 V/cm. Isopotential lines are 10 V/cm apart. **Panel B:** Map of second beat of ventricular tachycardia after defibrillation shock shown in panel A indicates origin of tachycardia adjacent to apical shock electrode. The potential gradient = 57 V/cm at this site; 10-msec isochronal lines. (Modified and reprinted with permission from Reference 19.)

Table 1
Defibrillation Thresholds for 5-ms Monophasic Truncated Exponential Waveforms

Study	Species	Energy (J)	Voltage (V)
Jones et al.[88]	Rabbit[a]	0.18 ± 0.13	51.7 ± 4.4
Chen et al.[37]	Dog[b]	6.8 ± 2.9	
	Dog[c]	10.9 ± 4.3	
	Dog[d]	6.4 ± 2.3	
Chen et al.[89]	Dog[e]	7.5 ± 4.2	
	Dog[f]	14.1 ± 5.7	
Dixon et al.[64]	Dog[g]	3.0 ± 1.6	191 ± 55
Chapman et al.[53]	Dog[h]	18	632
Saksena et al.[90]	Dog[i]	12.9 ± 5.1	691 ± 154
Jones et al.[59]	Pig[j]	27.2 ± 9.1	
	Pig[k]	16.5 ± 9.1	
Wyse et al.[91]	Human[l]	21.1 ± 9.3	516 ± 117

[a] RV [+], LV [−]; 1.1 cm² epicardial patches on isolated hearts; square wave
[b] RA [+], RV apex [−]; 4.5 cm² epicardial patches; 7% tilt
[c] LA [+], RV apex [−]; 4.5 cm² epicardial patches; 7% tilt
[d] RV apex [+], RA [−]; 4.5 cm² epicardial patches; 7% tilt
[e] RA [+], LV apex [−]; 4.5 cm² epicardial patches; 7% tilt
[f] RV base [+], LV base [−]; 4.5 cm² epicardial patches; 7% tilt
[g] LV [+], RV [−]; Contoured epicardial patches − RV [33 cm²], LV [39 cm²]
[h] Subcutaneous patch [13.9 cm²] on left thorax [+], catheter [4 cm² electrode 4 mm from tip] at RV apex [−]; Nonthoracotomy
[i] Subcutaneous patch [13 cm²] on left lateral thorax [+], catheter [6 cm²] at RV apex [−]; Nonthoracotomy
[j] Catheter at SVC [+], epicardial patch [2.5 cm²] at LV apex [−]; trapezoidal waveforms
[k] LV free wall [+], RV free wall [−]; 2.5 cm² epicardial patches
[l] Skin patch [50.4 cm²] in left axilla [+], catheter [4.26 cm²] at RV apex [−]; Nonthoracotomy; 65% tilt.

catheter patch electrode system, pulse durations of 5–15 msec were associated with the best combination of low initial voltage (596–632 V), low energy (18–25 J), and low average current (5–7 A).

Small improvements in defibrillation efficacy were found for sequential shocks with monophasic waveforms of the same magnitude, duration, and polarity that were separated in time (Figure 13).[53] The optimum separation between two shocks was approximately 85% of the activation rate during fibrillation.[39] Pulses have also been separated in both time and space to attempt to achieve a more uniform field and thus reduce defibrillation energy by summing this energy both temporally and spatially.[54]

Sequential pulses given through separate lead systems have resulted in lower DFTs than single pulses given simultaneously through the same lead systems.[55-59] When the separation time between shocks was between 0.2 and 1 msec, the effect of delivering sequential shocks was optimized, but the advantage disappeared if the shocks were separated by more than 10 msec.[60]

Four different electrode configurations were used to determine that a minimum potential gradient of 6–7 V/cm was needed for defibrillation with a 14-msec 16%–tilt monophasic waveform.[19] Another study found that a minimum potential gradient of approximately 6 V/cm was needed to defibrillate with a 10-msec truncated exponen-

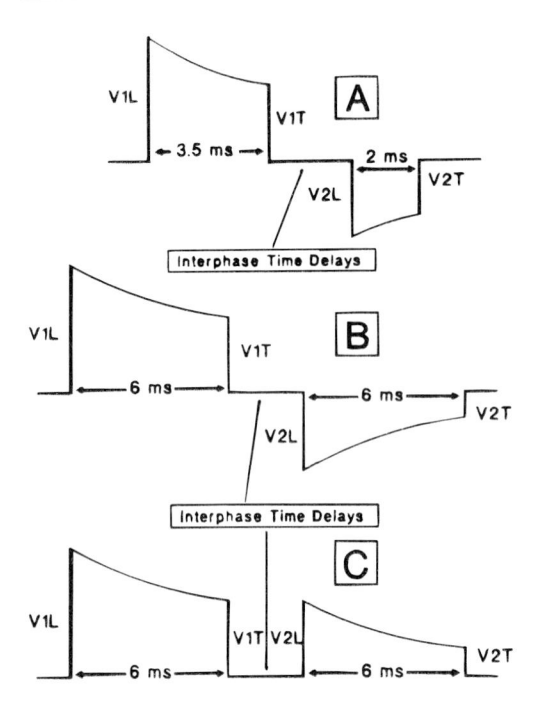

Figure 13. Monophasic and biphasic waveforms with time delays between phases. **Panel A:** Interphase time delays of 0, 1, 2, 3, 4, 6, 8, and 10 msec were used to separate a 3.5/2-msec biphasic waveform into two parts. **Panel B:** Interphase time delays of 0, 2, 3, 4, and 5 msec were used to separate a 6/6-msec biphasic waveform into two parts. **Panel C:** Two monophasic shocks were separated by time periods of 0, 5, 10, 15, 20, 25, 50, and 100 msec. For all waveforms, the leading edge voltage of phase 2 (V2L) was set equal to the trailing edge voltage of phase 1 (V1T). (Reprinted with permission from Reference 84.)

tial monophasic waveform.[20] In order to raise the minimum potential gradient of the heart to 6 V/cm, parts of the myocardium must be subjected to much higher potential gradients that can damage the myocardium and induce arrhythmias.[61] Conduction block occurred in dogs in regions where the potential gradient generated by a 10-msec truncated exponential monophasic waveform exceeded 64 ± 4 V/cm with longer periods of block occurring in regions with higher potential gradients.[7] Block occurred for as long as 15 seconds in regions exposed to a potential gradient of 148 ± 6 V/cm. Necrosis and other severe forms of damage probably occur in regions with high-potential gradients. The ratio of the potential gradient above which detrimental effects occurred to the minimum potential gradient needed for defibrillation, ie, the safety factor,[62] was approximately 10:1 (64:6 V/cm) for these monophasic waveforms.

Biphasic Truncated Exponential Waveforms

Monophasic waveforms of the same total duration (Table 2) or with equal phase durations (Table 3) as biphasic waveforms generally require more voltage and energy for internal ventricular defibrillation in animals and humans[63–68] and are also inferior to biphasics for external ventricular[69,70] and atrial defibrillation.[71] However, not all monophasic waveforms are inferior to all biphasic waveforms.[64,72–75] Biphasic waveforms that deliver more charge in the first versus the second phase are better since those that deliver more charge in the second phase require a higher voltage and more energy for defibrillation than do monophasic waveforms of the same total duration.[75] Internal ventricular, external ventricular, and internal atrial defibrillation all use different biphasic waveforms to achieve the lowest DFT.[69–71] Thus, there is not one single best biphasic waveform for all lead configurations and for both internal and external defibrillation.

One possible explanation for why biphasic waveforms are generally more effective than monophasics is that the undesirable effects found in the high-potential gradient regions are milder for biphasics. In a study by Yabe et al.,[7] epicardial patches on the RV and RA were used to deliver high-strength 10-msec monophasic and 5/5-msec biphasic shocks in which the leading edge voltage of the second phase was approximately 75% of the leading edge voltage of the first phase. Conduction block did not occur until a higher potential gradient (71 ± 6 V/cm) was reached for the biphasic shock than for the monophasic shock (64 ±

Table 2
Defibrillation Thresholds in Dogs for Monophasic and Biphasic Waveforms with Equal Total Durations

Study	Monophasic Time (msec)	Monophasic Energy (J)	Monophasic Voltage (V)	Biphasic Time (msec)	Biphasic Energy (J)	Biphasic Voltage (V)
[a] Daubert et al.[47]	3	4.14 ± 1.7	345 ± 78	2/1, S	2.9 ± 1.3	299 ± 73
[b] Feeser et al.[74]	7	1.43 ± 0.78	137.5 ± 35.4	3.5/3.5, S	0.75 ± 0.28	101.5 ± 18.9
	10.5	1.83 ± 0.65	149.4 ± 27.3	3.5/7.0, S	4.61 ± 2.33	228.7 ± 69.3
	10.5	2.36 ± 1.26	171.3 ± 42.4	7.0/3.5, S	0.98 ± 0.45	111.2 ± 23.2
	10.5	2.36 ± 1.26	171.3 ± 42.4	7.0/3.5, D	1.29 ± 0.57	98.5 ± 22.5
	14	4.01 ± 1.12	164.6 ± 44.8	3.5/10.5, S	6.30 ± 3.69	258.8 ± 83.6
	14	2.77 ± 1.14	177.8 ± 35.1	7.0/7.0, S	1.19 ± 0.40	116.9 ± 21.3
	14	2.77 ± 1.14	177.8 ± 35.1	7.0/7.0, D	1.99 ± 1.01	113.8 ± 29.3
	17.5	4.46 ± 1.54	184.8 ± 58.6	3.5/14.0, S	9.20 ± 4.53	315.1 ± 88.8
	17.5	2.44 ± 1.06	165.2 ± 37.0	7.0/10.5, S	2.37 ± 1.67	156.6 ± 55.7
	17.5	2.44 ± 1.06	165.2 ± 37.0	7.0/10.5, D	4.82 ± 2.89	167.8 ± 53.0
[c] Dixon et al.[64]	10	3.2 ± 1.9	159 ± 48	5/5, S	1.3 ± 0.4	106 ± 22
[d] Chapman et al.[86]	10	21.1	585	5/5	10.1	410
[e] Kavanagh et al.[63]	12	17.4 ± 8.0	424 ± 117	6/6, S	6.4 ± 2.6	266 ± 51
				6/6, D	18.0 ± 8.0	336 ± 76

S = 1-capacitor biphasic waveform
D = 2-capacitor biphasic waveform

[a] RV [+], LV [−]; 10 cm² epicardial patches; low tilt
[b] LV [+], RV [−]; Contoured epidcardial patches − RV [33 cm²], LV [39 cm²]; High tilt
[c] LV [+], RV [−]; Contoured epicardial patches − RV [33 cm²], LV [39 cm²]
[d] Subcutaneous patch [13.9 cm²] on left thorax [+], catheter [4 cm² electrode 4 mm from tip] at RV apex [−]; Nonthoracotomy
[e] Cutaneous R2 patch [113 cm²] on left thorax [+], catheters [3.7 cm² electrodes 5 mm from tip] in RV apex [−] and RV outflow tract [−]; Nonthoracotomy

4 V/cm). When a 5/5-msec biphasic waveform with a first phase leading edge voltage 10 times higher than the leading edge voltage of the second phase was tested, less conduction block occurred, but a higher voltage was required for the DFT. Thus, the effect of the high-potential gradient may not be the sole reason for the better performance of biphasic waveforms. When 850-V monophasic and biphasic shocks were given from the same mesh electrode adjacent to an array of recording electrodes, electrode sites located near the shocking electrode recovered sooner from the biphasic than from the monophasic shock (Figure 14). The higher tolerance that cardiac tissue has for biphasic shocks may explain the increased defibrillation efficacy since a biphasic waveform is less likely to cause block and reentry in the high-potential gradient area around the shocking electrode than a monophasic waveform with the same voltage. In a study by Cates et al.,[76] a 400-V (leading edge voltage) 5/5-msec biphasic shock was delivered to pigs through a defibrillating catheter in the RV and a cutaneous patch on the left lateral thorax. This biphasic shock induced postshock arrhythmias following successful shocks only 10% of the time, while it was able to defibrillate 80% of the time. An 800-V 10-msec monophasic shock also defibrillated 80% of the time, but induced

Table 3
Defibrillation Thresholds for Monophasic and Biphasic Waveforms with Equal Phase Durations

Study	Monophasic Time (msec)	Monophasic Energy (J)	Monophasic Voltage (V)	Biphasic Time (msec)	Biphasic Energy (J)	Biphasic Voltage (V)
Rabbit						
[a] Jones et al.[88]	5	0.18 ± 0.03	51.7 ± 4.4	5/5	0.12 ± 0.01	38.2 ± 2.2
Dog						
[b] Dixon et al.[64]	5	3.0 ± 1.6	191 ± 55	5/5, S	1.3 ± 0.4	106 ± 22
[c] Saksena et al.[90]	5	12.9 ± 5.1	691 ± 154	5/5, S	8.0 ± 3.2	488 ± 100
	5[d]	14.8 ± 4.9	717 ± 114	5/5, S	10.7 ± 3.4	543 ± 101
[e] Cooper et al.[84]				6/6, S	7.8 ± 1.1	307 ± 24
[f] Guse et al.[92]				6/6, S	7.2 ± 4.3	285 ± 63
				6/6, S[g]	8.5 ± 2.6	322 ± 52
				6/6, S[h]	7.0 ± 1.2	283 ± 27
				6/6, S[i]	3.2 ± 1.6	158 ± 32
				6/6, S[j]	8.0 ± 4.2	235 ± 51
Pig						
[k] Hillsley et al.[80]	6	5.62 ± 2.70		6/6	2.74 ± 1.26	
	16	8.41 ± 2.09		16/16	18.7 ± 12.3	
Human						
[l] Wyse et al.[91]	5	21.1 ± 9.3	516 ± 117	5/5	12.3 ± 5.3	407 ± 101
[m] Bardy et al.[68]	5.9	6.7 ± 4.9		5.7/5.7	4.8 ± 4.1	
	[n]8.6	20.0 ± 11.5		8.6/9.0	15.6 ± 7.2	
	[o]10.3	34.3 ± 10.4		10.2/10.4	23.4 ± 11.1	

S = 1-capacitor biphasic waveform

[a] RV [+], LV [−]; 1.1 cm² epicardial patches on isolated hearts; square wave

[b] LV [+], RV [−]; Contoured epicardial patches − RV [33 cm²], LV [39 cm²]

[c] Subcutaneous patch [13 cm²] on left lateral thorax [+], catheter [6 cm²] at RV apex [−]; V2L = 0.5 V1L; Nonthoracotomy

[d] Subcutaneous patch [13 cm²] on left lateral thorax [+], catheter [5 cm²] at SVC [+], catheter [6 cm²] at RV apex [−]; V2L = 0.5 V1L; Nonthoracotomy

[e] Cutaneous R2 patch [113 cm²] on left lateral thorax [+], catheter [6.17 cm² electrode] in RV apex [−]; Nonthoracotomy

[f] Cutaneous R2 patch [42 cm²] on left lateral thorax [+], catheter [5.4 cm² electrode] in LV apex [−]; Nonthoracotomy

[g] Cutaneous R2 patch [42 cm²] on left lateral thorax [+], catheter [5.4 cm² electrode] in RV apex [−]; Nonthoracotomy

[h] Cutaneous R2 patch [42 cm²] on left lateral thorax [+], catheters [5.4 cm² electrode] in RV apex [−] and RV outflow tract [−]; Nonthoracotomy

[i] Four cutaneous R2 patches [42 cm²], one each on left lateral, right lateral, anterior, and posterior thorax [+], catheter [5.4 cm² electrode] in LV apex [−]; Nonthoracotomy

[j] Four cutaneous R2 patches [42 cm²] one each on left lateral, right lateral, anterior, and posterior thorax [+], catheter [5.4 cm² electrode] in RV apex [−]; Nonthoracotomy

[k] Epicardial patch on RV [+], epicardial patch on LV [−]; square waves

[l] Skin patch [50.24 cm²] in left axilla [+], catheter [4.26 cm²] at RV apex [−]; Nonthoracotomy; 65% tilt

[m] Epicardial patch on RV [+], epicardial patch on LV [−]; 65% tilt

[n] Catheter in coronary sinus [+], catheter in RV apex [−]; 65% tilt; Nonthoracotomy

[o] Catheter in RV apex [+], chest patch on left lateral thorax [−]; 65% tilt; Nonthoracotomy

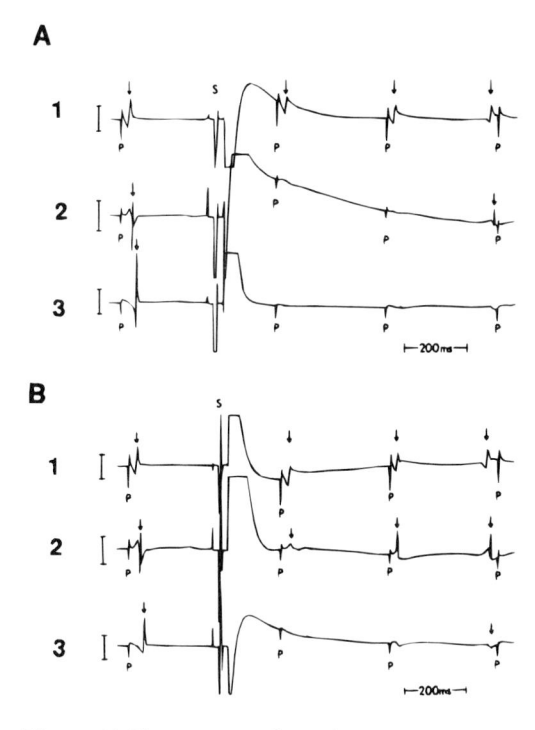

Figure 14. Electrograms from three selected electrode sites (1, 2, 3) following 850-V monophasic (Panel A1) and biphasic (Panel B1) shocks delivered through a mesh epicardial electrode adjacent to an array of recording electrodes. Site 3 was closest to the shocking electrode while site 1 was farthest away. The potential gradients during each shock were 54, 63, and 145 V/cm at sites 1, 2, and 3, respectively. **Panel A:** The third postshock cycle was spontaneous and occurred before the pacing stimulus, but did not propagate to site 3. The pacing stimuli did not result in activations at sites 2 and 3. **Panel B:** The third postshock cycle was also spontaneous after the biphasic shock and also occurred before the pacing stimulus. The second pacing stimulus resulted in activation at site 2. P: pacing artifacts; S: shock; arrows: activations; vertical bars: 10 mV. (Modified and reprinted with permisson from Reference 7.)

postshock arrhythmias in 45% of the successful defibrillation attempts.

Another possible hypothesis is that the minimum potential gradient required to defibrillate is lower for biphasic than for monophasic waveforms. In a study by Zhou et al.[20] (Figure 4), a minimum potential gradient of 5.4 ± 0.8 V/cm (measured at epicardial electrodes) was required for 10-msec monophasic shocks to defibrillate 80% of the time, while 5/5-msec biphasic shocks could defibrillate just as effectively with a potential gradient of only 2.7 ± 0.3 V/cm. Similar results occurred in another study that used 58 plunge needles (with a total of 116 recording electrodes) inserted transmurally through the ventricular walls of six dogs to determine the potential gradient in three dimensions.[77] This study found that the minimum potential gradient needed for defibrillation with a 6/6-msec biphasic waveform was 2.5 ± 0.5 V/cm. Both of these values for defibrillation with biphasic shocks are markedly less than the 4–9 V/cm that has been reported to be necessary for monophasic defibrillation.[18–20] The hypothesis that the minimum potential gradient required for biphasic defibrillation is lower is also supported by the finding that both the ULV and the DFT are lower for a 3.5/2-msec biphasic than for a 5.5-msec monophasic waveform.[78]

A third hypothesis that may explain the enhanced efficacy of biphasic shocks is that biphasic waveforms can stimulate myocardium better than monophasic waveforms. Long biphasic waveforms (≥ 20 msec in total duration) are inferior to monophasics for defibrillation (see the 16-msec monophasic and 16/16-msec biphasic waveforms under Hillsley et al. in Table 3). Biphasics are generally less able to excite myocardium than monophasics for total durations ≤ 12 msec even though such short biphasics are usually better able to defibrillate.[27] This finding has been confirmed by several different experiments. The effective refractory period was longer and the strength interval curve was shifted to the right for 3.5/2-msec biphasic versus 5.5-msec monophasic waveforms when epicardial defibrillation electrodes were used in dogs.[78]

The biphasic curve was also located to the right of the monophasic curve by 8 ± 4 msec (Figure 15) when field stimulation techniques were used to determine the strength duration curves for 2/1-msec biphasic and 3-msec monophasic waveforms. This indicates that the biphasic waveform

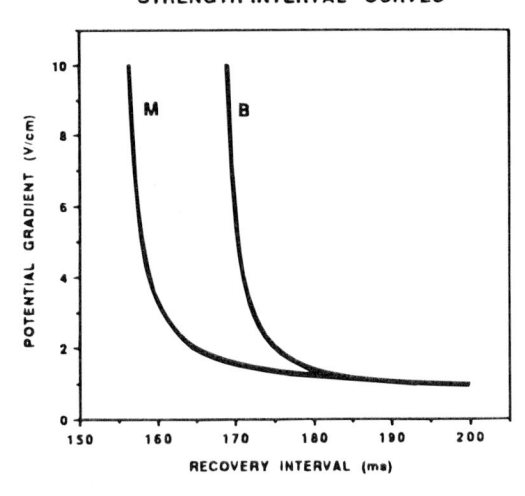

Figure 15. Monophasic and biphasic strength interval curves for a dog. Biphasic curve (B) is to the right of the monophasic (M) indicating the biphasic waveform is less able to directly excite relatively refractory myocardium. The absolute refractory period is the y-asymptote of the strength interval curve, and the diastolic threshold is the x-asymptote. The absolute refractory period was 155 msec for the monophasic and 168 msec for the biphasic curve. The monophasic diastolic threshold was 0.7 V/cm, and the biphasic diastolic threshold was 0.6 V/cm. (Reprinted with permission from Reference 47.)

was less able to excite refractory myocardium.[47] When 5-msec monophasic and 2.5/2.5-msec biphasic shocks were used to create a potential gradient of 5 V/cm at an in vivo site containing a microelectrode, the monophasic waveform had a larger effect on the action potential than did the biphasic waveform during premature stimulation (Figure 16).[25] The monophasic waveform caused more prolongation of the action potential and was better able to initiate a new one. The same results were found when biphasic and monophasic shocks were given during ventricular fibrillation.[26]

It is also possible that the first phase of a biphasic shock reactivates sodium channels so that the second phase can defibrillate more easily. This hypothesis implies that, within limits, delivering more energy in the first phase should reduce the charge needed in the second phase. Walker et al.[79] tested this implication in a study that used 25 different biphasic waveforms that had the same first phase, but short second phases (≤ 2 msec) with different durations and amplitudes. They found that for successful defibrillation, the charge required in the second phase increased as the charge delivered in the first phase decreased and that there was no significant difference in the sum of the charge of the two phases. The hypothesis that the first phase conditions the myocardium so that the second phase of a biphasic waveform can defibrillate more easily was supported by the reciprocal relationship between the amount of charge in the two phases that maintained a given total charge at the DFT.

Hillsley et al.[80] performed another test to determine whether the first or second phase of a biphasic waveform is the defibrillating phase. They compared three monophasic waveforms (an ascending ramp, A; a square wave, S; and a descending ramp, D) with six biphasic waveforms (three with A, S, or D in the first phase and a square wave in the second phase and three with a square wave in the first phase and A, S, or D in the second phase). The waveforms were ranked by mean current and energy at the DFT for 16-msec monophasic and 16/16-msec biphasic waveforms (Table 4). The biphasic waveforms that had the three different shapes in the second phase ranked in the same order for both mean current (A<S=D) and energy (A<S<D) as did the monophasic waveforms while the current and energy (S<A=D for both) for biphasic waveforms with the different shapes in the first phase differed. These results support the hypothesis that the second phase of a biphasic waveform is the defibrillating phase since changing the shape of the second phase had an effect on the DFT similar to the one that occurred when the shape of the monophasic waveform was changed. Although the ranking of current and energy requirements was similar, the actual values were higher at the DFT for the 16/16-msec biphasic waveforms than for the 16-msec

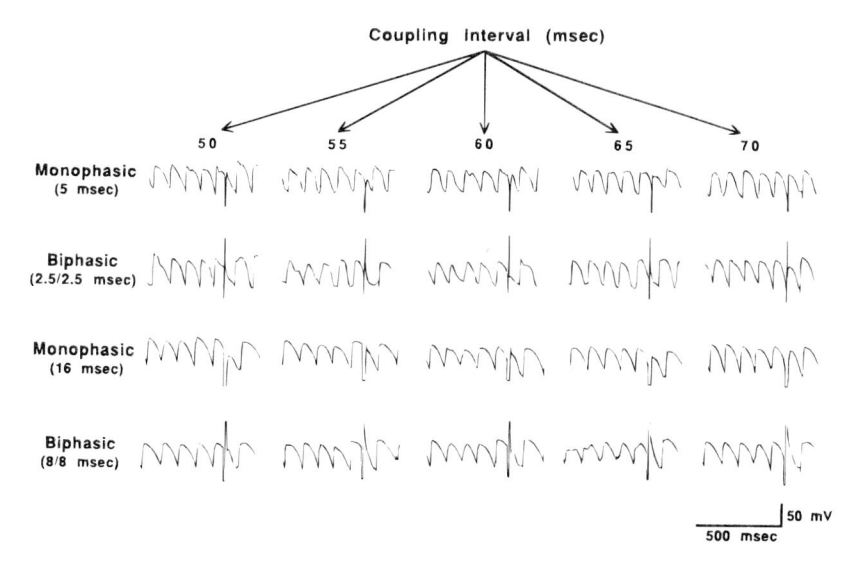

Figure 16. Examples of action potentials recorded before and after shocks during ventricular fibrillation. On the y axis are four different waveforms and on the x axis are the coupling intervals of 50 to 70 msec. Voltage and time scales are shown in the lower right corner. Action potential duration increased: 1) with an increase in coupling intervals for all shock waveforms; 2) for monophasic compared with biphasic waveforms of the same total duration; and 3) for longer compared with shorter waveforms of the same number of phases. (Reprinted with permission from Reference 26.)

monophasic ones (Hillsley et al., Table 3). When shorter and more clinically useful waveforms were used, the 6/6-msec biphasics had significantly lower DFTs than the 6-msec monophasics, but the rankings for current and energy no longer corresponded to the rankings of the monophasic waveforms when the tested shapes were in either the first or second phase of the biphasic waveforms. The hypothesis that the second phase of a biphasic waveform defibrillates was not supported for the more useful 6/6-msec waveform (which had lower DFTs than the 6-msec monophasic waveforms)

Table 4
Tank Defibrillation Threshold Orders by Mean Current and Energy

Duration	16 msec Mean Current	16 msec Energy	6 msec Mean Current	6 msec Energy
Monophasic	A < S = D	A < S = D	A < S = D	A = S < D
Biphasic-first phase	S < A = D	S < A = D	A = S = D	A = S = D
Biphasic-second phase	A < S = D	A < S < D	S = D < A	S = D < A

Ascending Ramp Square Descending Ramp
A S D

Modified and reprinted with permission from Reference 80.

even though it was supported for the longer, and less effective, 16/16-msec waveform (which had higher DFTs than the 16-msec monophasic waveforms).[80]

The hypothesis that the first phase, rather than the second of a biphasic waveform is the stimulating phase in defibrillation is consistent with the finding that biphasic shocks with low-tilt first phases and high-tilt second phases have low DFTs[81-83] because low-tilt monophasic waveforms have lower DFTs than high-tilt ones. Feeser et al.[74] determined strength-duration DFT voltage curves for monophasic waveforms that were 1–20 msec in duration and for biphasic waveforms with second phases that ranged from 1–20 msec and first phases that were held constant at either 3.5 or 7 msec.[74] For monophasic waveforms, the leading edge voltage remained relatively constant for all durations (Figure 17). For biphasic waveforms, the DFT increased markedly as the duration of the second phase increased. The energy and voltage at the DFT for monophasic waveforms were less than for biphasic waveforms of the same total duration when the duration of the second phase exceeded that of the first (Feeser et al., Table 2). When the second phase was 14 msec or longer, the leading edge voltage of the second phase at the DFT for the biphasic waveform was significantly higher than than of a monophasic waveform with the same duration as the second phase. This indicates that the preceding first phase actually made it more difficult to defibrillate.

Figure 17 shows that adding very small second phases, eg, a 1-msec second phase

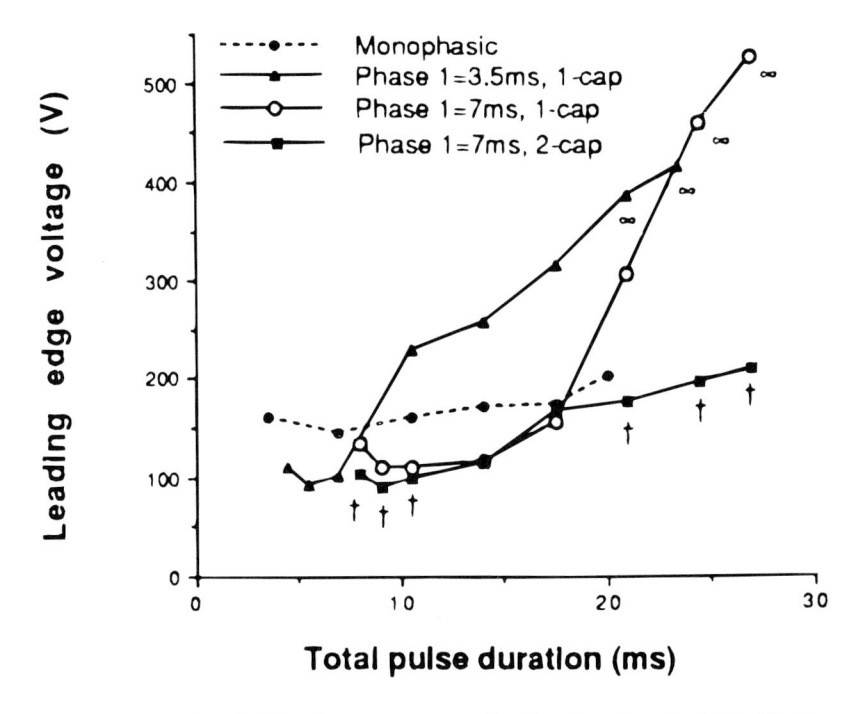

Figure 17. Defibrillation threshold voltage versus total pulse duration for high-tilt (time constant of 74–9 msec with tilt ranging from 10% to 90% depending upon phase duration) monophasic and biphasic waveforms. One-capacitor (1-cap) means leading edge voltage of second phase equals trailing edge voltage of first phase. Two-capacitor (2-cap) means leading edge voltage of second phase equals leading edge voltage of first phase. A ∞ indicates that some animals could not be defibrillated at the highest shock voltage. For biphasic waveforms with a 7-msec first phase leading edge voltage was lower for the 2-capacitor than the 1-capacitor waveform at all total durations except 14.0 and 17.5 msec († $P < 0.02$). (Reprinted with permission from Reference 74.)

to a 3.5-msec or 7-msec first phase, can lower the DFT. A 1-msec second phase does not last long enough to cause the second phase to reverse the polarity of the change in transmembrane potential[74] because of the membrane time constant. The membrane time constant to field stimulation is sufficiently long[28] that a 1-msec second phase is too short to depolarize the membrane in a region in which the transmembrane potential is hyperpolarized. Thus, the hypothesis that the first phase of a biphasic waveform conditions the heart so that the second phase can defibrillate more easily is either incorrect or is not the only mechanism at work in defibrillation. The actual mechanism is probably multifactorial for short clinically useful biphasic waveforms with the first factor being stimulation by the first phase and the second factor being the return of the transmembrane potential to a more physiological value by the second phase.

The effect on the DFT of the amplitude of the first versus the second phase was determined for 6/6-msec high-tilt biphasic waveforms in which the second phase was approximately 21%, 62%, 94%, and 141% of a constant value that was maintained for the first phase's leading edge voltage.[74] Increasing the second phase voltage first improved defibrillation efficacy, then decreased the percent success, and finally improved it again (Figure 18). Low-tilt (from 1% to 17% depending upon the duration of the pulse) biphasic waveforms gave the same results. These findings suggest that at least two mechanisms are effective during biphasic defibrillation. One mechanism is more effective for smaller, shorter second phases while another becomes more effective as the second phase increases in duration or amplitude. Stimulation may be the mechanism underlying the effectiveness of larger second phases and may be the same mechanism that explains effective monophasic shocks.

Another hypothesis that could explain why biphasic waveforms are generally superior to monophasics is that lower impedance during the second phase, due to elec-

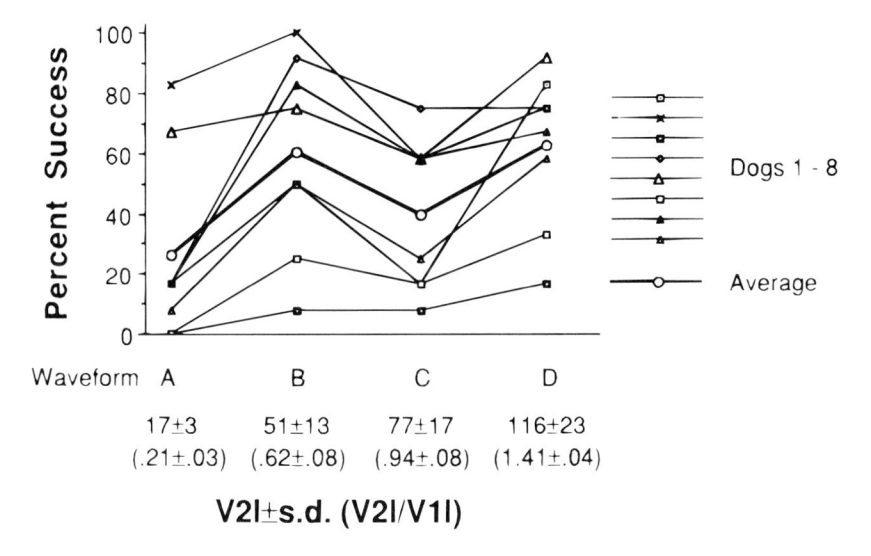

Figure 18. Defibrillation percent success versus second-phase leading edge voltage for 6/6-msec biphasic waveforms in which the first-phase voltage was held constant while the second-phase leading edge voltage was approximately 21% **(A)**, 62% **(B)**, 94% **(C)**, and 141% **(D)** of the first-phase leading edge voltage. V1L is first-phase leading edge voltage. V2L is second-phase leading edge voltage. As V2L increases from 21% to 141% of V1L, the percent success first increases ($P < 0.01$), then decreases ($P < 0.005$), and then increases again ($P < 0.02$). (Reprinted with permission from Reference 74.)

trode polarization in the first phase, could aid current flow during the polarity reversal between the two phases. However, impedance has been shown to decrease only slightly at the onset of the second phase of a biphasic shock, and this decrease is so small that it accounts for only a small part of the improved efficacy of biphasic compared with monophasic waveforms.[75] When the differences between effective monophasic and biphasic shocks are expressed in terms of voltage, current, and energy, these differences are much greater than can be accounted for by decreases in impedance.[75] Thus, this hypothesis does not explain why biphasic waveforms defibrillate at lower energies than monophasic shocks.

While the decrease in impedance that occurs during the second phase was not large enough to explain the improved efficacy of biphasic waveforms, it is possible that the large change in voltage that occurs between the first and second phases may account for the lower DFTs. This hypothesis has been tested in two experiments. Dixon et al.[64] determined DFTs for several biphasic waveforms that had total time courses of 10 msec, phases with different durations, and different voltage changes at phase reversal due to the exponential decay of the waveform. The DFT decreased as the duration of the second phase decreased and that of the first phase increased even though the amount of change in voltage between the two phases also decreased. In another study, various time delays were interposed between the two phases to interrupt the rapid voltage change between them (Figure 13).[84] Separating the phases by as much as 6 msec resulted in no changes in the voltage and energy required for defibrillation. Therefore, the large voltage change between the phases of biphasic waveforms is not a primary reason for why biphasic waveforms generally defibrillate better than monophasic ones.

Triphasic Truncated Exponential Waveforms

Because biphasic waveforms are generally better than monophasic ones, some investigators have tried to determine whether triphasic waveforms, which have a third phase the same polarity as the first (Figure 1), would be even more effective for defibrillation.[64,85,86] When compared to the results for a 5/5 biphasic waveform, no improvement was found in the energy required for defibrillating with a 5/5/2[64] and more energy was required (14.3 J versus 10.1 J) for a 2.5/5/2.5 triphasic waveform.[86] In both cases, the DFTs for triphasic waveforms were significantly lower than those for monophasics. Although triphasic waveforms do not lower the DFT, they have been shown to improve the ratio between the shock level that stimulates and the shock level that causes dysfunction (the safety factor) in cultured chick myocardial cells.[85] According to Jones et al., the first phase acts as a "conditioning prepusle" while the second "excites" or "defibrillates" and the third "heals." It is possible that triphasic waveforms may result in less dysfunction at the suprathreshold shock strengths which tend to be used in ICDs, but further work needs to be done to show that this is the case.

References

1. Grimm W, Flores BT, Marchlinski FE: Shock occurence and survival in 241 patients with implantable cardioverter defibrillator therapy. *Circulation* 87:1880, 1993.
2. Furman S, Kim SG: The present status of implantable cardioverter defibrillator therapy. *J Cardiovasc Electrophysiol* 3:602, 1992.
3. van Vleet JF, Tacker WA Jr, Geddes LA, et al: Sequential cardiac morphologic alterations induced in dogs by single transthoracic damped sinusoidal waveform defibrillator shocks. *Am J Vet Res* 39:271, 1978.
4. Babbs CF, Tacker WA Jr, van Vleet JF, et al: Therapeutic indices for damped sinusoidal defibrillator shocks: quantitation of effective, damaging, and lethal electrical doses. In: *Pro-*

ceedings of the 13th Annual AAMI Scientific Session. 1978, p. 14.
5. Jones JL, Jones RE: Postshock arrhythmias: a possible cause of unsuccessful defibrillation. *Crit Care Med* 8:167, 1980.
6. Ewy GA, Taren D, Bangert J, et al: Comparison of myocardial damage from defibrillator discharges at various dosages. *Med Instrum* 14:9, 1980.
7. Yabe S, Smith WM, Daubert JP, et al: Conduction disturbances caused by high current density electric fields. *Circ Res* 66:1190, 1990.
8. Lerman BB, Weiss JL, Bulkley BH, et al: Myocardial injury and induction of arrhythmia by direct current shock delivered via endocardial catheters in dogs. *Circulation* 69:1006, 1984.
9. Schuder JC, Stoeckle H, Gold JH, et al: Experimental ventricular defibrillation with an automatic and completely implanted system. *Trans Am Soc Artif Intern Organs* 16:207, 1970.
10. Mirowski M, Mower MM, Reid PR, et al: The automatic implantable defibrillator. *PACE* 5:384, 1982.
11. Geddes LA, Tacker WA Jr: Engineering and physiological considerations of direct capacitor-discharge ventricular defibrillation. *Med Biol Eng* 9:185, 1971.
12. Schuder JC, Stoeckle H, Keskar PY, et al: Transthoracic ventricular defibrillation in the dog with unidirectional rectangular double pulses. *Cardiovasc Res* 4:497, 1970.
13. Walker RG, Walcott GP, Smith WM, et al: Strength duration curves for short time constant truncated exponential monophasic waveforms (abstract). *PACE* 16:915, 1993.
14. Kroll MW: A minimal model of the monophasic defibrillation pulse. *PACE* 16:769, 1993.
15. Troup PJ: Implantable cardioverters and defibrillators. *Curr Prob Cardiol* 14:675, 1989.
16. Witkowski FX, Kerber RE: Currently known mechanisms underlying direct current external and internal cardiac defibrillation. *J Cardiovasc Electrophysiol* 2:562, 1991.
17. Ideker RE, Tang ASL, Frazier DW, et al: Ventricular defibrillation: basic concepts. In: *Cardiac Pacing and Electrophysiology.* Edited by N El-Sherif, P Samet. Orlando, FL: W.B. Saunders Co.; 1991, p. 713.
18. Witkowski FX, Penkoske PA, Plonsey R: Mechanism of cardiac defibrillation in openchest dogs with unipolar DC-coupled simultaneous activation and shock potential recordings. *Circulation* 82:244, 1990.
19. Wharton JM, Wolf PD, Smith WM, et al: Cardiac potential and potential gradient fields generated by single, combined, and sequential shocks during ventricular defibrillation. *Circulation* 85:1510, 1992.
20. Zhou X, Daubert JP, Wolf PD, et al: Epicardial mapping of ventricular defibrillation with monophasic and biphasic shocks in dogs. *Circ Res* 72:145, 1993.
21. Dillon SM: Optical recordings in the rabbit heart show that defibrillation strength shocks prolong the duration of depolarization and the refractory period. *Circ Res* 69:842, 1991.
22. Windisch H, Ahammer H, Schaffer P, et al: Optical monitoring of excitation patterns in single cardiomyocytes. Proceedings of the 12th Annual Conference of the IEEE Engineering in Medicine and Biology Society. 1990;12:1641.
23. Knisley SB, Blitchington TF, Hill BC, et al: Optical measurements of transmembrane potential changes during electric field stimulation of ventricular cells. *Circ Res* 72:255, 1993.
24. Tung L, Neunlist M: Regional depolarization of cardiac muscle adjacent to an epicardial stimulating anode (abstract). *Am Heart J* 124:834, 1992.
25. Zhou X, Knisley SB, Wolf PD, et al: Prolongation of repolarization time by electric field stimulation with monophasic and biphasic shocks in open chest dogs. *Circ Res* 68:1761, 1991.
26. Zhou X, Wolf PD, Rollins DL, et al: Effects of monophasic and biphasic shocks on action potentials during ventricular fibrillation in dogs. *Circ Res* 73:325, 1993.
27. Knisley SB, Smith WM, Ideker RE: Effect of intrastimulus polarity reversal on electric field stimulation thresholds in frog and rabbit myocardium. *J Cardiovasc Electrophysiol* 3:239, 1992.
28. Knisley SB, Smith WM, Ideker RE: Effect of field stimulation on cellular repolarization in rabbit myocardium: implications for reentry induction. *Circ Res* 70:707, 1992.
29. Plonsey R, Barr RC, Witkowski FX: One-dimensional model of cardiac defibrillation. *Med Biol Eng Comput* 29:465, 1991.
30. Sepulveda NG, Roth BJ, Wikswo JP Jr: Current injection into a two-dimensional anisotropic bidomain. *Biophys J* 55:987, 1989.
31. Krassowska W, Frazier DW, Pilkington TC, et al: Potential distribution in three-dimensional periodic myocardium: Part II. Application to extracellular stimulation. *IEEE Trans Biomed Eng* 37:267, 1990.
32. Trayanova NA, Pilkington TC, Henriquez CS: A periodic bidomain model for cardiac tissue. In: *Proceedings of the 13th Annual Conference of the IEEE Engineering in Medicine and Biology Society.* Edited by JH Nagel, WM Smith. Orlando, FL: IEEE, Inc.; 1991, p. 502.
33. Peleska B: Cardiac arrhythmias following

condenser discharges and their dependence upon strength of current and phase of cardiac cycle. *Circ Res* 13:21, 1963.
34. Zipes DP, Fischer J, King RM, et al: Termination of ventricular fibrillation in dogs by depolarizing a critical amount of myocardium. *Am J Cardiol* 36:37, 1975.
35. Chen P-S, Shibata N, Dixon EG, et al: Activation during ventricular defibrillation in open-chest dogs: evidence of complete cessation and regeneration of ventricular fibrillation after unsuccessful shocks. *J Clin Invest* 77:810, 1986.
36. Wiggers CJ: The physiologic basis for cardiac resuscitation from ventricular fibrillation: method for serial defibrillation. *Am Heart J* 20:413, 1940.
37. Chen P-S, Shibata N, Dixon EG, et al: Comparison of the defibrillation threshold and the upper limit of ventricular vulnerability. *Circulation* 73:1022, 1986.
38. Swartz JF, Jones JL, Jones RE, et al: Conditioning prepulse of biphasic defibrillator waveforms enhances refractoriness to fibrillation wavefronts. *Circ Res* 68:438, 1991.
39. Sweeney RJ, Gill RM, Reid PR: Characterization of refractory period extension by transcardiac shock. *Circulation* 83:2057, 1991.
40. Frazier DW, Wolf PD, Wharton JM, et al: Stimulus-induced critical point: mechanism for electrical initiation of reentry in normal canine myocardium. *J Clin Invest* 83:1039, 1989.
41. Rollins DL, Wolf PD, Ideker RE, et al: A programmable cardiac stimulator. In: *Proceedings of Computers in Cardiology*. Edited by A Murray, R Arzbaecher. Los Alamitos, CA: IEEE Computer Society Press; 1992, p. 507.
42. Ideker RE, Frazier DW, Krassowska W, et al: Experimental evidence for autowaves in the heart. In: *Mathematical Approaches to Cardiac Arrhythmias*. Edited by J Jalife. New York, NY: New York Academy of Sciences; 1990, p. 208.
43. Ideker RE, Chen P-S, Zhou X-H. Basic mechanisms of defibrillation. *J Electrocardiol* 23(suppl):36, 1991.
44. Chen P-S, Wolf PD, Ideker RE: Mechanism of cardiac defibrillation: a different point of view. *Circulation* 84:913, 1991.
45. Knisley SB, Afework Y, Li J, et al: Dispersion of repolarization induced by a nonuniform shock field. *PACE* 14:1148, 1991.
46. Knisley SB, Hill BC, Smith WM, et al: Implications of electrically-induced action potential prolongation for reentry induction in the heart. In: *Proceedings of the 14th Annual Conference of the IEEE Engineering in Medicine and Biology Society*. Edited by JP Morucci, R Plonsey, JL Coatrieux, S Laxminarayan. Paris, France: IEEE, Inc.; 1992, p. 633.
47. Daubert JP, Frazier DW, Wolf PD, et al: Response of relatively refractory canine myocardium to monophasic and biphasic shocks. *Circulation* 84:2522, 1991.
48. Kao CY, Hoffman BF: Graded and decremental response in heart muscle fibers. *Am J Physiol* 194:187, 1958.
49. Dillon SM: Synchronized repolarization after defibrillation shocks: a possible component of the defibrillation process demonstrated by optical recordings in rabbit heart. *Circulation* 85:1865, 1992.
50. Knisley SB, Hill BC: Optical recordings of the effect of electrical stimulation on action potential repolarization and the induction of reentry in two-dimensional perfused rabbit epicardium. *Circulation* 88:2402, 1993.
51. Chen P-S, Wolf PD, Melnick SB, et al: Comparison of activation during ventricular fibrillation and following unsuccessful defibrillation shocks in open chest dogs. *Circ Res* 66:1544, 1990.
52. Wessale JL, Boulard JD, Tacker WA, et al: Bipolar catheter defibrillation in dogs using trapezoidal waveforms of various tilts. *J Electrocardiol* 13:359, 1980.
53. Chapman PD, Wetherbee JN, Vetter JW, et al: Strength-duration curves of fixed pulse width variable tilt truncated exponential waveforms for nonthoracotomy internal defibrillation in dogs. *PACE* 11:1045, 1988.
54. Bourland JD, Tacker WA Jr, Wessale JL, et al: Sequential pulse defibrillation for implantable defibrillators. *Med Instrum* 20:138, 1986.
55. Jones DL, Klein GJ, Guiraudon GM, et al: Internal cardiac defibrillation in man: pronounced improvement with sequential pulse delivery to two different lead orientations. *Circulation* 73:484, 1986.
56. Jones DL, Klein GJ, Guiraudon GM, et al: Prediction of defibrillation success from a single defibrillation threshold measurement with sequential pulses and two current pathways in humans. *Circulation* 78:1144, 1988.
57. Bardou AL, Degonde J, Birkui PJ, et al: Reduction of energy required for defibrillation by delivering shocks in orthogonal directions in the dog. *PACE* 11:1990, 1988.
58. Jones DL, Klein GJ, Kallok MJ: Improved internal defibrillation with twin pulse sequential energy delivery to different lead orientations in pigs. *Am J Cardiol* 55:821, 1985.
59. Jones DL, Klein GJ, Rattes MF, et al: Internal cardiac defibrillation: single and sequential pulses and a variety of lead orientations. *PACE* 11:583, 1988.
60. Jones DL, Sohla A, Bourland JD, et al: Inter-

nal ventricular defibrillation with sequential pulse countershock in pigs: comparison with single pulses and effects of pulse separation. *PACE* 10:497, 1987.
61. Ideker RE, Hillsley RE, Wharton JM: Shock strength for the implantable defibrillator: can you have too much of a good thing? *PACE* 15:841, 1992.
62. Jones JL, Jones RE: Determination of safety factor for defibrillator waveforms in cultured heart cells. *Am J Physiol* 242:H662, 1982.
63. Kavanagh KM, Tang ASL, Rollins DL, et al: Comparison of the internal defibrillation thresholds for monophasic and double and single capacitor biphasic waveforms. *J Am Coll Cardiol* 14:1343, 1989.
64. Dixon EG, Tang ASL, Wolf PD, et al: Improved defibrillation thresholds with large contoured epicardial electrodes and biphasic waveforms. *Circulation* 76:1176, 1987.
65. Chapman PD, Vetter JW, Souza JJ, et al: Comparative efficacy of monophasic and biphasic truncated exponential shocks for nonthoracotomy internal defibrillation in dogs. *J Am Coll Cardiol* 12:739, 1988.
66. Winkle RA, Mead RH, Ruder MA, et al: Improved low energy defibrillation efficacy in man with the use of a biphasic truncated exponential waveform. *Am Heart J* 117:122, 1989.
67. Saksena S, An H, Krol RB, et al: Simultaneous biphasic shocks enhance efficacy of endocardial cardioversion defibrillation in man. *PACE* 14:1935, 1991.
68. Bardy GH, Troutman C, Johnson G, et al: Electrode system influence on biphasic waveform defibrillation efficacy in humans. *Circulation* 84:665, 1991.
69. Johnson EE, Hagler JA, Alferness CA, et al: Efficacy of short and long monophasic and biphasic waveforms in internal and external defibrillation (abstract). *Am Heart J* 124:836, 1992.
70. Walcott GP, Hagler JA, Walker RG, et al: Comparison of monophasic, biphasic, and the Edmark waveform for external defibrillation (abstract). *PACE* 15:563, 1992.
71. Cooper RAS, Alferness CA, Smith WM, et al: Internal cardioversion of atrial fibrillation in sheep. *Circulation* 87:1673, 1993.
72. Ideker RE, Cooper RAS, Wharton JM: New developments in implantable cardioverter-defibrillator electrodes and waveforms. In: *Sudden Cardiac Death: Strategies for the 1990's*. Edited by RM Luceri. Miami Lakes, FL: Peritus Corporation; 1991, p. 133.
73. Chapman PD, Vetter JW, Souza JJ, et al: Comparison of monophasic with single and dual capacitor biphasic waveforms for non-thoracotomy canine internal defibrillation. *J Am Coll Cardiol* 14:242, 1989.
74. Feeser SA, Tang ASL, Kavanagh KM, et al: Strength-duration and probability of success curves for defibrillation with biphasic waveforms. *Circulation* 82:2128, 1990.
75. Tang ASL, Yabe S, Wharton JM, et al: Ventricular defibrillation using biphasic waveforms: the importance of phasic duration. *J Am Coll Cardiol* 13:207, 1989.
76. Cates AW, Souza JJ, Hillsley RE, et al: Probability of defibrillation success and incidence of postshock arrhythmias as a function of shock strength (abstract). *J Am Coll Cardiol* 21:305A, 1993.
77. Kavanagh KM, Simpson EV, Wolf PD, et al: Minimum gradient required for biphasic defibrillation (abstract). *PACE* 16:916, 1993.
78. Wharton JM, Richard VJ, Murry CE Jr, et al: Electrophysiological effects of monophasic and biphasic stimuli in normal and infarcted dogs. *PACE* 13:1158, 1990.
79. Walker RG, Walcott GP, Swanson DK, et al: Relationship of charge distribution between phases in biphasic waveforms (abstract). *Circulation* 86:I-792, 1992.
80. Hillsley RE, Walker RG, Swanson DK, et al: Is the second phase of a biphasic defibrillation waveform the defibrillating phase? *PACE* 16:1401, 1993.
81. Walcott GP, Rollins DL, Smith WM, et al: Defibrillation efficacy of biphasic waveforms improved by raising phase 2 leading edge voltage (abstract). *PACE* 15:529, 1992.
82. Walcott GP, Rollins DL, Smith WM, et al: Effects of changing capacitors between phases of a biphasic shock on defibrillation efficacy (abstract). *J Am Coll Cardiol* 19:366A, 1992.
83. Walcott GP, Rollins DL, Smith WM, et al: Optimal capacitance value for a parallel-series defibrillator (abstract). *J Am Coll Cardiol* 21:307A, 1993.
84. Cooper RAS, Wallenius ST, Smith WM, et al: The effect of phase separation on biphasic waveform defibrillation. *PACE* 16:471, 1993.
85. Jones JL, Jones RE: Improved safety factors for triphasic defibrillator waveforms. *Circ Res* 64:1172, 1989.
86. Chapman PD, Wetherbee JN, Vetter JW, et al: Comparison of monophasic, biphasic, and triphasic truncated pulses for non-thoracotomy internal defibrillation (abstract). *J Am Coll Cardiol* 11:57A, 1988.
87. Frazier DW, Krassowska W, Chen P-S, et al: Transmural activations and stimulus potentials in three-dimensional anisotropic canine myocardium. *Circ Res* 63:135, 1988.
88. Jones JL, Swartz JF, Jones RE, et al: Increasing fibrillation duration enhances relative asym-

metrical biphasic versus monophasic defibrillator waveform efficacy. *Circ Res* 67:376, 1990.
89. Chen P-S, Wolf PD, Claydon FJ III, et al: The potential gradient field created by epicardial defibrillation electrodes in dogs. *Circulation* 74:626, 1986.
90. Saksena S, Scott SE, Accorti PR, et al: Efficacy and safety of monophasic and biphasic waveform shocks using a braided endocardial defibrillation lead system. *Am Heart J* 120:1342, 1990.
91. Wyse DG, Kavanagh KM, Gillis AM, et al: Comparison of biphasic and monophasic shocks for defibrillation using a nonthoracotomy system. *Am J Cardiol* 71:197, 1993.
92. Guse PA, Kavanagh KM, Alferness CA, et al: Defibrillation with low voltage using a left ventricular catheter and four cutaneous patch electrodes in dogs. *PACE* 14:443, 1991.

Chapter 8

Leads Technology

Peter R. Accorti, Jr.

Historical Perspective

Since the pioneering work conducted by Mirowski et al.[1] in the early 1970s, rapid advancement in implantable cardioverter-defibrillators (ICDs) and defibrillation electrode systems has occurred. Defibrillation lead systems have evolved in the following sequence: 1) transvenous leads; 2) endocardial spring and epicardial patch lead; 3) epicardial patch system; and 4) transvenous lead system with or without a subcutaneous patch.

One of the first defibrillation lead systems to be evaluated consisted of a right ventricular pressure/defibrillation lead and a subcutaneous electrode placed under the skin or on the anterior chest wall.[1] The early animal experiments conducted by Mirowski et al. were some of the first to suggest that implantable defibrillators were feasible. At the same time, Shuder et al.[2] successfully conducted experiments with a prototype automatic implantable defibrillator that used two chest wall patches and a capacitor discharge defibrillation waveform.

In 1972, Mirowski et al.[3] conducted experiments using a single transvenous lead with multiple distal electrodes and a saline soaked sponge located at the superior vena cava (SVC). This lead paved the way for a totally transvenous defibrillation electrode system consisting of proximal and distal ring electrodes. Rubin et al.[4] compared unipolar defibrillation using distal rings and chest wall patch to bipolar defibrillation using distal and proximal ring electrodes. In these experiments, the bipolar configuration produced lower defibrillation energies than the unipolar configuration.

The first human implants were conducted with a titanium spring positioned in the SVC and a titanium epicardial patch (Figure 1).[5] The electrogram sensing was accomplished from the high-voltage electrodes. However, oversensing prompted the use of a separate rate sensing lead, endocardial or epicardial (Figure 1).[6] Migration of the SVC spring electrode resulted in decreased defibrillation efficacy in some patients.[7,8] This problem led some to advocate a fully epicardial defibrillation lead system. Figure 2 is a schematic representing a fully epicardial defibrillation lead system. Figure 3 depicts two types of epicardial patches used in these systems. On the left is a titanium mesh patch representative of Telectronics model 040–107™ (Telectronics, Englewood, CO) electrode. The right patch electrode is a multicoil platinum (Pt) and iridium (Ir) lead used in Medtronic's defibrillator systems (models #6891, 6892, 6893, Medtronic, Minneapolis, MN). The Ventritex (Sunnyvale, CA) epicardial patch electrode is an oval patch with Pt/Ir mesh. Fig-

From Singer I, (ed.) Implantable Cardioverter-Defibrillator. Armonk, NY: Futura Publishing Company, Inc.; © 1994.

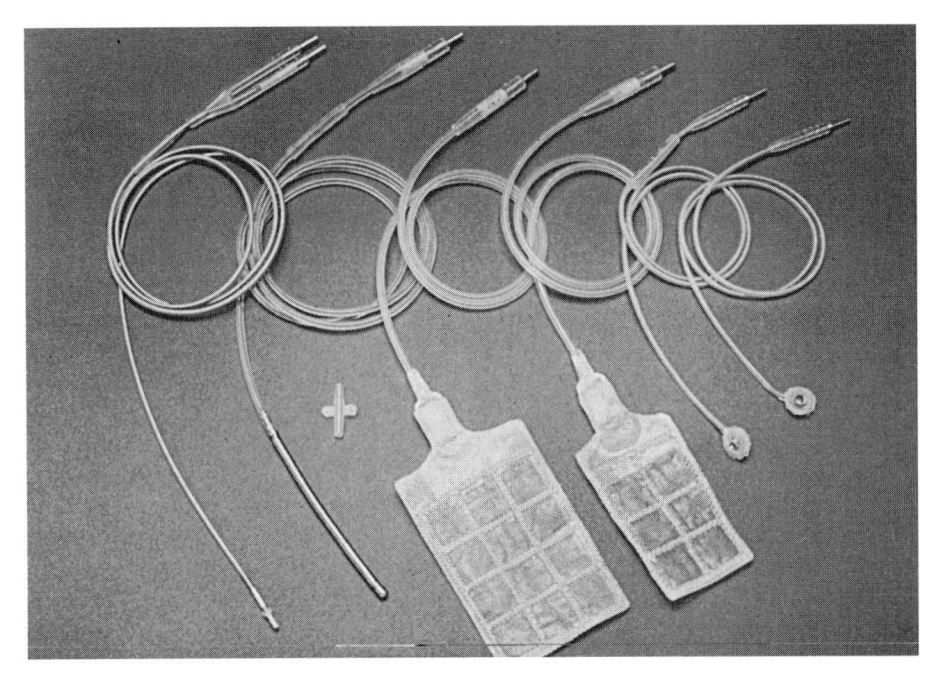

Figure 1. Early rate sensing, spring and epicardial patch lead system. (Courtesy of CPI, St. Paul, MN.)

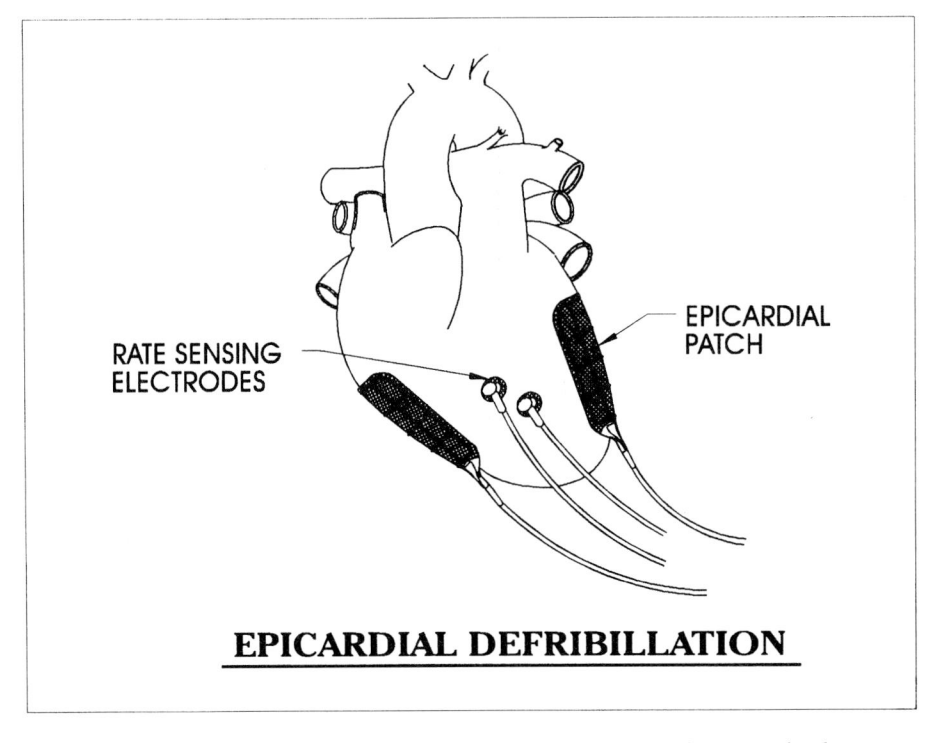

Figure 2. Schematic diagram of a complete epicardial patch and sensing lead system.

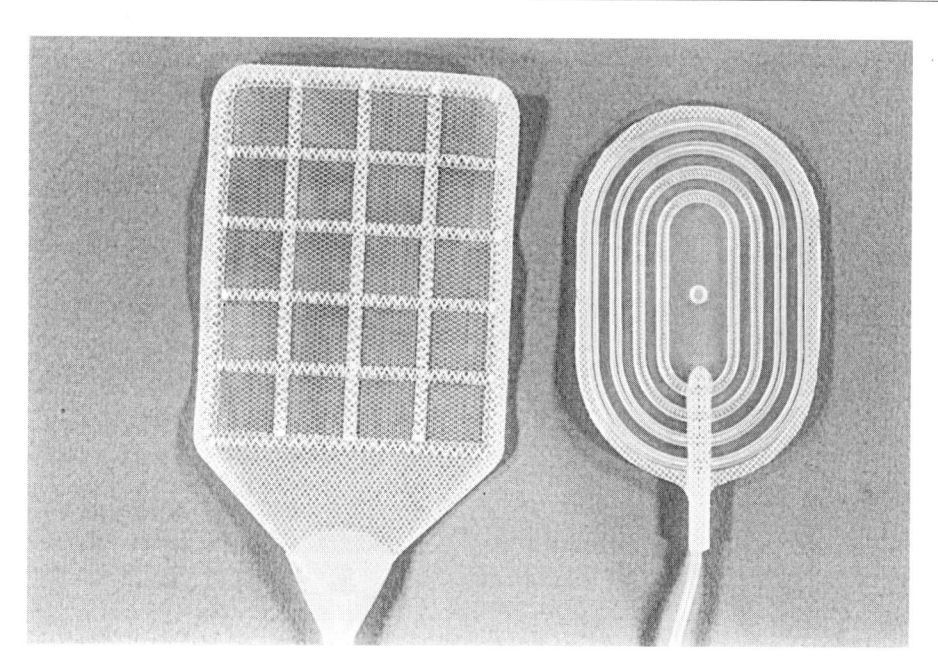

Figure 3. Telectronics model 040–107™ (Englewood, CO) and Medtronic model 6892™ (Minneapolis, MN) epicardial defibrillation patches.

ure 4 shows an epicardial rate-sensing lead. The lead consists of a unipolar platinum iridium helical screw that is used for epicardial pacing and sensing. Two unipolar electrodes are used to generate the bipolar sensing signal. The conductor is made of MP35N wire.

More progress occurred in catheter defibrillation in the early 1980s. Various investigators examined the feasibility of catheter defibrillation by using leads with distal and proximal ring electrodes.[9,10] Following these early investigations, Medtronic began conducting studies using the model 6880 and model 6882 transvenous leads. The leads consisted of two 125-mm² distal electrodes positioned in the right ventricular apex and two 125-mm² electrodes positioned in the right atrium-SVC junction.[11]

Temporary testing of a single pass defibrillation lead produced by Intec (Pittsburgh, PA) systems was conducted by Winkle et al.[12] The Intec catheter consisted of a three-electrode system. Pacing and sensing was accomplished from a 16-mm² distal platinum iridium tip. The lead consisted of a distal 4 cm² and a proximal 8 cm² helically wound titanium coils for defibrillation. This lead was the predecessor of CPI's Endotak™ (CPI, St. Paul, MN) defibrillation lead. Figure 5 shows the distal portion of the Endo-

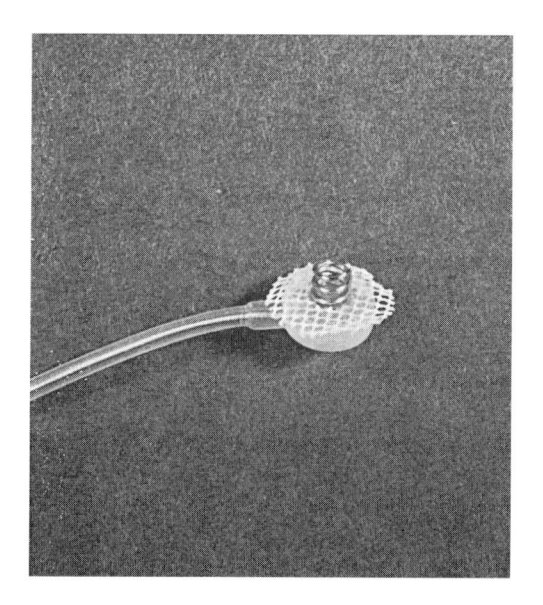

Figure 4. Daig model ML-151™ (Minnetonka, MN) epicardial pacing and sensing electrode.

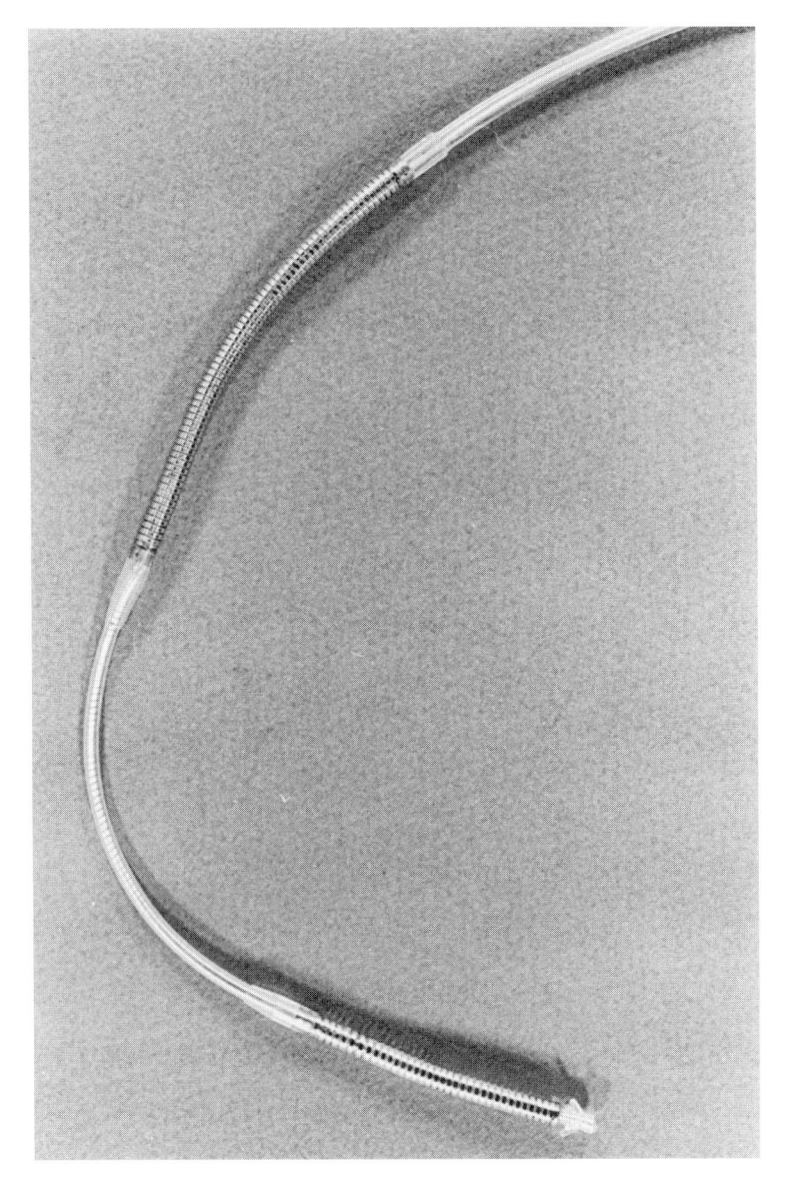

Figure 5. The distal portion of the CPI Endotak®-C (St. Paul, MN) single pass endocardial defibrillation lead.

tak lead. Since the first implants in 1988, the Endotak has undergone several modifications due to conductor fracture.[11] Currently, the lead consists of two Pt/Ir (proximal surface area [SA] = 295 mm^2, distal SA = 617 mm^2) ribbon coil electrodes for defibrillation, and a Pt/Ir pacing tip. The lead insulation is silastic and the high-voltage conductors are constructed from a drawn brazed strand. An optional subcutaneous patch may be used to obtain a three-electrode defibrillation configuration. The Endotak-C lead is the only fully market-released transvenous lead available at this time.

Three other manufacturers are conducting clinical trials with transvenous leads. The Medtronic Transvene™ lead system (model 6636 and 6933) consists of a tripolar ventricular lead and a unipolar SVC/CS (coronary sinus) lead. Pacing and sensing are separated from the defibrillation coil in the ventricular lead. Bipolar sensing is established from a distal helical screw (10 mm^2) and a Pt/Ir ring (37 mm^2). The defibrillation electrode is a single 5.0 cm long Pt/Ir coil with an SA of 426 mm^2.

Telectronics endocardial leads are undergoing clinical trials with a two-lead endocardial system, the EnGuard PFx®. The system consists of a bipolar ventricular and a bipolar atrial J lead. Pacing and sensing occurs between an 8-mm^2 Pt/Ir tip and the defibrillation electrode. The defibrillation electrodes are constructed from a 16-wire titanium braid. Currently, both leads use passive fixation tines for stability. Figure 6 shows the distal positions of the Endotak, Transvene, and the EnGuard defibrillation leads.

Intermedics (Angleton, TX) has recently begun clinical trials with an integrated bipolar defibrillation lead. The system consists of a single right ventricular active fixation lead. Pacing and sensing are accomplished between the electrically active screw and the defibrillation coil. The defibrillation electrode is made of titanium with a surface area of 48 cm^2. A tabulated summary of the characteristics and market availability (as of the completion of this manuscript) for epicardial and endocardial defibrillation leads is summarized in Table 1.

Design Considerations

One of the most important considerations in designing a defibrillation lead is biocompatibility and biostability. Materials used in the lead construction, both polymers and metals, must be inert in the body. This limits the choices available to lead designers to materials with known performance characteristics. The investigation of unproven new materials usually involves extensive (up to 2 years) biocompatibility testing in animals prior to human implants. Guidelines from the Food and Drug Admin-

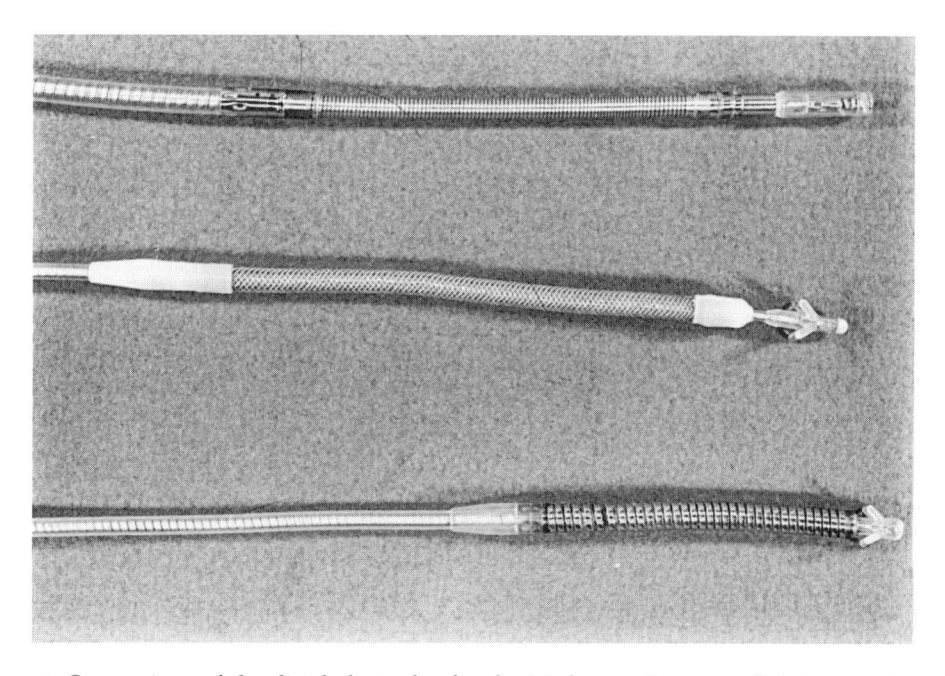

Figure 6. Comparison of the distal electrodes for the Medtronic Transvene™ (Minneapolis, MN), Telectronics EnGuard™ (Englewood, CO), and the CPI Endotak™ (St. Paul, MN) endocardial defibrillation leads.

Table 1
Summary of Defibrillation Lead Characteristics and Market Availability

Manufacturer	Lead Type	Model Number(s)	Insulation Material	Electrode Material/ Design	High-Voltage Conductor	Market Availability
CPI	Epicardial	L67, A67	Silicone	Titanium mesh	DBS	Yes
CPI	Endocardial	0060, 62, 64	Silicone	Platinum ribbon	DBS	Yes
CPI	Subcutaneous	0063	Silicone	Titanium mesh	DBS	Yes
Medtronic	Epicardial	6897	Silicone	Platinum/ iridium coils	DFT	Yes
Medtronic	Endocardial	6936, 6933	80A Polyurethane, Silicone	Platinum/ iridium coil	DFT	Yes
Ventritex	Epicardial	DP-5019, DP-5038	Silicone	Titanium mesh	DBS	Yes
Ventritex	Subcutaneous	SQ-701	Silicone	Titanium mesh	DFT	No
Ventritex	Endocardial	RV-1101, SV-1101	Silicone	Platinum/ iridium coils	DFT	No
Telectronics	Epicardial	040-105, 106, 107	Silicone	Titanium mesh	DBS	No
Telectronics	Endocardial	040-068, 069	55D Polyurethane	Titanium braid	DFT	No
Intermedics	Epicardial	497-01, 497-02, 497-11, 497-12, 497-15	Silicone	Titanium mesh	DBS	No
Intermedics	Endocardial	497-05	Silicone	Titanium coated with iroxide	DBS	No

istration (FDA) have suggested performing tripartite biocompatibility testing on blood contacting devices. The following tests are recommended: pyrogenicity hemolysis/ hemocompatibility, irritation, cytotoxicity, sensitivity, mutagenicity, acute toxicity, chronic toxicity, implant tests, and carcinogenicity. Some of these tests, specifically chronic stability and carcinogenicity, can take more than 2 years to complete. Usually, materials for the blood-contacting portions of the leads use either silastic or polyurethane for insulation and platinum, platinum alloy, or titanium for the stimulating electrodes.

Although the choice of materials may be limited, other design issues are not. The geometry and the connection scheme used for defibrillation electrodes is unique for each design.

Insulation Material

Recent concerns about the silastic and certain polyurethanes for permanent implants have made the choice of insulation material more difficult than originally anticipated.[13,14] Generally, one or more of the following insulation materials are used for de-

Table 2
Mean (Std) Bulk Properties of Dry, Unaged Silicone and Polyurethane[1]

Material	Young's Modulus (kg/cm^2)	Tear Strength (kg/cm^2)	Tensile Strength (kg/cm^2)	% Elongation	Resistivity (ohm/cm)
Silicone	43 (5)	>5.3	65 (6.5)	335 (19)	2×10^{17}
Polyurethane 80A	245 (16)	>33	440 (77)	650 (35)	4×10^{12}
Polyurethane 55D	1430 (96)	>46	600 (60)	440 (20)	6×10^{13}

Data derived from Stokes et al.[16]

fibrillation leads construction: silastic of various deurometers and polyurethane (either 55D or 80A hardness). Design considerations such as tensile strength, wear, dialetric properties, and stiffness must be examined. Tables 2 and 3 summarize the bulk properties for silicone and polyurethane in dry and wet environments.

Silicone rubber has many properties that make it a suitable material for insulation in leads. Specifically, the material is biostable, biocompatible, flexible, inert, and a good insulator. A summary of silicone chemistry and medical applications is beyond the scope of this chapter and may be found elsewhere.[15] Silicone rubbers are compounds consisting of a polymer, filler, and catalyst. Properties of the polymer, such as tensile strength and elongation are functions of the quantity ratios of the three components. The polymer backbone is based on polydimethylsiloxane. Medium to hard grades of silicone are produced by the copolymerization of dimethylsiloxane and small amounts of methylvinyl siloxane. Softer polymers are formed by the addition of phenylmethylsiloxane.

The filler used in silicone polymerization consists of very pure and fine (30 μm) silica particles. The filler particles give silicone its strength. Without them, the tensile strength is very low. There are two catalysts used in the polymerization process: dichlorobenzoyl peroxide and platinum. The terms "peroxide cured" or "platinum cured" are often used to describe the catalyst for polymerization.

Silicone rubber tubing used for leads is produced by a process known as extrusion. For example, extruded silicone tubing is used in the CPI Endotak lead. All defibrillation patches are made of molded silicone. One limitation of silicone tubing is that it has poor resistance to tearing. The tear strength of silicone can be almost an order of magnitude lower than that of polyurethane. Therefore, to counteract this deficiency, leads made with silicone tubing tend to be larger (ie, a greater diameter) than those made of polyurethane. An additional consideration with silicone leads is their degree of lubricity or the coefficient of friction. For instance, due to a higher coefficient of friction, two silastic leads tend to stick to-

Table 3
Mean (Std) Bulk Properties of Wet and Aged (7 days in Saline) Silicone and Polyurethane[1]

Material	Weight Change (%)	Tensile Strength (kg/cm^2)	% Elongation	Resistivity (ohm/cm)
Silicone	0.8 (0.15)	67 (13)	365 (23)	10^{17}
Polyurethane 80A	1.8 (0.28)	290 (27)	810 (30)	8×10^{10}
Polyurethane 55D	1.6 (0.22)	495 (39)	650 (35)	10^{12}

Data derived from Stokes et al.[16]

gether. This can present a technical challenge for two-lead implants.

Another insulation material of choice for defibrillation as well as for pacemaker leads is polyurethane. Polyurethane offers the advantage of high tear strength, elasticity, and low coefficient of friction. Because of the high tear strength, smaller diameter leads can be made. Also, once the lead is placed within blood, the polyurethane becomes more slippery. Therefore, placing two leads within one venous entry site becomes easier.

In general, polyurethane is the reaction product of three molecular monomers: the isocyanate, the macroglycol, and the chain extender. The reaction occurs in two phases. In the first phase, the isocyanate is reacted with the macroglycol. The second phase adds the chain extender to create a high molecular weight polyurethane. Generally, the terms soft and hard segments are used to describe polyurethane chemistry. The soft segments are composed of polytetramethylene oxide diol (PTMO), while the hard segments contain diphenylmethane diisocyanate (MDI)/butane diol (BD).[16] The degree of hardness for polyurethane depends on the ratio of soft to hard segments. For instance, pellathane 80A contains a higher percentage of soft segments than 55D, and as a result is more flexible and soft.

Recently, there has been much concern over the use of polyurethane in leads for pacemaker applications.[13] These issues will undoubtedly occur for defibrillation leads using polyurethane also. In some pacemaker leads using 80A polyurethane (eg, Medtronic model No. 6972), there have been reports of insulation failure. The mechanisms of these failures are believed to be due to either environmental stress cracking (ESC) or metal ion oxidation (MIO). Both mechanisms have been extensively tested by Stokes et al.[17,18]

Environmental stress cracking manifests itself in two ways. First, there can be small microscopic cracks at the site of stress, such as at the ligatures. The lead often has a cloudy appearance that is termed frosting or crazing. Because these cracks are small and superficial, the bulk molecular properties of the polymer are unaffected. However, in some cases ESC can result in a complete rupture of the insulation. The cracks often orient themselves at right angles to an identifiable strain vector. Some sources of strain include: direct suturing, sharp bends or kinks in the lead, areas where solvents are used to swell the polyurethane, or other areas where the polyurethane has been mechanically expanded. In most cases ESC can be minimized by proper handling of the lead at implant as well as by using new manufacturing techniques that minimize the stress imposed on the polymer due to processing.[19]

Conversely, MIO appears to be an oxidative degeneration of the polyurethane due to a complex interaction between hydrogen peroxide released from inflamatory cells and metal ions from the conductor coils. One ion thought to catalyze the process is silver, which is used extensively in defibrillation conductors such as drawn brazed strand or drawn filled tube. However, other data suggest that cobalt is the primary metal ion responsible for MIO.[18]

The insulator used for defibrillation and pacemaker leads will become a major concern for manufacturers and clinicians. Recently, Dow Corning, the manufacturer of pellathane, which is used for almost all leads, announced its intention to discontinue the material for medical implants. Also, a similar announcement was made for the use of silicone. This decision comes from the possible liability issues that may occur from silicone breast implants. Therefore, the future for insulation for leads will be dynamic, with new polymer materials and manufacturers entering into the market.

Defibrillation Electrodes

Perhaps the area of design with the most variability and possibilities for improved efficiency is the defibrillation electrode. In this regard, especially for transvenous leads, each manufacturer has produced a unique electrode design.

The choice of materials for the electrode is limited to high-conducting, low-corrosion, biocompatible and biostable metals. Therefore, metals such as silver, gold, and copper cannot be used because of their toxicity and corrosion in an aqueous environment. Most electrodes are manufactured with either platinum, platinum alloy, titanium, or in some investigational studies, carbon fibers. The bulk properties of some common electrode metals are found in Table 4.

Initially, leads, specifically epicardial patches, used titanium mesh as the defibrillation electrode. Titanium is considered a material of choice because of its biocompatibility, high conductivity, and good fatigue life.[20] However, certain aspects of titanium chemistry need to be understood when using it for delivery of high-voltage shocks, as well as for manufacturing processes. First, one of the reasons for titanium inertness in an aqueous environment is the fact that it forms no strong oxide layer. Typically, titanium oxide (TiO) forms on the metal in contact with air. Higher, more complex oxides can be formed by either changing the aqueous environment or by the delivery of a charge. The anode used for defibrillation often appears darkblue due to thick TiO buildup that can theoretically act as a semiconductor. Therefore, the efficiency of the shock may be due less to charging at the oxide layer. The oxidation of titanium provides challenges in manufacturing. For instance, welding of the titanium electrode requires reduction of the oxide layer. This is accomplished by performing the procedure in an atmosphere of nitrogen or by creating a vacuum. It is important to achieve good metal-to-metal contact, ie, the metals should be forged together or satisfactorily crimped in order to avoid gaps.

Another concern with titanium is the possibility that a phase charge can occur that will alter its crystalline structure. Normally, titanium used in medical applications is in the alpha phase and has a crystalline structure of body centered cubic (BCC). This crystalline structure gives titanium good fatigue characteristics. However, under certain conditions such as high temperatures, titanium may undergo a phase change to a beta phase resulting in a hexagonal closed pack (HCP) structure. Unlike the BCC, the HCP structure is brittle, ie, it does not have good fatigue properties. Therefore, care must be taken in the processing of titanium metal so that the transition temperature is not reached. This transition temperature under normal pH conditions is approximately 882°C.

Platinum or platinum-iridium (Pt/Ir) alloys are also used for defibrillation elec-

Table 4
Characteristics of Metals Typically Used for Defibrillation Electrodes and Conductors[1]

Material	Resistivity Ω-ft	Young's Modulus (10^6 psi)	Tensile Strength (10^3 psi)	% Elongation (minimum)
Platinum	2.544	25.0	35	3.0
90% Platinum 10% Iridium	6.016	21.3	95	3.0
Titanium	10.104	16.8	175	1.5
MP35N	24.840	33.76	275	2.0
DBS	2.520	28.60	185	1.5
DFT (25% Silver)	1.357	33.76	215	2.0

Information provided by Joseph B. Kain, Metallurgical Engineer, Ft. Wayne Metals Research Products Corporation, 9609 Indianapolis Road, Ft. Wayne, IN 46809.

trodes. Platinum is very resistant to corrosion in the body. Also, it is very conductive (has low resistance). Pt/Ir stimulation electrodes are used in the majority of pacemaker leads, and thus, have proven long-term reliability.

Pure platinum is very soft; therefore, processing of the metal wire into electrodes can be challenging. For instance, if the wire is to be coiled, the tension on the wire must be carefully controlled. Due to its softness, the wire has a high percent elongation and can be stretched, resulting in a nonuniform diameter. In most cases, a Pt/Ir alloy is used. The addition of iridium increases the hardness of the metal, simplifying the processing. However, increasing the iridium content may make the electrode stiffer and reduce its fatigue life.

Other materials are being investigated for defibrillation applications. Initial investigations of carbon fibers[21] are promising. It is believed that the increased surface area from the small fibers improves defibrillation efficacy. By its nature carbon is very biocompatible. However, issues such as long-term in vivo performance and manufacturability will need to be worked out before carbon can be widely used as a material for construction of defibrillation electrodes.

Areas of research for epicardial patches have concentrated on improved electrical field distribution. When passing a charge through any electrode, complex electrochemical reactions occur at the metal solution interface. The transition area between the electrode and the insulation results in a phenomenon called an edge effect. High-current densities result at the edge of the electrode. The higher than normal current densities result in less efficient energy delivery, as well as possible conduction disturbances and tissue damage in near proximity to the electrode.[22,23]

The first patches used by CPI included multiple "windows" of titanium mesh. This patch design is also used by Telectronics Pacing Systems. The windows act to yield uniform current densities by having multiple edges. Additionally, it is believed that the windowing will result in better mesh stability by anchoring tissue ingrowth at the Dacron instead of at the titanium. The Medtronic patch lead consists of multiple Pt/Ir coils connected at a central pin. The coils are tightly wound at the patch edge and have greater pitch near the center. It is believed that this design with a gradient of impedance (higher at the periphery, lower in the center) will result in an improved electrical charge distribution. Intermedics is investigating the use of contoured patches for defibrillation. These patches are designed to minimize the edge effects, and thus may improve defibrillation efficacy.[24] Early investigational data by Nathan et al.[25] show low defibrillation thresholds (DFTs). However, it is unclear whether the low DFTs were due to the patch design, or to the biphasic shock waveforms. An additional concern with large contoured patches is the possibility that they may insulate the heart from external defibrillation shocks.[26]

Endocardial defibrillation leads also have variable designs to improve defibrillation efficacy. For instance, the CPI Endotak lead uses a Pt/Ir ribbon as the defibrillation electrode. The ribbon provides a smooth surface and is quite strong mechanically. The surface area at the distal spring is 295 mm^2. In addition, the lead design incorporates a "shunted" electrode. In this context, shunting involves the connection of the distal and proximal portions of the electrode together with the high-voltage conductor. By doing this, the voltage drop-off that occurs due to the resistance of the wire is avoided. Therefore, high-current densities exist at both ends of the electrode. By minimizing the voltage drop, it is believed that better electrical fields exist, specifically near the ventricular apex. However, it may also be possible that high-current densities located near the sensing tip may result in postshock sensing abnormalities.[27] The electrogram changes appear to be minimized if the electrode is moved further away from the sensing tip.[28]

The Medtronic Transvene electrode uses a single wire Pt/Ir coil for defibrillation. Even though there is an impedance drop across the electrode, data suggest that there is good defibrillation efficacy.[29] There have been very few reports of electrogram sensing abnormalities with the Transvene electrodes.

Telectronics EnGuard defibrillation lead uses a 16-wire titanium braid for defibrillation. The braid design results in a large effective surface area with multiple edges. The multiple edges may result in a more uniform current distribution. Additionally, the interconnection of the wires minimizes the voltage drop phenomenon. The EnGuard is in phase I clinical trials (as of the time of this writing), and as a result, the data are too preliminary to make firm conclusions about its efficacy. Figure 7 is an idealized comparison of the three endocardial leads and the effect of the voltage drop-off.

Other manufacturers have just started or are anticipating beginning clinical trials of endocardial defibrillation lead(s) system. Most likely, these designs will incorporate new electrodes and possibly new materials.

The electrode designs are unique in regard to the hypothesized benefit of even electrical fields. However, all designs are developed with mechanical limitations in mind. There are multiple engineering trade-offs that make material and design issues more complex. The issues include: impedance, fatigue life, stiffness, and corrosion. Except for corrosion, which is addressed in the initial material choice, all other conditions are related to the design.

It can be argued that the most important design issue of the electrode is its fatigue performance. Although, the generator may last for 2.5–5 years, the lead system must remain viable for much longer. Therefore, the electrode/lead must be designed for improved fatigue performance. Fatigue life is a function of the material, wire diameter, radius of the electrode, number of wires, and the pitch angle of the coil. However, improved fatigue life generally comes at the expense of impedance and/or stiffness. This is summarized in Figure 8.

In designing the electrode for fatigue

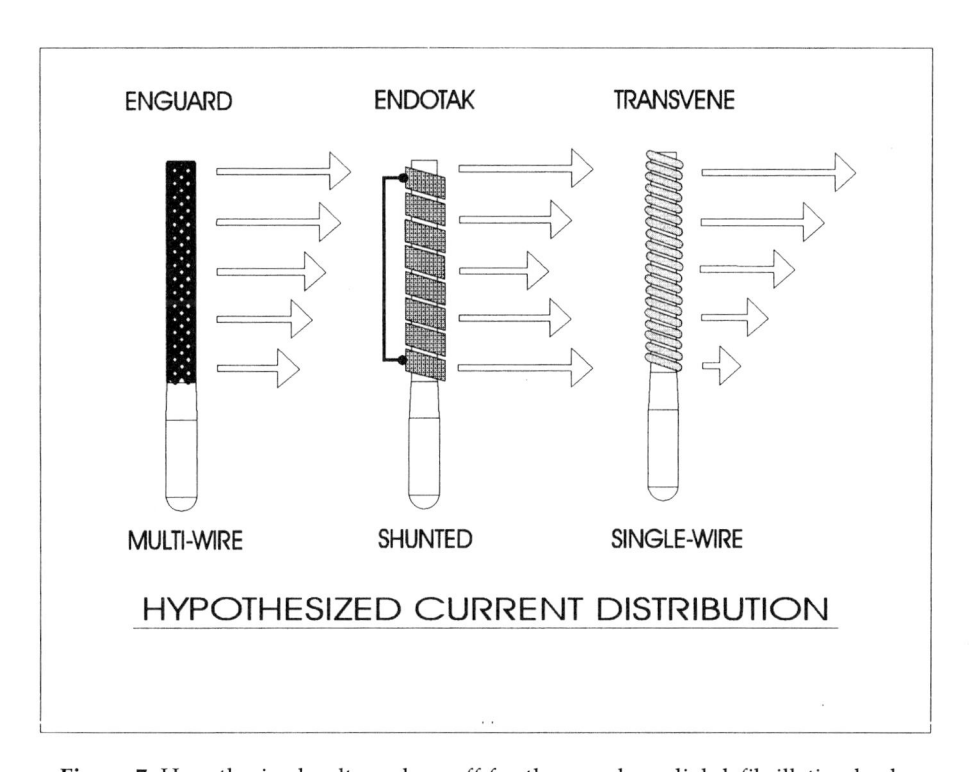

Figure 7. Hypothesized voltage drop-off for three endocardial defibrillation leads.

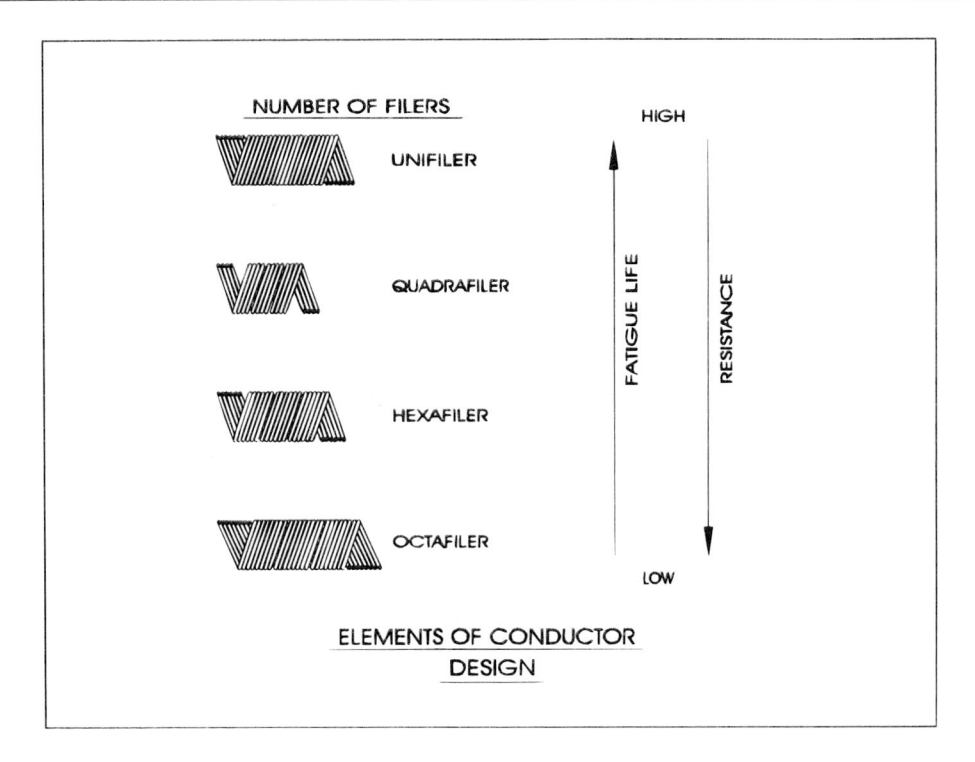

Figure 8. Resistance versus fatigue life: engineering design trade-offs for defibrillation conductors.

resistance, the ratio of the lead diameter to wire diameter must be as great as possible. This, in engineering terms, is called the "D-to-d" ratio. This is shown schematically in Figure 9. In general terms, a small wire diameter over a large lead body will result in improved fatigue life. However, such a design may not be practical due to high impedance of the wire, as well as the large size. The resistance of a wire is related to the following equation:

$$R = \frac{\rho l}{r^2}$$

R = Resistance
ρ = Resistivity of wire
l = Length of wire
r = Diameter of wire

The resistance is inversely related to the square of the wire diameter. Therefore, thicker wire is desired for impedance purposes. For defibrillation it is desirable to have the impedance as low as possible. As the diameter of leads gets smaller, thinner conductor wires with higher resistance will need to be used in order to obtain equivalent fatigue life. The high resistance may be minimized by using multiple conductors or other novel conductor designs. Multiple conductor or multifiler designs are also limited by fatigue. Specifically, an increase in the number of filers, ie, quadrifiler to hexafiler will decrease the fatigue life while improving the resistance. Table 5 summarizes the engineering trade-offs for electrode design.

High-Voltage Conductors

The choice of defibrillation conductors are influenced by the same design constraints as for electrodes. For defibrillation, low resistance and high fatigue life conductors are required. Currently, there are two conductors that are routinely used: drawn brazed strand and drawn filled tube. Most pacing leads use multifiler MP35N as the conductor. MP35N consists of 35% nickel, 35% colbalt, 20% chromium, and 10% molybdenum.[30] This wire has excellent fatigue

$$\frac{D}{d} > 5 \text{ (TYPICALLY)}$$

d = DIAMETER OF WIRE
D = DIAMETER OF ELECTRODE

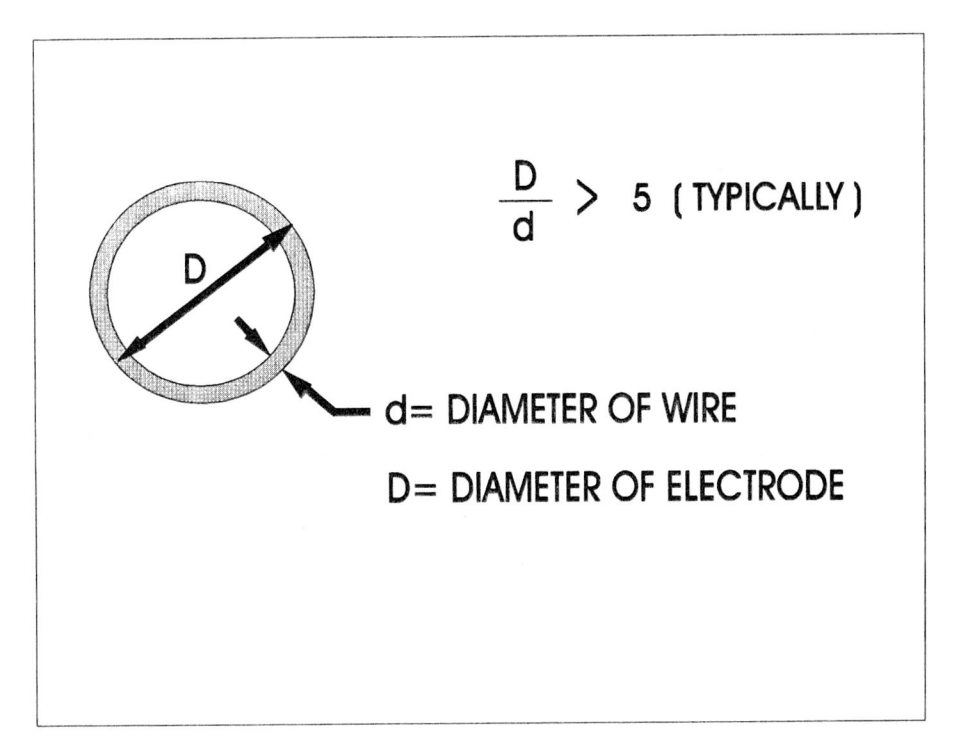

Figure 9. Lead body diameter to wire diameter ratio (D:d). Typically this value should be as large as possible in order to achieve improved fatigue life.

and corrosion resistance. However, the resistance is too high for defibrillation applications. Both drawn brazed strand and drawn filled tube contain MP35N for fatigue and manufacturing purposes. In addition to MP35N, the conductors incorporate silver to reduce the impedance. Figure 10 shows the cross section of drawn brazed strand and drawn filled tube wires.

Design of a robust conductor is especially critical for defibrillation leads. In addition to fatigue, there are two other areas of physical stress to be concerned with: 1) compression at the clavicle-first rib and 2) kinking of the lead within the defibrillator pocket. Typically, defibrillation leads are larger (greater diameter) than pacemaker leads. Therefore, their propensity to fracture due to the above forces is greater. A review of the forces imposed on lead systems due to implant locations were examined and reviewed by Jacobs et al.[31] and Magney et al.[32]

Most epicardial patches use a mul-

Table 5
Engineering Trade-Offs for Electrode and Conductor Designs

Increasing Variable (All Others Held Constant)	Resistance	Fatigue Life	Stiffness
Wire diameter	Decrease	Decrease	Increase
D/d ratio	Increase	Increase	Decrease
Number of wires	Decrease	Decrease	Increase
Wire spacing	Decrease	Decrease	Decrease

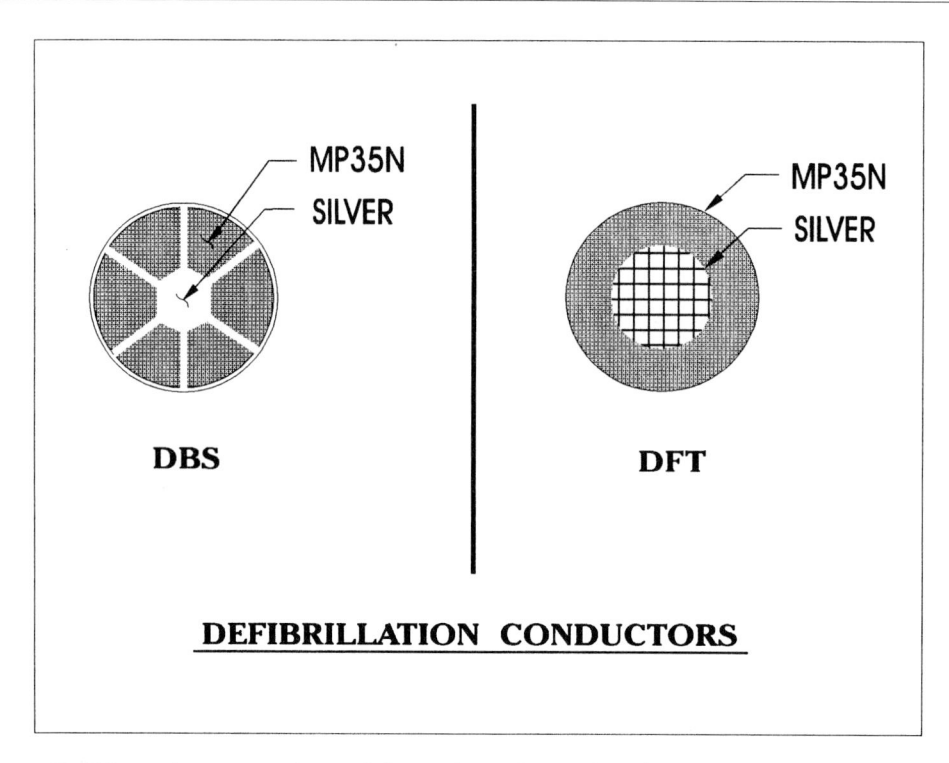

Figure 10. Schematic cross sections of drawn brazed strand and drawn filled tube defibrillation conductor wires.

tiwire drawn brazed strand cable for the conductor. In some cases, the drawn brazed strand cable is insulated with polytetrafluoroethylene (PTFE), ie, Teflon. The wires in the cable need to be small enough in order to achieve high fatigue life. Generally, the wire diameter is about 0.05 mm. In order to obtain low impedance, multiple wires are used. Connection of the drawn brazed strand wire to the titanium or platinum patch mesh, as well as to the stainless steel terminal pin, is usually performed by swaging and/or crimping of the cable. Welding is usually avoided due to the possibility of silver contamination outside of the weld joint.

Endocardial defibrillation leads use either drawn brazed strand conductor cables (Endotak) or drawn filled tube coils (Transvene and EnGuard). The Endotak construction is based on an extruded silicone tubing with three lumens. One lumen contains the MP35N pacing coil, while the other two contain the two high-voltage PTFE coated drawn brazed strand ropes. Therefore, in general terms, the conductor for the Endotak is similar to that used for epicardial patches. Both Transvene and EnGuard use multifiler drawn filled tube conductors.

The choice of the coil design offers additional complexities for manufacturing. First, because drawn filled tubes contain a core of silver (the thickness of the core can be variable and is determined by the manufacturer), welding of the wire is usually not performed. Therefore, crimping of the wire to the terminal pin and defibrillation electrode is the method of choice. This differs from pacemaker leads where the MP35N is typically welded. The crimp joint must be strong enough to withstand insertion/withdrawal forces at the defibrillator header. Figure 11 is a close-up view of the hexagonal crimp connection on the Transvene® lead.

Second, the resistance of the conductor needs to be as low as possible. For drawn

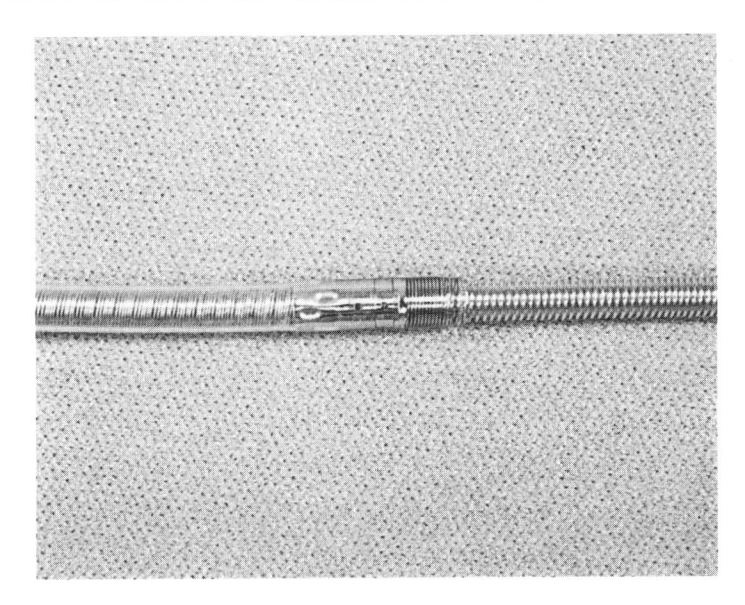

Figure 11. The hexagonal crimp connection on the Medtronic Transvene™ (Minneapolis, MN) defibrillation lead. The crimp connects the hexafiler drawn filled drawn filled tube conductor to the platinum iridium (Pt/Ir) defibrillation electrode.

filled tube conductors the resistance is a function of the wire diameter, percentage of silver, diameter of the coil and number of filers in the conductor. Conpte et al.[33] have determined that for maximal fatigue life, a quadrafiler coil should have a D:d ratio > 7. Additionally, increasing the number of wires in the coil reduces the fatigue life. The fatigue life of a coil can be related to the torsional stress.[34] Given the model of a simple spring (Figure 12), the equation for the torsional stress is given by:

$S = GdFK/\pi D^2$

where

- G = Torsional modules of elasticity (PSI) (material dependent)
- d = Cut wire diameter (in)
- F = Deflection (in) per effective coil
- K = Factor which compensates for increase in stress as the D/d ratio decreases
- D = Mean diameter of the coil
- T = Torsion of wire
- W = Weight or force applied load on the spring

Most of the strain associated with the wire occurs at the surface. Therefore, with a small silver core it may be negligible for evaluation of fatigue life. However, increasing the concentration of silver in the core may influence fatigue characteristics as well as pose additional challenges for corrosion if the insulation material is damaged or abraided.

The choice of drawn filled tube conductor wire depends heavily on the outer diameter of the lead. For instance, larger lead bodies can use larger wire because D:d ratio constraints will be avoided, whereas smaller French size leads must decrease wire diameter. Decreasing wire diameter comes at the cost of increased resistance. To offset this, the designer can either increase the silver concentration or increase the number of filers.

Smaller lead diameters will most likely become critical due to issues with clavicular "crush." The method of choice for implantation of transvenous leads continues to be subclavian vein puncture. Although cephalic insertion may be preferable for lead longevity, by minimizing the propensity for

$$T = WD/2$$

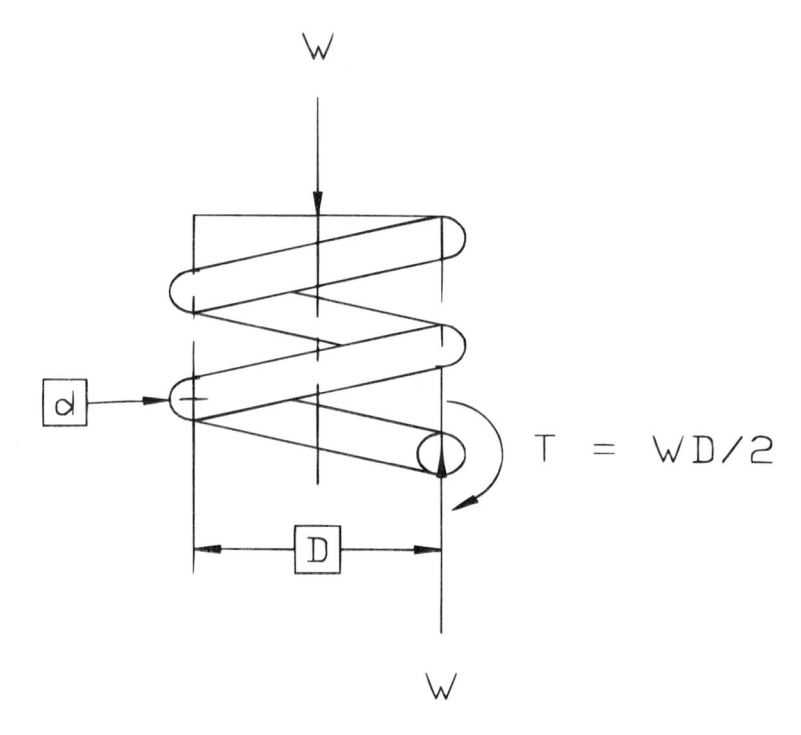

Figure 12. A simple spring model used for estimating fatigue life in a conductor coil.

lead fracture, the lead must be designed in such a way that it is capable of withstanding compression as much as possible.

Pacing and Sensing

Although the primary function of defibrillation leads is to deliver shocks, an equally important function is to reliably transduce the cardiac electrical signals. The lead must work in tandem with the defibrillation sense amplifier and detection algorithm to reliably detect and differentiate ventricular arrhythmias from the sinus rhythm. The pacing and sensing with endocardial defibrillation leads systems has come under scrutiny.[35] Helgura et al.[36] showed that when implanted properly, epimyocardial leads have similar performance as the endocardial leads. Pacing functions have generated less concern, since most patients are not pacer dependent and only require bradycardia support postshock. However, newer smaller ICDs may require improved pacing lead performance.

The sensing ability of leads, or the lack of, has been a focus of several manuscripts.[37-39] It is important to understand that the system's sensing ability depends on three factors: 1) the electrogram sensed by the lead; 2) the input amplifier characteristics (filtering, gain); and 3) the detection and classification algorithm. In this chapter only the signals sensed by the lead are examined. However, other variables are equally important (see Chapter 4).

Epicardial sensing is generally performed with two myocardial screw-in leads. The leads are positioned as close as possible to the parallel axis of propagation of the wave fronts. Morphological changes in the electrogram can occur due to lead positioning. Electrogram morphology changes due to epicardial positioning and design were examined by Accorti et al.[40] Figure 13 shows the electrode recording set-up and Figure 14 shows the electrograms recorded

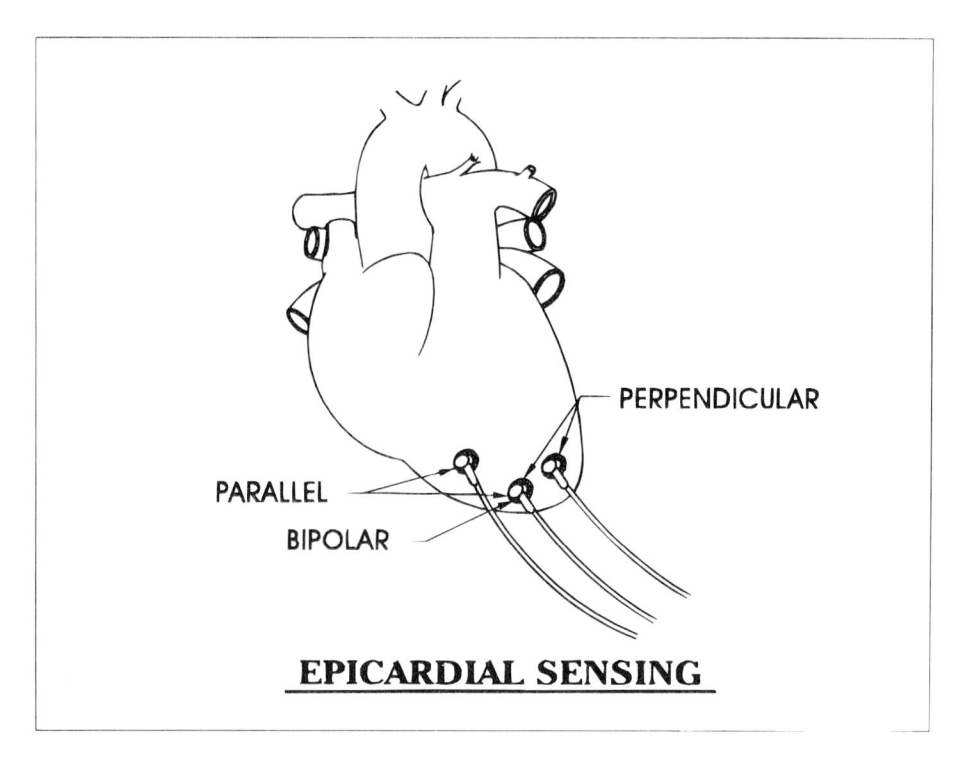

Figure 13. Electrode recording set-up used for comparing orientation to electrogram amplitude and morphology.

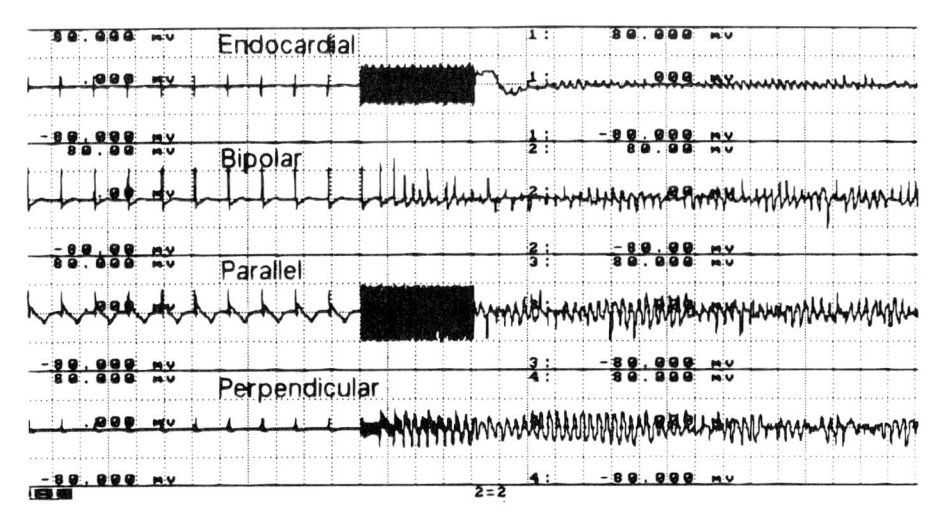

Figure 14. Multiple electrograms recorded from epicardial sensing leads: perpendicular, parallel, concentric bipolar, and an endocardial reference signal.

from multiple epicardial leads placed parallel and perpendicular to the axis of propagation. Also, recorded are signals from an investigational bipolar epimyocardial sensing lead developed by Possis Corporation. The morphology of the electrograms are different. How the morphology amplitude changes impact on the device sensing specificity depends on other factors, such as the sense amplifier characteristics and the detection algorithm. Table 6 summarizes the peak-peak amplitudes for sinus rhythm and ventricular fibrillation for the multiple epicardial sensing arrangements.

The biggest concern with using epicardial leads is their pacing performance. High pacing thresholds and exit block have been reported. In response to this, some investigators have suggested using only transvenous electrodes for sensing.[35] With the success of antitachycardia pacing reliable pacing functions become even more critical.

Most of the issues regarding electrogram sensing have involved endocardial defibrillation leads. There are two types of defibrillation leads used: true bipolar and integrated bipolar. The true bipolar lead consists of separate pace/sense electrodes similar to a standard pacemaker lead. The integrated bipolar lead uses the distal defibrillation electrode as the anode for pacing and sensing.

The electrograms from an integrated bipolar lead will appear to be more unipolar in appearance than a true bipolar lead. The large size of the anode band acts to average the propagating wave fronts. In the frequency domain, the integrated bipolar electrograms will have more power in the lower frequency band than the true bipolar lead. For example, Luceri et al.[41] investigated the use of a custom tripolar disposable defibrillation lead in the electrophysiology laboratory. During the study, true bipolar and integrated bipolar electrograms were simultaneously recorded from each patient. Figure 15 shows the catheter used in the study. Bipolar sensing occurred between the two sensing rings while integrated bipolar sensing occurred between the distal ring

Table 6
Unfiltered Peak to Peak Amplitudes for Sinus Rhythm and Ventricular Fibrillation for Multiple Epicardial Sensing Arrangements in the Canine

	Sinus Rhythm Concentric Bipolar	Sinus Rhythm Parallel Configuration	Sinus Rhythm Perpendicular Configuration	Ventricular Fibrillation Concentric Bipolar	Ventricular Fibrillation Parallel Configuration	Ventricular Fibrillation Perpendicular Configuration
Number of dogs	4	4	4	4	4	4
Number of Complexes Per Dog	50	50	50	30	30	30
Mean (Millivolts) Cummulative Electrograms	42.6	27.6*	19.1*	16.1	21.4*	21.0*
Standard Deviation (Millivolts) Cummulative Electrograms	8.8	12.3	2.7	3.7	2.6	0.9

* $P < 0.05$ compared with the concentric bipolar configuration

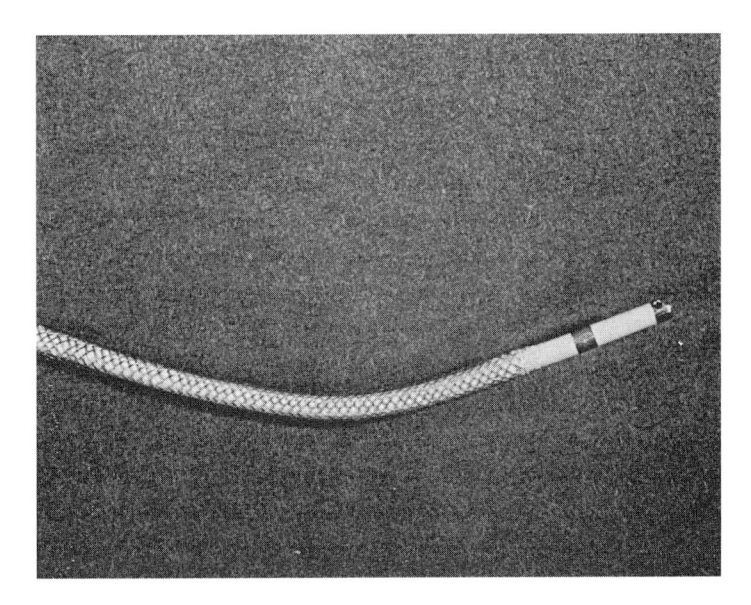

Figure 15. A custom tripolar catheter used to compare integrated and true bipolar electrograms.

and the proximal shocking electrode. Table 7 summarizes the comparison between the electrogram obtained with integrated bipolar and true bipolar sensing in this study. Typically, the integrated bipolar electrogram had more power in the lower frequency spectrum than the true bipolar signal. Figure 16 depicts normalized (to amplitude) power spectral density plot comparing the R waves for integrated bipolar and true bipolar electrograms obtained prior to defibrillation testing. Even though the frequency spectrum was different for the two bipolar pairs, the overall amplitudes for sinus rhythm and ventricular arrhythmias were not significantly different as shown in Table 7. It is important to note that the measurements made in Table 7 were performed on broadband (1–500 Hz) not high-pass filtered recordings. Signals with lower frequency content will appear attenuated when placed through a high-pass filter (eg, 30–200 Hz).

Interactions with recording systems and in some cases the sense amplifier can dramatically affect the electrograms for endocardial defibrillation leads. These effects can be more pronounced with integrated bipolar leads compared with true bipolar leads. In most pacemakers the sense ampli-

Table 7
Broad-Band Peak to Peak Amplitude Comparisons for Integrated and True Bipolar Electrograms for Sinus Rhythm and Ventricular Fibrillation

	Sinus Rhythm Integrated Bipolar	Sinus Rhythm True Bipolar	Ventricular Fibrillation Integrated Bipolar	Ventricular Fibrillation True Bipolar
Number of Eposides	58	58	8	8
Mean (millivolts)	5.4	6.4	2.7	2.5
Standard deviation (millivolts)	1.1	2.0	0.8	0.9
Significance	$P > 0.05$		$P > 0.05$	

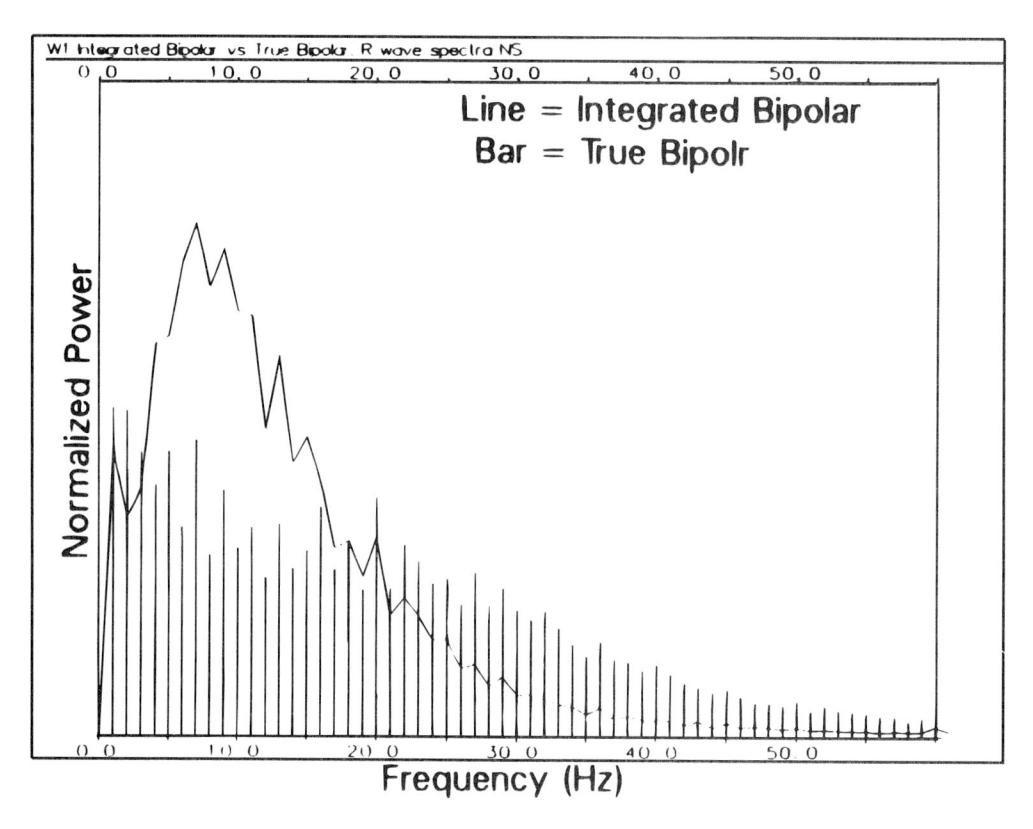

Figure 16. Mean normalized power spectral density comparing the R waves from integrated bipolar and true bipolar recordings.

fier is protected from high voltage by Zener diodes. The diodes function by short circuiting together the inputs to the amplifier once a critical voltage has been met (typically > 20 V). The voltage induced at the sense amplifier once the diodes have opened results in current flow along the lead. The magnitude of the current (shunt current) is limited by the conductor resistance. This chain of events is summarized in Figure 17.

Currents of up to or over 1 amp may be delivered through the pacing tip during shunting. The effect on the morphology of integrated bipolar electrograms due to current shunting is seen in Figure 18. The electrograms recorded in the laboratory show large ST segment changes along with a widening of the R wave after a shock of 700 V. The overall power of the electrogram is shifted to the lower frequencies. The effect of high-pass filtering the electrogram is shown in Figure 19. The postshock filtered R wave is dramatically reduced, whereas the unfiltered amplitudes are similar to the preshock values. For true bipolar sensing, this effect is minimized due to a lower potential difference of induced voltage and higher conductor impedance within the circuit.

Most of the new implantable defibrillators incorporate alternate modes of amplifier protection that result in open circuiting the inputs instead of short circuiting them. Therefore, the effect of current shunting is minimized.

Conduction disturbance due to high electrical fields have been reported by Yabe et al.[23] Certain voltage gradients can result in conduction block. Proximity of the defibrillation electrode to the sensing tip may result in conduction block during maximum shock delivery. This may become a

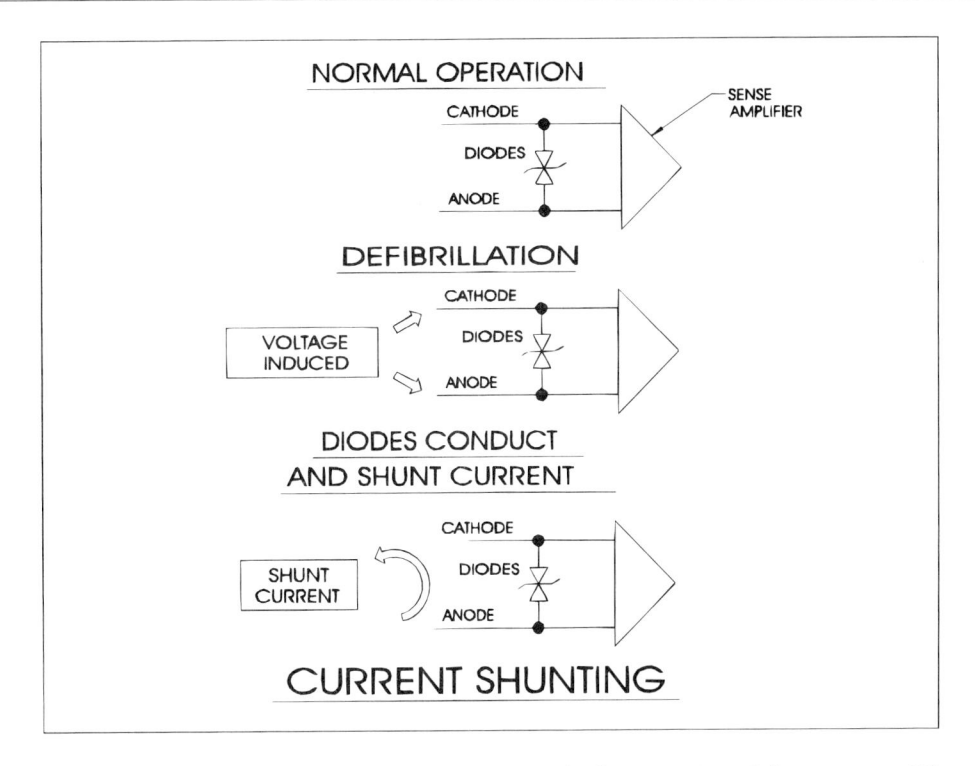

Figure 17. Current shunting chain of events due to diode protection of the sense amplifier.

concern for postshock detection of ventricular fibrillation.

Pacing thresholds and pacing efficiency have generally been secondary concerns for defibrillation leads. Recently, there have been reports of capture delay postdefibrillation shock using endocardial defibrillation leads. However, new lead systems will most likely use state-of-the art bradycardia lead technologies. These include low-

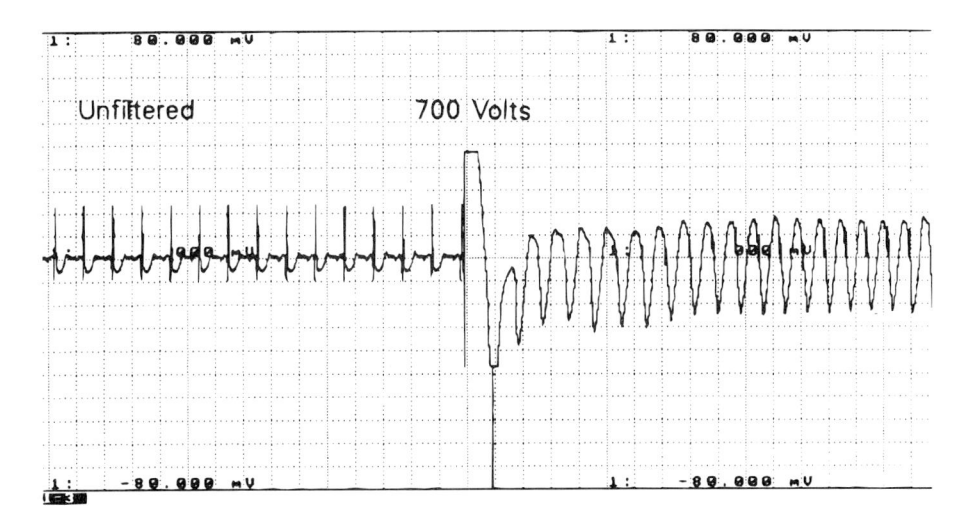

Figure 18. Electrogram morphology changes due to current shunting.

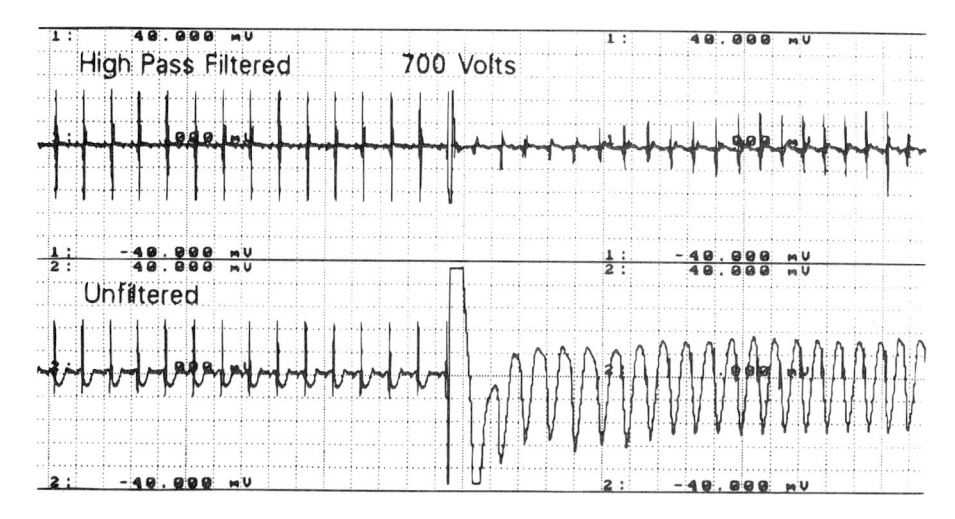

Figure 19. High-pass filtering (30–200 Hz) of the current shunted electrograms show significant amplitude reductions.

polarization small surface area tips and steroid elution. As the generators become smaller and incorporate smaller batteries, there will be more of a need to conserve battery charge. Thus, more efficient and stable pacing will need to be accomplished. Low-polarization methods, such as platinization and carbon and nitride deposition have been used in bradycardia applications.[42–44] The effective surface area is increased, allowing for smaller electrode macrosurface area leads, resulting in an increase in pacing impedance. However, the sensing impedance remains low due to the increased effective surface area. High-pacing impedance is desirable because it minimizes current drain. Polarization reduction at the electrode/tissue interface also improves pacing efficiency. Figure 20 compares a low-polarization platinized tip with a high-polarization smooth electrode.

The benefits of steroid elution have been well established for pacemaker leads.[45,46] The primary benefit from steroid elution is the decrease in pacing threshold peaking due to fibrotic encapsulation of the distal tip. Some data suggest that it may be possible to program pacing voltages to below 2.0 V. Currently, there are no market-released defibrillation lead systems that incorporate steroid elution. Only Medtronic has a market-released steroid elution pacemaker lead. Telectronics lead has been in clinical trials with a drug eluting collar.[47] Most likely, manufacturers with the capability of incorporating steroid elution will probably do so for future transvenous defibrillation leads. The benefits of steroid elution are also being explored with epicardial sensing leads.[48]

Additional Design Issues

Other areas of the lead system design include the terminations, adapters, and means of fixating the lead. These issues, although not usually discussed, are quite important for lead system design and performance.

In early defibrillation lead systems there was no standard for the terminations of the leads. The defibrillation electrodes tended to have 6-mm style terminations and the pace/sense inputs were unipolar 5-mm pins. Various standards are being actively discussed within the medical device industry for both the high-voltage and bipolar pace/sense terminations. Currently, there are only draft versions for the DF-1 (high

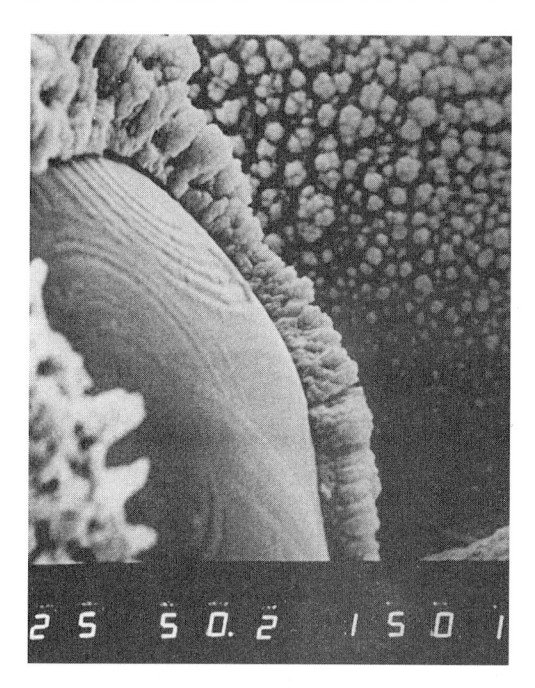

Figure 20. Magnification of a Telectronics (Englewood, CO) pacemaker electrode showing both a high surface area platinized portion and a smooth nonplatinized area.

voltage) and IS-1 (pace/sense) terminations. Figure 21 compares a draft DF-1 high-voltage terminal with a standard 6-mm terminal.

Therefore, most manufacturers' leads are only 100% compatible with their own generators. The trend is toward standardization in the industry. However, new multielectrode designs and/or the addition of special sensors may make standardization problematic in the future.

In many cases, especially when using multiple defibrillation electrodes or combining different lead systems, lead adapters must be used. The design of adapters must be performed with the same diligence as for the leads and generator density. Voltage breakdown of the sealing rings and current leakage across the seals must be understood and be within standard limits. Also, the method of stabilizing the lead in the adapter must be determined. Current methods include set-screws and spring-loaded rings. Failures of the adapter constitute failure of the system, and in most defibrillator patients this requires surgical intervention. A common adapter used for connecting two 6-mm unipolar pace/sense electrodes to an inline VS-1 bipolar connector is represented by Figure 22.

Fixation of the lead is accomplished in three ways: 1) at the distal tip to ensure lead stability within the heart; 2) at the venous puncture site; and 3) within the device pocket. To ensure lead body stability, distal fixation of the lead is accomplished in a similar fashion as with the pacemaker leads. In most cases the pacing tips and fixation mechanisms are identical to pacing electrodes. Either passive fixation tines or active fixation screws are used for lead stability. There are advantages and disadvantages to both systems. The long history of passive fixation tines has demonstrated their stability and performance. The main disadvantage of tine leads is the inability to place the lead in multiple locations. Placement can usually be made only in the ventricular apex or atrial appendage (if an atrial J lead is used). This results in limited possibilities of obtaining adequate R waves in some patients. Also, lead removal of tined leads, especially large defibrillation leads, may be quite difficult. Both the CPI Endotak and Telectronics EnGuard use passive fixation

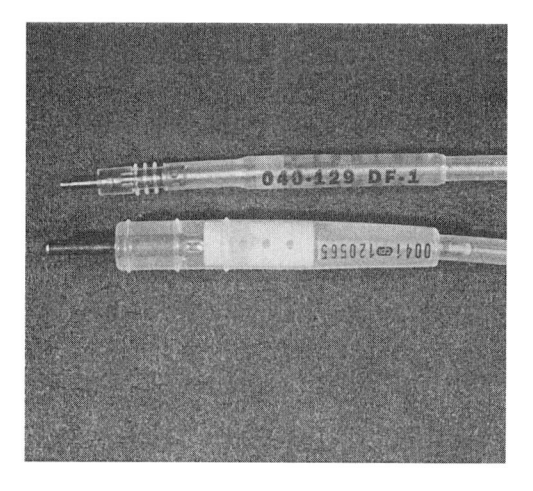

Figure 21. Comparison of a new DF-1 defibrillation terminal with a standard 6-mm connector.

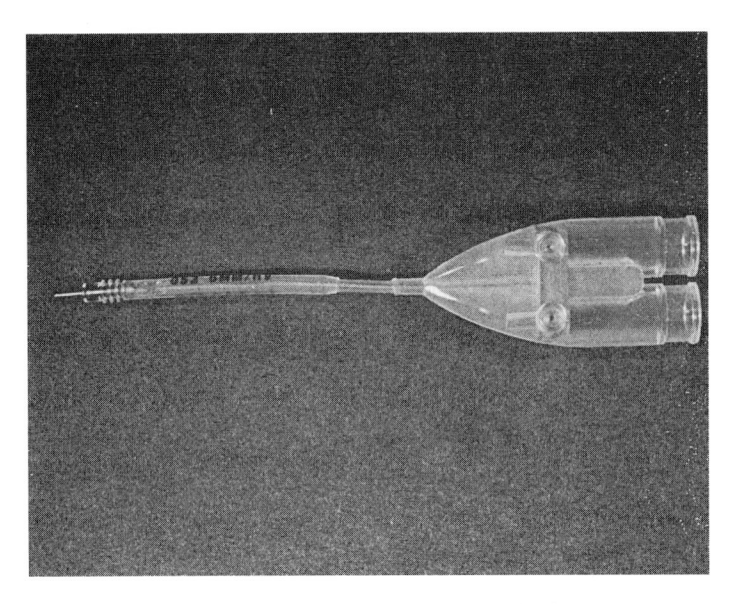

Figure 22. A 6-mm unipolar to VS-1 bipolar adapter. This type of adapter is necessary for generator replacements.

for lead stability. Active fixation leads generally incorporate a helical screw mechanism. Whether the screw can perform pacing and sensing depends on thespecific manufacturer's design. Currently Medtronic's Transvene and Intermedic's investigational lead incorporate active fixation. Active fixation leads have the advantage of being able to be positioned and secured in areas other than the right ventricular apex. In some patients, sensing from the right ventricular septum has been observed to be superior. However, formal studies designed to investigate this have not been published. Additionally, active fixation leads may be easier to remove chronically compared to passive fixation leads.

Lead anchoring is also very critical, especially for long transvenous leads where body movements and gravitational pressures from the device may precipitate lead migration and/or dislodgement. Lead migration has been a problem for leads placed free-floating in the SVC.[49] In many cases, additional suture sleeves are required to ensure lead stability. Loops placed proximal to the venous puncture site have also been recommended to minimize the stress imposed on the lead from body movements.

Due to their length (100–110 cm), the leads can easily be kinked within the defibrillator pocket. Excessive kinking of the lead can increase the propensity of connector fracture as well as insulation failure. Therefore, care should be taken to minimize lead kinking, either within the surgical pocket or within the tunnel region.

Summary and Future Directions

Because the lead is the interface between the patient and the device, its design and functionality is critical to the success of the ICD system. Unlike the device, the lead system must withstand millions of fatigue cycles and survive in the body for at least 10 years. Much of the technology used in defibrillation electrodes has been pioneered in pacemaker leads.

The electrode must be designed to withstand multiple fatigue cycles, have low resistance, and superior biocompatibility and biostability. The conductor design should be equally robust and must take into consideration the need for low impedance.

Sensing functions need to exceed pacemaker requirements. The signal sensed by the lead must be matched to the characteristics of the sense amplifier and the detection algorithm. Pacing functions will continue to improve with the incorporation of low polarization tips and steroid elution. Lead stability issues must be addressed through proper fixation mechanisms and suturing techniques. Finally, the choice of insulation material will become a paramount concern owing to the fact that major suppliers of the currently available materials plan to discontinue their supply to the medical device industry.

There will be new advances in defibrillation leads in the near future. Most of the changes will involve endocardial leads, since they are the method of choice for defibrillation therapy. The new advances will address the concerns with the current technology with respect to the physiology and functionality issues. Defibrillation leads, unlike pacemaker leads, tend to be larger and more traumatic to the surrounding tissues. The epicardial and the subcutaneous patches have been known to migrate or crumple due to tissue contraction.[50,51] These problems may lead to patch erosion, fibrotic scarring, tissue necrosis, and loss of defibrillation efficacy.[52] In most cases surgical intervention is necessary to correct the problem. The use of patch electrodes for defibrillation is decreasing due to the success of endocardial defibrillation. However, in some patients patch electrodes are used subcutaneously for multidirectional defibrillation in conjunction with endocardial leads. Early data from Obel[53] and more recently by Scott et al.[54] demonstrated defibrillation efficacy using catheter type electrodes in place of a subcutaneous patch. Recent clinical data with the CPI Subcutaneous Array lead demonstrated improved defibrillation performance with three ribbon electrodes placed subcutaneously.[55]

Endocardial leads have also resulted in increased fibrotic reactions within the heart. The fibrosis may result in new arrhythmogenic foci as well as a deterioration of the intracardiac electrogram.[56] Additionally, increased fibrosis in most cases will exacerbate lead removal.

New leads will be designed to minimize these concerns. Small flexible lead tips using low-polarization electrodes and steroid elution will be the norm rather than the exception. The benefits of small surface area pacing tips with steroid elution has been documented.[57] Additionally, stiffness at the distal portion of the lead should be minimized to avoid perforation, poor pacing, sensing, and fibrosis. These findings have been shown by Cumeron et al.[58] to be beneficial for pacemaker leads. In order to accomplish this, small-diameter leads will be used. The small diameter, by design, will result in a decreased defibrillation electrode surface area (the shadow surface area). Singer et al.[59] have shown that small surface area or low profile 6.5 French leads result in comparable defibrillation efficacy to the larger diameter leads currently in use.

Specificity of defibrillation therapy continues to be a concern. New lead systems, along with improved algorithms for arrhythmia detection will be used to address this concern. Much research has been devoted to using right ventricular pressure to differentiate hemodynamically tolerated and nontolerated ventricular arrhythmias.[60-62] In these cases improved specificity must be weighed against the new and as yet unforeseen complexities that may arise from the more complex lead system.

Another method studied by Khoury et al.[63] estimated changes in ventricular volume using intra-electrode impedance. This methodology may be incorporated into the existing lead systems. This is advantageous because special leads incorporating sensors do not have to be used.

Perhaps the easiest method to differentiate supraventricular tachyarrhythmias and sinus tachycardias from lethal ventricular arrhythmias is to incorporate atrial sensing into the detection algorithm. Schuger et al.[64] demonstrated that simple ventricular tachycardia criterion in tandem with atrioventricular interval tracking would have correctly classified 97% of ventricular tachycardias encountered in the study. However, studies examining atrial sensing with standard defibrillation electrodes are few.[65] Additional studies using defibrillation electrodes will need to be conducted to determine if postshock atrial sensing abnormalities are an issue.

There also has been a recent interest in the treatment of atrial fibrillation using endocardial leads. Powell et al.[66] demonstrated the efficacy of low-energy cardioversion of atrial fibrillation in sheep. Recent clinical data have also shown promise for low-energy atrial defibrillation.[67] Long-term studies on the safety and efficacy of such systems have not yet begun. Incorporation of atrial defibrillation capabilities into new devices will impose additional constraints on the lead system with respect to its functionality and design.

Along with device size, improved lead system designs will assist in driving the acceptance of arrhythmia control devices as a treatment of choice for ventricular arrhythmias. Prophylactic implantation of ICDs will become realizable when small nontraumatic lead systems with improved efficacy for both defibrillation and pacing are designed.

References

1. Mirowski M, Morton M, Mower MD, et al: Standby automatic defibrillator. *Arch Intern Med* 126:158, 1970.
2. Schuder JC, Stoeckle H, Gold JH, et al: Experimental ventricular defibrillation with an automatic and completely implanted system. *Trans Am Soc Artif Intern Organs* XVI:207, 1970.
3. Mirowski M, Mower MM, Gott VL, et al: Transvenous automatic defibrillator—preliminary clinical tests of its defibrillating subsystem. *Trans Am Soc Artif Intern Organs* XVIII:520, 1972.
4. Rubin L, Hudson P, Driller J, et al: Automatic defibrillation and pacing with a transvenous electrode. In: *Proceedings of the Fourth New England Bioengineering Conference.* Edited by S Saha. New York: Pergamon Press; 1976, p. 427.
5. Mirowski M, Mower MM, Reid PR, et al: Implantable automatic defibrillators: their potential in prevention of sudden coronary death. *Ann NY Acad Sci* 371, 1982.
6. Reid PR, Mirowski M, Mower MM, et al: Clinical evaluation of the internal automatic cardioverter defibrillator in survivors of sudden cardiac death. *Am J Cardiol* 51:1608, 1983.
7. Marchlinski FE, Flores BT, Buxton AE, et al: Automatic implantable cardioverter-defibrillator: efficacy, complications and device failures. *Ann Intern Med* 104:481, 1986.
8. Luceri RM, Thurer RJ, Palatianos GM, et al: The automatic implantable cardioverter-defibrillator: results, observations and comments. *PACE* 9:1343, 1986.
9. Ewy JA, Thomas E, Taren B: Electrode system for permanent implantable defibrillator: transvenous catheter and subcutaneous plate electrode. *Med Instrum* 12:296, 1978.
10. Mower MM, Mirowski M, Chier JS, et al: Patterns of ventricular activity during catheter defibrillation. *Circulation* 49:959, 1974.
11. Troup PJ: Implantable cardioverters and defibrillators. In: *Current Problems in Cardiology.* Edited by RA O'Rourke. Chicago, IL: Year Book Medical Publishers, Inc.; 1989, p. 679.
12. Winkle RA, Bach SM, Mead RH, et al: Comparison of defibrillation efficacy in humans using a new catheter and superior vena cava spring-left ventricular patch electrode. *J Am Coll Cardiol* 11:365, 1988.
13. Hanson JS: Sixteen failures in a single model of bipolar polyurethane-insulated ventricular pacing lead: a 44-month experience. *PACE* 7:389, 1984.
14. Cohney BC, Cohney TB, Hearne VA: Augmentation mammaplasty—a further review of 20 years using the polyurethane-covered prosthesis. *J Long-Term Effects Med Implants* 1(3):269, 1992.
15. van Noort R, Black MM: Silicone rubbers for medical applications. In: *Biocompatibility of Clinical Implant Materials.* Volume II. Edited by DF Williams. Boca Raton, FL: CRC Press, Inc.; 1981, p. 80.
16. Stokes K, Cobian K: Polyether polyurethanes for implantable pacemaker leads. *Biomaterials* 3:225, 1982.
17. Stokes KB: Polyether polyurethanes: biostable or not? *J Biomater Appl* 3:228, 1988.
18. Stokes K, Urbanski P, Upton J: The in vivo auto-oxidation of polyether polyurethane by metal ions. *J Biomater Sci Polymer Edn* 1(3):207, 1990.

19. Phillips R, Frey M, Martin RO: Long-term performance of polyurethane pacing leads: mechanisms of design-related failures. *PACE* 9:1166, 1986.
20. Tengvall P, Lundstrom I: Physico-chemical considerations of titanium as a biomaterial. *Clin Mater* 9:115, 1992.
21. Fotuhi P, Alt E, Callihan R, et al: Endocardial carbon braid electrodes: new approach to lowering defibrillation thresholds. *PACE* 16:1919, 1993.
22. Dillon SM, Wit AL: Voltage sensitive dye recordings from intact hearts using optical fibers (abstract). *Biophys J* 53:641a, 1988.
23. Yabe S, Smith WM, Daubert JP, et al: Conduction disturbances caused by high current density electric fields. *Circ Res* 66(5):1190, 1990.
24. Ideker RE, Wolf PD, Alferness C, et al: Current concepts for selecting the location, size and shape of defibrillation electrodes. *PACE* 14(1):227, 1991.
25. Barin ES, Elstob JE, Hakim MG, et al: Human defibrillation thresholds using biphasic waveforms and contoured epicardial patches. *PACE* 11:882, 1988.
26. Lerman BB, Deale OC: Effect of epicardial patch electrodes on transthoracic defibrillation. *Circulation* 81(4):1409, 1990.
27. Isbruch F, Block M, Wietholt D, et al: Reduction of the endocardial sensing signal of an integrated sense/pace/defibrillation lead after application of defibrillation shocks. *PACE* 15:562, 1992.
28. Jung W, Manz M, Pfeiffer D, et al: Failure of an implantable cardioverter-defibrillator to redetect ventricular fibrillation in patients with a nonthoracotomy lead system. *Circulation* 86(4):1217, 1992.
29. Mehra R, Norenberg MS, DeGroot P, et al: Multicenter clinical results with an implantable defibrillator utilizing transvenous leads. *PACE* 15:566, 1992.
30. Klingler LJ, Kurisky GA: MP35N alloy—the ultimate wire material. *Wire J* 13(7):68, 1980.
31. Jacobs DM, Fink AS, Miller RP, et al: Anatomical and morphological evaluation of pacemaker lead compression. *PACE* 16(1):434, 1993.
32. Magney JE, Flynn DM, Parsons JA, et al: Anatomical mechanisms explaining damage to pacemaker leads, defibrillator leads, and failure of central venous catheters adjacent to the sternoclavicular joint. *PACE* 16(1):445, 1993.
33. Comte P, Gysin E, Baehni T: Fatigue performances of stimulating electrodes. *Biomedizinische Technik Band* 28:19, 1983.
34. Juvinall RC: Springs. In: *Fundamentals of Machine Component Design*. New York: John Wiley & Sons; 1983, p. 351.
35. Krol R, Saksena S, Tullo NG, et al: Optimal pacing and sensing lead systems for implantable hybrid pacemaker-cardioverter-defibrillators. *J Am Coll Cardiol* 17(2):55A, 1991.
36. Helguera ME, Maloney JD, Woscoboinik JR: Long-term performance of epimyocardial pacing leads in adults: comparison with endocardial leads. *PACE* 16(I):412, 1993.
37. Almeida HF, Buckingham TA: Inappropriate implantable cardioverter defibrillator shocks secondary to sensing lead failure: utility of stored electrograms. *PACE* 16(I):407, 1993.
38. Sperry RE, Ellenbogen KA, Wood MA, et al: Failure of a second and third generation implantable cardioverter defibrillator to sense ventricular tachycardia: implications for fixed-gain sensing devices. *PACE* 15:749, 1992.
39. Callans DJ, Hook BG, Kleiman RB, et al: Unique sensing errors in third-generation implantable cardioverter-defibrillators. *J Am Coll Cardiol* 22(4):1135, 1993.
40. Accorti P, Callaghan F, et al: Concentric bipolar epimyocardial electrodes reduce amplitude modulation during ventricular fibrillation. *IEEE* 13(2):723, 1991.
41. Luceri R, Accorti P, Scott S, et al: Initial experience with a disposable custom electrophysiology/cardioverting/defibrillating catheter in patients with supraventricular or ventricular arrhythmias. *PACE* 15:596A, 1992.
42. Midel M, Jones B, Brinker J: A comparison of platinized grooved electrode performance with ring-tip electrodes. *PACE* 12:752, 1989.
43. Djordjevic M, Stojanov P, Velimirovic D, et al: Target lead-low threshold electrode. *PACE* 9:1206, 1986.
44. Thuesen L, Joern PJ, Vejby-Christensen H, et al: Lower chronic stimulation, threshold in the carbon-tip than in the platinum-tip endocardial electrode: a randomized study. *PACE* 12:1592, 1989.
45. Mond H, Stokes K: The electrode-tissue interface: the revolutionary role of steroid elution. *PACE* 15:95, 1992.
46. Stamato N, O'Toole MF, Fetter JG, et al: The safety and efficacy of chronic ventricular pacing at 1.6 volts using a steroid eluting lead. *PACE* 15:248, 1992.
47. Brewer G, Mathivanar R, Skalsky M, et al: Composite electrode tips containing externally placed drug releasing collars. *PACE* 11:1760, 1988.
48. Stokes K: Preliminary studies on a new steriod eluting epicardial electrode. *PACE* 11:1797, 1988.
49. Khastgir T, Lattuca J, Aarons D, et al: Ven-

tricular pacing threshold and time to capture postdefibrillation in patients undergoing implantable cardioverter-defibrillator implantation. *PACE* 14:768, 1991.
50. Siclari F, Klein H, Troster J: Intraventricular migration of an ICD patch. *PACE* 13:1356, 1990.
51. Block M, Borggrefe M, Schwammenthal E, et al: Long-term follow-up on defibrillation-patch-leads used for implantable cardioverter defibrillators (ICD). *PACE* 13:510, 1990.
52. Singer I, Hutchins G: Pathologic findings related to the lead system and repeated defibrillations in patients with the automatic implantable cardioverter-defibrillator. *J Am Coll Cardiol* 10(2):382, 1987.
53. Obel IWP: Electrode system for closed chest ventricular defibrillation. Cardiac Pacing & Electrophysiology Procedures of World Congress, Israel 1987, 465–472.
54. Scott S, Accorti P, Callaghan F, et al: Ventricular and atrial defibrillation using new transvenous tripolar and bipolar leads with 5 french electrodes and 8 french subcutaneous catheters. *PACE* 14:1893, 1991.
55. Swanson D, Lang D, et al: Improved defibrillation efficacy with separated subcutaneous wires replacing a subcutaneous patch. *Eur J Card Pacing Electrophysiol* 2(2):A106, 1992.
56. Epstein A, Anderson P, Kay GN, et al: Gross and microscopic changes associated with a nonthoracotomy implantable cardioverter defibrillator. *PACE* 15:382, 1992.
57. Schuchert A, Kuck K-H: Benefits of smaller electrode surface area (4 mm^2) on steroid-eluting leads. *PACE* 14:2098, 1991.
58. Camerson J, Mond H, Ciddor G, et al: Stiffness of the distal tip of bipolar pacing leads. *PACE* 13:1915, 1990.
59. Singer I, Maldonado C, Vance F, et al: Defibrillation efficacy using two low-profile endocardial electrodes. *Am J Med Sci* 302(2):82, 1991.
60. Beauregard L-A, Volosin K, Waxman HL: Differentiation of arrhythmias by measurement of intracardiac pressures in man. *PACE* 14:161, 1991.
61. Kapadia K, Wood M, Lub B, et al: A prospective study of changes in right ventricular dp/dt during ventricular tachycardia. *PACE* 14:1098, 1991.
62. Sharma A, Bennett T, Wilkoff B, et al: Right ventricular pressure during ventricular arrhythmias in humans: potential implications for implantable antitachycardia devices. *J Am Coll Cardiol* 15(3):648, 1990.
63. Khoury D, Mcalister H, Wilkoff B, et al: Continuous right ventricular volume assessment by catheter measurement of impedance for antitachycardia system control. *PACE* 12:1918, 1989.
64. Schuger C, Jackson K, Steinman RT, et al: Atrial sensing to augment ventricular tachycardia detection by the automatic implantable cardioverter defibrillator: a utility study. *PACE* 11:1456, 1988.
65. Block M, Isbruch F, et al: ECG's of defibrillation electrodes yield more information than ECG's of sensing electrodes. *Eur J Card Pacing Electrophysiol* 2(2):A122, 1992.
66. Powell A, Garan H, et al: Low energy conversion of atrial fibrillation in the sheep. *J Am Coll Cardiol* 20(3):707, 1992.
67. Tacker WA, Schoenlein WE, Janas W, et al: Catheter electrode evaluation for transvenous atrial defibrillation. *PACE* 16:853, 1993.

Chapter 9

A Logical Approach to Tiered-Therapy Implantable Cardioverter-Defibrillator Design

Eliot L. Ostrow

Introduction

The evolution of device therapy for lethal or potentially lethal ventricular tachyarrhythmias has followed a long and rather tortuous path. Pacemakers designed to detect ventricular tachycardia (VT), and to automatically treat the arrhythmia with antitachycardia pacing (ATP), first became available in the late 1970s.[1] However, the fear persisted that ATP, regardless of the method used or the extent of pre-implant testing, might accelerate a slow, well-tolerated VT to ventricular fibrillation (VF).[2-4] Thus, despite evidence that the overwhelming majority of slow VT episodes could be terminated with ATP,[5,6] these devices never achieved widespread acceptance. In fact, no antitachycardia pacemaker has ever been made commercially available in the United States for the treatment of VT.

Preliminary work was done in the late 1970s and early 1980s on an automatic implantable low-energy cardioverter for the treatment of VT.[7] Because such treatment had a success rate similar to that for ATP[8] and carried with it a similar risk of acceleration of VT to VF,[9] the implantable cardioverter suffered a comparable fate.

With the advent of the AICD™ (CPI, St. Paul, MN) in the early 1980s, physicians were given the means to terminate virtually any ventricular tachyarrhythmia. Yet the AICD proved to be a less than wholly satisfactory solution for those patients who had episodes of reasonably well-tolerated VT. High-energy shocks, while effective in terminating the arrhythmias, were not well perceived by relatively asymptomatic patients, particularly when the episodes occurred frequently.[2,4,10] In addition, some patients experienced troublesome bradycardia, which the device could not treat, after the delivery of a shock.[11]

To deal with these clinical situations, physicians began implanting various combinations of devices. Bradycardia pacemakers were implanted with ICDs,[12] as were antitachycardia pacemakers,[4,12] in an attempt to overcome the shortcomings of each of the devices alone. In extreme cases, a patient might receive a dual chamber bradycardia pacemaker, an antitachycardia pacemaker, and an ICD, resulting in an impressive array of hardware. Unfortunately, because these devices worked independently of one another, the possibility of unwanted interac-

---

From Singer I, (ed.) Implantable Cardioverter-Defibrillator. Armonk, NY: Futura Publishing Company, Inc.; © 1994.

tions existed.[12] For example, the ICD might sense the atrial and ventricular outputs of a dual-chamber pacemaker, as well as the evoked R wave, and misinterpret them as separate intrinsic ventricular events. After several such sequences, the ICD's rate detection criterion could be met, resulting in the delivery of an inappropriate shock to the patient. Similarly, if the bradycardia pacemaker's sensitivity were not sufficient to detect VF electrograms, the pacemaker would asynchronously pace into that rhythm. If the pacemaker outputs were detected by the ICD, and the ICD's automatic gain control circuitry adjusted to these large inputs, the ICD might be prevented from increasing its sensitivity to a level that would allow for detection of the VF electrograms. In such a case, the pacemaker's outputs could be incorrectly interpreted as a regular intrinsic rhythm, and therapy might be withheld.

Despite the limitations inherent in combining devices, such arrangements were, in fact, the first incarnations of tiered-device therapy for the treatment of ventricular tachyarrhythmias. These combinations highlighted the efficacy of tiered therapy, and the desirability of combining all of the antiarrhythmic therapies into a single device to prevent unwanted device interactions. In this chapter, clinical and engineering considerations inherent in the design of tiered-therapy ICDs are explored.

The Hierarchical Approach to the Treatment of Ventricular Arrhythmias

The conceptual basis of tiered-device therapy is the recognition that different arrhythmias may be most appropriately treated with different therapeutic modalities.[13] Antitachycardia pacing is clearly inappropriate for treating VF; similarly, treating a slow, well-tolerated VT with a 30- or 40-J shock is similar to shooting a mouse with an elephant gun. Simply stated, the goal of tiered therapy is to "make the punishment fit the crime."

Implicit in the concept of tiered therapy is the ability to distinguish between bradycardia, pace-terminable and nonpace-terminable VT, and VF, and to assign appropriate therapies to each arrhythmia class. Ideally, the device would also be able to alter its treatment approach based upon hemodynamic tolerance. Thus, one can think of the tiered-therapy device as embodying a pair of hierarchies: a classification hierarchy based on the clinical severity of the arrhythmia, and a response hierarchy that delivers an increasingly aggressive/increasingly uncomfortable/increasingly energy-consumptive series of therapies.

Rate Zones

All of the tiered-therapy ICDs available today, and those likely to find their way into clinical practice in the next few years, base their classification hierarchy on rate.[14] Figure 1A illustrates the simplest application of the hierarchical approach, in which the rate continuum is divided into three distinct segments: a bradycardia region, designated in this example to encompass any rhythm with a rate below 50 beats per minute in which bradycardia pacing would be provided; a normal sinus rhythm region, spanning a window from 50–150 beats per minute in which no therapy would be provided; and a tachyarrhythmia region in which any rhythm with a rate in excess of 150 beats per minute would be treated with high-energy shocks. Note that the zones are defined by the desire to apply a particular therapy, and do not necessarily match the clinical definitions of the rhythms implied by their names. Thus, a VT at a rate of 125 beats per minute would be classified as normal sinus rhythm in the example above, and no therapy would be delivered.

Figure 1B carries the hierarchical approach to its next logical step. The bradycardia and normal sinus regions are defined as before. However, the tachyarrhythmia re-

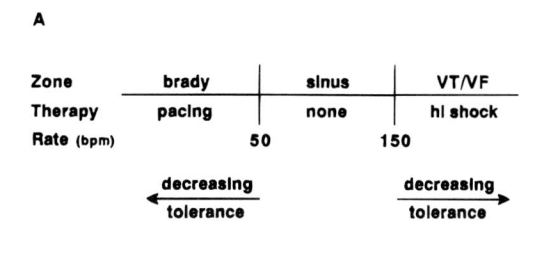

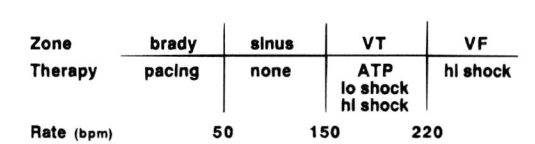

Tiered-Therapy Implantable Cardioverter-Defibrillator Design

A

Zone	brady	sinus	VT/VF
Therapy	pacing	none	hi shock
Rate (bpm)		50	150

← decreasing tolerance   decreasing tolerance →

B

Zone	brady	sinus	VT	VF
Therapy	pacing	none	ATP lo shock hi shock	hi shock
Rate (bpm)		50	150	220

Figure 1. Hierarchical approach to tiered-therapy automatic ICD design. **Panel A**: The rate continuum is divided into three regions based on rate: bradycardia (brady), normal sinus rhythm (sinus), and tachyarrhythmia (VT/VF). Rhythms with rates below 50 beats per minute are treated with bradycardia pacing. No therapy is delivered when the intrinsic rate is between 50 beats per minute and 150 beats per minute. Rates above 150 beats per minute are treated with high-energy shocks (hi shocks). Hemodynamic tolerance is assumed to diminish as cardiac rate decreases below 50 beats per minute or increases above 150 beats per minute. **Panel B**: The tachyarrhythmia region is subdivided into two subregions: ventricular tachycardia (VT) and ventricular fibrillation (VF). Arrhythmias in the VT region are treated with a hierarchy of therapies: antitachycardia pacing (ATP), low-energy cardioversion (lo shock), and high-energy cardioversion (hi shock). Arrhythmias above 220 beats per minute will be treated with high-energy shocks. Note: These conventions and abbreviations will be used in all figures to follow. No differentiation is made in the annotation of cardioversion and defibrillation; both are denoted as shocks.

gion is now divided into two subregions, designated VT and VF. Note that a simple therapy hierarchy has been assigned to the VT region, in which a sequence of ATP, low-energy cardioversion, and high-energy cardioversion will be applied in succession. Again, anything above 220 beats per minute, whether truly VF or simply a rapid VT, will be classified as VF, based upon the desire to treat fast (and, presumably, hemodynamically compromising) rhythms with high-energy shocks, regardless of the actual underlying mechanism.

It may, at times, be desirable to further subdivide the VT region, either to enhance therapy delivery or to allow for better arrhythmia discrimination. If the patient's ventricular tachycardias were to span a wide rate range, it might be appropriate to treat the faster, less hemodynamically stable arrhythmias with a more aggressive therapy. This could be accomplished by subdividing the VT region into two or more zones, with different therapies or therapy hierarchies applied to each. Figure 2 illustrates this concept. In this example, the VT region, which is defined as having a rate range of 150–220 beats per minute, is broken into two smaller (35 beats per minute) zones. Tachyarrhythmias in the first VT zone (VT-1), which will in this case be presumed to be well tolerated and pace-terminable, are treated with a succession of therapies. ATP-1, which might be a series of successively more aggressive autodecremental bursts,[15–17] is tried first. Should it prove unsuccessful, a series of scanned adaptive bursts (ATP-2) is attempted. If these do not successfully convert the patient to sinus rhythm, synchronized low-energy cardioversion shocks will be delivered, followed if necessary, by high-energy shocks. Tachyarrhythmias in the second VT zone (VT-2), which for this case are assumed to be non-pace-terminable and to result in fairly rapid hemodynamic decompensation, are treated with synchronized low-energy shocks followed by high-energy shocks. No pacing therapies are attempted; even in cases where ATP might be effective, the hemodynamic considerations would preclude their use.

At times, it may be desirable to subdivide the VT region to allow improved discrimination of arrhythmias, even if the same therapy hierarchy is applied to all of the resultant VT zones. For instance, sinus rate cross-over may exist, a circumstance in which the patient's fastest achievable sinus rate may exceed the slowest clinical VT. As discussed in an earlier chapter, this situa-

Zone	brady	sinus	VT-1	VT-2	VF
Therapy	pacing	none	ATP-1 ATP-2 lo shock hi shock	lo shock hi shock	hi shock
Rate (bpm)	50	150	185	220	

Figure 2 Subdivision of the ventricular tachycardia region into two zones, denoted as VT-1 and VT-2, for the purpose of allowing differentiation of therapies. See text for explanation. See legend for Figure 1 for conventions and abbreviations.

tion can often be addressed by including a sudden onset criterion in the detection algorithm, on the assumption that a sinus tachycardia will have a gradual onset, whereas a pathological VT will begin abruptly. Similarly, the patient may have atrial fibrillation with a ventricular response that falls within the low end of the VT region. A rate stability criterion may be added to the detection algorithm, based upon the concept that the cycle length of most reentrant VTs is relatively constant, while in many cases conducted atrial fibrillation results in an erratic ventricular rate. While including criteria such as sudden onset and rate stability in a detection algorithm increases the algorithm's specificity, it also results in a loss of sensitivity. Such a trade-off, which may prolong or prevent arrhythmia detection, may be acceptable in a lower rate range, where the tachycardia is likely to be well tolerated, but may not be appropriate in a higher rate range, where hemodynamic compromise is more likely.

Figure 3 provides an illustration of such a case. The hypothetical patient can achieve sinus rates of 140 beats per minute with maximum exertion. The patient's VT has been observed in the clinical setting to be as slow as 125 beats per minute when antiarrhythmic drug levels are at their peak, but may be considerably faster with lower drug levels or in a heightened catecholamine state. Moreover, the patient has atrial fibrillation with a ventricular response that never exceeds 135 beats per minute. The device could be configured as shown in Figure 3A, with a tachycardia region spanning rates from 120–200 beats per minute, and a fibrillation region for any rhythm above 200 beats per minute. The detection algorithm for the tachycardia region requires that the tachycardia be fast (above 120 beats per minute), abrupt in onset (to discriminate VT from sinus tachycardia), and have a stable beat-to-beat cycle length (to distinguish VT from atrial fibrillation), or a stable high rate

A

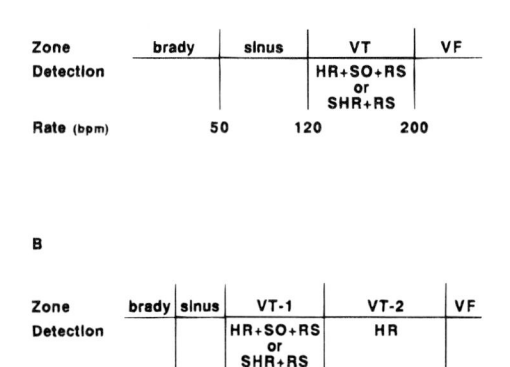

Zone Detection	brady	sinus	VT	VF
			HR+SO+RS or SHR+RS	
Rate (bpm)		50	120	200

B

Zone Detection	brady	sinus	VT-1	VT-2	VF
			HR+SO+RS or SHR+RS	HR	
Rate (bpm)		50	120	150	200

Figure 3. Subdivision of the ventricular tachycardia region for improved arrhythmia detection and discrimination. **Panel A**: Single VT zone. Therapies will be delivered only for rhythms that meet the assigned arrhythmia detection algorithm: (high rate [HR] + sudden onset [SO] + rate stability [RS]) or (sustained high rate [SHR] + rate stability). **Panel B**: A second VT zone is added, with different detection algorithms assigned to each. See text for further explanations. See legend for Figure 1 for conventions and abbreviations.

must be sustained for a long period of time (in case the sudden onset criterion is not met, possibly due to an exercise-induced VT). There are at least two potential clinical problems with a device configured in this manner. First, while the onset of the arrhythmia may, in fact, have been gradual if it were initiated by exercise, the transition from sinus tachycardia to VT could result in an arrhythmia at a rate of 180 beats per minute. However, since the sudden onset detection criterion would not have been met, the device would not deliver therapy until the sustained high-rate duration were exceeded, which could leave the patient in a hemodynamically unstable condition for a prolonged period of time.

The second potential problem that could arise with a device configured as shown in Figure 3A might be the emergence of a rapid, polymorphic VT with an unstable beat-to-beat cycle length. While this is clearly a rhythm that requires immediate attention, the rate stability criterion might preclude treatment entirely, because the device would consider the irregular rhythm to be most probably atrial fibrillation.

Both of these potential problems can be easily dealt with, if an additional tachycardia zone is added as illustrated in Figure 3B. The first tachycardia zone (VT-1) ranges from 120–150 beats per minute, to encompass both the sinus cross-over rates and the conducted atrial fibrillation rates. This zone would then be programmed to use the complex detection algorithm previously described. The second tachycardia zone (VT-2) is designed to detect and treat arrhythmias that by definition cannot be sinus tachycardia (because the lower boundary of VT-2 is above the patient's maximum achievable sinus rate) nor conducted atrial fibrillation (since VT-2's lower rate boundary is above the fastest rate at which the patient conducts atrial fibrillation). In this zone, where it is imperative to detect hemodynamically compromising arrhythmias quickly, the device can be programmed to use the simplest possible detection algorithm, high rate alone.

The flexibility of rate zone programming in the newer tiered-therapy ICDs allows the physician to define a simple device configuration when clinically appropriate, yet permits full use of the more complex detection and therapy features of the device, when necessary, without undue compromise.

Therapy Sequencing

Once rate zones have been established and appropriate detection algorithms assigned to each, the next priority is to decide on the sequence of therapies by which rhythms in each tachyarrhythmia zone are to be treated. This, again, is the overriding goal of the tiered-therapy concept: to provide the appropriate level of therapy for every tachyarrhythmia.

As previously alluded to, in cases where hemodynamic tolerance permits, more than one therapy may be applied in a given tachyarrhythmia zone. When this is the case, it is typical to begin with the least aggressive therapy, with subsequent therapies becoming more and more aggressive. Most tiered-therapy devices impose some form of such a therapy hierarchy, requiring that pacing therapies be attempted before shock therapies, and that lower energy shocks be delivered before higher energy shocks. This ensures that lower energy therapies, which are less battery consumptive and sometimes less uncomfortable for the patient, are used first.

Therapy sequencing becomes more complicated when multiple tachycardia zones are created (Figure 4). Note that a sequence of four therapies (two pacing therapies, low-energy cardioversion, and high-energy cardioversion) is assigned to the lower tachycardia zone, while only one pacing therapy is to be attempted before the initiation of shock therapies in the higher tachycardia zone. Three clinical scenarios may be considered: 1) a tachyarrhythmia that starts in the VT-1 zone, and is accelerated by the second pacing therapy into the

Zone	brady	sinus	VT-1	VT-2	VF
Therapy	pacing	none	ATP-1 ATP-2 lo shock hi shock	ATP-1 lo shock hi shock	hi shock
Rate (bpm)	50	120	150	220	

Figure 4. Therapy sequencing when a tachyarrhythmia moves between VT zones. See text for further explanation. See legend for Figure 1 for conventions and abbreviations.

VT-2 zone; 2) a VT that starts in the VT-2 zone, and is decelerated by low-energy cardioversion into the VT-1 zone; and 3) an arrhythmic episode in which ATP results in a sequence of accelerations and decelerations.

In the first scenario, the adaptive scanned decremental burst pacing therapy (ATP-2) accelerated a relatively slow arrhythmia into the higher tachycardia zone. What therapy should the ICD apply to the new, faster VT? Should the adaptive autodecremental burst pacing therapy (ATP-1), which failed to terminate the slower tachycardia, be attempted again since it has been programmed as the first therapy to be applied to VT-2 rhythms? One could argue that the failure of this ATP therapy to terminate the slower VT should not prevent its use on the faster VT because 1) it is an adaptive therapy, and will therefore be different from the therapy previously attempted; and 2) by the nature of the therapy having been programmed into the VT-2 zone, it must be presumed to be effective, at least some of the time, in terminating arrhythmias that fall into that region. Conversely, one could argue that because the patient has now been in tachycardia for a considerable period of time, ischemic changes are likely to have occurred that would make it desirable to bring the arrhythmic episode to a quick conclusion. Either of these arguments may be correct, depending upon the specifics of an individual patient's clinical picture, particularly his or her expected hemodynamic status after the acceleration of the arrhythmia. To allow the physician the ability to handle such a situation in the most clinically appropriate manner, a programmable therapy ratcheting feature[13] may be incorporated into an ICD. Such a feature would, when activated, enforce a rule whereby upon acceleration of the rhythm, subsequent therapies could not be less aggressive (ie, lower in the therapy sequence hierarchy) than the previous therapies delivered during the arrhythmic episode. Carried a step further, therapy ratcheting could dictate that upon arrhythmia acceleration, pacing therapies be terminated and shock therapies be delivered.

The second scenario, in which a low-energy cardioversion shock decelerates the arrhythmia from VT-2 to VT-1, presents a similar quandary. In some cases, one might choose to attempt ATP therapies on the now slow, well-tolerated VT; in other cases, it may be desirable to progress to shock therapies due to ischemic changes. To cover such situations, it is possible to incorporate a shock ratcheting feature into an ICD, such that once shock therapies are initiated, a less aggressive therapy (either an ATP therapy or a lower energy shock) may not be delivered, regardless of changes in the rate of the tachyarrhythmia. Such a feature might also be useful in cases where an arrhythmia in the VF region, accompanied by almost certain hemodynamic compromise and by ischemic changes is decelerated by a shock therapy into a VT zone. Carried to its extreme, this feature could be programmable by tachyarrhythmia zone, so that, for example, VF that decelerates to VT would be subject to the shock ratcheting rule, while a VT-2 arrhythmia that decelerates to VT-1 would not.

The third scenario considers the case in which an arrhythmia "ping-pongs" between two tachycardia zones, alternately accelerated by one pacing therapy, then decelerated by another. It is clearly desirable to prevent this sequence from going on indefinitely. One method of dealing with such a situation would be to limit the number of acceleration-deceleration sequences that could occur before pacing therapies are abandoned, and shock therapies instituted.

A programmable maximum time to shock, which may now be found in at least one tiered-therapy ICD,[18] could be used in lieu of or in conjunction with therapy ratcheting, shock ratcheting, and a deceleration limit. This additional feature would, as its name implies, abandon pacing therapies after a predetermined period of time, and initiate shock therapies. Ideally, the time period would be independently programmable for each VT zone, allowing more time for attempts at termination by ATP with slower, better tolerated arrhythmias, and progressing more quickly to shock therapies when the arrhythmias are more poorly tolerated.

Committed Versus Noncommitted Shocks

Once an ICD detects an arrhythmia, determines that a shock therapy is appropriate, and begins to charge, under what circumstances, if any, should delivery of the shock be withheld? This question underlies the controversy over whether a feature known as tachyarrhythmia reconfirmation is desirable or undesirable.

Most of the ICDs available are incapable of sensing while their high-energy capacitors are charging, due to the electrical interference generated by the charging circuit itself. This has led to the concern among clinicians that a patient could receive an unnecessary shock if a tachyarrhythmia were to spontaneously terminate during the charging cycle (which can last as long as 30 seconds). In response to that concern, some manufacturers have developed noncommitted devices, ie, devices that can withhold delivery of a shock if the arrhythmia is determined to have terminated during the charging process.[19] These ICDs incorporate algorithms that, at the end of the capacitor charging cycle, "look again" to reconfirm the continued presence of the arrhythmia.

Two principal arguments can be made against using reconfirmation schemes. First, because reconfirmation delays the delivery of appropriate shocks for as long as it takes to verify that the arrhythmia is still in progress, there is a concern that the efficacy of the shock therapy may be decreased because there is a reported correlation between the duration of a fibrillation episode and the defibrillation threshold. Second, and perhaps more important, is the recognition of the fact that the ability of today's devices to adequately detect arrhythmias, particularly fibrillation, is still less than perfect.[11,20] This leads to the concern that during the duration of the charging cycle, ischemic changes might result in a significant reduction in the amplitude of the fibrillation electrograms, causing undersensing of the fibrillation during the reconfirmation period. This could, in turn, result in the withholding of a shock from a patient in fibrillation. These two potential problems have led some to conclude that once an arrhythmia has been detected, and charging of the capacitors initiated, the device should be committed to deliver the shock, based on a guiding philosophy that it is better to give one shock too many than one too few.

The first concern, delaying the delivery of an appropriate shock while waiting for reconfirmation, is being addressed by advances in technology. At least one commercially available device has the ability to sense during capacitor charging,[11] and others will likely follow. This obviates the need for reconfirming the continued presence of an arrhythmia after charging is completed, because it allows for continuous confirmation throughout the course of the arrhythmic episode. In addition to the obvious advantage of preventing delivery of inappropriate shocks to the patient, being able to sense the spontaneous termination of the tachyarrhythmia during the charging cycle allows the device to abort its charging sequence mid-cycle, preventing the unnecessary battery consumption inherent when the decision to abort is made only after charging is completed.

Even with the ability to continuously confirm the presence of a tachyarrhythmia, the success of such algorithms is not ensured unless sensing is adequate, which as previously noted is not always the case. While continuous sensing during the charging cycle gives the ICD's automatic gain control time to adjust to ischemia-related diminution of electrogram amplitudes, not enough is known about the nature of these changes to completely dismiss concerns about them. This is even more true when the first delivered shock is unsuccessful at terminating the fibrillation episode, such that the duration of the episode is prolonged beyond the initial 20–30 seconds. To address such concerns, it is possible to devise a variety of semicommitted schemes. Among the potential options are to reconfirm on VT only, where sensing is more reliable, spontaneous termination is more likely, and an error will less often be catastrophic, or to allow a charging sequence to be aborted only once during a designated time period, precluding the possibility that borderline sensing would result in a prolonged sequence of detection failure.

Ultimately, some sort of sensor, hemodynamic or otherwise, may be used to assist in making the distinctions described above. Until 100% sensitivity and specificity can be guaranteed, the debate over committed versus noncommitted shock delivery is unlikely to be resolved.

Postshock Responses

The delivery of a 30- or 40-J shock directly to the myocardium produces transient changes that may affect the ICD's behavior for a short, but crucial period of time. This effect may be more pronounced in transvenous ICD lead systems, where the surface area of the shocking electrode coil is relatively small, and where the shock electrode may be in close proximity to, or even part of, the ICD's pacing and sensing system. As a result, it may be necessary or desirable to incorporate special postshock behaviors into ICD designs.

Postshock Sensing

The ability of an ICD to sense intrinsic cardiac signals has been shown to be diminished immediately after delivery of a shock, at least with some lead configurations.[21-23] Although it is not definitively known, possible explanations include stunning of the myocardium in the proximity of the shock electrodes,[22] a large buildup of polarization impedance,[22] and imperfect isolation of the ICD's sensing circuitry during and immediately after shock delivery. Some evidence exists to support each of these hypotheses.

The degree to which postshock sensing difficulties exist, and the duration for which these difficulties exist, seems to vary significantly from one manufacturer's device to the next, which would seem to lend some credence to the device design argument. However, since the vast majority of the ICD systems implanted to date have been composed of a device and leads from the same manufacturer (ie, limited mixing and matching of one manufacturer's leads with another's ICD), making it difficult, if not impossible, to separate the effects of device design from those that are lead system related.

Jung et al.[22] have shown that postshock sensing difficulties, at least with one system, are related to the distance between the sensing cathode and the shocking electrode, which also plays the role of the sensing anode in that system. Increasing this interelectrode distance was demonstrated to have a beneficial effect on both the magnitude and the duration of the changes in the postshock electrogram amplitude. It is possible that this relationship can be explained by polarization at the sensing cathode, which would be expected to diminish with increasing distance from the shock electrode. This might also explain the manufacturer-to-manufacturer differences previously noted, since the ICDs themselves may use more or less effective means for dissipating polarization charges.

Yee et al.[23] found that the postshock R wave amplitude in animals decreased significantly when bipolar recordings were taken from an electrode pair on the same catheter as the shock electrode; when shocks were delivered from sites remote from the sensing bipole, no such change in R wave amplitude was noted. Such observations lend credence to the hypothesis of myocardial stunning near the shock electrode site, which would have a profound impact on the relative positioning of the pacing/sensing and shock electrodes on transvenous ICD leads. However, polarization (and the device's ability to dissipate it) may also play a role in these observations.

While future research will likely shed additional light on this phenomenon, one might suspect that there will not be a single simple answer. Rather, it is most likely that a combination of factors, including those mentioned above, and perhaps others as well, will be found to contribute to the postshock sensing difficulties that are described in the literature today.

One of the challenges faced by the designers of ICD systems is to minimize the clinical impact of problems such as this, even when the mechanism of the problem is unclear. In the case of postshock undersensing, the potential for problems is twofold. First, following a shock that fails to terminate an episode of fibrillation, undersensing may result in a failure to detect the continuing nature of the episode or, at very least, in a delay in the delivery of subsequent shocks. If sensing problems persist long enough, the device might inappropriately conclude that sinus rhythm has been established. When the sensing problems eventually resolve, the device would then consider the detected fibrillation as an entirely new episode, and would deliver the lower energy shock that previously failed, rather than moving on to higher energy shocks. Given the now significant duration of the fibrillation episode, the defibrillation threshold is likely to have risen,[24] making success of the lower energy shock even less likely. Until the precise mechanisms of this undersensing are known, system designers will likely take steps to negate the hypothetical causes with changes to circuit design and lead systems, as well as to alter postshock sensing and detection algorithms in such a way as to minimize the likelihood of significant clinical consequences.

The second potential problem associated with postshock undersensing occurs when the delivered shock is successful in terminating the arrhythmic episode. In such a case, failure to sense the intrinsic activity may result in asynchronous pacing, which in this patient population, carries with it a significant risk of inducing a new arrhythmia. Since the electrograms of sinus beats are generally quite large, this form of undersensing is generally short lived, resolving itself within a few beats. Thus, a brief postshock pacing delay that gives the electrode/tissue interface changes time to at least partially resolve, and allows the automatic ICD's automatic gain control time to adjust, is most often all that is needed.

Postshock Pacing

Historically, approximately 10% of patients receiving ICDs have also had a concomitant need for bradycardia pacing.[25] Moreover, Platia et al.[26] have reported episodes of profound postshock bradycardia. Thus, the bradycardia pacing component of the tiered-therapy ICD can be expected to play a significant role in the treatment of patients receiving such devices.

Numerous studies have demonstrated

a rise in pacing thresholds immediately postshock, with transient loss of capture.[12,23,27] Some controversy exists as to whether this phenomenon is the result of the shock itself, or of ischemic changes related to the arrhythmic episode that preceded the shock.[27,28] Antiarrhythmic agents may also play a role in exacerbating this potential problem.[29] While the transient loss of capture rarely appears to have significant clinical consequences, it is clearly desirable that, if the ICD is going to pace after the delivery of a shock, capture be maintained. The obvious solution, from the clinician's standpoint, would be to program the bradycardia pacing output parameters (pulse amplitude and pulse width) to values that would ensure capture during the brief postshock period. However, for the pacemaker-dependent patient, this would mean pacing at an unnecessarily high output all of the time, when such an output is only necessary for a period of a few seconds to a few minutes immediately after a shock. This approach would result in a significant decrease in device longevity. For this reason, it is desirable to design an ICD such that the clinician could program the bradycardia pacing output to a higher value only for a predetermined time following a shock. Some devices being implanted today have such capabilities; more can be expected to have this feature in the future.

There may be times when a set of pacing parameters significantly different from that used for normal bradycardia pacing is desirable during the postshock period. For example, clinical cases might arise in which it would be beneficial to pace at a faster rate than usual during the postshock period to stabilize the electrophysiologic milieu and minimize refractory period dispersion. In other cases, it might be preferable to pace at a significantly slower rate, or to withhold pacing entirely, for a period of time after a shock because of the underlying electrophysiologic instability. For this reason, future devices may well incorporate the ability to program independent postshock and non-postshock bradycardia pacing parameters.

Post-Therapy Sinus Detection

After an antitachyarrhythmia therapy, whether ATP or a shock has been delivered, an ICD must then determine whether or not sinus rhythm has been reestablished. The ability to do so correctly is particularly crucial for proper sequencing of therapies when the delivered therapy is unsuccessful.

Early antitachycardia pacemakers used a single interval longer than that defined by the device as tachycardia to indicate a return to sinus rhythm. In many cases, this criterion proved to be less than satisfactory, especially in the ventricle where a burst of pacing often results in a compensatory pause before the tachycardia continues. Under such circumstances, the device would incorrectly determine that the first burst delivered had successfully terminated the episode. When, several beats later, the tachycardia were again detected, the device would consider it a new episode, which would again be treated with the first burst in the programmed sequence. In this way, the ICD would never progress beyond its first therapy.

Simply making the device sense multiple consecutive intervals within the sinus rhythm zone resolves the problem of prematurely considering a delivered therapy to be a success. However, as is usually the case, this increase in specificity results in a corresponding decrease in sensitivity. Take, for example, the case of a patient who emerges into a trigeminal rhythm after the successful termination of VT by a cardioversion shock. If the sinus detection criterion were set to three consecutive slow intervals, the device would not consider the VT episode terminated until the trigeminal rhythm resolved itself, because it would consistently see a slow-slow-fast sequence that would never meet its criterion. This would leave the device in limbo, with the rhythm being classified as neither sinus rhythm nor VT. Minutes, hours, or, potentially, days later, if the patient had another episode of VT, the device would classify it as a continuation of the previous episode, and would move on to the next step in its therapy sequence. This could have two potential consequences: one bothersome, the other dangerous.

In the situation described, the failure to detect sinus rhythm would result in the delivery of a more aggressive therapy than might be necessary at the onset of the second VT episode. Thus, the patient could receive a shock without ATP being attempted. This is clearly less than desirable, although not particularly dangerous. However, if one imagines the sequence described above being repeated over and over again, eventually the device will have exhausted its entire therapy sequence. Should another episode of VT occur, the device would not treat it at all, a condition that may be termed therapy runout.

Because no single sequence of intervals can adequately define sinus rhythm across the entire spectrum of patients, some of the newer ICDs incorporate a programmable "x out of y" criterion, similar in many ways to the type of algorithm often used to detect fibrillation. Thus, for the hypothetical patient described above, the clinician could choose a "2 out of 3" criterion (or some multiple thereof) that would allow the ICD to correctly identify trigeminy as the end of the arrhythmic episode, and a return to sinus rhythm.

One final consideration in the determination of posttherapy sinus detection is how to deal with posttherapy bradycardia pacing intervals. After the delivery of therapy, the device attempts to sense intrinsic activity so it can determine whether or not the therapy was successful. If the device does not detect any intrinsic activity during the subsequent bradycardia interval (or after the postshock pacing delay), it will deliver a bradycardia pacing pulse. However, it is impossible for the device to determine whether there was actually no intrinsic activity to be sensed, or whether its sensitivity setting was inadequate to detect activity that was actually there. This is most likely to occur if acceleration to VF has occurred, although it can happen under other circumstances as well. In order for the ICD to make the proper determination quickly, many systems incorporate features into their automatic gain control algorithm that result in a rapid increase in gain (ie, greater sensitivity) with pacing, so that any underlying intrinsic activity will be detected as quickly as possible. However, if maximum gain is achieved and intrinsic activity is still not sensed, the device must, by default, conclude that no underlying rhythm exists. It then concludes that the arrhythmic episode has been successfully terminated, and that sinus rhythm (in fact, bradycardia) has been established. While variations to the automatic gain control and/or detection algorithms have been proposed or attempted, none has yet proven wholly satisfactory. It may well take the incorporation of some sort of hemodynamic sensor into an ICD system to fully resolve this issue.

Engineering Considerations in ICD Design

As was mentioned in the introduction to this chapter, today's tiered-therapy ICDs are little more than the combination of bradycardia pacemakers, antitachycardia pacemakers, and the original shock-only defibrillators, combined into the same package and working together. On the surface, it would not appear to be a particularly difficult task to merge these technologies, which were available individually long before the first tiered-therapy ICDs were added to the physician's therapeutic armamentarium. However, the marriage of low-power and high-power circuitry into a single device is, in fact, a daunting engineering challenge, especially for an application such as this, which leaves little room for error. While it is beyond the scope of this chapter and this book to delve into the intricacies of circuit design, a general overview of the issues facing designers of ICD hardware is provided in the discussion that follows.

Combining High-Power and Low-Power Circuitry

The combination of high- and low-power electronic circuits into the same device raises a number of issues for ICD design teams. It influences the selection of a power source (see Chapter 5), the regulation and distribution of power to the various portions of the circuitry, the design and layout of the hybrid substrates upon which the integrated circuits and discrete components are mounted, and the placement of the discrete components themselves. Allowing the circuits to interact without interfering with one another is no small task.

The pacing, sensing, and logic circuits in an ICD are little different from those found in traditional bradycardia or antitachycardia pacemakers. Delivering a pacing pulse in the 1–10 V range (microjoules of delivered energy) creates a peak demand on the power source that may be measured in milliamperes. In stark contrast, the 700–800 V (30–40 J) shocks that may be delivered for cardioversion and defibrillation by the ICD's converter circuits may impose several amperes of peak current drain on the power source, a demand that is three orders of magnitude greater. These vastly different power requirements could be addressed to some extent by using two separate power sources, one for the high-voltage converter circuitry and another for everything else. While this would, in the perfect design, isolate the logic circuitry from the power fluctuations caused by capacitor charging, the implementation is not simple because the two circuits must still communicate with one another. Moreover, the use of dual power sources would likely necessitate an increase in size and weight, whereas the industry is striving to create smaller, lighter, pectorally implantable devices. For these reasons, most tiered-therapy ICD designs have avoided this approach.

The most significant consideration when a single power source is used for both high-power and low-power circuitry is to maintain an adequate voltage supply to the ICD's logic and control circuitry, even when the battery is nearing its end-of-service point and a full-energy shock is generated. Should the supply voltage to this circuitry dip below some minimum value, it is possible that control of the high-voltage circuit could be lost, with potentially clinically significant consequences. There are several possible methods for addressing this concern, some or all of which may be included in a particular ICD. One alternative might be to choose an end-of-service point that would guarantee, even with the demands imposed by a sequence of full-energy charges, that more than the minimum supply voltage to the logic and control circuitry would be maintained; another would be to incorporate additional circuitry to monitor supply voltage to these circuits, and prioritize power distribution in such a way as to maintain at least the minimum acceptable supply voltage. While each approach has its strengths and drawbacks, it is imperative that ICD design teams pay careful attention to this issue.

A second concern related to the combination of high- and low-power circuitry into a single device is the potential for internal interference. Such interference may, at times, manifest itself in an obvious manner. For example, it was previously stated that most of the current ICDs cannot sense during high-voltage capacitor charging. This limitation is most often the result of electrical noise generated by the charging circuitry, which interferes with the device's ability to sense intrinsic cardiac rhythm. Placement of components on the hybrid circuit plays a significant role in the degree to which such interference is likely to occur. New methods of shielding sensitive components may also aid in the avoidance of interference problems.

In other cases the interference may assume a much more subtle form. The substrate upon which the integrated circuits and discrete components of a hybrid circuit are mounted is typically a multilayered ceramic material, with metallized pathways running along and between layers to provide the interconnections among the various components and circuits. In the interest of conserving both space and energy, there is an obvious advantage to packing these traces, as they are known, as densely as possible. With only low-voltage/low-current circuitry, it is possible to maintain a very small intertrace distance. However, when high-voltage/high-power circuitry is incorporated as well, the possibility of inductive or capacitive coupling of current between traces goes up dramatically, and greater intertrace distances may be necessary if the device is to function appropriately. Careful layout of the ceramic substrate, which is now made somewhat easier with the advent of computer-assisted design (CAD) tools, allows for the optimization of intertrace spacing, thus minimizing size and current consumption while avoiding interference between traces.

Isolation and Protection

For years, bradycardia pacemakers have incorporated some form of protection against circuit damage due to occasional exposure to external high-voltage sources, such as external defibrillators. An ICD must protect its circuitry not only from these external high-voltage sources (to which exposure is more likely due to the nature of the disease that an ICD is designed to treat), but also from itself. The proximity of the high-voltage shock electrodes to the pacing/sensing electrodes provides a pathway by which the voltage resulting from a device-generated shock could be carried directly back to the low-voltage circuitry. A variety of passive and active means may be used, alone or in combination, to protect an ICD from external and self-generated high-voltage inputs. Regardless of the method chosen, careful consideration must be given to such protection, to ensure that it is adequate for the task at hand.

Software Corruption

Many, if not all, of the current generation of ICDs contain microprocessors, sophisticated computers that carry out a myriad of instructions every cardiac cycle. The ability of the ICD to perform appropriately is dependent upon the integrity of the instructions contained in its memory. The old computer adage, "garbage in, garbage out" is nowhere more applicable than here.

Some of the instructions that govern the actions of the microprocessor are contained in read only memory, or ROM, which is nonvolatile and subject to error only in the event of a hardware failure. However, much of the information that governs the device's actions must be alterable, based upon feedback regarding the patient's condition or instructions from an external programmer. As such, this information must be stored in random access memory, or RAM, which is, as its name implies, accessible and, therefore, changeable. The data stored in RAM may be corrupted in a variety of ways: external defibrillator shock energy coupled into the device may scramble the information contained in RAM; interruption of communication between the external programmer and the ICD, or electrical interference occurring during communications, may result in incomplete or incorrect reception of an instruction set by the ICD; or a brief drop in supply voltage to the microprocessor, as might occur if the high-voltage capacitors are charged when the battery is beyond its end-of-service point, could cause alteration of the memory state.

A variety of safety features are incorporated into the ICD to prevent the problems as described above; however, prevention is not always possible. Implantable cardioverter-defibrillator designers, taking after their pacemaking brethren, often include self-diagnostic software routines that are intended to detect software corruption, should it occur. In such an event, the device will typically go into some sort of a back-up or shut-down mode. This mode, the instructions for which are not subject to change barring a catastrophic hardware failure, is intended to bring the device to a safe state of operation. For a bradycardia pacemaker, it is relatively easy to identify a set of parameters that would generally be agreed to be safe. However, defining a single set of such parameters for a device that is intended to treat a variety of arrhythmias, under circumstances that vary greatly from one patient to the next, is virtually impossible. In a bradycardia-only device, it may be true that, "any pacing is better than no pacing at all"; for an ICD, that may not be the case. For that reason, the back-up mode for today's ICDs generally deactivates any form of antitachyarrhythmia therapy, leaving the patient unprotected in the event of a VT or VF episode. Therefore, the ideal design would ensure that the device goes into its back-up mode only when an irreversible software error has occurred, and when failure to revert to back-up presents a clearly greater risk to the patient than the reversion itself.

Conclusion

Today's tiered-therapy ICDs represent a huge leap forward in the treatment of the entire gamut of ventricular arrhythmias. They permit the clinician to tailor the device's responses to the particular needs of each patient, and to provide therapy commensurate with the severity of the arrhythmia. Designers of ICD systems have created devices that do a remarkably good job of automatically handling an enormously complex decision-making process in a nearly instantaneous fashion.

Yet much remains to be done. Better criteria than rate alone must be found for distinguishing between supraventricular and ventricular tachyarrhythmias, for assessing the patient's hemodynamic status, and for determining which therapy or sequence of therapies is most appropriate for dealing with the ever-changing physiological and electrophysiologic milieu in which the ICD operates. Better means of sensing the widely variable electrograms present during sinus rhythm, tachycardia, and especially, fibrillation must be devised, to eliminate the potential complications that can arise from underdetection of an arrhythmia, or from the fear of underdetection. New components, processes, and techniques must be developed to make the devices smaller, longer-lived, and even more reliable than they are today. These needs present daunting challenges to the designers of ICD systems, and to the researchers in the medical, academic, and industrial communities who support their efforts. If past history is any indicator, these obstacles will be overcome, allowing device therapy to gain even greater acceptance as the therapy of choice for the treatment of malignant ventricular arrhythmias.

References

1. Fisher JD, Furman S, Kim SG, et al: Tachycardia management by devices. In: *New Perspectives in Cardiac Pacing: 2.* Edited by SS Barold, J Mujica. Mount Kisco, NY: Futura Publishing Company; 1991, p. 359.
2. Bonnet CA, Fogoros RN, Elson JJ, et al: Long-term efficacy of an antitachycardia pacemaker and implantable defibrillator combination. *PACE* 14:814, 1991.
3. Fisher JD, Kim SG, Mercando AD: Electrical devices for treatment of arrhythmias. *Am J Cardiol* 61:45A, 1988.
4. Masterson M, Pinski SL, Wilkoff B, et al: Pacemaker and defibrillator combination therapy for recurrent ventricular tachycardia. *Cleve Clin J Med* 57:330, 1990.
5. Fisher JD, Mehra R, Furman S: Termination of ventricular tachycardia with bursts of rapid ventricular pacing. *Am J Cardiol* 41:94, 1978.
6. Fisher JD, Kim SG, Matos JA, et al: Comparative effectiveness of pacing techniques for termination of well-tolerated sustained ventricular tachycardia. *PACE* 6:915, 1983.

7. Zipes DP, Jackman WM, Heger JJ, et al: Clinical transvenous cardioversion of recurrent life threatening ventricular tachyarrhythmias: low energy synchronized cardioversion of ventricular tachycardia and termination of ventricular fibrillation in patients using a catheter electrode. *Am Heart J* 103:789, 1982.
8. Waspe LE, Kim SG, Matos JA, et al: Role of a catheter lead system for transvenous countershock and pacing during electrophysiologic tests: an assessment of the usefulness of catheter shocks for terminating ventricular tachyarrhythmias. *Am J Cardiol* 52:477, 1983.
9. Saksena S, Chandran P, Shah Y, et al: Comparative efficacy of transvenous cardioversion and pacing in patients with sustained ventricular tachycardia: a prospective, randomized, crossover study. *Circulation* 72:153, 1985.
10. Sharma AD, Bennett TD, Erickson M, et al: Right ventricular pressure during ventricular arrhythmias in humans: potential implications for implantable antitachycardia devices. *J Am Coll Cardiol* 15:648, 1990.
11. Mitchell JD, Lee R, Garan H, et al: Experience with an implantable tiered therapy device incorporating antitachycardia pacing and cardioverter/defibrillator therapy. *J Thorac Cardiovasc Surg* 105:453, 1993.
12. Calkins H, Brinker J, Veltri EP, et al: Clinical interactions between pacemakers and automatic implantable cardioverter-defibrillators. *J Am Coll Cardiol* 16:666, 1990.
13. Haluska EA, Whistler SJ, Calfee RJ: A hierarchical approach to the treatment of ventricular tachycardias. *PACE* 9:1320, 1986.
14. Sharma AD, Bennett TD, Erickson M, et al: Right ventricular pressure during ventricular arrhythmias in humans: potential implications for implantable antitachycardia devices. *J Am Coll Cardiol* 15:648, 1990.
15. Charos GS, Haffajee CI, Gold RL, et al: A theoretically and practically more effective method for interruption of ventricular tachycardia: self adapting autodecremental overdrive pacing. *Circulation* 73:309, 1986.
16. Waksman R, Pollack A, Berkovits BV, et al: Autodecremental pacing for the interruption of ventricular tachycardia and atrial flutter. *J Electrocardiol* 25:339, 1992.
17. den Dulk K, Kersschot IE, Brugada P, et al: Is there a universal antitachycardia pacing modality? *Am J Cardiol* 57:950, 1986.
18. Winkle RA: The implantable defibrillator: progression from first- to third-generation devices. In: *Cardiac Electrophysiology: From Cell to Bedside.* Edited by DP Zipes, J Jalife. Philadelphia, PA: W.B. Saunders Company; 1990, p. 963.
19. Klein LS, Miles WM, Zipes DP: Antitachycardia devices: realities and promises. *J Am Coll Cardiol* 18:1349, 1991.
20. Wilber DJ, Poczobutl-Johanos M: Time-dependent sensing alterations in implantable defibrillators: lessons from the Telectronics Guardian 4202/4203 (abstract). *PACE* 14(Part II):624, 1991.
21. Isbruch F, Block M, Hammel D, et al: Influence of defibrillation shocks on the endocardial sensing signals of an integrated sense/pace/defibrillation lead (abstract). *Eur Heart J* 12:1976, 1991.
22. Jung W, Manz M, Moosdorf R, et al: Failure of an implantable cardioverter-defibrillator to redetect ventricular fibrillation in patients with a nonthoracotomy lead system. *Circulation* 86:1217, 1992.
23. Yee R, Jones DL, Jarvis E, et al: Changes in pacing threshold and R wave amplitude after transvenous catheter countershock. *J Am Coll Cardiol* 4:543, 1984.
24. Winkle RA, Mead RH, Ruder MA, et al: Effect of duration of ventricular fibrillation on defibrillation efficacy in humans. *Circulation* 81:1477, 1990.
25. Winkle RA, Mead H, Ruder MA, et al: Long-term outcome with the automatic implantable cardioverter-defibrillator. *J Am Coll Cardiol* 13:1353, 1989.
26. Platia EV, Veltri EP, Griffith LSC, et al: Post defibrillation bradycardia following implantable defibrillator discharge (abstract). *J Am Coll Cardiol* 7:73A, 1986.
27. Slepian M, Levine JH, Watkins L Jr, et al: Automatic implantable cardioverter defibrillator/permanent pacemaker interaction: loss of pacemaker capture following ICD discharge. *PACE* 10:1194, 1987.
28. Reiter MJ, Lindenfeld J, Tyndal CM Jr, et al: Effects of ventricular fibrillation and defibrillation on pacing threshold in the anesthetized dog. *J Am Coll Cardiol* 13:180, 1989.
29. Singer I, Guarnieri T, Kupersmith J: Implanted automatic defibrillators: effects of drugs and pacemakers. *PACE* 11:2250, 1988.

Chapter 10

Implant Support Devices

Douglas J. Lang and Bruce H. KenKnight

Introduction

The occurrence and clinical management of spontaneous ventricular tachyarrhythmias has had great personal and economic impact on our society.[1-4] The mechanisms underlying these potentially lethal rhythm disorders are varied, ranging from different pathologies,[5-7] time-varying[8] or electrophysiologic triggering mechanisms,[9] and different clinical characteristics immediately preceding the event.[10] However, it is generally accepted that the terminal arrhythmia resulting in sudden cardiac death (SCD) is ventricular fibrillation (VF).[11,12] Early attempts to understand and treat this malady were fraught with frustration and somewhat discouraging results as a consequence of the frequent recurrence of the arrhythmia following the initial aborted arrest.[13,14] Although early hospital based, direct,[15,16] and transthoracic[17] capacitor discharge defibrillation therapies were quite effective at restoring sinus rhythm in patients fortunate enough to arrest in-hospital, they were usually unable to protect patients after release from the hospital.

This obvious limitation led to the concept of an implantable defibrillation system that could automatically terminate ventricular tachyarrhythmias with electric countershock.[18,19] Subsequent pioneering work by Mirowski and colleagues[20-25] and contributions by countless other investigators[26] have led to an impressive reduction in the incidence of SCD in patients known to be at high risk (see also Chapter 13).[27,28] For over a decade, automatic implantable cardioverter defibrillator (AICD™, CPI, St. Paul, MN) systems have been implanted in patients presenting with aborted SCD, unexplained syncope with inducible ventricular tachyarrhythmias, or drug refractory, life-threatening ventricular tachyarrhythmias.[22,25]

Intraoperative testing of implantable cardioverter-defibrillator (ICD) therapies has been performed since automatic implantable defibrillators were introduced[22] and remains a critical component of the implantation procedure (see Chapter 15).[29,30] Empiric verification that VF can be reliably terminated by the ICD is critical.[29] This is true not only during the final phases of the initial implantation procedure, but also at predischarge and occasionally at follow-up or after changes in concomitant drug therapy[31] to assess the stability of defibrillation requirements[32-34] and reprogram device output, if possible, to assure adequate performance.[35] Ventricular defibrillation can also be tested during generator replacement or after presentation of one or more device-related complications necessitating explant

From Singer I, (ed.) Implantable Cardioverter-Defibrillator. Armonk, NY: Futura Publishing Company, Inc.; © 1994.

and reimplant.[36,37] Defibrillation testing, although usually safe[38] is not devoid of risk.[30,39-41] Despite these risks, defibrillation testing must be performed in all patients; even in patients who have not experienced spontaneous episodes of VF,[42] since cardioversion thresholds are not predictive of defibrillation thresholds (DFTs).[29]

The original implant support devices were used to evaluate the patient's sensing characteristics and conversion requirements for defibrillation or cardioversion, providing therapies available in the implanted device. Recently introduced implant support systems include a diversity of implant tools ranging from external cardioverter defibrillators (ECD), instruments for electrophysiologic testing, and ICD programming capabilities for device based evaluation of therapies. These support system components, housed separately or together as a system, provide the increased sophistication to test the range of therapies offered by current ICD devices.

Fibrillation Testing Support Systems

Implant support systems play a key role in assuring the acute or chronic defibrillation efficacy of ICD systems. To fulfill this function, the support device must closely simulate the therapy delivered by the implanted system. Because manufacturers have implemented different waveforms and pulse delivery schema in their ICDs, support devices are supplied by each company as an integral part of their ICD system. This trend toward therapy diversity has moved the industry away from a universal VF implant support device toward a practice based on matched devices for support and therapy.

Another factor that has introduced diversity within the industry is the adoption of two different engineering methods for the delivery of a defibrillation pulse to the patient. These two methods differ primarily in the manner in which the pulse duration is determined: the first is a manual system, and the second automatic. While both systems are manual in the sense that shock intensity (energy or voltage) must be programmed, the latter shock delivery method automatically adjusts the duration of the pulse in accordance to the impedance of the patient's ICD lead system. Shock duration in devices implementing the former delivery method must be programmed at implant, and possibly at follow-up,[35] if patient impedance changes.[43]

Manual Implantable Cardioverter-Defibrillators

An ICD pulse generator with manually programmed shock duration controls delivery of the shock with a clock timer. After the shock is initiated, the device switches between shock phases of a biphasic waveform or ends the shock when the internal clock reaches the duration programmed by the user. This type of device is often referred to as a fixed pulse width device, referring to the fact that it will continue to deliver the same pulse width selected until it is reprogrammed. Shock intensities with these devices are typically calibrated in voltage or the initial energy stored on the ICD capacitors before the shock is given. One cannot directly program the amount of energy to be delivered to the heart, since the shape of the shock waveform and the amount of energy this type of ICD delivers will vary depending on the impedance of the patient's ICD system.[44]

The effect of impedance on pulse shape is due to the different discharge rates of the shock. If fixed pulse width ICDs were implanted using the same shock duration in a number of patients, these devices would deliver shocks with a range of different pulse shapes defined by their different system impedances. For patients with high impedance, the lower defibrillation current would discharge the ICD capacitors at a slower rate, resulting in higher trailing edge voltages when the clock finally terminates

MANUAL ICD

Waveform A
Waveform B

Programmed at Implant

AUTOMATIC ICD

Waveform C
Waveform D

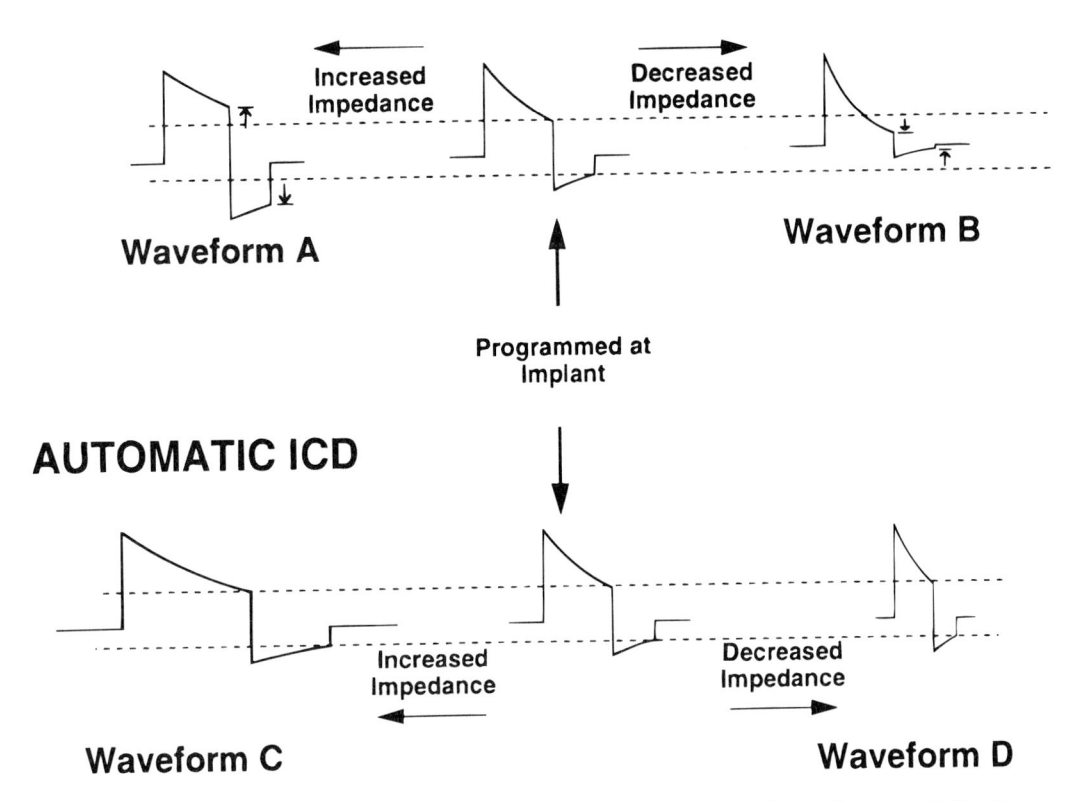

Figure 1. Impact of impedance changes on the wave shape of implantable cardioverter-defibrillator (ICD) shocks from manual and automatic ICDs. Manual ICDs use a fixed pulse width method of shock delivery that maintains the programmed pulse width when ICD system impedance changes. When impedance rises, the shock discharge rate is reduced, resulting in a higher trailing edge voltage at the end of the shock duration (waveform A). When impedance is reduced, the discharge is faster, causing the trailing edge voltage to be lower by the time the shock terminates (waveform B). Because the pulse width is fixed, the shape of the waveform (tailing edge voltage) will change as a result of changes in lead system impedance. Automatic ICDs use a variable pulse width method for shock delivery that maintains the final voltage constant for all ICD system impedances. When impedances rise, the slower discharge rate results in a longer duration pulse with the same trailing edge voltage at the end of the shock (waveform C). When impedance falls, the increased discharge rate yields a shorter shock duration with the same trailing edge voltage (waveform D). Because the trailing edge voltage is the same, the automatic ICDs deliver a constant energy to the patient. They also maintain a constant shock wave shape in the face of different impedances, avoiding waveform changes that could raise defibrillation thresholds.

the shock (waveform A, Figure 1). As the pulse shape becomes more rectangular, the energy remaining in the ICD at the end of the shock has increased, since the energy stored in the device (E_{stored}) is determined by its capacitance (C) and the charge voltage on the capacitor (V_{cap}; ie, $E_{stored} = 1/2\ CV^2_{cap}$). Thus, as a manual ICD encounters increased patient impedance, it will deliver less energy to the heart.

In contrast, low impedances will result in more triangular defibrillation pulse shapes at the same shock duration. The higher currents drawn from the device will increase the rate at which voltage is reduced on the capacitors, resulting in lower trailing edge voltages when the pulse is terminated (waveform B, Figure 1). Although the energy removed from the device has increased for these more triangular pulses, studies indicate that the DFT increases with highly spiked pulse shapes, possibly due to their low trailing edge voltages.[45]

Given the range of impedances found in ICD patients, the types of waveforms delivered by a fixed pulse width device could vary considerably, affecting shock efficacy. At implant, the impact of impedance on the shock waveform can be reduced by programming the proper shock duration for the patient's impedance. For monophasic waveforms, the optimal setting for the lowest DFT appears to be the shock duration that produces a specific pulse shape: the trailing edge voltage must be approximately 33% of the initial shock voltage.[46] This particular pulse shape and duration minimized defibrillation threshold (DFT) voltage, average current and delivered energy. For shorter programmed durations (more rectangular pulse shapes), DFT voltages rose and energies fell, consistent with the strength-duration relationships for defibrillation.[47] For longer durations (more triangular pulse shapes), defibrillation voltages and energies both rose, while average DFT currents reached a minimum.[46] The shock duration can be adjusted in each patient to minimize all shock parameters and obtain this particular pulse shape with 33% final voltage: longer durations for higher impedances, and shorter durations for lower impedances. Implant support devices for these fixed-duration devices typically provide a chart that can be used to select the charge voltage and pulse width to obtain the desired pulse shape and delivered energy for the patient's impedance.

Automatic Implantable Cardioverter-Defibrillators

The shock duration for the second type of ICD does not have to be programmed. The device automatically sets the pulse duration according to the patient's impedance by means of a voltage sensing circuit, rather than a timer.[48] After the shock is initiated, the device will switch shock phases or terminate the shock when the shock voltage reaches a percentage of the initial voltage predetermined by the manufacturer. These automatic ICDs are often referred to as variable pulse width devices, because the total duration of the shock is determined by the patient's impedance.[49] High impedances result in longer shock durations (waveform C, Figure 1), since the ICD will discharge its capacitor at a slower rate, extending the time required to reach the preset trailing edge voltage for shock termination. Patients with low impedances will experience shorter shock durations (waveform D, Figure 1), because the higher defibrillating currents increase the rate at which the ICD discharge approaches the final truncation voltage.

Although pulse durations will vary for automatic ICDs, these type of devices will always deliver the selected waveform shape because the ratio between the trailing and leading edge voltages is held constant. Currently, only one company (CPI) markets an automatic, variable pulse width ICD, using the name Automatic Implantable Cardioverter Defibrillator or AICD, to emphasize its automaticity features. Other ICDs that are currently market released are of the manual variety, using fixed pulse delivery techniques.

When CPI implemented monophasic waveforms in their present AICD pulse generators, they selected a final truncation point at a trailing edge voltage of 33%. This particular waveform represents the shock morphology that optimizes DFT voltages and delivered energies for the system.[46] While manual ICDs can be programmed at implant to yield this type of waveform once the patient's impedance is known, variable pulse width devices, like the AICD system, produce this optimal monophasic waveform automatically. In addition, these automatic pulse generators continue to deliver this waveform, even in the face of future changes in patient impedance.

For biphasic waveforms, the automatic design feature that yields a constant pulse shape applies to both voltage and timing ratios. Because the truncation voltages of both phases are expressed as percentages of the initial charge voltage, the transition voltage between phases and the relative amplitudes of the two phases are maintained. These voltage ratios also result in a fixed relationship between the durations of the two shock phases, eg, if an automatic ICD was preset to deliver biphasic shocks with a 60%:40% ratio between the durations of the first and second phases, it will deliver that waveform to all patients, independent of variations in patient impedance.

While manual ICDs can be adjusted at implant to yield biphasic waveforms with proper voltage and pulse duration ratios for the patient's impedance, this programmed waveform morphology cannot be guaranteed after implant, should the patient's impedance shift. The constant waveform characteristic of an automatic ICD may become a key feature for biphasic ICD systems, because it appears that DFTs are sensitive to the morphology of the biphasic waveform used.[50-53] If a manual ICD was programmed at implant with a biphasic waveform that minimized the DFT, a shift in waveform morphology could result in elevated thresholds and reduced device performance. Because automatic ICDs deliver similar shock morphologies for all patients, they not only simplify device programming at implant, but also provide security of consistent device function in the future.

Implant Support System Configurations

In the initial phases of the clinical trial for the original AICD, Mirowski and colleagues[24] soon recognized that not all patients who presented as candidates for ICD therapy would have defibrillation energy requirements that assured reliable conversion. Attempts to identify these high-threshold patients based on clinical characteristics have not been completely successful.[54]

Because some patients failed to meet implant criteria, device based testing prior to implant was not feasible. To circumvent this problem, an external cardioverter defibrillator (ECD™, Intec Systems, Inc., subsidiary of Marquest Medical Products, Engelwood, CO) was provided to evaluate DFT prior to implant. This battery powered support device permitted the selection of a wide range of shock energies for the assessment of a patient's conversion requirements. This simple tool became a standard addition to the array of support instruments for electrophysiologic testing. Enhanced versions of this original device (Ventak™ ECD [CPI, St. Paul, MN]) continue to provide this essential implant support function for the Ventak series of AICD systems from CPI. In addition to providing functions for patient diagnostics and therapy evaluation, the Ventak ECD also serves as a central implant device to which other support tools (eg, pacing system analyzer [PSA], fibrillation induction source, programmed electrical stimulator, and strip chart recorder) can be connected to the patient's lead systems.

This familiar implant support system can be used to develop a general model of the components and functions required in any implant support system. This will serve as a framework to discuss the currently available external implant support instruments. At this time, several models of implant support devices for ICD testing are being used: the Ventak ECD (Model 2805 monophasic, Model 2815 biphasic and monophasic [under clinical investigation in the United States]), the External Tachyarrhythmia Control Device (ETCD™, Model 5355, Medtronic, Inc., Minneapolis, MN), and the Ventritex High Voltage Stimulator (HVS™-02, Ventritex, Inc., Sunnyvale, CA). Implant support devices must be matched with the corresponding ICD system being implanted, because waveform, pulse delivery schema, ventricular electrogram sensing circuitry, and arrhythmia detection algorithms are substantially different for each ICD system.

One central subsystem of each of these external test devices is the system module responsible for delivering cardioversion and defibrillation therapies to the patient (the DEFIB therapy unit, Figure 2). This DEFIB module is programmed through various means, and can be manually triggered or set to deliver therapy automatically on

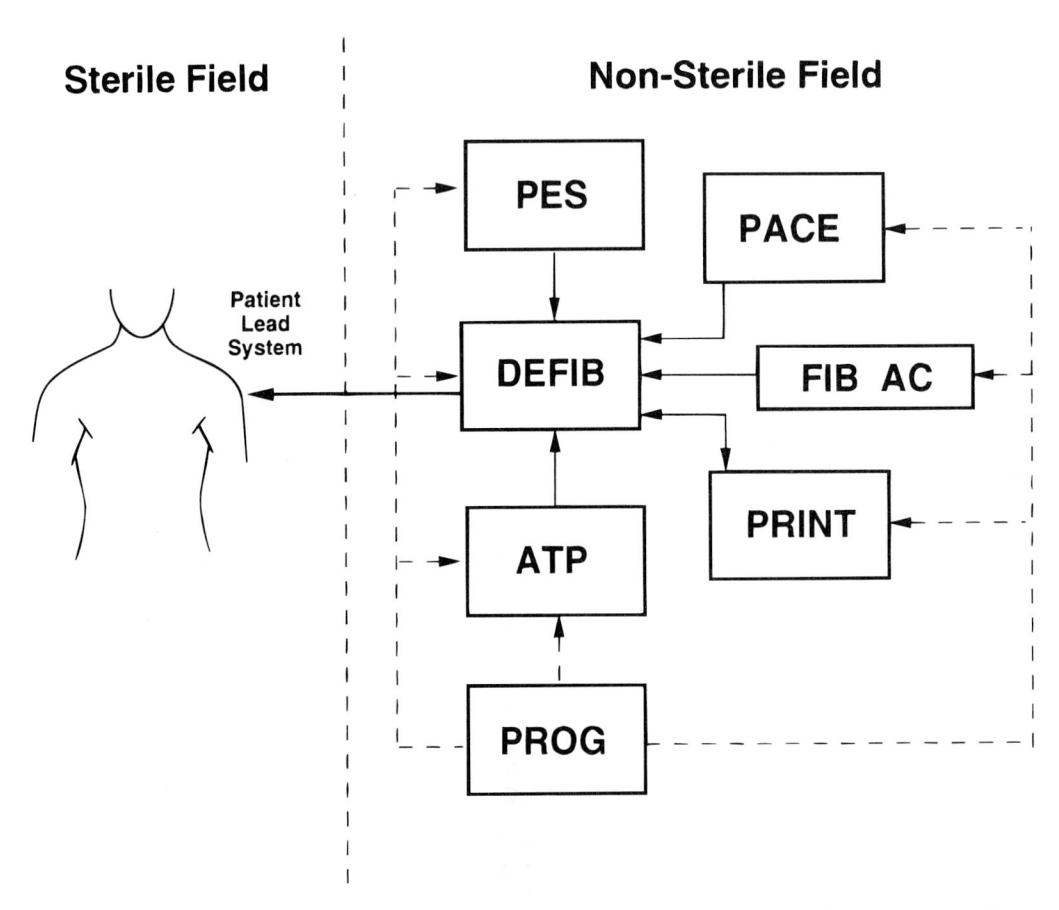

Figure 2. General schema of the various components of an implantable cardioverter-defibrillator (ICD) implant support system. Key subsystems for evaluation of ICD therapies include the following: a DEFIB unit (for testing cardioversion and defibrillation therapies); an ATP unit (for testing antitachycardia pacing therapies); a PES unit (for generating programmed electrical stimulation for electrophysiologic testing); a PACE unit (for single- or dual-chamber bradycardia pacing); a FIB AC unit (for inducing fibrillation with AC or other pulse stimulation); a PRINT unit (for printing therapy history summaries); and a PROG unit (for programming therapies in the implant support system or the implanted pulse generator). These various implant support modules are all available for implant support of the three commercially available ICD systems. Some support systems provide these features through external connections of common implant instruments to the central implant device using a pass-through mode, providing access to the patient's lead system. Other support systems incorporate several of these implant functions within one system. See Table 1 for a summary of these components as they are implemented in the three implant support systems currently available: the Ventak™ ECD system for supporting implant of the various Ventak AICD™ systems (CPI, St. Paul, MN); the ETCD™ system for supporting implant of the PCD™ Model 7217B (Medtronic, Minneapolis, MN); and the HVS-02™ system for support of the Cadence Model V-100 implant (Ventritex, Sunnyvale, CA).

Table 1

Characteristics	Ventak ECD™	ETCD™	HVS-02™
Separate PROG required?	NO	YES	NO
Program DEFIB shock?	From ECD	From PROG	From HVS-02
Trigger DEFIB shock?	Auto or manual from ECD	Manual from PROG	Manual from HVS-02
DEFIB waveform	Monophasic, biphasic*	Single path: monophasic, dual path: sequential, or simultaneous	Monophasic, biphasic
DEFIB delivery method	Automatic, variable pulse width	Manual, fixed pulse width	Manual, fixed pulse width
DEFIB shock settings	Delivered E	Stored E, pulse width	Peak V, pulse width
Display DEFIB shock parameters	On ECD	On ETCD	On HVS-02
PRINT DEFIB summaries?	YES from ECD	YES from PROG	NO
Deliver ATP therapies?	Via pass-through, or with device	YES, or with device	Via pass-through, or with device
EPS capabilities?	Via pass-through	YES with PROG	YES
PSA functions?	Via pass-through	Via pass-through	YES

* CPI's biphasic ECD system, Model 2815, is market-released in Europe and under clinical investigation in the United States.
E: energy; V: voltage.

arrhythmia detection. This subsystem could also permit the adjustment of waveform parameters, the selection of different waveform therapies, and the display of shock parameters, such as impedance, delivered energy, and peak voltage or current. Closely associated with this DEFIB therapy unit (Figure 2) are the components responsible for generating antitachycardia pacing therapy (ATP), programmed electrical stimulation for electrophysiologic testing (PES), bradycardia pacing (PACE), AC induction of fibrillation (FIB AC), and printed reports summarizing therapy history (PRINT). Some external systems require an ICD programming system to be included (PROG) for the tool to provide all therapeutic features. All implant support systems provide the capability of connecting other external support devices to provide any of these support functions to the patient (pass-through mode).

The similarities and differences between the three commercially available ICD implant support systems are summarized in Table 1. These devices will be discussed in the following sections with a brief overview of their features and specifications. These limited descriptions are not intended to be comprehensive instructions for use. Consult each manufacturer's user's manual before operating the devices discussed.

Ventak External-Cardioverter Defibrillator

The Ventak ECD system is used in the assessment of tachyarrhythmia conversion requirements for Ventak AICD systems (Figure 3). It is a portable, battery powered device that does not require interface with programmer systems. It can be used either as a stand-alone device, or as a central pass-through implant device in conjunction with other instruments that provide a variety of therapy tools (ATP, PES, external PACE, PSA, FIB induction, and recorder; see Table 1). The back panel of the Ventak ECD provides receptacles for the battery charger and all cables used with the system. These receptacles also constitute an electrical pass-through for attaching other implant support devices as part of an integrated system.

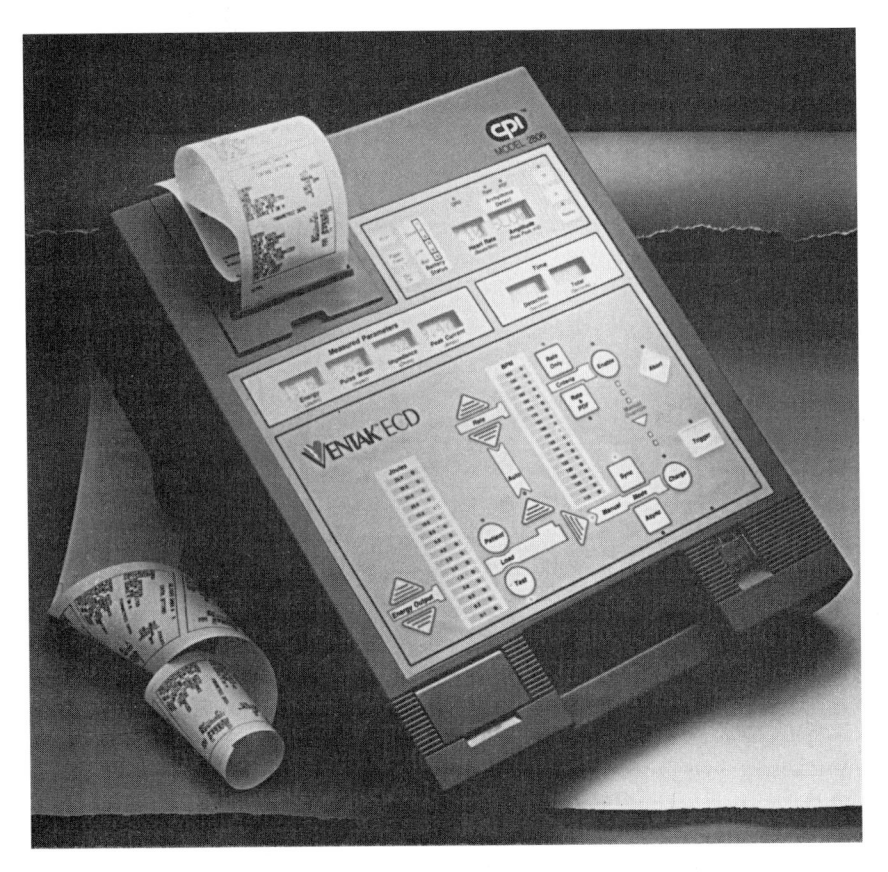

Figure 3. The Model 2805 Ventak™ External Cardioverter Defibrillator (CPI, St. Paul, MN) system for implant support of two devices from CPI's Ventak Automatic Implantable Cardioverter Defibrillator (AICD™) series: the Ventak P AICD system, and the Ventak PRx™ AICD system. The Model 2815 Ventak ECD system provides monophasic and biphasic waveforms for patient evaluation of two other Ventak AICD products: the Ventak P2 AICD system (under US clinical investigation), and the Ventak PRx-II AICD system (under US clinical investigation). The base of the Ventak ECD system is 1.1 feet wide and 1.3 feet deep. Refer to Table 1 for use of the Ventak ECD system in support of AICD implantation.

When external devices are used with the ECD in a pass-through fashion, the ECD remains fully functional.

The design intent of the Ventak ECD was to keep the front panel visually simple, uncluttered, and intuitive. It was ergonomically designed with a trapezoidal shape to place the front panel on a plane approximately orthogonal to the operator's line of sight when standing. Color codes also aid the operator during use by differentiating between manual and automatic modes of operation. Selections from the front panel during a normal test sequence flow from left to right (Figure 3): shock energy is first selected, then shock destination (patient or test load), and operational mode (automatic or manual shock delivery). In the manual mode, shocks can be given either synchronized to a sensed event or asynchronously. Prior to arrhythmia induction, the capacitors are manually charged by depressing the charge button. The current pulse is delivered to the patient or test load when the trigger button is depressed. Therapy can be aborted by pushing the abort key just above the trigger button. In the automatic mode, tachyarrhythmia detection algorithms, similar to those in the CPI Ventak P AICD pulse generator, automatically determine when therapy is needed based on programmable detection criteria (rate or rate and probability density function).[55] Once the selected rate criterion is met, the system will charge and deliver shock therapy. The detection parameters (heart rate, electrogram amplitude, detection criteria met, time for detection, and shock delivery) are displayed in real time on the front panel. The operator can also replay 10 seconds of the last recorded rhythm to adjust detection criteria without inducing another tachyarrhythmia. After the shock is delivered for either mode, important shock parameters are displayed on the front panel displays (delivered energy, pulse width, lead impedance and peak current). Therapy summaries including all shock and detection parameters can be printed from the ECD for patient records.

The Model 2805 Ventak ECD system delivers a monophasic truncated exponential pulse of up to 40 J of delivered energy and is protected from externally applied voltages from transthoracic defibrillators (up to 3,000 V). The newer Model 2815 Ventak ECD system has the same operating characteristics, but provides both biphasic and monophasic waveforms. This new model is commercially available in Europe, and is under clinical investigation in the United States.

External Tachyarrhythmia Control Device

The Medtronic Model 5355 ETCD is an external multiprogrammable device designed to assess the efficacy of electrical therapies for ventricular arrhythmias (Figure 4). The ETCD is not a stand-alone device because many of the implant support functions require the simultaneous use of a programmer and ETCD software module (Table 1). With the ETCD coupled to the telemetry head of the programming system, its operation is similar to the process of programming its corresponding ICD system, the Medtronic Pacer Cardioverter Defibrillator (PCD™ Model 7217B). Once programmed and placed in active mode, the ETCD can be used as a stand-alone device for VVI pacing and ventricular tachycardia (VT) detection and therapy with up to four adaptive VT overdrive therapies (burst or ramp). For other patient evaluation functions (PES for electrophysiologic testing and DEFIB for cardioversion and defibrillation therapies), the ETCD must be placed in the active mode with the programmer telemetry head attached for programmer control. If additional implant support tools are to be used with the system, the ETCD is placed in pass-through mode, which will connect external instruments (PSA, external PES, or AC FIB induction) attached to the side panel directly through to the patient cable. When external support devices are being used with the ETCD in the pass-through mode, the ETCD is disabled and cannot provide pacing, cardioversion, or defibrillation therapies; only programming and interrogation functions can be performed.

During a test sequence, the ETCD is primarily controlled by the programmer, much like the PCD Model 7217B. The front panel of the ETCD has control buttons for power, mode selection (standby, pass-through, and active), and viewing the ETCD display. All other parameters are set by telemetry through the programmer (Table 1). For cardioversion and defibrillation, the shock pulse width(s) and stored energy are programmed in addition to the pulsing scheme that is determined by the lead configuration implanted (single path with monophasic waveforms or dual paths with sequential or simultaneous monophasic pulse delivery). After fibrillating the patient in standby mode, the ETCD is placed in the active mode and defibrillation therapy is initiated by depressing the program key. At this point, the ETCD capacitors begin charging and therapy is delivered once the device is charged to the selected stored energy. Fol-

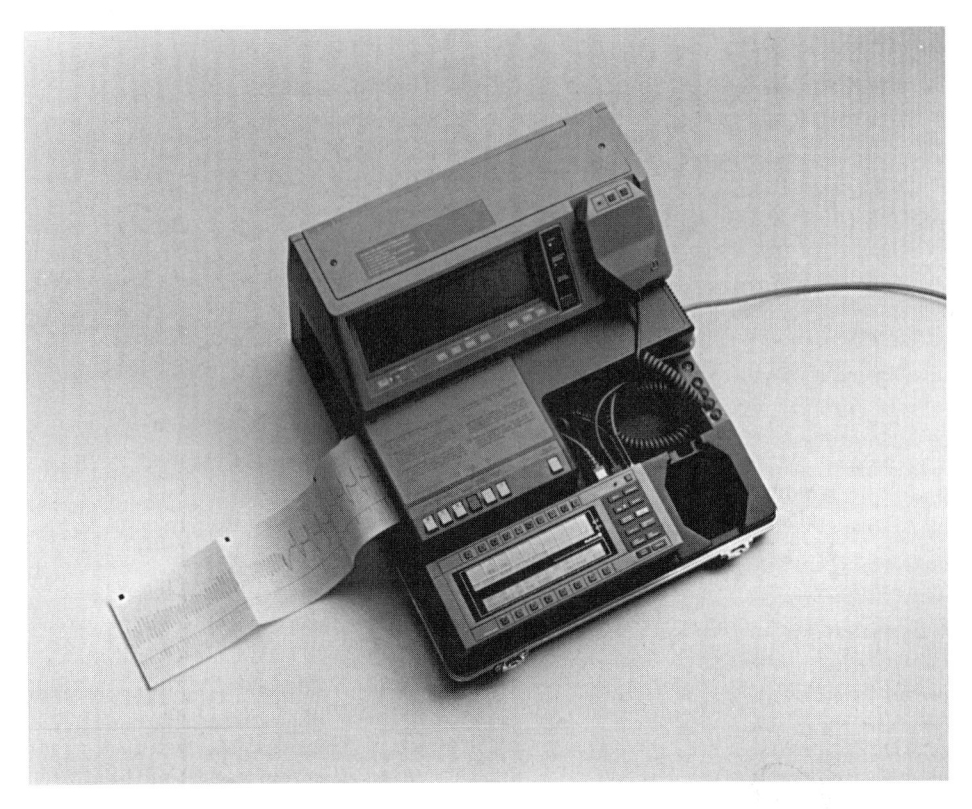

Figure 4. The Model 5355 External Tachyarrhythmia Control Device (ETCD™, Medtronic, Minneapolis, MN) for implant support of Medtronic's Pacer Cardioverter Defibrillator (PCD™) Model 7217B. When the ETCD sysem (1.4 feet wide and 0.7 feet deep) is combined with the Programmer, the base dimensions of the complete system is approximately 1.5 feet wide and 1.7 feet deep. Refer to Table 1 for use of the ETCD system as implant support of the PCD system. (Used with permission from Medtronic, Inc., St. Paul, MN)

lowing delivery of cardioversion or defibrillation therapy, the ETCD display presents summary information for the last therapy attempt (the pulse stored energy and energy actually delivered, peak voltage and current, and the resistance of the pulse pathway), as well as for each of the prior episodes retained in the ETCD memory. A printout of therapy history can also be obtained by interrogating the ETCD and printing the data on the programmer. Interrogation of the ETCD can also retrieve relevant programmed parameters associated with VT detection, VT pacing therapies and VVI pacing to be reviewed on the programmer display and printed using an external printer.

High-Voltage Stimulator

The Ventritex HVS-02 implant support device (Figure 5) is intended for use during electrophysiologic evaluation of patients for the Ventritex Cadence Tiered-Therapy Defibrillator System (Cadence™, Model V-100, Sunnyvale, CA). The HVS-02 device was designed to combine the functions of an ECD, a PES, and a PSA. The HVS-02 does not require a separate programmer to provide high-voltage therapies for VT and VF (Table 1).

Like the CPI Ventak ECD, the high-voltage stimulator portion of the device can be used to terminate induced tachyarrhythmias and to determine DFTs at the time of

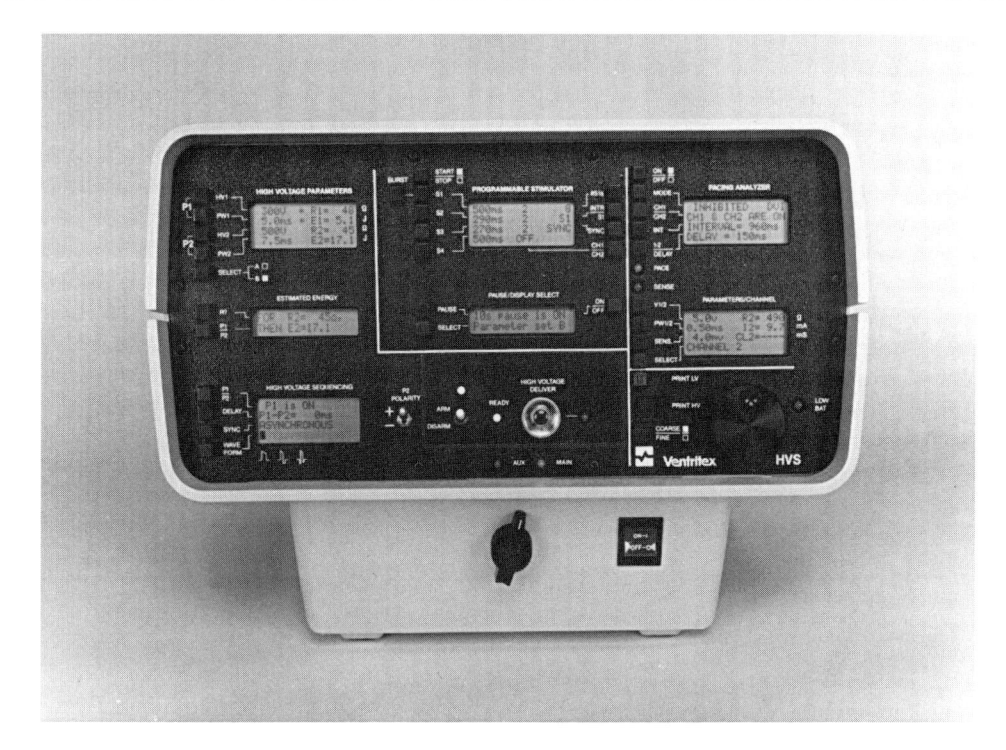

Figure 5. The High Voltage Stimulator (HVS-02™, Ventritex, Inc., Sunnyvale, CA) device for implant support of the Ventritex Cadence Tiered-Therapy Defibrillator System, Model V-100. The base of the HVS-02 system is 1.3 feet wide and 1.5 feet deep. Refer to Table 1 for use of the HVS-02 in support of the V-100 system. (Used with permission from Ventritex, Inc., Sunnyvale, CA)

implantation. Two separate, high-voltage output channels from two capacitor banks are provided. This feature allows the first channel to be used as the test shock and the second channel to be programmed for delivery of a rescue shock, in the event the first shock fails to convert the tachyarrhythmia. The PES portion of the HVS-02 can apply PES with a drive cycle of 1–99 S_1 and up to three extrastimuli (S_2, S_3, and S_4). Finally, the PSA section allows evaluation of pacemaker lead systems and provides back-up single- or dual-chamber pacing during electrophysiologic studies or during cardioversion/defibrillation testing.

To set up the HVS-02 for a test sequence, shock parameters are selected by depressing a red parameter button on the front panel corresponding to the feature to be programmed. Once illuminated, the value of this selected parameter can be changed by rotating the encoder dial on the front panel. The HVS-02 is capable of delivering several different pulse shapes: monophasic, biphasic single cycle, or biphasic 1½ cycles. Alternatively, the first and second phases of a biphasic waveform can be programmed independently, with the restriction that the first phase be set at a duration that is equal to or longer than the second phase. For example, to select the shock strength of a monophasic pulse to be delivered over channel 1, the HV1 button is depressed and the desired peak voltage is selected using the encoder dial. The duration of the pulse is programmed by selecting the PW1 button and adjusting the pulse width as desired. Once the device is charged and the arrhythmia induced, the therapy is initiated by depressing the high voltage deliver button. Peak voltage can be adjusted in 10-V increments from 50–990 V. Like the ETCD, the HVS-02 has a programmable pulse width. Once an HVS-02 pulse width is selected (0.1–20 msec, 0.1-msec increments) and programmed to provide the waveform tilt desired at implant, it remains fixed. Shock data (energy delivered, impedance) are displayed on the front panel after the shock is delivered. Printed therapy reports are not available from the HVS-02.

Programming Implantable Cardioverter-Defibrillator Systems Based on Ventricular Fibrillation Testing

The widely acknowledged success of ICDs is critically dependent on their ability to convert ventricular tachyarrhythmias over time. Implant support devices play a key role in assuring this long-term performance and reliability. To accomplish this goal, adequate testing procedures are required at the time of device implantation. From the assessment of the patient's defibrillation requirements, the implanted device is programmed to a shock strength sufficient to defibrillate the heart at implant and in the future.

One of the more common clinical tools for characterizing defibrillation efficacy is the DFT.[56,57] This method involves a test sequence of repeated fibrillation-defibrillation trials at successively increasing or decreasing energies using an ECD. If the initial energy is successful, subsequent defibrillation shock intensities are decreased in succeeding trials until conversion failure occurs. If the initial energy fails to defibrillate, subsequent shock levels are incremented until achieving a successful conversion. By either testing sequence, the DFT is defined as the minimum energy producing defibrillation success.

The concept of DFT implies that the slope of a curve relating defibrillation energy to conversion success is steep, permitting a clear division between effective and ineffective energies. Unfortunately, no sharp distinction between uniformly successful and unsuccessful energies can be shown experimentally.[58–61] Defibrillation requirements are best described by a dose-response curve relating the probability of successful conversion and shock strength[62] expressed as either energy, voltage, or current (Figure 6). Shock intensities located higher on the success curve have a higher likelihood of converting the arrhythmia. Intermediate level shocks near the sloping portion of the curve will defibrillate only part of the time, as dictated by their probability of success. When determining the actual defibrillation dose-response curve, many repeated defibrillation attempts are required at different shock intensities to adequately sample the conversion probabilities along this curve. Clinically, the determination of a defibrillation success curve is impractical and may be potentially hazardous.[30] However, the conceptual framework of a dose-response relationship has significant implications for the way in which testing methods are used to program the output of ICD systems.

To assure efficacy of implanted ICDs, defibrillation shock intensities must be programmed high enough above the DFT so that the ICD output is positioned beyond the defibrillation success curve, out on the patient's 100% conversion success plateau (E_{ICD}, Figure 6). In selecting the proper margin between the output of the device and the DFT, one must keep in mind that the DFT may not precisely determine the location of this defibrillation dose-response curve. Although the DFT is defined as the minimum shock intensity producing defibrillation success, the sequence of successes and failures at the end of the DFT protocol that identified this minimum is compatible with a range of dose-response curves (Figure 6). One possible curve that could have yielded the observed DFT sequence is a low-energy curve (curve A, Figure 6). In this case, the successful conversions in the DFT protocol occurred for shock strengths located on the patient's 100% success plateau and the conversion failure that ended the protocol resulted from a shock level on the

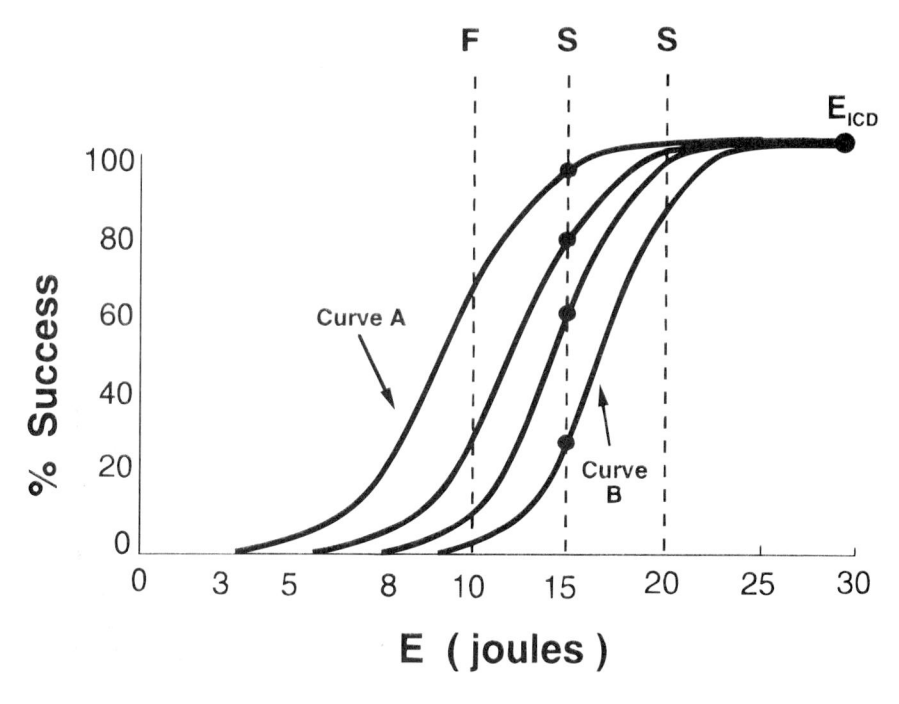

Figure 6. Range of possible defibrillation dose-response curves consistent with a step-down defibrillation threshold (DFT) of 15 J. The initial shock of the DFT sequence was at 20 J, which was a success. The next test shock at 15 J was also a success, which was followed by a failed conversion attempt at 10 J. This test sequence could be consistent with a low-energy dose-response curve (curve A), for which most of the DFT test shocks were above the curve out on the plateau. Due to the probability of defibrillation, the test sequence could also have been consistent with a high energy curve (curve B), for which the last two shocks were located along the sloping portion of the dose-response relationship. The patient's dose-response curve is bounded by the lowest curve A to the left and the highest, worst-case curve B to the right. Selection of ICD energies (E_{ICD}) should be based on the worst-case dose-response curve to assure adequate device performance for all patients.

high end of the curve's slope. With the probabilistic nature of defibrillation, however, this same DFT sequence could have resulted from a high-energy curve (curve B, Figure 6). Here, several of the successful conversions in the protocol could have occurred for shock energies located along the upper slope of the dose-response curve, with the energy yielding failure near the bottom of the curve. Unfortunately, with only a few conversion attempts, one does not know whether the patient's actual defibrillation dose-response curve is located near the high, middle, or low portion of the range of possible defibrillation success curve positions. This will have an impact on how large an output margin is required for an implanted ICD system. These programming guidelines are addressed in depth in a later section of this chapter.

As with any method that samples a probabilistic phenomenon, one becomes more certain as to the location of the dose-response curve with more comprehensive testing. However, since patient conditions limit the number of conversion attempts that can be given during operative testing, two types of testing methods have emerged in ICD medical practice—one aimed at verification, the other on assessment. The focus of the first class of methods is to verify that the ICD system can be programmed with an adequate margin between its output and the shock intensities tested at implant. While defibrillation failures can be encountered with these margin verification techniques, it is not their intent to extend testing until failures are found. The second class of testing protocols involves defibrillation testing at several shock levels with both conversion successes and failures observed. The goal of this type of method is to assess the actual defibrillation characteristics of the implanted system by continuing the protocol to obtain both possible conversion outcomes. Defibrillation threshold protocols are examples of this category. Because DFT protocols are somewhat open ended, they could result in a greater number of conversion episodes in some patients.

Margin Verification Protocols

The verification and assessment methods often involve a compromise between the amount of information obtained about the patient and the number of conversion attempts required. Margin verification techniques can involve fewer defibrillation episodes, but at the expense of knowing less about the position of the patient's defibrillation dose-response curve. The intent of these protocols is to confirm the adequacy of ICD programming through the observation of successful conversions at all shock levels studied. If no defibrillation failures are encountered, the verification protocol places an upper boundary on the position of the patient's defibrillation dose-response curve. While their defibrillation curve could be located near the successful test energies, it could also be located at much lower levels. The exact location of the curve is not of concern in this type of protocol, as long as it has an upper bound so that the ICD can be programmed to assure reliable conversion of spontaneous ventricular tachyarrhythmias.

One group of methods for verifying ICD implant margins is the repeated success protocols.[63] Under the straightforward guidelines of these methods, margins are evaluated by testing defibrillation success of a certain shock level with one, two or three conversion attempts, with no failures allowed (1S, 2S, or 3S protocols). If a failure is encountered, the selected margin might not be large enough, necessitating either the evaluation of a larger margin, the revision of the ICD system, or failure to implant. While the possibility of programming lower ICD output levels could be considered in performing these protocols, the repeated success methods are typically used when ICD systems are to be programmed to maximum output (eg, 34 J delivered energy). During operative testing, a lower level test shock is selected from the implant support device that represents a sufficient margin between the output of the ICD system and the test level.

Of the three repeated methods, the single success protocol (1S) requires the least amount of testing, but also yields the least amount of information for patient safety.[56] With additional successes at the test level, the double (2S) and triple (3S) repeated success protocols improve the accuracy of the estimated upper bound for the patient's defibrillation dose-response curve. This will provide more confidence that the output margin with which the ICD system is programmed will consistently defibrillate the patient.

A second type of method that can be used to verify ICD implant margins is the step-down success protocol. This testing technique can be viewed as a cross between the repeated success protocol and a standard DFT method. As with the DFT, the step-down success protocol involves a sequence of several defibrillation trials at successively lower shock levels delivered from the support device. Once a shock level is reached that is deemed to provide sufficient output margin for the ICD system, the testing protocol ends. As an example, assume a step-down success protocol began with an initial 20 J successful conversion and proceeded to 15 J, which was also a success. If testing was terminated at this point, the protocol places an upper bound for the DFT at 15 J. If testing had continued to 10 J and had failed, then 15 J would have been selected as the DFT, which is consistent with the step-down success result. Conversely, if the hypothetical test at 10 J was successful, the DFT would then be ≤ 10 J. This is still consistent with the step-down success result of DFT ≤ 15 J. With the ICD system programmed for a 15-J DFT, there is a potential that its actual output margin could be greater than the selected value if the DFT were lower than 15 J. In keeping with the philosophy of margin verification methods, the exact value of the DFT, and hence, the location of the dose-response curve, is not a concern in this protocol. The goal is to evaluate the patient sufficiently to program their ICD system to a safe output level.

The step-down success protocols have an advantage over the repeated success methods for margin verification in that they can be extended to lower shock levels if the situation permits. In this case, the step-down success protocol might involve three or four conversion attempts. If one of these additional tests resulted in failure, then the DFT has been defined. If these extra conversions were successful, one could place an even lower limit on the upper boundary for the DFT and the patient's dose-response curve. This additional information could result in margins that permit lower programmed shock levels for defibrillation and provides more precise information to assess changes in the patient's condition in the future.

Threshold Assessment Protocols

By extending the step-down success protocol to low enough shock strengths, defibrillation attempts will fail, changing the protocol into a standard DFT technique. The DFT protocols represent the assessment class of testing methods. Protocols in this second group involve defibrillation successes and failures at several shock levels. While this could possibly increase the number of conversion attempts for some patients, this has not been a hindrance to the clinical use of this protocol.[56] The advantage of assessment methods over the validation protocols is that they provide more detailed information on the defibrillation characteristics of the implanted system. This information can be invaluable in assessing the adequacy of programmed ICD margins at implant and managing the patient over time. These methods also identify the lowest shock strengths required for defibrillation, permitting the selection of initial defibrillation shocks with lower strength. This strategy may reduce charge time, energy consumption,[48] therapy discomfort, and potential effects of high-intensity shocks on the myocardium.[64]

These assessment protocols share several distinct characteristics: 1) they involve a test sequence of repeated fibrillation-defibrillation trials at successively increasing or decreasing shock strengths, and 2) they are recursive; shock strength selections after the first attempt are based on the outcome of the previous attempt. However, despite these obvious similarities, they also possess significant differences. The most notable of these differences is the precision for locating the position of the defibrillation dose-response curve. The ideal method for evaluating a patient's defibrillation requirements would identify a critical shock strength that is an absolute upper bound for the patient's dose-response curve, ie, this critical shock strength and all shocks with higher intensities have a 100% probability for successful defibrillation. Unfortunately, the large number of shocks required to accurately identify this critical level are not compatible with clinical practice. Because clinical considerations limit the number of observations, precision is also significantly reduced.

Each assessment protocol ultimately identifies an intermediate range of shock strengths that lie somewhere along the sloping portion of the defibrillation dose-response curve—shocks that have intermediate probabilities for success. Some assessment protocols could place the DFT anywhere along the curve,[59] while others could isolate the DFT position to a narrow region near the top.[60] The extent of the DFTs distribution along this curve will determine the accuracy with which a specific DFT protocol locates the defibrillation curve. This range of positions will be influenced by the conversion sequence within the DFT protocol near the vicinity of the sloping portion of the dose-response curve. This sequence is governed by the conversion probabilities at each shock level, the order in which these levels are sampled, the size of the step increments in the protocol, and the width of the defibrillation dose-response curve.[30,59,63]

Simple DFT protocols are the least precise for locating the patient's defibrillation curve. These protocols involve either an increasing or decreasing sequence of shock strengths with the DFT defined as the minimum energy producing defibrillation success. These single DFT protocols can be classified into three groups based on the relative position of their starting point with respect to the mid-point of the defibrillation dose-response curve.[59] A DFT protocol starting at higher shock strengths to the right of the curve will step-down to reach it, initially sampling shock levels near the upper part of the curve. This protocol, called the step-down DFT, has a great probability of encountering a failed attempt before reaching the lower part of the curve. The DFT would then be located one step back up the curve at the minimum successful shock. This typically places the step-down DFT somewhere along the upper three fourths of the dose-response curve.[58–61,63]

Defibrillation thresholds beginning at low-shock intensities to the left of the curve will step-up to meet the curve, initially sampling the sloping portion near the bottom. As these step-up DFT methods progressively sample shock levels along the slope, they will most likely encounter a successful conversion (ie, the DFT) before reaching the upper portion of the curve. The step-up method tends to keep the distribution of possible locations for the step-up DFT along the lower three fourths of the curve, with the typical location approximately one third up from the bottom.[59,60]

Finally, a mid-point DFT protocol, which begins at a shock level near the middle of the dose-response curve, has an equal chance of moving shock levels up or down after the first test. If a success was initially observed, shock levels are decreased until a failure is encountered, which will occur before reaching the lower part of the curve.[59] Failed attempts for the first shock, lead to increasing shock intensities until a success is observed, typically before reaching the upper portion of the curve. Thus, DFTs measured with this mid-point protocol will tend to be distributed along the middle half of the dose-response curve.[59]

Given the limited number of shocks involved with these single DFT protocols, the possible locations for the DFTs can be spread over a wide portion of the defibrillation success curve. This lack of precision will have an impact on how well the DFT acts as an upper bound for the position of the patient's defibrillation curve. If a single DFT determination is used as the sole measure to determine an acceptable output margin for the ICD, one may need to choose a slightly larger margin than for more comprehensive methods, due to the low precision of the DFT. The selection of these margins is addressed in the following sections.

One approach that has been recommended for improved precision of threshold assessments is to determine the mean threshold after repeating the DFT protocol several times. Animal studies evaluating this multiple DFT technique indicate that three replicates are optimum to gain the greatest improvement in accuracy and precision with the lowest number of conversion attempts.[65,66] The mean triplicate DFT in this study was an accurate, unbiased predictor of the mid-point of the defibrillation dose-response curve, since the group mean DFT was not significantly different from the mean energy at 50% success (E_{50}). In addition, this multiple DFT approach evidenced a coefficient of variation, and hence, a precision comparable to that of the "gold standard" logistic estimate of E_{50}, which required more fibrillation episodes.[66]

One reason the triplicate DFT may have

been such a good estimator of the E_{50} was that the DFT technique used to obtain the replicates was similar to the mid-point DFT protocol. The DFT starting point in these studies was comparable to the mean mid-point energy.[66] Studies of the mid-point DFT technique indicate that it closely estimates the mid-point shock strength.[59] Thus, with additional mid-point DFT replicates, the precision would have improved as the standard error of the mean steadily decreased, while the true accuracy of the mid-point DFT in measuring E_{50} became more evident.

If higher or lower energy starting points had been consistently chosen for this study, the precision of the triplicate DFT would still have been evident, but the mean DFTs would no longer have been an unbiased estimate of the mid-point. If step-up DFTs were consistently used, the mean triplicate DFT would have underestimated E_{50}, whereas step-down DFTs would have resulted in an overestimate.[59] Both of these other DFT methods are unbiased estimators for other points on the defibrillation curve, but not for the mid-point shock strength. As investigators consider triplicate DFT methods for defibrillation research in animals or humans, they should consider what part of the dose-response curve is being characterized by the DFT protocol in use. This may have an impact on the size of the output margin that is programmed for the ICD system.

A simplified variation of this multiple DFT approach has been proposed which involves the average of only two DFT-type test sequences.[67] One of the sequences is a step-up DFT, which would be the first level to succeed, approaching from below. The second testing sequence included in the average is determined with a step-down DFT protocol, but instead of the DFT, the energy level used in the average is the first shock intensity that failed, one step below the DFT. The average of these two measures is an unbiased estimator of the mid-point shock strength, since the processes involved in the two sampling techniques are symmetric about the mid-point of the defibrillation success curve.[67]

A third technique that provides an unbiased measure of the mid-point with minimal testing could be considered an extension of the dual measurement approach above. This alternate involves a four-episode, up-down algorithm for the conversion test sequence.[68] The direction in which shock strength is incremented in this up-down approach is dictated by the outcome of the prior attempt. If the last attempt were a success, the next shock is set one step lower. While if the last shock were a failure, the next test would occur at the next higher shock strength. This four-shock up-down sequence is similar to the dual approach described above with the two sequences performed in series. Once the four tests are complete, the unbiased estimator is derived from the average of all four energy levels plus the next level that would have been performed, had the protocol continued to a fifth shock. This up-down measure was slightly more precise than a single DFT technique (less variability), but was much better at predicting the mid-point.[68] The final protocol recommended by the authors was a delayed four-episode, up-down approach to minimize the sensitivity to changes in the initial starting point. This delayed protocol begins counting the four episodes after the first reversal of conversion success. The predictable accuracy and improved precision compared to the DFT makes this algorithm attractive for certain clinical studies that require rigorous comparisons between treatments.[69]

For patients with high DFTs (≥ 20 J), the variability of the normal assessment protocols alone could have a significant impact on the adequacy of programmed output margins for the ICD system. These situations require enhanced assessment protocols that have greater accuracy and precision.[60] One enhanced method that requires minimal extra testing is the augmented DFT. This protocol involves performing one or possibly two additional defibrillation trials at the measured DFT energy to clarify where the DFT could be located on the dose-response curve.[70]

If the first additional conversion test is successful, the outcome is described as a DFT+. If two extra conversion tests are successful at the DFT, then that energy is indicated as a DFT++. With each extra success that is encountered at the DFT (DFT+ or DFT++), there is greater confidence that the observed DFT is only located higher on the curve.[30,60,63,70] This would reduce the size of the output margins that are needed to provide consistent performance for the implanted device.

These enhanced protocols do not allow any failures to be seen at the DFT. If any of these additional tests fails (eg, a DFT−, or possibly a DFT±, which represents a mixed outcome with one success and one failure), one is not able to limit the extent of the DFT distribution to the top portion of the curve. The margins would therefore be the same as required for the single DFT alone. For the case of the high-threshold patient, it may not be possible to program the ICD system to an output that would provide the margin dictated by the single DFT measure. If this situation occurs, it is recommended that the ICD system be revised with a new lead or waveform, or a higher output device be selected.

Programming Defibrillation Energy Margins

Once a defibrillation testing protocol has been completed, the information derived from this test must be used to program the output of the ICD system to a shock intensity that is high enough to be effective at implant and safe for continued performance in the future. To assure consistent defibrillation at implant, shock strengths from the ICD device must be programmed to a level that has 100% probability for success. The minimum level that would satisfy this efficacy requirement would be the shock intensity at the top corner of the defibrillation dose-response curve (E_{100}). Of course, shocks stronger than this would also perform consistently at implant. To assure continued safety of device performance if the dose-response curve possibly shifted to less favorable positions at higher energies, the output of the device could be programmed out on the 100% success plateau beyond the location of the patient's dose-response curve at implant. Although animal and human data suggest that defibrillation curves for patch lead systems do not shift substantially over time, between generator replacements,[34,71,72] other factors may influence thresholds. Factors that might contribute to an upward shift in defibrillation requirements might stem from disease progression, alterations in certain antiarrhythmic drugs, ischemia, prolonged fibrillation duration, or other as yet undetermined mechanisms.

One significant factor, for example, may be the duration of VF.[73–75] Anecdotal and preliminary data[76–78] suggest that prolonged VF duration due to unsuccessful initial conversion is associated with an increase in the defibrillation energy requirements. For example, one study indicated that energy thresholds after 30–40 seconds of VF increased approximately 50% compared to thresholds for the durations of 5–10 seconds.[76] This duration of VF would correspond to the length of arrhythmia encountered by the ICD when delivering later shocks in a multishock sequence for VF therapies (third to fifth shock in a five-shock sequence). In practice, this would dictate that ICD energy margins for subsequent shocks from the device later in a VF episode should be selected to provide at least 50% higher energies than the upper end of the efficacy margin. Patients with high thresholds (≥ 20 J) may require more extensive testing (eg, DFT+ or DFT++) to verify that safety margins for the later shocks are sufficient to accommodate the potentially larger margin required for prolonged VF.

When programming for efficacy and safety, the location of the patient's defibrillation dose-response curve serves as the basis for defining the appropriate ICD output. Because clinical defibrillation protocols have limited precision for locating this curve, there will be a range of dose-response curves compatible with the observed testing outcome (Figure 6). If the patient's curve happened to be low in this range (curve A, Figure 6), the location of the DFT along the sloping portion of this curve would be near the top corner (DFT = E_{100}). An ICD output programmed above this high-positioned DFT would place the ICD shock intensities out on the plateau of this curve. The size of the output margin above the DFT (E_{ICD}-DFT) would represent the width of the plateau between the ICD output and the minimum shock strength for consistent defibrillation (E_{100}). The width of this plateau is defined as the safety margin for the device (E_{ICD}-E_{100}). The safety margin should be large enough to accommodate possible shifts in the defibrillation curve, while still maintaining device efficacy.

The selection of ICD safety margins, however, is complicated by the probabilistic nature of defibrillation. In the above example, the observed DFT sequence could easily have been consistent with a defibrillation curve near the top of its range of potential dose-response curves (curve B, Figure 6). For this "worst-case" example, the DFT is located far down on the curve's slope at the lowest probable location dictated by the testing protocol. The worst-case output margin (E_{ICD}-DFT) will now overestimate the actual safety margin for the patient. In this situation, the measured output margin consists of two components: the true safety margin (E_{ICD}-E_{100}, Figure 7) and an "effi-

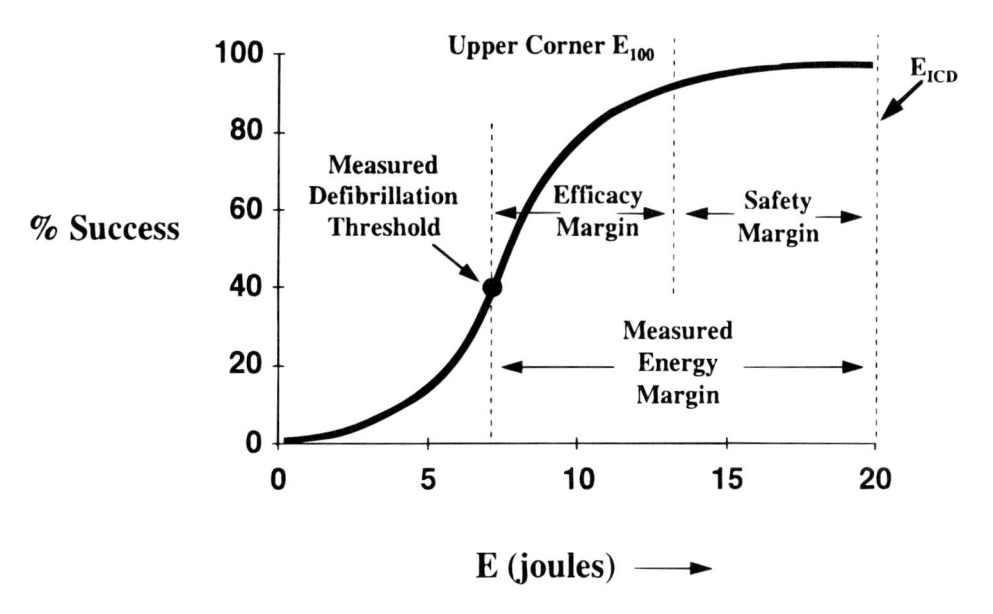

Figure 7. Percent probability for successful defibrillation versus shock energy. The measured implantable cardioverter-defibrillator (ICD) output margin is the energy difference between the lowest conversion success (defibrillation threshold [DFT]) and the programmed ICD energy: output margin = E_{ICD} − DFT. The output margin consists of two components: the efficacy margin and the safety margin. The ICD efficacy margin is the energy difference between the lowest conversion success (DFT) and the upper corner of the dose-response curve, ie, the lowest energy required for 100% success at implant: efficacy margin = E_{100} − DFT. An adequate efficacy margin is required to assure consistent device efficacy at implant. The ICD safety margin is the energy difference between the lowest energy required for 100% success at implant (E_{100}) and the programmed ICD energy: safety margin = E_{ICD} − E_{100}. The safety margin is important to assure continued device function should the dose-response curve ever shift to higher energies. (Reproduced with permission from Reference 30.)

cacy" margin, which is defined as the energy required to move up the curve from the low-positioned DFT to shocks strengths that yield consistent defibrillation efficacy (E_{100}-DFT, Figure 7).

Since the clinical defibrillation protocols do not indicate whether the DFT is high or low on the curve, one must make the conservative worst-case assumption that the DFT is at the lowest possible position when programming margins. Setting everyone's output margin equal to the size required for the worst-case patient will assure proper margins for all ICD patients. Because most of the patients have DFTs located above the worst-case position on the curve, a general rule for setting everyone's output margin based on the worst-case patient will provide much larger safety margins for the average patient.

To derive suggested output margins for the various types of defibrillation testing protocols, one must consider the worst-case position along the defibrillation curve for that testing method. Most of the analysis in this area has focused on DFT protocols. Numerical modeling has demonstrated that standard step-down DFT protocols using 10% voltage decrements (20% energy steps) were distributed asymmetrically toward the upper end of the dose-response curve, with the most probable location near 75% defibrillation success (range 30% to 100% success).[59] Defibrillation thresholds measured with a step-up protocol with similar step sizes were distributed asymmetrically toward the lower end of the dose-response curve, with the probable location near 30% defibrillation success (range 1% to 73% success).[59] A DFT protocol starting near the mid-point of the curve resulted in DFTs that were evenly distributed about the 57% success mark (range from 26% to 90%).[59]

These theoretical predictions of DFT positions along the defibrillation dose-response curve have been validated in animal studies.[58,60,61] In one study, the mean value for the $DFT_{step-down}$ was 10 ± 3.4 J, with a range of DFTs along the curve ranging from 25% to 88% success (mean 71% $\pm$ 26%).[61] Thus, both numerical and experimental models suggest that for step-down protocols, the probable DFT location is approximately one fourth down from the top of the energy success curve, with DFT energies ranging from approximately E_{25}–E_{100}.

With a worst-case $DFT_{step-down}$ of E_{25}, the efficacy margin to reach E_{100} for this method is three fourths of the defibrillation curve width.[58,59] Translating this efficacy margin into energy requires information on the width of the defibrillation success curve. For dogs,[58] the full width of the defibrillation curve expressed in terms of energy ($E_{100} - E_0$) is approximately $1.0 \times E_{50}$,[a] or equivalently in terms of other energies on the curve: full width = $2.0 \times E_0 = 1.3 \times E_{25} = 0.8 \times E_{75}$.[a] Based on this information,

---

[a] Davy et al. reported a partial curve width (pCW) in dogs equal to $E_{80} - E_{20} = (0.85 \pm 0.27) \times E_{20}$. Since E_{50} is in the middle of this partial curve segment ($E_{50} = E_{20} \pm 0.5 \times$ pCW, or equivalently $E_{20} = E_{50} - 0.5 \times$ pCW), the partial curve width can be expressed in terms of the mid-point energy as follows: pCW = $0.85 \times E_{20} = 0.85 \times (E_{50} - 0.5 \times$ pCW). Solving this expression for pCW, results in the relation: pCW = $E_{80} - E_{20} = (0.6 \pm 0.2) \times E_{50}$.

The full curve width (fCW) of the defibrillation curve ($E_{100} - E_0$) can be obtained by extrapolating the linear mid-section of the defibrillation curve ($E_{80} - E_{20}$) to the upper and lower bounds at 100% and 0%. Since this full width spans the full 100% range of defibrillation probabilities compared to the partial curve (80% $-$ 20% = 60% span), the full curve width will be proportionately larger: fCW = (100%/60%) $\times$ pCW = $1.67 \times (0.6 \pm 0.2) \times E_{50} = (1.0 \pm 0.3) \times E_{50}$.

This expression can also be written in terms of other energies by linear interpolation using this curve width relation. For example, since E_{25} is one fourth down the curve from E_{50}, E_{25} can be expressed as a function of E_{50} as follows: $E_{25} = E_{50} - 0.25 \times$ fCW $= E_{50} - 0.25 \times (1.0 \times E_{50}) = 0.75 \times E_{50}$. In a similar manner, $E_0 = E_{50} - 0.5 \times$ fCW $= 0.5 \times E_{50}$, and $E_{75} = E_{50} \pm 0.25 \times$ fCW $= 1.25 \times E_{50}$. Solving for E_{50} in these expressions results in the following energy relations: $E_{50} = 2.0 \times E_0$, $E_{50} = 1.33 \times E_{25}$, and $E_{50} = 0.8 \times E_{75}$. These can be used to define the full curve width in terms of several energies on the dose-response curve: fCW = $(1.0 \pm 0.3) \times E_{50} = (2.0 \pm 0.6) \times E_0 = (1.3 \pm 0.4) \times E_{25} = (0.8 \pm 0.24) \times E_{75}$.

the efficacy margin required for the worst-case $DFT_{step-down} = E_{25} = 0.75 \times$ full width $= 0.75 \times (1.3 \times E_{25}) = 1.0 \times E_{25}.^{30}$) Thus, one would have to deliver shock energies at $2 \times DFT_{step-down}$ to assure 100% conversion for all subjects, since $E_{100} = E_{25} \pm$ efficacy margin $= E_{25} \pm [(1.0 \pm 0.3) \times E_{25}] = (2.0 \pm 0.3) \times E_{25}$. This closely agrees with the efficacy margins required in pigs to consistently defibrillate all animals based on the step-down DFT protocol (1.7 $\times DFT_{step-down}$).[61]

Although these margins are based on numeric and animal models, they show very close consistency with clinical work using single DFT measurements.[79] The DFT protocol in this clinical study began with a shock energy approximately in the center of the defibrillation success curve, using 20% energy steps. Since the $DFT_{mid-point}$ protocol has a similar minimum DFT position as the step-down protocol (E_{25}), the numeric and animal models would predict that test shock energies in this clinical study would have to be increased to at least $2.0 \times DFT$ for the worst-case patient, before 100% defibrillation success is observed for everyone in the study. This agrees directly with the clinical results, ie, 100% success for all patients was achieved for shock energies between $2.0–2.6 \times DFT$, depending on the lead system.[79] Thus, for both mid-point or step-down DFT protocols, efficacy margins dictate that approximately two times the DFT energy are required to assure consistent defibrillation success in all patients.[63,79]

Since the efficacy margin factor is based on the worst-case position for the DFT (< 5% to 7% of the population),[58] a shock energy of $2 \times DFT$ for most patients would be located out on the 100% plateau to the right of the defibrillation curve with adequate safety margins. From their numerical model, McDaniel and Schuder[59] predict that most of the time (88% of patients), the step-down DFT will lie above the mid-point of the curve (E_{50}), yielding even greater safety margins with the "2 $\times$ DFT" rule. If the DFT were at the mid-point, a $2 \times DFT$ energy margin would place the ICD output beyond the curve with a safety margin 33% $> E_{100}$.[b] Since most (88%) patients have DFTs placed higher than E_{50}, they will have safety margins larger than 33%. For example, the safety margin for the average $DFT_{step-down}$ (near E_{75})[58,59,61] would result in an ICD output 67% greater than the upper corner of the defibrillation dose-response curve.[c] Since half of the patients have step-down DFTs located above E_{75}, they will have even larger safety margins, ranging from 67% to 200%.

For patients with DFTs ≥ 20 J, it may not be possible to provide the patient with the size of energy margin dictated by the low placement of the DFT measure alone. While the up-down and repeated DFT protocols increase the precision of the testing method, their output margins will not be significantly smaller than the $2 \times DFT$ recommendation for single DFTs, since these alternate protocols are intended to accurately estimate the mid-point of the curve (E_{50}), resulting in similar lower bounds on the curve as the single DFT. While these protocols provide more precise estimates of E_{50}, their capability to reduce margins is determined by their ability to raise the lower extent of their distributions on the defibrillation curve. Since their mean is near E_{50}, one can surmise that their lower extent is no higher than E_{40} or E_{30}, in which case the

---

[b] The shock energy for consistent defibrillation (E_{100}) for a DFT at E_{50} equals $E_{100} = E_{50} \pm 0.5 \times$ full curve width $= E_{50} \pm 0.5 \times (1.0 \times E_{50}) = 1.5 \times E_{50}$. Using the $2 \times DFT$ output margin for this DFT at the mid-point energy, the output of the device would equal $E_{ICD} = 2 \times E_{50}$, which is out on the plateau to the right of the upper corner of the curve. The safety margin for this relatively low-positioned DFT equals the ratio between $E_{ICD}/E_{100} = (2.0 \times E_{50})/(1.5 \times E_{50}) = 1.33$, which corresponds to a safety margin of 33%.

[c] The energy required for consistent defibrillation for a DFT $= E_{75}$ can be expressed as follows: $E_{100} = E_{75} \pm 0.25 \times$ full curve width $= E_{75} \pm 0.25 \times (0.8 \times E_{75}) = 1.2 \times E_{75}$. With the output of the device at $E_{ICD} = 2 \times E_{75}$, the safety margin ($E_{ICD}/E_{100} = 2.0/1.2 = 1.67$) would be 67%.

efficacy margins would be 1.7–1.9 × DFT, rather than 2 × DFT.[d]

The augmented DFT protocols (DFT+ and DFT++) appear to be more effective at reducing the size of the required energy margins while minimizing the number of additional tests. The sole purpose of evaluating the DFT with one or two additional tests is to limit the possible extent of the DFT distribution down the defibrillation curve. These extra shocks will allow implant with smaller energy margins, which is a key requirement for implanting high-threshold patients. In addition, augmented DFT protocols may also be needed if the ICD energy is to be programmed to a lower energy that might reduce the ICD output margin.

Lang et al.[60] have shown that the lowest DFT position for a DFT+ outcome is E_{50} and for a DFT++, it is E_{75}. The DFT+ efficacy margin, consistent with a DFT = E_{50}, is 1.5 × DFT, while for DFT++, it is 1.2 × DFT. If the additional tests fail (DFT− or DFT±), the distribution for the augmented protocol is identical to that of the single DFT alone (E_{25} curve minimum). Since this requires the full 2 × DFT, there may not be enough output margin for device implant. In this case, it is strongly recommended that the ICD lead system or waveform be revised, or an ICD be selected that can provide higher delivered energy.

Historically, a recommended energy margin of 10–15 J has been a criterion for device implantation. This rule of thumb has provided adequate efficacy and safety margins for the Ventak AICD systems, since they have demonstrated a very low incidence of sudden death mortality (DFTs 1–20 J, maximum shock output 30–35 J).[25] The efficacy and safety margins for these 30–35 J devices are consistent with the new 2 × DFT recommendation for patients with step-down DFTs ≤ 15 J. For higher threshold patients (DFT+ = 20 J), a 30-J device provides an energy margin of 1.5 × DFT, which provides device efficacy for even the worst-case patient (E_{100} = 1.5 × E_{50}). Because most patients have DFTs located above this minimum DFT+, this 10-J rule of thumb also provides VF safety margins for the majority of patients. The use of higher output devices that deliver 34 J will assure an efficacy margin and even larger safety margin for all patients with 20-J DFTs (34 J = 1.7 × DFT energy margin).

As new leads and waveforms are introduced, which yield lower DFTs, the rule by which ICD shock energies are programmed to assure adequate efficacy and safety margins may be based on some multiple of the DFT, rather than this fixed-energy 10–15 J recommendation. For higher threshold patients (DFTs ≥ 20 J), enhanced DFT protocols should be used to assure adequate efficacy and safety margins.

If the patient's condition limits the amount of testing so that assessment protocols are not possible, efficacy and safety margins can also be assessed with verification protocols (2S, 3S, and step-down success protocols).[63] The single test protocols (1S) are not recommended for implant testing, because they require very large output margins and provide limited information about the patient.[58] For the two success protocol, the lowest position a 2S energy (E_{2S}) could have on the defibrillation curve is approximately 25% success, since two shocks each with a 25% probability of success would only have a 6% chance of both succeeding = 0.25 × 0.25. This lower limit is similar to that for the step-down DFT, thus, an efficacy margin would dictate that the device be programmed to at least 2 × E_{25}. To provide safety margins for the majority of patients, an extra 33% to 50% could be added to this 2S margin, since the E_{2S} distribution is not inherently skewed to the upper regions of the curve like the step-down DFT. This skewed nature provided extra safety margin for most patients with

---

[d] The shock energy for consistent defibrillation (E_{100}) for a DFT at E_{30} equals E_{100} = E_{30} ± 0.7 × full curve width = E_{30} ± 0.7 × (1.25 × E_{30}) = 1.9 × E_{30}, in keeping with the analysis in footnote a. For E_{40}, E_{100} = E_{40} ± 0.6 × full curve width = E_{40} ± 0.6 × (1.11 × E_{40}) = 1.7 × E_{40}.

the 2 × DFT guideline. For the 2S, the output margin may need to be programmed to 2.3–2.5 × E_{2S} to provide both efficacy and safety for the patient.

If the first conversion attempt in the 2S protocol is successful, but the second trial failed (1S, 1F), the test energy could lie anywhere on the defibrillation curve (from E_0–E_{100}). The output margins for this extensive distribution along the curve are very large (3.0–3.5 × E_{1S1F}),[30] similar in size to those for the 1S outcome. With this outcome, the system should either be revised, reevaluated for output margins that are acceptable, or replaced with a system with higher output energies.

A greater precision could be obtained with three test shocks at one energy. The lowest possible location on the defibrillation curve for an energy yielding three successful conversions (3S) is 40% success, since the probability of three consecutive successes at 40% is $0.4^3 = 6\%$. An ICD output of 1.7 × E_{40} will provide the minimum efficacy margin for a 3S evaluation (see footnote d). Allowing for 33% to 50% safety margins, since the 3S distribution is not skewed to the top of the curve like the step-down DFTs, the ICD should be programmed to energies $\geq 2.2 \times E_{3S}$ for adequate energy margins for all patients. As with the other testing methods, this output margin is based on the worst-case patient. Since this is a verification protocol, the exact position of the dose-response curve is not known. As the defibrillation curve is located further to the left of the 3S test energy, the actual efficacy and safety margins with this 2.2 × E_{3S} rule will be larger.

These efficacy methods provide an alternative to regular DFT testing. As more conversions are observed at the test energy (1S, 2S, or 3S), the upper boundary for the defibrillation curve becomes more accurately defined, allowing smaller efficacy margins to assure 100% defibrillation success. This trend is also seen for other DFT methods. The adequacy of an ICD energy margin becomes more apparent as the amount of testing increases (DFT, DFT+ to DFT++). For both methods, if higher thresholds yield energy margins that are too small, a few extra conversion tests at the DFT or the test energy are needed to assure adequate efficacy and safety margins for the patient. If adequate energy margins cannot be verified with the enhanced protocols, the ICD system should be revised or not implanted.

Future Testing Regimens

The most widely used methods for testing ICD therapies require multiple inductions of VF and delivery of many high-strength countershocks. Without this testing, the selection of appropriate therapy sequences is difficult and could jeopardize patient safety.[56] However, patient safety can also be threatened by excessive testing that provokes central nervous system abnormalities as a consequence of the cumulative effects of cerebral ischemia from hemodynamic collapse during the test session.[39,40,80] Future testing regimens that incorporate fewer episodes of VF and possibly a reduced number of shocks may be less traumatic and require significantly less time. Such techniques are currently being studied in animal models and in an increasing number of human studies.

In the past, the practices of defibrillation testing have varied widely, primarily dependent on the investigator's preferences, clinical protocol requirements (if applicable), and the hemodynamic status of the patient both before and during testing. Despite the diversity of implant testing techniques, long-term SCD survival apparently has remained unaffected by these differences.[27,25] The driving goal in adapting a testing technique to the patient is to establish a balance between the need to minimize the impact of testing on the patient,[30] and the selection of a therapeutic regime that is highly effective. The proper resolution of these issues may be especially difficult when one considers the possibility that future ICD therapy may be provided on a prophylactic basis in high-risk patient groups.[35] Patients that present with severe tachyarrhythmia-related symptoms will probably better tolerate the rigors of electrophysiologic and device implant testing, compared to high-risk patients that have never experienced such symptoms. Thus, all future and present ICD patients would welcome and benefit from a less traumatic means of verifying the safety and efficacy of ICD therapy.

One low-impact alternative to the current approach of ICD implant testing involves a sequence of therapy tests performed during the vulnerable time period of the cardiac cycle in sinus or paced rhythms. This method could potentially reduce the number of VF inductions during operative testing. Based on the concept of the cardiac vulnerable period during the T wave,[81] theoretical predictions,[82] and experimental data[83] suggest that shocks above a certain critical strength given during this period will no longer induce fibrillation. The minimum shock strength that does not induce VF above this critical level is called the ventricular upper limit of vulnerability (ULV). A correlation between the ULV and the requirements for defibrillation would make the ULV testing protocol an inviting alternative to current ICD test techniques.

As these initial ULV studies were performed, it was discovered that the ULV mechanism was also probabilistic.[84] The induction of VF by shocks near the ULV is characterized by a probability, similar to the probability governing defibrillation success. As the ULV protocol samples the ULV probability dose-response curve, it will experience the same limitations for locating this curve as the defibrillation assessment protocols.[30,58–63] This may result in the same type of energy margin specifications for programming ICD output using the ULV protocol (eg, $E_{ICD} \geq 2 \times ULV$), as described earlier in this chapter for implant margins based on defibrillation techniques.

Animal data reported by Chen et al.[83] and more recently by others[84–87] suggests that the ULV energy is well correlated to the DFT. Chen et al.[83] found that the ULV energy correlated to the mid-point (E_{50}) of the defibrillation dose-response curve. Souza et al.[84] and Malkin[86] suggest that the best correlation between the ULV and defibrillation dose-response curves occurs at a point higher on the defibrillation curve, near 97% defibrillation probability. While the majority of ULV/DFT comparisons have been obtained from animal models,[83–88] several recent clinical studies have also reported correlations between the ULV and defibrillation requirements.[69,89–91]

While these preliminary results in humans support the use of ULV testing during ICD implants,[69] the specific protocol that should be used for best correlation with the DFT has not been determined. One suggestion for the ULV protocol uses a fixed coupling interval with shocks given at the same point during the T wave. The initial shock strength is set above the ULV, with successive shocks decreasing in strength until fibrillation is induced.[69,89] The ULV is defined as the lowest energy shock that did not induce fibrillation. An alternate ULV protocol also starts with initial shock strengths above the ULV, but before decrementing the shock strength, successive shocks of the same energy are given at different coupling intervals, scanning the T wave.[84,90,91] The lowest energy that did not produce fibrillation at any point during the scan of the T wave is defined as the ULV. These two protocols may yield different relationships between the ULV and portions of the defibrillation dose-response curve.

A logical step for ICD implant testing is to combine the ULV and DFT protocols to increase the information gained about the patient.[69,86] The ULV testing can be used to assess the patient's ULV energy during sinus or paced rhythms, while also serving as the method for inducing VF. Once the arrhythmia is initiated, the DFT or other defibrillation protocol can be used to terminate it. Thus, by interweaving both protocols, one obtains both ULV and DFT assessments for the patient. Based on the correlation between the ULV and DFT energies for the protocol selected, these dual measures could provide a better assessment of curve location with fewer VF inductions.

Another approach for improving the precision of implant testing, while reducing the number of VF inductions, is to incorporate prior clinical experience about DFTs in prior patients with the same ICD system. This method takes advantage of the ICD patient population to improve the estimate of the location of the defibrillation dose-response curve. Malkin et al.[92] proposed a statistical approach based on prior information of the population's defibrillation curve characteristics to direct test levels during the defibrillation protocol and to calculate the estimated shock strength that would yield 95% defibrillation success. Using Bayesian estimation theory, they were able to provide estimates of the upper corner of the defibrillation success curve (E_{95}) using 2–4 episodes with far greater precision than the standard DFT protocols.[92] This approach may allow smaller margins to be programmed for the devices. A clinical extension of this method has been proposed by Penzotti et al.[93] using the DFTs observed in prior patients as the historical sample data for the Bayesian estimate of E_{95}. Further work in this area will demonstrate whether these statistical methods will provide greater power in defibrillation assessment, while avoiding exposure to multiple shocks.

This Bayesian estimation approach can also be used to analyze the defibrillation requirements from a combined ULV/DFT method.[86] By combining both DFT and ULV test shocks and using prior information about defibrillation and ULV characteristics from the population, this estimation analysis produced an estimate of the location of the upper corner of the defibrillation dose-response curve that was more accurate than DFT or ULV testing alone.[86] This estimate of E_{95} could then be used to program the desired safety margin for the device.

In summary, intraoperative and follow-up testing of defibrillation therapy efficacy could be improved by reducing both the number of high-strength shocks and the cumulative time during which the patient is exposed to systemic hypotension. Present test methods require larger margins due to their inherent lack of precision at locating the defibrillation dose-response curve. New techniques that use information about correlations between ULV and DFT alone or in combination with prior threshold information from the population may be implemented in the future. However, additional data and carefully designed clinical studies are needed from larger cohorts of patients to conclusively demonstrate the clinical viability of these new testing regimens.

Summary and Future Role of Implant Support Devices

The use of implant support devices during ICD implant, follow-up, or replacement has become an indispensable part of the ICD therapy application. Proper implant techniques have contributed to the favorable long-term therapeutic outcomes by assuring ICD output margins. Implant support devices have undergone tremendous change as the complexity of new ICDs has increased. Collectively, these implant support systems possess features such as: 1) automatic arrhythmia detection; 2) arrhythmic event play-back; 3) detection parameter adjustment; 4) ventricular tachycardia therapy such as defibrillation, cardioversion, or ATP regimens; 5) single or dual pathway shock delivery capabilities; 6) different defibrillation waveforms; 7) PES; and 8) PSA.

The importance of implant support testing becomes amplified when the need to reduce ICD volume is met by introduction of limited output (< 30 J) ICDs. With these new devices, accurate determination of energy margins will be even more critical since it is expected that most,[94] but not all patients will be eligible for implant.[54]

Future device designs may take advantage of recent and expected advances in ergonomics, interfacial engineering, expert systems and data transmission. As technologies evolve, implant support devices and systems will become more transportable and flexible. As they evolve, implant systems will become even more automatic. Algorithms that automatically determine optimum therapy parameters and recommend suitably patient-tailored therapy hierarchies for multiprogrammable implantable pacer/defibrillators may be developed. In addition, improvements in patient data management are foreseen. Computerized networks could be accessed with special hardware and software provided by the implant support device to quickly and efficiently update hospital and medical databases without the need for tedious manual data entry.

Finally, while the primary emphasis of this review has been directed toward the use of implant support devices for evaluation of implantable ventricular tachyarrhythmia therapies, supraventricular tachyarrhythmia therapy testing may soon become necessary as well.[95] Efficacy of internal atrial defibrillation with clinically relevant lead configurations has recently been reported by Cooper et al.[96] and others.[97,98] These reports demonstrate that conversion of atrial fibrillation in the acute sheep model is possible with reasonably low shock strengths (1–2 J) compared to transthoracic requirements.[99] In addition to atrial defibrillation therapy, it is conceivable that atrial flutter[100] and possibly atrial fibrillation[101] could be controlled via atrial site-specific pacing.

The need to control atrial tachyarrhythmias has been rather controversial.[102] However, there is mounting evidence that maintenance of normal sinus rhythm delays hemodynamic degradation of patients with congestive heart failure.[103] And, as a consequence of the rather disappointing results of pharmacological agents,[104] an implanted device that could terminate paroxysms of atrial flutter or fibrillation may have some promising clinical utility.[95] Just like ventricular therapies for tachyarrhythmia treatment, atrial therapies will also need to be carefully evaluated at time of implant. However, the consequences of failed atrial therapies (nonconversion, without proarrhythmia) are trivial compared to the life-threatening result of failed ventricular tachyarrhythmia therapy. For this reason, the criteria, method and devices used for evaluation of atrial therapies may be markedly different from those presently used during evaluation of ventricular therapies. Most notably, for atrial defibrillation, 100% conversion is not required for all shock attempts, since severely compromised hemodynamic states are not typically seen with this arrhythmia. Any atrial therapy (pacing or low-strength cardioversion) that has some probability of success and can be well tolerated by the patient can be attempted repeatedly, until a normal rhythm has been restored. Using this approach, atrial defibrillation shock strengths can be intentionally programmed to "sub-DFT" values to minimize discomfort.

Certainly, methods and devices for evaluating atrial tachyarrhythmia therapies will continue to evolve. Even though there appears to be a compelling need for electric therapies to help maintain normal atrial rhythms, there are limitations to the concept of the implantable atrial cardioverter/defibrillator such as efficacy, pain, automatic rhythm discrimination, and proarrhythmia need to be carefully addressed.[95] Most likely, atrial therapy systems will be merged with ventricular therapy systems to provide a "whole-heart" cardioverter/defibrillator.

Thus, future implant support systems are likely to incorporate features that provide means to test both ventricular and atrial therapies using protocols that minimize a patient's exposure to hemodynamically unstable rhythms and high-strength shocks. Proper assessment of the efficacy of ICD therapies will continue to hold a central role in the implant procedures in the future. Implant support systems, whether external or centered in the implanted device, are destined to remain an integral part of this ICD therapy implementation.

References

1. Lown B: Sudden cardiac death: the major challenge facing contemporary cardiology. *Am J Cardiol* 41:313, 1979.
2. Gillum RF: Sudden coronary death in the United States, 1980–1985. *Circulation* 79:756, 1989.
3. Goldberg J: Declining out-of-hospital sudden coronary death rates: additional pieces of the epidemiologic puzzle. *Circulation* 79:1369, 1989.
4. Myerburg RJ, Kessler KM, Castellanos A: Sudden cardiac death: structure, function and time dependence of risk. *Circulation* 85(suppl I):I2, 1992.
5. Myerburg RJ, Kessler KM, Interian A, et al: Clinical and experimental pathophysiology of sudden cardiac death. In: *Cardiac Electrophysiology: From Cell to Bedside*. Edited by DP Zipes, J Jalife. Philadelphia, PA: WB Saunders Co.; 1990, p. 666.
6. Roberts WC, Jones AA: Quantitation of coronary arterial narrowing at necropsy in sudden coronary death. Analysis of 31 patients and comparison with 25 controls. *Am J Cardiol* 44:39, 1979.
7. Warnes CA, Roberts WC: Sudden coronary death: relation of amount and distribution of coronary narrowing at necropsy to previous symptoms of myocardial ischemia, left ventricular scarring and heart weight. *Am J Cardiol* 54:65, 1984.
8. Muller JE, Tofler GH, Stone PH: Circadian variation and triggers of onset of acute cardiovascular disease. *Circulation* 79:733, 1989.
9. Willich SN, Maclure M, Mittleman M, et al: Sudden cardiac death: support for a role of triggering in causation. *Circulation* 87(5):1442, 1993.
10. Bardy GH, Olson WH: Clinical characteristics of spontaneous-onset sustained ventricular tachycardia and ventricular fibrillation in survivors of cardiac arrest. In: *Cardiac Electrophysiology: From Cell to Bedside*. Edited by DP Zipes, J Jalife. Philadelphia, PA: WB Saunders Co.; 1990, p. 778.
11. Lown B, Wolf M: Approaches to sudden death from coronary heart disease. *Circulation* 44:130, 1971.
12. Julian DG: Toward preventing coronary death from ventricular fibrillation. *Circulation* 54(3):360, 1976.
13. Myerburg RJ, Conde CA, Sung RJ, et al: Clinical, electrophysiologic and hemodynamic profile of patients resuscitated from pre-hospital cardiac arrest. *Am J Med* 68:568, 1980.
14. Cobb LA, Werner JA, Trobaugh GB: Sudden cardiac death: I. A decade's experience with out-of-hospital resuscitation. *Mod Concepts Cardiovasc Dis* 49:31, 1980.
15. Mackay RS, Leeds SE: Physiologic effects of condenser discharges. *J Appl Physiol* 6:67, 1953.
16. Edmark KW, Thomas GI, Jones TW: DC pulse defibrillation. *J Thorac Cardiovasc Surg* 51(3):326, 1966.
17. Peleska B: Cardiac arrhythmias following condenser discharges and their dependence upon strength of current and phase of cardiac cycle. *Circ Res* 13:21, 1963.
18. Mirowski M, Mower MM, Staewen WS: Standby automatic defibrillator: an approach to prevention of sudden coronary death. *Arch Intern Med* 126:158, 1970.
19. Schuder JC, Stoeckle H, Gold JH, et al: Experimental ventricular defibrillation with an automatic and completely implanted system. *Trans Am Soc Artif Organs* 16:207, 1970.
20. Mirowski M, Mower MM, Gott VL, et al: Feasibility and effectiveness of low-energy catheter defibrillation in man. *Circulation* 57:79, 1973.
21. Mirowski M, Mower MM, Langer A, et al: A chronically implanted system for automatic defibrillation in active conscious dogs: experimental model for treatment of sudden death from ventricular fibrillation. *Circulation* 58:90, 1978.
22. Mirowski M, Reid PR, Mower MM, et al: Termination of malignant ventricular arrhythmias with an implanted automatic defibrillator in human beings. *N Engl J Med* 303:322, 1980.
23. Mirowski M, Mower MM, Reid PR, et al: The automatic implantable defibrillator. *PACE* 5:384, 1982.
24. Mirowski M, Reid PR, Watkins L, et al: Clinical treatment of life-threatening ventricular tachyarrhythmias with the automatic implantable defibrillator. *Am Heart J* 102:265, 1981.
25. Nisam S, Mower MM, Thomas A, et al: Patient survival comparisons in three generations of automatic implantable cardioverter defibrillators: review of 12 years, 25,000 patients. *PACE* 16(2):174, 1993.
26. Coumel P: Historical milestones of implanted defibrillation. *PACE* 15(4):598, 1992.
27. Winkle R, Mead R, Ruder M, et al: Long-term outcome with the automatic implanta-

ble cardioverter defibrillator. *J Am Coll Cardiol* 13:1353, 1989.
28. Akhtar M, Avitall B, Jazayeri M, et al: Role of implantable cardioverter defibrillator therapy in the management of high-risk patients. *Circulation* 85(1):I131, 1992.
29. Winkle RA, Bach SM, Echt DS, et al: Defibrillation/cardioversion energy requirements using the implantable apical patch-superior vena caval spring leads. *Circulation* 69:766, 1984.
30. Singer I, Lang DJ: Defibrillation threshold: clinical utility and therapeutic implications. *PACE* 15(6):932, 1992.
31. Jung W, Manz M, Lüderitz B: Effects of antiarrhythmic drugs on defibrillation threshold in patients with the implantable cardioverter defibrillator. *PACE* 15(4):645, 1992.
32. Bardy GH, Buono G, Troutman CL, et al: Subacute changes in defibrillation threshold following multiprogrammable defibrillation implantation in man (abstract). *J Am Coll Cardiol* 17:344A, 1991.
33. Venditti FJ, Vassolas G, Martin D: Chronic defibrillation thresholds in an implanted transvenous cardioverter defibrillator system. *Circulation* 86(4):I-441, 1992.
34. Frame R, Brodman R, Furman S, et al: Long-term stability of defibrillation thresholds with intraepicardial defibrillation patches. *PACE* 16(1):208, 1993.
35. Bardy GH, Hofer B, Johnson G, et al: Implantable transvenous cardioverter-defibrillators. *Circulation* 87(4):1152, 1993.
36. Bakker PFA, Hauer RNW, Wever EFD: Infections involving implanted cardioverter defibrillator devices. *PACE* 15:654, 1992.
37. Brooks R, McGovern BA, Garan H, et al: Comparison of two different nonthoracotomy cardioverter-defibrillator systems: analysis of 74 patients at one center. (abstract) *J Am Coll Cardiol* 21(2):155A, 1993.
38. Frame R, Brodman R, Furman S, et al: Clinical evaluation of the safety repetitive intraoperative defibrillation threshold testing. *PACE* 15(6):870, 1992.
39. Singer I, Edmonds HL, vander Laken C, et al: Is defibrillation testing safe? *PACE* 14:1899, 1991.
40. Singer I, Edmonds H, Slater D, et al: Cerebral hypoperfusion is an important factor to consider when programming implantable defibrillators (abstract). *PACE* 15(4):530, 1992.
41. Stoddard MF, Redd RR, Buckingham TA, et al: Effects of electrophysiologic testing of the automatic implantable cardioverter-defibrillator on left ventricular systolic function and diastolic filling. *Am Heart J* 122:714, 1991.
42. Echt DS, Lee JT, Hammon JW: Implantation and intraoperative assessment of antitachycardia devices. In: *Electrical Therapy for Cardiac Arrhythmias*. Edited by S Saksena, N Goldschlager. Philadelphia, PA: W.B. Saunders Co.; 1990, p. 489.
43. Schwartzman D, Jadonath R, Estepo J, et al: Serial patch-patch impedance values in an epicardial defibrillation system (abstract). *PACE* 16(4):916, 1993.
44. Troup PJ: Implantable cardioverters and defibrillators. *Curr Prob Cardiol* 14(12):675, 1989.
45. Schuder JC, Rahmoeller GA, Stoeckle H: Transthoracic ventricular defibrillation with triangular and trapezoidal waveforms. *Circ Res* 19:689, 1966.
46. Chapman PD, Wetherbee JN, Vetter JW, et al: Strength-duration curves of fixed pulse width variable tilt truncated exponential waveforms for nonthoracotomy internal defibrillation in dogs. *PACE* 11:1045, 1988.
47. Wessale JL, Bourland JD, Tacker WA, et al: Bipolar catheter defibrillation in dogs using trapezoidal waveforms of various tilts. *J Electrocardiol* 13(4):359, 1980.
48. Bach SM, Shapland JE: Engineering aspects of implantable defibrillators. In: *Electrical Therapy for Cardiac Arrhythmias*. Edited by S Saksena, N Goldschlager. Philadelphia, PA: W.B. Saunders Co.; 1990, p. 489.
49. Lawrence JH, Brin KP, Halperin HR, et al: The characterization of human transmyocardial impedance during implantation of the automatic internal cardioverter defibrillator. *PACE* 9:745, 1986.
50. Tang ASL, Yabe S, Wharton JM, et al: Ventricular defibrillation using biphasic waveforms: the importance of phasic duration. *J Am Coll Cardiol* 13:207, 1989.
51. Feeser SA, Tang ASL, Kavanagh KM, et al: Strength-duration and probability of success curves for defibrillation with biphasic waveforms. *Circulation* 82:2128, 1990.
52. Dixon EG, Tang ASL, Wolf PD, et al: Improved defibrillation thresholds with large contoured epicardial electrodes and biphasic waveforms. *Circulation* 76:1176, 1987.
53. Cooper RAS, Ideker RE, Feeser SA, et al: Optimum waveform morphology for defibrillation. In: *The Implantable Cardioverter/Defibrillator*. Edited by E Alt, H Klein, JC Griffin. Berlin: Springer-Verlag; 1992, p. 97.
54. Epstein AE, Ellenbogen KA, Kirk KA, et al: Clinical characteristics and outcome of patients with high defibrillation thresholds. *Circulation* 86:1206, 1992.
55. Langer A, Heilman MS, Mower MM, et al: Considerations in the development of the

automatic implantable defibrillator. *Med Instrum* 10(3):163, 1976.
56. Lehmann MH, Steinman RT, Schuger CD, et al: Defibrillation threshold testing and other practices related to AICD implantation: do all roads lead to Rome? *PACE* 12:1530, 1989.
57. Bourland JD, Tacker WA, Geddes LA: Strength-duration curves for trapezoidal waveforms of various tilts for transchest defibrillation in animals. *Med Instrum* 12(1):38, 1978.
58. Davy JM, Fain ES, Dorian P, et al: The relationship between successful defibrillation and delivered energy in open-chest dogs: Reappraisal of the "defibrillation threshold" concept. *Am Heart J* 113:77, 1987.
59. McDaniel WC, Schuder JC: The cardiac ventricular defibrillation threshold-inherent limitations in its application and interpretation. *Med Instrum* 21:170, 1987.
60. Lang DJ, Cato EL, Echt DS: Protocol for evaluation of internal defibrillation safety margins (abstract). *J Am Coll Cardiol* 13(2):111A, 1989.
61. Rattes MF, Jones DL, Sharma AD, et al: Defibrillation threshold: a simple and quantitative estimate of the ability to defibrillate. *PACE* 10:70, 1987.
62. Schuder JC, McDaniel WC: Defibrillation threshold-normal distribution initial shock. In: *Proceedings of the 38th Annual Conference on Engineering in Medicine and Biology*. 1985, 27:316.
63. Lang DJ, Swanson DK: Safety margin for defibrillation. Presented at 2nd International Congress on Rate Adaptive Cardiac Pacing and Implantable Defibrillators, October 10–13, 1990, Munich, Germany.
64. Yabe S, Smith WM, Daubert JP, et al: Conduction disturbances caused by high current density electric fields. *Circ Res* 66:1190, 1990.
65. Jones DL, Fujimura O, Klein GJ: Minimum replications to estimate average threshold energy for defibrillation. *Med Instrum* 22:298, 1988.
66. Jones DL, Irish WD, Klein GJ: Defibrillation efficacy—comparison of defibrillation threshold versus dose-response curve determination. *Circ Res* 69:45, 1991.
67. Church T, Martinson M, Kallok M, et al: A model to evaluate alternative methods of defibrillation threshold determination. *PACE* 11:2002, 1988.
68. McDaniel WC, Schuder JC: An up-down algorithm for estimation of the cardiac ventricular defibrillation threshold. *Med Instrum* 22:286, 1988.
69. Chen PS, Feld GK, Kriett JM, et al: The relationship between the upper limit of vulnerability and the defibrillation threshold in humans. *Circulation* 88:186, 1993.
70. Schuder JC, McDaniel WC: Improving the significance of cardiac defibrillation threshold determinations by means of algorithms involving one or two additional episodes (abstract). Proceedings of AAMI 22nd Annual Meeting, 1987, p. 58.
71. Deeb GM, Griffith BP, Thompson ME, et al: Lead systems for internal ventricular defibrillation. *Circulation* 64:242, 1981.
72. Mead RH, Ruder M, Schmidt P, et al: Improved defibrillation efficacy with chronically implanted defibrillation leads (abstract). *Circulation* 74:II-110, 1986.
73. Echt DS, Barbey JT, Black NJ: Influence of ventricular fibrillation duration on defibrillation energy in dogs using bidirectional pulse discharges. *PACE* 11:1315, 1988.
74. Fujimura C, Jones DL, Klein GJ: Effects of time to defibrillation and subthreshold preshocks on defibrillation success in pigs. *PACE* 12:358, 1989.
75. Jones JL, Swartz JF, Jones RE, et al: Increasing fibrillation duration enhances relative asymmetrical biphasic versus monophasic defibrillator waveform efficacy. *Circ Res* 67:376, 1990.
76. Bardy GH, Stewart RS, Ivey TD, et al: Potential risk of low energy cardioversion attempts by implantable cardioverters (abstract). *J Am Coll Cardiol* 9:168A, 1987.
77. Bardy GH, Ivey TD, Allen M, et al: A prospective, randomized evaluation of effect of ventricular fibrillation duration on defibrillation thresholds in humans. *J Am Coll Cardiol* 13:1362, 1989.
78. Bardy GH, Ivey TD, Johnson G, et al: Prospective evaluation of initially ineffective defibrillation pulses on subsequent defibrillation success during ventricular fibrillation in survivors of cardiac arrest. *Am J Cardiol* 62:718, 1988.
79. Jones DL, Klein GJ, Guiraudon GM, et al: Prediction of defibrillation success from a single defibrillation threshold measurement with sequential pulses and two current pathways in humans. *Circulation* 78:1144, 1988.
80. Konstadt SN, Blakeman B, Wilber D, et al: The effects of normothermic hypoperfusion on processed EEG in patients. *Anesth Analg* 70:213, 1990.
81. Wiggers CJ, Wegria R: Ventricular fibrillation due to single, localized inductions and condenser shocks applied during the vulnerable phase of ventricular systole. *Am J Physiol* 128:500, 1940.

82. Winfree AT: Sudden cardiac death—a problem of topology. *Sci Am* 248:144, 1983.
83. Chen PS, Shibata N, Dixon EG, et al: Comparison of the defibrillation threshold and the upper limit of ventricular vulnerability. *Circulation* 73(5):1022, 1986.
84. Souza JJ, Malkin RA, Smith WM, et al: Relationship between upper limit of vulnerability and defibrillation threshold in a nonthoracotomy pig model (abstract). *PACE* 16:888, 1993.
85. Kavanagh KM, Harrison JH, Dixon EG, et al: The correlation of the defibrillation threshold and the upper limit of vulnerability using catheter-patch defibrillating electrodes (abstract). *J Am Coll Cardiol* 15:73A, 1990.
86. Malkin RA; *Estimating Defibrillation Efficacy Using Upper Limit of Vulnerability Testing.* Durham, NC: Duke University; 1993. Doctoral dissertation.
87. Wharton JM, Richard VJ, Murry CE, et al: Electrophysiological effects of monophasic and biphasic stimuli in normal and infarcted dogs. *PACE* 13:1158, 1990.
88. Chen PS, Feld GK, Mower MM, et al: Effects of pacing rate and timing of defibrillation shock on the relation between the defibrillation threshold and the upper limit of vulnerability in open chest dogs. *J Am Coll Cardiol* 18:1555, 1991.
89. Chen PS, Feld GK, Kriett JM, et al: The relationship between the upper limit of vulnerability and the defibrillation threshold in humans (abstract). *PACE* 15(2):530, 1992.
90. Stanton MS, Mehra R, Morris J, et al: Relationship between defibrillation threshold and upper limit of vulnerability in humans (abstract). *PACE* 15(4):563, 1992.
91. Bacon ME, Vitullo RN, Kasell JH, et al: Upper limit of vulnerability and its relationship to defibrillation threshold in humans (abstract). *PACE* 15(4):530, 1992.
92. Malkin RA, Burdick DS, Johnson EE, et al: Estimating the 95% effective defibrillation dose. *IEEE Trans Biomed Eng* 40(3):256, 1993.
93. Penzotti JE, Malkin RA, Pilkington TC: A new high performance designer of optimal defibrillation experiments. *Computers in Cardiology* IEEE Computers Society Press; 1992, p. 487.
94. Block M, Dieter H, Böcker D, et al: Subcutaneous array lead for internal defibrillation—a new lead configuration. *PACE* 16(2):896, 1993.
95. Levy S, Camm AJ: An implantable atrial defibrillator: an impossible dream? *Circulation* 87(5):1769, 1993.
96. Cooper RAS, Alferness CA, Smith WM, et al: Internal cardioversion of atrial fibrillation in sheep. *Circulation* 87(5):1673, 1993.
97. Alferness CA, Ilina MI, Wagner DO, et al: Comparison of a dual to a single lead system for transvenous atrial defibrillation (abstract). *PACE* 16(4):854, 1993.
98. Tacker WA, Schoenlein WE, Janas W, et al: Catheter electrode evaluation for transvenous atrial defibrillation (abstract). *PACE* 16(4):853, 1993.
99. Lown B, Perlroth MG, Kaidbey S, et al: "Cardioversion" of atrial fibrillation. A report on the treatment of 65 episodes in 50 patients. *N Engl J Med* 269:325, 1963.
100. Josephson ME: Atrial flutter and fibrillation. In: *Clinical Cardiac Electrophysiology: Techniques and Interpretations.* Edited by M Josephson. Philadelphia, PA: Lea & Febiger; 1993, p. 275.
101. Allessie MA, Kirchhof C, Scheffer GJ, et al: Regional control of atrial fibrillation by rapid pacing in conscious dogs. *Circulation* 84:1689, 1991.
102. Kerr CR, Chung DC: Atrial fibrillation. Fact, controversy and future. *Clin Prog Electrophysiol Pacing* 3:319, 1985.
103. Kannel WB, Abbott RD, Savage DD, et al: Epidemiologic features of chronic atrial fibrillation: Framingham study. N Engl J Med 306:1018, 1982.
104. Pai SM, Torres V: Atrial fibrillation: new management strategies. *Curr Prob Cardiol* 18(4):235, 1993.

Chapter 11

Device Telemetry

Igor Singer

Implantable cardioverter-defibrillators (ICDs) have evolved from relatively simple devices capable of administering committed cardioversion/defibrillation shocks for ventricular tachycardia (VT) or ventricular fibrillation (VF) to more complex noncommitted devices capable of delivering tiered-therapy responses.[1] Inclusion of complex antitachycardia pacing algorithms, low-energy cardioversion, and bradycardia pacing to defibrillation has further increased the complexities of device programming and patient evaluation expanding the need for data storage and retrieval capabilities. Telemetered data provides information about the battery status, lead system integrity, and diagnostic data that are essential for assessment of device/lead system function.

System Evaluation

Assessment of Battery Integrity

The most fundamental of the measurements is the determination of the battery status. The early devices (AID™, AID-B™, AID-BR™, Intec, Pittsburgh, PA) and (Ventak C™, CPI, St. Paul, MN) used lithium vanadium pentoxide (LiV$_2$O$_5$) battery. This type of battery has a relatively constant voltage under low-current loads. Therefore, the only way to assess the battery status is to test it under the load conditions. This is done by measuring the capacitor charge time. This measurement requires capacitor reforming followed by a charge cycle. The determination of elective replacement indicator (ERI) was cumbersome, as well as wasteful of energy.

Current generation ICDs (PCD™, Medtronic Inc., Minneapolis, MN; Cadence™, Ventritex, Sunnyvale, CA; Guardian ATP™ 4211, Telectronics, Inc., Englewood, CO; PRX™, CPI, Inc.) use lithium silver vanadium pentoxide (LiAgV$_2$O$_5$). The open circuit voltage with this battery reflects the remaining voltage capacity. A direct measurement of the battery voltage, an indicator of whether ERI has been reached, may be obtained by a simple device interrogation. Another third-generation ICD (Res-Q™, Intermedics, Inc., Angleton, TX) uses a different lithium chemistry whose open circuit voltage may not be indicative of the remaining battery capacity.

The ERI voltage recommendations of various manufacturers are summarized in Table 1. A second, end-of-life (EOL) voltage, is sometimes also specified. When this voltage is reached, the device may no longer be capable of functioning within the manufacturer's specifications and should be replaced immediately.

From Singer I, (ed.) Implantable Cardioverter-Defibrillator. Armonk, NY: Futura Publishing Company, Inc.; © 1994.

Table 1
Elective Replacement Indicators for ICDs

ICD	Manufacturer	ERI
Ventak P™	CPI	33% increase in charge time
Cadence™	Ventritex	5.10 V preshock
PCD™	Medtronic	4.97 V preshock
Guardian™	Telectronics	5% remaining capacity
Res-Q™	Intermedics	8.15 V preshock

ICD: implantable cardioverter-defibrillator; ERI: elective replacement indicator

Assessment of the Lead Integrity

Lead integrity is essential for successful system operation. Two separate lead systems are required for ICD function: 1) pace/sense leads and 2) defibrillation (high-voltage) leads.

The integrity of the pace/sense leads may be assessed by the pacing threshold margin and by measuring the lead impedance. Pacing threshold may be evaluated automatically with some devices (eg, Guardian ATP 4210 and 4211; Figure 1.) Lead impedance measurement is typically 300–1,000 Ω. Decrease in lead impedance suggests insulation breakdown, while increase in impedance suggests conductor fracture.

To evaluate defibrillation lead integrity a shock must be delivered through the defibrillating electrodes. If a defibrillation lead problem is suspected a shock may be delivered to the patient synchronously in sinus rhythm under controlled conditions (in the electrophysiology laboratory) to determine the defibrillation lead impedance (Figure 2). Typically, impedance for defibrillating leads is 20–100 Ω. Impedance is influenced by the surface area of the electrodes, the size of the heart, the lead geometry, and possibly by other as yet undetermined physiological variables.[2]

Some devices (eg, PRX) have output pulse width that varies with the lead impedance (see Chapter 10). Other devices (eg, Guardian; Cadence) deliver fixed pulse width, which is programmable, and automatically measure voltage and impedance. Other devices (eg, PCD 7217B; Res-Q) cannot noninvasively telemeter the defibrillation lead impedance. Future models of these devices will likely incorporate this capability.

Some devices, eg, Cadence; P-2 are capable of real-time electrogram storage and retrieval. Guardian ATP 4211 has the capability of storing 1-second electrogram snapshots before and after administering therapy. Other devices (eg, PCD 7217B and Guardian 4211) are capable of storing R-R interval history prior to and following therapy. Evaluation of electrograms and R-R interval history is useful to confirm the ar-

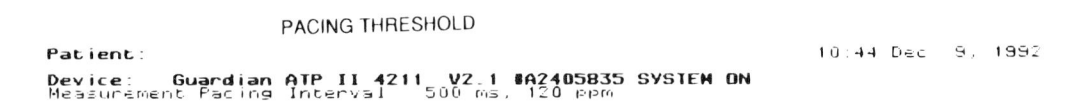

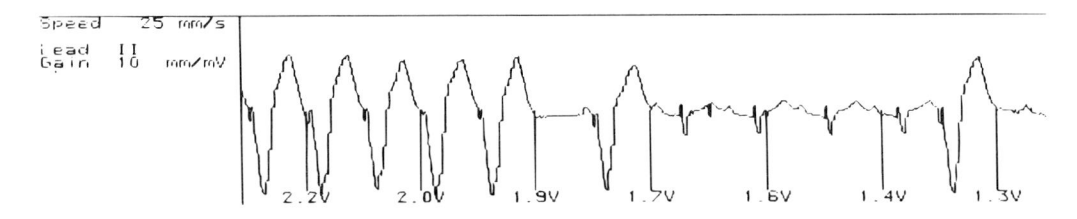

Figure 1. Automatic threshold determination (Guardian ATP™ 4210, Telectronics, Englewood, CO).

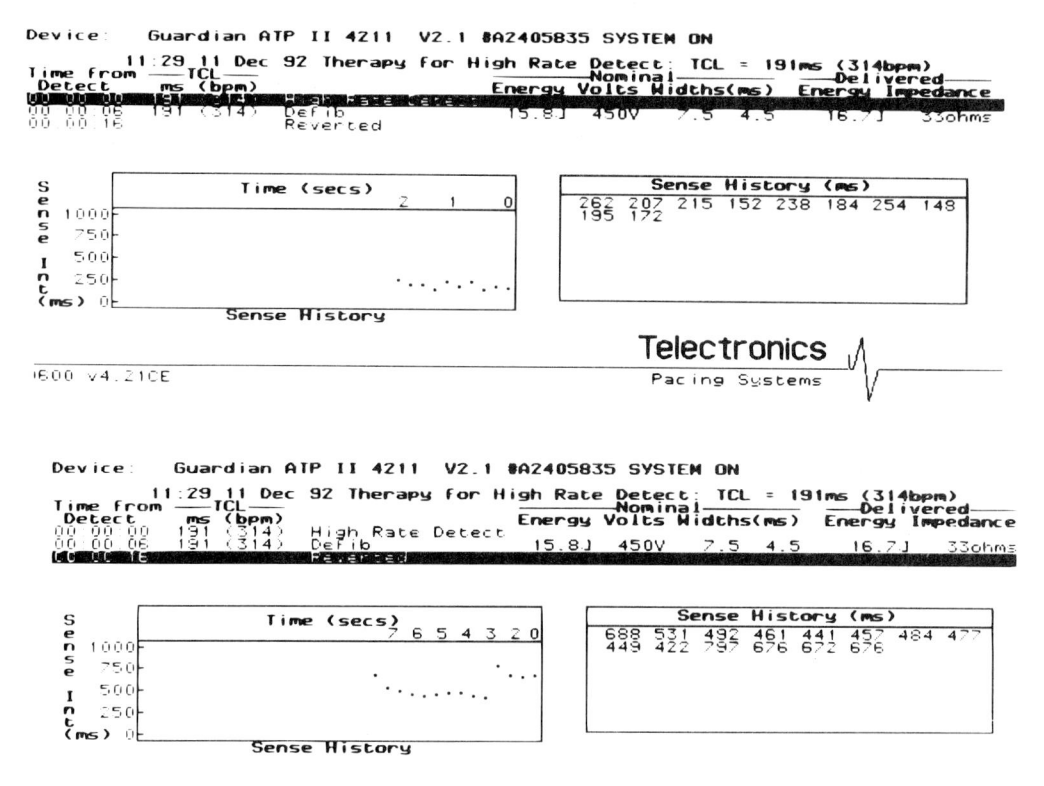

Figure 2. Telemetry displaying an episode of ventricular fibrillation, followed by a defibrillation shock of 16.7 J and reversion to sinus rhythm. The patch-to-patch lead impedance is measured to be 33 Ω. On the left is a plot of R-R intervals over time, on the right the actual R-R interval measurements. The top and bottom panels are continuous (Guardian ATP™ 4211, Telectronics, Englewood, CO).

rhythmia occurrence and to diagnose potential lead or device malfunction (see also Chapters 21 and 22).

Capacitor Reformation

Implantable cardioverter-defibrillators use electrolytic capacitors to store charge prior to shock delivery (see Chapter 5). These types of capacitors have a relatively high current leakage if they are not periodically charged. "Reforming" the capacitors reduces the current leakage, which can potentially result in unacceptably prolonged charge times. Capacitors reformation is required every 2–6 months, depending on the capacitor type, circuit design, the battery type, and time from the prior shock delivery. Recommended capacitor reformation times are summarized in Table 2.

If the capacitors are not reformed periodically it is possible that the charge time may become excessive. When the battery is close to the EOL, it is possible that a shock may not be delivered because most ICDs

Table 2
Recommended Capacitor Reformation Intervals

ICD	Manufacturer	Interval
Ventak P™	CPI	2 months manual
Guardian™	Telectronics	2 months automatic
PCD™	Medtronic	3 months manual
Res-Q™	Intermedics	4 months manual
Cadence™	Ventritex	6 months automatic

ICD: implantable cardioverter-defibrillator.

are designed to abort shock delivery if the capacitor cannot be charged within a specified time. Conversely, reforming capacitors with excessive frequency may result in premature battery depletion.

Treatment History Evaluation

Retrieval of the stored data is helpful for complete patient evaluation facilitating follow-up. The first-generation devices (AID, AID-B, AID-BR), provided only the most rudimentary information regarding the device therapy. Advance in the shock counters would alert the physician to delivery of therapy by the ICD. These early devices also were capable of measuring the capacitors charge times, an indirect measure of the battery status.

The second-generation devices (Ventak C and Ventak P) provided minimal incremental improvement in the available stored information. With these devices one could obtain the cumulative shock count, number of test shocks used to test the capacitor charge times, and capacitor reformation times. Minimal programmability was available in these devices, ie, the rate detection, detection algorithm, inclusion or exclusion of probability density function (PDF), delay of up to 5 seconds for detection to exclude the nonsustained VTs, and the choice of 26- or 30-J output for the initial shock (Ventak-P; Figure 3).

No electrograms could be stored or retrieved, therefore, no information regarding the arrhythmic events could be obtained beyond the knowledge that a shock had occurred. Clinical information could not be supplanted by electrogram retrieval.

Ingenious methods to detect and document ICD sensing problems were devised using the phonocardiographic methods. By recording the amplified sounds emitted by the automatic ICD, the so-called "beepograms"[3] could be recorded (Figure 4). The Ventak series of AICDs emit high-frequency sounds synchronous with ventricular depo-

```
****************
    VENTAK P
    MODEL 1600
  PULSE GENERATOR
****************
PRESENT PARAMETERS
―――――――――――――――
MODE       ACTIVE
RATE       175 BPM
PDF        OFF
DELAY
  1ST        5 SEC
  2-5      2.5 SEC
SHOCK ENERGY
  1ST      30 JOULES
  2-5      30 JOULES
―――――――――――――――
CHARGE TIME
           6.6 SEC
LEAD IMPEDANCE
          TEST OHMS
PG BATTERY STATUS
       EVALUATE ERI
CAPACITOR FORM
          33.0 SEC
COUNT
  1ST SHOCK      7
  2-5 SHOCK      7
  TOTAL PATIENT 14
  TEST SHOCK   18
****************
```

Figure 3. An example of the telemetered data that can be retrieved from Ventak™ P device (CPI, St. Paul, MN). Limited programmability and simple digital readouts of the number of shocks administered, capacitor reformation, and charge times is available only.

larization when a doughnut magnet is applied over the device. Thus, one could occasionally document T wave oversensing, or in some patients with concurrently implanted pacemakers, pacemaker artifact oversensing by recording emitted sounds synchronous with T waves or pacemaker artifacts (Figure 5.) Thus, only crude evaluation of sensing could be inferred from these devices.

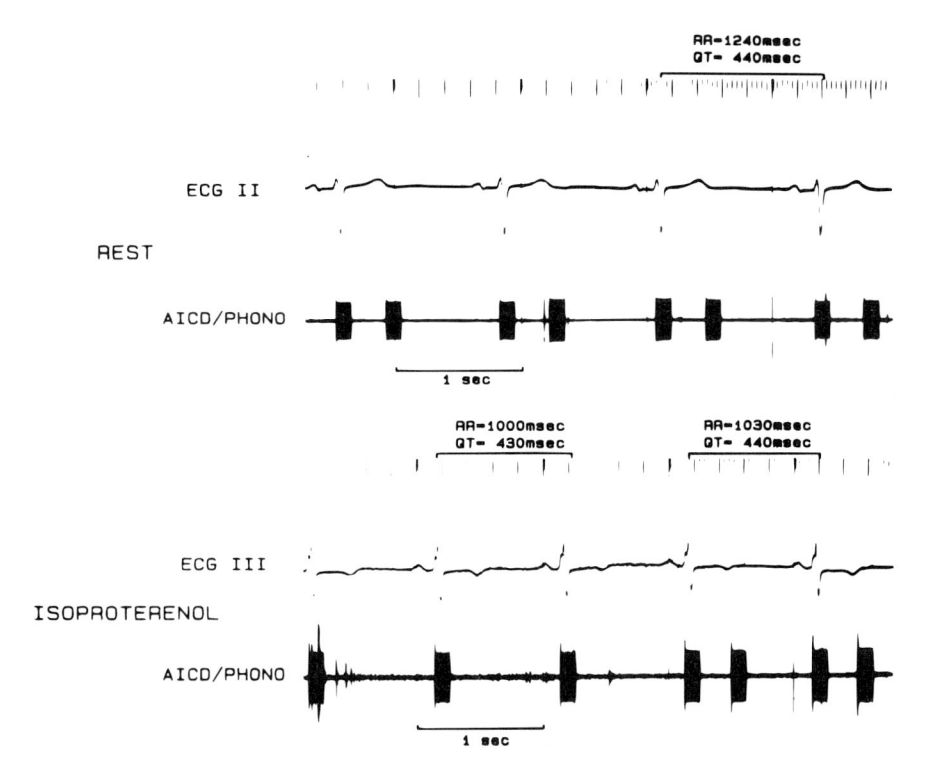

Figure 4. Double counting due to inappropriate T wave sensing by Ventak™ (CPI, St. Paul, MN) is noted at rest. With isoproterenol infusion, double counting becomes intermittent due to shortening of the QT interval. (Reproduced from permission from Reference 4.)

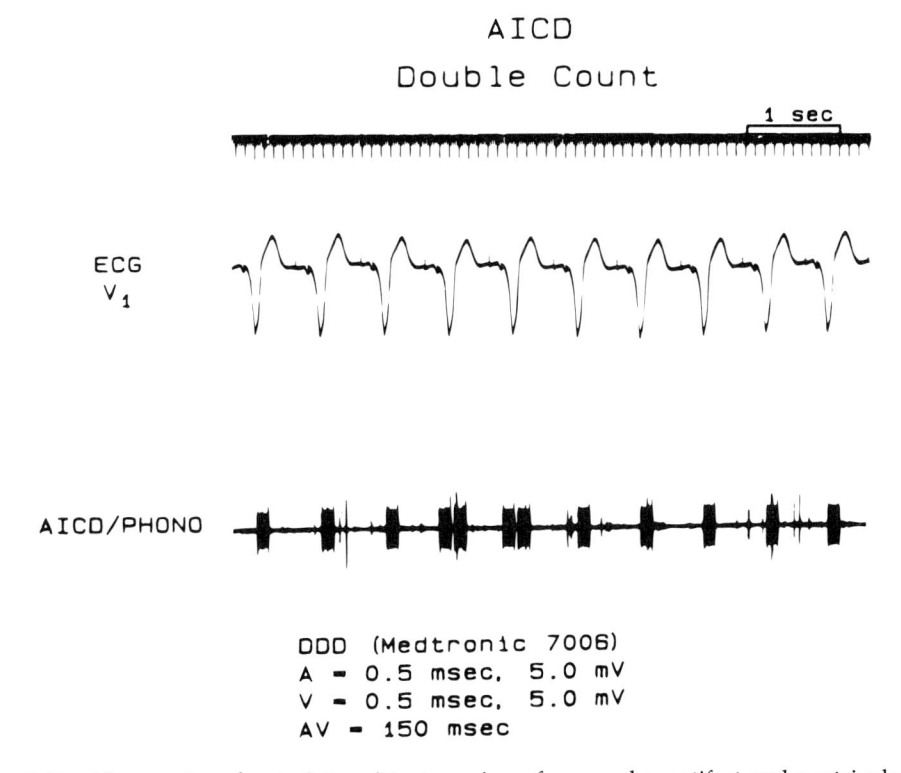

Figure 5. Double counting due to intermittent sensing of pacemaker artifact and ventricular electrogram by Ventak™ (CPI, St. Paul, MN). (Reproduced from permission from Reference 4.)

The earlier ICDs were not microprocessor based. Hence, only a limited memory was available at a cost of a large current drain. Third-generation devices are all microprocessor controlled. It is now possible to record large amounts of discrete information. Patient data such as implant date, the leads used, ICD programming, diagnostic data, including tachyarrhythmia detections, therapies, and outcomes are readily retrievable (Figure 6). Information regarding battery status, lead impedance, and defibrillation electrode integrity can now be stored and easily retrieved by noninvasive telemetry.

The quantity of continuous analog data that can be stored is, however, limited because the amount of data storage depends on the precision, the resolution and the duration of therapies stored. The number of data bits in each sample of analog data and the number of samples per second determine the resolution. Therefore, the duration of data stored is determined by the memory size divided by the word length and the number of samples recorded per second. Data of individual events may be stored as interval samples (R-R interval history) or real-time electrograms. Only a limited information is available from the R-R interval history. In general, relatively constant R-R intervals during uniform monomorphic tachycardia or during sinus rhythm suggest appropriate sensing (Figure 2). Erratic R-R interval history suggests atrial fibrillation or flutter. If the intervals are unphysiologically short or short-long-short (short interval being < 150 msec), this may be due to undersensing, oversensing, or both (Figure 7). Some devices can store R-R intervals in a numeric or graphic format and also provide a brief "snapshot" of the detected electrograms prior to and/or following arrhythmia detection and therapy (Figure 8).

Analog data (electrograms) are more helpful. Direct electrogram telemetry permits more accurate analysis of sensing, tachyarrhythmia history, and therapy efficacy (Figure 9). It is anticipated that in the future faster data processing may improve further the scope and the volume of data collected and stored. The need for further data retrieval and faster data processing will become even greater with incorporation of hemodynamic sensors, dual-chamber pacing, sensing, and defibrillation functions in the next generations of ICDs anticipated in the future.

Analysis of stored episodes of tachyarrhythmias is extremely valuable for determination of the appropriateness of detection parameters and therapy "prescription" for the ICD. These data are also useful for assessment of the therapeutic efficacy of antiarrhythmic drugs, which are frequently used to suppress or modify VT. Frequency, duration and cycle lengths of recorded tachycardia episodes may be used to assess efficacy of the antiarrhythmic and device therapy and potentially adverse drug-device interactions (Figure 10).

The type and the format of recorded data varies for deferent devices and manufacturers. Each ICD can only be interrogated or programmed using the manufacturer-specific programmer and software. Therefore, in a clinical center where more than one type of device is implanted, or where patients with different types of devices are being followed, multiple programmers from various manufacturers must be readily available.

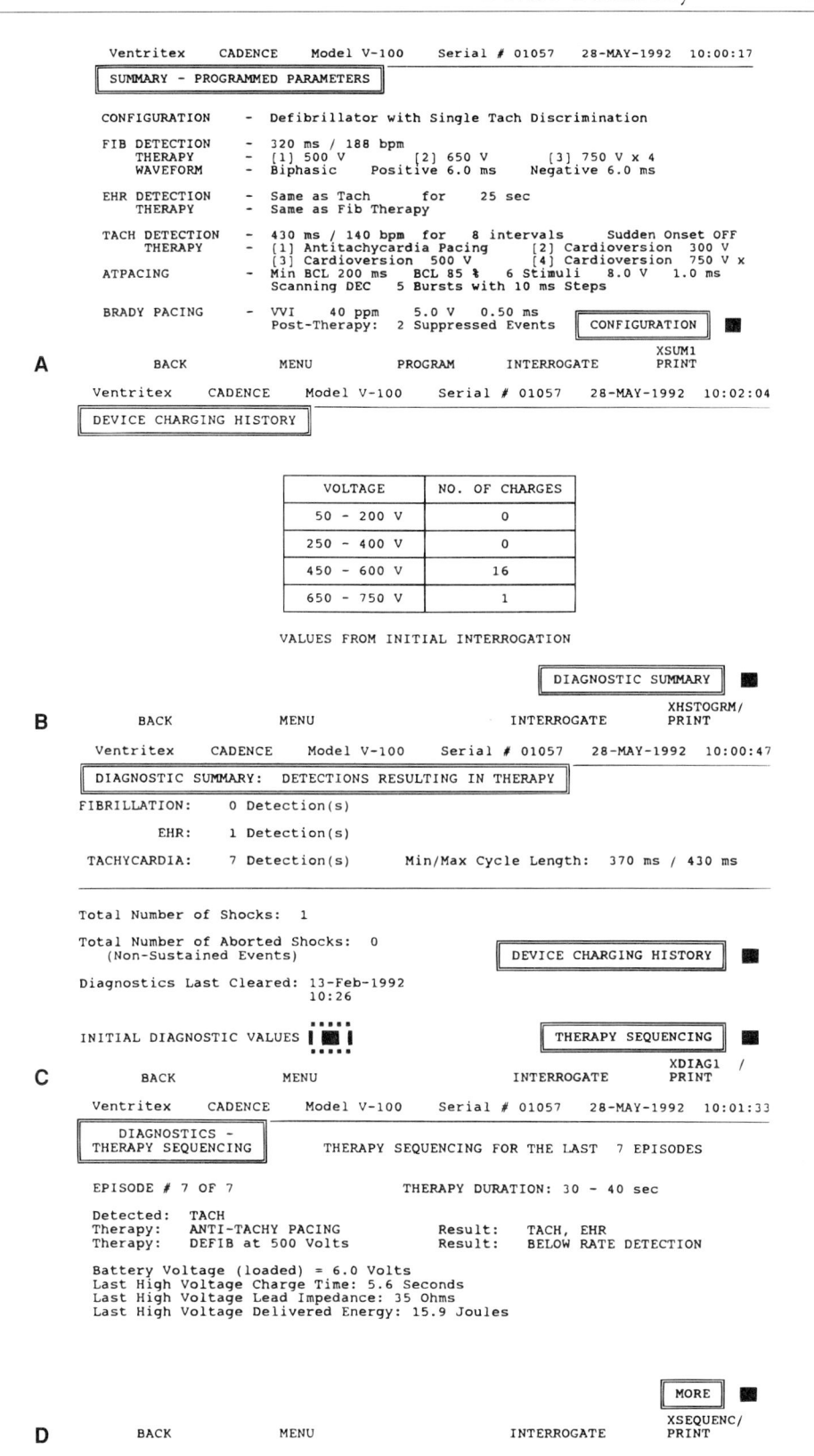

```
Ventritex    CADENCE    Model V-100    Serial # 01057    28-MAY-1992  10:00:17
  SUMMARY - PROGRAMMED PARAMETERS

    CONFIGURATION    - Defibrillator with Single Tach Discrimination
    FIB DETECTION    - 320 ms / 188 bpm
         THERAPY     - [1] 500 V          [2] 650 V          [3] 750 V x 4
         WAVEFORM    - Biphasic    Positive 6.0 ms    Negative 6.0 ms
    EHR DETECTION    - Same as Tach      for      25 sec
         THERAPY     - Same as Fib Therapy
    TACH DETECTION   - 430 ms / 140 bpm  for   8 intervals    Sudden Onset OFF
         THERAPY     - [1] Antitachycardia Pacing    [2] Cardioversion  300 V
                       [3] Cardioversion 500 V       [4] Cardioversion  750 V x
    ATPACING         - Min BCL 200 ms    BCL 85 %    6 Stimuli   8.0 V   1.0 ms
                       Scanning DEC   5 Bursts with 10 ms Steps
    BRADY PACING     - VVI    40 ppm    5.0 V   0.50 ms
                       Post-Therapy:  2 Suppressed Events      CONFIGURATION
                                                                      XSUM1
         BACK          MENU           PROGRAM     INTERROGATE          PRINT
    Ventritex    CADENCE    Model V-100    Serial # 01057    28-MAY-1992  10:02:04
     DEVICE CHARGING HISTORY
```

VOLTAGE	NO. OF CHARGES
50 - 200 V	0
250 - 400 V	0
450 - 600 V	16
650 - 750 V	1

```
                    VALUES FROM INITIAL INTERROGATION

                                                  DIAGNOSTIC SUMMARY
                                                                   XHSTOGRM/
         BACK          MENU                      INTERROGATE        PRINT
    Ventritex    CADENCE    Model V-100    Serial # 01057    28-MAY-1992  10:00:47
     DIAGNOSTIC SUMMARY:  DETECTIONS RESULTING IN THERAPY
    FIBRILLATION:    0 Detection(s)
            EHR:     1 Detection(s)
    TACHYCARDIA:     7 Detection(s)    Min/Max Cycle Length:  370 ms / 430 ms

    Total Number of Shocks:   1
    Total Number of Aborted Shocks:  0
      (Non-Sustained Events)                   DEVICE CHARGING HISTORY
    Diagnostics Last Cleared: 13-Feb-1992
                              10:26

        INITIAL DIAGNOSTIC VALUES                  THERAPY SEQUENCING
                                                                   XDIAG1 /
         BACK          MENU                      INTERROGATE        PRINT
    Ventritex    CADENCE    Model V-100    Serial # 01057    28-MAY-1992  10:01:33
      DIAGNOSTICS -
     THERAPY SEQUENCING      THERAPY SEQUENCING FOR THE LAST  7 EPISODES

    EPISODE # 7 OF 7                    THERAPY DURATION: 30 - 40 sec

    Detected:   TACH
    Therapy:    ANTI-TACHY PACING       Result:    TACH, EHR
    Therapy:    DEFIB at 500 Volts      Result:    BELOW RATE DETECTION

    Battery Voltage (loaded) = 6.0 Volts
    Last High Voltage Charge Time: 5.6 Seconds
    Last High Voltage Lead Impedance: 35 Ohms
    Last High Voltage Delivered Energy: 15.9 Joules


                                                          MORE
                                                                   XSEQUENC/
         BACK          MENU                      INTERROGATE        PRINT
```

Figure 6. Summary of programmed parameters (**A**), noninvasive measurements (**B**), diagnostic summary (**C**), and history of therapy (**D**), which can be obtained by a simple interrogation (Cadence®, Ventritex, Sunnyvale, CA).

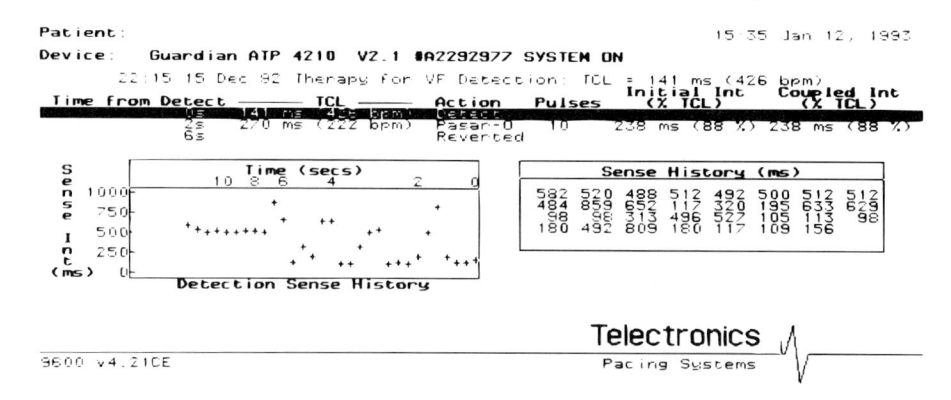

Figure 7. Datalog demonstrating oversensing and possible undersensing by Guardian ATP® 4210 device (Telectronics, Englewood, CO). Note the erratic R-R intervals (plotted left) and in a numeric printout (right). The long and short intervals that are alternating (some are < 100 msec) are clearly nonphysiological and demonstrate a sensing problem.

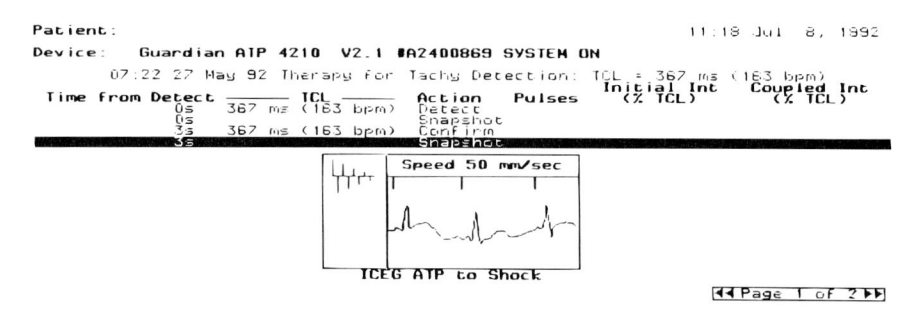

Figure 8. Detection of tachyarrhythmia, with "snapshot" recording of the actual ventricular electrogram (Guardian ATP™ 4210, Telectronics, Englewood, CO).

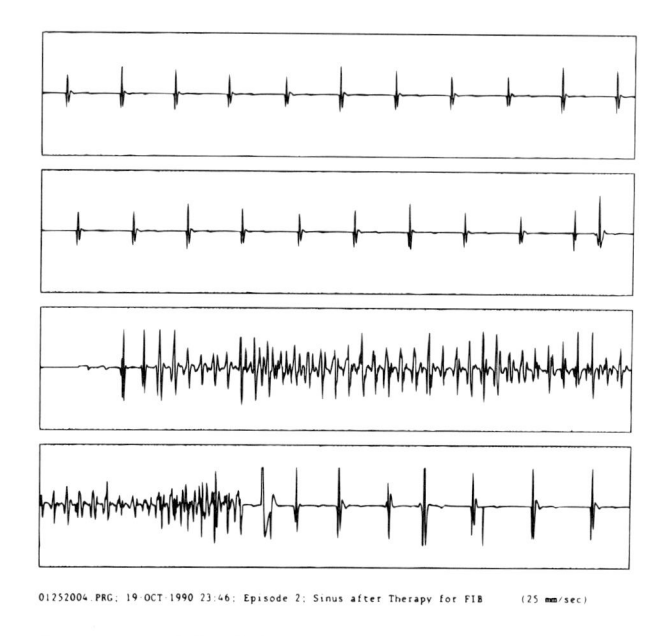

Figure 9. Real-time electrograms (EGMs) demonstrating induction of ventricular fibrillation at electrophysiologic study (Cadence™, Ventritex, Sunnyvale, CA).

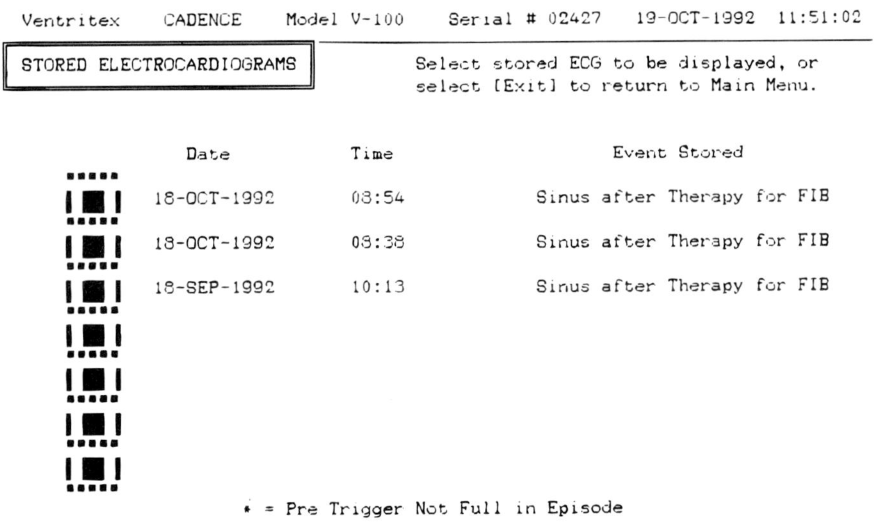

```
Ventritex    CADENCE    Model V-100    Serial # 02427    19-OCT-1992  11:51:02

┌─────────────────────────────┐
│ STORED ELECTROCARDIOGRAMS   │    Select stored ECG to be displayed, or
└─────────────────────────────┘    select [Exit] to return to Main Menu.

              Date           Time           Event Stored
  ▪▪▪▪▪
  │▪│     18-OCT-1992       08:54       Sinus after Therapy for FIB
  ▪▪▪▪▪
  │▪│     18-OCT-1992       08:38       Sinus after Therapy for FIB
  ▪▪▪▪▪
  │▪│     18-SEP-1992       10:13       Sinus after Therapy for FIB

  │▪│
  ▪▪▪▪▪
  │▪│
  ▪▪▪▪▪
  │▪│
  ▪▪▪▪▪
  │▪│

              • = Pre Trigger Not Full in Episode
```

Figure 10. An example of stored information that may be retrieved by telemetry. Treatment log demonstrates three episodes of ventricular fibrillation that were treated successfully by defibrillation (Cadence™, Ventritex, Sunnyvale, CA).

Device Programming

Evaluation of ICDs may be performed in an outpatient setting. Trained personnel, continuous ECG recording, and resuscitative equipment must be readily available. During each visit event history and delivered therapies are retrieved. Each event is evaluated for 1) appropriateness of sensing; 2) therapy effectiveness; and 3) ICD system performance. Routinely, pacing thresholds, sensing during sinus rhythm (Figure 11) and lead impedance are checked. Implantable cardioverter-defibrillator programming may be changed based on the analysis of recorded arrhythmia history and other relevant patient data. Major changes in therapy, however, such as reprogramming of antitachycardia pacing routines or alterations of voltage for cardioversion and defibrillation, require further electrophysiologic testing to ensure the effectiveness of the therapy prescriptions. Minor adjustments, such as increase in the pacing voltage, may be accomplished in the outpatient setting.

Appropriate detection criteria depend on the cycle length (rate) and hemodynamic stability of VT. These parameters may change over time due to the changing clinical substrate (disease progression) or changes in antiarrhythmic drug therapy or fluctuating serum levels. For example, if a patient is on an antiarrhythmic drug with a long half-life ($t_{1/2}$), eg, amiodarone, the cumulative pharmacological effect of the drug may not be realized for up to 6 months. Ventricular tachycardia rate is likely to change (become slower), requiring reprogramming of the rate cutoff. Characteristics of VT may render antitachycardia therapy previously effective less effective or ineffective.[4] Some antiarrhythmic drugs (eg, Class IC or amiodarone) are known to increase defibrillation thresholds (DFTs).[5-14] This may result in ineffective defibrillation if the initial energies are programmed too low. Event history indicating a failure of the initial energy shock to cardiovert or defibrillate, which is subsequently followed by a successful defibrillation on the subsequent, higher energy shocks, suggests inadequate safety margins, or increase in DFTs.[15]

Some drugs (Class IC and some Class III antiarrhythmics) increase pacing thresholds.[16] This may lead to inability to capture, requiring reprogramming of the pacing voltage or pulse width.

Reprogramming of cardioversion and defibrillation energies and/or antitachycardia pacing therapies requires retesting of the patient in the electrophysiology laboratory. The availability of the noninvasive programmed stimulation in the third-generation devices simplifies the ICD electrophysiologic testing.

Remote Follow-Up

Currently transtelephonic follow-up of patients with implanted ICDs is not available. Therefore, patients with implanted ICDs must be followed periodically in the physician's office. The frequency of follow-up is in part, dictated by the need to manually reform capacitors of some devices (Table 2), but periodic reassessment of the ICD therapy effectiveness, device antiarrhythmic drug interactions, and other clinical variables is required.

The future holds promise with regard to transtelephonic (T™) data transmission for remote patient follow-up. When available, transtelephonic telemetry transmission could simplify greatly the follow-up of patients with implanted ICDs who live at remote or inaccessible sites.

Value of Telemetered Information for Device Troubleshooting

Extensive discussion of troubleshooting, follow-up, and complications of ICDs may be found in Chapters 25 and 26. However, a brief discussion of the value of telemetered electrograms for diagnosis of ICD system-related problems is presented here.

Value of Electrograms for Diagnosing Lead Fracture

Appropriate sensing is fundamental for proper ICD function. Frequent, seemingly clinically inappropriate shocks, eg, shocks which occur at rest or during trivial activity and unaccompanied by symptoms ("dizziness," presyncope, syncope, or palpitations) should be suspected to be potentially inappropriate. Sensing problems may result from inadequate signal amplitude or slew rates, lead insulation break, conductor fracture, or a lead-to-connector "noise."

Lead fracture may be associated with abnormally high pacing thresholds or loss of capture (Figure 12) and increase in lead impedance (Figure 13). Datalog may reveal multiple tachyarrhythmia detections that "spontaneously" terminate or result in inappropriate therapy (Figure 14). Fluoroscopic and radiographic data are only occasionally helpful, although they should always be obtained since gross displacement of intracardiac leads or pin-to-device disconnection from the ICD header may be simply diagnosed by this method.

Defibrillation lead fractures may be manifested by a failure to defibrillate (Figure 15), high-defibrillation lead impedance postshock (usually > 1,800 Ω) (Figure 16), and/or by radiographic evidence of lead fracture (Figure 17).

Device Telemetry • 263

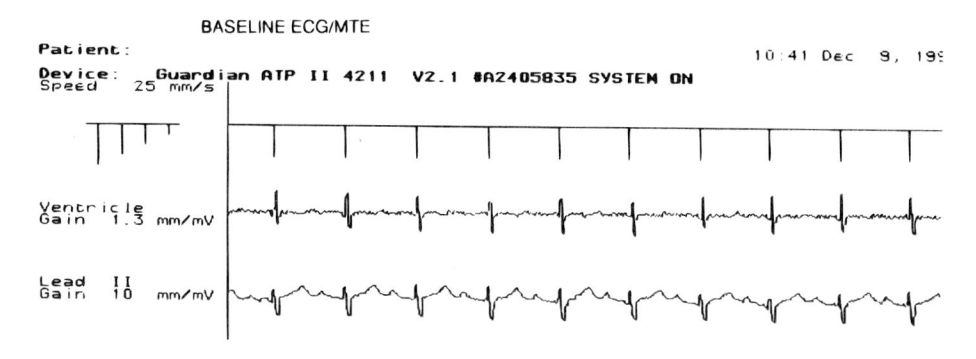

Figure 11. Sensing in sinus rhythm. Main timing events (MTE) markers (top), intracardiac electrograms (EGMs) and surface lead II are displayed.

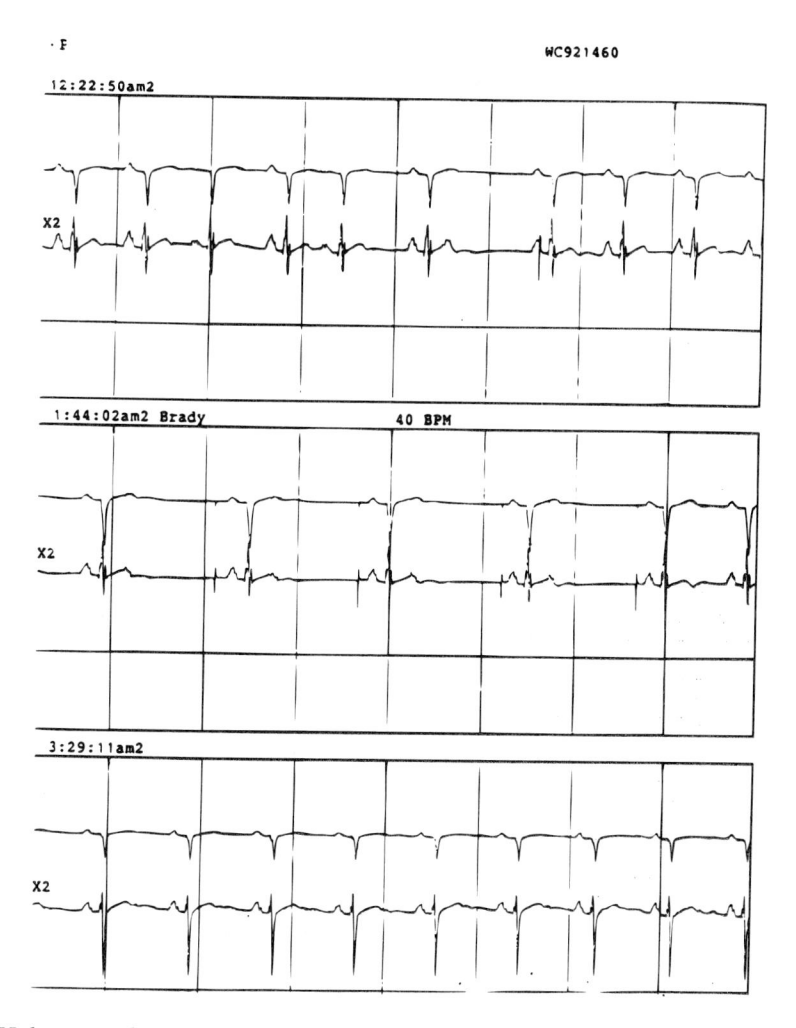

Figure 12. Holter recording of a patient with implanted third-generation implantable cardioverter-defibrillator (ICD) demonstrating failure to capture and sense due to lead fracture. Interrogation revealed high endocardial lead impedance (see Figure 13).

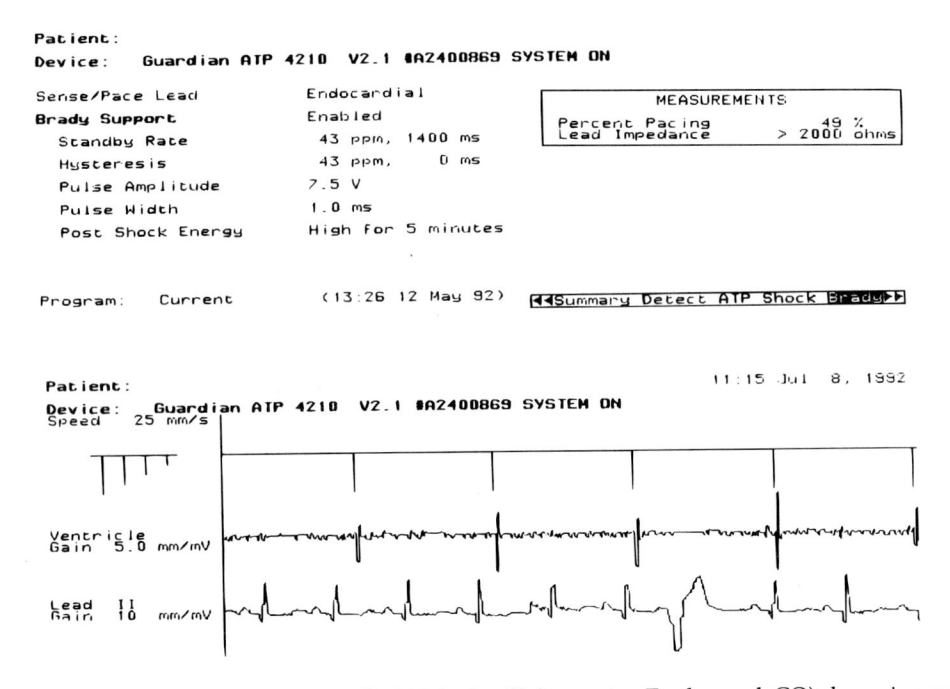

Figure 13. Telemetry of Guardian ATP™ 4210 device (Telectronics, Englewood, CO) shows increased impedance (> 2,000 Ω) suggesting lead conductor fracture (**top panel**) and failure to sense (**bottom panel**).

Figure 14. Telemetry demonstrates multiple tachyarrhythmia "detections" with extremely short R-R intervals (98–113 msec) that revert "spontaneously." These data suggest oversensing, which may be seen with "noise" secondary to lead fracture.

Device Telemetry • 265

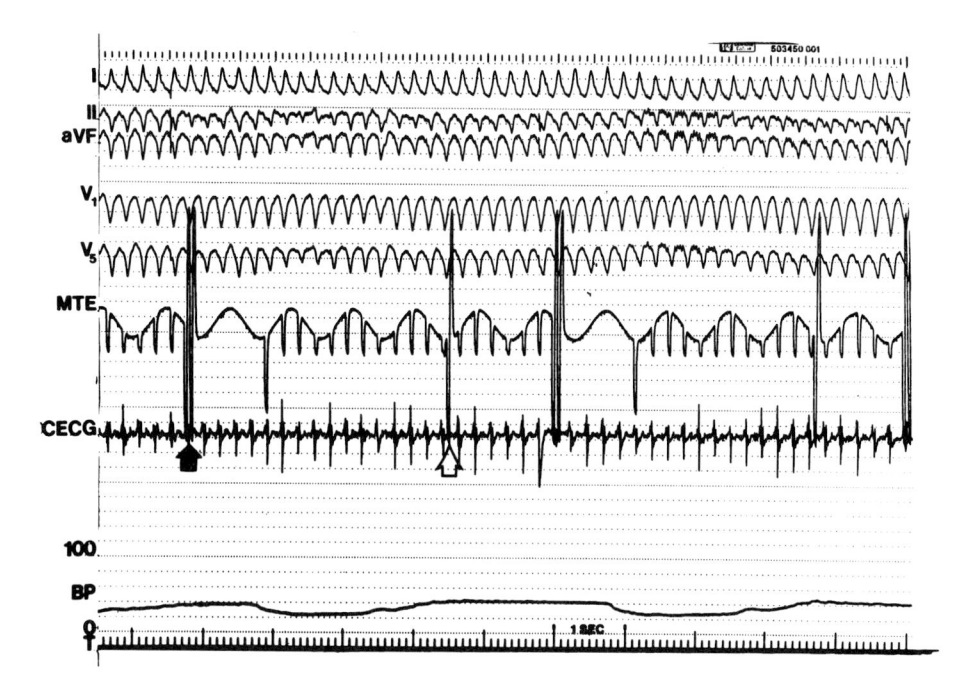

Figure 15. Failure of multiple shocks to terminate ventricular fibrillation due to endocardial defibrillation lead fracture (Accufix DF™ lead, Telectronics, Englewood, CO). From top to bottom: surface leads I, II, AVF, V_1, V_5, main timing events (MTE), intracardiac ECG (ICECG), blood pressure (BP), and time lines (T). Dark arrow denotes an unsuccessful shock; open arrow denotes charging of the capacitors.

Figure 16. Telemetry of the recorded event (see Figure 15). Note appropriate detection, followed by the implantable cardioverter-defibrillator (ICD) shock delivery of 36.1 J (three times) with an actual delivery of 1.0, 0.5, and 0.5 J and lead impedance > 500 Ω, indicative of a defibrillation lead fracture.

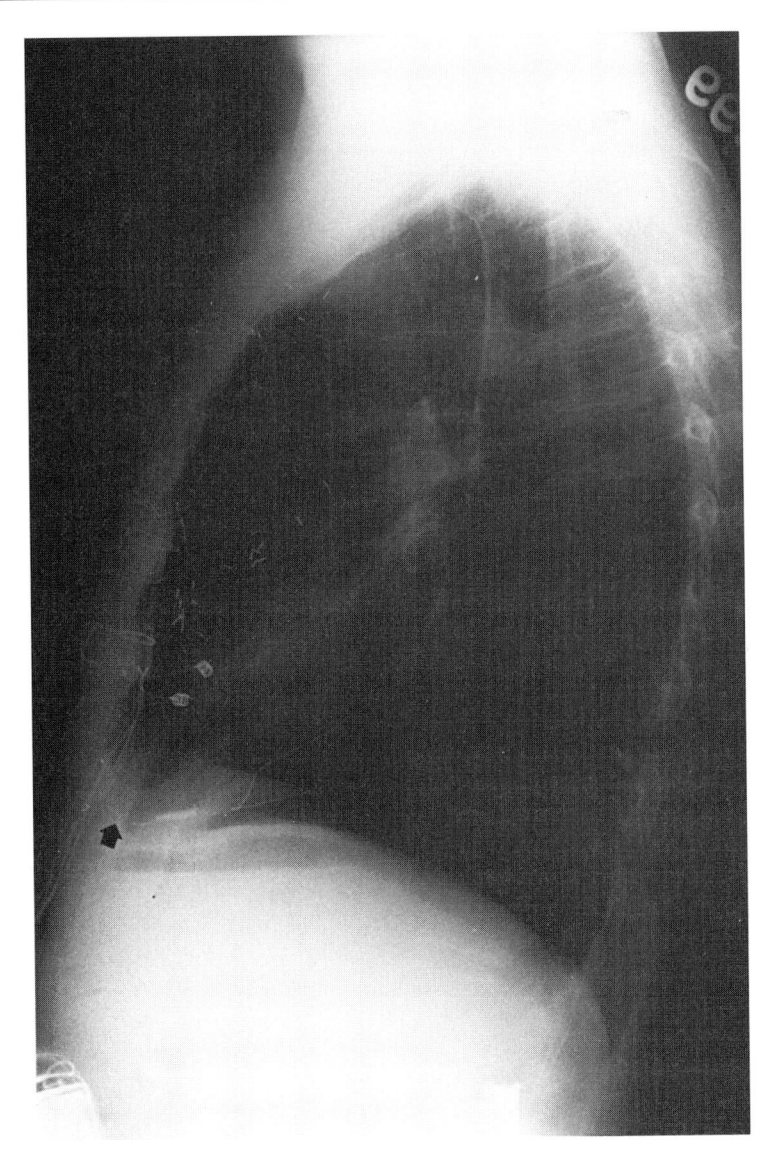

Figure 17. Radiograph demonstrating a patch lead fracture (dark arrow) (CPI, St. Paul, MN).

Oversensing and Undersensing

Oversensing and undersensing is seen rarely with devices that use automatic gain control.[3] However, undersensing and oversensing are not uncommon with ICDs that use fixed gain sensitivity, even when the sensitivity is automatically doubled when VF is detected.[17] Oversensing may be diagnosed when telemetry demonstrates multiple tachyarrhythmia detections and the datalog of each episode demonstrates long-short-long R-R sequences where R-R intervals fall within the range of noise detections (100 msec), or where the so-called VF detections (tachycardia cycle length < 250 msec) are followed by frequent "spontaneous" reversions (Figure 14).

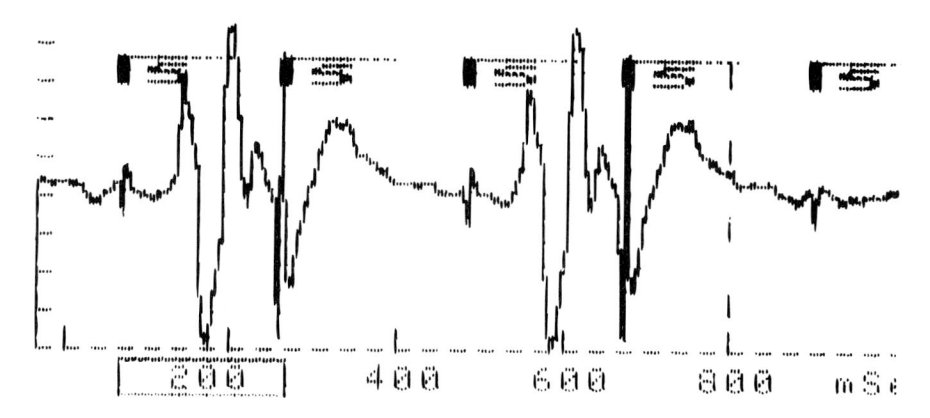

Figure 18. T wave sensing with implanted Res-Q™ device (Intermedics, Angleton, TX).

Fixed gain sensing is inappropriate and potentially dangerous for ICDs in the authors opinion, due to the continuously changing amplitudes and slew rates of the ventricular bipolar signal during VT and particularly during VF that could result in VF nondetection.[17] Intermittent oversensing may also occur, although infrequently, with automatic gain control devices under certain circumstances (Figure 5).[3] The cause of oversensing may be changing QT interval or T wave amplitudes secondary to antiarrhythmic drugs that may prolong the QT interval or alter the T wave amplitude or

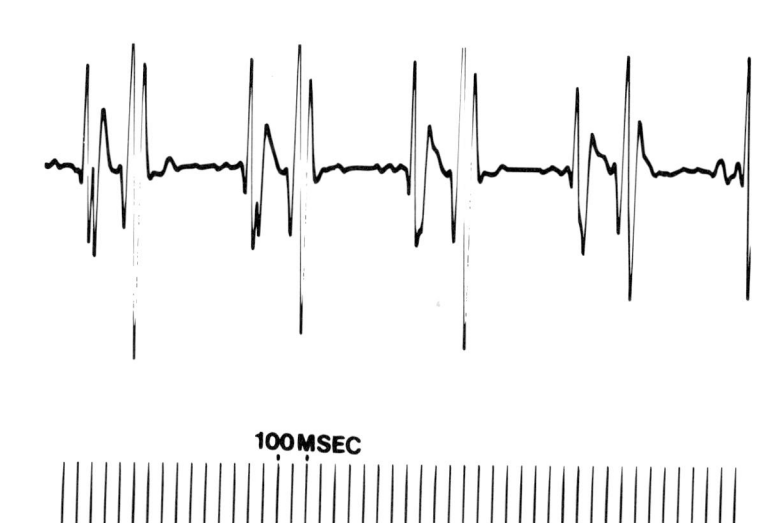

Figure 19. Real-time electrograms demonstrate atrial and ventricular sensing by the displaced endocardial lead. Proximal displacement of the endocardial lead to the tricuspid valve area is suggested by atrial and ventricular electrograms of similar amplitudes. This was later confirmed by fluoroscopy (Cadence™, Ventritex, Sunnyvale, CA).

morphology, electrolyte abnormalities (eg, hyperkalemia) that may exaggerate the T wave amplitude, or other factors that alter QRS-T relationship.

Some devices (eg, Res-Q) permit testing for T wave sensing and automatic gain adjustments, a desirable feature in selected situations. This device currently uses a pseudobipolar sensing from the endocardial right ventricular pace/sense lead cathode to the epicardial patch lead. Therefore, it is more likely to sense far field signals, including the repolarization wave fronts (T wave; Figure 18). Closely spaced bipolar electrodes (endocardial or epicardial) are less likely to sense the far field signals.

Double sensing may also be seen with endocardial lead displacement. When the lead migrates proximally, real-time electrograms may demonstrate both atrial and ventricular sensing due to the proximity of the bipolar electrodes to the right atrium and ventricle (Figure 19). Lead displacement is easily confirmed by fluoroscopy.

Future Developments

Diagnostic information provided by the telemetered data is invaluable for device programming and follow-up. It is possible, even likely, that hemodynamic sensors will be incorporated in future ICDs. Hemodynamic data may be used to enhance and refine arrhythmia detection and to stratify therapy based on the hemodynamic consequences of tachyarrhythmias.

Analysis and storage of arrhythmia trends, heart rate variability, and ST segment analysis may be useful for ischemia detection. Analysis of pressure signal (dP/dt), cardiac output, or oxygen saturation may provide additional parameters for assessment of circulatory consequences of tachyarrhythmias.

Fundamental to the expansion of telemetry capabilities is increase in the computational powers of the microprocessor and increase in the memory capacity. The use of parallel processing and/or other newer computer technologies is likely to accelerate these trends.

Overview

Implantable cardioverter-defibrillator telemetry provides an invaluable diagnostic tool to guide therapy, assess battery longevity, ICD function, troubleshoot device/leads malfunction, and assess device antiarrhythmic drug interactions.

References

1. Winkle RA: State of the art of the AICD. *PACE* 14:961, 1991.
2. Shibata N, Chen PS, Dixon EG, et al: Endocardial activation after unsuccessful defibrillation shocks in dogs. *Am J Physiol* 255:H902, 1988.
3. Singer I, De Borde R, Veltri EP, et al: Automatic cardioverter defibrillator: T wave sensing in the newest generation. *PACE* 11:1584, 1988.
4. Singer I, Guarnieri T, Kupersmith J: Implantable automatic defibrillators: effects of drugs and pacemakers. *PACE* 11:2250, 1988.
5. Fain ES, Dorian P, Davy JM, et al: Effects of encainide and its metabolites on energy requirements for defibrillation. *Circulation* 73:1334, 1986.
6. Reiffel JA, Coromilas J, Zimmerman JM, et al: Drug-device interactions: clinical considerations. *PACE* 8:369, 1985.
7. Frame LH, Sheldon JH: Effect of recainam on the energy required for ventricular defibrillation in dogs as assessed with implanted electrodes. *J Am Coll Cardiol* 12:746, 1988.
8. Dorian P, Fain ES, Davy JM, et al: Lidocaine causes a reversible, concentration-dependent increase in defibrillation energy requirements. *J Am Coll Cardiol* 8:347, 1986.
9. Marinchak RA, Friehling TD, Line RA, et al: Effect of antiarrhythmic drugs on defibrillation threshold: case report of an adverse effect of mexiletine and review of the literature. *PACE* 11:7, 1988.
10. Haberman RJ, Veltri EP, Mower MM: The

effect of amiodarone on defibrillation threshold. *J Electrophysiol* 2:415, 1988.
11. Fain ES, Lee JT, Winkle RA: Effects of acute intravenous and chronic oral amiodarone on defibrillation energy requirements. *Am Heart J* 114:8, 1987.
12. Kentsch M, Kunze KP, Bleifeld W: Effect of intravenous amiodarone on ventricular fibrillation during out-of-hospital cardiac arrest (abstract). *J Am Coll Cardiol* 7:82A, 1986.
13. Fogoros RN: Amiodarone-induced refractoriness to cardioversion. *Ann Intern Med* 100: 699, 1984.
14. Guarnieri T, Levine JH, Veltri EP: Success of chronic defibrillation and the role of antiarrhythmic drugs with the automatic implantable cardioverter/defibrillator. *Am J Cardiol* 60:1061, 1987.
15. Singer I, Lang D: Defibrillation threshold: clinical utility and therapeutic implications. *PACE* 15(6):932, 1992.
16. Guarneri T, Datorre SD, Bondke H, et al: Increased pacing threshold after an automatic defibrillator shock in dogs: effects of Class I and Class II antiarrhythmic drugs. *PACE* 11: 1324, 1988.
17. Singer I, Adams L, Austin E: The potential hazards of fixed sensitivity and tachyarrhythmia detection algorithm for implantable cardioverter/defibrillators. *PACE* 16(5): 1070, 1993.

Chapter 12

Antitachycardia Pacing

Berndt Lüderitz, Werner Jung, and Matthias Manz

Introduction

The two primary pathological mechanisms causing clinical tachycardias are circus movement (reentry) and triggered activity. Reentry is caused by pathological changes in conduction and refractoriness in the myocardial tissues.[1] Ectopic focal impulse formation results from local disturbances of depolarization and repolarization of the cell membranes.[2,3] The pioneering work of Wellens[4] and Josephson and coworkers[5] have shown that in patients with recurrent sustained ventricular tachyarrhythmias this arrhythmia can be safely and reproducibly terminated by programmed electrical stimulation (PES) of the heart in the catheterization laboratory.[6]

Mechanisms of Antitachycardia Pacing

Antitachycardia pacing (ATP) is most effective for termination of reentry tachycardias. The following conditions have to be fulfilled for reentry to occur: 1) unidirectional block of an impulse in one or more than one region of the heart; 2) slow passage of an impulse via an alternative pathway; 3) delayed excitation of the tissue distal to the blocked site; and 4) reexcitation of the tissue proximal to the site of block.[4,7] The perpetuation of the tachycardia demands a refractory period shorter than the time needed for conduction of the activation wave around a loop. In mathematical terms: $RP < \int 1/V \, dl$. That is, the refractory period must be less than the circle integral 1 over V (V = conduction velocity in the pathway) multiplied by the differential length of the pathway (dl). The reentrant tachycardia is terminated if the refractory period exceeds the conduction time around the loop. A schematic illustration is given in Figure 1 using the example of an antegrade right bundle branch block. A reentry tachycardia can be terminated by: 1) prolongation of the refractory period in the pathological pathway (eg, by drugs or appropriate electrical stimulation); 2) increase in conduction velocity in the pathological pathway; and 3) decreased radius of the pathological reentry pathway and external depolarization of the excitable gap by properly timed electrical stimulation. Reentry has been hypothesized as the primary mechanism of ventricular tachycardias (VTs), although this is far more difficult to prove than in the atria. Reentry pathways may consist of bundle branches, Purkinje fibers with or without the surrounding muscle cells, as well as the infarcted or fibrotic muscle cells.[7] A relatively long duration of the action potential and re-

---

From Singer I, (ed.) Implantable Cardioverter-Defibrillator. Armonk, NY: Futura Publishing Company, Inc.; © 1994.

$$RP < \oint \frac{1}{V} dl$$

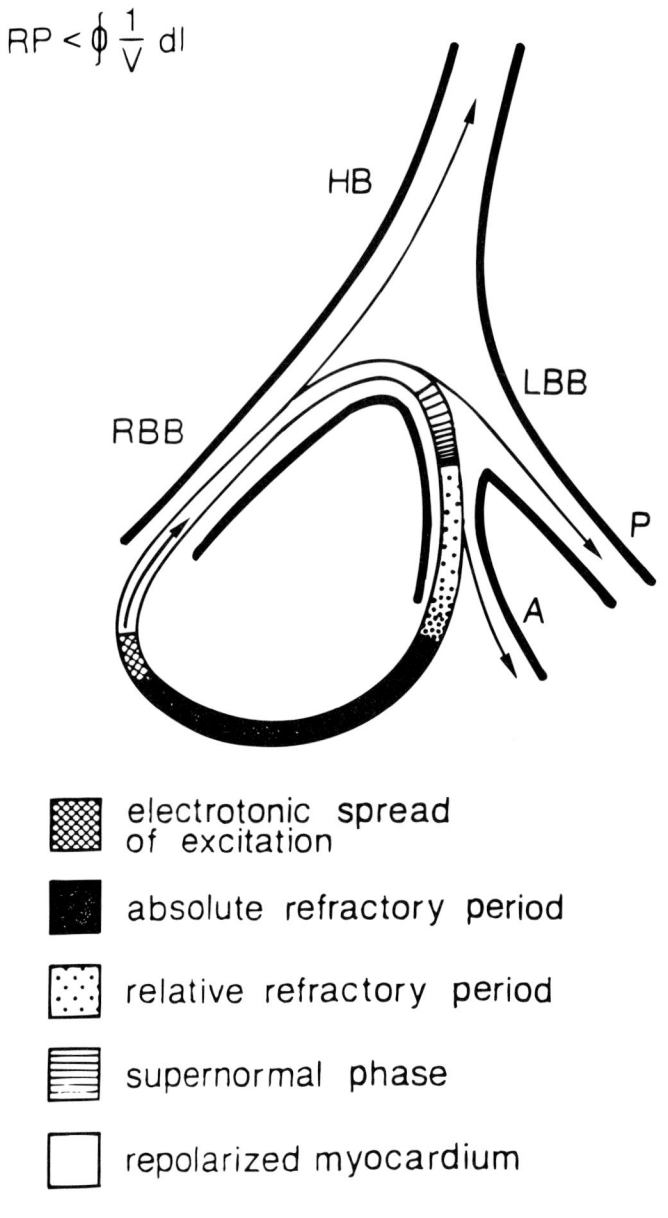

Figure 1. Complete right bundle branch block with bundle branch reentry tachycardia. Arrows indicate possible pathways for a reentry ventricular tachycardia (VT) via the bundle branches. HB: His bundle; RBB: right bundle branch; LBB: left bundle branch; A: anterior fascicle; P: posterior fascicle; RP: refractory period; V: conduction velocity; dl: differential length of the pathway.

fractory period in the ventricles may suggest a large reentry pathway, ie, macroreentry. It could also be shown that in case of the block at the site of transition from Purkinje fibers to muscle cells a marked abbreviation of the action potential occurs in the Purkinje fibers.[8,9] This favors microreentry at the peripheral transitions from the Purkinje fibers to the ventricular muscle cells. In addition, a decrease in conduction velocity may play an important role in reentry phenomena.[10,11]

Mechanisms of Antitachycardia Pacing in Ventricular Tachycardias

Termination of tachycardias by properly timed premature stimulation has been regarded as being indicative of the existence of reentry mechanism.[7] The termination of tachycardia assumes that the artificial additional impulse depolarizes the excitable gap of the pathological reentry pathway, which in turn becomes refractory to the circling excitation. On the basis of theoretical considerations as well as the more recent findings from the animal experiments, however, it has become doubtful again whether success or failure of electrical stimulation can serve as a differential diagnostic criterion to distinguish between focal or reentry tachycardia. One could, for instance, argue that the artificial impulse might perhaps not reach the site of the reentry if the distance between the electrode and the site of the circus movement is too long or if the conduction velocity is too slow. Furthermore, the chances of terminating the circus movement by an additional impulse becomes less promising if an anatomically very small circus pathway is present. Ultimately the circus could be just as short as the wavelength of the excitation itself. Thus, there would be no excitable gap for an additional artificial stimulus between the beginning and the end of the excitation wave front. This leads to the conclusion that a failure of pacemaker therapy to terminate tachycardia does not exclude reentry as the underlying mechanism just as much as the success does not necessarily contradict triggered activity as the underlying mechanism (see Chapter 2).[12-14] Several different modes of cardiac pacing are currently used to suppress or terminate VTs.

Antitachycardia Pacing Modes (Table 1)

Rapid Ventricular Stimulation

Supraventricular reentry tachycardias may be terminated by short-term rapid ventricular stimulation, provided that there is sufficient retrograde conduction. Rapid stimulation has to be used in special circumstances. Occasionally, very short bursts of pacing are sufficient to terminate the tachycardia (Figure 2).

Table 1
Cardiac Pacing in Ventricular Tachyarrhythmias

Indication	Method
Ventricular extrasystoles	Rapid ventricular stimulation Overdrive pacing
Ventricular tachycardia	Coupled stimulation Programmed stimulation: 1. Fixed rate stimulation 2. Stimulation with progressive coupling intervals 3. Rate related interval stimulation

Overdrive Pacing

Increasing the pacing rate in order to suppress ventricular or supraventricular ectopic activity is termed overdrive pacing.[15] The stimulation rate has to be faster than the spontaneous rate, but it may be markedly slower than the ectopic rate that is to be suppressed. Often a rate just slightly above the spontaneous rate is sufficient. This type of stimulation is particularly successful for suppression of extrasystoles. Overdrive pacing can also be used in emergencies for hours or even days. It is particularly useful for postoperative patients or patients with myocardial infarction suffering from drug resistant extrasystoles causing hemodynamic embarrassment (Figure 3). The precise electrophysiologic mechanism of overdrive suppression is still unclear. In this context, not only the rate but also the site of stimulation are important.[16]

Programmed Stimulation

The following pacing modes are used: single and multiple premature stimuli, un-

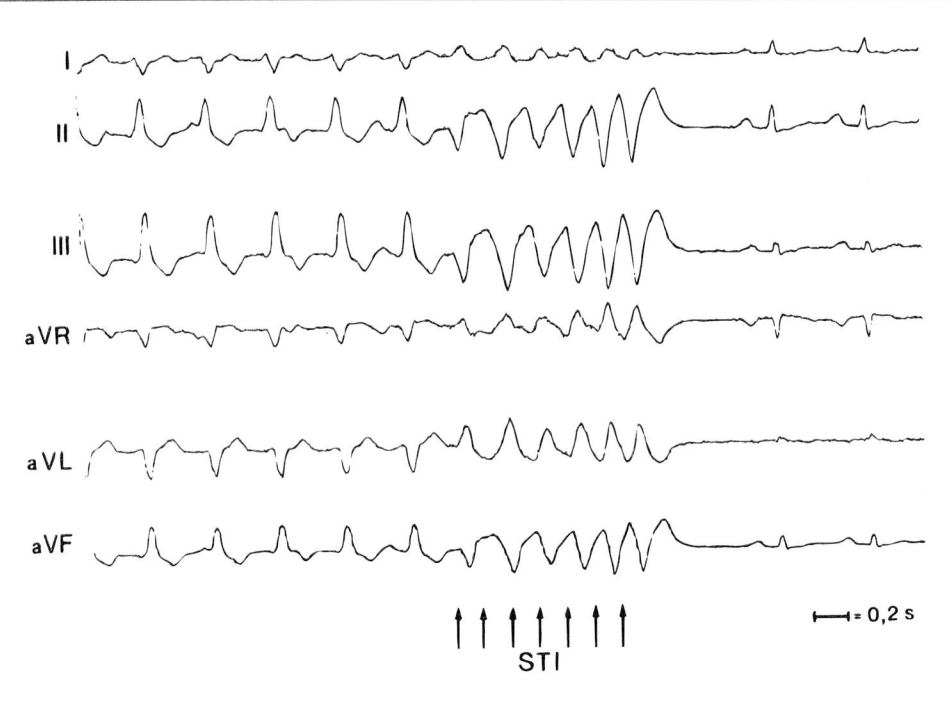

Figure 2. Termination of a sustained ventricular tachycardia (163 per minute) by rapid ventricular stimulation (STI) applied to the right ventricle. Seven impulses were elicited at a rate of 400 per minute according to a stimulation interval of 150 msec. After pacemaker intervention a normal sinus rhythm is reestablished.

derdrive, and burst pacing. Precisely timed single premature stimuli may terminate VT. Pacing at a rate clearly below the rate of tachycardia may terminate the arrhythmia. Both methods, however, are usually only effective when the rate of the VT is relatively slow (< 180 per minute).[17] Overdrive pacing is accomplished by pacing the ventricles for a variable period of time at a rate up to 30 beats per minute faster than the rate of VT. If this method fails, timed double or triple premature stimuli or ultimately burst pacing (pacing rate > 30 beats per minute faster than tachycardia rate) may terminate the arrhythmia. An example of programmed stimulation is shown in Figure 4.

Recently it has been reported that an increase of stimulus current strengths may increase the likelihood of tachycardia termination,[18] as well as the addition of one or two premature extrastimuli to the end of the train of overdrive burst pacing.[19] The more aggressive the stimulation protocol necessary for termination, the more likely it is that the VT may degenerate to ventricular fibrillation (VF). This is shown in Figure 5. The reported incidence of acceleration by programmed stimulation is 7% to 50%.[20-22] Most patients in whom ATP is used for VT termination require concomitant use of antiarrhythmic drug therapy to slow the tachycardia rate sufficiently to permit success of the pacing techniques. Furthermore, the antitachycardia pacemaker function may become ineffective due to spontaneous changes in the patient's tachycardia rates and/or the excitation patterns. The latter problem may be partly overcome by more sophisticated pacing algorithms.[6]

Programmed Rate-Related Stimulation

Precisely timed premature stimulation may be achieved by programmed rate-related interval stimulation (orthorhythmic pacing).[23,24] The delivery of an electric im-

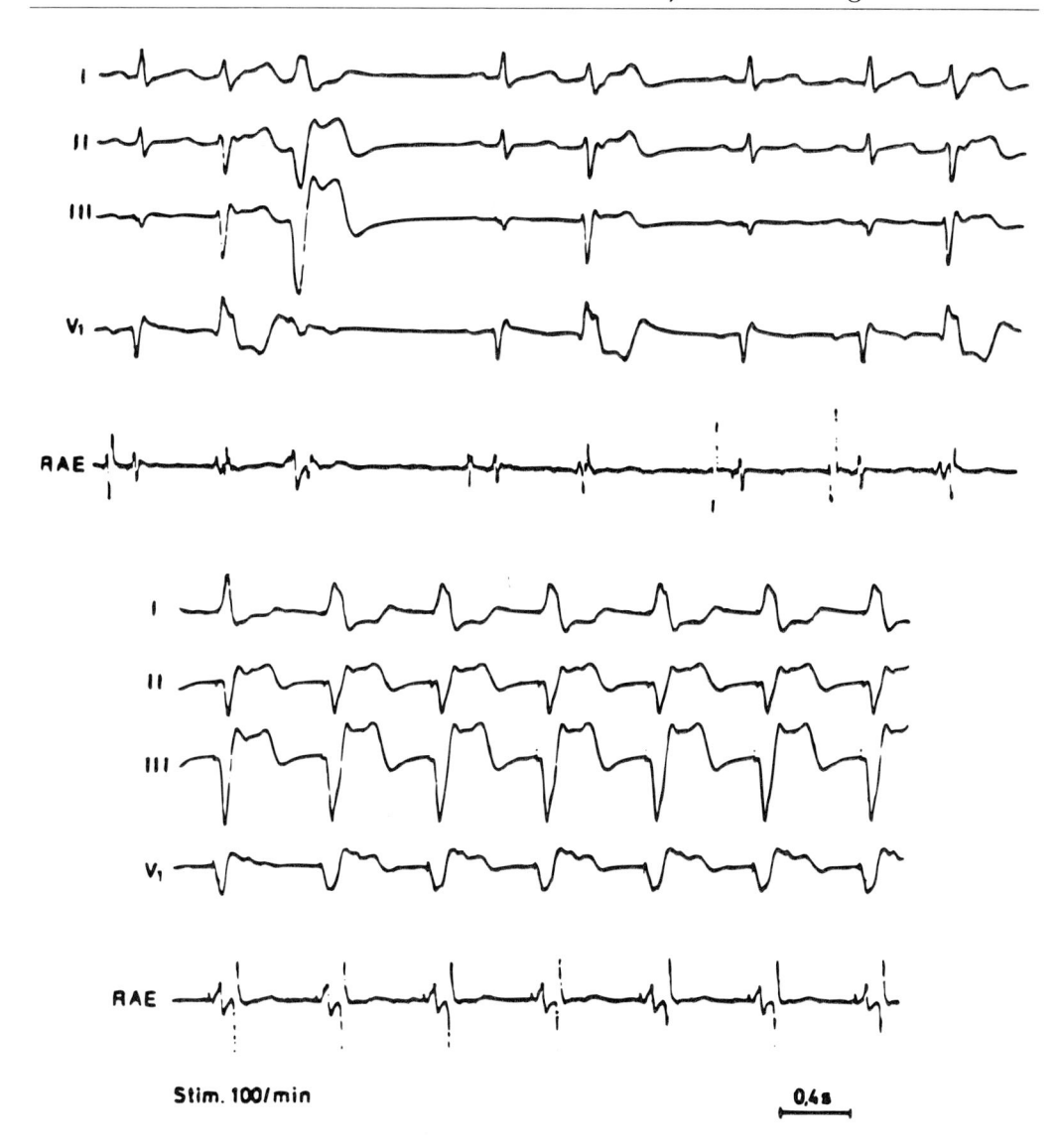

Figure 3. A 42-year-old female patient suffering from myocarditis. Suppression of ventricular premature beats by increasing the electrically paced ventricular rate (100 beats per minute) by overdrive pacing. RAE: right atrial electrogram.

pulse is determined by the preceding interval of atrial or ventricular depolarization. Therefore, this pacing mode is automatically rate dependent (Figure 6). Rate-related pacing is characterized by programmable demand pacing with escape intervals related to the length of the preceding cardiac cycle. Whereas conventional demand pacemakers operate at a fixed escape interval, the so-called orthorhythmic system possesses a variable hysteresis: the pacemaker takes into consideration the exact time of the extrasystole and produces a response delay that automatically varies as a function of the premature beat interval. The variable response delay (stimulation interval) may be identical to the premature beat interval. The ratio of these two intervals can, however, be modified. The orthorhythmic system consists of an external pacemaker that

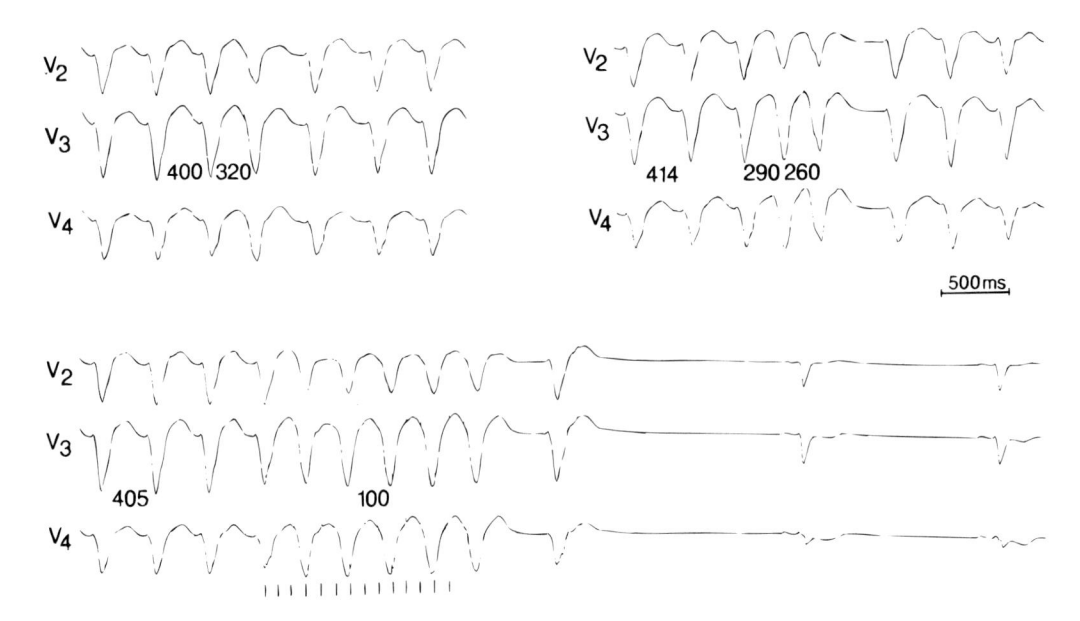

Figure 4. Interruption of ventricular tachycardia (VT) by programmed ventricular stimulation. In all three panels unipolar leads V$_2$, V$_3$, and V$_4$ are shown. **Top panel left**: Single premature stimuli shorten the R-R interval but do not stop tachycardia. **Top panel right**: Double premature stimuli are also ineffective. **Bottom panel**: A series of 14 stimuli at an interval of 100 msec terminates the tachycardia.

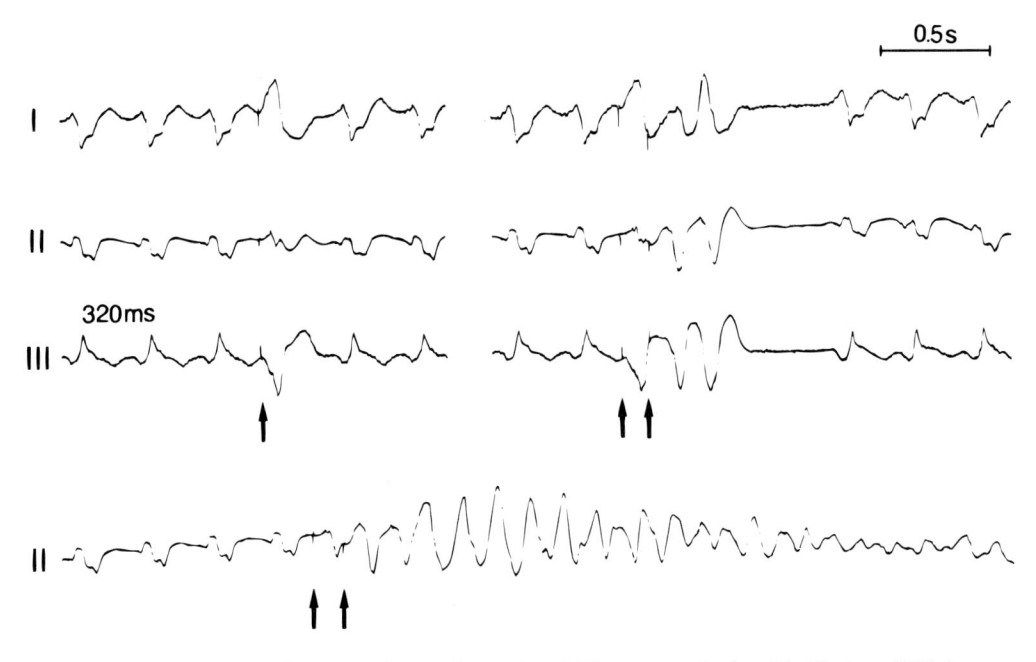

Figure 5. Degeneration of ventricular tachycardia (VT) to ventricular fibrillation (VF) by programmed stimulation. Records of leads I, II, and III are shown. **Top panel left**: Application of single premature stimulus, ineffective. **Top panel right**: Application of double premature stimuli, followed by one extra beat and, thereafter, persistence of tachycardia. **Bottom panel**: Increasing the prematurity of the second premature stimulus, VF is induced.

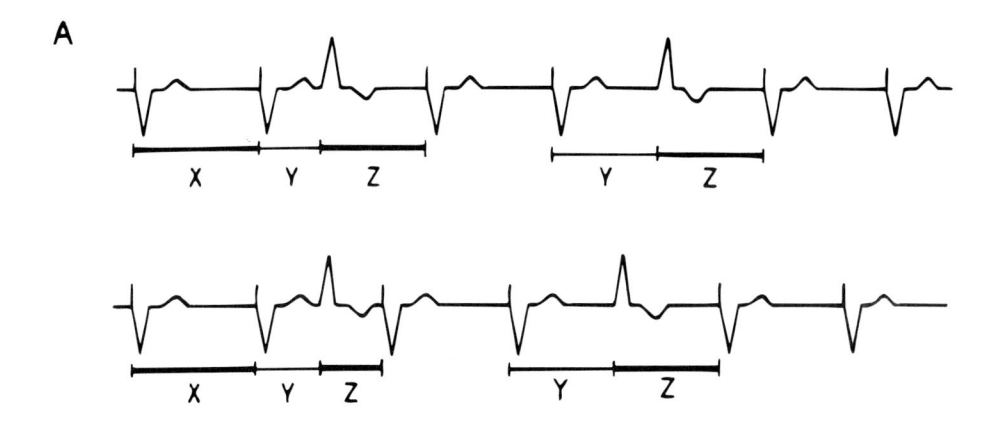

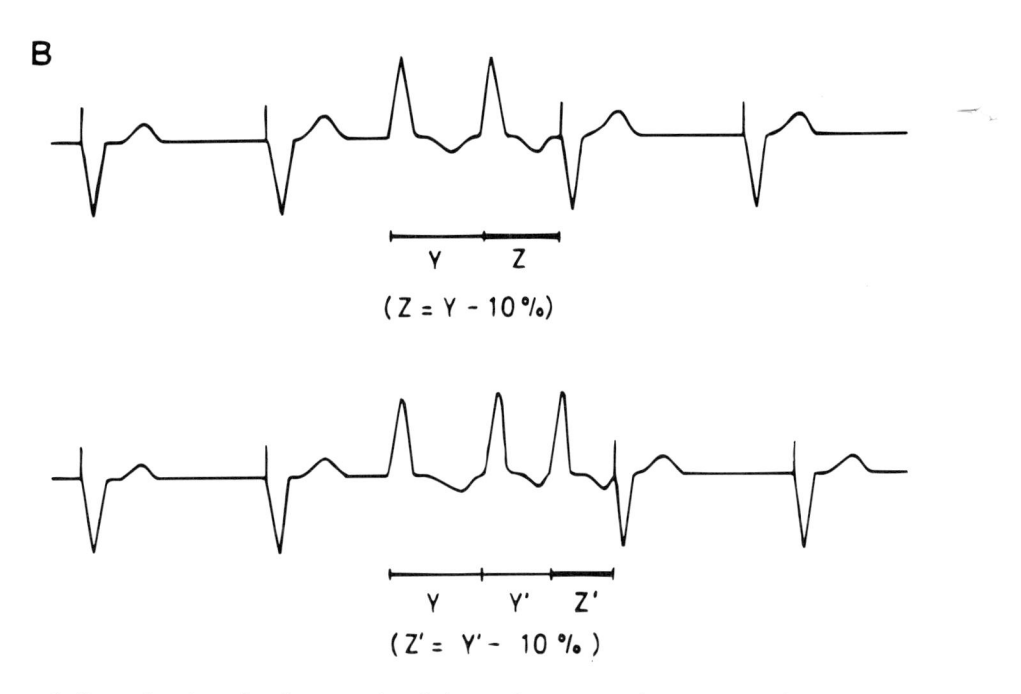

Figure 6. Operational mode of conventional demand pacing and programmed rate-related pacing following premature beats. X: basic cycle; Y: stimulation interval; Z: postextrasystolic interval. **A.** After extrasystoles with varying prematurity (upper tracing), demand pacemakers will keep the same invariable delay (Z) before delivering the next impulse. Applying rate-related stimulation (lower tracing), the moment of delivery of impulse after the extrasystole can be modified as a function of Y:Z = (f)Y. **B.** Rate-related pacing at repetitive extrasystoles. In two consecutively occuring extrasystoles (upper tracing), the stimulation interval Z is determined by the distance Y between these two extrasystoles. In this case, Z is 10% shorter than Y. The electrically induced premature beat anticipates a possibly emerging third extrasystole. If consecutive extrasystoles occur with increasing prematurity (lower tracing), rate-related pacing automatically takes into account the altered interval (Y′) between the last two extrasystoles.

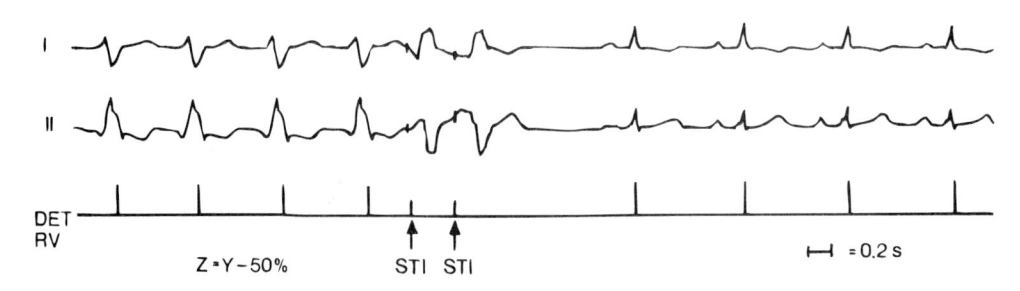

Figure 7. Termination of ventricular tachycardia (VT) by rate-related stimulation. Two stimuli according to the program $Z = Y - 50\%$, ie, the stimulation interval is half as long as the preceding R-R interval. DET: detection channel; RV: right ventricle.

is connected to temporary endocardial electrodes. Temporary epicardial electrodes may be used after the open heart surgery. The power source consists of two 9-V alkaline batteries. Orthorhythmic pacing can be applied to the atria or to the ventricles. It can be performed with single or repeated stimulations delivered in accordance with a program that takes into account the spontaneous or stimulated heart rate. This type of stimulation, which is controlled by sensing of the intrinsic intracardiac signals from either the atrium or the ventricle, provides the possibility of consecutive stimulation such as paired, triple, or quadruple pulses in very rapid salvos. This on-demand stimulation coupled to the preceding cardiac depolarizations can be applied for bradycardias as well as various types of tachycardias (Figure 7).[24,25] When applied in drug resistant, spontaneously occurring ventricular extrasystoles or recurrent tachycardias in 56 patients, programmed rate-related stimulation, either by single or multiple extrastimuli was effective in interrupting the tachycardia in 54% of cases (Table 2). In most cases the ventricular tachyarrhythmias were terminated after several attempts with rate-related stimulation.[26,27]

Programmed rate-related stimulation was also applied in ventricular extrasystoles or recurrent tachycardias in 74 patients with chronic ischemic coronary disease. Rate-related stimulation was effective in 40 patients by terminating the tachycardia. In four patients the tachycardia occurred within 24 hours after admission to the coronary care unit for acute myocardial infarction. In three patients the tachycardia could not be terminated by programmed stimulation (Table 3). The rate-related stimulation technique was effective only in one case (Figure 8).

While programmed rate-related stimulation is effective in dysrhythmias due to chronic coronary disease, this mode of pacing is generally unsuccessful for therapy of ventricular tachyarrhythmias following acute myocardial infarction. This finding suggests that the mechanism of VTs during acute myocardial infarction differs from the chronic recurrent type of VT. The complica-

Table 2
Success of Rate-Related Stimulation in Ventricular Tachyarrhythmias

	%	Patients (n)
Spontaneous	54	56
During cardiac catheterization	21	20

Table 3
Efficiency of Rate-Related Stimulation in Ventricular Tachyarrhythmias

Condition	Total No. of Patients	Termination Achieved
Chronic coronary heart disease	74	40
Acute myocardial infarction	4	1

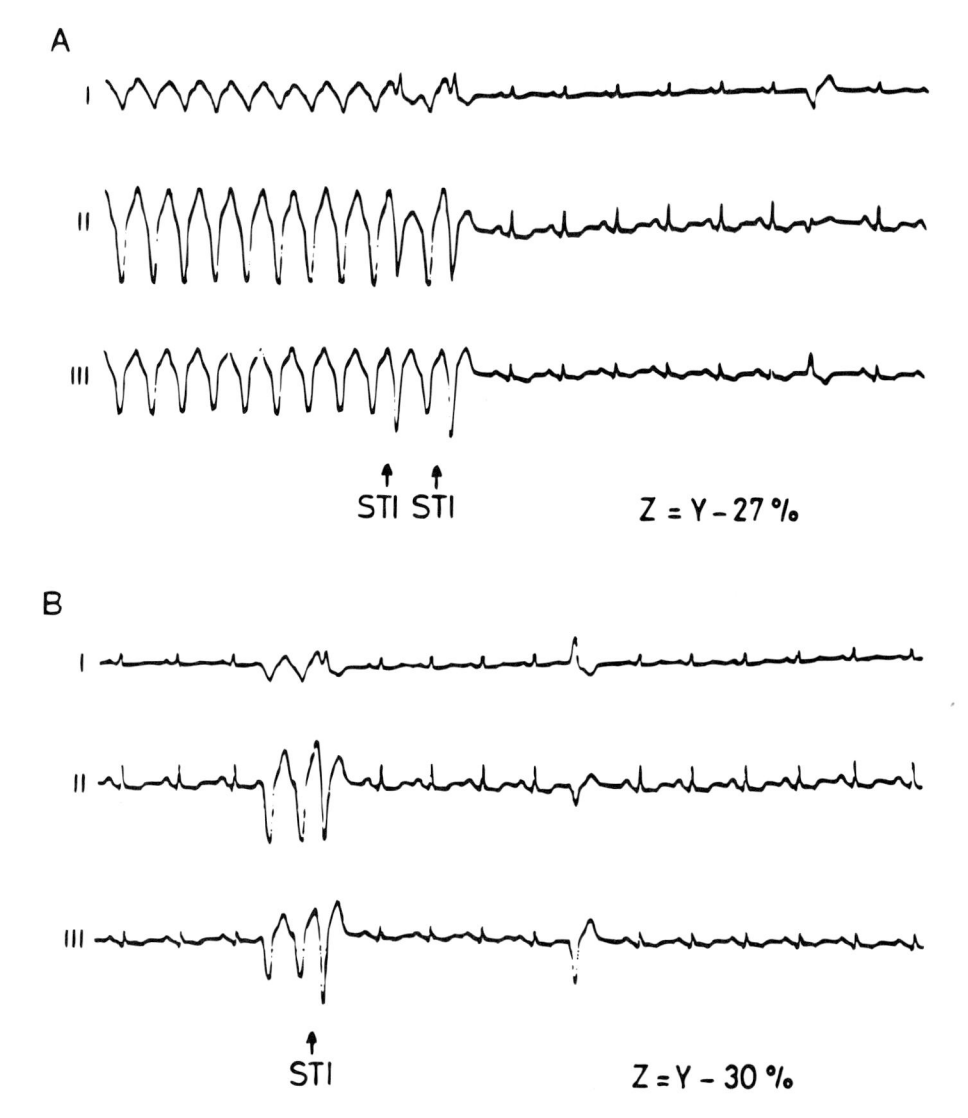

Figure 8. Suppression of ventricular dysrhythmias by programmed stimulation. **A**: Ventricular tachycardia (VT) is terminated by the second electrical intervention according to the program Z = Y − 27%. **B**: Two ventricular premature beats that may indicate the beginning of a ventricular tachycardia. One properly timed impulse elicited by the program Z = Y − 30% immediately terminates the arising tachycardia.

tions resulting from permanent antitachycardia pacemaker therapy is shown in Table 4.

The risk of antitachycardia therapy is acceleration of the tachycardia or degeneration to VF. Thus, an implantable cardioverter-defibrillator (ICD) is mandatory when an antitachycardia pacemaker is used for

Table 4
Complications of the Treatment of Tachyarrhythmias With Implanted Pacemakers

—Change of the excitation pattern (2/13)
—Acceleration of the tachycardia (1/13)
—Degeneration to ventricular fibrillation (−)
—Side effects of the drug therapy (1/13)

VT therapy. Implantation of an antitachycardia pacemaker should be avoided in cases in which no reproducible excitation pattern can be found, invasive diagnostic electrophysiologic study is not possible, no suitable clinical follow-up can be maintained, or when a patient is unable or unwilling to cooperate.[28]

Combination of Antitachycardia Pacemaker and Implantable Cardioverter-Defibrillator for Management of Ventricular Tachyarrhythmias

The use of antitachycardia pacemakers with ICDs as two separate devices is now mostly obsolete due to the development of the third-generation ICDs that incorporate ATP and bradycardia pacing functions with cardioversion and defibrillation. It must be emphasized that the frequency of VT and the discomfort to the patient produced by the defibrillation shocks can limit treatment with an ICD. Conversely, ATP for VT is associated with possible acceleration of VT. Therefore, the combined use of ATP and ICD therapy may be combined logically to enhance advantages and to avoid the disadvantages of either therapies.

We described this type of treatment in 1986 by evaluating 6 of 54 patients (mean age 57 ± 11 years) in whom an ICD was implanted for therapy of VT that could be terminated by temporary overdrive pacing (Table 5). In the automatic mode, the antitachycardia pacemaker, Tachylog™ (Siemens Pacesetter, Inc., Sylmar, CA), functioned as a bipolar ventricular inhibited (VVI) device with antitachycardia burst stimulation: 2–5 stimuli, interval 260–300 msec, one or two interventions. During follow-up of 47 ± 24 months, the Tachylog reliably terminated VT 50–505 times per patient. In five patients, acceleration of VT occurred during burst stimulation but could be reliably terminated by automatic ICD discharges (Figures 9 and 10). It is concluded that drug resistant VT can be terminated by an antitachycardia pacemaker while avoiding undue discomfort. Acceleration of VT can be terminated by the ICD shock.[31,32] The more recent, third-generation ICDs provide bradycardia support, which may be useful for patients with sick sinus

Table 5
Combined Use of Automatic Implantable Cardioverter-Defibrillator (AICD™) and Antitachycardia Pacemaker (Tachylog™) in Ventricular Tachyarrhythmias

Pt.	Age (yr) and Sex	Diagnosis	Rate of VT (min^{-1})	Pacing Mode; No. of Stimuli; Interval	Tachylog™ (n)	AICD™ (n)	Months
1	66 M	CAD	171	Burst; 5; 260 msec ‡ (stimulation no longer effective)	50	57	46*‡
2	53 M	CMP	160	Burst; 2; 270 msec	444	91	47*
3	70 M	CAD	162	Burst; 4; 300 msec	286	22	28‡
4	59 M	CAD	188	Burst; 5; 4× 300 msec, 1× 280 msec	505	19	29†
5	63 M	CAD	182	Burst; 3; 300 msec	346	30	41‡
6	50 M	CAD	200	Burst; 4; 300 msec	0	8	1¼‡

* AICD replacement 2 times.
† AICD replacement 1 time.
‡ Deceased.
CAD: Coronary artery disease; CMP: congestive cardiomyopathy; n: number of interventions.
AICD™ (CPI, Inc., St. Paul, MN); Tachylog™, (Siemens Pacesetter, Inc., Sylmar, CA).

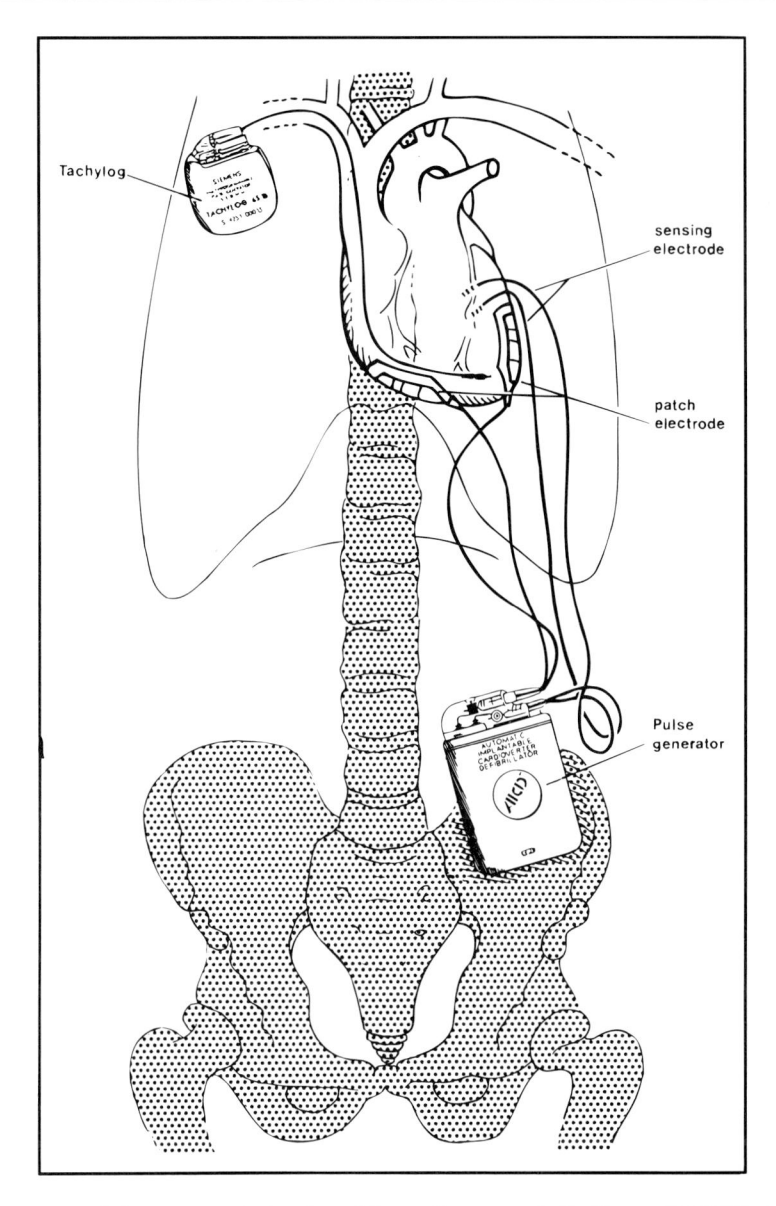

Figure 9. Diagram of the automatic implantable cardioverter-defibrillator (AICD™, CPI, St. Paul, MN) in combination with the antitachycardia pacemaker (Tachylog™, Siemens Pacesetter, Inc., Sylmar, CA). Two screw-in leads were positioned near the anterobasal portion of the left ventricle for rate detection by the AICD. For defibrillation of the heart, two flexible patch electrodes were placed over the anterior and inferior parts of ventricles. The bipolar electrode of the antitachycardia pacemaker was advanced transvenously to the apex of the right ventricle.

syndrome or in patients with conduction disturbances. In addition, more sophisticated ATP algorithms are available (Table 6).

For example, at the Bonn University Hospital until June 1993, 176 cardioverter/defibrillators were implanted in 140 patients (36 unit replacements). Third-generation ICD-ATP devices were implanted in 87 patients (Table 7). In 68 patients the transvenous/subcutaneous implantation technique was chosen for surgical access, whereby the postoperative recovery time was shortened and the perioperative complications rates reduced.[33]

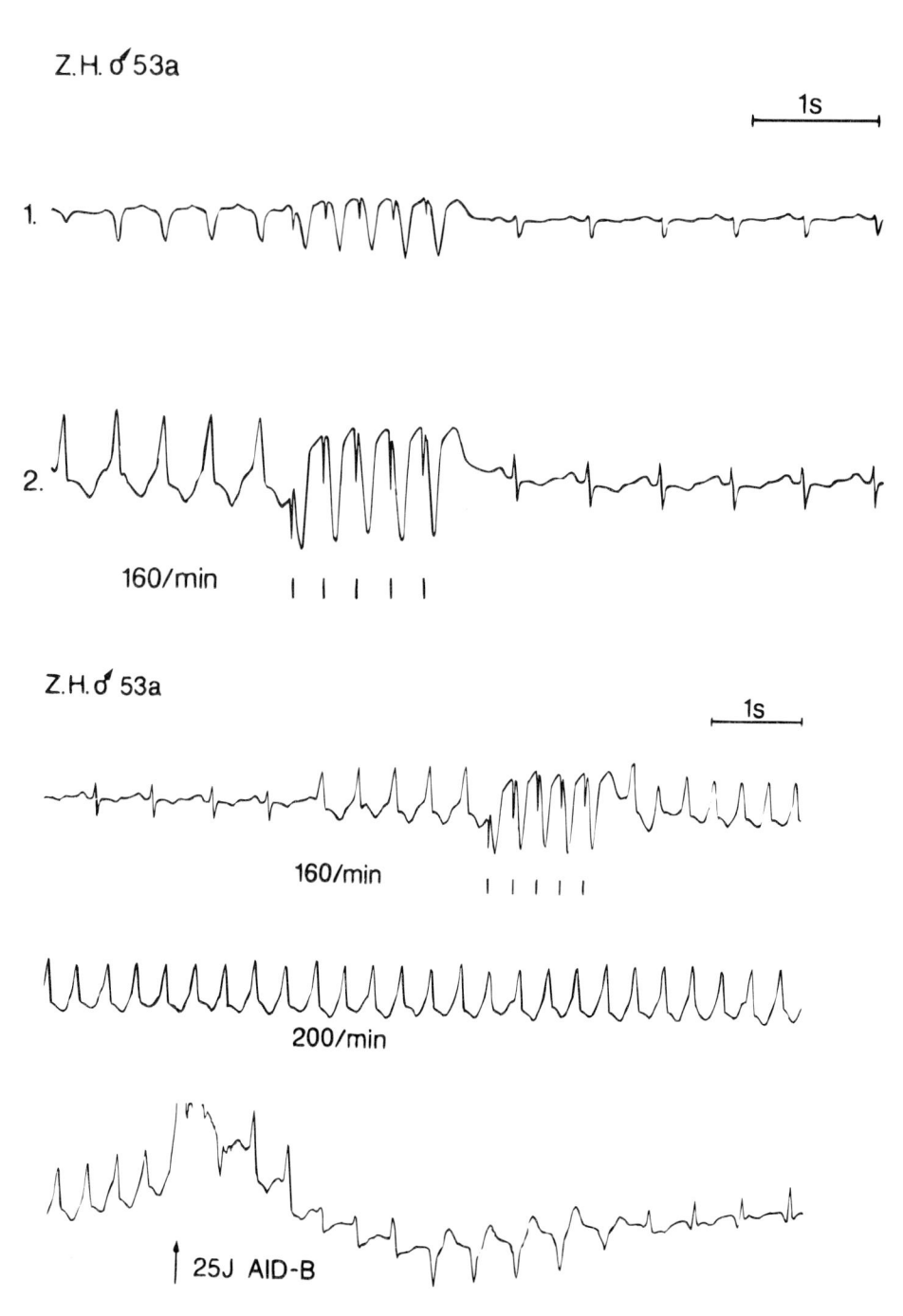

Figure 10. A 53-year-old male patient with persistent ventricular tachycardia (VT). (**Top**) successful termination of a VT by burst stimulation with five impulses from the implanted antitachycardia pacemaker (Tachylog™, Siemens Pacesetter, Inc., Sylmar, CA) (two-channel Holter recording). (**Bottom**) ECG of the same patient. After the first intervention by the Tachylog system with a stimulation burst, the VT accelerates. This activates the ICD system (AICD™, CPI, St. Paul, MN), which terminates the VT with an automatic application of shock (25 J).

Table 6
ATP-ICD Pulse Generators: Third Generation

	CPI Ventak™ P2	CPI PRx™ I	CPI PRx™ II	Intermedics RES-Q™	Silemens Silecure™	Telectronics Guardian™	Ventritex Cadence™	Medtronic 7217™	PCD Jewel™
Antitachycardia pacing	−	+	+	+	+	+	+	+	+
Bradycardia pacing	+	+	+	+	+	+	+	+	+
Programmable rate/energy	+	+	+	+	+	+	+	+	+
Waveforms	M,B	M	M,B	B	M	M	M,B	M,S	M,B
Tiered therapy	−	+	+	+	+	+	+	+	+
Noninvasive EPS	+	+	+	+	+	+	+	+	+
Weight (grams)	240	220	220	220	200	270	237	200	132

M = monophasic; B = biphasic; S = sequential.
EPS: electrophysiological study.

Although a wide variety of pacing algorithms have been used to terminate clinical tachycardias, they fall into three general groups: 1) scanning modalities in which the coupling interval of 1, 2, or 3 extrastimuli are individually decreased to terminate the arrhythmia; 2) burst pacing at fixed cycle lengths less than the tachycardia are introduced (usually at progressively shorter cycle lengths for a fixed or incremental number of intervals); and 3) autodecremental methods in which sequential extrastimuli are delivered at progressively shorter coupling intervals.[34,35] All of these pacing modalities may be initiated using specific preset coupling intervals or paced cycle lengths. However, it is more appropriate for each of these pacing modalities to be introduced as a percentage of the tachycardia cycle length (ie, adaptive mode) since tachycardia cycle length may vary or multiple tachycardias may be present in an individual patient. This allows the ATP device to respond to spontaneous or induced variations in tachycardia cycle lengths. Various types of pacing modalities have been described by Fisher et al.[36,37] Table 8 provides

Table 7
ICD-ATP

Patients:	87 (m: 74, f: 13)
Age:	56 +/− 9
Diagnosis:	
—CAD	61
—CMP	16
—MYOCARDITIS	1
—ARVD	3
—IDIOPATH. VF	6
PCD™ (35), PCD™ II (4), Res-Q™ (21), PRx-I™ (17), PRx-II™ (4), Cadence™ (2), Guardian™ ATP™ II 4211 (4)	
Transvenous Approach:	72
Shocks:	11 +/− 13
ATP:	45 +/− 13
Months:	21 +/− 18

CAD: coronary artery disease; CMP: cardiomyopathy; ARVD: arrhythmogenic right ventricular dysplasia; VF: ventricular fibrillation.

Table 8
Antitachycardia Pacing Modalities

- Single capture techniques
  Underdrive stimulation, programmed extrastimuli, ultrarapid stimulation
- Complex capture techniques
  a) Burst stimulation:
     Fixed or adaptive burst pacing, shifting bursts
  b) Scanning modes:
     Scanning burst (concertina), incremental
     —decremental scan
  c) Autodecremental methods:
     Ramp pacing, changing ramps, autodecremental pacing, adaptive pacing with changes in the number of stimuli
- Newer pacing techniques
  Subthreshold stimulation

the information about the most important ATP algorithms.

Underdrive Pacing (Figure 11, Ia)

Underdrive or slow asynchronous pacing during tachycardia is performed if the heart rate moves below or above prescribed limits and the latter becomes active only during tachycardia. A fixed cycle length between successive stimuli competing with the faster tachycardia will gradually scan the tachycardia cycle length, unless the tachycardia is exactly twice, three times, etc., the rate of the underdriving stimuli. This approach is relatively simple, with a low risk of acceleration.[38] However, successful application requires a relatively slow, well-tolerated tachycardia susceptible to single capture termination, conditions

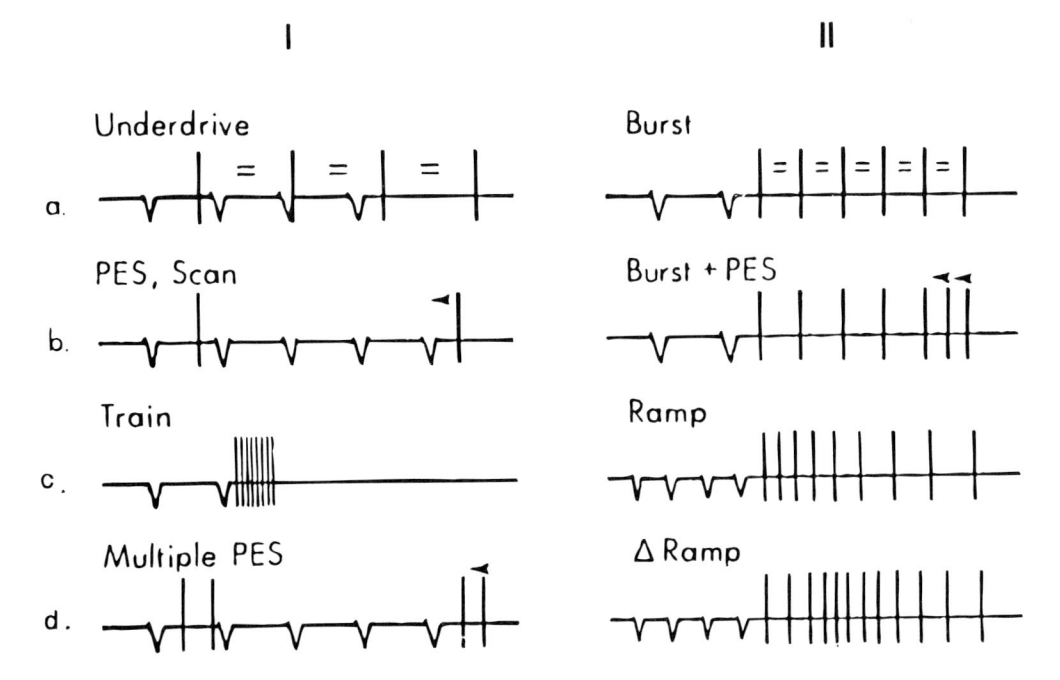

Figure 11. Basic stimulation patterns for tachycardia termination. In this figure, as well as in Figures 12 and 13, spontaneous atrial or ventricular depolarizations are represented by a V-like deflection from the baseline, and pacer stimuli by vertical lines. The small arrowheads at the top of the pacer stimulation lines represent the direction of changes in timing of successive stimuli. Tachycardia depolarizations are omitted after termination has occurred, or when they might obscure the stimulation pattern. **Ia. Underdrive**: Competitive pacing at rates slower than the tachycardia will terminate tachycardia with a wide termination zone. This is an inherently inefficient technique, although it does have the virtue of simplicity and can be attempted using virtually any pacing system. **Ib. PES**: Timed single extrastimuli can probably terminate reentrant tachycardias if other conditions are met. **Ic. Train Stimulation**: Delivery of ultra-rapid trains of stimuli with frequencies up to 100 Hz to obtain a single ventricular capture at the end of ventricular refractoriness. **Id. Multiple PES**: Double and triple programmed extrastimuli have been used, but are mostly inefficient, and offer few advantages over rapid pacing. **IIa. Burst**: A fixed burst is characterized by an equal-interval set of pulses and is introduced at a predetermined coupling interval. **IIb. Burst + PES**: A burst is followed by one or more programmed extrastimuli. **IIc.** A ramp sequence consisting of a decreasing or increasing interval set of pulses. In this example, each subsequent interval in the ramp sequence is incremented from the preceding interval by a programmable value. **IId. Changing ramp**: The rate of a ramp is changed from slower to faster and again to slower. PES: programmed extrastimulus (Reproduced with permission from Reference 36.)

that uncommonly prevail in patients with VTs.

Programmed Extrastimuli or Scanning Methods (Figure 11, Ib)

The timing of successive stimuli is altered in an orderly fashion with respect to the tachycardia cycle length, a quantum increase in efficiency compared to the underdrive approach. Some implantable devices retain the timing of the extrastimulus that terminated the tachycardia and use the same interval for subsequent initial termination attempts. This method may be more effective in terminating VT than supraventricular tachycardia, because the latter frequently changes substantially in rate and timing of a termination zone with alterations in posture, sympathetic tone, etc. For example, this pacing method is implemented in the Guardian™ ICD system (Telectronics, Inc., Englewood, CO).

Ultrarapid Train Stimulation (Figure 11, Ic)

For most tachycardia susceptible to single capture termination, the termination zone begins immediately after the effective refractory period.[39] Thus, a train of ultrarapid stimuli (cycle lengths 10–20 msec, equivalent to 3,000–6,000 beats per minute) beginning during the refractory period but of a duration resulting in single capture should result in termination upon the first attempt. Because trains are calculated to begin during the refractory period and cover a fairly broad zone during a single tachycardia cycling, the method is relatively immune to changes of the tachycardia cycle length or the timing of the termination zone. However, trains of sufficient duration to cause multiple captures will therefore drive the heart to the maximum possible rate and appear to increase the risk of acceleration. The efficacy of this technique appears limited, resulting in termination of approximately 50% to 60% of tachycardias reported.

This pacing algorithm is implemented in the Res-Q™ system (Intermedics Inc., Angleton, TX).

Multiple Programmed Extrastimuli (Figure 11, Id)

Two, three, or more extrastimuli can be programmed with some devices. The timing of these extrastimuli are in some instances independently programmable so that multiple variations of coupling intervals are possible. For instance, the Guardian ATP device offers this pacing mode.

Burst Pacing (Figure 11, IIa)

Stimuli are delivered at fixed cycle length, faster than the tachycardia.[22] It is desirable to keep both the number of stimuli and the burst rate as low as possible to minimize the risk of VT acceleration. The risk of acceleration for multiple capture techniques is higher than for single capture methods even for slow, well-tolerated tachycardias. This pacing mode may be implemented in all future ICDs.

Burst Plus Programmed Electrical Stimulation (Figure 11, IIb)

Burst stimulation is followed by one or more programmed electrical stimulation (PES). Termination of the VT can sometimes be achieved with a slower burst rate when PES is added.

Ramp Pacing (Figure 11, IIc)

The rapid pacing rate is continuously altered from faster to slower (tune down) as shown in Figure 11, IIc, or in the opposite direction. Ramping from faster to slower rates is less likely to result in acceleration than straight burst pacing. Both the PCD™ (Medtronic Inc., Minneapolis, MN), and the Res-Q™ have implemented this pacing technique. Ramp pacing is one of the most successful ATP modalities available.

Changing Ramps
(Figure 11, IId)

The rate of the ramp is changed from slower to faster to slower (as shown in Figure 11, IId) or in the reverse order. The gradual acceleration to rapid rate followed by deceleration in the pacing rate may be less "jolting" than very rapid bursts.

Adaptive Bursts
(Figure 12, Ia, Ib)

In this case, the burst cycle length is determined by a percentage of the tachycardia cycle length. This method, therefore, provides changing burst rates to accommodate changes in tachycardia cycle lengths. Thus, in Figure 12, panels Ia and Ib, there is a change in the tachycardia cycle length, but the burst rate remains at a fixed percentage of the tachycardia cycle length.[40,41] Pacing modalities in which pacing bursts are introduced as a percentage of the sensed tachycardia cycle length are superior to modalities with predetermined coupling intervals or pacing cycle lengths. Adaptive modes lessen the significance of spontaneous variations in tachycardia cycle lengths or changes in tachycardia rate induced by pacing.

Shifting Bursts
(Figure 12, Ic, Id)

The burst rate is fixed, but the timing of the first stimulus is progressively decre-

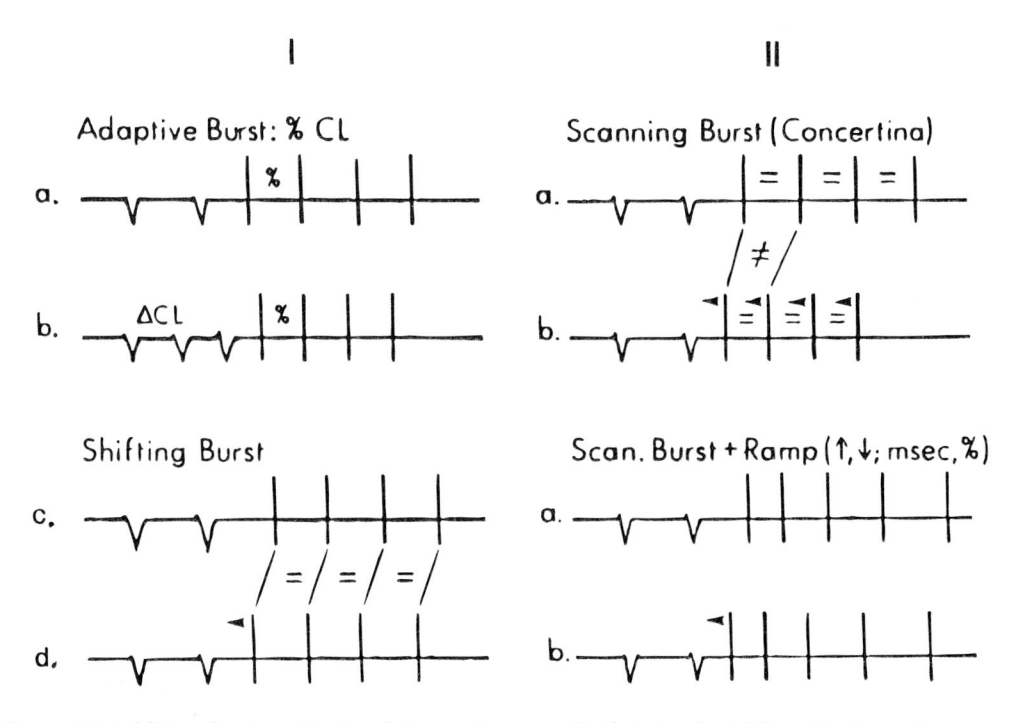

Figure 12. Additional automatic stimulation patterns available in implantable antitachycardia pacers. Conventions as for Figure 11. **Ia + Ib. Adaptive burst**: The burst cycle length is a percentage of the tachycardia cycle length. If there is a change in tachycardia cycle length, the burst rate remains a fixed percentage of the tachycardia cycle length. **Ic + d. Shifting burst**: A fixed burst is delivered, but the timing of the first stimulus is progressively decreased. **IIa + b. Scanning burst**: The timing of the first stimulus decreases with successive attempts and in addition, the cycle length of the successive bursts also decreases. **IIc + d. Scanning burst + ramp**: A ramp with the timing of the first beat of the ramp decreasing during successive termination attempts. CL: cycle length. (Reproduced with permission from Reference 36.)

mented with reference to the previous tachycardia beat. Thus, the coupling interval of the first stimulus to the tachycardia cycle length is continuously altered.

Scanning Burst (Concertina/Accordion) (Figure 12, IIa, IIb)

As with the shifting burst, the timing of a first stimulus decrements with successive attempts, but in this case, the cycle length of successive bursts also decreases.[42] This pacing technique is one of the most successful pacing modalities and is available in almost all newer ICDs. Experience has been gained with this pacing mode with antitachycardia pacemakers used for termination of supraventricular tachycardias (Intertach™, Intermedics Inc., Angleton, TX).

Scanning Burst With Ramp Pacing (Figure 12, IIc, IId)

A further variation of scanning bursts, this is actually a ramp with the timing of the first beat of the ramp changing during successive termination attempts. Sometimes, the ramp can be incremented or decremented with the changes determined in milliseconds, or as a percentage of the tachycardia cycle length (adaptive).

Incremental-Decremental (Centrifugal) Scan (Figure 13, Ia-Id)

In this variation, the timing of the burst stimulus (S_2) increments with successive termination attempts with the variation in timing of the burst stimulus programmable in milliseconds or as a percentage of the tachycardia cycle length (adaptive). A single extrastimulus may be used, or stimuli may be added to form the equivalent of multiple extrastimuli or burst pacing. These in turn can be programmed independently to increment or decrement upon successive attempts.[43] This pacing algorithm has been used with the antitachycardia pacemakers (Tachylog and Intertach).

Adaptive Pacing With Changes in the Number of Stimuli (Figure 13, IIa-IIe)

This approach has been described as the "universal" antitachycardia stimulation mode.[44] The first extrastimulus is delivered at a programmed percentage of the tachycardia cycle length. If the arrhythmia persists, a second extrastimulus is delivered at a slightly smaller percentage of the cycle length, a third extrastimulus at a still smaller percentage of the cycle length is delivered if necessary. If the tachycardia continues, successive stimuli may be delivered either without further decrement, as shown in this figure, or with further decrement in the percentage of the tachycardia cycle length.

Autodecremental Pacing

By programming autodecremental mode, it is possible to automatically decrease the pulse-to-pulse cycle length within a burst by either a fixed or an adaptive value.[45] The first results obtained using autodecremental pacing are favorable. Therefore, this pacing mode has been implemented in almost all third-generation ICDs.

Subthreshold Pacing

Subthreshold pacing is among the more unusual methods of pacing. It may be effective in some instances for tachycardia termination. Subthreshold stimulation has been shown to inhibit premature atrial and ventricular depolarizations and has also been shown to cause termination of reentrant and sustained uniform VTs in humans.[46] This technique is limited by the requirement for application of subthreshold stimulation in close proximity to the reentrant circuit.

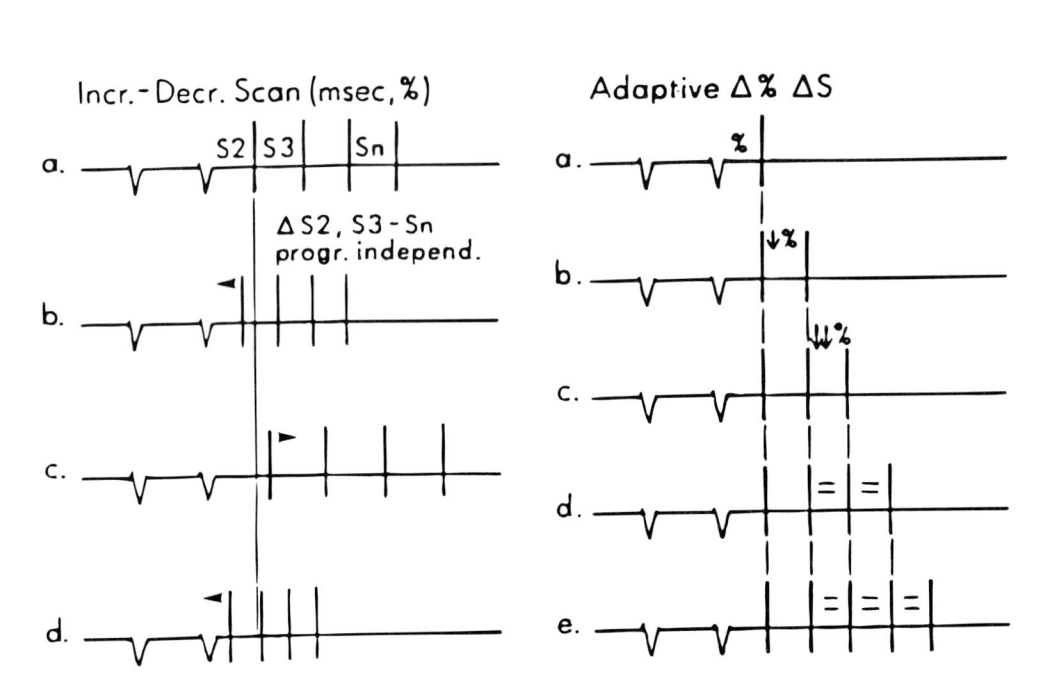

Figure 13. Complex stimulation patterns. Conventions as for Figures 11 and 12. **Ia-d. Incremental/decremental scan**: If an increment-decrement scanning pattern is programmed, scanned intervals are alternately lengthened and shortened causing the burst to search for a termination window near the center starting point. **IIa-e.** In this adaptive pacing mode, an extrastimulus is introduced as a percentage of the sensed tachycardia cycle length. In the next attempt, a second extrastimulus is added with a preselected decremental value. Further extrastimuli are automatically added sequentially, at coupling intervals that are preset percentages of the tachycardia cycle length, until termination occurs. Decr.: decremental; Incr.: incremental; S: stimulus. (Reproduced with permission from Reference 36.)

Efficacy of Antitachycardia Pacing

As stated previously, ATP is an important method for VT termination and is most useful for patients with recurrent monomorphic VTs. Because most instances of VF are preceded by VT, even in patients with VF as the "primary" rhythm disturbance, VT may be the primary target of therapy.[47] Although ATP can reliably terminate most monomorphic VTs due to reentry, this modality will not be effective in all patients and in every instance. There are several causes for the failure of ATP to terminate VT: 1) the reentrant circuit may be so short that the excitable gap cannot be penetrated by the depolarizing wave front; 2) the site of stimulation may be too distant from the reentrant circuit; 3) the induced wave front will depolarize the excitable gap and reset the VT; 4) ATP may accelerate VT or even induce VF; 5) the electrophysiologic determinants of VT may change under the influence of the autonomic nervous system or due to the underlying cardiac disease, thus leaving the chosen ATP mode ineffective; and 6) initiation of the clinical VT may not be possible so that appropriate pacing modes cannot be selected.

Considering these previously mentioned limitations, the efficacy of ATP will depend on the electrophysiologic characteristics of the arrhythmia and on the underlying cardiac disease, as well as on the pacing modes provided by the antitachycardia program.

Termination of the persistent VT by ATP depends on the presence of an excitable gap.[48] Transient entrainment may be used to demonstrate presence of an excitable gap. By using this technique in a prospective series of 27 consecutive patients with sustained VT induced by programmed stimulation, transient entrainment could be documented in 79% of the patients and in 76% of the tachycardia episodes.[49] Of note, the pacing site of rapid ventricular pacing was critically important for the demonstration of the excitable gap. The latter prerequisite cannot be realized in every patient during chronic ICD therapy. According to these data, most patients with sustained VT induced by PES have a reentrant basis for their arrhythmia. Reentrant circuits can also be documented during intraoperative mapping in the intact human ventricle.[50] If an excitable gap is present, as in most patients with sustained VT, the depolarizing wave front of ATP has to penetrate the reentrant circuit. This phenomenon can be demonstrated by entrainment or by the resetting response after electrical stimulation.[51,52] In patients with hemodynamically tolerated VT, the response patterns during electrical stimulation indicate reentrant circuits with relatively long resetting intervals favoring the mechanism of reentrant circuits, which are at least in part anatomically defined in the majority of these tachycardias.[52]

Efficacy of Different Pacing Modes

If single ventricular extrastimuli are applied, resetting of the VT can be seen in two thirds of the cases. Termination of VT occurs in a minority of patients only. Naccarelli et al.[53] investigated 57 patients with 89 episodes of induced sustained VT. Pacing successfully terminated VT in 18% using single stimulus, 42% using double extrastimuli, and 61% using burst right ventricular pacing.[53] In a similar study with 58 VTs, single right ventricular extrastimuli terminated the VTs in 9%, double ventricular extrastimuli in 36%, and rapid ventricular pacing in 48% of the episodes.[54] Thus, greater number of extrastimuli is necessary to interact with the reentrant circuit for termination of VT. Aside from the number of extrastimuli chosen, the relation of the pacing rate and the rate of VT determines the efficacy of ATP. With decreasing cycle length of the stimulating train in relation to the cycle length of VT, the efficacy of the therapy increases. With a shorter cycle length of the pacing train, however, acceleration of VT becomes more likely. Figure 14 demonstrates the relationship between the efficacy of the stimulation train and pacing rate in a series of 90 VT episodes.[54]

Comparison of Fixed Burst Versus Decremental Burst Pacing

Clinically available ICDs use two primary ATP techniques: 1) burst pacing (a train of pulses with identical coupling intervals) and 2) decremental burst pacing (a train of stimuli with decreasing coupling intervals within the sequence). Whereas the coupling intervals of fixed burst pacing can remain close to the VT cycle length during the initial attempts at ATP, the decremental burst pacing introduces comparably short pacing cycles from the beginning of the stimulation process. In a prospective study of 44 patients with inducible sustained VT, fixed burst pacing had a success rate of 70%, acceleration rate of 21%, and failure rate of 9%. The corresponding rates for decremental burst pacing were 72%, 18%, and 10%, respectively (Table 9).[55] Thus, no significant difference with these two pacing modes could be found. In addition, both pacing modes were significantly more effective for VTs with cycle lengths of > 300 msec (Fig-

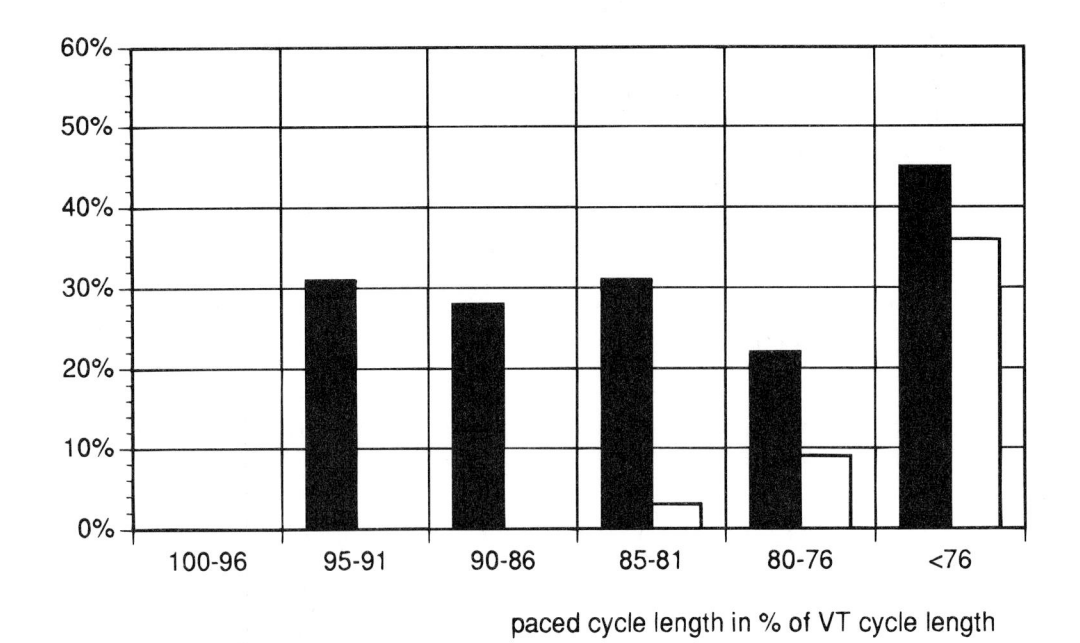

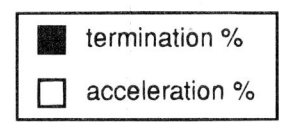

Figure 14. The efficacy of antitachycardia pacing (ATP) depends on the relation between the rate of VT and rate of the stimulating train. With a stimulating train of higher than 95% of the ventricular tachycardia (VT) cycle length, no VT episode was terminated. Trains with shorter cycle lengths interrupted the VT episodes in the range of 22% to 45%. However, the risk of acceleration increased with shorter intervals of the pacing train.

ure 15). The mean number of stimuli from each pacing mode was approximately 5.[55]

In a similar investigation, autodecremental overdrive pacing with 5-msec decrement was compared to 10-msec decrement and fixed burst pacing of 90% to 80% of the cycle length of VT. Autodecremental pacing with the shorter decrement of 5 msec appeared to be less effective than the decrement of 10 msec (efficacy rate 28% versus 75%). Compared to the fixed burst, autodecremental pacing with a decrement of 10 msec had the same success rate for VT termination (77% and 75%, respectively). A mean of 2.8 ± 2 pacing attempts was necessary.[56]

In a further randomized trial, ramp pacing was compared to a scanning protocol in 65 VT episodes during invasive electrophysiologic studies carried out in 29 patients. The ramp mode consisted of an eight-beat burst with the first beat-to-beat interval

Table 9
Comparison of Fixed Burst Versus Decremental Burst Pacing for Termination of VT.

	VT episodes	Success	Acceleration	Failure
Fixed burst pacing	57	70%	21%	9%
Decremental burst pacing	57	72%	18%	10%

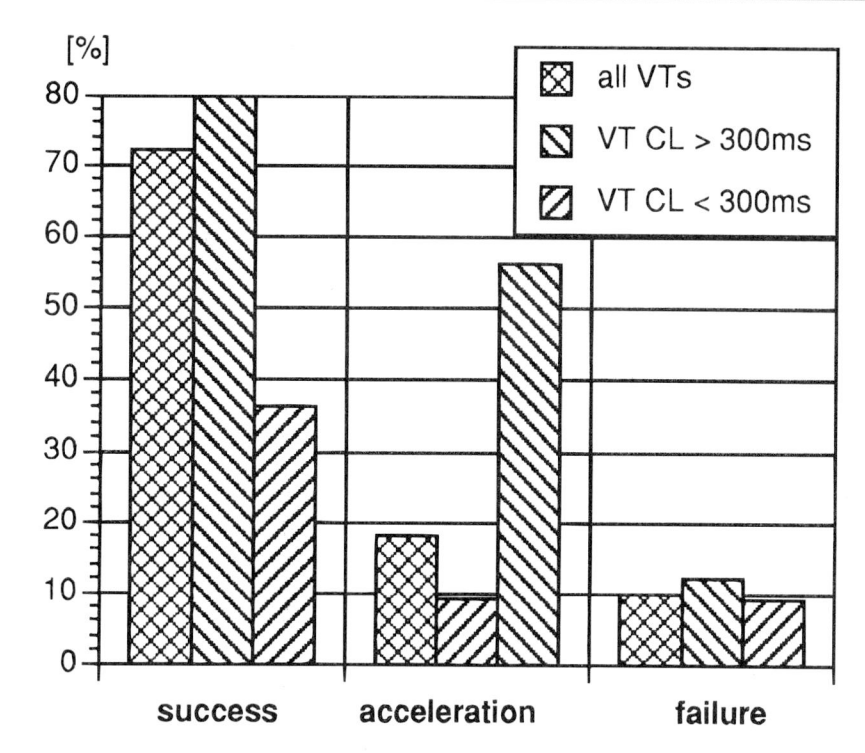

Figure 15. The efficacy of decremental burst pacing in 57 ventricular tachycardia (VT) episodes is demonstrated. The overall termination rate was 72%; 18% of VT episodes were accelerated, and 10% were unchanged. The effectiveness of decremental burst pacing was greater for VTs with a longer cycle length (> 300 msec). (Reproduced with permission from Reference 55.)

of the first attempt adapted to 90% of VT cycle length. There was a 3% decrement within the eight beats of the burst. The scan protocol used an eight-beat ATP drive with a constant interval throughout the burst. As for the ramp algorithm, the first beat-to-beat interval was progressively decreased from 90% to 75% of VT cycle length. Conversion to sinus rhythm occurred in 85% of scan versus 90% of ramp protocols.

Tachycardia acceleration during pacing was registered in 11% of the episodes. Acceleration of VT and failure to convert VT was associated with shorter VT cycle length.[57] In electrophysiologically induced VT an efficacy rate of ATP in the range of 70% can be expected by different pacing modes. Fixed burst pacing and autodecremental pacing do not differ significantly with respect to the efficacy in VT termination. Consecutive application of these pacing modes does not improve efficacy substantially.[56]

Because efficacy of VT termination depends on the rate of VT, antiarrhythmic drugs may be used to slow the VT rate, to improve the chance of ATP termination of VT, in most cases. In a minority of patients, however, more aggressive termination techniques are required with the concomitant use of antiarrhythmic drugs.[53]

Comparison of Efficacy of Antitachycardia Pacing With Cardioversion

The comparative efficacy of transvenous cardioversion and ATP in patients with sustained VT was initially evaluated in the electrophysiology laboratory. The two techniques were compared in 15 patients with organic heart disease. The termination sequence consisted of sequential shocks of 0.5, 1.1, and 2.7 J, and sequential bursts of rapid ventricular pacing with 10–15 stimuli at 90%, 75%, and 65% of VT cycle length. The success rate for termination of VT with transvenous cardioversion was 83%, and with rapid ventricular pacing 80%. The incidence of acceleration of VT episodes was 11% for cardioversion and 6% for ATP. Aside from patient discomfort from cardioversion in 57% of patients, the most significant difference was the occurrence of transient supraventricular tachyarrhythmias in 23% after cardioversion compared to 3% after ATP. Thus, after transvenous cardioversion there is a higher incidence of postcardioversion arrhythmias and poorer patient tolerance. For long-term treatment with electrical devices, rapid ventricular pacing techniques offer superior patient tolerance. According to these data, ATP should be considered the primary electrical therapy for the implanted ICDs.[58] A similar investigation using sequential pacing or intermediate high-energy shocks for faster sustained VTs, demonstrated a 30% risk of acceleration of VT, or induction of VF with 5- and 15-J shocks. High-energy shocks (25 J) reproducibly terminated sustained VT without acceleration to VF.[59] These data suggest that overdrive pacing is expected to be highly successful for termination of sustained VT with lower rates (cycle length > 300 msec). Intermediate energy shocks should be avoided because they are accompanied by a high propensity for acceleration to VF and for induction of atrial tachyarrhythmias. The combination of rapid ventricular pacing with high-energy shocks may reduce patient exposure to painful shocks and facilitate patient management when treated with ICDs.

The following practical aspects for ATP therapy can be summarized: 1) stable VT with a cycle length of > 300 msec should be the target for ATP; 2) either fixed burst pacing with 95% to 75% of VT cycle length and decrements of 10 msec or autodecremental pacing should be selected; 3) the length of the train should begin at five stimuli; 4) by slowing the rate of VT antiarrhythmic drugs improve efficacy of ATP for the majority of patients; 5) ATP and low-energy cardioversion are comparable in efficacy for termination of VT with improved patient acceptance and lower incidence of induced atrial arrhythmias with ATP; 6) to cope with the acceleration of VT, relatively high-energy cardioversion shocks should back up the ATP therapies.

Clinical Experience With Antitachycardia Pacing After Implantable Cardioverter-Defibrillator Implantation

With third-generation devices a hierarchical approach to the treatment of VTs has been implemented. In these devices up to four different arrhythmia zones can be defined. For each classified arrhythmia several therapies may be programmed and sequentially delivered. Thus, ATP can be applied for VT episodes with defined rates, leaving high-rate VT and VF for high-energy cardioversion or defibrillation.[60] At present, limited data regarding efficacy of ATP with these multiprogrammable antitachycardia devices is available. Preliminary experience with long-term ATP therapy has been obtained in a study of 16 patients with a third-generation device. Programmed electrical stimulation was used to induce monomorphic VT in 12 patients. Antitachycardia pacing alone was reliably successful in induced VT termination in 5 of 15 patients and low-energy shocks in 2 of 15 patients. During a follow-up of 2 to 12 months, 96 VT episodes occurred in 7 patients. Antitachycardia pacing was successful in 81% of the VT episodes. Two patients demonstrated inappropriate ATP during sinus rhythm. Reprogramming for ATP was necessary in two patients.[61]

The integrated antibradycardia/antitachycardia pacemaker-cardioverter-defibrillator system was evaluated in a total of 41 patients. During acute testing, 173 episodes of monomorphic VT were observed in 35 patients. Antitachycardia pacing was effective in terminating VT in 73% of the episodes. With antiarrhythmic drugs, the cycle length of VT lengthened. Thus, the efficacy of VT termination could be improved with success in 86% of VT episodes. Acceleration of VT by ATP was observed in 4% of the episodes and in another 10% ATP alone was ineffective. Fixed burst pacing was selected in 6 cases, based on the results of the electrophysiologic testing and autodecremental overdrive pacing in 25 patients. The mean number of stimuli were 6, the interval of the burst was 90% of the ventricular cycle length, and the ATP routines were repeated up to five times. During a follow-up of 8.4 months, 147 VT episodes could be documented in 18 patients, and ATP alone was effective in 89% of the episodes, 3 episodes ended spontaneously, and 13 episodes by low-energy cardioversion. The cycle length of the spontaneous VT was 367 ± 51 msec longer than the induced VT (305 ± 31 msec). Acceleration by ATP was not observed, but incessant VT in two patients rendered ATP ineffective. Antitachycardia pacing during atrial fibrillation induced VT in another two patients.[62]

Leitch and co-workers[63] tested 46 consecutive patients who presented with VT (35 patients) and VF (9 patients). During electrophysiologic study, monomorphic VT could be induced in 38 of 46 patients. At predischarge evaluation, sustained monomorphic VT was induced in 26 patients. Antitachycardia pacing was successful in 32 of 36 episodes (89%). Acceleration to VF occurred in 2 cases (6%) and inefficacy of ATP alone in another 6%. During the follow-up period of 6.1 months, 25 patients experienced spontaneous arrhythmic events. Decremental pacing was used as primary therapy in 38 patients, burst pacing in 2 cases. Of 909 tachycardia episodes treated by ATP, 840 were successfully terminated (92%). Pacing-induced acceleration of VT was estimated to have occurred 39 times (4.3%) in 5 patients. One of these accelerations was accompanied by syncope. Antitachycardia pacing was ineffective in 30 episodes (3%). There were no cardiac deaths related to ATP during follow-up.[63]

In a systematic evaluation burst pacing and autodecremental ramp pacing were randomly investigated in 28 of 42 patients, who received the Ventak PRx™ 1700/1705 (CPI, Inc., St. Paul, MN).[64] During preoperative and postoperative electrophysiologic studies hemodynamically stable VT could be induced in 31 patients (74%). Antitachycardia pacing terminated VT in 28 patients. Acceleration occurred in 2 patients, atrial tachyarrhythmias were induced during ATP in 3 patients. During the follow-up period of 6.3 ± 2 months, 15 patients were treated by ATP because of 236 spontaneous episodes. Ventricular tachycardia could be terminated by ATP alone in 83% of the episodes. Antitachycardia pacing was not successful in 22 VTs (9%) in 5 patients. Ventricular tachycardia acceleration occurred in 7 episodes (3%) in 3 patients. In 7 patients atrial tachyarrhythmias activated the ATP mode, however, induction of VT did not occur during delivery of ATP in these patients. The sudden onset criterion was programmed in 3 and the rate stability criterion in 6 patients (16 msec in 2 patients, 23 msec in 3 patients, and 39 msec in 1 patient). After activation of these detection algorithms, further inappropriate therapies could be prevented in 5 of 7 patients during 4.5 ± 8 months without indication of undetected sustained VT episodes.[64]

In 50 cardiac arrest survivors, ATP was selected as the primary treatment in 26 patients (52%) based on the results of the electrophysiolog testing.[65] Self-adaptive burst pacing or autodecremental overdrive pacing was used. In these patients 623 episodes were deemed to be due to VTs. Antitachycardia pacing therapies were successful in 498 episodes (80%). Low-energy cardioversion (< 1 J) was effective in an additional 78 (13%) of the VT episodes. High-energy cardioversion was required in 32 of the 623 VT episodes (5%). A total of 15 episodes of true VT (2%) were not terminated by the device (5 terminated spontaneously, 5 accelerated to VF by VT cardioversion therapy, 5 were incessant and required antiarrhythmic drug therapy). Aside from the rate criteron, rate stability was used to help discriminate atrial fibrillation from VT in 11 patients (22%). The interval stability parameter was selected with an interval 40 or 60 msec. In addition to the stability criteria, detection of VT was improved by increasing the number of consecutive intervals for tachycardia detection from 20 to 24. The selection of ATP had no negative impact on the overall survival in this study.[65]

In a multicenter study of 102 patients, 38 patients were treated by ATP during a follow-up period of 9.4 ± 5.8 months. The overall efficacy rate of ATP in this group was 92%. In 3% of the episodes ATP was ineffective. The remaining VT episodes were treated by cardioversion. The actuarial survival rate at 12 months was 91%. One sudden arrhythmic death occurred unrelated to the ATP therapy.[66] Although this study did not allow for detailed evaluation of the ATP therapy, it is important in that it documented the overall survival for patients with third-generation devices comparable to the survival seen with earlier devices that delivered shock therapy only.

In an investigation by Siebels and coworkers,[67] a predefined universal ramp pacing mode with 81% tachycardia coupling interval, 3 initital pulses, 10-msec decrement per pulse, 200-msec minimum coupling interval, and 5 sequences was evaluated during predischarge testing and during follow-up of 14 ± 11 months. At the predischarge ICD testing, 94 episodes of monomorphic VT could be induced in 26 of 38 patients. The termination rate of VT episodes was 78%, the acceleration rate 17%, and no effect was seen in 5%. Of note, patients with and without inducible VT were considered for chronic ATP. In the chronic phase ATP was effective in 94.9% of the VT episodes. Acceleration was documented in 0.4% and no effect in 4.7% of the episodes. Acute testing of ATP had a low predictive value for the efficacy during the chronic phase of the study.[67]

At present, the experience with ATP in patients after ICD implantation is still limited. In most instances ATP was selected as the primary therapy only if monomorphic VT could be induced during electrophysiologic testing or if an effective sequence of stimuli could be selected. Under these conditions, the comparable high efficacy rate of ATP in the range of 80% to 95% of the VT episodes was found (Table 10). This ap-

Table 10
Efficacy of ATP during Chronic ICD Therapy

Study	Patients	ATP	Follow-up Months	Efficacy (VT episodes, %)	Acceleration (VF episodes, %)	No effect (VT episodes, %)
Saksena et al.[61] 1991	16	15	2–12	78/96 (81%)	—	
Schmitt et al.[62] 1991	41	31	8.4 (1–24)	131/147 (89%)	—	(2 pts)
Leitch et al.[63] 1991	46	38	6.1	840/909 (92%)	39/909 (4.3%)	30/909 (3%)
Bardy et al.[65] 1992	50	26	15 ± 5	498/623 (80%)	5/623 (1%)	5/623 (1%)
Fromer et al.[66] 1992	102	38	9.4 ± 5	1114/1204 (92%)	—	39/1204 (3%)
Siebels et al.[67] 1992	51	51	14 ± 11	1184/1248 (94.9%)	5/1248 (0.4%)	59/1248 (4.7%)
Wietholt et al.[64] 1993	42	28	6.3 ± 2	218/236 (83%)	7/236 (3%)	22/236 (9%)

proach overestimates the efficacy rates of ATP because it relies on the event counter of the devices. The following shortcomings have to be considered: 1) the device does not distinguish between ongoing and separate episodes, therefore, acceleration to VF can only be estimated; 2) the system will address nonsustained VT as well as sustained VT; and 3) sinus tachycardia or atrial fibrillation may fulfill the VT criteria. In the newest implantable defibrillators, stored ventricular electrograms for arrhythmia classification are provided. With these systems a more accurate evaluation of the role of ATP in long-term ICD therapy will be possible in the future. With stored electrograms available the additional detection criteria such as "sudden onset" and "rate stability" have to be analyzed systematically because there are presently few cases with these programmed features that have been systematically analyzed.

Complications Associated With Antitachycardia Pacing Therapy

Antitachycardia pacing therapy as a component of the ICD therapies proved to be highly effective with respect to VT termination. The interaction of ATP with the arrhythmia is a time-consuming process. Tachycardia detection by the ICD has thus far relied entirely on ventricular electrogram analysis, which unfortunately is of limited value in determining the hemodynamic consequences, or a patient's tolerance to tachyarrhythmia. Persistence of VT despite ATP may produce impairment of cardiac, hemodynamic, and consequently metabolic functions. It may lead to myocardial ischemia, further deterioration of already reduced cardiac output, and systemic hypoperfusion. Depending on the length of time required to terminate VT syncope may result. In the worst case, the defibrillation threshold may rise rendering subsequent defibrillation shocks ineffective. In the previously conducted studies (Table 10) ATP was programmed conservatively. In most instances, ATP was programmed based on the results of electrophysiologic evaluation. The number of therapies delivered were limited. Under these conditions the inclusion of ATP as a therapeutic option did not affect the overall outcome in a negative way. There are several documented complications of ATP, however, including:

1. ATP therapy may lead to acceleration of the VT, transforming a slow, hemodynamically well-tolerated VT to a tachyarrhythmia with a short cycle length, which may induce hemodynamic collapse. One possible mechanism of acceleration is modification of electrophysiologic properties of the reentrant circuit with the development of alternative conduction pathways, or with doubling the reentrant wavelength within the same circuit. In addition, greater dispersion of refractoriness in both ventricles could be induced by rapid pacing. Acceleration of VT has to be expected in up to 9% of the VT episodes (Table 10). Therefore, high-energy cardioversion is mandatory to back up ATP and to prevent sudden cardiac death. Nevertheless, the longer termination process, including ATP and defibrillation, can lead to syncope in some patients.[63]

2. If atrial tachyarrhythmias fulfill the VT detection criteria, ATP can induce VT; this has been documented in some patients.[62] Since the rate cutoff for ATP is typically lower than for defibrillation, the likelihood of inappropriate ATP therapy is higher. Potentially, therefore, inadvertent induction of VT by inappropriate ATP therapy followed by cardioversion and defibrillation shocks becomes more likely.

3. During ATP therapy for VT, atrial flutter or fibrillation may be in-

duced due to the longer period required for termination of VT with repeated pacing trains.[64] One possible mechanism causing atrial tachyarrhythmias during ATP may be hemodynamic instability due to the persistent arrhythmias. Atrioventricular dissociation during the VT, retrograde atrial depolarization, and the influence of the autonomic nervous system could further contribute to the occurrence of atrial tachyarrhythmias. Compared with cardioversion shocks, the incidence of atrial tachyarrhythmias caused by ATP therapy is lower.[58]

4. Complications related to transvenous lead placement, which is generally preferred for ATP because of lower pacing thresholds than for epicardial leads and the long-term stability, are uncommon in clinical studies. One potential problem relates to the intracavity shock delivery when the pacing and the shocking electrodes are located on the same lead. High-energy intracavity shocks may be associated with increased pacing thresholds, which may lead to ineffective antibradycardia pacing as well as ATP.[68] Furthermore, the intracavity shock discharges may influence the amplitude of the endocardial electrograms, which may impair reliable detection of the ventricular electrograms under certain conditions.[69] The reduction of the amplitude of the intracardiac electrogram may be a function of the proximity of the sense/pace electrode and defibrillating coil electrodes. With the awareness of this interaction, the design of the endocardial lead systems may be modified in order to improve the reliability of the detection signals.[70]

Considering the data of ATP in "unselected" patients this feature of electrical treatment of VT can be considered highly effective and safe for patients with implanted ICDs.[67]

References

1. Mines GR: On circulating excitations in heart muscles and their possible relation to tachycardia and fibrillation. *Trans R Soc Can* 3(4.8):43, 1914.
2. Aronson RS, Cranefield PF: The effect of resting potential on the electrical activity of canine cardiac Purkinje fibers exposed to Na-free solution or to ouabain. *Pflügers Arch* 347:101, 1974.
3. Lüderitz B: Electrophysiology related to cardiac pacing techniques. In: *Fundamentals of Cardiac Pacing*. Edited by HJTh Thalen, CC Meere. The Hague/Boston/London: Martinus Nijhoff Publishers; 1979, p. 79.
4. Wellens HJJ: *Electrical Stimulation of the Heart in the Study and Treatment of Tachycardias*. Leiden: Stenfort Kroese; 1971.
5. Josephson ME, Horowitz LN, Farshidi A, et al: Recurrent sustained ventricular tachycardia. I. Mechanisms. *Circulation* 57:431, 1978.
6. Steinbeck G, Naumann d'Alnoncourt Ch, Lüderitz B: Treatment of ventricular tachyarrhythmias—pacing. In: *Cardiac Pacing*. Edited by K Steinbach, et al. Darmstadt: Steinkopff Verlag; 1983, p. 779.
7. Wellens HJJ, Schuilenburg RM, Durrer D: Electrical stimulation in patients with ventricular tachycardia. *Circulation* 46:216, 1972.
8. Mendez C, Mueller WJ, Meredith J, et al: Interaction of transmembrane potentials in canine Purkinje fibers and of Purkinje-fiber muscle junctions. *Circ Res* 24:361, 1969.
9. Sasyniuk BI, Mendez C: A mechanism for reentry in canine ventricular tissue. *Circ Res* 28:3, 1971.
10. Cranefield PF, Klein HO, Hoffman BF: Conduction of the cardiac impulse I: delay, block, and one-way block in depressed Purkinje fibers. *Circ Res* 28:199, 1971.
11. Wit AL, Cranefield PF, Hoffman BF: Slow conduction and re-entry in the ventricular conduction system II: single and sustained circus movement in networks of canine and bovine Purkinje fibers. *Circ Res* 30:11, 1972.
12. Wit AL, Cranefield PF: Triggered activity in

cardiac muscle fibers of the simian mitral valve. *Circ Res* 38:85, 1976.
13. Cranefield PF, Aronson RS: Initiation of sustained rhythmic activity by single propagated action potentials in canine cardiac Purkinje fibers exposed to sodium-free solution or ouabain. *Circ Res* 34:477, 1974.
14. Lüderitz B, Saksena S (eds): *Interventional Electrophysiology*. Mount Kisco, NY: Futura Publishing Company, Inc.; 1991.
15. Sowton E, Leatham A, Carson P: The suppression of arrhythmia by artificial pacing. *Lancet* 1098 (2), 1964.
16. Barold SS: Therapeutic use of cardiac pacing in tachyarrhythmias. In: *His Bundle Electrocardiography and Clinical Electrophysiology*. Edited by OS Narula. Philadelphia, PA: FA Davis; 1975, p. 407.
17. Wellens HJJ, Bär FW, Borgels AP, et al: Electrical management of arrhythmias with emphasis on tachycardias. *Am J Cardiol* 41:1025, 1978.
18. Waxman HL, Cain ME, Greenspan AM, et al: Termination of ventricular tachycardia with ventricular stimulation: salutary effect of increased current strength. *Circulation* 65:800, 1983.
19. Gardner MJ, Waxman HL, Buxton AE, et al: Termination of ventricular tachycardia. Evaluation of a new pacing method. *Am J Cardiol* 50:1338, 1982.
20. Roy D, Waxman HL, Buxton AE, et al: Termination of ventricular tachycardia: role of tachycardia cycle length. *Am J Cardiol* 50:1346, 1982.
21. Josephson ME, Horowitz LN: Electrophysiologic approach to therapy of recurrent sustained ventricular tachycardia. *Am J Cardiol* 43:631, 1979.
22. Fisher JD, Mehra R, Furman S: Termination of ventricular tachycardia with bursts of rapid ventricular pacing. *Am J Cardiol* 41:94, 1978.
23. Guize L, Zacouto F, Lenègre J: Un nouveau stimulateur du coeur: le pacemaker orthorhythmique. *Presse Méd* 79:2071, 1971.
24. Zacouto F, Guize L: Fundamentals of orthorhythmic pacing. In: *Cardiac Pacing: Diagnostic and Therapeutic Tools*. Edited by B Lüderitz. Berlin: Springer; 1976.
25. Lüderitz B, Steinbeck G, Zacouto F: Significant reduction of recurrent tachycardias by programmed rate-related premature stimulation. In: *Cardiac Pacing*. Edited by Y Watanabe. Amsterdam: Excerpta Medica; 1977.
26. Lüderitz B (ed): *Cardiac Pacing: Diagnostic and Therapeutic Tools*. Berlin: Springer; 1976.
27. Benchimol A, McNally EM: Atrial pacing during selective coronary angiography. *Br Heart J* 29:767, 1967.
28. Lüderitz B, Naumann d'Alnoncourt Ch, Steinbeck G, et al: Therapeutic pacing in tachyarrhythmias by implanted pacemakers. *PACE* 5:366, 1982.
29. Lüderitz B, Gerckens U, Kirchhoff PG, et al: Automatic implantable cardioverter/defibrillator (AICD) and antitachycardia pacemaker (Tachylog) in ventricular tachyarrhythmias. *New Trends Arrhythmias* 1:185, 1986.
30. Mirowski M, Reid PR, Watkins L, et al: Clinical treatment of life-threatening ventricular tachyarrhythmias with the automatic implantable defibrillator. *Am Heart J* 102:265, 1981.
31. Manz M, Gerckens U, Lüderitz B: Erroneous discharge from an implanted automatic defibrillator during supraventricular tachyarrhythmia induced ventricular fibrillation. *Am J Cardiol* 57:343, 1986.
32. Manz M, Gerckens U, Funke HD, et al: Combination of antitachycardia pacemaker and automatic implantable cardioverter/defibrillator for ventricular tachycardia. *PACE* 9:676, 1986.
33. Lüderitz B, Jung W, Manz M: Automatic implantable antitachycardia cardioverter/defibrillator: guidelines to the selection of candidates. In: *Proceedings of the International Symposium on Progress in Clinical Pacing*. Edited by M Santini, M Pistolese, A Alliegro. Mount Kisco, NY: Futura Media Services Inc.; 1992.
34. Rosenthal ME, Josephson ME: Current status of antitachycardia devices. *Circulation* 82:1889, 1990.
35. Klein LS, Miles WM, Zipes DP: Antitachycardia devices: realities and promises. *J Am Coll Cardiol* 18:1349, 1991.
36. Fisher JD, Johnston DR, Kim SG, et al: Implantable pacers for tachycardia termination: stimulation techniques and long-term efficacy. *PACE* 9:1325, 1986.
37. Fisher JD, Kim SG, Mercando AD: Electrical devices for treatment of arrhythmias. *Am J Cardiol* 61:45A, 1988.
38. Fisher JD, Kim SG, Matos JA, et al: Comparative effectiveness of pacing techniques for termination of well-tolerated sustained ventricular tachycardia. *PACE* 6:915, 1983.
39. Fisher JD, Ostrow E, Kim SG, et al: Ultrarapid single- capture train stimulation for termination of ventricular tachycardia. *Am J Cardiol* 51:1334, 1983.
40. Charos GS, Haffajee CI, Gold RL, et al: A theoretically and practically more effective method for interruption of ventricular tachycardia: a self-adapting autodecremental overdrive pacing. *Circulation* 73:309, 1986.
41. Holt P, Crick JCP, Sowton E: Antitachycardia

pacing: a comparison of burst overdrive, self searching and adaptive table scanning programs. *PACE* 9:490, 1986.
42. Jung W, Mletzko R, Manz M, et al: Long-term therapy of antitachycardia pacing for supraventricular tachycardia. *PACE* 15:179, 1992.
43. Jung W, Mletzko R, Manz M, et al: Clinical results of chronic antitachycardia pacing in supraventricular tachycardia. In: *Interventional Electrophysiology*. Edited by B Lüderitz, S Saksena. Mount Kisco, NY: Futura Publishing Company, Inc.; 1991, p. 197.
44. den Dulk K, Kersschot IE, Brugada P, et al: Is there a universal antitachycardia pacing mode? *Am J Cardiol* 57:950, 1986.
45. Jung W, Mletzko R, Manz M, et al: Comparison of two antitachycardia pacing modes in supraventricular tachycardia. *PACE* 14:1762, 1991.
46. Shenasa M, Cardinal R, Kus T, et al: Termination of sustained ventricular tachycardia by ultrarapid subthreshold stimulation in humans. *Circulation* 78:1135, 1988.
47. de Luna Bayés A, Coumel P, Leclercq JF: Ambulatory sudden cardiac death: mechanisms of production of fatal arrhythmia on the basis of data from 157 cases. *Am Heart J* 117:151. 1989.
48. Josephson ME, Horowitz LN, Farshidi A, et al: Recurrent sustained ventricular tachycardia. *Circulation* 57:431, 1978.
49. Kay GN, Epstein AE, Plumb VJ: Incidence of reentry with an excitable gap in ventricular tachycardia: a prospective evaluation utilizing transient entrainment. *J Am Coll Cardiol* 11:530, 1988.
50. Downar E, Harris L, Mickleborough LL, et al: Endocardial mapping of ventricular tachycardia in the intact human ventricle: evidence for reentrant mechanisms. *J Am Coll Cardiol* 11:783, 1988.
51. Almendral JM, Gottlieb C, Marchlinski FE, et al: Entrainment of ventricular tachycardia by atrial depolarization. *Am J Cardiol* 56:298, 1985.
52. Almendral JM, Stamato NJ, Rosenthal ME, et al: Resetting response patterns during sustained ventricular tachycardia: relationship to the excitable gap. *Circulation* 74:722, 1986.
53. Naccarelli GV, Zipes DP, Rahilly GT, et al: Influence of tachycardia cycle length and antiarrhythmic drugs on pacing termination and acceleration of ventricular tachycardia. *Am Heart J* 105:1, 1983.
54. Almendral J, Arenal A, Villacastin JP, et al: The importance of antitachycardia pacing for patients presenting with ventricular tachycardia. *PACE* 16:535, 1993.

55. Calkins H, El-Atassi R, Kalbfleisch S, et al: Comparison of fixed burst versus decremental burst pacing for termination of ventricular tachycardia. *PACE* 16:26, 1993.
56. Cook JR, Kirchhoffer JB, Fitzgerald TF, et al: Comparison of decremental and burst overdrive pacing as treatment for ventricular tachycardia associated with coronary artery disease. *Am J Cardiol* 70:311, 1992.
57. Newman D, Dorian P, Hardy J: Randomized controlled comparison of antitachycardia pacing algorithms for termination of ventricular tachycardia. *J Am Coll Cardiol* 21:1413, 1993.
58. Saksena S, Chandran P, Shah Y, et al: Comparative efficacy of transvenous cardioversion and pacing in patients with sustained ventricular tachycardia: a prospective, randomized, crossover study. *Circulation* 72:153, 1985.
59. Lindsay BD, Saksena S, Rothbart ST, et al: Prospective evaluation of a sequential pacing and high-energy bidirectional shock algorithm for transvenous cardioversion in patients with ventricular tachycardia. *Circulation* 76:601, 1987.
60. Haluska EA, Whistler SJ, Calfee RJ: A hierarchical approach to the treatment of ventricular tachycardias. *PACE* 9:1320, 1986.
61. Saksena S, Mehta D, Krol RB, et al: Experience with a third-generation implantable cardioverter-defibrillator. *Am J Cardiol* 67:1375, 1991.
62. Schmitt C, Brachmann J, Saggau W, et al: Integrated antibradycardiac/antitachycardiac pacemaker-cardioverter-defibrillator systems in patients with recurrent ventricular tachyarrhythmias. *Z Kardiol* 80:665, 1991.
63. Leitch JW, Gillis AM, Wyse G, et al: Reduction in defibrillator shocks with an implantable device combining antitachycardia pacing and shock therapy. *J Am Coll Cardiol* 18:145, 1991.
64. Wietholt D, Block M, Isbruch F, et al: Clinical experience with antitachycardia pacing and improved detection algorithms in a new implantable cardioverter-defibrillator. *J Am Coll Cardiol* 21:885, 1993.
65. Bardy GH, Troutman C, Poole JE, et al: Clinical experience with a tiered-therapy, multiprogrammable antiarrhythmia device. *Circulation* 85:1689, 1992.
66. Fromer M, Brachmann J, Block M, et al: Efficacy of automatic multimodal device therapy for ventricular tachyarrhythmias as delivered by a new implantable pacing cardioverter-defibrillator: results of a European multicenter study of 102 implants. *Circulation* 86:363, 1992.

67. Siebels J, Rüppel R, Schneider MAE, et al: Antitachycardia pacing regardless of acute testing results in patients with an implanted defibrillator. In: *The '92 Scenario On Cardiac Pacing*. Edited by E Adornato, A Galassi. Edizioni Luigi Pozzi 1992, p. 96.
68. Yee R, Jones DL, Klein GJ: Pacing threshold changes after transvenous catheter countershock. *Am J Cardiol* 53:503, 1984.
69. Jung W, Manz M, Moosdorf R, et al: Failure of an implantable cardioverter-defibrillator to redetect ventricular fibrillation in patients with a nonthoracotomy lead system. *Circulation* 86:1217, 1992.
70. Jung W, Manz M, Pfeiffer D, et al: Substantial improvement in redetection of ventricular fibrillation with a new nonthoracotomy lead system. *Circulation* 86:I-791, 1992.

Part 3

Clinical Aspects of Implantable Cardioverter-Defibrillator Therapy

Chapter 13

Indications for Implantable Cardioverter-Defibrillator Therapy

Theofilos M. Kolettis and Sanjeev Saksena

Introduction

Sudden cardiac death is a major public health problem in developed nations. Approximately 400,000 people die suddenly in the United States every year, accounting for about half of all cardiac mortality.[1] In most instances, the initiating mechanism is a malignant ventricular tachyarrhythmia causing circulatory collapse. Emergency medical systems, consisting of mobile intensive care units, have reduced this death toll,[2,3] however, the most optimistic figures for successful out-of-hospital resuscitation do not exceed 30% of all victims.[4] Poorer results are quite common. Thus, recent investigative effort has been devoted to primary prevention of cardiac arrest.

The management of cardiac arrest survivors remains difficult and controversial. If untreated, the prognosis for such patients is generally poor, with recurrence rates at the range of 50% for the first 2 years.[5,6] Antiarrhythmic drug selection guided by programmed electrical stimulation is one accepted practice, but an effective antiarrhythmic drug regimen can be identified in only approximately one third of all patients.[7,8] The prognosis of patients, whose arrhythmia is suppressed in the electrophysiology laboratory by type I or type III antiarrhythmic agents, has been reported to be more favorable, compared with patients who are not suppressed,[9] however, considerable controversy still exists in this area.[10]

The advent of implantable cardioverter-defibrillators (ICDs) offers a significant therapeutic option in the secondary prevention of sudden death in high-risk patients; a number of clinical trials[11-14] have demonstrated a low incidence of sudden arrhythmic death in device-treated patients. These data indicate that ICDs are a safe and effective therapy and they have now been considered by some expert authorities as first-line therapy for the prevention of sudden cardiac death. This chapter discusses the currently accepted indications for ICD therapy.

Early Evolution

The first ICD was implanted by Mirowski and colleagues[15] at Johns Hopkins University Hospital in 1980, in a patient with two prior cardiac arrests. For the next 2 years, ICD therapy was reserved only for patients with documented cardiac arrest due to ventricular fibrillation (VF) and implantation was restricted to only a few centers. In 1985, the Food and Drug Adminis-

From Singer I, (ed.) Implantable Cardioverter-Defibrillator. Armonk, NY: Futura Publishing Company, Inc.; © 1994.

tration (FDA), after reviewing the investigational data, released the device for commercial use. More importantly, the indications were extended[16]: the ICD could now be implanted in patients with previous cardiac arrest or in patients with recurrent sustained ventricular tachyarrhythmias that were not suppressed by drugs in the electrophysiology laboratory.

Current Indications

During 1991, two expert panels, reflecting the experience of several investigators, published their reports on updated indications for ICD implantation: one from the North American Society of Pacing And Electrophysiology[17] and the other from the American College of Cardiology/American Heart Association task force.[18] The recommendations of both authorities were similar in their content; in both reports, the indications have been classified into three major categories: Class I: ICD therapy is indicated, based upon consensus; Class II: ICD therapy is a therapeutic option, but consensus does not always exist; and Class III: ICD therapy is not justified based upon consensus.

Class I Conditions

Patients With Drug-Refractory Ventricular Fibrillation or Sustained Ventricular Tachycardia

In patients with spontaneous VF or sustained ventricular tachycardia (VT), persistent inducibility of clinically relevant sustained VT or VF at electrophysiologic study on best available drug therapy constitutes an indication for ICD therapy. In carefully selected patients, VT surgery or catheter ablation are alternative approaches. However, in view of the excellent long-term results of ICD therapy,[11–14] such treatment is the preferred approach in the majority of patients.

Late Drug Failure

Spontaneous recurrence(s) of sustained VT or VF in a patient whose arrhythmia was previously suppressed by antiarrhythmic medications guided by electrophysiologic study or by continuous electrocardiographic recording is an indication for ICD implantation. This involves a potentially large subgroup of patients, because nonfatal recurrences occur in a substantial proportion of these patients.[19,20] Recent data from the Electrophysiologic Study Versus Electrocardiographic Monitoring (ESVEM) study showed recurrence rates of over 40% for type I agents and over 20% for sotalol within the first year of follow-up.[21]

Patients With Ventricular Fibrillation or Sustained Ventricular Tachycardia and Intolerance to Drugs

Sustained VT or VF in a patient in whom antiarrhythmic drug therapy is limited by intolerance or noncompliance is another indication for ICD therapy. This also involves a large category of patients because side effects are commonly observed with antiarrhythmic medications: approximately 20% to 40% of patients treated with type I agents discontinue treatment during the first year because of intolerance to medication.[22,23] Long-term amiodarone treatment is occasionally associated with serious side effects, such as interstitial pneumonitis, hyper- and hypothyroidism, or liver toxicity.[24] In a recent report, 86% of patients experienced significant side effects, and 37% discontinued amiodarone therapy in a 5-year follow-up.[25]

Cardiac Arrest Victims With No Inducible Arrhythmias

The initial FDA guidelines in 1985, restricted ICD implantation only to patients who were inducible and not suppressed in the electrophysiology laboratory. This was based on the premise that all noninducible patients (usually 25% tp 30% of all VF/VT patients) had a relatively good prognosis.[26] Subsequent reports,[27,28] however, demonstrated that some of these patients may also be at a high risk of ventricular tachyarrhythmia recurrences, particularly when advanced left ventricular dysfunction or dilated cardiomyopathy is present. In current guidelines, ICD therapy is indicated in patients with one or more episodes of spontaneous sustained VT or VF, in whom sustained ventricular tachyarrhythmias are not inducible at electrophysiologic testing, and spontaneous ventricular arrhythmias, such as runs of nonsustained VT, couplets and premature ventricular contractions are not frequent enough to be used accurately to predict efficacy of drug therapy. These recommendations were confirmed by the results of a recent study[29] examining the outcome of survivors of out-of-hospital cardiac arrest with and without inducible arrhythmias. This study reported a high incidence of ventricular tachyarrhythmia recurrences in both groups of patients; furthermore, when the outcome of those treated with and without an ICD was compared, ICD therapy was shown to significantly lower mortality from sudden cardiac death, although no difference in overall survival was demonstrated.

Class II Conditions

The conditions under Class II include patients in whom there is a history of syncope, where medical evaluation fails to reveal another cause, but during electrophysiologic study clinically relevant sustained VT or VF is induced, which is either resistant to antiarrhythmic drug therapy, or the patient is intolerant or noncompliant to such treatment. Table 1 summarizes all current indications for ICD therapy.

Contraindications

Patients With Cardiac Arrest or Ventricular Tachycardia Due to Reversible Triggering Factors

Every potential ICD recipient should undergo extensive noninvasive and invasive evaluation, as discussed in Chapter 14. Potentially reversible triggering factors that are important to the genesis of VT and VF need to be excluded before ICD implantation is considered. Patients in whom such factors are identified usually have no ventricular arrhythmias induced in the electrophysiology laboratory and can be effectively managed without the use of antiarrhythmic treatment.[30]

Ventricular tachyarrhythmias associated with acute myocardial infarction are a common example of transient or reversible etiology. Clinical decision making, however, can sometimes be problematic, because many cardiac arrest patients have secondary myocardial injury. Electrolyte abnormalities (eg, severe hypokalemia) or

---

Table 1
Indications for ICD Therapy

Class I
1) One or more episodes of spontaneous sustained VT or VF in a patient in whom electrophysiologic testing and/or spontaneous ventricular arrhythmias cannot be used accurately to predict the efficacy of other therapies.
2) Recurrent episodes of spontaneous sustained VT or VF in a patient despite antiarrhythmic drug therapy (guided by electrophysiologic testing or noninvasive methods).
3) Spontaneous sustained VT or VF in a patient in whom antiarrhythmic drug therapy is limited by intolerance or noncompliance.
4) Persistent inducibility of clinically relevant sustained VT or VF at electrophysiologic study, on best available drug therapy or despite surgical/catheter ablation, in a patient with spontaneous sustained VT or VF.

Class II
Syncope of undetermined etiology in a patient with clinically relevant sustained VT or VF induced at electrophysiologic study in whom antiarrhythmic drug therapy is limited by inefficacy, intolerance, or noncompliance.

Table 2
Contraindications for ICD Therapy

1) Sustained VT or VF mediated by acute ischemia/infarction or toxic/metabolic etiology amenable to correction or reversibility.
2) Recurrent syncope of undetermined etiology in a patient without inducible sustained ventricular tachyarrhythmias.
3) Incessant VT or VF
4) VF secondary to atrial fibrillation in Wolff-Parkinson-White syndrome, in a patient whose bypass tract is amenable to surgical or catheter ablation.
5) Surgical, medical, or psychiatric contraindications.

evidence of toxic or metabolic causes need to be excluded during baseline evaluation. Finally, patients with Wolff-Parkinson-White syndrome, who present with VF secondary to atrial fibrillation should not be treated with an ICD if their bypass tract is amenable to surgical or catheter ablation (Table 2).

Other Conditions

Incessant VT or frequent runs of nonsustained VT that cannot be controlled by pharmacological treatment may cause excessive device activation and, therefore, constitute a relative contraindication to device implantation. Device therapy should also be avoided in patients with supraventricular tachycardia or atrial fibrillation with a fast ventricular response, especially if uncontrolled with medical treatment. Radiofrequency ablation of the atrioventricular conduction system is a therapeutic alternative; in third-generation ICD devices, on-demand ventricular pacing is available and can be activated after ablation. However, in patients requiring dual-chamber pacing, additional implantation of a pacemaker will be required; in these patients, specific attention to avoid adverse device-device interactions is necessary. Patients with VT or VF and severe concurrent illnesses that are expected to limit their survival to < 6 months are not suitable candidates for ICD therapy.

Significant behavioral changes such as anxiety neurosis, device dependence, or social withdrawal have been described in ICD patients.[31] Therefore, ICD therapy should be used very cautiously in psychologically unstable patients, such as patients with severe anxiety disorders, uncontrolled depression, or substance abuse (Table 2).

Implantable Cardioverter-Defibrillator Therapy in Specific Disease States

The ICD patient population consists mainly of coronary artery disease patients and patients with dilated cardiomyopathy. Other diagnoses, such as hypertrophic cardiomyopathy, valvular heart disease (usually associated with ventricular hypertrophy or dilatation), long QT syndrome, mitral valve prolapse, arrhythmogenic right ventricular dysplasia, sarcoidosis, etc., are much less common. In Central and South America, chronic Chagasic myocarditis is an important cause of sustained VT.[32] No apparent structural heart disease can be found in approximately 10% of patients with sustained VT.[7,8] Although the etiology of VT may have an important impact on prognosis,[33,34] it is not clear whether the underlying diagnosis bears any relationship to the clinical decision to implant an ICD. Therefore, the guidelines issued by both AHA/ACC and NASPE do not relate the results of electrophysiologic study to the underlying heart disease.

Patients With Coronary Artery Disease

These patients constitute the vast majority of ICD recipients, ranging from 70% to 80% in most series.[11–14] Most of these patients have a history of previous myocardial infarction and compromised left ventricular function. The scarred myocardium appears to provide the substrate for reentrant ventricular tachyarrhythmias and sudden death in the absence of further acute myocardial ischemia.[35] Risk stratification techniques identify high-risk patients after a myocardial infarction, who are most likely to benefit from antiarrhythmic treatment.[36]

The optimal pharmacological treatment of coronary artery disease patients with ventricular tachyarrhythmias remains controversial. With increasing scepticism focusing on the potential proarrhythmic effects of long-term antiarrhythmic therapy,[37] the use of nonpharmacological therapy is expected to increase.

Dilated Cardiomyopathy

Dilated cardiomyopathy is frequently associated with ventricular tachyarrhythmias and an increased risk of sudden death.[38] It has been shown that the results of primary electrophysiologic study, as well as serial drug testing are less reliable in these patients.[39] Cardiac arrest in a patient with dilated cardiomyopathy now constitutes an indication for ICD implantation due to the inefficacy or unreliability of drug therapy.

The Long QT Syndrome

The long QT syndrome is characterized by a predisposition to malignant ventricular arrhythmias. These arrhythmias are characterized by the rapid polymorphic configuration known as torsade de pointes, which can cause syncope or may degenerate into VF. If treatment with β blockers, and/or permanent pacing[40-42] fails to prevent recurrent syncope, left-sided stellate ganglionectomy or implantation of an ICD system should be considered.[43]

Mitral Valve Prolapse

Mitral valve prolapse is frequently associated with ventricular arrhythmias. Although these arrhythmias generally carry a benign prognosis, sudden death has been described in some patients. Malignant ventricular tachyarrhythmias can occasionally be induced by programmed stimulation, although their prognostic significance is unclear.[44,45] In patients who have experienced cardiac arrest or have symptomatic sustained VT refractory to antiarrhythmic drugs, however, implantation of an ICD can be considered.

Hypertrophic Cardiomyopathy

Hypertrophic cardiomyopathy is frequently associated with malignant ventricular arrhythmias that may lead to syncope or sudden death.[46] This mode of death may occur in previously asymptomatic individuals or in patients with an otherwise stable course.[47] β-adrenoceptor blockade or calcium antagonists are frequently used in the treatment of this condition, although their protective effect from sudden cardiac death has not been definitively established. Amiodarone has been reported to be effective in suppressing ventricular tachyarrhythmias and early data suggest that it may be effective in preventing sudden death.[48]

High-risk patients are identified by clinical history and invasive and noninvasive diagnostic methods. These include patients with a history of cardiac arrest or syncope, inducible VT at electrophysiologic study, spontaneous VT on Holter monitoring, or a family history of sudden death. Such individuals should be considered for ICD therapy in conjunction with pharmacological treatment.[49]

Arrhythmogenic Right Ventricular Dysplasia

Arrhythmogenic right ventricular dysplasia can be an important cause of ventricular arrhythmias in children and young adults with an apparently normal heart, as well as in some older patients.[50] In patients with drug-refractory ventricular arrhythmias, life-threatening recurrences are common; in such patients, ICD treatment is safe and effective and may improve long-term prognosis.[51]

Discussion

How Does the Presenting Arrhythmia Affect Clinical Decision Making?

The clinical presentation of the potential ICD patient varies widely and can range between resuscitated cardiac arrest and sustained VT associated with presyncope or syncope. In coronary artery disease patients, the cardiac arrest population appears to have higher recurrent sudden death and total mortality rates, compared to patients with sustained VT.[52,53] Despite these differences, both groups are considered to be at high risk for sudden death.

There is evidence to suggest that, in selected patients with coronary artery disease and VF, surgical coronary revascularization may abolish inducible arrhythmias, with good long-term prognosis.[54] In patients with stable monomorphic VT, coronary revascularization has little effect on the spontaneous or induced arrhythmia. Although concomitant ICD implantation in every patient with VT or VF who undergoes revascularization surgery has been suggested,[55] at present, there are no firm data to support such an indication.

What Consists Failure of Alternative Therapies?

Considerable variation exists among different institutions, regarding the definition of noninducibility on drug restudy, or the number of drug trials required. Recent reports confirm the clinical impression that finding a successful drug after two or three unsuccessful drug trials is minimal.[56] Our current practice is to consider ICD implantation in a patient in whom two agents of different antiarrhythmic classes have been proven unsuccessful. Other alternative approaches to ICD implantation would include catheter ablation or VT surgery.

Some success has been observed in patients without coronary artery disease, such as in patients with automatic ventricular arrhythmias, or in ablation of the right bundle branch in patients with bundle branch reentry. However, catheter ablation of VT has been associated with limited success rates in patients with coronary artery disease.[57–59]

Ventricular tachycardia surgery presents a more "curative" form of therapy. Its feasibility, however, in a large number of patients is limited by the need for careful patient selection and the requirement for highly specialized equipment and personnel; as a result, this form of therapy is now being used with decreasing frequency.[60,61] It has been most successful in patients with coronary artery disease and inducible monomorphic VT. The arrhythmia has to be hemodynamically tolerated during pre- and intraoperative mapping. Patients undergoing VT surgery usually have a discrete left ventricular aneurysm and/or clinical indications for revascularization surgery. Intraoperative map-guided subendocardial resection, cryoablation, or laser ablation is performed.[62–64] In patients with multiple VT configurations, when intraoperative mapping is considered unsatisfactory, or, in general, in patients thought to be at risk for postoperative VT recurrences, prophylactic epicardial patches can be considered.[65]

Implantable Cardioverter-Defibrillator or Class III Antiarrhythmic Agents?

Sotalol, an antiarrhythmic agent with both Class II and Class III properties, was recently approved by the FDA for clinical use. Clinical experience shows that this drug is well tolerated and effective in selected patients, particularly in those, who demonstrate suppression of VT induction in the electrophysiology laboratory.[66] However, direct comparison between treatment with this agent and ICD therapy is lacking.

Similarly, the role of amiodarone is not

well clarified. Such treatment may favorably alter the prognosis of survivors of cardiac arrest,[67] or even of lower risk patients such as survivors of an acute myocardial infarction.[68] However, to date, there are no firm data comparing ICD treatment with amiodarone therapy. In an attempt to provide controlled data two groups[69,70] have conducted retrospective studies that matched patients who received ICDs with similar patients who received amiodarone without ICD treatment. From these studies, it appears that ICD patients have a significantly lower sudden cardiac death, although the effect of such treatment on total mortality may be much less pronounced. However, because neither of these trials were randomized, it is possible that factors not examined or recognized by the authors could have differentially affected the comparisons. Therefore, a number of prospective randomized clinical trials are in progress.[71] In the Canadian Implantable Defibrillator Study (CIDS), patients with VF arrest or sustained VT with syncope are randomized to amiodarone or ICD therapy. This study started screening patients in the fall of 1990 and the enrollment period will be approximately 4 years.

The Cardiac Arrest Study of Hamburg (CASH) trial screens patients admitted to hospitals in Hamburg, Germany. Patients with cardiac arrest and inducible VT or VF are randomized to ICD treatment or one of three drug treatments each with a different mechanism of action: propafenone, metoprolol, or amiodarone. Preliminary interim analysis[72] showed no significant differences among the populations treated with amiodarone, metoprolol, or ICD. A significantly higher cardiac arrest recurrence and total mortality was found in the propafenone arm, when compared to the ICD arm. As a result, the propafenone arm was discontinued after 11 months of follow-up.

A large-scale prospective clinical trial (Antiarrhythmics Versus Implantable Defibrillators [AVID]), coordinated by the National Institutes of Health is now under way and it randomly assigns patients to ICD therapy or one of two antiarrhythmic drugs (sotalol or amiodarone). Total mortality, sudden death and other cardiovascular events as well as quality of life will be the end points.

How Does the Status of Left Ventricular Function Affect Clinical Decision Making?

In patients with ventricular tachyarrhythmias, depressed left ventricular function is associated with high sudden death rates and cardiac mortality. Thus, left ventricular function is one of the most important clinical variables that predicts survival in these patients.[5,6,28] Furthermore, patients with different underlying diagnoses, but similar degree of left ventricular dysfunction, have comparable incidences of device utilization, sudden death rates, and total mortality.[73] Identification of effective antiarrhythmic drugs is reduced in the presence of a low ejection fraction. In addition, such patients even on electrophysiologically guided antiarrhythmic treatment, continue to be at higher risk for recurrent sudden death.[74] Thus, it may be justified to attempt more extensive drug testing in the higher (> 40%) ejection fraction population, but ICD therapy may be favored in patients with lower (< 25%) ejection fraction.[75,76]

Concurrent Illnesses

Severe concurrent illnesses, that significantly shorten prognosis are considered a contraindication to ICD treatment (Table 2). Medical conditions, such as chronic obstructive pulmonary disease, chronic renal failure, or very poor left ventricular function[77] increase perioperative mortality and, therefore, constitute relative contraindications. In addition, the risk of device infection is higher in diabetic patients. However, implantation of an ICD using a nonthoracotomy lead system lowers perioperative mortality significantly,[78] and is expected to become the procedure of choice in such high-risk patients.

Implantable Cardioverter-Defibrillators in Elderly Patients?

Although a higher perioperative mortality can be expected in elderly patients, it seems likely that this may not be related to the ICD implantation procedure, but rather to a higher rate of concomitant surgery (revascularization surgery or subendocardial resection). Complications due to ICD implantation per se have been reported to be similar in elderly and younger patients.[79] Furthermore, the benefit in prevention of sudden cardiac death appears comparable in the elderly and younger population.[79] As a result, current indications do not discuss age limitations for ICD implantation; decision making has to be individualized and take into account the entire clinical picture as well as socio-economic aspects.

Impact of New Technology on Implantable Cardioverter-Defibrillator Indications

Implantable cardioverter-defibrillator systems constitute an area of continuous clinical and experimental research. In the future, considerable improvements in technology can be expected to greatly improve implantation procedures, performance and follow-up of ICD devices. Such improvements are anticipated to make ICD therapy more attractive and widely applicable.[80]

Nonthoracotomy lead systems reduce perioperative implant risk and increase patient acceptance. With the use of tiered therapy, the number of shocks will be reduced. This will reduce psychological distress from frequent shocks and could prolong battery life. Biphasic shocks, present in fourth-generation devices, have been shown to be a more effective waveform[81] and thus permit nonthoracotomy implantation in patients with high defibrillation thresholds. Continuing improvement of implantation techniques may produce a more acceptable cosmetic result.[82] More importantly, the new technological advances are anticipated to lower the energy required for defibrillation; this would lead to smaller capacitor and generator size. Pectoral implantation can then be used, enhancing patient acceptance and simplifying surgical implant procedures.[80]

Possible Future Expansion of Implantable Cardioverter-Defibrillator Indications

Implantable Cardioverter-Defibrillators for Primary Prevention of Sudden Death

Currently, implantation of an ICD is indicated only in patients who have had either cardiac arrest or sustained VT. However, there is a large category of patients who have not experienced such an event, but are believed to be at a high risk in the future. Such patients have poor left ventricular function and/or electrical instability, as evidenced by runs of nonsustained VT.[83,84] In these patients, opinions differ as to whether prophylactic antiarrhythmic treatment is warranted. Nonetheless, it seems that patients with spontaneous nonsustained VT and inducible sustained VT at electrophysiologic study are at high risk for future events.[85] Three trials are now in progress,[71] comparing prophylactic ICD placement with conventional therapy in such patients. These trials are the Multicenter Automatic Defibrillator Implantation Trial (MADIT), the Multicenter Unsustained Tachycardia Trial (MUSTT), and the CABG- PATCH study. These trials will provide information whether ICD therapy is beneficial in asymptomatic "high-risk" patients.

References

1. Gillum RF: Sudden coronary death in the United States: 1980–1985. *Circulation* 79:756, 1989.
2. Pantridge JF, Geddes JS: A mobile intensive-care unit in the management of myocardial infarction. *Lancet* 2:271, 1967.
3. Cobb LA, Conn RD, Samson WE, et al: Prehospital coronary care: the role of a rapid response mobile intensive coronary care system. *Circulation* 43(suppl II):139, 1971.
4. Cobb A, Hallstrom AP: Community-based cardiopulmonary resuscitation: what have we learned? *Ann NY Acad Sci* 382:330, 1982.
5. Baum RS, Alvarez H III, Cobb LA: Survival after resuscitation from out-of-hospital ventricular fibrillation. *Circulation* 50:1231, 1974.
6. Cobb LA, Baum RS, Alvarez H III, et al: Resuscitation from out-of-hospital ventricular fibrillation: 4 years follow-up. *Circulation* 51:223, 1975.
7. Spielman SR, Schwartz JS, McCarthy DM, et al: Predictors of the success or failure of medical therapy in patients with chronic recurrent sustained ventricular tachycardia: a discriminant analysis. *J Am Coll Cardiol* 1:401, 1983.
8. Swerdlow CD, Gong G, Echt DS, et al: Clinical factors predicting successful electrophysiologic-pharmacologic study in patients with ventricular tachycardia. *J Am Coll Cardiol* 1:409, 1983.
9. Rae AP, Greenspan AM, Spielman SR, et al: Antiarrhythmic drug efficacy for ventricular tachyarrhythmias associated with coronary artery disease as assessed by electrophysiologic studies. *Am J Cardiol* 55:1494, 1985.
10. Hallstrom AP, Cobb LA, Yu BH, et al: An antiarrhythmic drug experience in 941 patients resuscitated from an initial cardiac arrest between 1970 and 1985. *Am J Cardiol* 68:1025, 1991.
11. Thomas AC, Moser SA, Smurka ML, et al: Implantable defibrillation: eight years experience. *PACE* 11:2053, 1988.
12. Winkle RA, Mead RH, Ruder MA, et al: Long-term outcome with automatic implantable cardioverter-defibrillator. *J Am Coll Cardiol* 13:1353, 1989.
13. Fogoros RN, Fielder SB, Elson JJ: The automatic implantable cardioverter-defibrillator in drug-refractory ventricular tachyarrhythmias. *Ann Intern Med* 107:635, 1987.
14. Kelly PA, Cannom DS, Garan H, et al: The automatic implantable cardioverter-defibrillator: efficacy, complications and survival in patients with malignant ventricular arrhythmias. *J Am Coll Cardiol* 11:1278, 1988.
15. Mirowski M, Reid PR, Mower MM, et al: Termination of malignant ventricular arrhythmias with an implanted automatic defibrillator in human beings. *N Engl J Med* 303:322, 1980.
16. US Food and Drug Administration, 50 Fed Reg. 47276, 1985.
17. Lehman MH, Saksena S: Implantable cardioverter defibrillators in cardiovascular practice: report of the Policy Conference of the North American Society of Pacing and Electrophysiology. NASPE policy Conference Committee. *PACE* 14:969, 1991.
18. Dreifus LS, Fisch C, Griffin JC, et al: Guidelines for implantation of cardiac pacemakers and antiarrhythmia devices: a report of the American College of Cardiology/American Heart Association task force on assessment of diagnostic and therapeutic cardiovascular procedures (committee on pacemaker implantation). *J Am Coll Cardiol* 18:1, 1991.
19. Skale BT, Miles EM, Heger JJ, et al: Survivors of cardiac arrest: prevention of recurrence by drug therapy as predicted by electrophysiological testing or electrocardiographic monitoring. *Am J Cardiol* 57:113, 1986.
20. Mitchell LB, Duff HJ, Manyari DE, et al: A randomized clinical trial of the noninvasive and invasive approaches to drug therapy for ventricular tachycardia. *N Engl J Med* 317:1681, 1987.
21. Mason JW, on behalf of the ESVEM (Electrophysiologic Study Versus Electrocardiographic Monitoring) Investigators: A comparison of seven antiarrhythmic drugs in patients with ventricular tachyarrhythmias. *N Engl J Med* (in press).
22. Jelinek MV, Lehrbauer L, Lown B: Antiarrhythmic drug therapy for sporadic ventricular ectopic arrhythmias. *Circulation* 49:659, 1974.
23. Podrid PJ, Schoenberger A, Lown B: Congestive heart failure caused by oral disopyramide. *N Engl J Med* 302:614, 1980.
24. Mason JW. Amiodarone. *N Engl J Med* 316:455, 1987.
25. Herre JM, Sauve MJ, Malone P, et al: Long-term results of amiodarone therapy in patients with recurrent sustained ventricular tachycardia or ventricular fibrillation. *J Am Coll Cardiol* 13:442, 1989.
26. Benditt DG, Benson DW Jr, Klein GJ, et al: Prevention of recurrent cardiac arrest: role of provocative electropharmacologic testing. *J Am Coll Cardiol* 2:418, 1983.
27. Eldar M, Sauve MJ, Scheinmann MM: Electrophysiologic testing and follow-up in pa-

tients with aborted sudden death. *J Am Coll Cardiol* 10:291, 1987.
28. Wilber DJ, Garan H, Finkelstein D, et al: Out-of-hospital cardiac arrest: use of electrophysiologic testing in the prediction of long-term outcome. *N Engl J Med* 318:19, 1988.
29. Crandall BG, Morris CD, Cutler JE, et al: Implantable cardioverter-defibrillator therapy in survivors of out-of-hospital sudden cardiac death without inducible arrhythmias. *J Am Coll Cardiol* 21:1186, 1993.
30. Zheutlin TA, Steinman RT, Mattioni TA, et al: Long-term arrhythmic outcome in survivors of ventricular fibrillation with absence of inducible ventricular tachycardia. *Am J Cardiol* 62:1213, 1988.
31. Fricchione GL, Olson LC, Vlay SC: Psychiatric syndrome in patients with the automatic internal cardioverter defibrillator: anxiety, psychological dependence, abuse and withdrawal. *Am Heart J* 117:1411, 1989.
32. Mendoza I, Camardo J, Moleiro F, et al: Sustained ventricular tachycardia in chronic Chagasic myocarditis: electrophysiologic and pharmacologic characteristics. *Am J Cardiol* 57:423, 1986.
33. Trappe H-J, Brugada P, Talajic M, et al: Prognosis of patients with ventricular tachycardia and ventricular fibrillation: role of underlying etiology. *J Am Coll Cardiol* 12:166, 1988.
34. Brugada P, Talajic M, Smeets J, et al: Risk stratification of patients with ventricular tachycardia or ventricular fibrillation after myocardial infarction: the value of the clinical history. *Eur Heart J* 10:747, 1989.
35. Wit AL, Rosen M: Pathophysiologic mechanisms of cardiac arrhythmias. *Am Heart J* 106:798, 1983.
36. Bigger JT Jr, Steinberg JS: Risk stratification for arrhythmic death after myocardial infarction. In: *Cardiac Pacing and Electrophysiology*. Edited by N El-Sheriff, P Samet. W.B. Saunders Company; 1991, p. 303.
37. Echt DS, Liebson PR, Mitchell LB, et al: Mortality and morbidity in patients receiving encainide, flecainide or placebo. The Cardiac Arrhythmia Suppression Trial. *N Engl J Med* 324:781, 1991.
38. VonOlshausen K, Schafer A, Mehmel HC, et al: Ventricular arrhythmias in idiopathic dilated cardiomyopathy. *Br Heart J* 51:195, 1984.
39. Milner PG, DiMarco JP, Lerman BB: Electrophysiological evaluation of sustained ventricular tachyarrhythmias in idiopathic dilated cardiomyopathy. *PACE* 11:562, 1988.
40. Schwartz PJ, Locati E: The idiopathic long QT syndrome: pathogenetic mechanisms and therapy. *Eur Heart J* 6(suppl D):103, 1985.
41. Schwartz PJ, Locati EH, Moss AJ, et al: Left cardiac sympathetic denervation in the therapy of congenital long QT syndrome. A worldwide report. *Circulation* 84:503, 1991.
42. Eldar M, Griffin JC, Abbott JA, et al: Permanent cardiac pacing in patients with the long QT syndrome. *J Am Coll Cardiol* 10:600, 1987.
43. Leenhardt A, Coumel P, Slama R: Torsade de pointes. *J Cardiovasc Electrophysiol* 3:281, 1992.
44. Rosenthal ME, Hamer A, Gang ES, et al: The yield of programmed ventricular stimulation in mitral valve prolapse patients with ventricular arrhythmias. *Am Heart J* 110:970, 1985.
45. Morady F, Shen E, Bhandari A, et al: Programmed electrical stimulation in mitral valve prolapse: analysis of 36 patients. *Am J Cardiol* 53:135, 1984.
46. Maron BJ, Roberts WC, Edwards JE, et al: Sudden death in patients with hypertrophic cardiomyopathy. Characterization of 26 patients without functional limitation. *Am J Cardiol* 41:803, 1978.
47. Shah PM, Adelman AG, Wigle ED, et al: The natural (and unnatural) history of hypertrophic obstructive cardiomyopathy. *Circ Res* 34/35(suppl II):11, 1974.
48. McKenna WJ, Oakley CM, Krikler DM, et al: Improved survival with amiodarone in patients with hypertrophic cardiomyopathy and ventricular tachycardia. *Br Heart J* 53:412, 1985.
49. Tripodi D, McAreavy D, Epstein ND, et al: Impact of the implantable defibrillator in hypertrophic cardiomyopathy patients at high risk for sudden death. *J Am Coll Cardiol* 21:352A, 1993.
50. Dungan WT, Garson A, Gillette PC Jr: Arrhythmogenic right ventricular dysplasia. A cause of ventricular tachycardia in children with apparently normal hearts. *Am Heart J* 102:745, 1981.
51. Wichter T, Block M, Bocker D, et al: Cardioverter-defibrillator therapy in a high-risk subgroup of patients with arrhythmogenic right ventricular disease. *J Am Coll Cardiol* 21:127A, 1993.
52. Saxon LA, Uretz EF, Denes P: Significance of the clinical presentation in ventricular tachycardia/fibrillation. *Am Heart J* 118:695, 1989.
53. Rodriguez LM, Smeets J, O'Hara GE, et al: Incidence and timing of recurrences of sudden death and ventricular tachycardia during antiarrhythmic drug treatment after myocardial infarction. *Am J Cardiol* 69:1403, 1992.
54. Kelly P, Ruskin JN, Vlahakes GJ, et al: Surgical coronary revascularization in survivors of prehospital cardiac arrest: its effect on in-

ducible ventricular arrhythmias and long-term survival. *J Am Coll Cardiol* 15:267, 1990.
55. The CEDARS Investigators: Comprehensive evaluation of defibrillators and resuscitative shocks (CEDARS) study: does concomitant revascularization surgery affect the incidence of recurrence in survival of sudden death? *J Am Coll Cardiol* 21:278A, 1993.
56. Kavanagh KM, Wyse DG, Duff HJ, et al: Drug therapy for ventricular tachyarrhythmias: how many electropharmacologic trials are appropriate? *J Am Coll Cardiol* 17:391, 1987.
57. Belhassen B, Miller HI, Geller E, et al: Transcatheter electrical shock ablation of ventricular tachycardia. *J Am Coll Cardiol* 7:1347, 1986.
58. Morady F, Scheinman MM, DiCarlo LA, et al: Catheter ablation of ventricular tachycardia with intracardiac shocks: results in 33 patients. *Circulation* 75:1037, 1987.
59. Klein LS, Hue-Teh S, Hackett FK, et al: Radiofrequency catheter ablation of ventricular tachycardia in patients without structural heart disease. *Circulation* 85:1666, 1992.
60. Ostermeyer J, Borggrefe M, Breithardt G, et al: Direct operations for the management of life-threatening ischemic ventricular tachycardia. *J Thorac Cardiovasc Surg* 94:848, 1987.
61. Saksena S, Hussain SM, Wasty N, et al: Long-term efficacy of subendocardial resection in refractory ventricular tachycardia: relationship to site of arrhythmia origin. *Ann Thorac Surg* 42:685, 1986.
62. Horowitz LN, Harken AH, Kastor JA, et al: Ventricular resection guided by epicardial and endocardial mapping for treatment of recurrent ventricular tachycardia. *N Engl J Med* 302:589, 1980.
63. Miller JM, Kienzle MG, Harken AH, et al: Subendocardial resection for ventricular tachycardia: predictors of clinical success. *Circulation* 60:624, 1984.
64. Saksena S: Laser energy for tachycardia ablation. *N Engl J Med* 87:881, 1990.
65. Manolis AS, Rastegar H, Estes NAM III: Prophylactic automatic implantable cardioverter-defibrillator patches in patients at high risk for postoperative ventricular tachyarrhythmias. *J Am Coll Cardiol* 13:1367, 1989.
66. Rancin AC, Smith PN, Hamilton L, et al: Long-term efficacy and tolerance of oral sotalol in patients with drug-refractory ventricular arrhythmias. *J Am Coll Cardiol* 17(Suppl): 32A, 1991.
67. Burkart F, Pfisterer M, Kiowski W, et al: Effect of antiarrhythmic therapy on mortality in survivors of myocardial infarction with asymptomatic complex ventricular arrhythmias: Basel Antiarrhythmic Study of Infarct Survival (BASIS). *J Am Coll Cardiol* 16:1711, 1990.
68. Ceremuzynski L, Kleczar E, Krzeminska-Pakula M, et al: Effect of amiodarone on mortality after myocardial infarction: a double-blind, placebo controlled, pilot study. *J Am Coll Cardiol* 20:1056, 1992.
69. Fogoros RN, Fiedler SB, Elson JJ: The automatic implantable cardioverter-defibrillator in drug-refractory ventricular tachyarrhythmias. *Ann Intern Med* 107:635, 1987.
70. Newman D, Sauve MJ, Herre J, et al: Survival after implantation of the cardioverter defibrillator. *Am J Cardiol* 69:899, 1992.
71. Bigger JT Jr: Future studies with the implantable cardioverter defibrillator. *PACE* 14:883, 1991.
72. Siebels J, Cappato R, Ruppel R, et al: ICD versus drugs in cardiac arrest survivors: preliminary results of the cardiac arrest study Hamburg. *PACE* 16:552, 1993.
73. Lessmeier T, Lehmann M, Fromm B, et al: How does the outcome of implantable cardioverter-defibrillator therapy for ventricular fibrillation survivors compare between patients with idiopathic dilated cardiomyopathy versus coronary artery disease? *PACE* 15:541, 1992.
74. Ip JH, Winters SL, Camunas J, et al: Incidence of sudden cardiac death in patients with sustained ventricular arrhythmias treated with antiarrhythmics versus implantable defibrillator. Role of left ventricular function. *J Am Coll Cardiol* 21:126A, 1993.
75. Kim SG: Management of survivors of cardiac arrest: is electrophysiologic testing obsolete in the era of implantable defibrillators? *J Am Coll Cardiol* 16:756, 1990.
76. Akhtar M, Garan H, Lehmann MH, et al: Sudden cardiac death: management of high-risk patients. *Ann Intern Med* 114:449, 1991.
77. Kim SG, Fisher JD, Choue CW, et al: Influence of left ventricular function on outcome of patients treated with implantable difibrillators. *Circulation* 85:1304, 1992.
78. Saksena S, Mehta D, The PCD Investigators & Participating Institutions: Long-term results of implantable cardioverter- defibrillators using endocardial & epicardial leads: a worldwide experience. *PACE* 15:505, 1992.
79. Manolis AS, Rastegar H, Wang PJ, et al: Implantation of the automatic defibrillator system in elderly and younger patients: comparative results. *J Am Coll Cardiol* 21:212A, 1993.
80. Kolettis TM, Saksena S: Implantable cardioverters defibrillators for prevention of sudden death. *J Arrhythmia Management* Fall:3, 1992.
81. Saksena S, An H, Mehra R, et al: Prospective

comparison of biphasic and monophasic shocks for implantable cardioverter-defibrillators using endocardial leads. *Am J Cardiol* 70:304, 1992.
82. Kolettis TM, Saxena A, Krol RB, et al: Submammary implantation of a cardioverter-defibrillator using a nonthoracotomy lead system. *Am Heart J* (in press).
83. Bigger JT, Weld FM, Rolnitzky LM: Prevalence, characteristics and significance of ventricular tachycardia (three or more complexes) detected with ambulatory electrocardiographic recording in the late hospital phase of acute myocardial infarction. *Am J Cardiol* 43:815, 1981.
84. Bigger JT, Fleiss JL, Kleiger R, et al: The relationships among ventricular arrhythmias, left ventricular dysfunction and mortality in the two years after myocardial infarction. *Circulation* 69:250, 1984.
85. Wilber DJ, Olshansky B, Moran JF, et al: Electrophysiological testing and nonsustained ventricular tachycardia: use and limitations in patients with coronary artery disease and impaired ventricular function. *Circulation* 82:350, 1990.

Chapter 14

Evaluation of a Prospective Patient for Implantable Cardioverter-Defibrillator Therapy

Michael Block and Günter Breithardt

Evaluation of a prospective patient for the implantation of a cardioverter-defibrillator (ICD) should take into account several parameters. Indications for ICD implantation should be clearly established, according to the published guidelines[1,2] (see Chapter 13). Alternative therapies such as antiarrhythmic drugs, catheter ablation, or antitachycardia surgery should be considered.[3] Finally, evaluation should include a general assessment, particularly of the respiratory and the cerebrovascular systems.

Once an ICD implantation is determined to be the therapy of choice, the most appropriate device, lead system, and surgical approach should be chosen. Equally important is the timing of ICD implantation and especially the need for additional cardiac surgery.

Based on the initial evaluation of the arrhythmia history and the results of the noninvasive and electrophysiologic studies performed prior to the ICD implantation, individualized programming of tachycardia detection and therapy can be determined. Careful documentation of historical and clinical data is mandatory, especially for patients presenting with cardiac arrest, syncope, and documented ventricular tachycardia or ventricular fibrillation. Based on this evaluation, the need for additional antiarrhythmic drug therapy,[4] catheter ablation,[3] or cardiac surgery may be decided.

Evaluation of a prospective patient for ICD therapy should yield sufficient information to guide the operative procedure and program the implanted device. A single procedure like the baseline electrophysiologic study might be conducted at a point in time when the implantation of an ICD is still unlikely and serial antiarrhythmic drug testing is being considered. However, at the initial study, information pertinent to the operative procedure (eg, mode of termination of induced ventricular tachycardias by pacing) or programming of the device (eg, fast atrioventricular [AV] conduction time) should be collected.

Major steps in evaluation are shown in Figure 1. Mandatory and optional studies prior to the ICD implantation are shown in Table 1, those that help reduce risk of the implantation in Table 2, and those that yield the information needed for programming of the ICD in Table 3. Tests used to identify noncardiac causes of syncope are not listed in Table 1, but should be considered in pa-

From Singer I, (ed.) Implantable Cardioverter-Defibrillator. Armonk, NY: Futura Publishing Company, Inc.; © 1994.

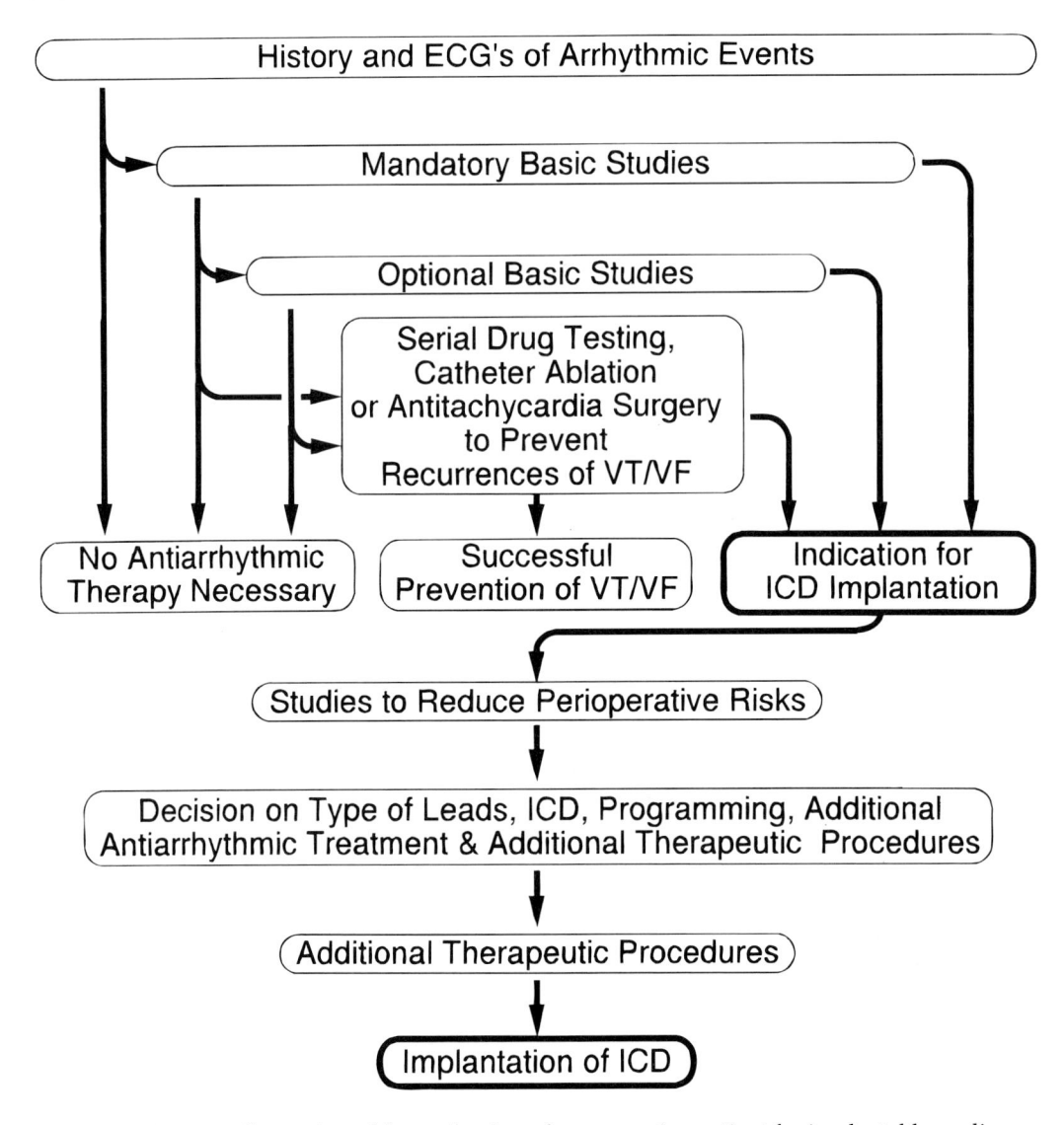

Figure 1. Schematic illustration of the evaluation of a prospective patient for implantable cardioverter-defibrillator (ICD) therapy. ECG: electrocardiogram; VF: ventricular fibrillation; VT: ventricular tachycardia.

tients presenting with syncope with inducible but undocumented spontaneous ventricular tachycardia, in absence of underlying cardiac disease.[5]

Arrhythmia History and Electrocardiograms of Arrhythmic Events

Arrhythmia history should consider the extent of the underlying cardiac disorder, propensity to develop ischemia, the rate and duration of the tachycardia, its hemodynamic stability, and the frequency of arrhythmic episodes. Acute myocardial infarction should be excluded as a cause. Sustained ventricular tachyarrhythmia occurring more than 48–72 hours after the onset of acute myocardial infarction should be considered as chronic arrhythmia.[6]

Anginal symptoms unrelated to exertion, unexpected pulmonary edema, palpi-

Table 1
Tests and Studies that are Mandatory or Optional Before a Decision on ICD Therapy

Mandatory	Optional
ECG at rest	Tilt table test
ECG during exercise	Right heart catheterization
Holter ECG	Myocardial perfusion imaging
Echocardiography	Gated blood pool
Coronary arteriography	Right ventricular angiography and biopsy
Left ventriculography	Magnetic resonance imaging
Electrophysiological study	Tests to identify noncardiac causes of syncope

ECG: electrocardiogram; ICD: implantable cardioverter-defibrillator.

Table 2
Tests and Studies That Help to Reduce the Risks of ICD Implantation

Test or Study	Risk
Ultrasound of subclavian and jugular veins	Thrombosis of the vein used to insert endocardial leads
Carotid artery sonography	Cerebral ischemia during DFT tests
Noninvasive tests of respiratory function	Perioperative pulmonary dysfunction
Tests excluding bleeding disorders	Perioperative bleeding
Exclusion of hidden infections	ICD infection

DFT: defibrillation threshold; ICD: implantable cardioverter-defibrillator.

Table 3
Tests and Studies that Yield Information to Program the ICD

Test or Study	Information
ECG during exercise	Maximal heart rate
Holter ECG	Minimal and maximal heart rate; rate, frequency and duration of runs of SVT and VT
Electrophysiologic study	Rate and hemodynamic consequence of induced VTs; Induced VTs terminated by antitachycardia pacing?
Coronary arteriography	Risk of aggravation of a sustained VT due to myocardial ischemia
Left ventricular angiography	Risk of syncope during a sustained VT due to low EF

ECG: electrocardiogram; EF: left ventricular ejection fraction; ICD: implantable cardioverter-defibrillator; SVT: supraventricular tachycardia; VT: ventricular tachycardia.

tations, or sensation of rapid heartbeat represent diverse symptoms that may be caused by ventricular tachycardia. In some cases, the onset of ventricular tachycardia may be abrupt, causing an immediate circulatory collapse, syncope, or cardiac arrest. The longer the time period between the loss of consciousness and an effective resuscitative intervention, the greater the likelihood that the initial arrhythmia was an organized ventricular tachycardia. The initiating tachyarrhythmia should be differentiated from the tachyarrhythmia seen during hemodynamic collapse,[7] or after the drug intervention, which may modify the morphology or the rate of the tachycardia. Symptoms preceding the arrhythmic event might be absent, sometimes because of the retrograde amnesia following the cardiac arrest. In these circumstances an eyewitness account may be especially helpful.

Analysis of historical clues may be helpful. For example, if a patient experiences syncope without any warning symptoms, an ICD that warns the patient as soon as a tachycardia is detected, eg, by an audible tone, might be useful in avoiding injuries. Palpitations felt by the patient prior to loss of consciousness suggest a slow ventricular tachycardia preceded a fast ventricular tachyarrhythmia. Frequent palpitations outside the documented event might be due to nonsustained ventricular or supraventricular tachycardias. In these patients, only a noncommitted ICD should be considered. Vigorous exercise and/or angina pectoris immediately preceding the arrhythmic event suggest myocardial ischemia as a possible etiology or a contributing factor. In patients presenting with syncope, but without documented ventricular tachyarrhythmias, other causes of syncope should be considered (eg, bradyarrhythmias).

All previous documentation of ventricular tachyarrhythmias should be reviewed. An attempt to document the ventricular tachycardia by a 12-lead ECG is important in order to assess the QRS morphology.[8,9] Spontaneous ventricular tachyarrhythmias should be classified as: 1) ventricular fibrillation; 2) torsade de pointes; 3) fast hemodynamically poorly-tolerated ventricular tachycardia; and 4) slow hemodynamically well-tolerated monomorphic or pleomorphic ventricular tachycardias. Rate and stability of these tachycardias should be determined. Decision as to which ICD to implant and how to program the ICD is partly based on this information. If the primary arrhythmia is a monomorphic ventricular tachycardia, its origin may be mapped and catheter ablation or antitachycardia surgery considered as therapeutic options or alternatives. In case of primary ventricular fibrillation, myocardial ischemia should be considered as a possible cause. If torsade de pointes is documented, careful search for a congenital or acquired (drug-induced) long QT syndrome is indicated.

A list of antiarrhythmic drugs, their dosages, and relationship to the arrhythmic event(s), as well as documentation of drug effect on ventricular arrhythmias (suppression and proarrhythmic events) are all important points in clinical history that help to guide future antiarrhythmic drug selection. Electrolytes measured prior to the arrhythmic event may help rule out electrolyte imbalance as the causative or contributing factor to the arrhythmic event. ECGs recorded before the arrhythmic event might show ST segments or T wave changes indicative of myocardial ischemia or infarction. Recording of these changes after the arrhythmic event may not be as helpful because these changes might be caused by compromised myocardial perfusion secondary to the arrhythmia. Erroneously, an acute myocardial infarction might be diagnosed as the cause of a ventricular tachyarrhthmia if a patient with an anterior wall aneurysm presents with an elevated creatine kinase after external defibrillation.

Resting Electrocardiogram

A 12-lead electrocardiogram (ECG) may reflect the underlying cardiac disorder (previous myocardial infarction), but it may also show nonspecific ST-T changes or be normal. An accessory pathway may be present and identified only intermittently, suggesting relatively long anterograde effective refractory period. In the presence of constant preexcitation, short refractory period of the accessory pathway is likely.[10] If present, catheter ablation of the accessory pathway is indicated. However, even if ventricular fibrillation is unrelated to preexcitation, catheter ablation of the accessory pathway should be performed prior to ICD implantation to avoid inappropriate activation of the device by recurrent AV reciprocating tachycardias.

Diagnosis of congenital long QT syndrome as a cause of ventricular tachyarrhythmias is based on prolonged QT interval recorded on a 12-lead ECG. QT interval prolongation may occur intermittently.[11] Therefore, all available ECGs should be examined, especially those that were recorded immediately before or after the arrhythmic event. If an ICD is implanted for congenital long QT syndrome, additional therapy with β-blocking drugs should be considered.

Electrocardiograms recorded immediately before the arrhythmic event may show signs of transient myocardial ischemia. Coronary artery spasm may cause ischemia-induced ventricular fibrillation, a rare but frequently undiagnosed entity.[12] Relative role of coronary artery spasm as a cause of sudden cardiac death is unknown.

Conduction abnormalities may also cause syncope. Presence of conduction abnormalities may, however, be coincidental and lead to a false conclusion that they are the causative factor of syncope. In patients with syncope and conduction abnormalities, but without documented ventricular arrhythmias, implantation of a permanent pacemaker should be considered. Furthermore, in patients with ventricular tachyarrhythmias conduction abnormalities may limit the use of antiarrhythmic drugs known to prolong the ventricular refractory period, because they may also aggravate the existing conduction abnormalities.

Other diagnoses may be suggested by the 12-lead ECG, eg, right or left ventricular (LV) hypertrophy or hypertrophic cardiomyopathy. However, these diagnoses may be more readily established by other cardiac imaging techniques (eg, two-dimensional echocardiography).

Exercise Electrocardiography

Most candidates for ICD implantation should undergo exercise testing to assess maximal heart rate during exercise, propensity to develop ischemia, and to exclude exercise-induced supraventricular tachyarrhythmias. If myocardial ischemia is identified, revascularization should be considered prior to ICD implantation, to avoid the risk of inducing ischemia during intraoperative testing or subsequent spontaneous episodes of ischemia. Rarely, myocardial ischemia might trigger sustained ventricular tachyarrhythmias during exercise stress testing, indicating that revascularization might be the adequate strategy to prevent recurrences of ventricular tachyarrhythmias.

In patients with exercise-induced ventricular tachycardia without concomitant myocardial ischemia, arrhythmogenic right ventricular cardiomyopathy should be considered as possible etiology. Most commonly, the tachycardia is characterized by left bundle branch block and right axis morphology. There is usually only a small increase in rate when ventricular tachycardia starts during exercise. Similarity in the rates of ventricular and sinus tachycardia may cause problems for tachycardia detection and differentiation for the ICD.

Maximal heart rate during exercise is an important variable to consider in any patient. The work capacity immediately after ICD implantation is usually submaximal. Therefore, maximal heart rate should be determined before ICD implantation. However, since patients are often confined to a monitoring unit for several days prior to ICD implantation, heart rates achieved during exercise testing are still likely to be submaximal. This should be taken into account during predischarge programming and reevaluated at the outpatient clinic visit. If the maximal heart rate overlaps with spontaneous or induced ventricular tachycardia rates, β-blocking drugs and/or programming of the sudden onset detection criterion should be considered.

Holter Recording

Holter recordings are of limited value for the evaluation of prospective patients for ICD implantation because sustained ventricular arrhythmias are rarely recorded during monitoring. Nonsustained ventricular tachycardias are more frequently documented. They may have prognostic value. Nonsustained ventricular tachycardia is currently being evaluated as one of the clinical variables to predict sudden cardiac death in a subset of patients with impaired LV function. Prophylactic ICD indications are currently investigated in the MUSTT and the MADIT trials[13–15] (see Chapter 26).

Holter recordings may yield some useful information for the programming of the

ICD. The maximal heart rate during regular activity or atrial fibrillation fortuitously observed during Holter recording may be comparable to the exercise data. Atrial fibrillation is a common cause of inappropriate shocks.[16] If intermittent atrial fibrillation is detected, antiarrhythmic drugs are prescribed to prevent and/or slow AV conduction during atrial fibrillation. Alternatively, programming of R-R interval stability or sudden onset criteria should be considered.[17,18] Using an ICD without the stability detection criterion should be discouraged in this case, since overlaps in rates during atrial fibrillation and during ventricular tachycardia may cause inappropriate ICD discharges.

Nonsustained episodes of ventricular tachycardia that satisfy the programmed ventricular tachycardia detection criteria may occur so frequently that they initiate detections and result in frequent shocks by committed ICDs, or in case of noncommitted devices cause multiple internal charge dumps leading to premature battery depletion.[19] Frequency of nonsustained ventricular tachycardia episodes influences device selection, programming, and concurrent use of antiarrhythmic drugs. If frequent episodes of ventricular tachycardia cannot be controlled by antiarrhythmic drugs, ICD may be an inappropriate therapeutic choice. In that case, catheter ablation of ventricular tachycardia should be considered before ICD implantation. Detection of nonsustained episodes or sustained supraventricular tachycardia on Holter would cause similar concerns.

Echocardiography

Two-dimensional echocardiography may provide additional diagnostic information. For example, intraventricular thrombus, which would interfere with mapping techniques, may be readily detected by two-dimensional echocardiography or transesophageal echocardiography. Marked myocardial hypertrophy, primary or secondary, is readily detected by echocardiographic techniques. Presence of hypertrophy may alert the physician to anticipate careful fluid management in the preoperative period to maintain adequate preload. In the case of hypertrophic obstructive cardiomyopathy,[20] primary myectomy may be preferred to ICD therapy, based on our recent, although limited experience.[21] Rarely, echocardiographic diagnosis of mitral valve prolapse as an isolated abnormality may be detected in patients presenting with ventricular tachyarrhythmias.[22,23]

Marked dilatation of the right atrium and/or ventricle suggests that selection of a longer distance between the proximal and distal defibrillation coils for a single lead endocardial defibrillation system (Endotak™, CPI, St. Paul, MN) is preferable. In most instances, however, the size of the cardiac chambers and ventricular contractility are best evaluated by contrast angiography.

Coronary Arteriography and Left Ventriculography

Normal contraction pattern and size of the left ventricle associated with high-grade coronary artery stenosis, especially of the left main coronary artery, suggests that the tachyarrhythmic event may be due to myocardial ischemia, amenable to coronary revascularization.[24] If coronary stenosis coexists with abnormal LV function, the cause of the tachyarrhythmic event is more likely to be due to the myocardial scar rather than to primary ischemia. In this case, it is more difficult to establish sufficient evidence that revascularization alone would prevent ventricular tachyarrhythmias. Definite myocardial ischemic zone must be present, which is amenable to complete revascularization. In that case, clinical signs of ischemia should precede the onset of spontaneous ventricular tachyarrhythmia. Ventricular tachycardia that is inducible at the baseline electrophysiologic study would be expected to be noninducible after revascularization if ischemia is the primary mechanism. If these criteria are not met, and especially if ventricular tachycardia remains inducible after revascularization, reentry mechanism related to myocardial scarring is suspected. In these patients ICD should be implanted.[25-27]

Critical narrowing of major coronary arteries supplying the noninfarcted myocardium should be carefully considered for revascularization independent of the occurrence of angina pectoris. During ventricular tachycardia, myocardial ischemia could aggravate arrhythmia, possibly leading to ventricular fibrillation. Revascularization may be accomplished by percutaneous transluminal coronary angioplasty or by surgical coronary revascularization.

Percutaneous transluminal angioplasty may be performed before the ICD implantation. If coronary artery bypass surgery is performed, the standard approach has been to implant an ICD at the end of the bypass procedure while the patient is still on partial cardiopulmonary bypass. Some European centers (including ours, as of July 1991) have changed their approach by performing a two-stage procedure.[28] Implantable cardioverter-defibrillator implantation with nonthoracotomy leads instead of the epicardial approach, is used about 1 week after the coronary artery bypass surgery, when the patient has recovered from the initial operation. This approach is preferred because nearly 100% defibrillation efficacy may be achieved with endocardial leads in combination with the fourth-generation ICDs capable of biphasic waveform defibrillation.[29] Furthermore, epicardial leads may interfere with a subsequent reoperation should this become necessary. Management of a possible ICD infection is also more difficult with the thoracotomy approach. The data from the literature suggest that perioperative mortality for the combined procedures is higher than for the ICD implantation using the endocardial lead systems, following coronary artery bypass graft (CABG) surgery.[30,31] Whether ICD implantation increases the perioperative mortality of the CABG surgery is controversial. Results of the ongoing CABG-PATCH trial will answer this question.[14]

Finally, if the LV angiogram shows a marked anterior wall aneurysm with good contractility of the remaining myocardium, and CABG has to be performed, surgery directed toward the primary cure of ventricular tachycardia (eg, subendocardial resection combined with aneurysmectomy) should be considered as an alternative to the ICD implantation[32,33] (see Chapter 29).

Electrophysiologic Study

The single most important study in the evaluation of a prospective patient for ICD therapy is the electrophysiologic study. Electrophysiologic study should be performed at baseline, without antiarrhythmic drugs. If the patient is already receiving amiodarone, but amiodarone has failed to control ventricular arrhythmias, it should be stopped at least 3 weeks before the evaluation. Amiodarone has been shown to increase intraoperative defibrillation thresholds (DFTs) significantly, and may make ventricular fibrillation hard to terminate.[34] If the patient is in sinus rhythm and not in atrial fibrillation, electrophysiologic study should always include programmed atrial stimulation and assessment of AV and ventriculoatrial (VA) conduction to exclude supraventricular tachycardias as a cause of spontaneous tachyarrhythmias, and concealed accessory pathways as a potential cause of inappropriate ICD discharges.

In the case of fast AV conduction time and rate overlaps between supraventricular tachycardia and ventricular tachycardia, implantation of an ICD with a single tachycardia detection zone without additional detection criteria of R-R interval stability and sudden onset is now obsolete.[17,18,35] Administration of digitalis, verapamil, and/or β-blocking drugs before ICD implantation should be considered. In cases of abnormally slow AV conduction or abnormal sinus node function, ICDs with pacing function should be used.

If a narrow QRS complex tachycardia is inducible, especially if associated with wide QRS complexes, careful consideration of the AV node reentry tachycardia with bundle branch block, AV reciprocating tachycardias, atrial flutter, and other possible etiologies of narrow QRS complex tachycardias must be considered as a potential cause of spontaneous arrhythmic events.[20,36] Discovery of a concealed or manifest accessory pathway conduction during electrophysiologic study requires elicitation of the antegrade conduction properties of the accessory pathway.[10] Evaluation of the conduction time during catecholamines administration is important. If narrow QRS complex tachycardias are induced in addition to the ventricular tachyarrhythmias, their rate and R-R interval stability should be carefully documented and compared to the rate and the R-R intervals of spontaneous and induced ventricular tachycardias. If a rate overlap exists, additional detection criteria such as sudden onset or R-R interval stability might not distinguish narrow QRS complex tachycardias from ventricular tachycardia, since both are generally regular and usually have sudden onset. For AV node reentry and AV reciprocating tachycardias, catheter ablation or antiarrhythmic drug therapy might be considered. Catheter ablation should preferably be performed prior to the ICD implantation, to avoid endocardial lead dislodgment and iatrogenic infection of the leads.

If ventricular tachyarrhythmias are not inducible by programmed ventricular stimulation, the success of antiarrhythmic drugs in preventing recurrences of ventricular tachyarrhythmias cannot be assessed by serial electrophysiologic testing. In that case, ICD therapy is preferred.[37] Additional induction methods such as burst pacing, high-frequency stimulation, or catecholamines administration, might be used to induce ventricular tachyarrhythmia during electrophysiologic study to gain information helpful for selection and programming of the ICD. Especially in patients with arrhythmogenic right ventricular cardiomyopathy, additional induction modes, including catecholamine administration, are frequently required.[38]

If ventricular tachyarrhythmias are inducible by programmed ventricular stimulation, therapeutic interventions to prevent recurrences of ventricular tachyarrhythmias by antiarrhythmic drugs, catheter ablation, and antitachycardia surgery should be considered. During electrophysiologic study, information should be obtained for selection and programming of the ICD. For example, if a slow, hemodynamically well-tolerated ventricular tachycardia is inducible, only ICDs that have antitachycardia pacing (ATP) capabilities and provide additional detection criteria, such as sudden onset and R-R interval stability, should be used.[17,18,35] The rate and stability of the induced ventricular tachycardia may be determined and the efficacy of ATP tested during the electrophysiological study. Instead of suppressing ventricular tachycardias completely, antiarrhythmic drugs may alter their rate, hemodynamic impact, and susceptibility to ATP. Testing of the antiarrhythmic drug effects on the DFT should be delayed until the predischarge ICD test.[4]

Optional Studies

Additional studies may be useful in selected situations. The tilt table test may be used to identify noncardiac causes of syncope.[39] If noninvasive studies, LV angiography, and coronary arteriography do not demonstrate underlying cardiac disease, right ventricular angiography, myocardial biopsy and magnetic resonance imaging should be performed to exclude arrhythmogenic right ventricular cardiomyopathy.[40] This diagnosis should be suspected if exercise-induced ventricular tachycardia or frequent premature ventricular contractions with left bundle branch block pattern and negative T waves in the right precordial leads are present, and/or localized right ventricular contraction abnormalities are noted on two-dimensional echocardiogram.

Right heart catheterization and gated blood pool imaging may be used to assess cardiac performance at rest and during exercise. Poor cardiac performance during exercise may be due to ventricular aneurysm. Presence of normal contractility of the remaining myocardial segments favors map guided antitachycardia surgery combined with aneurysmectomy.[32] Very poor cardiac systolic function (ejection fraction ≤ 20%) associated with generalized LV hypokinesis favors ICD therapy or heart transplantation.

Myocardial perfusion imaging may be used to differentiate hibernating and infarcted myocardium in patients in whom the LV angiogram demonstrates hypokinesis or akinesis, but history and 12-lead ECG do not indicate myocardial infarction. Identification of hibernating myocardium helps identify patients with myocardial ischemia who may be adequately treated by revascularization. In contrast, identification of a large transmural infarction, especially of the anterior wall, supports antitachycardia surgery as an alternative to ICD implantation.

Tests and Studies Required Before the Operative Procedure

Endocardial lead systems are preferred for ICD implantation.[29,41] Because central venous lines are frequently used in critically ill patients, such as those resuscitated from cardiac arrest, thrombosis of the subclavian or jugular veins should be excluded by ultrasound techniques prior to ICD implantation. In rare instances, an angiogram of the superior vena cava and its inflow may be required.

Defibrillation threshold testing may cause prolonged episodes of cerebral ischemia in the anesthetized patient. Doppler sonography of the carotid arteries should be performed in all patients. In case of a severe internal carotid artery stenosis, online electroencephologram monitoring should be performed during DFT testing.[42] If the patient has suffered transient ischemic attacks or strokes, a complete neurological evaluation prior to the surgery is appropriate. If the patient has not shown complete neurological recovery from the preceding cardiac arrest, ICD implantation should be delayed until the neurological deficits have resolved.

Noninvasive tests of respiratory function are of somewhat lesser significance when nonthoracotomy lead systems are used. Patients who have received amiodarone prior to ICD implant require careful evaluation, including measurement of pulmonary diffusing capacity. Some institutions have reported higher incidence of adult respiratory distress syndrome in the immediate postoperative period in these patients.[43] In patients with a limited pulmonary reserve, puncture of the subclavian vein should be avoided, since it may cause pneumothorax. The cephalic vein approach is preferred (see Chapter 15).

Coagulation studies should be routinely obtained prior to any surgical procedures. With nonthoracotomy leads, bleeding may be associated with a subcutaneous patch placement and may cause perioperative morbidity.[44] Pre- and postoperative management of antiplatelet and anticoagulant therapy is controversial. Cessation of aspirin early before implantation is considered mandatory by some investigators, while others use vigorous anticoagulation to avoid thrombi on the endocardial leads while accepting the risk of bleeding.[41,45]

Although exclusion of occult infection prior to the ICD implant is a sound clinical practice, no data are available to show that ICD infections are related to bacteremia from a hidden source rather than from a direct infection acquired during ICD surgery.[44,46,47]

Conclusion

The purpose of the evaluation of a prospective patient for ICD implantation is to assess the need for therapy, elicit data to optimize programming, and assess the role of concomitant or alternative therapeutic modalities. Combination of noninvasive and invasive tests are carefully selected to optimize therapy and minimize cost, thus maximizing the therapeutic benefits of ICD therapy.

References

1. ACC/AHA Task Force: Guidelines for implantation of cardiac pacemakers and antiarrhythmia devices. *J Am Coll Cardiol* 18:1, 1991.
2. Task Force of the Working Groups on Cardiac Arrhythmias and Cardiac Pacing of the European Society of Cardiology: Guidelines for the use of implantable cardioverter defibrillators. *Eur Heart J* 13:1304, 1992.
3. Breithardt G, Borggrefe M, Wietholt D, et al: Role of ventricular tachycardia surgery and catheter ablation as complements or alternatives to the implantable cardioverter defibrillators in the 1990s. *PACE* 15:681, 1992.
4. Block M, Lubienski A, Bocker D, et al: The use of antiarrhythmic drugs in patients with antitachycardia - cardioverter - defibrillator systems. In: *Progress in Clinical Pacing*. Edited by M Santini, M Pistolese, A Alliegro. Mount Kisco, NY: Futura Publishing Company, Inc.; 1993, p. 95.
5. Epstein E, Dailey S, Shepard RB, et al: Inability of the signal-averaged electrocardiogram to determine risk of arrhythmia recurrence in patients with implantable cardioverter defibrillators. *PACE* 14:1169, 1991.
6. Goldberg RJ, Gore JM, Haffajee CI, et al: Outcome after cardiac arrest during acute myocardial infarction. *Am J Cardiol* 59:251, 1987.
7. Bayes-de-Luna A, Torner P, Guindo J, et al: Holter ECG study of ambulatory sudden death. Review of 158 published cases. *New Trends Arrhythmias* 1:293, 1985.
8. Miller JM, Marchlinski FE, Buxton AE, et al: Relationship between the 12-lead electrocardiogram during ventricular tachycardia and endocardial site of origin in patients with coronary artery disease. *Circulation* 77:759, 1988.
9. Coumel P: Diagnostic significance of the QRS wave form in patients with ventricular tachycardia. *Cardiol Clin* 5:527, 1987.
10. Torner-Montoya P, Brugada P, Smeets J, et al: Ventricular fibrillation in the Wolff-Parkinson-White syndrome. *Eur Heart J* 12:144, 1991.
11. Moss AJ, Schwartz PJ, Crampton RS, et al: The long QT syndrome. Prospective longitudinal study of 328 families. *Circulation* 84:1136, 1991.
12. Dubuc M, Lalonde G, Page P, et al: Variant angina and sudden death: use of an implantable defibrillator. *J Electrophysiol* 3:81, 1989.
13. Wilber DJ, Olshansky B, Moran JF, et al: Electrophysiological testing and nonsustained ventricular tachycardia. Use and limitations in patients with coronary artery disease and impaired ventricular function. *Circulation* 82:350, 1990.
14. Moss AJ: Prospective antiarrhythmic studies assessing prophylactic pharmacological and device therapy in high risk coronary patients. *PACE* 15:694, 1992.
15. MADIT Executive Committee: Multicenter automatic defibrillator implantation trial (MADIT): design and clinical protocol. *PACE* 14:920, 1991.
16. Grimm W, Flores B, Marchilinski FE: Complications of implantable cardioverter defibrillator therapy: follow-up of 241 patients. *PACE* 16:218, 1993.
17. Weitholt D, Block M, Isbruch F, et al: Clinical experience with antitachycardia pacing and improved detection algorithms in a new implantable cardioverter defibrillator. *J Am Coll Cardiol* 21:885, 1993.
18. Bardy GH, Troutman C, Poole JE, et al: Clinical experience with a tiered-therapy multiprogrammable antiarrhythmia device. *Circulation* 85:1689, 1992.
19. Saksena S, Poczobutt-Johanos M, Castle LW, et al: Long-term multicenter experience with a second-generation implantable pacemaker-defibrillator in patients with malignant ventricular tachyarrhythmias. *J Am Coll Cardiol* 19:490, 1992.
20. Fananapazir L, Epstein SE: Hemodynamic and electrophysiologic evaluation of patients with hypertrophic cardiomyopathy surviving cardiac arrest. *Am J Cardiol* 67:280, 1991.
21. Borggrefe M, Martinez-Rubio A, Block M, et al: Hypertrophic cardiomyopathy—electrophysiologic findings and management of survivors of cardiac arrest (abstract). *Eur Heart J* 10(Suppl):316, 1989.
22. Corrado D, Thiene G: Sudden death in children and adolescents without apparent heart disease. *New Trends Arrhythmias* 7:209, 1991.
23. Boudoulas H, Schaal SF, Stang JM, et al: Mitral valve prolapse: cardiac arrest with long term survival. *Int J Cardiol* 26:37, 1990.

24. Borggrefe M, Roithinger F, Block M, et al: Effects of myocardial revascularization by either PTCA or bypass surgery on the inducibility of ventricular tachycardia or ventricular fibrillation (abstract). *J Am Coll Cardiol* 19:282A, 1992.
25. Morady F, DiCarlo LA, Krol RB, et al: Role of myocardial ischemia during programmed stimulation in survivors of cardiac arrest with coronary artery disease. *J Am Coll Cardiol* 9:1004, 1987.
26. Kron IL, Lermann BB, Hainer DE, et al: Coronary artery bypass grafting in patients with ventricular fibrillation. *Ann Thorac Surg* 48:85, 1989.
27. Cernaianu AC, Cilley JH, Libby JA, et al: Implantation of a cardioverter-defibrillator after coronary artery bypass surgery. *ASAIO J* 38:M257, 1992.
28. Hammel D, Block M, Konertz W, et al: Implantable cardioverter/defibrillator and open-heart surgery—concomitant surgery or staged procedure using non-thoracotomy lead systems? *Z. Herz-,Thorax-,GefaBchir* 7:12, 1993.
29. Block M, and the European P2 Investigators: Combination of endocardial leads with a new ICD capable of biphasic shocks—first results of a multicenter study (abstract). *PACE* 16:874, 1993.
30. Edel TB, Maloney JD, Moore SL, et al: Analysis of death in patients with an implantable cardioverter/defibrillator. *PACE* 15:60, 1992.
31. Saksena S, and the PCD Investigators and Participating Institutions: Defibrillation thresholds and perioperative mortality associated with endocardial and epicardial defibrillation lead systems. *PACE* 16:202, 1993.
32. Ostermeyer J, Borggrefe M, Breithardt G, et al: Direct operations for the management of life threatening ischemic ventricular tachycardia. *J Thorac Cardiovasc Surg* 6:848, 1987.
33. Selle JG: Definitive surgery for postinfarction ventricular tachycardia. *Coronary Artery Dis* 3:204, 1992.
34. Block M, Hammel D, Isbruch F, et al: High defibrillation thresholds (DFT) with transvenous-subcutaneous defibrillation leads (abstract). *J Am Coll Cardiol* 19:243, 1992.
35. Fromer M, Brachmann J, Block M, et al: Efficacy of automatic multimodal device therapy for ventricular tachyarrhythmias as delivered by a new implantable pacing cardioverter-defibrillator. *Circulation* 86:363, 1992.
36. Wong Y, Scheinman MM, Chien WW, et al: Patients with supraventricular tachycardia presenting with aborted sudden death: incidence, mechanisms and long term follow-up. *J Am Coll Cardiol* 18:1711, 1991.
37. Andresen D, Steinbeck G, Bruggeman T, et al: Inaccurate risk stratification for sudden cardiac death using programmed ventricular stimulation alone. *New Trends Arrhythmias* 8:135, 1992.
38. Wichter T, Borggrefe M, Haverkamp W, et al: Efficacy of antiarrhythmic drugs in patients with arrhythmogenic right ventricular disease. Results in patients with inducible and noninducible ventricular tachycardia. *Circulation* 86:29, 1992.
39. Benditt DG, Asso A, Remole S, et al: Tilt-table testing and syncope. *Curr Opin Cardiol* 7:37, 1992.
40. Breithardt G, Borggrefe M, Wichter T: Catheter ablation of idiopathic right ventricular tachycardia. *Circulation* 82:2273, 1990.
41. Block M, Hammel D, Isbruch F, et al: Results and realistic expectations with transvenous lead systems. *PACE* 15:665, 1992.
42. Singer I, van der Laken J, Edmonds HL, et al: Is defibrillation testing safe? *PACE* 14:1899, 1991.
43. Greenspan AJ, Kidwell GA, Hurley W, et al: Amiodarone-related postoperative adult respiratory distress syndrome. *Circulation* 84:III-407, 1991.
44. Lindemans FW, van Binsbergen E, Conolly D: *Clinical Evaluation Report of the European PCD™ Study—Patients with Transvene™ Lead Systems.* Maastricht: Medtronic Bakken Research Center; 1991.
45. Jung W, Fehske W, Manz M, et al: Incidence of floating vegetations on tranvenous defibrillation leads: impact of anticoagulant therapy (abstract). *PACE* 16:916, 1993.
46. *Clinical Summary Report of the Endotak™ Lead System, Phase II.* St.Paul, MN: Cardiac Pacemakers, Inc., 1992.
47. Bakker PFA, Hauer RNW, Wever EFD: Infections involving implanted cardioverter defibrillator devices. *PACE* 15:654, 1992.

Chapter 15

Operative Techniques for Implantation and Testing of Implantable Cardioverter-Defibrillators

Erle Austin and Igor Singer

Operative Techniques

A variety of techniques for implantable cardioverter-defibrillator (ICD) implantation has evolved since the first successful implant by Mirowski and associates in 1980.[1] Although early conceptions of ICD therapy envisioned total transvenous placement of both sensing and defibrillating electrodes, the success of currently approved devices has relied until recently on the surgical placement of at least one patch electrode directly on the heart or pericardium. The objective of electrode placement is to achieve defibrillation thresholds (DFTs) that are sufficiently low to ensure successful defibrillation with pulses of 30 J or less. Recent improvements in transvenous electrodes have reintroduced the concept of ICD implantation without thoracotomy. Preliminary results from the recent clinical trials evaluating nonthoracotomy approaches are encouraging and will be reviewed, but the epicardial approach must be considered the "gold standard" for ICD implantation against which the endocardial approaches should be compared. Knowledge and familiarity with the various epicardial approaches will always be important for surgeons who are performing implantations and who will undoubtedly encounter patients in whom sufficiently low DFTs can only be achieved by thoracotomy.

The Epicardial Approach

Historically, the first clinical ICD implantations were performed using a median sternotomy or left thoracotomy.[2] While median sternotomy remains the approach of choice for combination open heart surgery and ICD implantation, the subxiphoid and subcostal approaches have been developed to diminish the morbidity of isolated ICD implantation (Figure 1).

Whichever approach is used, the goal is to achieve low DFTs by placing defibrillating patches around the heart. The first clinical implants involved an epicardial cup electrode on the ventricular apex and an intravascular helical spring electrode in the superior vena cava.[2] Subsequent experience with displacement of the superior vena cava electrode and problems with high DFTs lead to the preference for two epicardial patch electrodes.[3] The patches can be placed either inside or outside the pericardium, but most surgeons prefer extrapericardial placement to avoid bleeding from epicar-

From Singer I, (ed.) Implantable Cardioverter-Defibrillator. Armonk, NY: Futura Publishing Company, Inc.; © 1994.

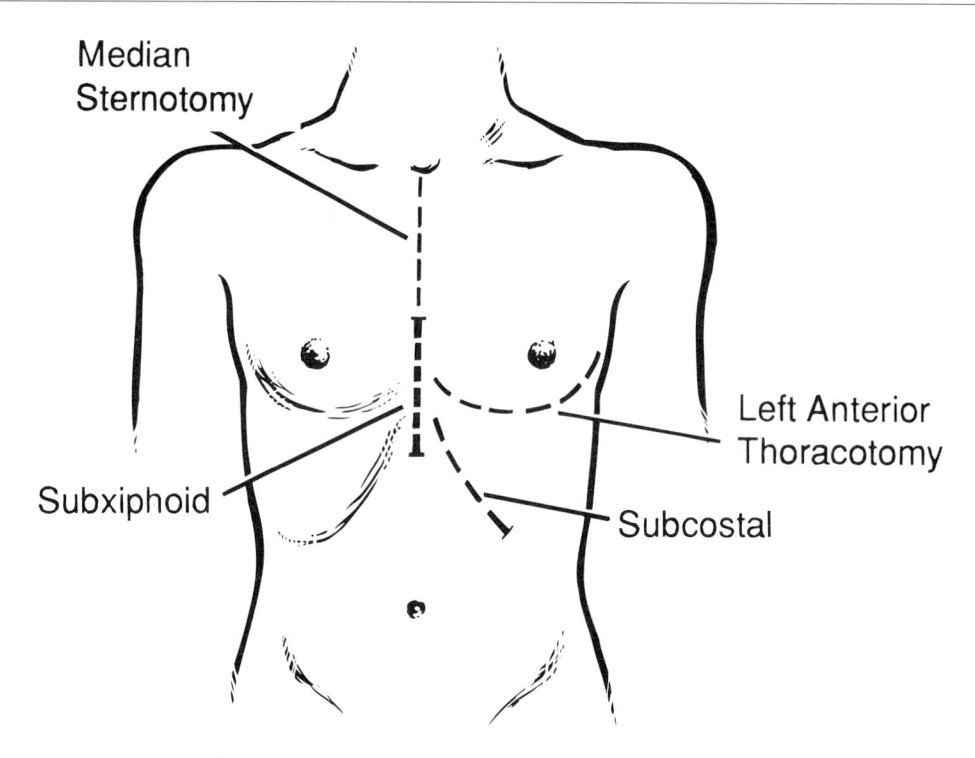

Figure 1. The epicardial approaches for implantable cardioverter-defibrillator (ICD) implantation.

dial blood vessels and to prevent epicardial scarring and adhesions.

The shape of the patches depends on the manufacturer of the ICD device. The greatest experience has been obtained with the rectangular Cardiac Pacemakers, Inc. (CPI) patches (Figure 2), although the oval Medtronic, Inc. (Figure 3), and elliptical Ventritex patches (Figure 4) appear to conform more easily to the cardiac surface. Intermedics, Inc. has developed separate patch electrodes for each ventricle (Figure 5). All manufacturers provide patches in more than one size to allow adjustment to different sized hearts and available surface areas. The objective of patch placement is to encompass as large a surface area as possible with each patch, while at the same time including the largest possible amount of myocardium between the two diametrically opposed patches. The patches, however, should not touch or overlap one another to avoid short circuiting when the pulse is applied. In most cases, the placement of a large patch posteriorly behind the left ventricle and another patch (as large as possible) anteriorly over the right ventricle will achieve a low DFT. Rate sensing leads must also be placed. The epicardial approach for patch lead placement also permits access for the placement of epicardial rate sensing leads. If the patches have been placed outside the pericardium, however, a small incision in the pericardium is necessary to expose viable myocardium. Two sutureless screw-in leads (Figure 2) are placed next to one another and R wave amplitude and pacing thresholds are measured. Because endocardial leads tend to provide better sensing characteristics and long-term performance than epicardial leads, an endocardial lead may be preferable to these epicardial leads. If an endocardial rate sensing lead is used, it is most easily introduced through the left subclavian or cephalic vein and fluoroscopically guided into the right ventricle. After being firmly affixed, the endocardial lead is then subcutaneouly tunneled to the device

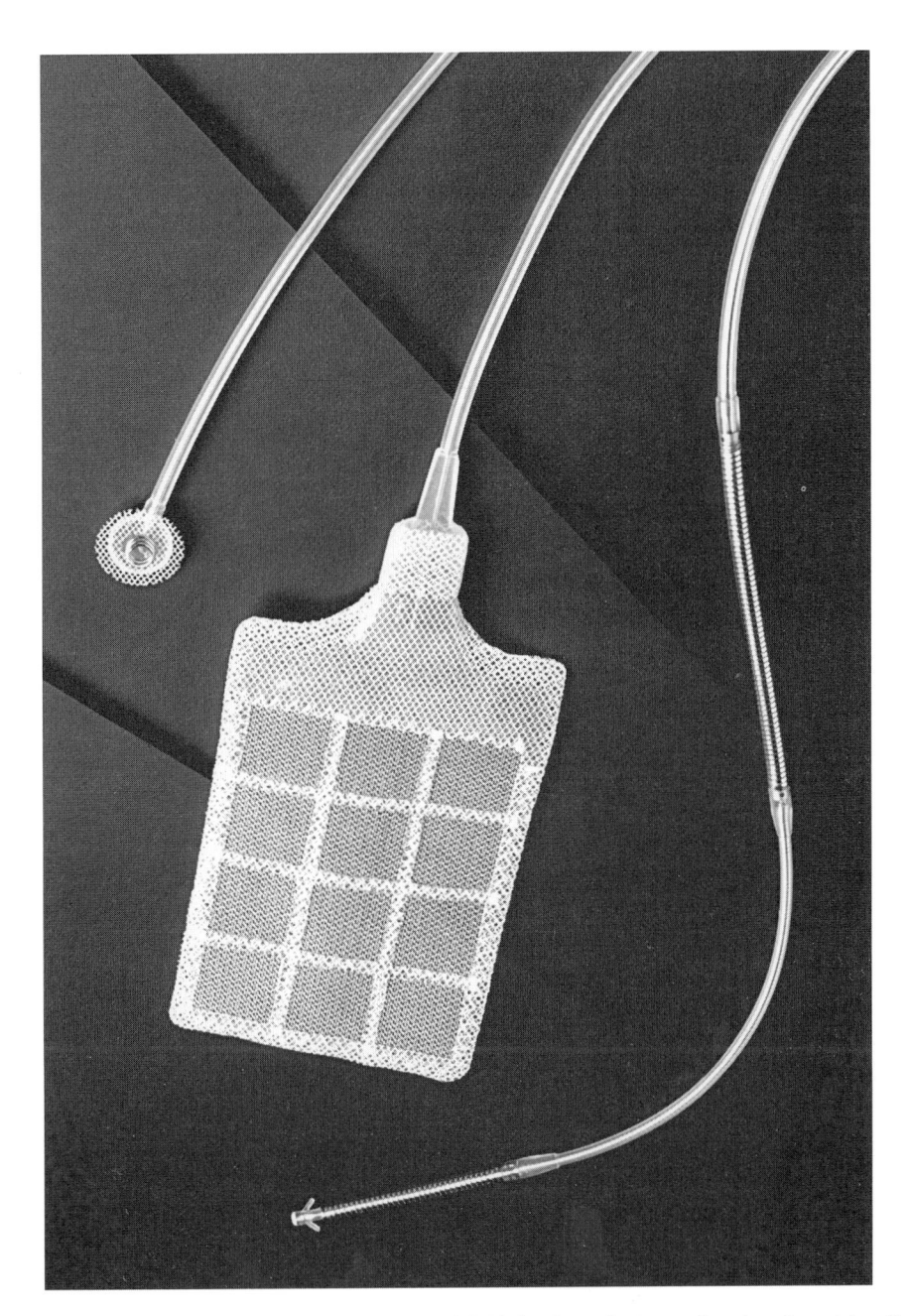

Figure 2. Implantable cardioverter-defibrillator (ICD) leads and electrodes developed by Cardiac Pacemakers, Inc. **Left**: the Endotak-C™ (CPI, St. Paul, MN) transvenous lead. **Center**: a rectangular CPI epicardial patch electrode. **Right**: an epicardial screw-in rate sensing electrode. (Figure courtesy of CPI, Inc., St. Paul, MN.)

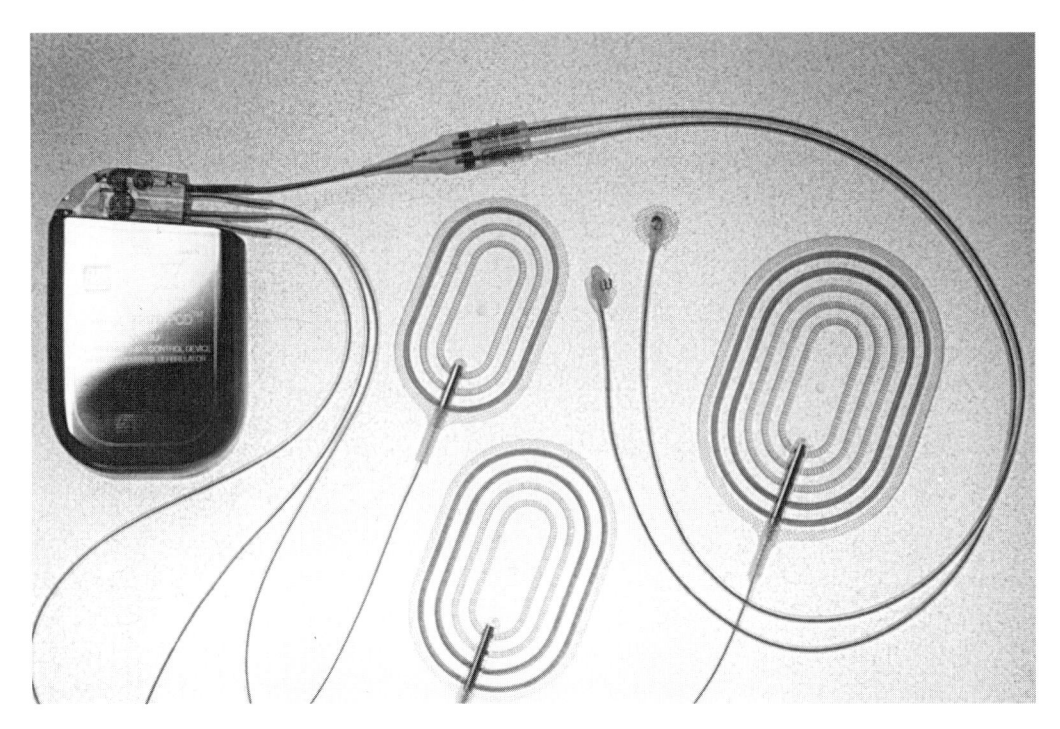

Figure 3. The oval epicardial patch electrodes developed by Medtronic, shown connected to the PCD™ (Medtronic, Minneaplis, MN) device. Also shown are attached epicardial screw-in leads. (Figure courtesy of Medtronic, Inc., Minneapolis, MN.)

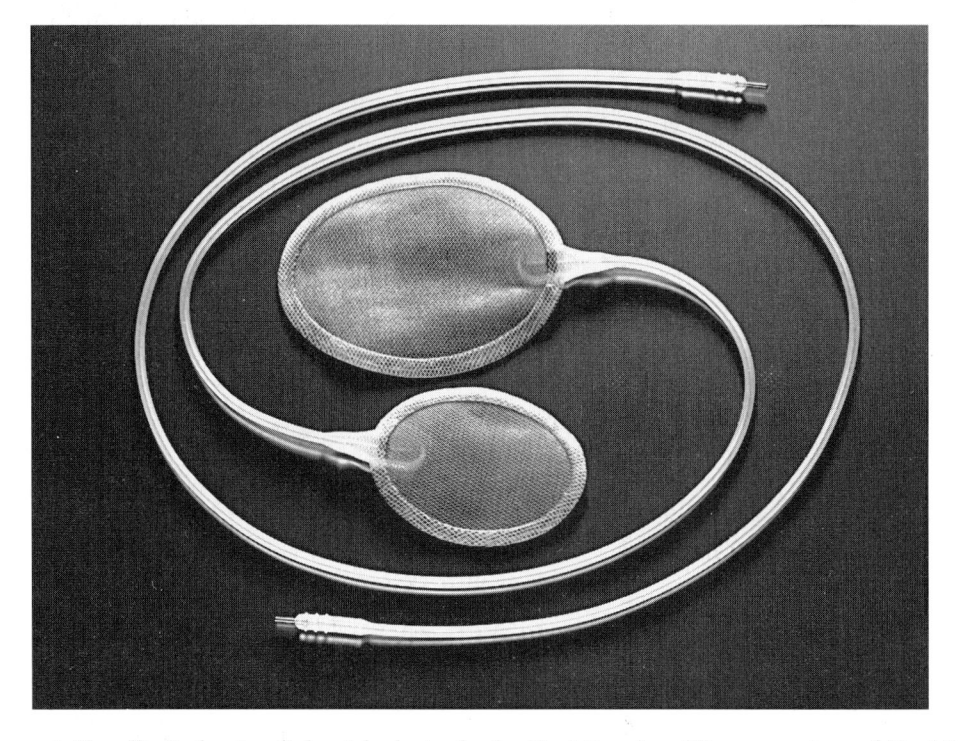

Figure 4. The elliptical epicardial patch electrodes by Ventritex, Inc. (Figure courtesy of Ventritex, Inc., Sunnyvale, CA.)

the internal and external oblique fascia (Figure 6). Subrectus placement is usually less noticeable cosmetically and is more comfortable to the patient than a subcutaneous position. Furthermore, the potential for device extrusion is minimized. The device is positioned at the level of the umbilicus to avoid patient discomfort encountered during bending should the device ride underneath the costal margin or impinge upon the iliac crest. Care must be taken to ensure hemostasis before inserting the device since the formation of a hematoma markedly increases the risk of infection.

These principles of electrode placement and pocket creation are similar for all epicardial approaches. Which approach is used must be chosen by the surgeon performing the implantation based on the need for concomitant cardiac surgery, a history of previous cardiac surgery, and the comfort that the surgeon has with each approach. Although morbidity may be lessened by the more limited subxiphoid or subcostal approaches, the surgeon must be certain that patch positioning and resulting DFT is not compromised by inadequate exposure.

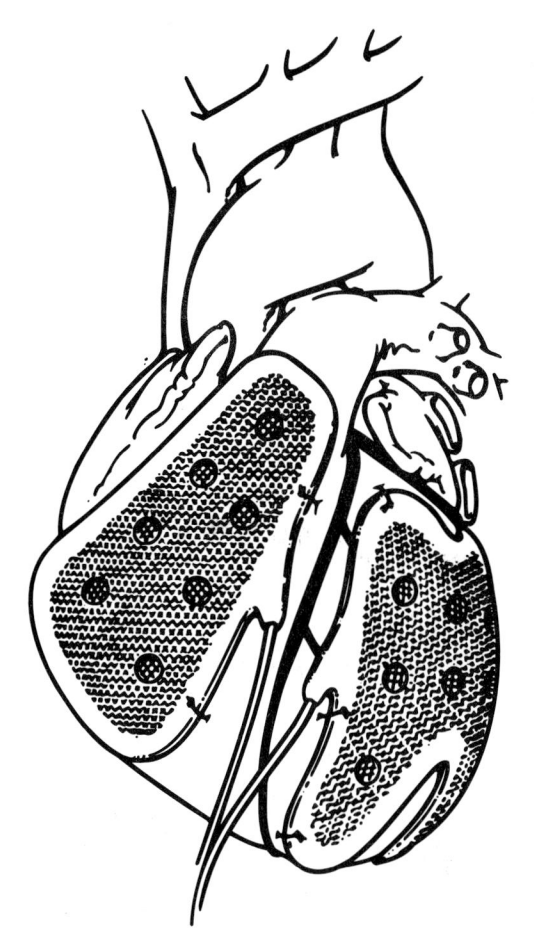

Figure 5. Patch electrodes developed by Intermedics to conform to left ventricular apex and anterior surface of right ventricle. (Figure courtesy of Intermedics, Inc., Angleton, TX.)

Median Sternotomy

Median sternotomy (Figure 7) is commonly used by cardiovascular surgeons because it provides the greatest access to all areas of the heart. For patients undergoing concomitant ICD implantation and open heart procedures such as coronary revascularization, valve replacement, or endocardial resection, median sternotomy is the only suitable choice.

In these cases, placement of defibrillation patches is performed at the conclusion of the cardiac procedure but prior to discontinuing cardiopulmonary bypass. Ideally, two large patches are positioned. The first patch is placed behind the left ventricle outside of the pericardium. Rightward traction of stay sutures placed on the free edge of the opened pericardium will allow exposure of

pocket. Tunneling of leads to the pocket can be performed using any specially designed tunneling instrument, but we have found that a large Crafoord clamp and a 36F chest tube perform this maneuver quite easily.

The significant size of currently available ICD pulse generators limits the number of sites for its implantation. A pocket formed in the left abdominal wall has generally been the preferred site for device placement. Although a subcutaneous pocket may be adequate in patients with a thick layer of adipose tissue, in most cases it is preferable to create a pocket deep to the rectus muscle, extending it laterally beneath

ICD PLACEMENT

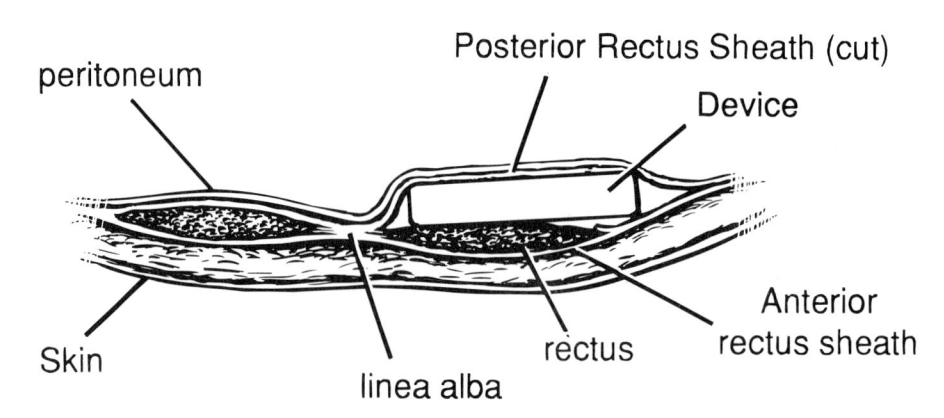

Figure 6. Cross section of abdominal wall demonstrating placement of implantable cardioverter-defibrillator (ICD) device posterior to left rectus abdominis muscle. Size of device usually requires extending pocket laterally beneath confluence of external and internal oblique fascia.

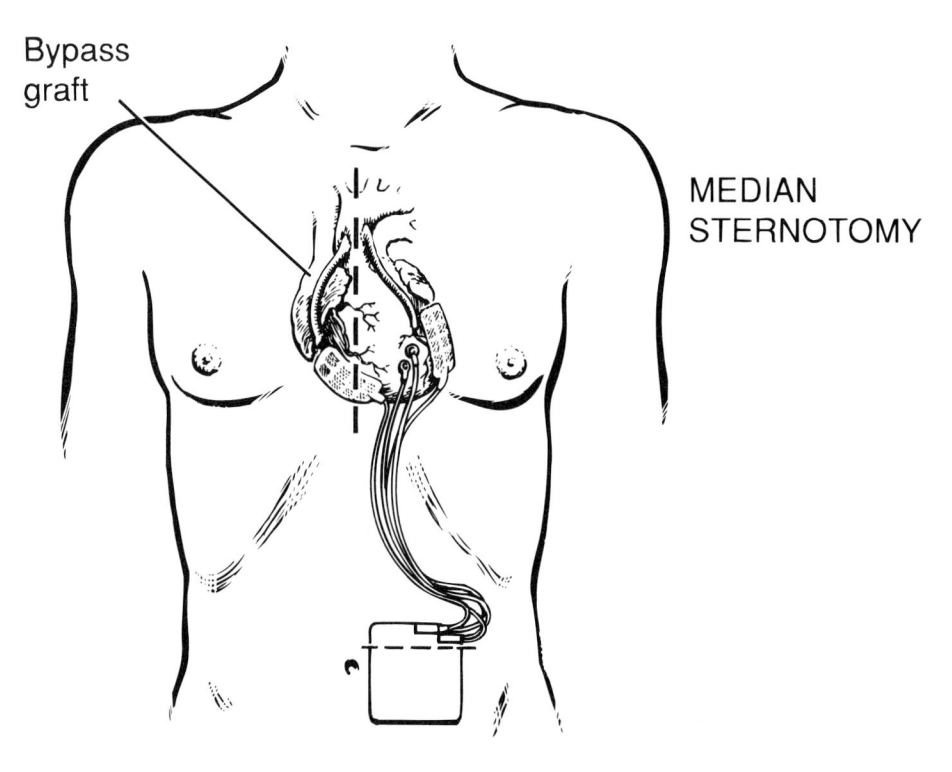

Figure 7. Median sternotomy approach commonly used for concomitant open heart surgery and implantable cardioverter-defibrillator (ICD) implantation.

this posterior pericardial surface. The phrenic nerve and pulmonary hilum are easily visualized. Excision of some pericardial fat often facilitates patch placement. Performing this part of the ICD implantation while on cardiopulmonary bypass permits excellent exposure because the left lung can be deflated and the cardiac apex can be retracted without inducing hemodynamic instability. Four nonabsorbable sutures fix the patch electrode to the pericardium, taking care not to injure the phrenic nerve or underlying vein grafts or coronary vessels. Once the posterior patch has been placed, two rate sensing epicardial electrodes are screwed into the surface of the heart. The inferior aspect of the right ventricle provides an accessible surface that usually is free of coronary vessels. These two electrodes should be placed close to one another to optimize bipolar sensing. A second patch electrode is now placed on the surface of the right ventricle. It is often necessary to use a smaller patch in this position since there is less surface area for attachment. Careful placement of sutures in the epicardium can successfully affix this patch in place. Alternatively, attaching the patch to the inside of the pericardium may be preferable if the epicardium appears friable. By this time, the patient is weaned from cardiopulmonary bypass. Once the heparin is reversed, a pocket is made in the left paraumbilical region and the four electrode leads (two patch and two rate sensing) are tunneled from the mediastinum to the pocket.

Median sternotomy is usually well tolerated and felt to engender less pain than a thoracotomy. Some surgeons prefer this approach even for isolated ICD implantation.[4] Conversely, this approach is avoided in patients that have had previous median sternotomy for cardiac surgery because repeat sternotomy risks injury to underlying cardiac structures or bypass grafts.

Left Anterior Thoracotomy

Left anterior thoracotomy (Figure 8) is the approach most commonly used for patients that have had previous cardiac surgery. Since it provides excellent exposure of both the anterior and posterior surfaces of the heart and pericardium, many surgeons prefer this approach for all ICD placements.[4]

After general anesthesia is induced and a double lumen endotracheal tube is inserted (optional), the patient is positioned almost supine on the operating table. The left chest is elevated 20°–30° by placing a rolled sheet under the left scapula. The left arm is positioned beside the patient. The patient is prepped from the neck to the waist allowing access to both infraclavicular areas to permit placement of transvenous leads. A curvilinear incision is then made in the inframammary crease and the left pleural space is entered through the fifth interspace. The intercostal muscle is incised far posteriorly but the skin incision can be minimized. A large patch electrode can generally be placed extrapericardially over the posterior surface of the left ventricle. Minimal dissection between the pericardium and the sternum permits placement of an anterior patch. In patients that have had previous cardiac surgery, dissection anteriorly must be carefully performed to avoid injuring bypass grafts or inadvertently entering the right ventricle. Should it not be possible to place two separate patches from this approach, a transvenous helical (spring) electrode can be introduced via the left subclavian vein and fluoroscopically guided into the superior vena cava. Satisfactory DFTs can usually be achieved with various combinations of electrode placement with this approach. Rarely, a limited right anterior thoracotomy via the fourth interspace is necessary to provide additional exposure to position a patch electrode on the right side of the heart.

Although the most versatile of incisions for ICD placement, the anterior thoracotomy imposes the most postoperative discomfort. Atelectasis and pleural effusions are common although self-limited. A more lateral approach[5] that avoids dividing the latissimus dorsi muscle may diminish some

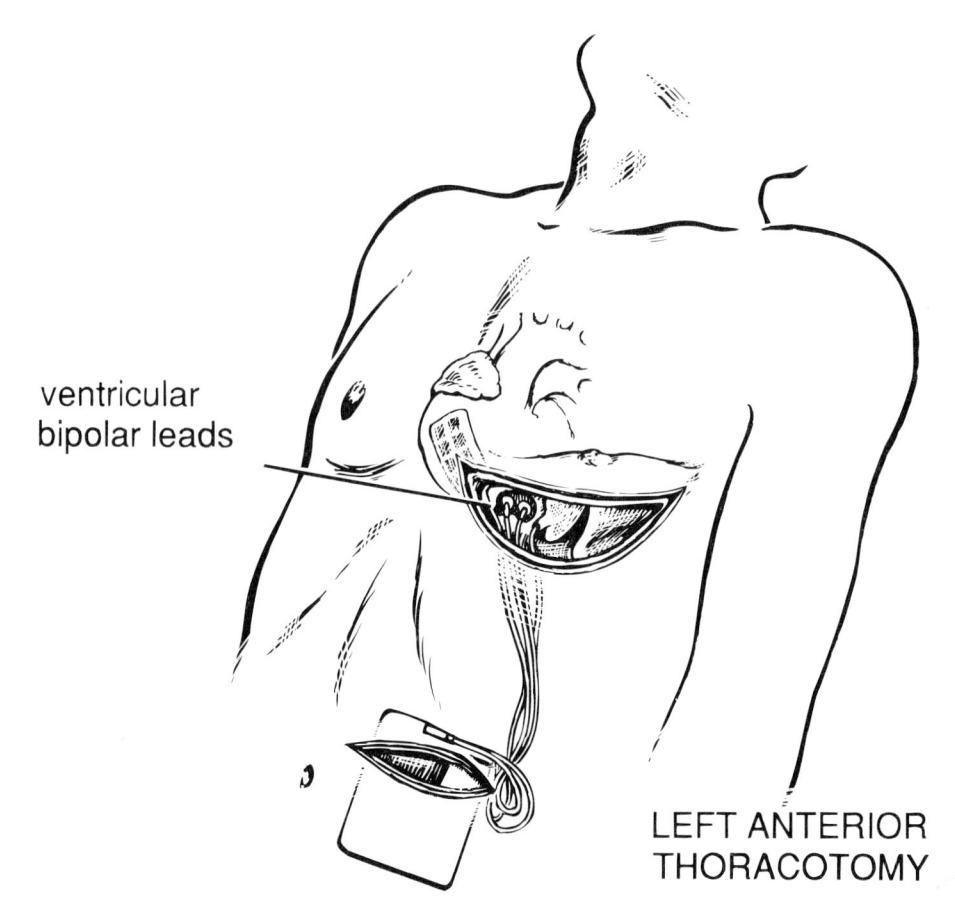

Figure 8. Left anterior thoracotomy provides excellent exposure for implantable cardioverter-defibrillator (ICD) implantation at the expense of increased postoperative pain, atelectasis, and effusion.

of the postoperative pain but transvenous access for inserting rate sensing or additional defibrillation leads is compromised.

The Subxiphoid Approach

The subxiphoid approach (Figure 9) was developed by Watkins and associates[6] to decrease the morbidity of the median sternotomy and thoracotomy approaches. Although this approach has been used successfully in patients after previous coronary bypass surgery,[7] it is primarily reserved for those patients undergoing isolated ICD implantation who have not had and are unlikely to need cardiac surgery.

With the patient in the supine position, a mid-line incision from just above the xiphisternal junction to 5–6 cm caudally is made. The linea alba in incised and the xiphoid is split or excised. The pericardium is identified and incised anteriorly and horizontally as upward traction is placed on the sternum. Through this limited exposure, one patch lead is placed intrapericardially beneath the diaphragmatic surface of the heart near the ventricular apex. A second patch is placed over the right anterior surface of the heart. Both patches are secured by attachment to the pericardium. Epicardial rate sensing leads can also be inserted by this approach. A generator pocket can be fashioned by a subcutaneous or subfascial extension of subxiphoid incision or more commonly created through a separate incision in the left paraumbilical area.

SUBXIPHOID

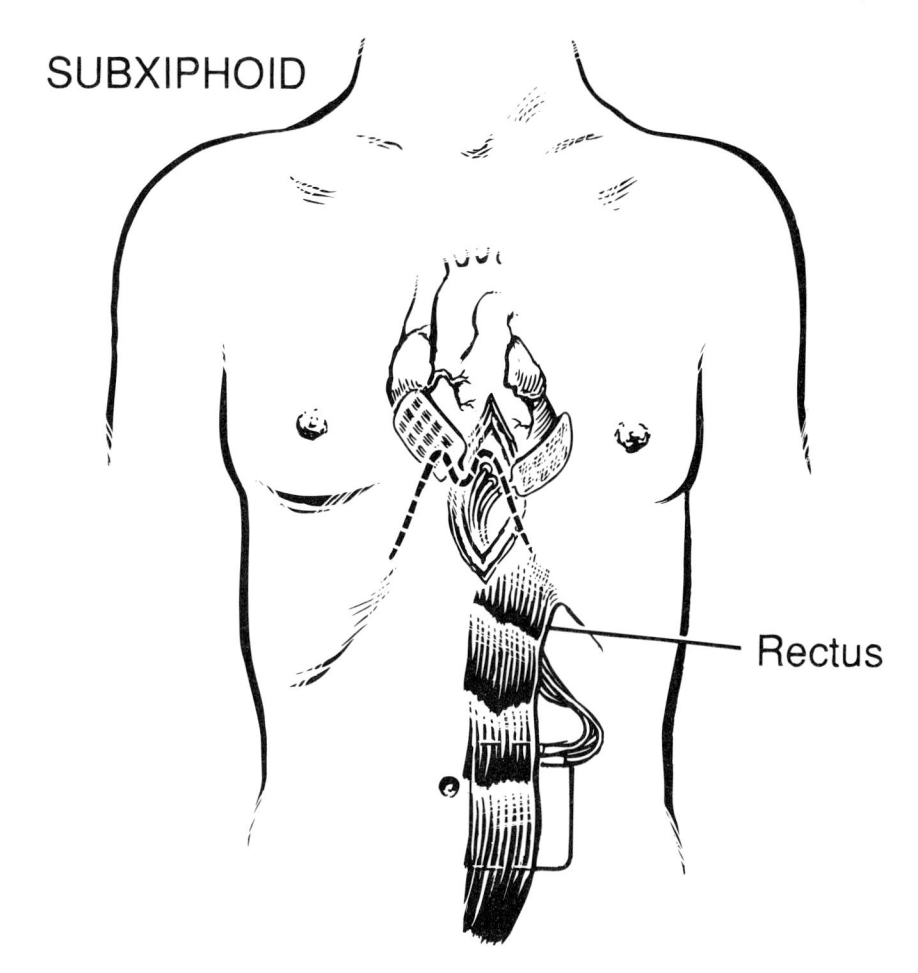

Rectus

Figure 9. Subxiphoid approach minimizes postoperative pulmonary complications, but provides limited exposure.

A recent comparison of the subxiphoid method to median sternotomy or thoracotomy demonstrated a decrease in postoperative hospital stay but a slight increase in DFTs.[8] This approach may well improve postoperative discomfort and morbidity, but many surgeons are uncomfortable with the limited exposure.

Left Subcostal Approach

Like the subxiphoid approach, the left subcostal technique (Figure 10) represents a method originally developed for inserting epicardial pacing leads that has been modified for the implantation of ICD patches. Lawrie and associates[9] have developed and advocated this approach to provide adequate exposure with minimal morbidity.

With the patient supine, a left subcostal incision is performed dividing the rectus muscle but leaving the posterior rectus sheath intact. Blunt dissection directly beneath the costal margin provides exposure of the pericardium. An upper hand retractor placed underneath the costal margin greatly facilitates exposure. Dissection can be extended outside the pericardium permitting extrapericardial placement of patch electrodes in patients with or without previous cardiac surgery. Through the same incision, a subrectus pocket can be made for placement of the pulse generator.

SUBCOSTAL

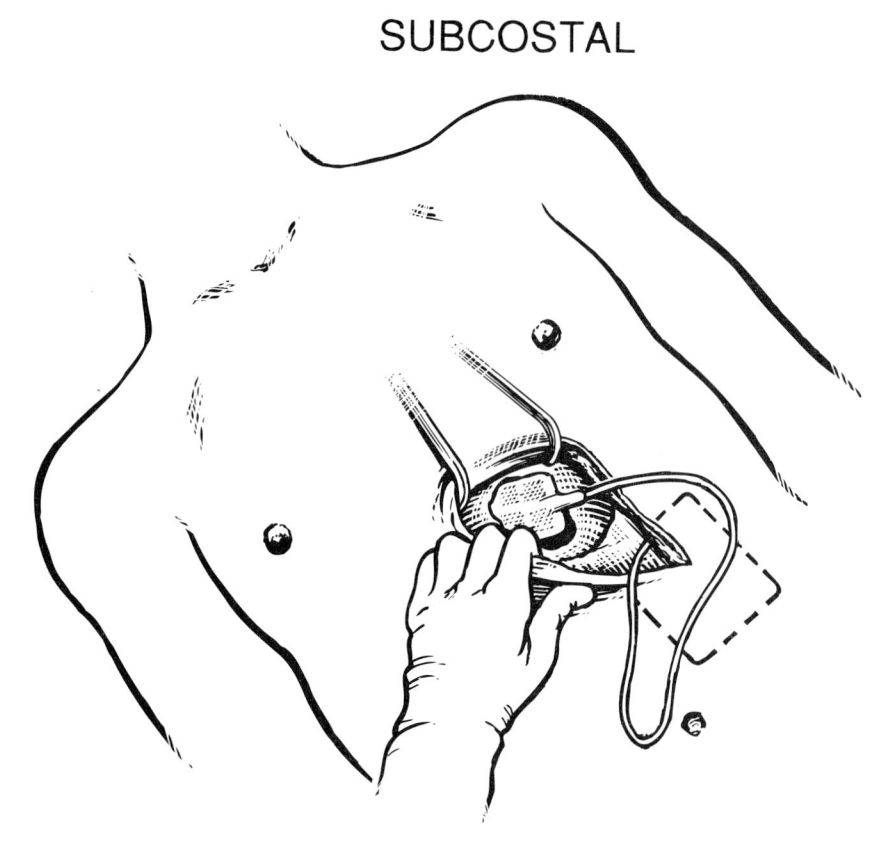

Figure 10. Subcostal approach improves exposure of subxiphoid approach while minimizing pulmonary problems. In addition, implantable cardioverter-defibrillator (ICD) device can be inserted through same incision.

Similar to the subxiphoid method, the left subcostal approach minimizes the pulmonary complications of thoracotomy, but the division of the rectus muscle may increase the postoperative discomfort. Nevertheless, this approach may improve on the limited exposure provided by the subxiphoid technique yet decrease the morbidity that occurs with sternotomy or thoracotomy.

Other Approaches

A transdiaphragmatic approach has been described that entails a longitudinal epigastric extraperitoneal incision with access to the heart through an incision in the central tendon of the diaphragm.[10] This approach is very similar to the subcostal method but does not appear to have many advocates.

Thoracoscopic placement of ICD patches has recently been reported[11,12] (Figure 11). With this technique, the defibrillation patches are introduced into the left pleural space through a very small incision and with thoracoscopic guidance attached to the surface of the pericardium. This approach avoids thoracotomy or sternotomy and may have the lowest morbidity of all epicardial approaches. Until more experience has been obtained with this approach, however, its safety and efficacy cannot be fairly compared to the other techniques described. Nevertheless, studies evaluating this technique are warranted as it may represent the least invasive epicardial approach.

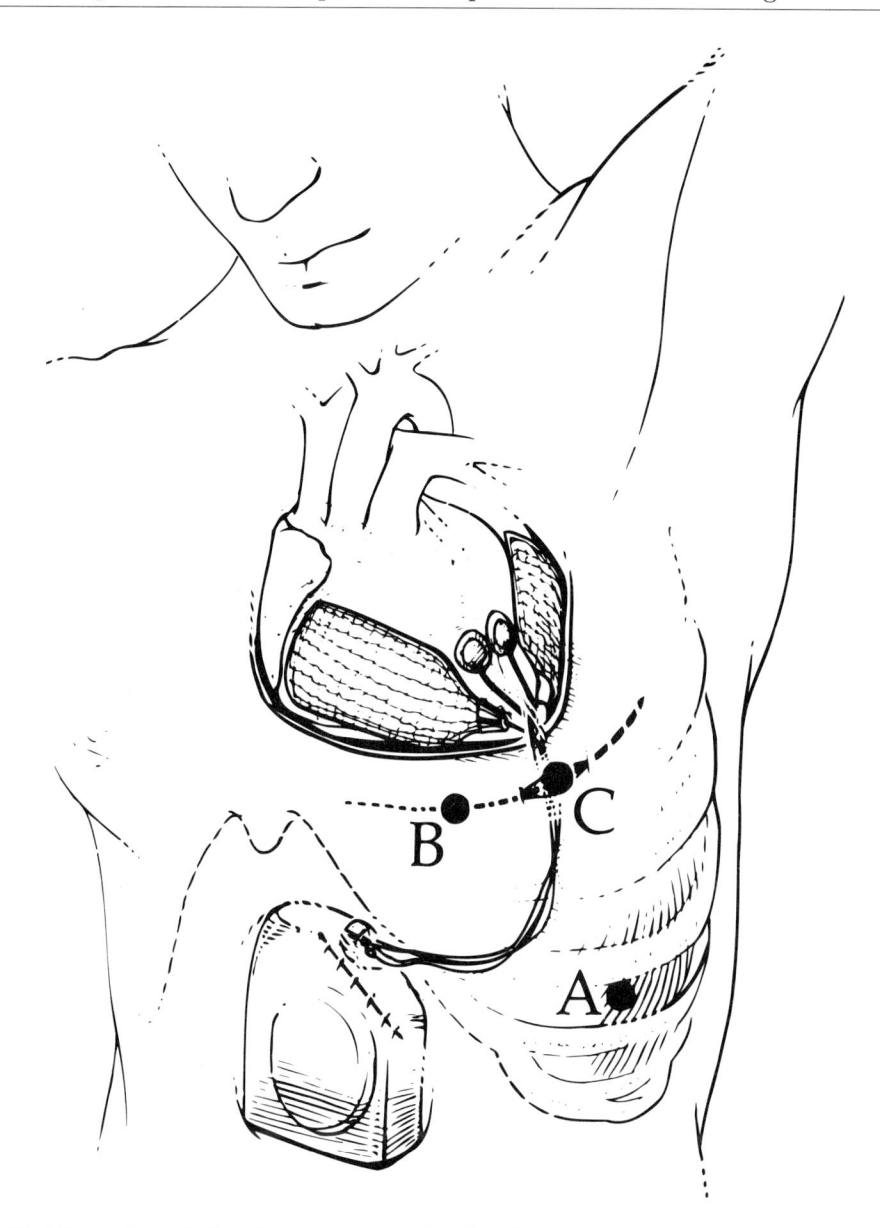

Figure 11. Illustration of sites for trocar insertion for thoracoscopic implantation of implantable cardioverter-defibrillator (ICD). Thoracoscope is placed through site A, grasping forceps through site B, and incision for insertion of patches and sensing electrodes through site C. (Reproduced with permission from Reference 12.)

Endocardial Approach

The possiblity of defibrillating the heart with a transvenous catheter has been known for years,[13,14] but because of high DFTs, endocardial leads were not considered suitable for ICD therapy. In 1987, an endocardial lead system (Endotak™ [CPI, St. Paul, MN) was implanted in a small number of patients, but a series of lead fractures forced a discontinuation of that study.[15] Redesign of the Endotak lead (Endotak-C) (Figures 2 and 12) as well as the development of tranvenous leads by other

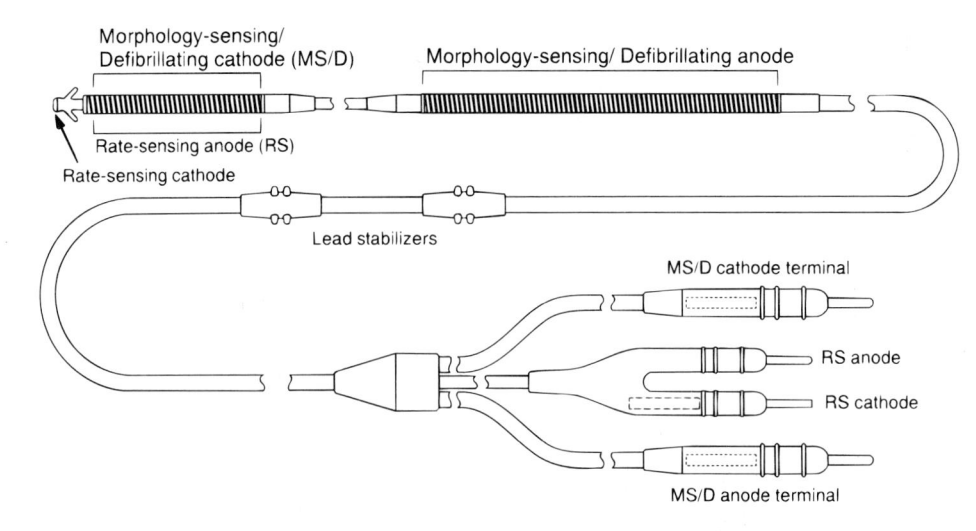

Figure 12. Diagrammatic illustration of the Endotak-C™ (CPI, St. Paul, MN) lead. Electrodes for rate and morphology sensing and two defibrillating electrodes are combined into a single lead. (Reproduced with permission from CPI, Inc., St. Paul, MN.)

manufacturers (Medtronic, Inc., Telectronics, Intermedics, Ventritex, Inc.) has renewed interest in the endocardial approach for ICD implantation. Over the past 3–4 years, clinical trials have been ongoing in Europe and the United States evaluating the safety and efficacy of nonthoracotomy ICD systems. In the majority of these trials, the transvenous endocardial electrode has been combined with a patch electrode that is implanted subcutaneously in the chest wall over the cardiac apex or elsewhere. More recently CPI has introduced into clinical trials a subcutaneous array as a substitute for the subcutaneous patch.

Technique

When the endocardial approach is elected, the patient should be positioned and prepared for easy conversion to an epicardial approach (most commonly a left anterior thoracotomy) so that reprepping and redraping is unnecessary. Thus, the patient is placed in the supine position with the left chest elevated 20°–30° and with the left arm by the side. Once the patient is positioned the operating table can be tilted 20°–30° to bring the patient's shoulders to the horizontal plane.

Insertion of transvenous defibrillation and/or rate sensing leads follows the same principles used when inserting permanent pacemaker leads (Figure 13). A subclavian introducer technique greatly facilitates lead insertion. The left subclavian vein is preferred because of accessibility and the occasional need to combine the endocardial electrode with a left-sided subcutaneous electrode. The right infraclavicular area, however, should be included in the operative field should access be unobtainable from the left side. Supraclavicular and internal jugular approaches should be avoided because passage of the lead over the clavicle threatens the security of the lead tip position in the right ventricle.

With the patient in deep Trendelenburg, the needle is introduced just beneath the mid-point of the clavicle aiming about 1 cm above the sternal notch in a line that is parallel with the deltopectoral groove. The left subclavian vein is punctured with gentle aspiration on the syringe. This can be done percutaneously or through a limited infraclavicular incision. A vigorous gush of blood generally indicates successful needle

Operative Techniques for Implantation and Testing • 339

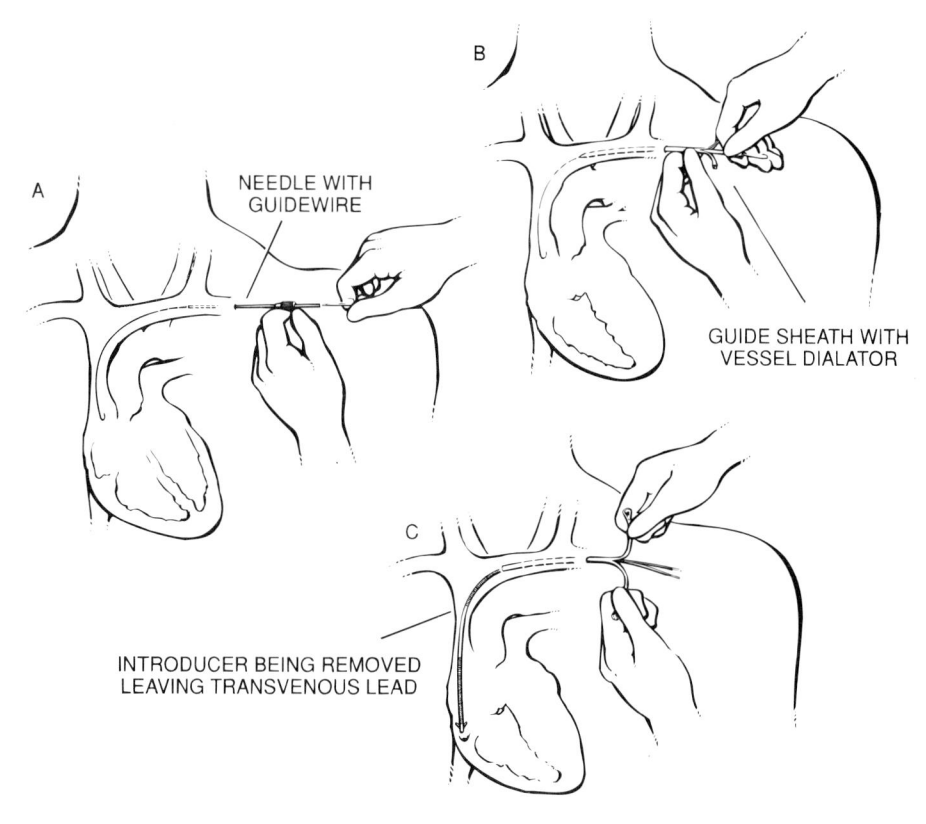

Figure 13. Technique of inserting transvenous leads for implantable cardioverter-defibrillator (ICD) implantation. See text for discussion.

placement. If the subclavian artery has been encountered, however, the needle is withdrawn and pressure applied for several minutes. Once the needle is positioned in the suclavian vein, the flexible J guidewire is advanced through the needle and positioned with fluoroscopic guidance in the inferior vena cava. An introducer sheath is advanced over the guidewire (12–14F) and the guidewire and the introducer removed. The sheath is pinched between the thumb and the forefinger to prevent air aspiration, and the endocardial lead advanced to the atrial-superior vena caval junction. The introducer sheath is then peeled off. With the Endotak-C the tip of the lead is positioned in the right ventricular apex. In case of the Transvene™ (Medtronic, Minneapolis, MN) or EnGuard™ (Telectronics, Englewood, CO) endocardial leads, the proximal and the distal defibrillation coils are located on two separate leads, thus, one electode is positioned into the right ventricular apex and the other in the superior vena caval-atrial junction (Figure 14). Some patients receiving the Medtronic system have a defibrillating lead placed in the coronary sinus (Figure 15). With the Telectronics system (EnGuard) the superior vena caval electrode is located on an atrial passive tined electrode analogous to a pacing atrial lead. The tip of the atrial J is positioned in the atrial appendage. Once the endocardial lead(s) is positioned, the satisfactory R wave sensing and pacing thresholds assured, the lead(s) should be carefully and securely fixed to the pectoralis fascia at the point where they exit the muscle. Defibrillation thresholds can now be determined. If the endocardial lead(s) alone provide satisfactory defibrilla-

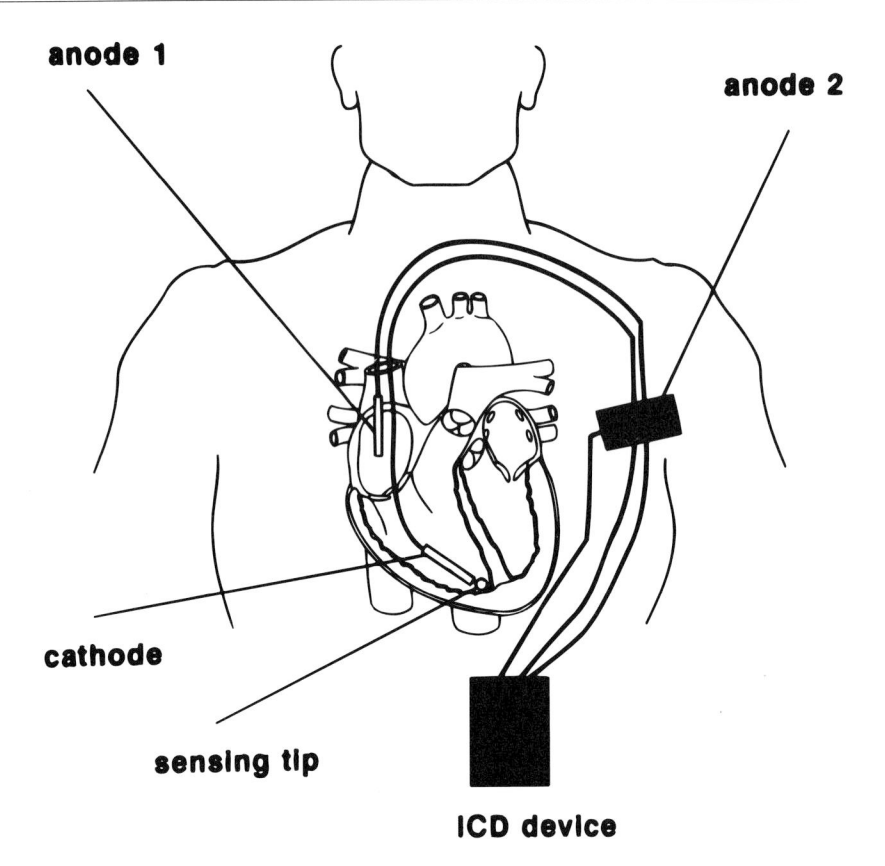

Figure 14. Placement of two separate transvenous defibrillating leads with one electrode in the right ventricular apex and the other at the superior atriocaval junction as performed with Medtronic or Telectronics lead systems. A subcutaneous patch lead may be necessary to achieve a safe defibrillation threshold. (Reproduced with permission from Reference 18.)

tion, the lead(s) is then tunneled subcutaneously to the already created left-sided paraumbilical device pocket. A small loop of the lead should be left where the lead exits the pectoralis fascia to relieve tension.

When endocardial leads alone fail to provide a satisfactory DFT, a subcutaneous electrode is added. This patch electrode is inserted through a small anterior chest incision that is placed in the left inframammary crease in line with what might have to be extended into an anterior thoracotomy. A subcutaneous pocket is developed up toward the axilla. The patch electrode is then fixed to the fascia of the chest wall with interrupted nonabsorbable sutures. Defibrillation thresholds are again obtained, and, if satisfactory, this lead is tunneled subcuta-

neously to the device pocket (Figure 16). If a CPI endocardial system is being implanted, a subcutaneous array may serve as the additional electrode. This array consists of three flexible electrode leads that are designed to fan out along the contour of the left chest wall (Figures 17, 18, and 19). The three leads come together into a single lead that serves as the additional electrode. Insertion of the array requires a small incision along the inframammary crease just to the left of the sternal border with dissection down to the chest wall fascia. A blunt-tipped malleable stylet is used to create a pathway for each limb of the array. Once a pathway is created along the chest wall an introducer sheath is placed over the stylet and the stylet and introducer are positioned

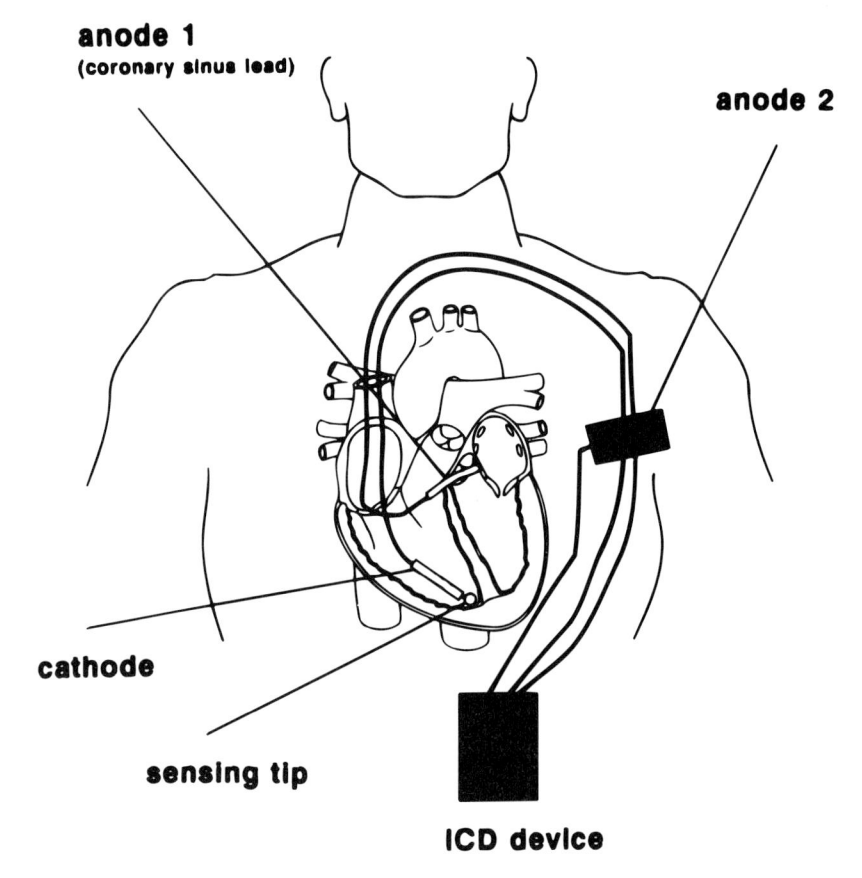

Figure 15. With the Medtronic transvenous lead system one of the defibrillating leads may be placed in the coronary sinus. (Reproduced with permission from Reference 18.)

in the pathway. The stylet is then removed and the limb of the array is inserted into the sheath. The split sheath is then carefully removed as the array limb is held in position. This maneuver is repeated for the other two limbs of the array. The three limbs of the array should be placed so that they roughly follow the course of the fourth, fifth, and sixth intercostal spaces (Figure 19). The hub of the array is then fixed to the chest wall fascia and the lead is tested and then tunneled to the device pocket.

Alternative methods to enhance defibrillation efficacy with endocardial leads are being explored. One such approach is to use a single defibrillation electrode, positioned in the right ventricular apex, and the can of the ICD in the pectoral pocket as two defibrillation electrodes (Medtronic Jewel™).

In those cases in which satisfactory DFTs cannot be achieved with a combination of endocardial and subcutaneous electrodes, an epicardial approach must be used. Conversion to an anterior thoracotomy is easily performed by extending the incision already made for the subcutaneous electrode and entering the chest through the fifth intercostal space.

Current Results

Several recent reports describe initial experiences with transvenous defibrillation systems. Yee and associates[16] described their experience with 14 patients using

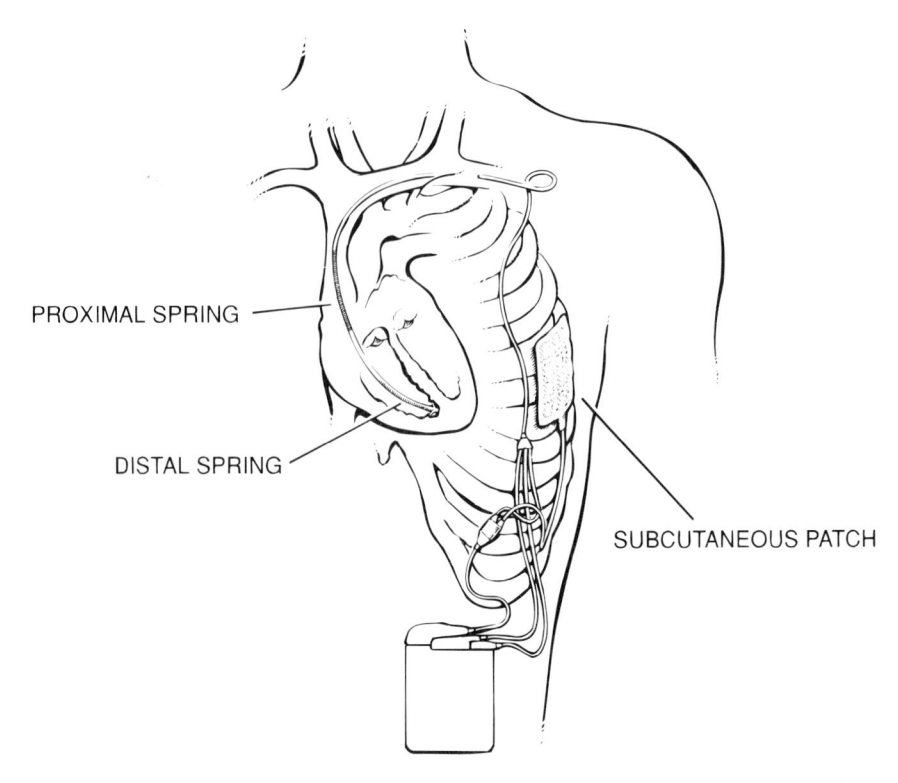

Figure 16. Final appearance after satisfactory placement of Endotak™-C (CPI, St. Paul, MN) lead and subcutaneous patch electrode.

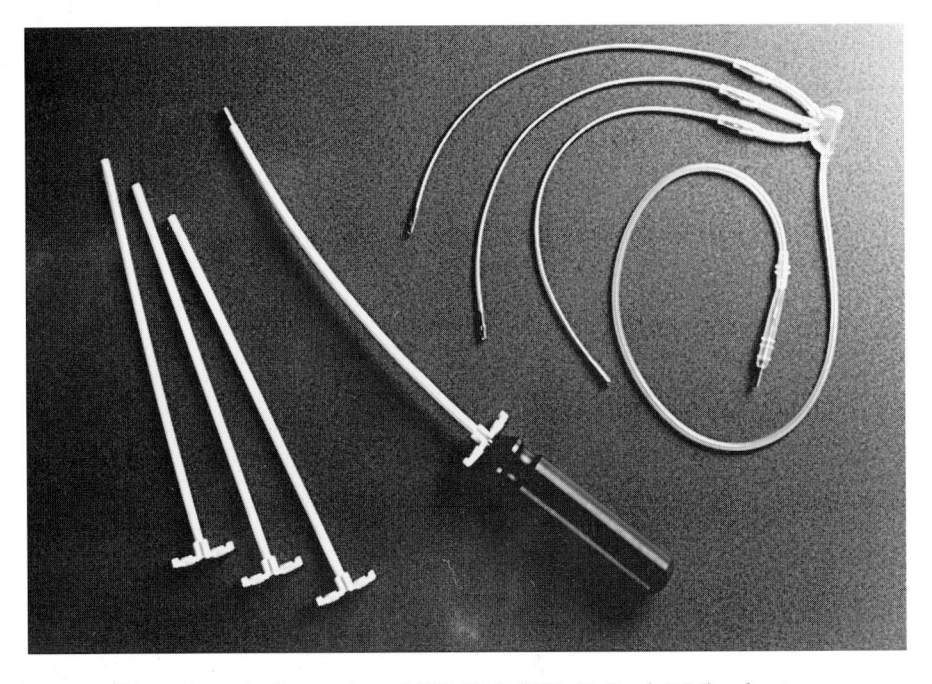

Figure 17. Diagrammatic illustration of CPI SQ™ (CPI, St. Paul, MN) subcutaneous array.

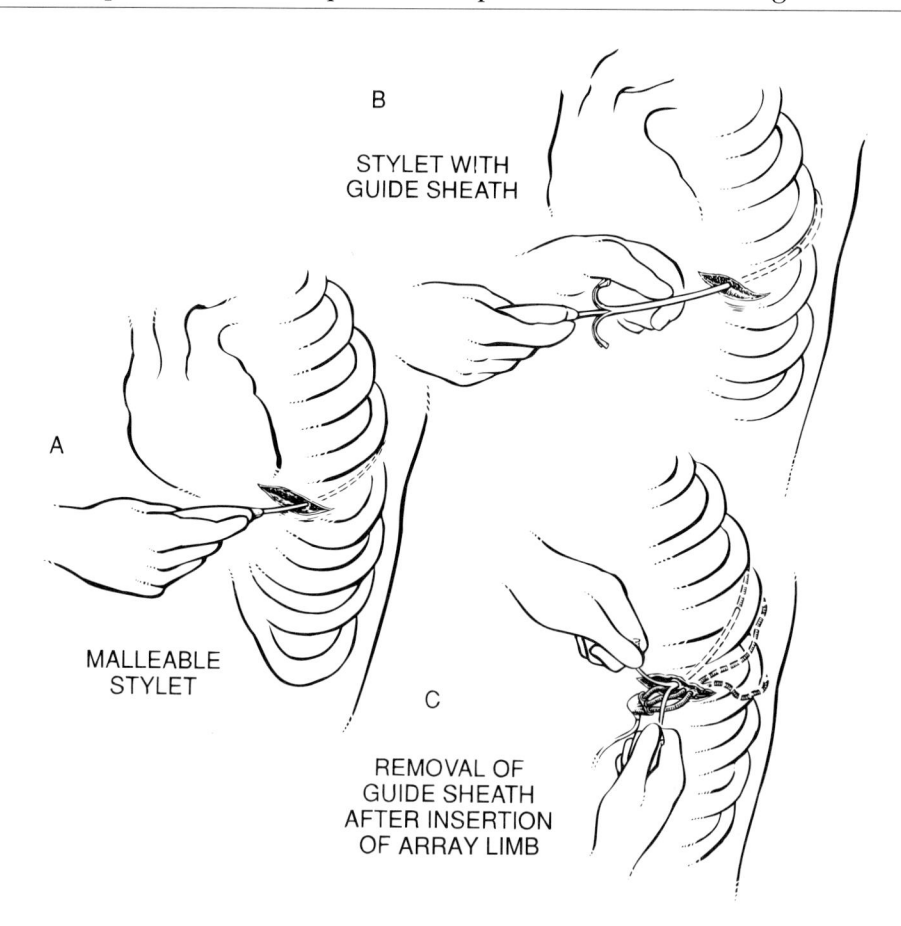

Figure 18. The limbs of the CPI SQ™ (CPI, St Paul, MN) subcutaneous array are inserted along the chest wall using a malleable stylet and split guide sheaths.

leads designed by Medtronic. In this study a totally transvenous system (no subcutaneous patch) was achieved in 7 patients and a partial transvenous system (including a subcutaneous patch) was achieved in 4 patients. Three patients (21%) required thoracotomy to place epicardial electrodes. Trappe and associates[17] attempted endocardial lead systems using the Endotak lead and a subcutaneous patch in 47 patients. Only 8 patients (17%) required thoracotomy and epicardial patch implantation to achieve satisfactory DFTs. Complications occurred in 2 of the 47 patients (4%). Two other successful reports indicate successful transvenous lead implantation in 80% to 90% of patients.[18,19] These two reports, however, also indicate that the transvenous approach is not without morbidity. Hammel and associates[18] reported an overall complication rate of 14% that included postoperative bleeding, generator pocket hematoma, and a subcutaneous patch pocket infection. Frame and associates[19] reported on 34 patients, 3 of whom developed pulmonary edema and low-output postoperatively, 2 developed hematoma, and 1 a pneumothorax. Of particular note in this report was the prolonged testing time used for the nonthoracotomy lead systems in comparison to the thoracotomy systems. None of these reports has cited any lead fractures in the short-term follow-up, although lead dislodgment did occur in two patients in the report by Frame et al.

The initial experience with endocardial

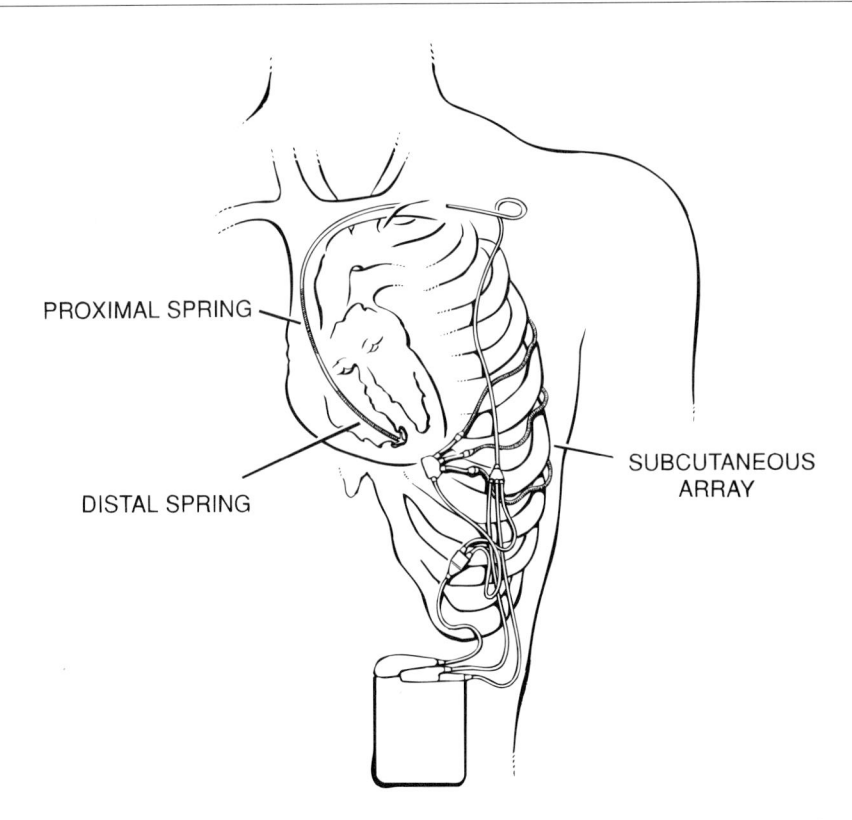

Figure 19. Final appearance after satisfactory placement of Endotak™-C (CPI, St. Paul, MN) lead and subcutaneous array.

implantation of ICDs is encouraging because over 80% of patients have avoided thoracotomy with this approach. If additional experience confirms these early reports, the endocardial approach to ICD implantation will become the preferred technique with the epicardial approach reserved for those patients in whom this technique fails to achieve safe DFTs.

Intraoperative Testing of the Implantable Cardioverter-Defibrillator System

The goal of intraoperative testing is to ensure proper ICD function. Toward that end, a number of steps are taken to optimize the system performance, minimize intraoperative time, and enhance patients' safety.

Preoperative Preparation

Patient selection is discussed in Chapters 13 and 14. Preoperative evaluation should include assessment of the cardiovascular system, peripheral circulation, pulmonary function, and neurological status. Cerebrovascular circulation is assessed in patients with prior history of cerebrovascular accidents by noninvasive and invasive techniques, if necessary. Since transient circulatory arrest accompanies DFT testing, intraoperative quantitative EEG (QEEG) and transcranial Doppler flow monitoring may be useful adjunctive techniques to minimize the risk of intraoperative cerebrovascular accidents.[20]

Implantable cardioverter-defibrillator system infection is a serious potential complication with devastating consequences. Therefore, all care must be taken to prevent or minimize its risk. The role of prophylactic antibiotics for this purpose has not been systematically evaluated. It is our current practice, based on empiric considerations only, to use prophylactic parenteral antibiotics 1 hour prior to surgery and to continue the antibiotics in the most immediate postoperative period (24–48 hours). We usually administer Vancomycin or another systemic drug effective for penicillinase resistant and sensitive staphylococcal prophylaxis, since these organisms are most commonly implicated in the perioperative ICD system infections. Prophylactic antibiotic administration does not supplant or compensate for poor aseptic technique. In the operating room we limit the number of personnel to the minimum required, and strongly discourage spectators and personnel traffic in and out of the operating room once the implant procedure has begun.

Another possible source of sterile field contamination is the fluoroscopic equipment, which is often moved in and out of the position when the transvenous leads are manipulated. We insist that all exposed surfaces are draped with a sterile cover. Continuous surveillance of the operative and ancillary personnel and procedural methods used in the operating room is essential to ensure that a breakdown in sterile technique does not occur.

Intraoperative Patient Monitoring

Careful monitoring is a standard component of all operative procedures. Implantable cardioverter-defibrillator implantation is no exception. Some unique considerations apply to ICD surgery. For example, during DFT testing repeated episodes of transient circulatory arrest occur. Although these episodes are relatively short (10–20 seconds), at times they are more prolonged, particularly when the initial shock fails to defibrillate. At times, the circulatory arrest may be 30–60 seconds, or longer. The defibrillator shock may cause transient cardiac stunning and the circulatory arrest may cause transient or prolonged episodes of cerebral ischemia. Continuous monitoring of intraarterial pressure is therefore mandatory throughout the procedure. We also advocate continuous QEEG and transcranial Doppler monitoring to minimize the potential for cerebral ischemia or injury.[20,21]

Central venous access is ensured by the placement of an internal jugular venous catheter (6F or 7F). We generally avoid placement of a Swan-Ganz pulmonary artery catheter in patients undergoing transvenous lead placement for a number of reasons: 1) pulmonary artery pressure monitoring is not absolutely necessary; 2) lead entanglement and lead displacement are an ever present danger; and 3) the potential for nosocomial infection is enhanced with temporary transvenous catheters, particularly those that may be in contact with transvenous leads. Therefore, after anesthesia induction, the pulmonary arterial catheter is withdrawn prior to transvenous lead placement and positioning.

Equipment and Personnel

The minimum necessary equipment and personnel requirements are listed in Tables 1 and 2. A checklist of equipment is

---

Table 1
Recommended Equipment Requirements for ICD Implantation

- Implant support system (ISS)—manufacturer specific
- Sterile high-voltage cables (2)
- Sterile pace/sense cables (2)
- Physiological, multichannel recorder
- Programmable stimulator
- External defibrillator with sterile external paddles and internal paddles.
- A back-up external defibrillator
- AC fibrillator
- Sterile magnet (doughnut)
- Sterile wand for communication with ICD via the external programmer (2)
- Imaging equipment (fluoroscopy)
- Standard instrument tray for thoracotomy
- Introducers and guidewires (10F–14)-multiple
- Multiple endocardial and epicardial leads, adapters, wrenches-manufacturer specific
- ICD (2)

Table 2
Personnel Requirements for ICD Implant and Testing

- Cardiothoracic surgeon
- Anesthesiologist
- Electrophysiologist
- Technical support personnel (engineer, technician or an EP-trained cardiovascular nurse)

recommended prior to an implant. All reusable accessories required for an implant (eg, cables, sterile programmer wand) should be available with back-up component for each, since inadvertent contamination of cables or component malfunction may occur during an implant. Therefore, back-up equipment must always be available.

The staff requirements are listed in Table 2. A cardiovascular surgeon familiar with all aspects of ICD implant techniques and treatment alternatives, an electrophysiologist,[22,23] anesthesiologist, and supporting personnel constitute a team whose members must interact harmoniously to achieve the best possible results.

Intraoperative Electrophysiologic Measurements

Surgical techniques for hardware implantation have already been described. The purpose of intraoperative testing is to ensure proper positioning of pace/sense and defibrillation leads, adequate defibrillation safety margins for the implanted ICD system, and to demonstrate appropriate ICD programming and function. Therefore, testing is conducted in three stages: 1) testing of pace/sense leads; 2) DFT testing; and 3) ICD testing.

Testing of Pace/Sense Leads

It is fundamental for proper ICD function to differentiate normal sinus rhythm from tachyarrhythmias. Current devices (including the investigational devices) accomplish this goal primarily by rate differentiation (see Chapter 4). With some devices (Ventak™ series [CPI, St. Paul, MN]) morphological characteristics of the transmyocardial electrogram from the shocking leads may be used to complement detection based on the rate analysis exclusively.

Effective sensing involves proper interaction between the depolarizing myocardium, the lead, and the sensing amplifier. The spectral content of electrograms is important because sense amplifiers have bandpass filters that are designed to select frequencies characteristic of electrograms while rejecting the unwanted signals, eg, T waves, myopotentials, and pacing pulse polarization artifacts. Electrode location is also important. Sensing electrodes detect the amplitude of the depolarization wave front as it moves toward and away from the electrodes. A bipolar electrode that lies on the parallel plane to the advancing wave front receives the same potential at each electrode simultaneously, providing no potential difference. Therefore, small or no signal is detected. Conversely, if the signal is perpendicular to the wave front, the potential difference is maximized. Signal detection and processing are discussed extensively in Chapters 4 and 8.

It may be intuitively obvious that the larger the signal amplitude, and the faster the rate of change of the signal voltage (ie, the slew rate) in sinus rhythm, the more likely it is that the signal amplitude and slew rate characteristics will be more easily detected during ventricular tachycardia, but especially fibrillation. This may not always be so, however, because the activation sequence during ventricular tachycardia and fibrillation are significantly different from that which is detected during sinus rhythm, but this "rule of thumb" generally holds true. Nevertheless, signal amplitude and sensing during ventricular tachycardia and fibrillation must be tested.

The R wave amplitude in sinus rhythm is determined by direct pacing system analyzer measurement, electronic measurement via an implant support device, or by direct printout from a physiological recorder. We use all three of the above methods and always insist on "paper recordings" and measurements to exclude a potential for electronic noise and extraneous signal detections (eg, pacemaker artifact or other electronic signals). In general, the greater the R wave amplitude in sinus rhythm, the better. The minimum acceptable R wave amplitude detected from the pace/sense leads is ≥ 5 mV. If the R wave is < 5 mV, the sensing lead(s) needs to be repositioned. In the case of epicardial pace/sense leads, "mapping" of the best potential sites is useful prior to attaching the epicardial screw-in leads. This may be accomplished by continuous recording of the signal characteristics while the surgeon sequentially positions the leads on alternate epicardial surface sites. When the best site is identified, epicardial leads are screwed-in and sensing characteristics reconfirmed. In the case of an endocardial lead, suboptimal R wave characteristics should prompt repositioning of the lead.

Slew rate is the first derivative of a waveform. How amplitude and slew rate relate to sensing depends on the sense amplifier characteristics. The precise relationship between amplitude, slew rate, and the spectral content of an electrogram depends on the morphology of the specific electrogram. Assuming a constant intrinsic deflection amplitude, increasing slew rate increases the high-frequency content of the waveform. Conversely, assuming constant morphology, slew rate and amplitude are directly proportional. The correlation, however, is relatively weak due to large variability in electrogram morphology.[24] Slew rate may be used to provide further assurance that a specific waveform will be sensed. In general, slew rates ≥ 0.75 V/s are desirable, although signal amplitude in sinus rhythm has been regarded as the more important of the two measurements.

Intracardiac R wave duration of < 100 msec is generally associated with optimal sensing, although signal durations > 100 msec are not uncommon when underlying bundle branch block is present and/or when antiarrhythmic drugs that prolong the ventricular depolarization are used for arrhythmia therapy.

Bipolar sensing only is used for ICDs. This is because unwanted, far-field signals other than cardiac depolarization are rejected more efficiently by this mode of sensing. When epicardial sensing is used, it is important to position the electrode pair close together (within 1–2 cm) to ensure that true bipolar sensing occurs. In the case of endocardial electrodes, the electrode pair distance is determined by the lead design. With endocardial (NTL) leads, sensing occurs between the distal tip (cathode) and the distal defibrillation coil (anode) (Figure 12).

Pacing thresholds are routinely measured and ideally should be < 1 V at the pulse width of 0.5 msec for endocardial leads. However, thresholds of up to 1.5 V are acceptable. For epicardial leads, the thresholds are generally somewhat higher, though thresholds above 2 V should not be accepted for acute leads. If the leads are used only for sensing, ie, if the ICD does not have antitachycardia pacing (ATP) capabilities, optimization of pacing thresholds is less critical. In general, we advocate endocardial lead placement when ATP function is used (ie, for third-generation ICDs) and favor endocardial leads in most other cases, except when risks outweigh the potential benefits, or when placement of endocardial lead is impractical (ie, in a patient undergoing simultaneous cardiac surgery and ICD placement via a median sternotomy where the approach to the subclavian veins is difficult or impossible).

Pacing lead impedance is determined routinely. It is usually found to be in the range of 200–1,000 Ω. Pacing impedance typically changes with time after the implant, and typically drops after the first week. It then increases with time to a value of about 10% to 20% below the impedance at implant.[25]

Typically, the pacing thresholds, impedance, and R wave amplitude are measured at the time of pace/sense lead placement, and the measurements are repeated after lead tunneling. This later step is important, since tunneling of the lead(s) may cause gross lead dislodgment (transvenous endocardial lead), or damage to insulation of the leads may occur due to rough handling during subcutaneous tunneling.

Shocking lead characteristics should also be measured. When probability density function or its digital counterpart, turning point morphology, are used for rhythm differentiation (eg, Ventak) the sensing characteristics of the shocking leads are important to determine. Amplitudes > 1 mV are generally recommended, but clearly, the greater the amplitude of the signal in sinus rhythm, the more likely it is that the signal will be sensed appropriately during ventricular tachycardia and fibrillation. Durations of up to 150 msec is acceptable for the morphology (patch leads).

Patch (shocking electrode) impedance is measured using the implant support device and is generally acceptable if it is in the range of 20–100 Ω. Typically, the impedance is measured between 30–60 Ω. In the case of NTL systems, the shocking coils on the transvenous leads subserve the function of the patch leads. Shocking coil impedance measurments are similar to the epicardial patch lead impedance measurements.

Defibrillation Threshold Testing

The subject of DFT testing is discussed extensively in Chapter 10. However, several points are worth emphasizing here. The ability of an ICD to terminate spontaneous episodes of ventricular fibrillation is fundamental to its widely acknowledged success in preventing sudden tachyarrhythmic cardiac death. To accomplish this goal, adequate testing is required at the time of device implantation. Assessment of DFT is required to optimize device function and to assure adequate safety margins. To accomplish this goal, a test sequence of repeated fibrillation-defibrillation trials at successively decreasing or increasing energies using an external cardioverter-defibrillator (ECD) support device is required. The DFT is defined as the minimum energy producing defibrillation success.

Defibrillation threshold implies that the slope of a curve relating defibrillation energy to conversion success is steep, permitting a clear distinction between effective and ineffective energies. However, a dose-response curve relating probability of success to shock energy, voltage, or current best expresses this relationship (Figure 20). To define this curve experimentally, multiple defibrillation attempts are required at different energy levels to adequately define the point along this curve. In clinical practice, however, this approach is impractical and potentially hazardous. The conceptual framework, however, is important to understand, since this relationship has significant clinical implications.

To assure efficacy of implanted ICDs, defibrillation shock intensities must be programmed so that ICD output is positioned on the 100% conversion success plateau (E_{ICD}) (Figure 20). Because of the probabilistic nature of defibrillation, one becomes more certain as to the location of the dose responsive curve with more extensive testing, ie, the number of conversion attempts. Generally two types of testing methods have been used in clinical practice: 1) aimed at verification of the safety margin; and 2) DFT assessment.

The goal of the first type of testing is to verify that an ICD can be programmed with an adequate margin between its output and the tested energy levels. In general, this type of testing can be used when a limited number of fibrillation-defibrillation sequences can only be used, due to clinical factors which may make more extensive testing hazardous. In this case a test energy, say 20 J is tested two or three times (2S or 3S protocols), and if successful, the ICD may be programmed to an energy output of 30 J. This rule of thumb, programmed energy of 10 J plus the defibrillation success energy,

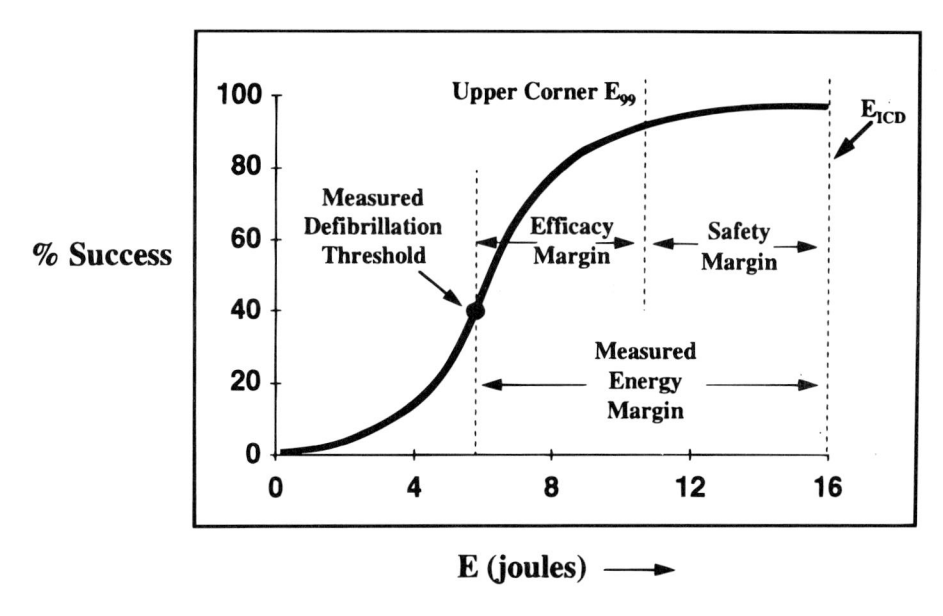

Figure 20. Percent probability for successful defibrillation versus shock energy. The implantable cardioverter-defibrillator (ICD) safety margin is the energy difference between the lowest energy required for 100% success at implant (E_{100}) and the programmed ICD energy. For discussion see text.

has been proven clinically effective. The weakness of this approach is that the true DFT may be considerably less, hence, unnecessarily wasteful high energies must be programmed, increasing patient's discomfort and limiting the device longevity. The arbitrary energy of 20 J is selected largely for historical reasons, since the Ventak device, which was the first market-released device, has a maximum energy output of 30 J (except for the high-energy Ventak 1555).

The second type of testing involves defibrillation testing at several shock levels with both conversion successes and failures. The purpose of this method is to assess the actual defibrillation characteristics of the implanted system. Defibrillation threshold protocols are examples of this category. The most common technique used clinically is the step-down success method. The step-down success protocol involves a sequence of several defibrillation trials at successively lower energy levels delivered from the implant support device. Once a sufficient energy level is reached, which is considered adequate to provide sufficient safety margin for the ICD, the testing protocol ends. Commonly, the sequence is begun at 20 J. With successful conversion at 20 J, the next attempt is at 15 J. If this too is successful, the next attempt would be at 10 J. If at this point a failure occurs, the DFT is said to be ≤ 15 J. If the success occurred at 10 J, the DFT would be ≤ 10 J. With a device capable of delivering 30 J output, no further testing would be required to further assess the actual DFT, since an adequate safety margin can be programmed. If, however, the clinical situation permits, the testing sequence may be extended until a failure is encountered.

The advantage of assessment protocols over the validation protocols is that they provide more detailed information on the defibrillation characteristics of the implanted system, which may be helpful in managing patients over time.

If adequate safety margins cannot be demonstrated, the shocking leads should be repositioned (epicardial leads) or a different lead configuration tried (using a larger patch, moving the patch position, or adding a third patch electrode for epicardial systems). In general, one aims to encompass the greatest possible myocardial mass between the electrodes. In case of NTL systems, a subcutaneous electrode may be added (Endotak, Transvene, EnGuard) and various lead polarities and combinations tested.

The use of biphasic pulses generally decreases the DFT requirements. Biphasic shock waveforms are discussed in detail in Chapter 7. Alternatively, sequential shocks may be tried (PCD™, Medtronic, Minneaplis, MN). Moving the subcutaneous electrode to a more anterior position or to the mid-axillary positions may also be helpful. Alternatively, a coronary sinus electrode or a right ventricular outflow tract electrode may be tried.

An important cautionary note with respect to duration of ventricular fibrillation prior to shock is worth emphasizing. Since the duration of ventricular fibrillation episodes affects the success of defibrillation,[26-31] it is important that the duration of ventricular filbrillation be comparable for each fibrillation-defibrillation attempt. We generally use 10 seconds of ventricular fibrillation per episode. Ventricular fibrillation is most efficiently induced with alternating current (AC) or it may also be induced by rapid ramp pacing. With more modern implant support devices (ECDs) ramp pacing may be delivered from the ECD either via the shocking or the pace/sense leads. Alternatively, ventricular fibrillation may be induced by direct cardiac stimulation (by epicardial wires or endocardial catheter). Failure of the initial shock to terminate the ventricular fibrillation episode is usually followed by a rescue shock from the ECD at 30–40 J and if unsuccessful, by external shock via an ECD at maximum output (360–400 J) or internal paddles (during open heart surgery 40–50 J). Adequate resting periods between the fibrillation-defibrillation attempts should be ensured, so that vital signs stabilize and the electrocardiogram returns to baseline. We also routinely monitor cerebral blood flow and QEEG and await return of EEG and blood flow parameters prior to resumption of testing.[20,21] Thus, a variable rest period of 1–5 minutes may be required between the successive tests.

Table 3*
Effects of Antiarrhythmic Drugs on Cardiac Defibrillation (DFT)

Increase	No Change	Decrease
Encainide	MODE	Amiodarone
ODE	Quinidine	(acute)
Flecainide	Procainamide	Clofilium
Recainam	Bretylium	Sotalol
Lidocaine		NAPA
Mexiletine		Isoproterenol
Amiodarone		
(chronic)		

* Adapted with permission from Reference 32.

Once the defibrillation testing has been completed, the information derived from the testing is used to program the output of the ICD. To assure consistent performance over time the ICD must be programmed to a level that has 100% probability of success (E_{100}) plus the safety margin. Several factors may conspire to increase DFTs over time. These include antiarrhythmic drugs (Table 3),[32] ischemia, prolonged fibrillation duration,[26-31] or other, as yet undetermined mechanisms.

Testing of the Implantable Cardioverter-Defibrillator Generator

After intraoperative lead and DFT testing, the surgeon tunnels the leads to an ICD pocket, generally in the left upper quadrant of the patient's abdomen, in either a subcutaneous or a subrectal location. The lead testing (signal amplitude, pacing thresholds and impedance) should be repeated after tunneling and prior to ICD connection to ensure that dislodgment of the leads or damage to the insulation did not occur during tunneling. Integrity of shocking leads and proper connections should be checked by administering a synchronized low-energy shock in sinus rhythm to measure the shocking lead impedance. At this point, poor lead connection or insulation damage to the leads is readily detected without exposing the patient to a possibility of conversion failure during ICD testing.

After the ICD generator is connected, and prior to ventricular fibrillation induction, sensing in sinus rhythm should be checked (Figure 21). We also check the pacing thresholds by noninvasive methods (Figure 22). Sensing of ICDs that lack telemetry (eg, Ventak 1600) should be checked by placing a doughnut magnet over the device to listen to emitted "beeps" synchronized with the QRS complex. Double, triple, and multiple sensing due to multiple signal detections may be picked up by this simple method. These devices are likely to be phased out from the clinical use as more sophisticated devices with telemetry become commonplace. Ventricular fibrillation is then induced by the noninvasive programmed stimulation from the implanted device or by AC current application when ICD lacks this facility (eg, Ventak). Once ventricular fibrillation is induced, the device is activated either automatically (eg, Cadence™ [Ventritex, Sunnyvale, CA], Guardian™ ATP [Telectronics, Englewood, CO], PCD) or manually (eg, Ventak). Appropriate sensing during ventricular fibrillation and defibrillation is verified (Figure 23). Back-up external cardioversion must be on standby, should a failure to convert ven-

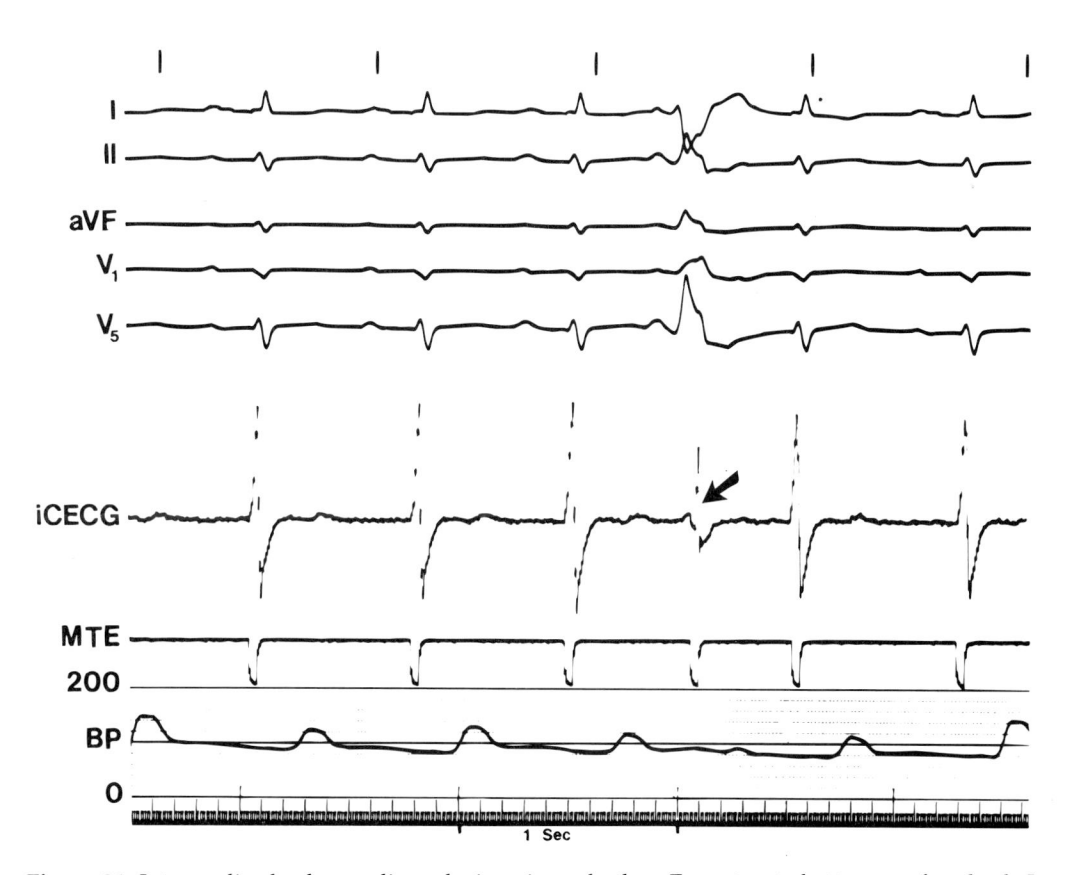

Figure 21. Intracardiac lead recordings during sinus rhythm. From top to bottom: surface leads I, II, aVF, V_1 and V_5, intracardiac ECG (ICECG) form the bipolar sensing lead, main timing events (MTE), and blood pressure (BP). Note appropriate sensing of sinus rhythm and ventricular ectopic beat (arrow).

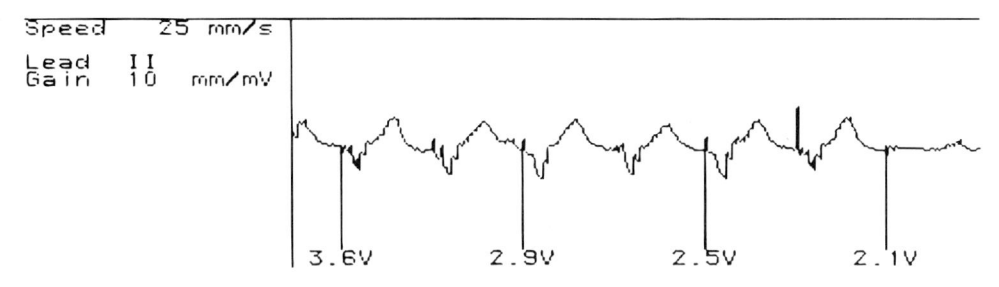

Figure 22. Automatic threshold test (Guardian™ ATP 4211, Telectronics, Englewood, CO). The threshold is measured to be 2.5 V at the pulse width of 0.5 msec.

tricular fibrillation occur. It is important to switch off electrocautery during testing to prevent interference with sensing of the ICD. Newer ICDs have telemetry capabilities to enable direct examination of electrograms and telemetry markers during ventricular fibrillation induction. These are valuable for recognition of sensing problems (oversensing and undersening). Some devices (eg, Cadence, P2™ [CPI]) are capa-

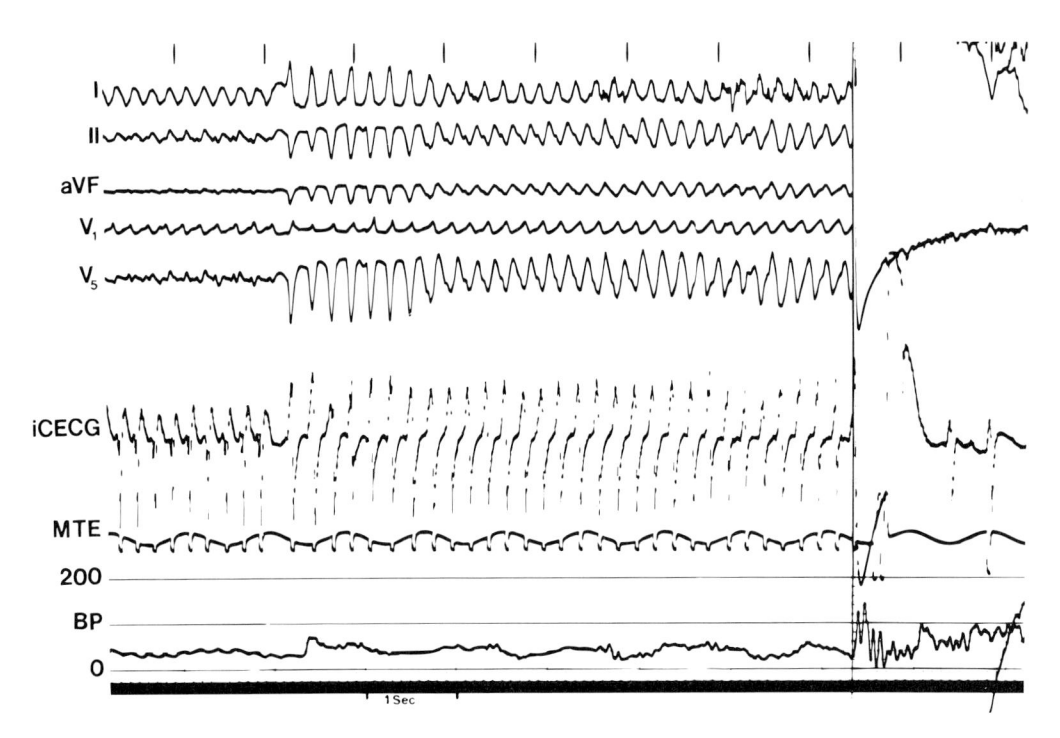

Figure 23. Polymorphous ventricular tachycardia/ventricular fibrillation followed by implantable cardioverter-defibrillator (ICD) shock and conversion to sinus rhythm, by Guardian™ ATP 4211 and nonthoracotomy EnGuard™ system (Telectronics, Englwood, CO). Note appropriate sensing during the episode. From top to bottom: surface leads I, II, aVF, V_1 and V_5, intracardiac electrogram (ICECG), main timing events (MTE), and blood pressure (BP).

ble of real-time electrogram recordings from the rate sensing or morphology lead(s).

The device is generally deactivated prior to the pocket closure to allow the surgeon to use electrocautery. At the end of the operation and before leaving the operating room we rountinely activate the ICD. Antitachycardia pacing functions are generally turned off, with only defibrillation and bradycardia pacing functions turned on. The ATP function is turned on only after thorough testing of ATP at predischarge electrophysiologic study (see Chapter 19). We recommend programming a "high" rate cutoff postoperatively (eg, 200 beats per minute) to ensure that the device does not become activated by atrial fibrillation or nonsustained tachyarrhythmias, which are common in the postoperataive period. At the same time, however, the patient is protected from ventricular fibrillation.

Implantable Cardioverter-Defibrillator and Lead Testing for Pulse Generator Replacements

Implantable cardioverter-defibrillator generators need to be replaced when the end-of-life indicator has been reached. We generally perform this procedure in the operating room to minimize the potential for infection. Availability of general anesthesia is an additional advantage. Some investigators perform this procedure in the electrophysiology laboratory using local anesthesia and parenteral sedation. The advantages and the disadvantages of either approach could be debated, however, the most important elements of safety and efficacy must be ensured: 1) absolute sterility (infections are more common with generator replacements); 2) ability to revise leads if necessary; and 3) access to immediate anesthesia and surgical back-up.

The ICD pocket is opened with careful dissection and due care to not injure the leads. The ICD is then disconnected from the leads and electrophysiologic measurements performed analogous to the initial implant with pace/sense, shocking leads testing, and DFT measurements. If the testing yields acceptable values, the new ICD generator is connected to the existing lead system, and the ICD tested as for the original implant.

With third-generation devices incorporating electrophysiologic testing capabilities, ventricular fibrillation can be induced with ramp pacing or ventricular burst stimulation at ultrashort cycle lengths of 50–100 msec. When devices that lack these capabilities are tested, an external AC current may be delivered by means of screwdrivers placed in the shocking lead set-screw ports, and connected to the external AC current generator by means of an electrical cable with alligator clips. Once ventricular fibrillation is induced, the screw drivers are disconnected (to prevent current shunting) and the device activated. Successsful conversion to sinus rhythm is then observed. The pocket is generally irrigated with antibiotic solution (eg, Bacitracin or equivalent) and the pocket closed in the routine manner with absorbable suture material.

Troubleshooting Problems at Cardioverter-Defibrillator Implantation

Failure of the Implantable Cardioverter-Defibrillator to Deliver Therapy

If the ICD fails to deliver therapy, sensing problems (eg, undersensing) or inappropriate programming should be suspected. Is there a signal dropout on the marker channel? Was the device activated? Is the rate cutoff of ventricular fibrillation or ventricular tachycardia above the rate measured? Is there external interference (eg, electrocautery)? Are the leads properly connected? (Check sensing in sinus rhythm) Has the sensing lead dislodged? (Check sensing in sinus rhythm and lead impedance, look at the sensing lead position on fluoroscopy)

The Implantable Cardioverter-Defibrillator Delivers Shocks, But the Shock Fails to Defibrillate

Potential causes include: 1) inadequate programmed safety margin or incomplete DFT testing protocol; 2) dislodgment or displacement of the transvenous defibrillation leads; 3) patch lead displacement or folding; 4) current shunting due to surgical retractors (during open thoracotomy); and 5) poor shocking lead connection or damage to the leads. If the impedance is high (> 150 Ω) fracture or poor lead connection is likely, or if low (< 20 Ω) an insulation break is suggested. Lead position, connections, and programming should be reviewed.

Inappropriate Shocks

Inappropriate shocks in sinus rhythm may occur due to oversensing (poor sensing lead connection due to a loose set screw or lead fracture) or due to external electrical interference (electrocautery). Certain devices that use fixed gain control (Guardian 4202, 4203, and 4210) may also oversense due to fixed gain sensing amplifier control. However, oversensing of T waves, P waves, and myopotentials may also occur with automatic gain control amplifiers. For a more exhaustive discussion of troubleshooting, see Chapter 21.

Conclusion and Overview

Implantation and testing of ICDs require an integrated approach involving the cardiac surgeon, the electrophysiologist, and the anesthesiologist. Familiarity with a range of devices and available surgical options is essential to allow flexibility and to optimize device performance. With advances in technology, reduction in the device size and volume, further refinement of nonthoracotomy lead systems is anticipated. In the future, it is likely that most ICD implants not requiring concomitant surgical procedures could be done in the electrophysiology laboratory, with surgical back-up (see Chapter 16). For pectoral ICD generator placement it is entirely possible that the implantation will be simplified to the point where the implantation technique will be no more complex than the current implantation techniques for permanent pacemakers, though selection, testing, and management of such patients would still be relatively more complex (see Chapter 17). With NTL systems the morbidity, mortality, and the duration of hospitalization are likely to be dramatically reduced. Still, for some patients thoracotomy will be necessary when DFTs are too high, or when concomitant cardiac surgery is required.

References

1. Mirowski M, Reid PR, Mower MM, et al: Termination of malignant ventricular arrhythmias with an implanted automatic defibrillator in human beings. *N Engl J Med* 303:322, 1980.
2. Watkins L Jr, Mirowski M, Mower MM, et al: Automatic defibrillation in man—the initial surgical experience. *J Thorac Cardiovasc Surg* 82:492, 1981.
3. Troup PJ, Chapman PD, Olinger GN, et al: The implanted defibrillator: relation of defibrillating lead configuration and clinical variables to defibrillation threshold. *J Am Coll Cardiol* 6:1315, 1985.
4. Shepard RB, Goldin MD, Lawrie GM, et al: Automatic implantable cardioverter defibrillator: surgical approaches for implantation. *J Cardiac Surg* 7:208, 1992.
5. Slater D, Singer I, Stavens C, et al: Lateral thoracotomy for automatic defibrillator. *Arch Surg* 126:778, 1991.
6. Watkins L Jr, Mirowski M, Mower MM, et al: Implantation of the automatic defibrillator: the subxiphoid approach. *Ann Thorac Surg* 34:515, 1982.
7. Beckman DJ, Crevey BJ, Foster PR, et al: Subxiphoid approach for implantable cardioverter defibrillator in patients with previous coronary bypass surgery. *PACE* 15:1637, 1992.
8. Flaker G, Boley T, Walls J, et al: Comparison of subxiphoid and traditional approaches

for ICD implantation. *PACE* 15:1531, 1992.
9. Lawrie GM, Griffin JC, Wyndham CRC: Epicardial implantation of the automatic implantable defibrillator by left subcostal thoracotomy. *PACE* 7:1370, 1984.
10. Shapira N, Cohen AI, Wish M, et al: Transdiaphragmatic implantation of the automatic implantable cardioverter defibrillator. *Ann Thorac Surg* 48:371, 1989.
11. Frumin H, Goodman GR, Pleatman M: ICD implantation via thoracoscopy without the need for sternotomy or thoracotomy. *PACE* 16:257, 1993.
12. Ely SW, Kron IL: Thoracoscopic implantation of the implantable cardioverter defibrillator. *Chest* 103:271, 1993.
13. Hopps JA, Bigelow WG: Electrical treatment of cardiac arrest: a cardiac stimulator/defibrillator. *Surgery* 36:833, 1954.
14. Mirowski M, Mower MM, Gott VL, et al: Feasibility and effectiveness of low energy catheter defibrillation in man. *Circulation* 47:79, 1973.
15. Saksena S, Parsonnet V: Implantation of a cardioverter/defibrillator without thoracotomy using a triple electrode system. *JAMA* 259:69, 1988.
16. Yee R, Klein GJ, Leitch JW, et al: A permanent transvenous lead system for an implantable pacemaker cardioverter defibrillator: nonthoracotomy approach to implantation. *Circulation* 85:196, 1992.
17. Trappe H, Klein H, Fieguth H, et al: Initial experience with a new tranvenous defibrillation system. *PACE* 16:134, 1993.
18. Hammel D, Block M, Konertz W, et al: Surgical experience with defibrillator implantation using nonthoracotomy leads. *Ann Thorac Surg* 55:685, 1993.
19. Frame R, Broadman R, Gross J, et al: Initial experience with transvenous implantable cardioverter defibrillator lead systems: operative morbidity and mortality. *PACE* 16:149, 1993.
20. Singer I, van der Laken, Edmonds HL Jr, et al: Is defibrillation testing safe? In: *Proceedings of IXth World Symposium on Cardiac Pacing and Electrophysiology*. *PACE* 14:11, 1991.
21. Singer I, Edmonds H Jr: Cerebrovasomotor reactivity predicts tolerance to tiered therapy with implantable cardioverter-defibrillators. In: *Proceedings of Euro-Pace '93—6th European Symposium on Cardiac Pacing*. Edited by AE Aubert, M. Ector, R Strobandt. Bologna, Italy: Monduzzi Editore; 1993, p. 559.
22. Flowers NC, Abildskov JA, Armstrong WF, et al: ACC Policy Statement. Recommended guidelines for training in adult clinical cardiac electrophysiology. *J Am Coll Cardiol* 18:637, 1991.
23. Scheinman M, Akhtar M, Brugada P, et al: Teaching objectives for fellowship programs in clinical electrophysiology. Report for the Ad Hoc Committee of the North American Society of Pacing and Electrophysiology. *J Am Coll Cardiol* 12:255, 1988.
24. Hurzeler Ph, DeCaprio V, Furman S: Endocardial electrograms and pacer sensing. In: *Advances in Pacemaker Technology*. Edited by M Schaldach, S Furman. New York: Springer-Verlag; 1975, p. 307.
25. Sedney MI, Rodrigo FA, Buis B, et al: Behavior of stimulation resistance and stimulation threshold of pacemaker leads during and after implantation (abstract). In: *Cursus Pacemakers*. Nederlandse Werkgroep Hartstimulatie; p 10, October 1982.
26. Echt DS, Barbey, JT, Black NJ: Influence of ventricular fibrillation duration on defibrillation energy in dogs using bidirectional pulse discharges. *PACE* 11:1315, 1988.
27. Fujimura C, Jones DL, Klein GJ: Effects of time to defibrillation and subthreshold preshocks on defibrillation success in pigs. *PACE* 12:358, 1989.
28. Jones JL, Swartz JF, Jones RE, et al: Increasing fibrillation duration enhances relative asymmetrical biphasic versus monophasic defibrillator waveform efficacy. *Circ Res* 67:376, 1990.
29. Bardy GH, Stewart RS, Ivey TD, et al: Potential risk of low energy cardioversion attempts by implantable cardioverters. *J Am Coll Cardiol* 9:168A, 1987.
30. Bardy GH, Ivey TD, Allen M, et al: A prospective, randomized evaluation of effect of ventricular fibrillation duration on defibrillation thresholds in humans. *J Am Coll Cardiol* 13:1362, 1989.
31. Bardy GH, Ivey TD, Johnson G, et al: Prospective evaluation of initially ineffective defibrillation pulses on subsequent defibrillation success during ventricular fibrillation in survivors of cardiac arrest. *Am J Cardiol* 62:718, 1988.
32. Singer I, Lang D: Defibrillation threshold-clinical utility and therapeutic implications. *PACE* 15:6, 1992.

performed in the electrophysiology or cardiac catheterization laboratory with the results of the procedure when performed in a traditional operating room environment.[19,20] These studies have demonstrated a similar rate of procedural complications such as lead dislodgment and infection for both operative settings. The only objective advantage of pacemaker implantation in the cardiac catheterization or electrophysiology laboratory that has been demonstrated has been the lower costs associated with the procedure. Perhaps because of this factor, but more likely because patients are usually evaluated by cardiologists before they are referred to cardiac or general surgeons, most pacemakers are now implanted outside the operating room.

Before carrying the analogy of ICD implantation to that of permanent pacemaker implantation any further, it is imperative that the differences in these procedures be recognized. First, patients requiring ICD implantation are more ill than those requiring permanent pacemakers. The vast majority of these patients have important structural heart disease, often with poor left ventricular function and advanced coronary artery disease. Many patients suffering from ventricular tachycardia and fibrillation also have important pulmonary dysfunction. Second, although most pacemakers can be implanted using local anesthesia alone, some method of general anesthesia is always required for implantation and testing of an ICD. Third, several features of ICD implantation involve a much greater amount of surgical dissection than for pacemaker implantation. The much larger size of the presently available ICD pulse generators (> 180 g) requires implantation in the subcutaneous (or submuscular) planes of the abdominal wall. In contrast, implantation of a permanent pacemaker (< 40 g) requires minimal dissection. Although most transvenous ICDs can be implanted with a lead-only system, achievement of an acceptable defibrillation threshold may require the use of a subcutaneous defibrillating patch electrode[12–15,17,21–23] or array.[24,25] In addition, a transvenous lead must be tunneled from the subclavian or cephalic vein entrance site to the abdominal pocket.

Anesthesia for Implantable Cardioverter-Defibrillator Implantation

Although implantation of a transvenous lead-only ICD system may not require extensive surgical dissection, a subcutaneous electrode patch or array may be necessary to achieve an acceptable defibrillation threshold.[12–15,17,21–25] Because intraoperative defibrillation threshold testing is required to ensure optimal electrode placement, general anesthesia is necessary for ICD implantation. Several centers have used intravenous sedation with the combination of a narcotic (fentanyl, meperidine, or morphine) and a benzodiazepine for implantation of a transvenous lead-only ICD system. During tunneling of the lead to the abdominal pocket or during subcutaneous or submuscular dissection for implantation of an axillary patch electrode or array, sedation may be supplemented with short-acting intravenous barbiturates such as methohexital. The alternative approach is to use intravenous narcotics and sedative-hypnotics with standard endotracheal intubation and mechanical ventilation.

Although there are no studies, to our knowledge, that have assessed the effects of anesthetics on the defibrillation threshold in humans, the effects of several have been examined in animal models, and the influence is inconsistent. Wang and Dorian[26] reported that the energies required for 50% and 80% success for defibrillation in dogs were approximately 28% to 36% lower with fentanyl than with pentobarbital or enflurane. Gill et al.[27] found no difference in the defibrillation threshold when measured in the presence of pentobarbital, halothane, or isoflurane. Furthermore, since anesthetics may alter the inducibility of ventricular tachycardia[28,29] and fibrillation,[30] the defibrillation threshold may also be affected. Thus, anesthetics that may increase the defibrillation threshold are best avoided.[26,31]

In the opinion of the authors, there are several important advantages to endotracheal intubation. First, the operator is relieved of the distractions required to monitor the adequacy of ventilation with intravenous sedation alone. Second, the airway is protected throughout the procedure by endotracheal intubation in a controlled setting prior to start of the procedure. Because defibrillation testing may require repeated induction and termination of ventricular fibrillation, the hemodynamic state of the patient may consequently deteriorate.[32-34] The added control of the airway and the adequacy of ventilation ensure that these factors do not contribute to deteriorating hemodynamics. In addition, elective intubation minimizes the consequences of emergency intubation, including aspiration, hypoxemia, and airway trauma. Because of these concerns, it is our practice to perform ICD implantation in the electrophysiology laboratory with routine, elective endotracheal intubation and mechanical ventilation supervised by a cardiac anesthesiologist. The adequacy of ventilation is assessed by continuous monitoring of transcutaneous oxygen saturation and end-expired carbon dioxide concentration with periodic measurement of arterial blood gases. Arterial pressure is monitored by the use of a radial arterial catheter and the central venous pressure is monitored by the use of a multiple lumen catheter placed in the right internal jugular vein. For patients with poor left or right ventricular function, a pulmonary artery catheter may also be used for hemodynamic monitoring, although it may interfere with placement of the permanent transvenous defibrillation, sensing and pacing electrode catheters. Although such an approach may add to the cost of the procedure, the safety of ICD implantation may be enhanced, and in some circumstances, cost may be even decreased by decreasing complications.

The Environment of the Electrophysiology Laboratory for Implantable Cardioverter-Defibrillator Implantation

In many ways the electrophysiology laboratory is ideally suited to ICD implantation. First, the technicians and nurses are experienced in the care of patients with arrhythmias.[35] Hemodynamic and electrophysiologic monitoring are routinely performed in the electrophysiology laboratory. Perhaps most importantly, fluoroscopic equipment is available that usually far surpasses that available in the operating room. Equipment for inserting electrophysiologic catheters, temporary pacemakers, programmable stimulators, physiological recorders, and high-energy external defibrillators are routinely available. If angiographic recordings are required, such facilities are available as well as the operators experienced in these techniques. Such factors are considerable advantages for ICD implantation.

The electrophysiology laboratory, however, may have several disadvantages in comparison to the operating room. First, the sterility of the room may not be suitable for the implantation of the large amount of foreign materials of an ICD system. It is thus imperative that the sterile environment not be compromised. The air supply to the room must be filtered, with the airflow directed toward the operating table. With this standard configuration, the airflow carries airborne particles away from the operative field and is collected at the sides of the room. The air pressure within the room must exceed that in the hallways outside the room to avoid the influx of untreated air. The lighting must be adequate to ensure visibility with a light source for the operative field that is adjustable by the operators without compromising sterility. The availability of oxygen for mechanical ventilators and suction facilities should not be inferior to those in the operating room.

Preoperative Preparation and General Considerations

The preoperative preparation of the patient undergoing ICD implantation should be the same regardless of where the procedure is performed. It is our practice to have patients bath with an antimicrobial soap (Hibiclens) the night prior to the procedure at least twice and preferably three times. Prophylactic antibiotics are given intravenously beginning the night before the procedure, typically a combination of vancomycin and a fourth-generation cephalosporin. This approach ensures adequate tissue levels of antibiotics at the time the skin is incised.[36] Intravenous diphenhydramine is given on call as a mild sedative. Operative sterility is emphasized throughout the procedure. The incisions, tunnel, and pocket are all irrigated with antibiotic solution containing either polymyxin B and methicillin,[6] or polymyxin B and bacitracin.

Implantation of Transvenous Defibrillating Leads

Although either the right or left subclavian or cephalic veins can be used for access to the heart, from a surgical perspective, a left-sided approach is preferred because the large transvenous leads pass with greater ease from the left than from the right. Whenever the cephalic vein accommodates the transvenous lead or leads, it should be used to decrease the risk of pneumothorax and "clavicular crush".[37-39] We have used an internal jugular approach on one occasion when neither subclavian nor cephalic approaches were feasible. It is our observation that the tip of the right ventricular electrode, whether it be part of a composite lead (Cardiac Pacemakers, Inc., St. Paul, MN) or not (Medtronic, Inc., Minneapolis, MN; Intermedics, Inc., Angleton, TX; Ventritex, Sunnyvale, CA), should be as close to the right ventricular apex as possible for both stability and optimization of the defibrillation threshold. Conversely, the second transvenous electrode should be as high in the superior vena cava as possible, or even in the innominate vein. This positioning maximizes the shock vector to incorporate as much of the interventricular septum and left ventricle as possible that is thought to be important for minimizing the energy required for defibrillation. These observations are in keeping with those of Saksena et al.[40] who observed that for intermediate energy shocks, the optimal defibrillation pathway was between the right ventricular apex and the left axilla. Indeed, if a right-sided approach were used, this shock trajectory would be impossible to achieve. We are unaware of any data comparing the defibrillation threshold using right or left-sided approaches.

After confirmation of an adequate defibrillation threshold, with either a totally transvenous system, or incorporating a subcutaneous electrode of some kind, the lead must be tunneled to the upper abdominal quadrant for attachment to the ICD. New generation, smaller ICDs will be prepectoral and not have such a requirement.[16,17] Tunneling of the lead can be accomplished with either a trochar or blunt dissection and "pulling through" of the lead(s) within a Penrose drain.[6] For this procedure, a way-incision is required halfway in between the subclavian incision and the abdominal pocket at which the pull-through is carried out in a two-stage process. The tunnel diameter must allow passage of the drain and leads without tension.

Prior to the development of ICDs providing pacing capabilities, combined device systems were not infrequently required for bradycardia support and for antitachycardia pacing. Although new generation ICDs with both shock and pacing capabilities are available, there are instances where a permanent pacemaker is still required, for example to provide atrial synchrony. Also, current ICD battery technology is not yet at a stage that allows for continual pacing without a tremendous cost to device longevity. As previously, complications attributable to adverse device-device interactions can be avoided by paying special attention to positioning of the ICD sensing/pacing leads relative to the permanent pacing lead(s).[41–43] With nonthoracotomy ICDs, it is usually advisable to implant the ICD first so that the distal defibrillating lead can be positioned at the right ventricular apex for optimization of the defibrillation threshold. Thereafter, active fixation pacing leads can be positioned at locations (eg, the right ventricular outflow tract, or atrium) distant from the ICD sensing circuit.[43]

Implantation of Subcutaneous and Submuscular Electrodes

With the advent of more effective defibrillation waveforms and prepectoral ICD devices, the use of a subcutaneous or submuscular electrode to decrease the defibrillation threshold should decrease in frequency. However, when required, a subcutaneous or submuscular lead can spare the patient from thoracotomy. In keeping with the work of Saksena et al.,[40] our practice has been to implant the extrathoracic electrode toward the axilla and posteriorly. Some have even chosen a subscapular location, but the long-term effect of scapular pressure on these leads is unknown.

A most exciting innovation in lead technology is the SQ Array™ lead (CPI, St. Paul, MN). This lead is comprised of three electrically common multifilar coil elements joined at a molded yoke by insulated cable to be used as part of the defibrillation circuit.[24,25] It is implanted subcutaneously or submuscularly over the left thorax in place of the more commonly used subcutaneous or submuscular patch. A 3- to 4-cm incision is made perpendicular to the ribs to the left of the sternum where the yoke and suture sleeves will be located. A tunneler is used with peel-away sheaths to position the three filaments along the left thorax in a posterior location. We have found it useful to have the three filaments widely spaced with the most superior one coursing posteriorly in the axilla. Again, this location is in keeping with the findings of Saksena et al.[40] showing lower defibrillation energy requirements with electrodes in the axillary location. Using this approach we have had no failures to defibrillate with monophasic shocks using an intravascular catheter with this new lead.

Intraoperative Defibrillation Threshold Testing

Defibrillation threshold testing is an integral part of ICD implantation. Although it has been shown that patients with high defibrillation thresholds may still benefit from ICD therapy, their proportional incidence of arrhythmic death is greater than in patients with lower defibrillation thresholds.[44] An adequate defibrillation threshold is even more important than with epicardial lead systems since defibrillation energy requirements are higher with nonthoracotomy systems than with epicardial ones, and unlike with epicardial systems there may be an increase in the defibrillation threshold with time[45–47] thereby necessitating a wider margin of safety at implantation to ensure an adequate margin of safety later on. If the defibrillation threshold is unsatisfactory and a thoracotomy is then planned, the latter should be undertaken on a separate day since operative mortality is increased if the anesthesia and operation are extended on the same day after multiple defibrillations.[32–35,48]

Construction of the Abdominal Pocket

There is no difference in construction of the abdominal pocket whether it is done in the operating room or in the electrophysiology laboratory. Although pockets may be constructed subcutaneously anterior to the rectus sheath, intramuscularly within the rectus muscle, or under the rectus muscle, we have most recently chosen to implant the generators deeply overlying the abdominal fascia in the subrectus position. This leads to an improved cosmetic result (the device is further removed from the skin surface resulting in a smaller external bulge) and perhaps a lower incidence of infection because of superior lymphatic drainage from the deeper location. Such deeper incisions, however, may have a greater chance for intraperitoneal perforation, a complication we have fortunately not encountered. Special care is taken to avoid damage to the perforating arteries to the skin so that healing can be optimal.

Postoperative Care of the Implantable Cardioverter-Defibrillator Patient

Patients are usually extubated in the electrophysiology laboratory after the procedure. It is our practice to allow patients to recover for 1–4 hours before transfer to a telemetry unit. Antibiotics are administered intravenously for 24 hours postoperatively. The following morning patients are encouraged to ambulate in the hallway. If the patient is recuperating normally, all intravenous lines and in-dwelling urinary catheters are removed by 24 hours after the operation. This approach greatly minimizes the risk of nosocomial infections. Patients typically undergo a postoperative electrophysiologic study to confirm appropriate sensing, pacing, cardioversion, and defibrillation thresholds of the implanted system. For this procedure, patients are given the choice of whether or not to receive intravenous sedation. Many in fact are interested in experiencing a shock in this controlled environment to be aware of the sensation before they experience a spontaneous event. If the recovery period has been uneventful, patients may be discharged from the hospital as early as 48 hours after their operation. Usually, however, we keep patients longer to complete their intravenous antibiotic course and to perform postoperative electrophysiologic study.

Summary

The development of transvenous defibrillating electrodes, biphasic shock waveforms, and the decreasing size of the ICD pulse generator have allowed implantation of the ICD within the electrophysiology laboratory. Although ICD implantation has become less traumatic for the patient with these advances, the safety and efficacy of these procedures must not be compromised by a change in the implantation setting. As devices become smaller and incorporate the pulse generator case into the defibrillating electrodes it is likely that the majority of ICDs will be implanted outside the operating room.

References

1. Watkins L, Mower MM, Reid PR, et al: Surgical techniques for implanting the automatic implantable defibrillator. *PACE* 7:1357, 1984.
2. Cannom DS, Winkle RA: Implantation of the automatic implantable cardioverter defibrillator (AICD): practical aspects. *PACE* 9:793, 1986.
3. Thurer RJ, Luceri RM, Bolooki H: Automatic implantable cardioverter-defibrillator: techniques of implantation and results. *Ann Thorac Surg* 42:143, 1986.
4. Watkins L, Taylor E: The surgical aspects of automatic implantable cardioverter-defibrillator implantation. *PACE* 14:953, 1991.
5. Frank G, Lowes D: Implantable cardioverter defibrillators: surgical considerations. *PACE* 15:631, 1992.
6. Shepard RB, Goldin MD, Lawrie GM, et al: Automatic implantable cardioverter defibrillator: surgical approaches for implantation. *J Cardiac Surg* 7:208, 1992.
7. Mirowski M, Mower M, Staewen WS, et al:

Ventricular defibrillation through a single intravascular catheter electrode system (abstract). *Clin Res* 19:328, 1971.
8. Schuder JC, Stoeckle H, West JA, et al: Ventricular defibrillation with catheter having distal electrode in right ventricle and proximal electrode in superior vena cava (abstract). *Circulation* 43–44:99, 1971.
9. Mower M, Mirowski M, Pitt B, et al: Ventricular defibrillation with a single intravascular catheter system having distal electrode in left pulmonary artery and proximal electrode in right ventricle or right atrium (abstract). *Clin Res* 20:389, 1972.
10. Mirowski M, Mower MM, Staewen WS, et al: The development of the transvenous automatic defibrillator. *Arch Intern Med* 129:773, 1972.
11. Mirowski M, Mower MM, Gott VL, et al: Feasibility and effectiveness of low-energy catheter defibrillation in man. *Circulation* 47:79, 1973.
12. Saksena S, Parsonnet V: Implantation of a cardioverter/defibrillator without thoracotomy using a triple electrode system. *JAMA* 259:69, 1988.
13. Saksena S, Tullo NG, Krol RB, et al: Initial clinical experience with endocardial defibrillation using an implantable cardioverter/defibrillator with a triple-electrode system. *Arch Intern Med* 149:2333, 1989.
14. Bardy GH, Allen MD, Mehra R, et al: Transvenous defibrillation in humans via the coronary sinus. *Circulation* 81:1252, 1990.
15. Bardy GH, Hofer B, Johnson G, et al: Implantable transvenous cardioverter-defibrillators. *Circulation* 87:1152, 1993.
16. Bardy GH, Johnson G, Poole JE, et al: A simplified, single-lead unipolar transvenous cardioversion-defibrillation system. *Circulation* 88:543, 1993.
17. Camuñas J, Mehta D, Ip J, et al: Total pectoral implantation: a new technique for implantation of transvenous defibrillator lead systems and implantable cardioverter defibrillator. *PACE* 16:1380, 1993.
18. Gross JN, Ben-Zur UM, Furman S, et al: Transvenous ICD implantation: feasibility of implantation by cardiologists in a cardiac catheterization laboratory environment (abstract). 16:902, 1993.
19. Parsonnet V, Bernstein AD, Lindsay B: Pacemaker-implantation complication rates: an analysis of some contributing factors. *J Am Coll Cardiol* 13:917, 1989.
20. Bernstein AD, Parsonnet V: Survey of cardiac pacing in the United States in 1989. *Am J Cardiol* 69:331, 1992.
21. McCowan R, Maloney J, Wilkoff B, et al: Automatic implantable cardioverter-defibrillator implantation without thoracotomy using an endocardial and submuscular patch system. *J Am Coll Cardiol* 17:415, 1991.
22. Hauser RG, Kurschinski DT, McVeigh K, et al: Clinical results with nonthoracotomy ICD systems. *PACE* 16:141, 1993.
23. Winter J, Vester EG, Kuhls S, et al: Defibrillation energy requirements with single endocardial (Endotak™) lead. *PACE* 16:540, 1993.
24. Jordaens L, Vertongen P, van Belleghem Y: A subcutaneous lead array for implantable cardioverter defibrillators. *PACE* 16:1429, 1993.
25. Baker JH, Epstein AE, Voshage L, et al: The SQ array: a new non-thoracotomy implantable cardioverter defibrillator lead that reduces the defibrillation threshold. *J Am Coll Cardiol* (in press).
26. Wang M, Dorian P: Defibrillation energy requirements differ between anesthetic agents. *J Electrophysiol* 3:86, 1989.
27. Gill RM, Sweeney RJ, Reid PR: The defibrillation threshold: a comparison of anesthetics and measurement methods. *PACE* 16:708, 1993.
28. Hunt GB, Ross DL: Comparison of effects of three anesthetic agents on induction of ventricular tachycardia in a canine model of myocardial infarction. *Circulation* 78:221, 1988.
29. Hief C, Borggrefe M, Chen X, et al: Effects of enflurane on inducibility of ventricular tachycardia. *Am J Cardiol* 68:609, 1991.
30. Saini V, Carr DB, Hagestad EL, et al: Antifibrillatory action of the narcotic agonist fentanyl. *Am Heart J* 115:598, 1988.
31. Natale A, Jones DL, Kim Y-H, et al: Effects of lidocaine on defibrillation threshold in the pig: evidence of anesthesia related increase. *PACE* 14:1239, 1991.
32. Singer I, van der Laken J, Edmonds HL, et al: Is defibrillation testing safe? *PACE* 14:1899, 1991.
33. Frame R, Brodman R, Furman S, et al: Clinical evaluation of the safety of repetitive intraoperative defibrillation threshold testing. *PACE* 15:870, 1992.
34. Ware DL, Atkinson JB, Brooks MJ, et al: Ventricular defibrillation in canines with chronic infarction, and effects of lidocaine and procainamide. *PACE* 16:337, 1993.
35. Lehmann MH, Saksena S: Implantable cardioverter defibrillators in cardiovascular practice: report of the Policy Conference of the North American Society of Pacing and Electrophysiology. *PACE* 14:969, 1991.
36. Mounsey JP, Griffith MJ, Gold RG, et al: Antibiotic prophylaxis reduces re-operation rate for infective complications following permanent cardiac pacemaker implantation:

a prospective randomized trial (abstract). *Circulation* 88:I-19, 1993.
37. Fyke FE: Infraclavicular lead failure: tarnish on a golden route. *PACE* 16:373, 1993.
38. Jacobs DM, Fink AS, Miller RP, et al: Anatomical and morphological evaluation of pacemaker lead compression. *PACE* 16:434, 1993.
39. Magney JE, Flynn DM, Parsons JA, et al: Anatomical mechanisms explaining damage to pacemaker leads, defibrillator leads, and failure of central venous catheters adjacent to the sternoclavicular joint. *PACE* 16:445, 1993.
40. Saksena S, DeGroot P, Krol RB, et al: Low-energy endocardial defibrillation using an axillary or a pectoral thoracic electrode location. *Circulation* 88:2655, 1993.
41. Epstein AE, Kay GN, Plumb VJ, et al: Combined automatic implantable cardioverter-defibrillator and pacemaker systems: implantation techniques and follow-up. *J Am Coll Cardiol* 13:121, 1989.
42. Epstein AE, Shepard RB: Permanant pacemakers and implantable cardioverter defibrillators: potential interactions. In: *Automatic Implantable Cardioverter Defibrillators: A Comprehensive Text*. Edited by P Wang, NAM Estes, A Manolis. New York, NY: Marcel Dekker, Inc.; (in press).
43. Epstein AE, Wilkoff BL: Pacemaker-defibrillator interactions. In: *Clinical Cardiac Pacing*. Edited by KA Ellenbogen, GN Kay, BL Wilkoff. Philadelphia, PA: WB Saunders Company; (in press).
44. Epstein AE, Ellenbogen KA, Kirk KA, et al: Clinical characteristics and outcome of patients with high defibrillation thresholds: a multicenter study. *Circulation* 86:1206, 1992.
45. Kallock MJ, Wibel FH, Bourland JD, et al: Catheter electrode defibrillation in dogs: threshold dependence on implant time and catheter stability. *Am Heart J* 109:821, 1985.
46. Hsia HH, Flores BT, Marchlinski FE: Early postoperative increase in defibrillation threshold with nonthoracotomy lead system in man (abstract). *Circulation* 86:I-451, 1993.
47. Venditti FJ, Martin DT, Vassolas G, et al: Rise in chronic defibrillation thresholds in nonthoracotomy implantable defibrillator. *Circulation* 89:216, 1994.
48. Lehmann MH, Mitchell LB, Saksena S, et al: Operative (30-day) mortality with transvenous vs. epicardial ICD implantation: an intention-to-treat analysis. *Circulation* 86:I-656, 1992.

Chapter 17

Unipolar Defibrillation Systems

Gust H. Bardy, Merritt H. Raitt, and Greg K. Jones

Introduction

The use of a nonthoracotomy lead (NTL) implantable cardioverter-defibrillators (ICDs) demands a high degree of technical expertise compared with pacemaker therapy. The complexity of NTL ICDs arises in part from the need to frequently test multiple lead configurations and pulsing methods, from the size of the ICD that usually require implantation in the abdomen, and/or from the use of long transvenous leads (110 cm) that must be tunneled from their cephalic or subclavian vein insertion sites subcutaneously along the chest and over the costal margin to the abdominal pocket. These long leads together with the need for an abdominal pocket, increase the complexity of the implant procedure, require two, and sometimes three incisions if a subcutaneous patch is needed, and may lead to complications like lead dislodgment, lead fracture, and pocket infections.[1,2] Consequently, the utility of NTL ICDs in preventing sudden cardiac death is offset by their complexity and resultant morbidity. A simpler ICD might provide all the benefits of protection from ventricular tachycardia (VT) or ventricular fibrillation (VF) without the drawbacks of what remains a major surgical procedure.

A Unipolar, Single Electrode Pectoral Transvenous Defibrillation System

Converting the shell of a relatively small 80-cc volume ICD into an active electrode to be used in conjunction with a single transvenous right ventricular (RV) defibrillation electrode system, has been shown to greatly simplify ICD use.[3] The pulse generator of this relatively small device (Medtronic model 7219C, Minneapolis, MN) has been designed for pectoral implantation (Figure 1). The active "can" is a titanium shell that contains the pulse generator and acts as a large surface area electrode. The large surface area electrode of the ICD can, coupled to a 65% tilt biphasic pulse, has been demonstrated to improve defibrillation efficacy substantially. This unipolar system has been tested in 102 consecutive patients undergoing standard NTL defibrillator implantation at our institution. In 100 patients (98%) the defibrillation threshold (DFT) was < 24 J (Figure 2) with the mean DFT being 9.8 ± 6.6 J.

Comparison of the defibrillation efficacy and ease of implantation of this system with a standard NTL system using two transvenous electrodes and a subcutaneous patch lead system has been favorable. As

From Singer I, (ed.) Implantable Cardioverter-Defibrillator. Armonk, NY: Futura Publishing Company, Inc.; © 1994.

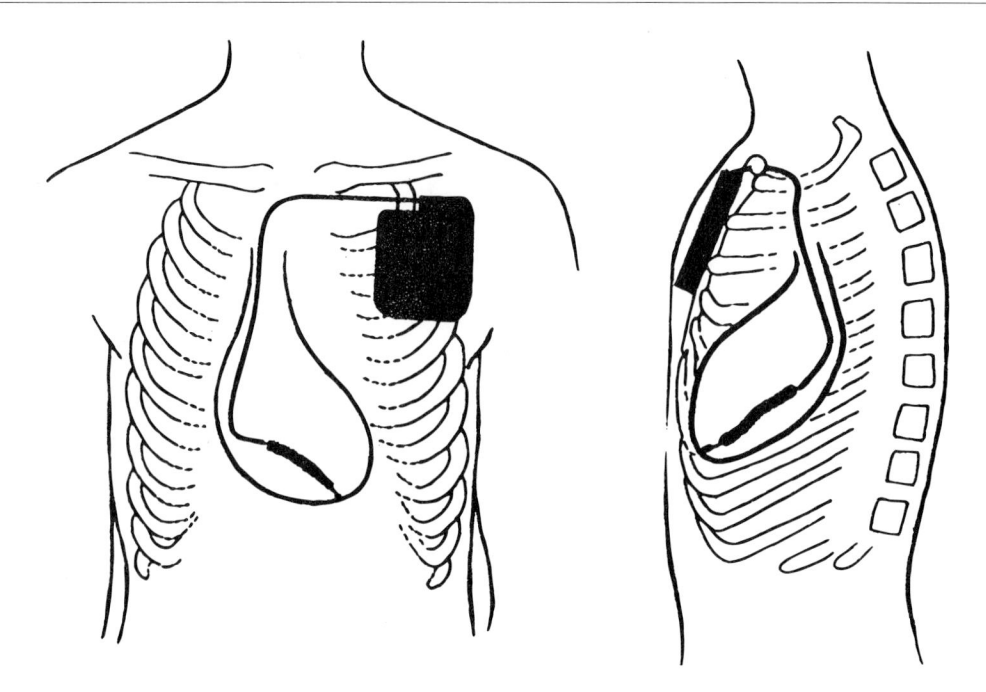

Figure 1. Schematic representation of the unipolar single electrode transvenous defibrillation system. The pulse generator, an active "can" titanium shell, is the cathode for defibrillation and the coil electrode in the right ventricular apex is the anode. The large surface area of the can electrode and the inferior-to-superior and right-to-left orientation of the defibrillation pulse probably contribute significantly to the low energy required for defibrillation using this system. (Reprinted with permission from Reference 3.)

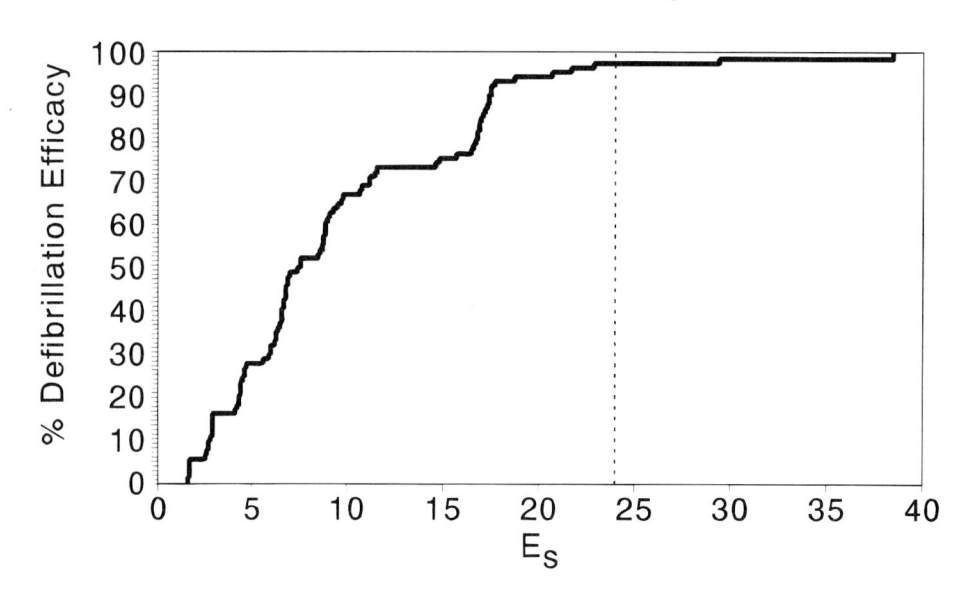

Figure 2. Percent efficacy curve for the single electrode transvenous defibrillation system in 102 consecutive patients. The percent of patients with successful defibrillation at each stored energy level is plotted. At an energy of ≤ 24 J, 98% of patients had successful defibrillation as indicated by the vertical dotted line.

mentioned above, the DFT for the unipolar, active can system was 9.8 ± 6.6 J while the DFT for the best configuration tested of the standard NTL system was 12.0 ± 5.2 J ($P < 0.0001$). To identify the optimal standard NTL system with such a relatively low DFT, 3.2 ± 2.0 pulsing methods were tested involving 6.9 ± 2.5 VF inductions. The standard NTL system consequently compared poorly in this regard to the single configuration unipolar system where only 3.4 ± 0.9 VF inductions were required to determine the DFT, $P < 0.0001$. Moreover, a corresponding implant time savings for the single lead, single incision unipolar system was observed, 108 ± 128 minutes, compared to the 183 ± 19 minutes for the standard NTL approach.[3] This system, therefore, appears to be nearly as simple to implant as a single lead pacemaker with a 98% implantation success rate assuming the need for at least a 10-J safety margin above the DFT. Such a system may have profound implications for ICD reliability, safety and cost, and for ICD use.

Why the unipolar single lead system performs so well is not completely clear. Part of its performance can be explained by the use of an efficient biphasic defibrillation pulse.[4] Other factors may also be responsible for its efficacy. The large surface area of the pectoral can electrode probably increases the electric field gradient that the heart experiences by decreasing impedance at the electrode/tissue interface thereby allowing more current to enter the thorax. In addition, the inferior to superior and right to left vectors of the defibrillation pulse may optimize cardiac electric field distribution in at least two of three dimensions. Finally, making the RV lead (the electrode closest to the heart) anodal is probably the best configuration to maximize defibrillation efficacy.[5,6]

Implantation Technique

The method of implantation of the unipolar defibrillation system will ultimately depend on anatomy and body habitus. For most people, the 80-cc active can system can be inserted via a subcutaneous or subpectoral approach in the left infraclavicular area. In very small people, a traditional abdominal implantation site would be required and the unipolar system would not be useful in this instance. Similarly, if the left shoulder area is inaccessible, then an alternative ICD system is indicated. If the active can is placed in the right shoulder area or the abdomen, the current vector from RV to an active pectoral can would be suboptimal or ineffective. In these instances, use of more traditional lead systems, such as a superior vena cava, subcutaneous patch, or coronary sinus lead system, in conjunction with an RV lead, would be more appropriate.

Insertion of the 10.5F RV endocardial lead that is part of the unipolar defibrillation system is possible with either Seldinger cannulation of the left subclavian vein or direct venotomy of the left cephalic vein. It is recommended that the cephalic vein be used whenever possible to avoid crush injury in the first rib-clavicular space of the RV lead. When inserting the RV lead, care must be taken to position the RV lead coil such that it does not interfere with the active can electrode. Figure 3 shows the RV lead entering the cephalic vein. It is anchored to the underlying fascia in such a manner that the lead makes a gentle clockwise curve sufficient to curl about the ICD and enter a medially oriented connector block. If the subclavian vein is used (Figure 4), the 10.5F lead should be inserted into the left subclavian vein at a site more lateral than usual to minimize the likelihood of first rib-clavicular crush syndrome. Regardless of cephalic or subclavian vein use, as the lead exits the vein, the lead should encircle the can in a clockwise direction. This allows the lead to enter the portals of the connector block without undue torsion or convolution of the lead. Moreover, it avoids location of the lead body either above or beneath the ICD, a location that might interfere with defibrillation current transmission. This position-

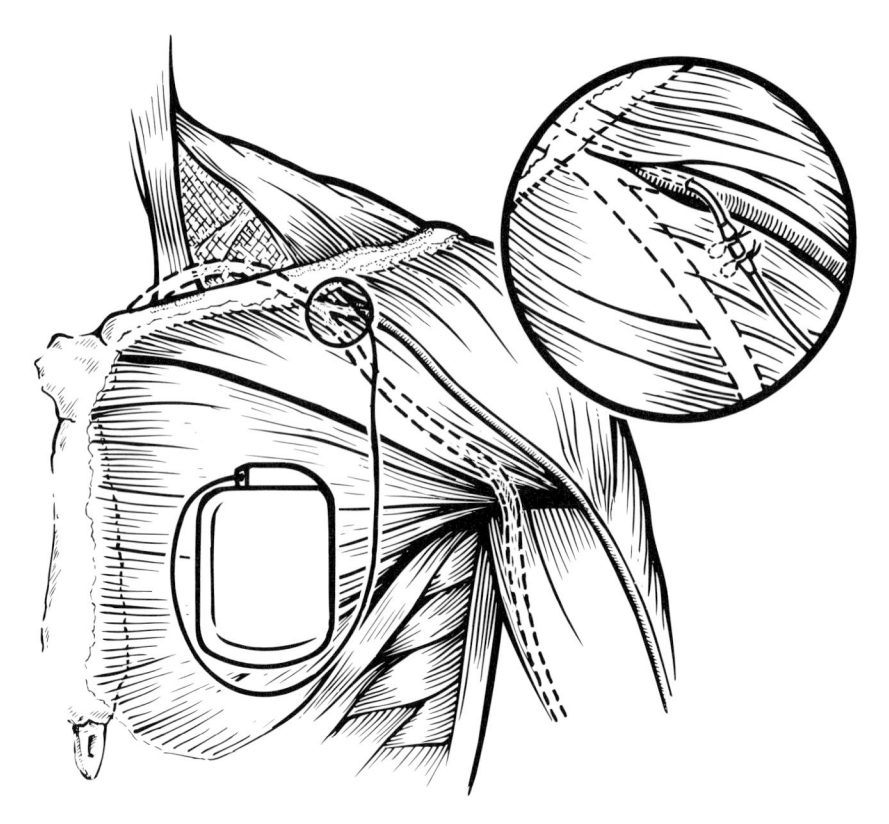

Figure 3. Visualization of the right ventricular (RV) lead entering the cephalic vein. It is recommended that the cephalic vein be used whenever possible to avoid crush injury of the 10.5F RV lead in the first rib-clavicular space. The lead is then anchored such that it forms a gentle clockwise curve that will enable the lead to curl about the implantable cardioverter-defibrillator (ICD) and enter a medially oriented connector block without undue torsion or convolution of the lead. Moreover, it avoids location of the lead body either above or beneath the ICD. This lead location might interfere with current transmission between tissues and the can. Appropriate lead positioning requires that lead length be estimated reasonably accurately prior to insertion to ensure that the lead is long enough. Three interrupted 1-O sutures firmly applied to the anchoring sleeve is usually sufficient to secure the RV lead.

ing of the lead coil requires that lead length be estimated reasonably accurately prior to ICD surgery to ensure that lead length is sufficient.

The unipolar ICD can be inserted subcutaneously rather than subpectorally in most patients (Figure 5). We prefer this location because it is similar to a pacemaker implant and also because of the ease of ICD replacement should it become necessary. For the subcutaneous approach, it will often be necessary to invert the engraving side of the ICD to better accommodate the lead. In addition, care should be taken to position and anchor the can sufficiently medial to the left humeral head to avoid interference with left shoulder motion, in particular, left upper arm abduction.

Subpectoral insertion of the active can (Figure 6 is best reserved for patients without sufficient subcutaneous fat or space to accommodate this relatively large pulse generator. In such patients, the subpectoral approach can eliminate the type of pocket tension that would be observed with a subcutaneous insertion but this approach re-

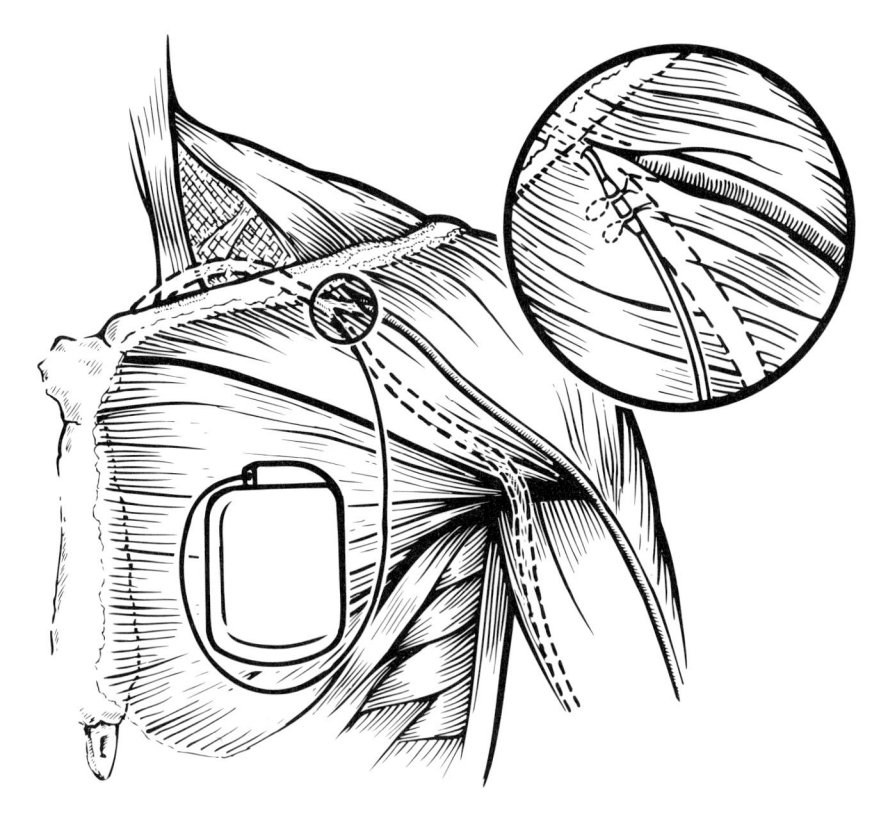

Figure 4. Illustration of the 10.5F right ventricular (RV) lead inserted into the left subclavian below the clavicle and positioned more laterally than usual to avoid first rib-clavicular crush.

quires more surgery. For this procedure, a dissection is required to the pectoralis fascia where the fibrous band that separates the inferior (sternal) portion of the pectoralis major muscle from its clavicular head can be identified (Figure 6A). The two portions of the pectoralis major muscle can then be separated with a combination of sharp and blunt dissection (Figures 6A and 6B). Usually, a modest initial interruption of the fibrous band between the two heads of the pectoralis major muscle with scissors will allow a finger to be inserted for separation of the muscle bundles along the connecting fibrous plane. Note that the caudal segment of the pectoralis major muscle descends obliquely underneath the clavicular segment for approximately 1–2 cm before the submuscular space can be entered and that the thoraco-acromial neurovascular bundle descends vertically on the underbelly of the pectoralis major muscle (Figure 6B). A cross section of the overlapping bundles of the pectoralis major (Figure 6C), reveals the oblique orientation of the two sections of the pectoralis major when viewed in the sagittal plane. Once the muscle is separated, the submuscular space is fully and easily accessible (Figure 6D), revealing intercostal muscles, the pectoralis minor muscle, the thoraco-acromial neurovascular bundle, and ribs whose periosteal tissues can serve as an anchoring site for the ICD. If possible, the thoraco-acromial neurovascular bundle should be left intact as its interruption will result in the loss of pectoralis major muscle mass and forward power of the left shoulder.

Figure 6E shows the ICD positioned beneath the pectoralis major muscle and con-

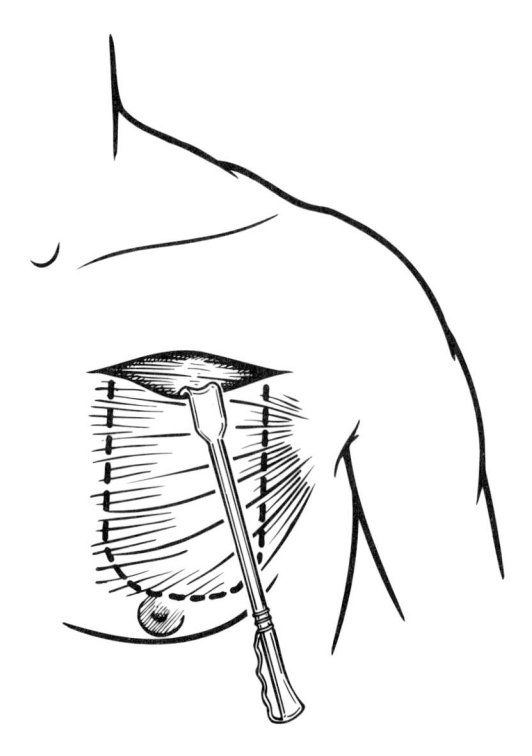

Figure 5. Subcutaneous location of the active can implantable cardioverter-defibrillator (ICD). The unipolar ICD can be inserted subcutaneously in most patients. This location is preferred because it is similar to a pacemaker implant and also because of the ease of ICD replacement should it become necessary. For the subcutaneous approach, it will often be necessary to invert the engraving side of the ICD to better accommodate the lead. In addition, care should be taken to position the ICD sufficiently medial to the left humeral head to avoid interference with left shoulder motion, in particular upper arm abduction. The ICD should also be anchored to the underlying pectoralis fascia to avoid caudad drift.

nected to the RV lead as it exits the cephalic vein. Note the pulse generator is oriented differently than with the subcutaneous approach to better accommodate the lead as it descends through the pectoralis muscle between the clavicular and sternal muscle bundles. Usually, longer lead length is needed for submuscular ICD placement. Ultimately, the direction of the connector block will best be guided by the amount of redundant lead remaining and the natural curve of the lead.

An alternative subpectoral approach is via a lateral reflection of the clavicular head of the pectoralis major (Figure 7). This portion of the pectoralis major muscle is especially accessible during left cephalic vein insertion of the RV lead.

The process of anchoring the RV lead is similar to standard pacemaker lead system anchoring rather than NTL system anchoring. The problems with lead dislodgment that occur with 110-cm NTL systems are less likely to occur with the unipolar system's shorter RV lead because this lead does not need to be tunneled to the abdomen, a location that subjects the longer leads of I systems to repetitive flexion and torsion as the patient conducts their normal activities. Consequently, the anchoring process need not be as extensive. Three interrupted 1-O sutures firmly applied to the anchoring sleeve and underlying fascia is usually sufficient to secure the RV lead.

The final part of the procedure regards anchoring the ICD to the underlying pectoralis fascia. The 80-cc Medtronic 7219C ICD is relatively large and may prove prone to caudad drift. There are anchoring portals in the ICD connector block that can be used to secure the pulse generator to the underlying pectoralis fascia (or rib fascia when inserted subpectorally). The suture should not be tightly applied to allow some modest motion of the ICD when the patient assumes the upright posture. This will avoid tenting of the skin over the cephalad portion of the ICD pocket when the patient is sitting or standing. It is important, however, to prevent significant caudad drift or this might adversely alter the electric field during shocks.

Reliability

The unipolar transvenous defibrillation system is in its infancy. However, it may well lead to improved reliability through two main mechanisms. First, the lower average DFT, compared to a standard NTL system, allows for a larger DFT safety margin. This larger safety margin may

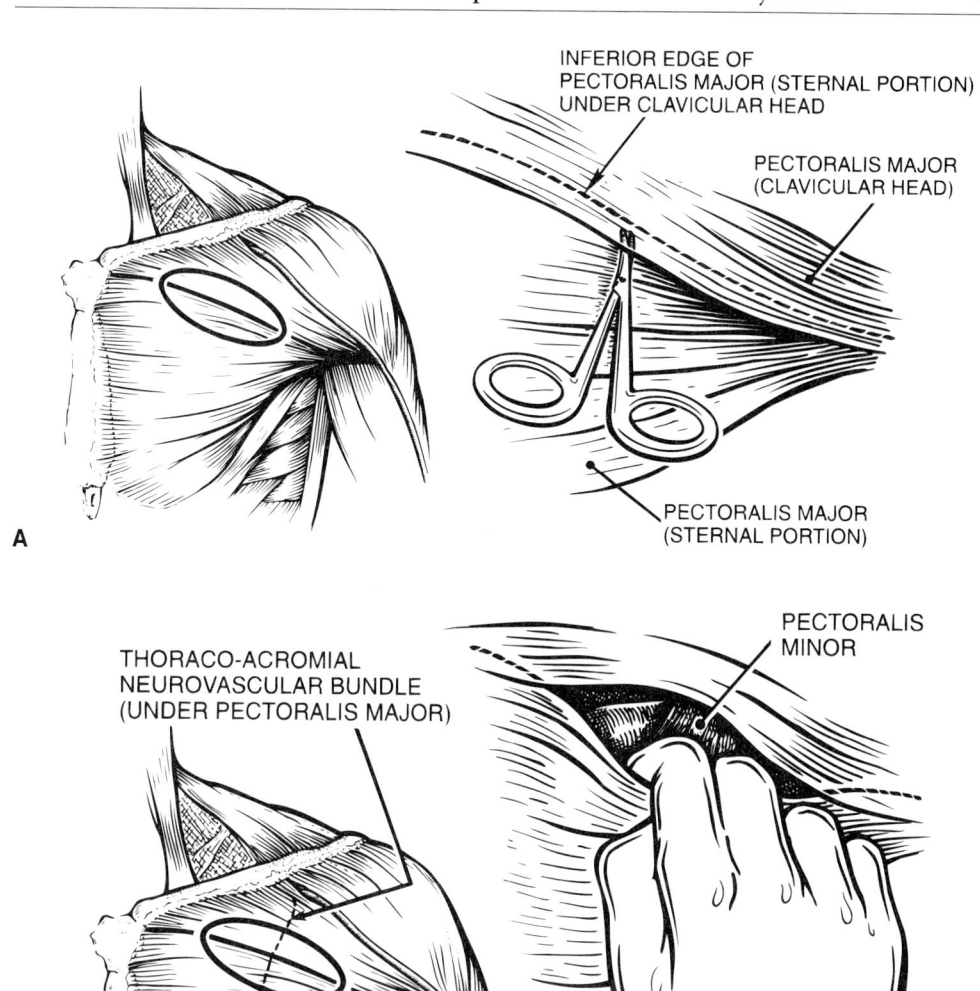

Figure 6. Subpectoral location of the active can. This location is best reserved for patients without sufficient subcutaneous fat to accommodate this relatively large pulse generator. In such patients, a subpectoral location may minimize the likelihood of implantable cardioverter-defibrillator (ICD) erosion. As shown in panel **A**, the subpectoral approach requires a dissection down to the superficial pectoralis fascia with identification of the fibrous band (encircled) that separates the inferior portion of the pectoralis major muscle from its clavicular head. Shown in the associated enlargement and in accompanying panels **B** and **C**, the two portions of the pectoralis major muscle can be separated with blunt dissection. Usually, a slight horizontal spreading of the fibrous band initially with scissors will allow a finger, panels B and C, to be inserted for separation of the muscle bundles. Note that the inferior segment or sternal portion of the pectoralis major muscle descends underneath the clavicular segment for approximately 1–2 cm before the submuscular space can be entered. This overlap is shown as a dotted line in panels A and B. A cross section of the overlapping leaves of the pectoralis major, panel C, reveals the orientation of these two sections of the pectoralis major. Once the muscle is separated, the submuscular space is easily accessible (**panel D**) revealing intercostal muscles, the pectoralis minor muscle, and the ribs whose periosteal tissues can serve as a suture

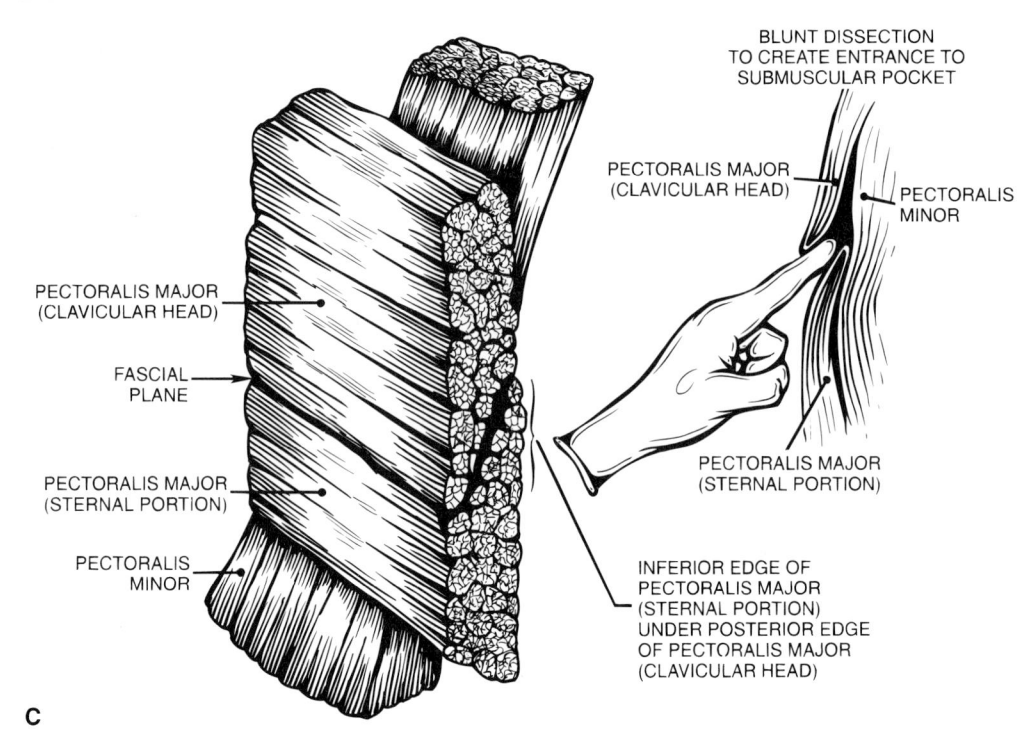

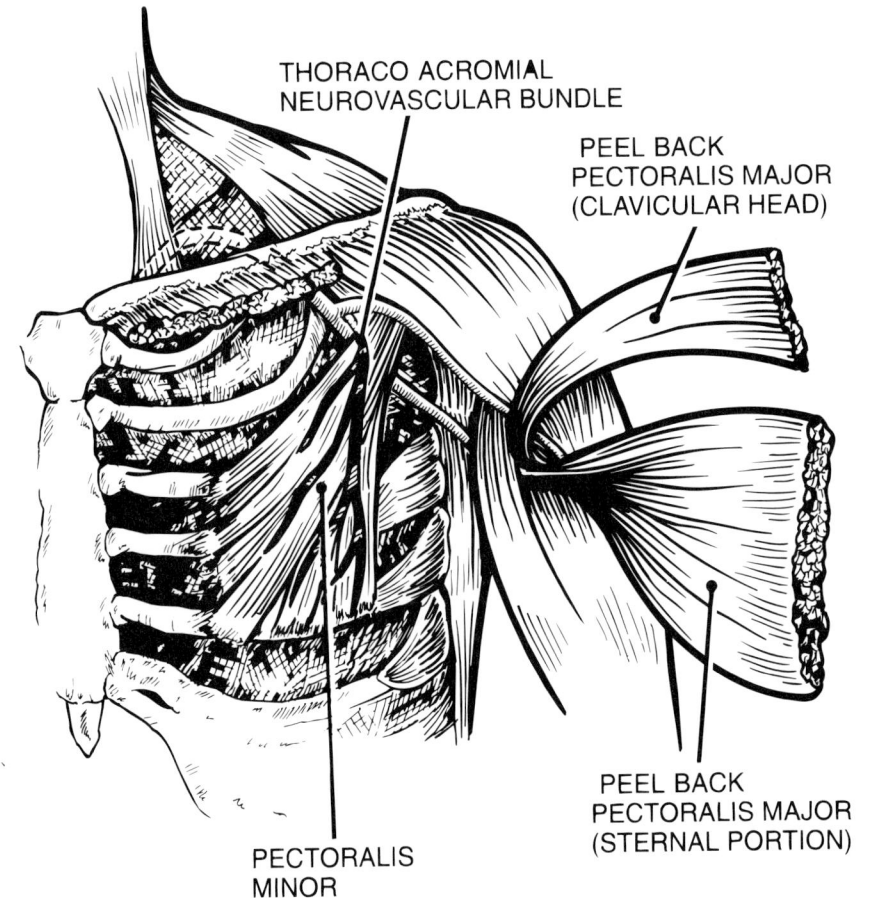

Figure 6. *(Continued)*

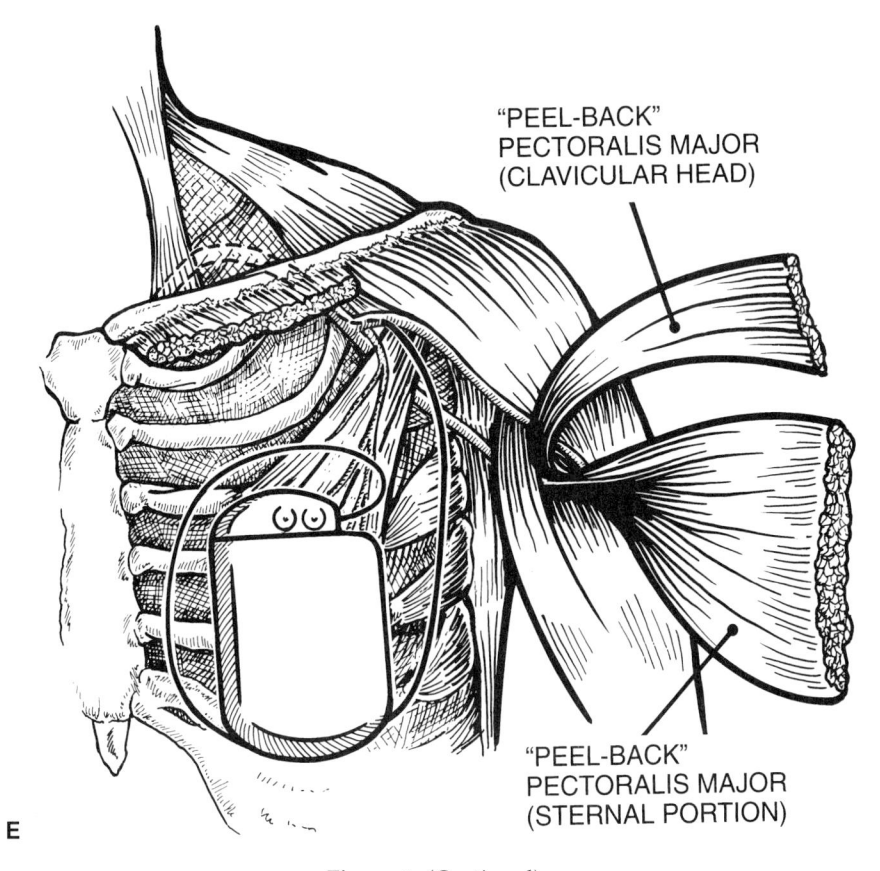

Figure 6. *(Continued)*
anchoring site for the ICD. Throughout the dissection, care must be taken to avoid severing the thoraco-acromial neurovascular bundle as it traverses vertically on the underbelly of the pectoralis major muscle, shown in panel B. Too vigorous a manual dissection of the subpectoral space may tear the vessels. One should not ligate this neurovascular bundle, if feasible, as it is the major nerve supply to the pectoralis major muscle. Loss of this nerve function will reduce forward power of the left upper arm, a problem in some athletic patients. **Panel E** shows the ICD positioned beneath the pectoralis major muscle and connected to the right ventricular (RV) lead as it exits the cephalic vein. Note the pulse generator is oriented differently than with the subcutaneous approach to better accommodate the lead as it descends through the pectoralis muscle. Usually, longer lead length is needed for submuscular ICD placement. The direction of the connector block, ultimately, will best be guided by the amount of redundant lead remaining.

make treatment failure less likely than occurs presently and may allow for the development of lower output and therefore smaller ICDs. Second, unipolar pectoral implantation has the potential to decrease the incidence of complications like lead dislodgment and fracture. Although survival with standard NTL ICDs has been excellent in our experience (Figure 8), lead system problems have been worrisome. Both lead dislodgment and fracture remain significant long-term concerns in epicardial and NTL systems.[1,2,7–9] Lead fracture has led directly to the death of one of our patients and at least one other as reported in the literature.[1] Because the unipolar ICD system requires only a single lead of a standard length (58–65 cm versus 110 cm) this lead is not likely to be subjected to the same degree of stress that a lead will be when tun-

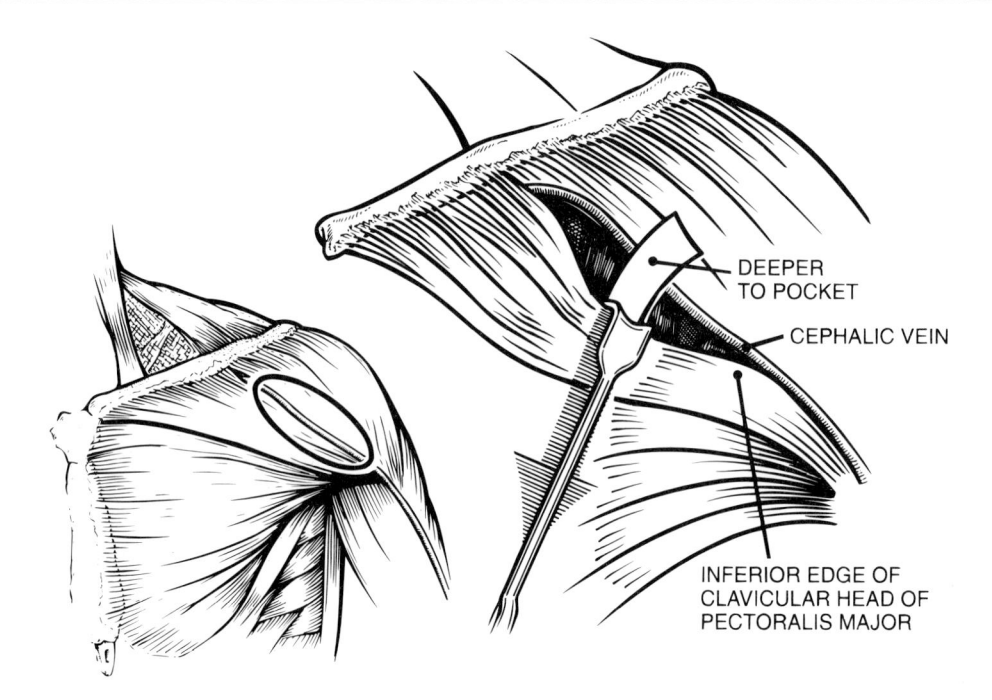

Figure 7. Submuscular approach via a lateral reflection of the clavicular head of the pectoralis major. This approach will depend upon ease of separation of the tissues, venous access site, and ability to position the implantable cardioverter-defibrillator (ICD) sufficiently medial as to not interfere with abductor motion of the left humeral head.

neled along the chest wall and across the costal margin, shorter leads, therefore should improve longevity. In addition, the fewer the leads used, the less likely fracture and lead dislodgment will probably be. Thus, low defibrillation energy requirements and a simpler lead system hold promise for increased reliability for the ICD systems.

Safety

Beyond the increased safety afforded by improved defibrillation reliability, other aspects of this new system may make it safer than standard NTL systems. First, by reducing the number of defibrillations and the anesthesia time required for implantation, operative morbidity and mortality for defibrillator implantation may be improved. Second, as a consequence of reducing operating room time, reducing the number of incisions from two or three to one, and eliminating tunneling and subcutaneous patch placement, ICD infections may prove less common. Finally, the abovementioned decrease in operating room times, the lower number of VF inductions, and the elimination of tunneling will likely allow the procedure to be done under local anesthesia in the electrophysiology laboratory, thereby eliminating the risk associated with general anesthesia. In such a procedure, the pain caused by a shock during defibrillation testing could avoided by using short-acting anesthesia, as in a standard transthoracic cardioversion procedure.

Cost

Short operative times, the use of a local anesthetic, and the ability to implant this

Cumulative Percent Surviving: TTx ICD

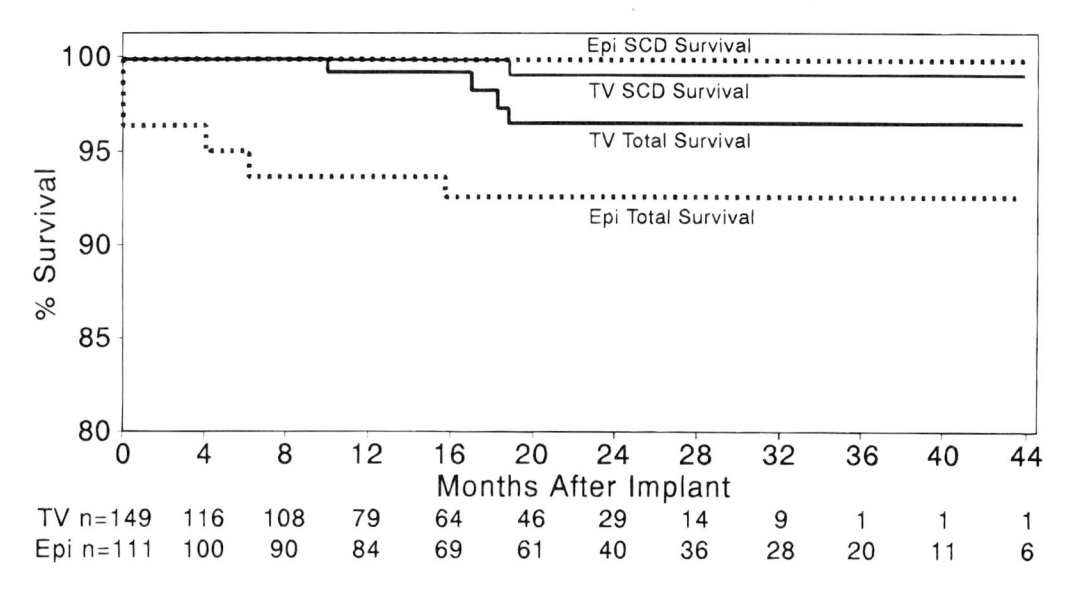

	0	4	8	12	16	20	24	28	32	36	40	44
TV n=149		116	108	79	64	46	29	14	9	1	1	1
Epi n=111		100	90	84	69	61	40	36	28	20	11	6

Figure 8. The graphs show survival curves for patients with a history of life-threatening ventricular arrhythmia after nonthoracotomy (NTL) (n = 160) and epicardial (EPI) (n = 111) defibrillation systems were implanted at our institution.

system in the electrophysiology laboratory by a cardiologist alone, in the fashion of a pacemaker, without surgical assistance, should significantly reduce the cost associated with ICD use. This cost reduction, combined with what may be a lower operative morbidity and mortality, could substantially increase the cost effectiveness of ICDs.

Utilization

If this new unipolar defibrillation system realizes its potential to be a more reliable, safer, more cost-effective alternative to epicardial or standard NTL ICDs, the indications for ICD use may be expanded. Not only may more patients with a history of ventricular arrhythmias receive ICD therapy but prophylactic ICD therapy may become a medically reasonable and cost-effective therapeutic alternative in high-risk patients who have not yet had VT or VF. There are several ongoing studies designed to test the hypothesis that mortality may be reduced by prophylactic defibrillator implantation in specific high-risk groups.[10] In these studies, operative mortality and device reliability will be key factors in determining the utility of prophylactic defibrillator implantation. The single lead unipolar defibrillation system described in this chapter, with its potential for decreased operative morbidity and mortality, increased reliability, and lower implantation cost, may be ideal for such studies investigating the role of prophylactic defibrillators.

Acknowledgments: The authors wish to thank Pete Dolan and Robin Close for their illustration work and Joan McDaniel for secretarial assistance.

References

1. Tullo NG, Saksena S, Krol RB, et al: Management of complications associated with a first-generation endocardial defibrillation lead system for implantable cardioverter-defibrillators. *Am J Cardiol* 66:411, 1990.
2. Allmassi GH, Olinger GN, Wetherbee JN, et al: Long-term complications of implantable cardioverter defibrillator lead systems. *Ann Thorac Surg* 55:888, 1993.
3. Bardy GH, Johnson G, Poole JE, et al: A simplified, single-lead unipolar transvenous cardioversion-defibrillation system. *Circulation* 88:543, 1993.
4. Bardy GH, Ivey TD, Allen MD, et al: A prospective, randomized evaluation of biphasic vs monophasic waveform pulses on defibrillation efficacy in humans. *J Am Coll Cardiol* 14:728, 1989.
5. Bardy GH, Ivey TD, Allen MD, et al: Evaluation of electrode polarity on defibrillation efficacy. *Am J Cardiol* 63:433, 1989.
6. O'Neill PG, Boahene KA, Lawrie GM, et al: The automatic implantable cardioverter-defibrillator: effect of patch polarity on defibrillation threshold. *J Am Coll Cardiol* 17:707, 1991.
7. Bardy GH, Hofer B, Johnson G, et al: Implantable transvenous cardioverter-defibrillators. *Circulation* 87:1152, 1993.
8. Stambler BS, Wood MA, Damiano RJ, et al: Prospective study of sensing/pacing lead complications with a third generation implantable cardioverter defibrillator (ICD): implications for national lead database (abstract). *Circulation* 86(Suppl I):I-59, 1992.
9. Daoud EG, Lewis RR, Siddique AH, et al: Incidence of internal cardioverter defibrillator sensing lead fracture (abstract). *Circulation* 86(Suppl I):I-452, 1992.
10. Klein H, Trappe HJ, Fieguth HG, et al: Prospective studies evaluating prophylactic ICD therapy for high risk patients with coronary artery disease. *PACE* 16:564, 1993.

Chapter 18

Interactions of Implantable Cardioverter-Defibrillators With Antiarrhythmic Drugs and Pacemakers

Igor Singer and David A. Slater

During the past decade, implantable cardioverter-defibrillators (ICDs) have evolved from nonprogrammable devices capable of only administering a cardioverting or defibrillating shock to multiprogrammable tiered-therapy devices with antitachycardia pacing (ATP), low-energy cardioversion, defibrillation, and bradycardia support capabilities. The way that we approach ventricular arrhythmias has evolved along with these technological advances. Implantable cardioverter-defibrillators are no longer used as the treatment of last resort, but thought of instead as an essential component of a multidisciplinary approach used to treat malignant tachyarrhythmias. For example, antiarrhythmic drugs are frequently used in patients with implanted devices to: 1) suppress the emergence of sustained ventricular tachycardia (VT); 2) decrease the frequency of nonsustained episodes of VT; 3) to modify the tachycardia characteristics (increase the cycle length of VT), thus rendering the arrhythmia more amenable to ATP or low-energy cardioversion and improving the hemodynamic tolerance for the arrhythmia; 4) for therapy of supraventricular arrhythmias, especially atrial fibrillation; and 5) to modify atrioventricular node conduction, thus preventing overlaps in ventricular rates during sinus rhythm and VTs.

Antiarrhythmic Drugs

Clinical experience supports the use of antiarrhythmic drug therapy with ICDs. A recent report revealed that over 80% of patients with implanted third-generation tiered-therapy devices were treated concomitantly with antiarrhythmic drugs.[1,2] The clinical rationale for concomitant drug therapy is to reduce the frequency of nonsustained VT, to slow VT so that the less aggressive therapies may be used (eg, ATP or low-energy cardioversion), thus reducing the frequency of higher energy shocks, prolonging the battery longevity, and improving the quality of life.

Arrhythmia Suppression

Antiarrhythmic drug therapy is usually based on the results of previous electrophysiologic drug testing. Those antiarrhythmic drugs most effective in suppressing VT or slowing the rate are most com-

---

From Singer I, (ed.) Implantable Cardioverter-Defibrillator. Armonk, NY: Futura Publishing Company, Inc.; © 1994.

Table 1
Possible Interactions Between Antiarrhythmic Drugs and ICDs

1. Alterations in DFT
2. Increase in latency, PR interval or conduction leading to double counting
3. Change in QRS morphology resulting in satisfaction of PDF criteria for VT
4. Increase or decrease in VT cycle length
5. Change from sustained to nonsustained VT, resulting in inappropriate shocks during nonsustained VT
6. Alteration in post-shock excitability
7. Increase in pacing thresholds

Adapted with permission from Singer I, et al: Implanted Automatic Defibrillators: Effects of Drugs and Pacemakers. *PACE* 11:2250, 1989.

monly chosen. Because noninducibility is not an essential therapeutic objective, less stringent end points may be used. However, the ICD function and drug-device interactions must be tested for in the electrophysiology laboratory to demonstrate not only the drug efficacy, but also the appropriateness of device programming.

Suppression of supraventricular arrhythmias with appropriate antiarrhythmic therapy can help prevent inappropriate shocks. A recent report has emphasized that over 20% of patients have received shocks for rhythms other than the VT.[3] Potential interactions between antiarrhythmic drugs and ICDs are listed in Table 1.

Effects of Antiarrhythmic Drugs on Defibrillation Threshold

Antiarrhythmic drugs may alter the defibrillation threshold (DFT). One possible mechanism by which antiarrhythmic drugs modulate the DFTs is by their effects on the transmembrane currents.[4] Most of the published data of drug effects on the DFTs are derived from canine experiments. A summary of known drug effects on the DFT are presented in Table 2. The effect of antiarrhythmic drugs may be to increase or decrease DFTs, or they may have no significant effect on the DFTs.

Antiarrhythmic Drugs That Increase Defibrillation Thresholds

Antiarrhythmic drugs that exert their major effect by sodium channel blockade also increase the energy requirements for defibrillation. Several drugs have been demonstrated to increase DFTs. Class IC drugs, such as encainide, its metabolite O-dimethyl-encainide (ODE), flecainide, Class IB drugs such as lidocaine, mexiletine, and other pure sodium channel blockers, phenytoin, propafenone, and recainam have also been demonstrated to increase the DFTs. Fain et al.[5] examined the effect of intravenous encainide and its two major metabolites, ODE and 3-methoxy-ODE

Table 2
Effects of Antiarrhythmic Drugs on Defibrillation Thresholds

Increase	No Change	Decrease
Encainide[5]	MODE[5]	Amiodarone[11,12] (acute)
ODE[5]	Quinidine[18]	Ciofilium[21]
Flecainide[6]		
Lidocaine[7]	Procainamide[19]	Isoproterenol[22]
Amiodarone[13,14] (chronic)	Bretylium[20,21]	d-Sotalol[4]
Phenytoin[4]		N-acetyl Procainamide[4]
Propoferone[4]		
Recainam[9,10]		

Adapted with permission from Singer I, et al: Implanted automatic defibrillators: effects of drugs and pacemakers. *PACE* 11:2250, 1989.

(MODE), on DFTs in the canine model. Encainide and ODE increased the E_{50}, the energy required to achieve 50% success of defibrillation, by 129% and 76%, respectively. No significant increase in E_{50} was observed after administration of MODE. Another Class IC drug, flecainide, is known to increase the DFTs in the canine model.[6]

Lidocaine, a Class IB antiarrhythmic drug, has also been demonstrated to increase defibrillation energy. Dorian et al.[7] demonstrated in phenobarbital anesthetized dogs that lidocaine increased the E_{50}. Lidocaine caused a reversible, concentration-dependent increase in the energy requirements for successful defibrillation. There is anecdotal evidence suggesting that another orally administered Class IB drug, mexiletine, also may increase the DFTs.[8] Other Class I drugs with pure sodium channel blockade have also been demonstrated to increase the DFTs.[8-10]

The data on amiodarone are somewhat conflicting and controversial. Fain et al.[11] demonstrated that DFTs are decreased by acute intravenous administration of amiodarone. The clinical experience to some extent supports these experimental findings. For example, it has been observed that intravenous administration of amiodarone bolus acutely to patients with out-of-hospital cardiac arrest due to ventricular fibrillation, makes subsequent defibrillation more likely.[12]

Clinical data suggest that long-term administration of amiodarone increases the DFTs. Fogoros[13] has described a case where amiodarone was presumably responsible for DFT elevation in a patient, with return of the DFT to acceptable levels on amiodarone discontinuation. Guarnieri et al.[14] demonstrated doubling of DFTs with implanted AICD™ (CPI, St. Paul, MN) at replacement of the generator. The mean DFT increased from 10.9 to 20 J. In contrast, DFT decreased in patients not on antiarrhythmic drugs or on Class I drugs.

Therefore, the amiodarone data suggest a bimodal effect. The differences demonstrated with short- and long-term administration of amiodarone may be due to its metabolite desethylamiodarone, and the cumulative tissue burden of amiodarone, since the drug is not excreted to a significant extent and accumulates in the tissues over time.[15,16] The elimination half-life of amiodarone is in the order of 40 days. The elimination of the metabolite desethylamiodarone is even longer. High concentrations of the parent compound and its metabolite are found in the tissue samples. The high concentrations of amiodarone and its metabolite in the myocardium long term may help explain the delayed onset of the drug's antiarrhythmic action and may also explain its bimodal effect on the DFTs in vivo.

Drugs That Do Not Alter Defibrillation Threshold

In clinically acceptable concentrations Class IA drugs appear to have no significant effect on DFTs. Babbs et al.[17] studied the effects of quinidine on the peak threshold current and found a mean increase of 70% and an increase in the delivered energy of 172%. This change, however, occurred immediately after the bolus administration. In contrast, Dorian et al.[18] found no significant effect on DFTs after quinidine infusion. Therefore, it appears that in clinically relevant concentrations, quinidine has no consistent demonstrable effect on the DFTs. Similarly, another Class IA antiarrhythmic drug, procainamide, was also found to have no significant effects on DFTs either in the canine or in the pig model.[19]

Antiarrhythmic drug bretylium has been studied by a number of investigators.[18-20] Using different experimental models bretylium was demonstrated to have insignificant effect on the DFTs. However, Tacker et al.[21] found that DFTs were lowered after an intravenous bolus of bretylium in dogs. The observed decrease was 31% for the energy and 16% for the current. These apparent differences in the experimental results may be due to the diverse methodologies used for the determination of DFTs. The term DFT is really a misnomer, since the relationship of the probability of successful defibrillation and energies is sigmoidal rather than a straight line function. Therefore, the apparent minor differences may also be related to the methodology used for calculating the DFTs.

Drugs That Decrease Defibrillation Thresholds

In general, antiarrhythmic drugs whose predominant effect is to prolong the repolarization, Class III drugs, have been found to decrease the DFTs. These drugs include clofilium,[21] N-acetyl-procainamide, and d-sotalol.[22] This effect is most likely due to the blockade of the outward potassium channel.[4]

Catecholamines facilitate ventricular defibrillation in animals. Ruffy et al.[23] examined the effects of β-adrenergic blockade and stimulation in anesthetized dogs. They demonstrated that isoproterenol decreased the DFTs. This beneficial effect was blocked by administration of propranolol. The clinical significance of this effect is that in the clinical situations where the initial attempts to defibrillate are unsuccessful, the administration of the bolus doses of cathecolamines, eg, epinephrine, may facilitate subsequent defibrillation attempts by lowering the DFT.

Effects of Antiarrhythmic Drugs on Arrhythmia Recognition by Implantable Cardioverter-Defibrillators

Antiarrhythmic drugs have other clinically important effects that may affect arrhythmia recognition by the ICD. Antiarrhythmic drugs may increase latency, prolong PR interval, cause QRS widening, and affect the repolarization, thus prolonging or shortening the QT interval. Widening of the QRS may result in morphology that is indistinguishable from VT during supraventricular tachycardia or atrial fibrillation. Although the most commonly used detection criteria in the presently available ICDs use the rate of the tachycardia as the main detection criterion, some (AICD) are capable of using morphological criterion in conjunction with the rate criterion. This additional detection criterion was conceived as a way to distinguish the narrow complex, supraventricular tachycardias from the wide complex, VTs. Unfortunately, either because of coexisting bundle branch block or because of the QRS widening secondary to the antiarrhythmic drug effect, PDF has not fulfilled its initial anticipated benefit.

Another beneficial effect of antiarrhythmic drugs is to slow the rate of VT. If, however, the rate decreases to below the programmed rate minimum, it would result in failure to deliver therapy for VTs below the programmed rate. This problem may occur especially in patients taking amiodarone, where the onset of drug action is delayed for several weeks and may peak at 3–6 months after the drug initiation.

Another potentially beneficial effect of antiarrhythmic drugs is to convert a previously sustained VT to a nonsustained rhythm. Spontaneous termination of arrhythmia though clinically desirable, may lead to inappropriate shocks from a committed ICD, or even from a noncommitted ICD if the reconfirmation algorithm is not met (Figure 1). Antiarrhythmic drugs may alter postshock excitability leading to prolonged pauses postdefibrillation. The newer devices can overcome this problem by the use of high-energy output postshock (eg, Guardian ATP™ 4211, Telectronics, Englewood, CO; Cadence™, Ventritex, Sunnyvale, CA).

Another possible problem may occur when the QRS prolongation is extreme, or when the QT interval is prolonged excessively. Double counting may occur due to the "double" signal detection when both QRS and T waves are sensed, leading to inappropriate shocks when the rate artifactually exceeds the programmed rate (Figure 2).

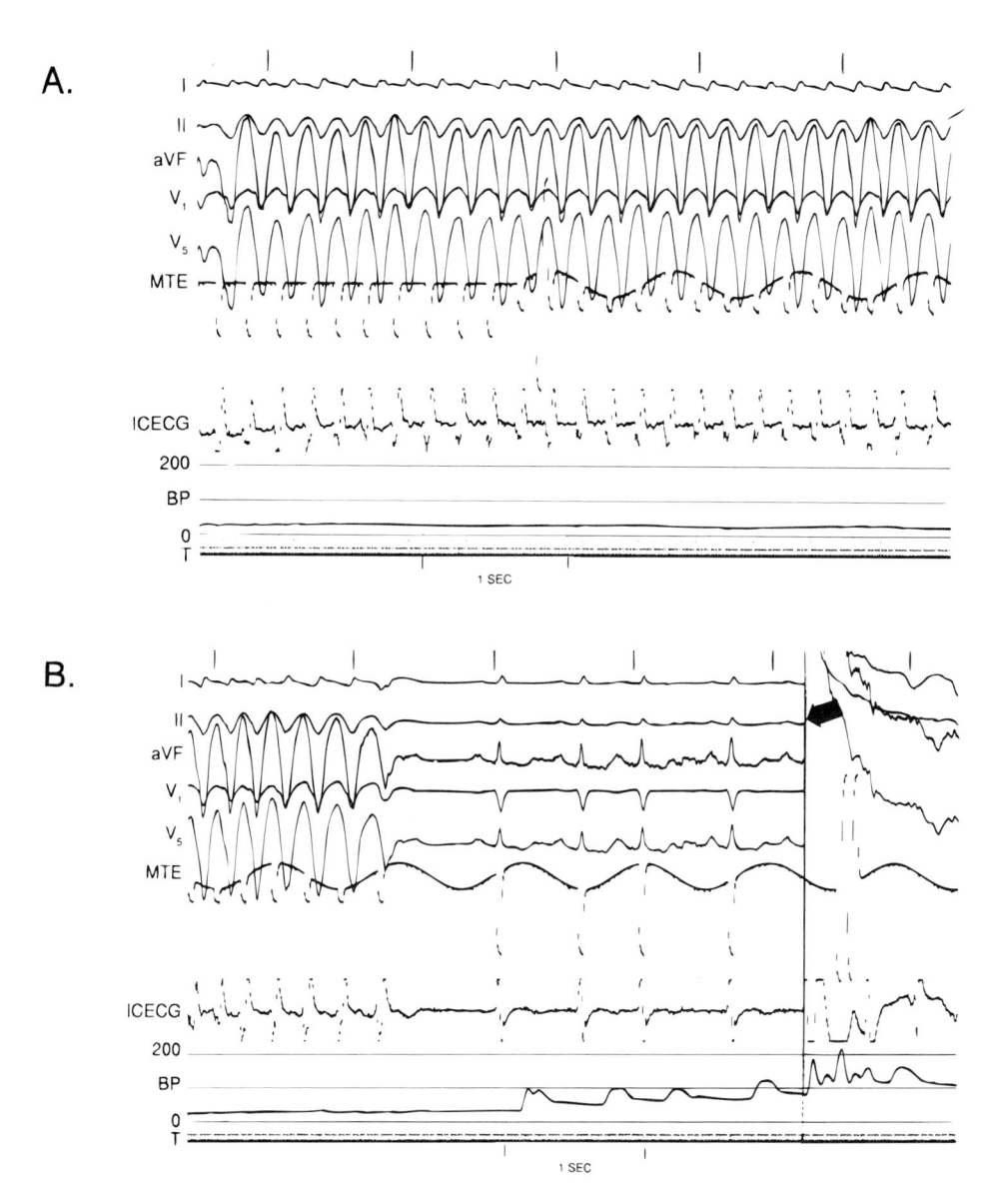

Figure 1. Ventricular tachycardia (VT) is detected by the Guardian™ ATP 4211 (Telectronics, Englewood, CO) third-generation implantable cardioverter-defibrillator (ICD), which has a reconfirmation algorithm prior to the shock delivery. This algorithm uses 6 of 10 intervals for reconfirmation, which must be below the cycle length for rate detection. In this case, although the criteria for reconfirmation are met, the arrhythmia terminates prior to the shock delivery. However, at this stage, the ICD is already committed and delivers the shock nevertheless. From top to bottom: surface leads I, II, aVF, V_1, V_5, main timing events markers (MTE); intracardiac electrogram (ICECG); blood pressure (BP); time lines (T). A and B are continuous strips.

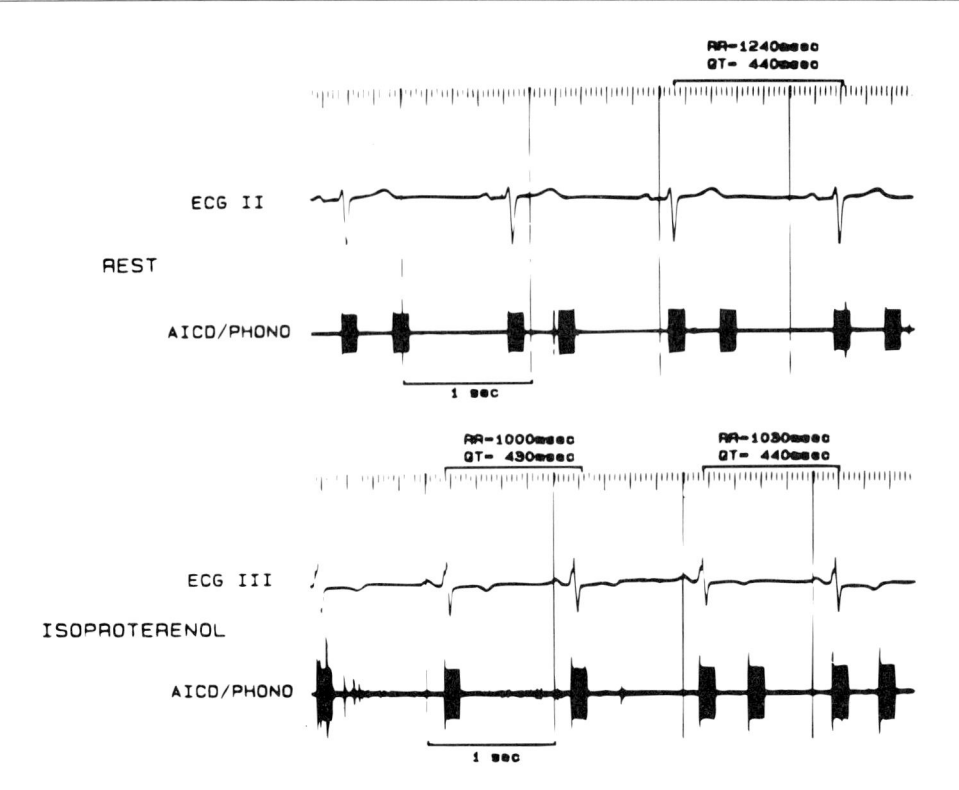

Figure 2. Double counting at rest by the AICD™ (CPI, St. Paul, MN). Displayed are the surface ECG (II) and the phonocardiographic trace. The cycle length was 1,240 msec with a QT interval of 440 msec. The bottom panel shows the surface ECG lead III and the tones emitted from the device during isoproterenol infusion. Note that in the early stages of the infusion as the cycle length varies from 1,000–1,030 msec there is variable T wave sensing. This demonstrates that subtle changes in the cycle length and QT interval may produce double sensing involving the T wave. (Reproduced with permission from Reference 48.)

Proarrhythmia

An increase in arrhythmia frequency, new brady- and tachyarrhythmias arising as a result of antiarrhythmic therapy is referred to as proarrhythmia. Proarrhythmic propensity is exacerbated by electrolyte abnormalities (hypokalemia and hypomagnesemia), toxic plasma levels of antiarrhythmic drugs, poor left ventricular function,[25] bradycardia,[26,27] and excessive plasma concentrations of digitalis.

Proarrhythmia due to Class IC drugs was, for example, responsible for increased mortality of patients in the antiarrhythmic drug treated group in the CAST trial.[28] Class IC drugs have also been implicated as a cause of incessant VT, which are difficult to cardiovert.[29,30]

Class III drugs prolong action potential duration and QT interval. Excessive prolongation in repolarization may result in triggered activity due to early or late afterdepolarizations and result in torsade de pointes.[31,32]

Postdefibrillation asystole, sinus bradycardia, and chronotropic incompetence may result from treatment with amiodarone, sotalol, β-blocking drugs, or digitalis, singly or in combination. Because the current generation of ICDs are capable of providing only the VVI support, in some patients with poor ventricular function ventricular pacing may result in pacemaker syndrome, due to reduction of the cardiac output, loss of atrioventricular synchrony and loss of rate adaptation during activity. In some patients therefore, implantation of a dual chamber pacemaker in addition to the ICD is required to optimize the hemodynamics and ameliorate symptoms resulting from bradyarrhythmias.

Potential Interactions of Implantable Cardioverter-Defibrillators With Pacemakers

Potential and recognized interactions between ICDs and pacemakers are listed in Table 3. Concomitant implantation of pacemakers and ICDs was commonplace in the earlier stages of the development, when the device lacked bradycardia support capabilities (Ventak™, CPI, St. Paul, MN; AID™ Intec, Pittsburgh, PA; and AICD). Since some of these devices are still being implanted as of the time of this writing (Ventak 1600, 1550, and 1555), the need for concomitant implantation of single or dual chamber pacemakers will arise in the foreseeable future. In addition, there are many patients with implanted permanent pacemakers and ICDs who are currently being followed worldwide. The following interactions may occur between implanted pacemakers and ICDs: 1) the effect of defibrillation shock on the pacemaker and the lead system; 2) the effect of defibrillation on the pacing thresholds acutely; 3) sensing problems related to the pacemaker artifacts; and 4) interactions between the ICD and antitachycardia pacemaker. Concomitant implantation of ICD and a permanent pacemaker requires an understanding of the functioning of both devices and their potential interactions.

Effect of Defibrillation on the Pacemaker

Pacemaker damage or reprogramming was documented to occur with external DC countershock.[33-37] However, although the theoretical possibility exists that the discharge of an internal defibrillator may cause damage to the implanted pacemaker, thus far such permanent damage has not been reported. To reduce the potential for such damage to occur, the manufacturers have incorporated circuits to shield the electronic components from massive surges in energy resulting from defibrillation. The protective circuits are designed to shunt excessive energy away from the sensitive electronics of the pulse generator to the pacing electrode. Because the lead constitutes a relatively low-resistance pathway, large amounts of energy shunted to the endocardium may result in the endocardial damage, leading to acute and chronic rises in stimulation thresholds and possibly loss of pacing.[38,39]

Alteration of Stimulation Threshold After Cardioversion

Bradycardia and asystole following ICD defibrillation are not uncommon.[40] Occasionally bradycardia and asystole are prolonged and require immediate back-up pacing. Slepian et al.[39] reported on a patient who demonstrated a failure to sense and capture after the shock from an AICD. Guarnieri et al.[41] examined this question sys-

---

Table 3
Potential Pacemaker and ICD Interactions

I. Pacemaker-ICD Interactions
  1. VF-non-detection due to pacemaker stimuli (especially true with unipolar pacemakers)
  2. Double, triple and multiple counting resulting in false positive shocks
II. ICD-Pacemaker Interactions
  1. Pacemaker reprogramming by the defibrillation discharge
  2. Sensing/capture failure post-defibrillation
III. ICD-Antitachycardia Interactions
  1. Antitachycardia pacing triggering ICD discharge

Adapted with permission from Singer I, et al: Implanted automatic defibrillators: effects of drugs and pacemakers. PACE 11:2262, 1989.

tematically using the canine model. A transient loss of capture was observed post-ICD shock, the duration of the capture loss was related to the current strength of the pacemaker. During endocardial pacing at threshold current the mean time to capture was 4.9 seconds, while at current values twice the threshold, the mean time to capture was 2.2 seconds. No significant difference was found between endocardial and epicardial pacing. Flecainide significantly increased the mean time to capture, to 14.9 seconds at the threshold value ($P < 0.01$), and to 5.6 seconds at twice the threshold ($P < 0.05$). No significant difference was seen with the β-blocking drug propranolol.

These data indicate that there is an immediate transient increase in the pacing thresholds post-ICD shock. The duration of the capture loss is current dependent and is significantly exacerbated by Class IC antiarrhythmic drugs. These considerations have been recognized by the manufacturers, and high-output pacing after the ICD shock was incorporated as a programmable feature of some third-generation ICDs.

Antitachycardia Pacemaker Interactions

Antitachycardia pacing has been demonstrated to be very efficacious in terminating relatively slow, monomorphic VTs.[42-44] The ability to terminate VT is determined by several factors including the tachycardia cycle length, the number of extrastimuli, the distance of the reentry circuit from the site of the stimulation and the hemodynamic tolerance of therapy. Antiarrhythmic drugs have beneficial effects by slowing the conduction, increasing the cycle length of the VT, by prolonging the refractoriness of the ventricular tissue and thereby prolonging the excitable gap available for ATP termination.

With first- and second-generation devices there was a need to implant antitachycardia pacemakers in conjunction with ICDs, as two separate devices. Third-generation ICDs have largely superseded this need by incorporating the ATP capabilities within the ICD. Thus, the potential interactions of ATP and cardioverter/defibrillators have steadily diminished. Nevertheless, a number of patients with implanted antitachycardia pacemakers and ICDs are still being followed, hence an understanding of potential interactions is still important. The understanding of sequential role of pacing therapies and cardioversion/defibrillation is very important to optimally program the tiered-therapy devices. Antitachycardia pacing techniques use most frequently a series of extrastimuli at either fixed coupling intervals or in a decremental ramp. Other more elaborate modes for tachycardia termination have been described, including a combination of incremental and decremental bursts, combination of timed extrastimuli and decremental ramp pacing, and so on. Whatever the method of pacing used, the principles on which VT termination is based are the same. The proposed mechanism by which ATP terminates the tachycardia is that the extrastimuli capture in the excitable gap, creating a temporary tissue refractoriness to conduction and interrupting the tachycardia. The size of the excitable gap is dependent on the conduction velocity around the reentry circuit, refractoriness of the tissue in the reentry circuit, and the size of the reentry circuit. The distance of the site of stimulation from the reentry zone is another important variable.

Pacing techniques are generally ineffective for polymorphous VT and uniformly ineffective for ventricular fibrillation. Although effective in terminating monomorphic VT, aggressive pacing algorithms may result in arrhythmia acceleration and ventricular fibrillation. Therefore, ATP techniques should never be used as a stand-alone method for terminating VTs without a back-up cardioversion/defibrillation.

Prior to the incorporation of ATP algorithms in the ICDs antitachycardia pacemakers were implanted separately in addition to an implanted ICD. The constraints of the second-generation devices often limited

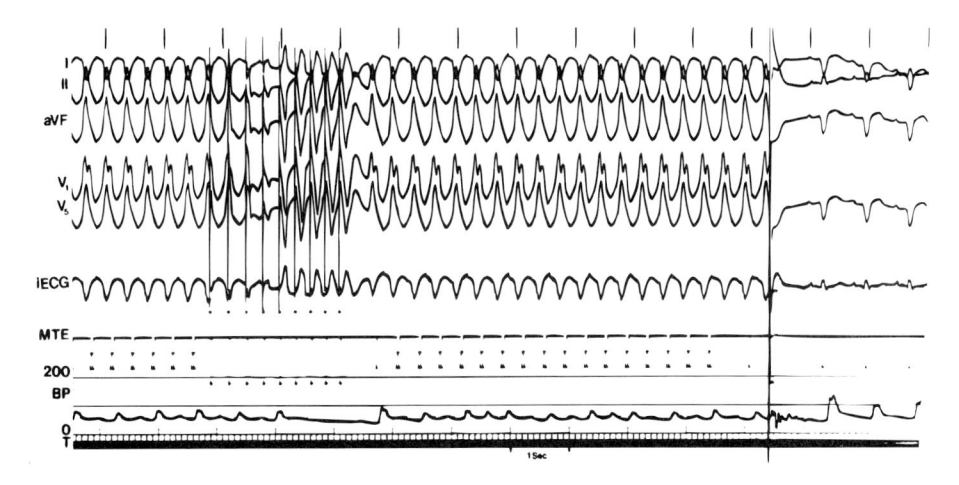

Figure 3. Antitachycardia pacing is unsuccessful in terminating the ventricular tachycardia (VT), which is followed by cardioversion, which restores the sinus rhythm. The device is the PCD™ (Medtronic, Minneapolis, MN). From top to bottom: surface leads I, II, aVF, V_1, V_5; intracardiac electrogram (IECG); main timing events (MTE); blood pressure (BP); time lines (T).

the ATP options, because of the restricted sensing time window available for the ICD, which limited the duration of the pacing trains.

The use of the combined devices is now of historical interest primarily. Currently available ICDs provide the capability to program up to two independent tiers of ATP therapy. Failure of ATP to terminate VT is then followed by cardioversion or defibrillation (Figure 3).

Device-Device Interactions

The fundamental function of an ICD is to detect VT and fibrillation and to deliver effective therapy. To accomplish this task ICDs use primarily the rate detection of the ventricular endocardial signal with additional detection enhancements, such as suddenness of onset, tachycardia stability, duration, and so on. It is readily apparent then, that the current generation of ICDs lack specificity, since the conditions set for VT detection using these criteria, may also be satisfied by the supraventricular tachycardias under certain circumstances (see also Chapters 12 and 22). The sensing algorithm must be capable of distinguishing ventricular from atrial depolarization, ventricular repolarization, myopotentials, or other external electrical noise.

Presence of an electronic signal other than the QRS, for example the pacemaker artifact, further complicates this situation. If the pacemaker artifacts are sensed in addition to the ventricular depolarization (ie, the QRS complex), double counting may result. If the rate exceeds the ICD rate cutoff, it may result in inappropriate shocks (Figure 4). Worse still, pacemaker artifact detection during an episode of ventricular fibrillation may cause the automatic gain amplifier to lock on the pacing signal, thus ignoring the ventricular fibrillation, resulting in no therapy delivery, with potentially fatal consequences.[45,46]

The following interactions may occur between the ICD and implanted pacemaker: 1) detection inhibition; (2) double or multiple counting; and 3) cardioversion shock-induced loss of sensing by the pacemaker leading to asynchronous pacing.[47]

Detection inhibition may occur with temporary or permanent atrial or ventricular pacemakers. If the patient develops VT or ventricular fibrillation the pacemaker may not sense the signal appropriately and continue to pace as if asystole were present.

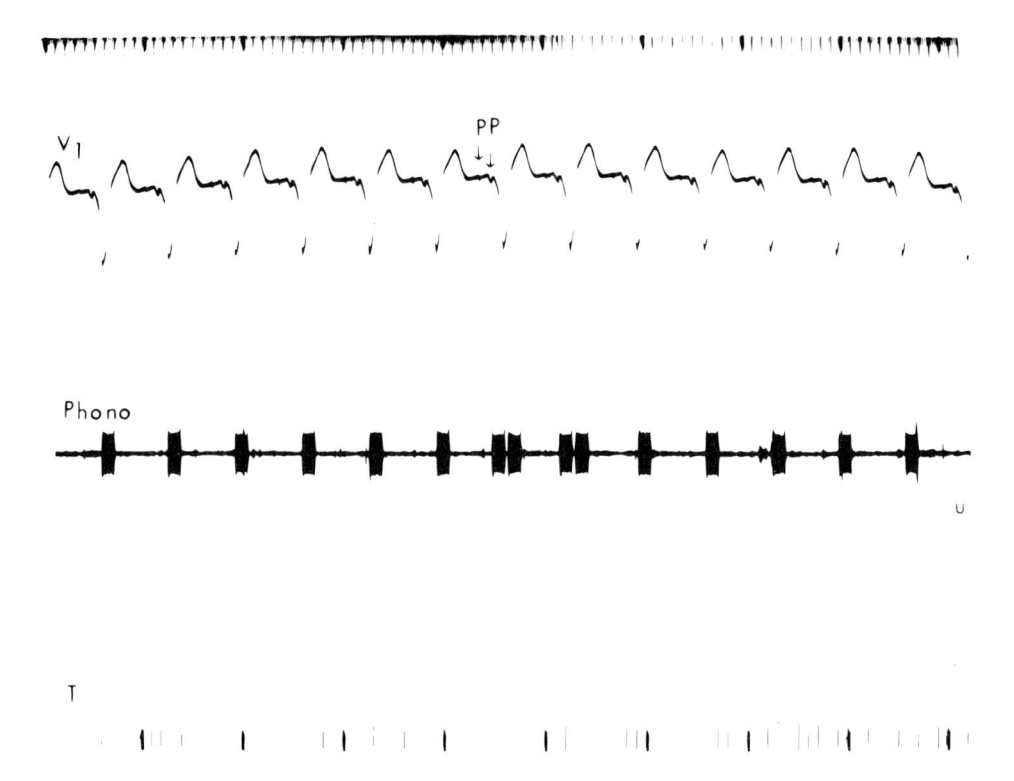

Figure 4. Double sensing occurs with Ventak™ (CPI, St. Paul, MN) device due to the sensing of pacemaker artifact and the ventricular depolarization. Top tracing: lead V₁; bottom tracing phonocardiogram. Note the intermittent double counting.

Under these conditions if the pacemaker signal is detected by the ICD and interpreted as ventricular depolarization, ICD may be inhibited and fail to deliver the lifesaving shock.[46]

Following cardioversion, the pacemaker may experience a transient loss of sensing due to the shock and operate in the asynchronous mode. The ICD input bipolar signals then consists of the transcardiac depolarizations and asynchronous pacemaker artifacts. If large enough, these artifacts may be detected by the ICD and misinterpreted as the ventricular depolarizations. Double counting could then result in therapy delivery if the rate criteria are met. Diastolic T wave sensing has also been described.[48] Antiarrhythmic drugs which slow the ventricular rates and prolong the QT interval, such as amiodarone, are particularly prone to cause this phenomenon.

Recommendations Regarding the Use of Pacemakers and Implantable Cardioverter-Defibrillators

Although the combined use of pacemakers and ICDs is largely of historical interest since the currently available and investigational ICDs now combine these functions in the same device, the need to use two separate devices may still arise under certain circumstances. These include the following possible scenarios: 1) a patient who requires concomitant dual chamber pacing and ICD; 2) a patient who requires rate adaptive pacing; and 3) loss of ventricular capture due to exit block in a patient with implanted ICD who is pacemaker dependent, but where ICD lead revision is difficult or impractical. Finally, there are a number of patients with implanted dual systems. Therefore, understanding of potential device-device interactions is essential for optimal therapy.

The following recommendations may be made if a combination of ICD and a pacemaker is contemplated: 1) unipolar pacemakers are contraindicated in patients with ICDs; 2) potential for nondetection of ventricular fibrillation should be tested for at the time of the implant. This may be accomplished by programming the pacemaker to VOO or DOO mode during ventricular fibrillation induction; 3) ICD sensing electrode(s) should be positioned as far as possible away from the pacemaker electrodes to minimize the potential for pacemaker artifact detection, and 4) sensing in sinus rhythm with pacing should be carefully examined either by inspection of the endocardial channel (devices that have noninvasive telemetry available), or by the use of a doughnut magnet for Ventak devices, which lack the noninvasive telemetry. A further practical point can be made with respect to interrogation of the pacemakers in patients with both a pacemaker and an ICD. The ICD should be temporarily disabled during magnet testing of the pacemaker, because the asynchronous pacing may result in double counting and unintentional triggering of the ICD.

References

1. Winkle, RA, Fain ES, Sweeney MB, et al: Survival in patients with ventricular tachyarrhythmias treated with programmable tiered therapy implantable defibrillators (abstract). *J Am Coll Cardiol* 19:209A, 1992.
2. Dorian P, Feindel C, Lipton I: Usefulness of sotalol in conjunction with automatic implanted defibrillators in man (abstract). *PACE* 13:517, 1990.
3. Grimm W, Flores BF, Marchlinski FE: ECG-documented unnecessary, spontaneous shocks in 106 patients with implantable cardioverter-defibrillators (abstract). *J Am Coll Cardiol* 19:287A, 1992.
4. Echt DS, Black JN, Barbey JT, et al: Evaluation of antiarrhythmic drugs on defibrillation energy requirements in dogs: sodium channel block and action potential prolongation. *Circulation* 79:1106, 1989.
5. Fain ES, Dorian P, Davy JM, et al: Effects of encainide and its metabolites on energy requirements for defibrillation. *Circulation* 73:1334, 1986.
6. Reiffel JA, Coromilas J, Zimmerman JM, et al: Drug-device interactions: clinical considerations. *PACE* 8:369, 1985.
7. Dorian P, Fain ES, Davy JM, et al: Lidocaine causes a reversible, concentration-dependent increase in defibrillation energy requirements. *J Am Coll Cardiol* 8:327, 1986.
8. Marinchak RA, Friehling TD, Kline RA, et al: Effect of antiarrhythmic drugs on defibrillation threshold: case report of an adverse effect of mexiletine and review of the literature. *PACE* 11:7, 1988.
9. Peters W, Gang ES, Solingen S, et al: Acute effects of intravenous propafenone on the internal ventricular defibrillation energy requirements in the anesthetized dog (abstract). *J Am Coll Cardiol* 17:129A, 1991.
10. Frame LH, Sheldon JH: Effects of recainam on the energy required for ventricular defibrillation in dogs as assessed with implanted electrodes. *J Am Coll Cardiol* 12:746, 1988.
11. Fain ES, Lee JT, Winkle RA: Effects of acute intravenous and chronic oral amiodarone on defibrillation energy requirements. *Am Heart J* 114:8, 1987.
12. Kentsch M, Kunze KP, Bleifeld W: Effect of intravenous amiodarone on ventricular fibrillation during out-of-hospital cardiac arrest (abstract). *J Am Coll Cardiol* 7:82A, 1986.
13. Fogoros RN: Amiodarone-induced refractoriness to cardioversion. *Ann Intern Med* 100:699, 1984.
14. Guarnieri T, Levine JH, Veltri EP: Success of chronic defibrillation and the role of antiarrhythmic drugs with the automatic implantable cardioverter/defibrillator. *Am J Cardiol* 60:1061, 1987.
15. Holt DW, Tucker GT, Jackson PR, et al: Amiodarone pharmacokinetics. *Am Heart J* 106:840, 1983.
16. Barbieri E, Conti F, Zampieri P, et al: Amiodarone and desethylamiodarone distribution in the atrium and adipose tissue of patients undergoing short- and long-term treatment with amiodarone. *J Am Coll Cardiol* 8:210, 1986.
17. Babbs CF, Yim GKW, Whistler SJ, et al: Elevation of ventricular defibrillation threshold in dogs by antiarrhythmic drugs. *Am Heart J* 98:345, 1979.
18. Dorian P, Fain ES, Davy JM, et al: Effect of quinidine and bretylium on defibrillation energy requirements. *Am Heart J* 112:19, 1986.

19. Deeb GM, Hardesty RL, Griffith BP, et al: The effects of cardiovascular drugs on the defibrillation threshold and the pathological effects on the heart using an automatic implantable defibrillator. *Ann Thorac Surg* 4:361, 1983.
20. Kerber RE, Pandian NG, Jensen SR, et al: Effect of lidocaine and bretylium on energy requirements for transthoracic defibrillation: experimental studies. *J Am Coll Cardiol* 7:397, 1986.
21. Tacker WA, Nieballer MJ, Babbs CF, et al: The effect of newer antiarrhythmic drugs on defibrillation threshold. *Crit Care Med* 8:177, 1980.
22. Wang MJ, Dorian P: DL and D sotalol decrease defibrillation energy requirements. *PACE* 12:1522, 1989.
23. Ruffy R, Schechtuan K, Moaje E, et al: B-adrenergic modulation of direct defibrillation energy in anesthetized dog heart. *Am J Physiol* 248(17):H674, 1985.
24. Ruffy R, Lal R, Kouchoukos NT, et al: Combined bipolar dual chamber pacing and automatic implantable cardioverter/defibrillator. *J Am Coll Cardiol* 7:933, 1986.
25. Slater W, Lampert S, Podrid PJ, et al: Clinical predictors of arrhythmia worsening by antiarrhythmic drugs. *Am J Cardiol* 61:349, 1988.
26. Keren A, Tzivoni D, Gavish D, et al: Etiology warning signs and therapy of torsades de pointe. A study of ten patients. *Circulation* 64:1167, 1981.
27. Schlepper M: Cardiodepressive effects of antiarrhythmic drugs. *Eur Heart J* 10(Suppl E):73, 1989.
28. Echt DS, Liebson PR, Mitchell LB, et al: Mortality and morbidity in patients receiving encainide, flecainide, or placebo: the Cardiac Arrhythmia Suppression Trial. *N Engl J Med* 324:781, 1991.
29. Duff HJ, Roden DM, Carey EL, et al: Spectrum of antiarrhythmic response to encainide. *Am J Cardiol* 56:887, 1985.
30. Winkle RA, Mason JW, Griffin, et al: Malignant ventricular tachyarrhythmias associated with the use of encainide. *Am Heart J* 102:857, 1981.
31. Jackman WM, Friday KJ, Anderson JL, et al: The long QT syndromes: a critical review, new clinical observations and a unifying hypothesis. *Prog Cardiovasc Dis* 31:115, 1988.
32. Coumel PH, LeClercq JF, Leenhardt A: Arrhythmias as predictors of sudden death. *Am Heart J* 114:929, 1987.
33. Aylward P, Blood R, Tonkin A: Complications of defibrillation with permanent pacemaker in situ. *PACE* 2:462, 1979.
34. Gould L, Patel S, Gomes GI, et al: Pacemaker failure following external defibrillation. *PACE* 4:575, 1981.
35. Giedwoyn JO: Pacemaker failure following external defibrillation. *Circulation* 44:293, 1971.
36. Palac RT, Hwang MH, Klodnycky ML, et al: Delayed pulse generator malfunction after DC countershock. *PACE* 4:163, 1981.
37. Das G, Eaton J: Pacemaker malfunction following transthoracic countershock. *PACE* 4:487, 1981.
38. Levine PA, Barold SS, Fletcher RD, et al: Adverse acute and chronic effects of electrical defibrillation and cardioversion on implanted unipolar cardiac pacing systems. *J Am Coll Cardiol* 6:1413, 1983.
39. Slepian M, Levine JH, Watkins L, et al: The automatic implantable cardioverter defibrillator-permanent pacemaker interaction: loss of pacemaker capture following AICD discharge. *PACE* 11:1194, 1987.
40. Platia EV, Griffith LSC, Reid PR, et al: Post-defibrillation bradycardia following implantable defibrillator discharge (abstract). *J Am Coll Cardiol* 7:144A, 1986.
41. Guarnieri T, Datorre SD, Bondke H, et al: Increased pacing threshold after an automatic defibrillator shock in dogs: effects of Class I and Class II antiarrhythmic drugs. *PACE* (in press).
42. Roy D, Waxman HL, Buxton AE, et al: Termination of ventricular tachycardia: role of tachycardia cycle length. *Am J Cardiol* 50:1346, 1982.
43. Naccarelli GV, Zipes DP, Rahilly GT, et al: Influence of tachycardia cycle length and antiarrhythmic drugs on pacing termination and acceleration of ventricular tachycardia. *Am Heart J* 105:1, 1983.
44. Keren G, Muira DS, Somberg JC: Pacing termination of ventricular tachycardia: influence of antiarrhythmic-slowed ectopic rate. *Am Heart J* 107:638, 1984.
45. Kim SG, Furman S, Waspe LE, et al: Unipolar pacer artifacts induced failure of an automatic implantable cardioverter/defibrillator to detect ventricular fibrillation. *Am J Cardiol* 57:880, 1986.
46. Cohen AI, Wish MW, Fletcher RD, et al: The use and interaction of permanent pacemakers and the automatic implantable cardioverter defibrillator. *PACE* 11:704, 1988.
47. Bach JM: *AID-B Cardioverter-Defibrillator: Possible Interactions with Pacemakers*. Intec Systems Technical Communication 1983, Document 1650095.
48. Singer I, DeBorde R, Veltri EP, et al: The automatic implantable cardioverter defibrillator: T wave sensing in the newest generation (abstract). *PACE* 11:485, 1988.

Chapter 19

Postoperative Care and Follow-up of Implantable Cardioverter-Defibrillator Patients

Igor Singer and Lesa Adams

Postoperative care and follow-up of impantable cardioverter-defibrillator (ICD) patients are important for successful therapy. Postoperative care of a patient with ICDs begins in the operating room and extends to hospital discharge. The patient then enters a follow-up phase. This chapter is organized in three parts: 1) the postoperative period; 2) predischarge electrophysiologic study; and 3) follow-up.

The Postoperative Period

A thoracotomy is required when concomitant cardiac surgery, eg, coronary revascularization, valve, or arrhythmia directed surgery is performed in addition to the ICD implantation. Current clinical practice is to implant nonthoracotomy lead (NTL) systems when only an ICD is required, and to resort to a thoracotomy when defibrillation thresholds (DFTs) are unsatisfactory.[1,2]

The clinical profile of a typical patient undergoing ICD implantation places the patient in Goldman multifactorial risk category II or III.[3] In this category, the expected cardiac mortality rate is 1% to 4%. This is closely mirrored by the reported operative mortality rates of 0.7% to 4.7%.[4–8] Many factors may impact adversely on the operative mortality and morbidity rates. These include, but are not limited to the following: 1) poor left ventricular ejection fraction (LVEF < 30%)[6,7,9–11]; 2) concomitant cardiac surgery[6–8]; 3) amiodarone, which has been reported to increase DFTs[12] and frequency and severity of postoperative pulmonary complications[13,14]; and 4) surgical techniques used for ICD implantation, with less invasive techniques, eg, subxiphoid[15] or subcostal approaches[16] having a somewhat smaller postoperative morbidity (see also Chapter 15).

Postoperative complications include: 1) cardiac nonarrhythmic; 2) arrhythmic; 3) pulmonary; 4) infective; and 5) systemic. These are dealt with in detail in Chapter 20. However, in discussing the immediate postoperative phase one must consider all of these potential risks. These risks are not exclusively related to the thoracotomy per se, but are also encountered with NTL systems implants, albeit less frequently.

Postoperative Management

Patients are managed postoperatively in an intensive care environment for 24–72

From Singer I, (ed.) Implantable Cardioverter-Defibrillator. Armonk, NY: Futura Publishing Company, Inc.; © 1994.

hours. Postthoracotomy patients may require ventilatory support in the immediate postoperative period. Patients are extubated as soon as is practical. Prolonged intubation is undesirable and may compound or precipitate other complications. Extended use of central venous catheters is strongly discouraged. Whenever possible invasive monitoring catheters are removed within 24–48 hours. The risk of nosocomial infections is significantly increased by the use of central venous and arterial catheters. Furthermore, invasive monitoring confines the patient to the bed unnecessarily, delaying mobilization.

Fluids and Pressors

In the immediate postoperative period, careful fluid management is required. Patients may be fluid overloaded intraoperatively. Judicious diuresis, while maintaining adequate preload in patients with left ventricular dysfunction, is required to optimize cardiac output. In severely ill patients, continuous pulmonary artery and intra-arterial pressure monitoring is helpful for optimal management.

In general, we avoid the use of pressors whenever possible. When unavoidable, cardioselective agonists with minimal arrhythmogenic potential (eg, dobutamine or low-dose dopamine in the minimum effective doses) are used. It should be remembered that sympathetic agonists increase the potential for arrhythmias and may precipitate arrhythmic "storms."

Most often, combination of preload and afterload reduction in combination with diuresis is sufficient for the management of congestive heart failure. Electrolyte abnormalities are corrected aggressively. Potassium and magnesium levels should be monitored frequently. Vigorous diuresis may lead to hypokalemia and/or hypomagnesemia, which may precipitate or potentiate ventricular arrhythmias.

Postoperative Pain Management

A thoracotomy is a particularly painful operation. A lateral or anterior thoracotomy is probably more painful than the median sternotomy or subxiphoid approach. Nonthoracotomy lead system implantation causes less discomfort. The need for adequate postoperative analgesia cannot be overemphasized. Postoperative pain may be deleterious in several ways: 1) it leads to reflexive chest splinting and poor inspiratory effort resulting in atelectasis; 2) pain slows patient mobilization; and 3) severe discomfort may be demoralizing to the patient and family, resulting in negative attitude to the ICD and interfering in subsequent follow-up and compliance.

Advice of the pain management team is often helpful. The use of regional epidural block is extremely helpful when lateral or anterior thoracotomy approaches are used. Continuous patient regulated intravenous morphine administration or equivalent is another excellent alternative. Adequate analgesia helps to institute vigorous pulmonary toilet and early mobilization.

The removal of pleural and mediastinal chest tubes reduces the demand for analgesia. Therefore, the removal of chest and mediastinal tubes is encouraged at the earliest possible time. Vigorous physiotherapy and encouragement is vital for smooth postoperative recovery.

Wound Care

Meticulous attention to wound care is essential. Most infections are acquired at the time of the ICD system implantation, ie, in the operating room. However, secondary infections are possible particularly with intravenous and intra-arterial vascular catheters. All incision and intravenous sites should be inspected daily. Redness or swelling at the incision site should be carefully scrutinized. Intravascular catheters used for invasive monitoring should be removed as soon as practical. Although common in the immediate postoperative period (24–48 hours), elevations in temperature should be aggressively investigated. We routinely use prophylactic antibiotics preoperatively (eg, vancomycin) 1 hour before surgery and continue the antibiotic for 24 hours postoperatively.

The management of device and lead infections is discussed in Chapter 20. Device and lead infection, although relatively rare complications of ICD surgery (1% to 2%),[3,5,11,17,18] are devastating and almost always necessitate device and/or lead system removal. Therefore, prevention of infection is essential.

Management of Postoperative Arrhythmias

The most frequent arrhythmia after epicardial patch leads placement is atrial fibrillation. It is reported as occurring in up to 19% of patients postoperatively.[5,10,17,18] Atrial fibrillation is also common after other types of cardiac surgery and may occur independently of the epicardial patch leads. Rapid ventricular response during atrial fibrillation may trigger ICD discharges if the detection criteria are met because currently available devices cannot reliably distinguish supraventricular from ventricular tachycardias. Sudden onset and rate stability criteria may be valuable in differentiating monomorphic ventricular tachycardia from atrial fibrillation. However, these detection criteria are less reliable in differentiating polymorphous ventricular tachycardia from atrial fibrillation (Figure 1). Rate control with digoxin, β-adrenergic and calcium channel blocking drugs is helpful to increase atrioventricular (AV) nodal block. Atrial fibrillation may have other undesirable consequences. Decrease in cardiac output due to loss of AV synchrony, absence of atrial systole, and decrease in diastolic filling time may precipitate pulmonary edema or congestive heart failure.

Therefore, atrial fibrillation should be treated aggressively. Class IA or Class III drugs may be used with electrical cardioversion. These drugs are discontinued after 6–8 weeks, unless they are also administered for the concomitant treatment of other arrhythmias, eg, ventricular tachycardia, or if atrial fibrillation is unrelated to and antedates ICD surgery.

Ventricular tachyarrhythmias may become more frequent in the immediate postoperative period.[5,10,17,18] The etiology of increased frequency and severity of ventricular dysrhythmias is probably multifactorial. Causes may include perioperative ischemia, electrolyte abnormalities, fluctuating serum levels of antiarrhythmic drugs, congestive heart failure, increased sympathetic tone, pressor drugs, ventricular irritability due to patch lead placement, or other poorly understood factors. Because of the increased risk of postoperative ventricular tachycardia, we recommend turning the ICD on when the patient leaves the operating room. The rate cutoff should be programmed high (eg, 200 beats per minute) for the initial 72–96 hours to prevent inappropriate shocks due to atrial fibrillation. The device is turned off only if frequent or incessant ventricular tachycardia develops.

The fine-tuning of the device is postponed until the postoperative electrophysiologic study when steady-state serum levels of orally administered antiarrhythmic drugs are present. Class IA, IC, or III drugs are administered either singly or in combination to decrease frequency, abort nonsustained ventricular tachycardia episodes, or slow ventricular tachycardia rate and improve antitachycardia pacing (ATP) efficacy. Third-generation ICDs that are capable of ATP can terminate episodes of ventricular tachycardia with ATP, thus decreasing patient discomfort due to cardioverting/defibrillating shocks and extending the life of the pulse generator (Figure 2).

Nonthoracotomy Lead Systems

Operative mortality is reduced with NTL systems. For the Transvene™ system

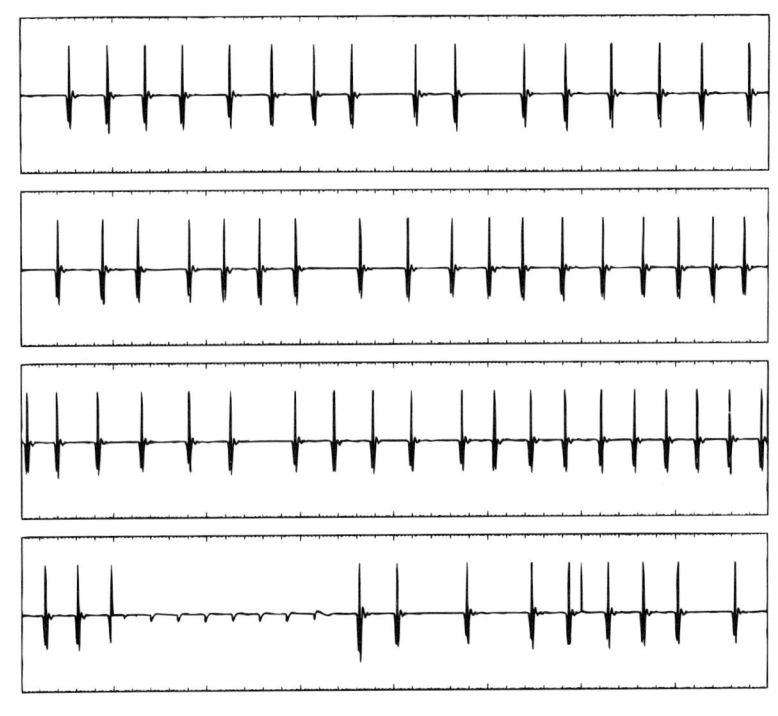

01232013.PRG; 03-DEC-1992 07:56; Episode 3; Sinus after Therapy for TACH A   (25 mm/sec)

Figure 1. Inappropriate therapy for atrial fibrillation. Electrogram recordings (strips 1 to 4) are continuous (Cadence™, Ventritex, Sunnyvale, CA). Note irregular R-R intervals suggesting that the rhythm is most likely atrial fibrillation. Antitachycardia therapy (ATP) is given (fourth strip) that predictably does not terminate the arrhythmia (note that R-R intervals remain irregular). Figure courtesy of Ventritex, Sunnyvale, CA.

(Medtronic, Minneapolis, MN) it was reported to be 1.6%[19] and for Endotak™ (CPI, St. Paul, MN) it was reported to be 1.7%.[20] The postoperative hospital course is shorter and morbidity reduced, with a decrease in pulmonary and cardiac complications.[21] This is not surprising because thoracotomy and concomitant cardiac surgery increase operative and perioperative risks. Some complications, however, may be more frequent with NTL leads. For example, lead displacement or dislodgment, lead fractures, subcutaneous patch hematoma, or patch crimping are more common with NTL systems.[19–21]

Predischarge Electrophysiologic Testing

The purpose of the predischarge electrophysiologic testing is to: 1) assure proper ICD function in a clinically safe environment where resuscitative equipment and trained medical personnel are available; 2) optimize device programming; 3) assess hemodynamic consequences of induced arrhythmias and therapy prescription.

Although it could be argued that most goals of the predischarge electrophysiologic testing may be accomplished at the ICD implant (see Chapters 10, 15, and 16), the operating room differs significantly from the clinical environment. For example, the effects of anesthesia on arrhythmia inducibility must be considered. Clinical ventricular tachycardia may not be inducible in the operating room. The rigors of the surgical procedure often preclude repeated ventricular tachycardia inductions to test ATP efficacy. Finally, antiarrhythmic therapy is often modified postoperatively. In turn,

01043015.PRG; 25-APR-1992 13:25; Episode 1; Sinus after Therapy for TACH A (25 mm/sec)

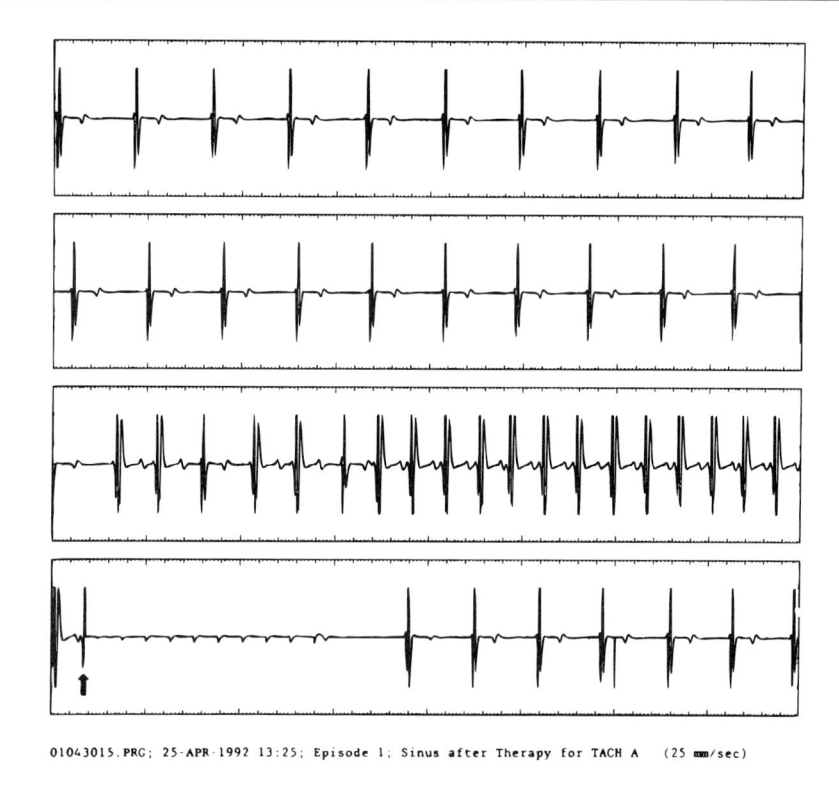

Figure 2. Antitachycardia pacing (ATP) therapy for ventricular tachycardia (Cadence™, Ventritex, Sunnyvale, CA). Analog signals replay shows onset of ventricular tachycardia (third strip from the top). Ventricular tachycardia is sensed appropriately and terminated by ATP pacing (arrow) with resumption of sinus rhythm. Figure courtesy of Ventritex, Sunnyvale, CA.

antiarrhythmic drugs may alter the cycle length of the ventricular tachycardia, rendering ventricular tachycardia noninducible, or they may affect ICD efficacy by altering electrogram morphology, repolarization, by increasing DFTs, AV block, or by altering hemodynamics.[22] Therefore, programming that may have been effective initially may subsequently become less effective or ineffective.

Other factors may conspire to alter effective ICD function. For example, patch leads may fold, crimp, or move resulting in ineffective defibrillation. The development of a significant pericardial effusion may increase DFTs. Lead connections may be loose, or endocardial leads may displace, causing failure to sense or pace, or inability to defibrillate. High DFTs at implant may result in inability to reliably defibrillate subsequently. This is particularly true when the defibrillation safety margin is < 10 J.[23] Although detection of device malfunction at predischarge electrophysiologic study is uncommon, some investigators have noted significant incidence of failure to defibrillate on predischarge electrophysiologic study.[24]

Electrophysiologic Study

Generally, patients are sedated with intravenous midazolam (Versed™, Roche Laboratories, Nutley, NJ) or equivalent, but awake. Arterial pressure is routinely monitored. A central venous access is usually ensured with a 7F femoral venous sheath. Although electrophysiologic study may be performed without invasive access with third-generation ICDs, there are several advantages to this approach. First, recognition of the hemodynamic effects of ventricular tachycardia are important. Second, the safety of the patient is maximized by continuous hemodynamic monitoring. Finally, in the event that rapid administration of intravenous fluids, pressors, or antiarrhythmic drugs become necessary due to hemodynamic collapse, ready central venous access is available. When ventricular tachycardia or ventricular fibrillation are not inducible by noninvasive programmed stimulation, or when ICD lacks noninvasive programmed stimulation capabilities (eg, Ventak™, CPI, St. Paul, MN), an endocardial electrode catheter is required for programmed ventricular stimulation or ventricular fibrillation induction.

We routinely monitor arterial saturation by means of a pulse oximeter. Transcranial Doppler and quantitative EEG (QEEG) are also used in our laboratory to evaluate cerebral perfusion in response to induced ventricular tachycardia and ventricular fibrillation and to optimize device programming[25] (Figures 3 and 4). These techniques are investigational, but yield useful information in the assessment of the adequacy of device programming.[25,26]

Assessment of Sensing and Pacing Functions

Electrograms are recorded during spontaneous or paced rhythm (Figure 5), during induced ventricular tachycardia (Figure 6), and during ventricular fibrillation (Figure 7). Pacing thresholds are tested

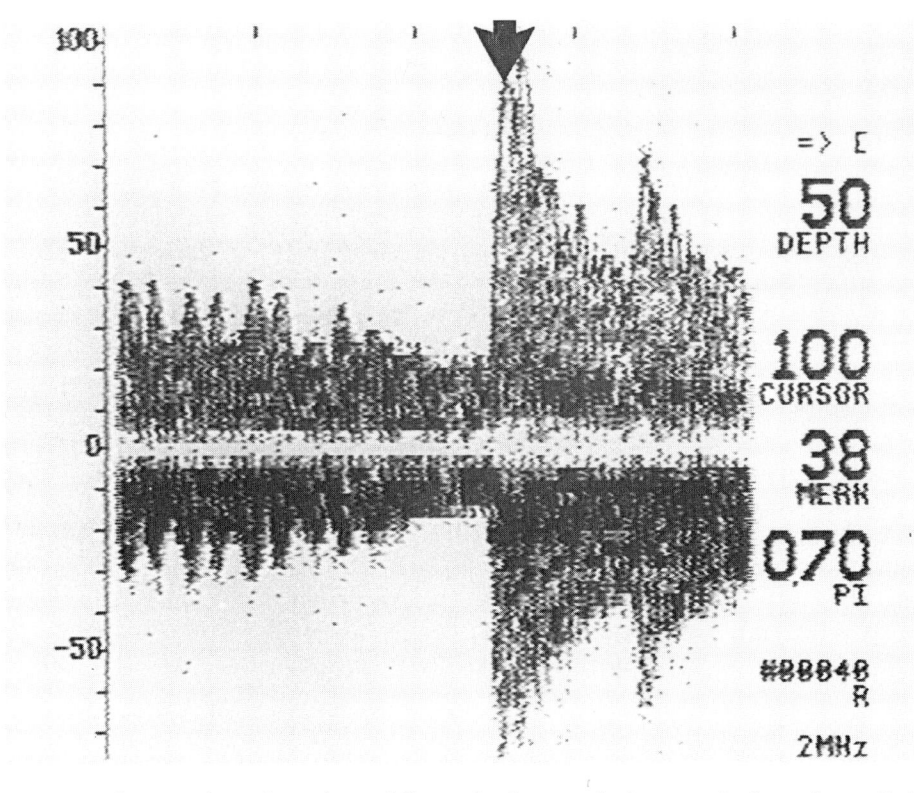

Figure 3. Doppler recordings from the middle cerebral artery during ventricular tachycardia induction in the electrophysiology laboratory. Note a profound decrease in cerebral perfusion during ventricular tachycardia, and rebound hyperemia after termination (first beat postventricular tachycardia termination is indicated by the arrow).[26]

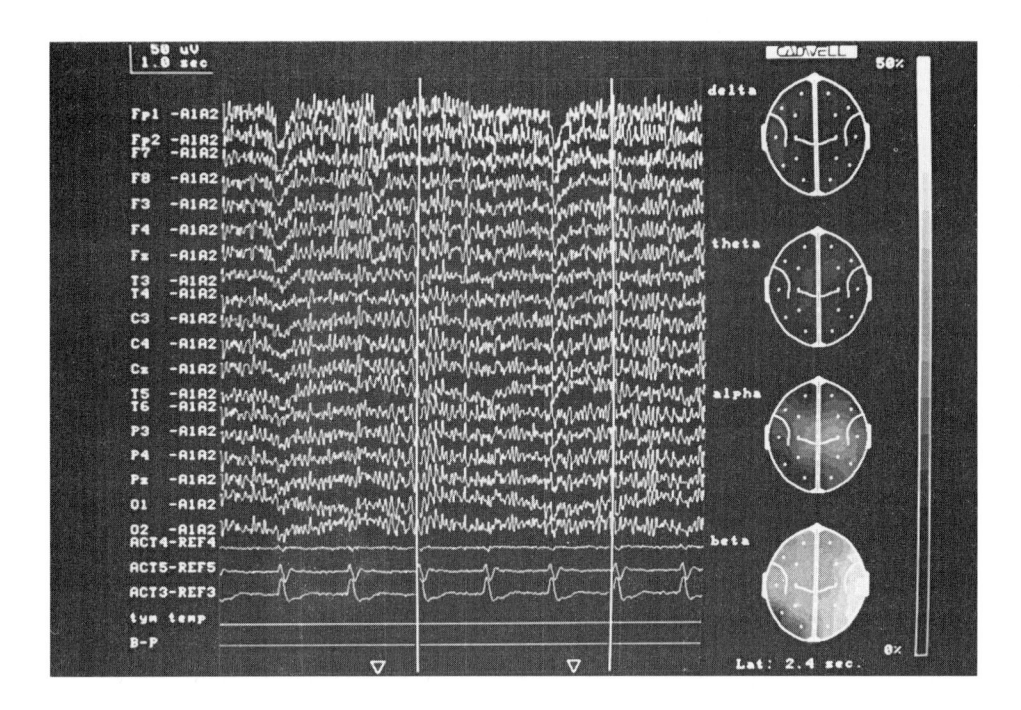

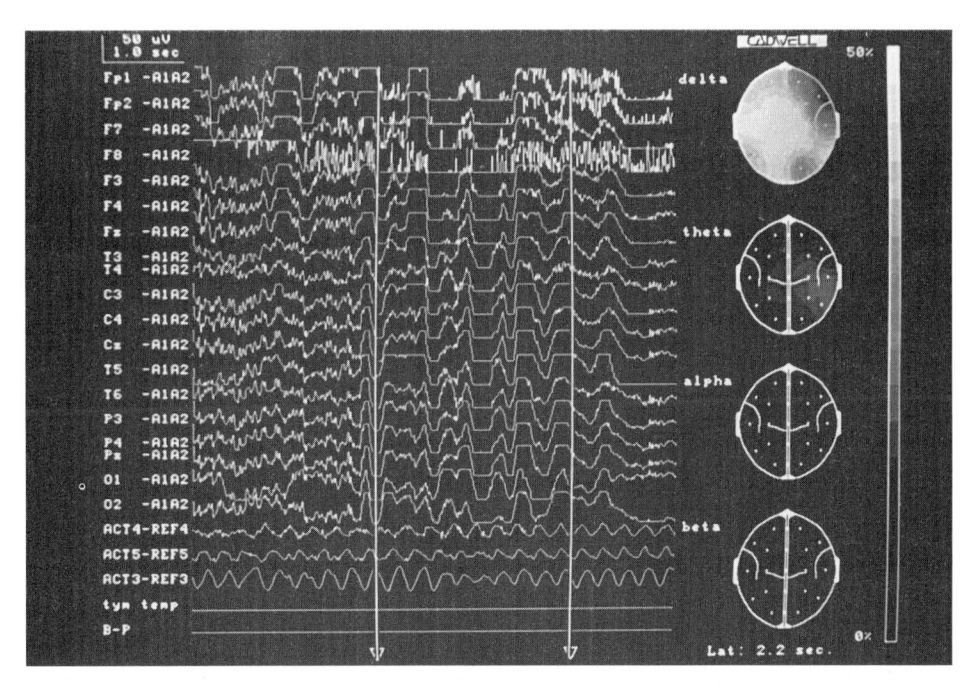

Figure 4. Quantitative electroencephalographic (QEEG) recordings during normal sinus rhythm (**top**) and ventricular fibrillation (**bottom**). Left panel shows analog signals, right panel shows schematized heads viewed from above, demonstrating EEG frequency distribution (beta, alpha, theta, delta from bottom to top). Note that during sinus rhythm, EEG is in the normal (beta range). During ventricular fibrillation, frequency shift occurs in the QEEG to the delta range indicating cerebral ischemia.

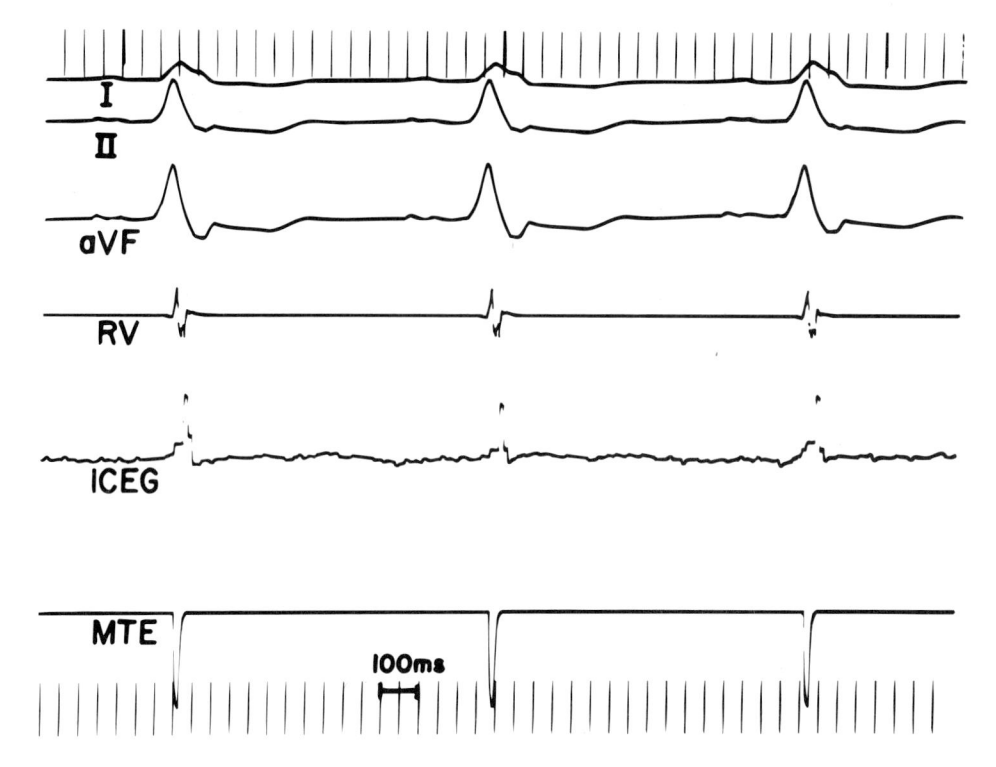

Figure 5. Intracardiac electrogram recordings during sinus rhythm (Guardian™ ATP 4210, Telectronics, Englewood CO). From top to bottom: surface leads I, II, aVF, intracardiac electrode in the right ventricular apex position (RVA), intracardial electrogram (ICECG) and main timing events (MTE). Note appropriate QRS sensing during sinus rhythm.

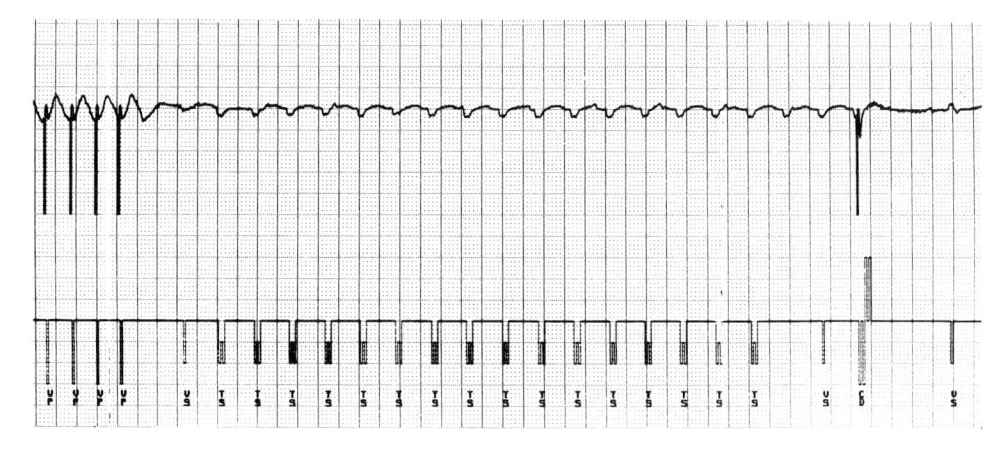

Figure 6. Ventricular tachycardia induction by noninvasive programmed stimulation. Appropriate sensing and ventricular tachycardia termination by shock (CD) is observed (PCD™ 7217B, Medtronic, Minneapolis, MN). **Top tracing:** surface lead; **bottom tracing**; main timing events. VP: ventricular paced event; VS: ventricular sensed event; TS: tachycardia sensing; CD: cardioversion/defibrillation.

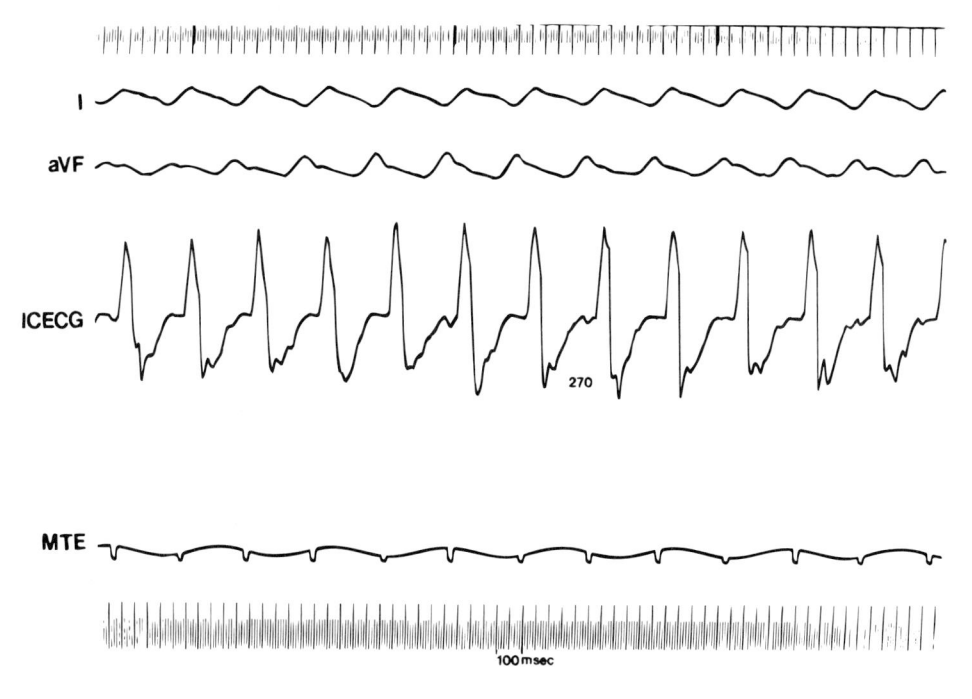

Figure 7. Ventricular flutter. From top to bottom: surface lead I and aVF, intracardiac electrogram (ICECG), main timing event (MTE). Note appropriate sensing of ventricular flutter by Guardian™ ATP 4210 (Telectronics, Englewood, CO.) (Reproduced from Singer I, et al. *PACE*, 1993, with permission).

and appropriate safety margins programmed (Figure 8). Occasionally, pacing thresholds may be high immediately after surgery due to edema, lead displacement, or lead perforation of the ventricle. If thresholds remain unacceptably high, resulting in loss of capture, the endocardial rate sensing lead may need to be repositioned.

Lead impedance is also measured. Causes of altered lead impedance are carefully assessed. High lead impedance sug-

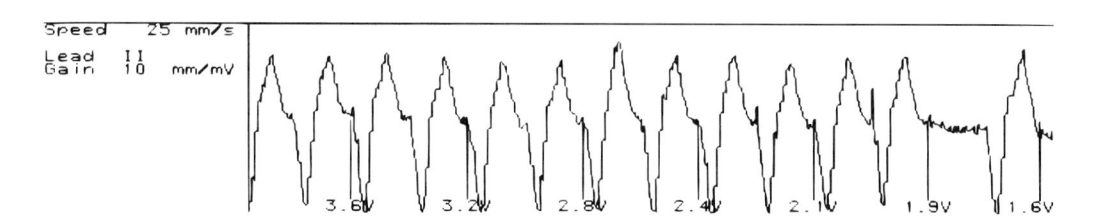

Figure 8. Automatic threshold testing (Guardian™ ATP 4210, Telectronics, Englewood, CO). Note appropriate capture at 2.1 V, but failure to capture at 1.9 V.

gests lead fracture or perforation of the ventricle. Low impedance suggests insulation breakdown or a gross lead displacement.

Induction of Ventricular Tachycardia

Third-generation ICDs have noninvasive programmed stimulation capabilities. Therefore, ventricular tachycardia and ventricular fibrillation may be induced noninvasively. The goal of programmed electrical stimulation (PES) is to ascertain if ventricular tachycardia is inducible, and if so, to program ICD therapy optimally.

The sequence of PES is similar to a routine electrophysiologic study. At least two cycle lengths are tested (eg, 600 and 400 msec) with single, double, and triple extrastimuli and ventricular burst stimulation. Multiple inductions of the clinical ventricular tachycardia are necessary to ascertain the efficacy of the programmed ATP or tiered-therapy response (Figure 9).

Detection algorithms are programmed to fit the clinical situation. Rate detection criteria for monomorphic ventricular tachycardia should be programmed at least 15–20 beats per minute below the ventricular tachycardia rate, but above the maximal exercise heart rate (that may be determined by treadmill exercise testing or Holter monitoring). If there is a rate overlap between the exercise-induced sinus tachycardia and clinical ventricular tachycardia, β-blocking drugs, digitalis or calcium channel blocking drugs are used to slow AV nodal conduction. If atrial flutter or fibrillation are a concomitant clinical problem, additional rate detection criteria may be programmed (eg, sudden onset detection, rate stability, or both).

Noncommitted devices (eg, Cadence™, Ventritex, Sunnyvale, CA or Guardian™ ATP 4211, Telectronics, Englewood, CO) are preferred when repeated episodes of nonsustained ventricular tachycardia are a problem, since these ICDs require reconfirmation of ventricular tachycardia prior to shock. However, committed ICDs (eg, Ventak) may deliver therapy even when ventricular tachycardia is nonsustained. This may result in repeated shocks for nonsustained ventricular tachycardia. The detection criteria may be altered to increase the sensing time required for ventricular tachycardia recognition prior to detection (eg, Ventak P). Though imperfect, this may be

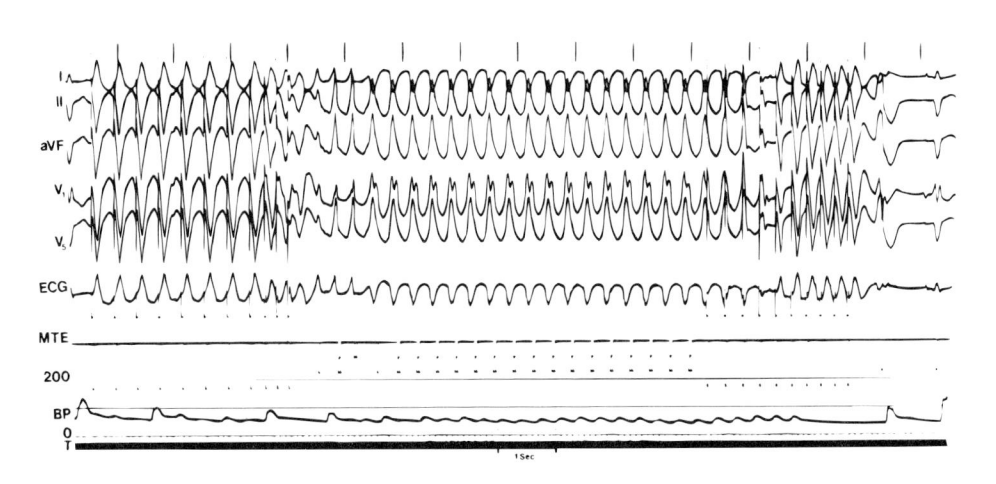

Figure 9. Induction and termination of ventricular tachycardia during electrophysiologic testing (PCD™ 7217B, Medtronic, Minneapolis, MN). From top to bottom: surface leads I, II, aVF, V_1, and V_5, surface electrogram (ECG), main timing events (MTE), blood pressure (BP), time lines (T). Note induction, followed by monomorphic ventricular tachycardia and termination by antitachycardia pacing.

adequate if nonsustained episodes are relatively short.

Occasionally, more than one clinical ventricular tachycardia is present. Some third-generation devices allow multiple zones of arrhythmia detection and therapy (eg, Guardian ATP 4211, Cadence, and PRx™ [CPI, St. Paul, MN). Independent zones for detection and therapy can then be "prescribed" for specific ventricular tachycardias.

Antitachycardia pacing is a subject that is discussed in detail in Chapters 9 and 12. However, some comments are pertinent to the present discussion. Antitachycardia pacing is generally effective for stable, monomorphic ventricular tachycardias. In our experience, the most effective ATP therapy, consists of an autodecremental burst ramp (Figure 10) or ventricular burst pacing (Figure 11). Scanning of ventricular tachycardia by multiple extrastimuli is generally ineffective unless the ventricular tachycardia is slow (rates 110–130 beats per minute) and

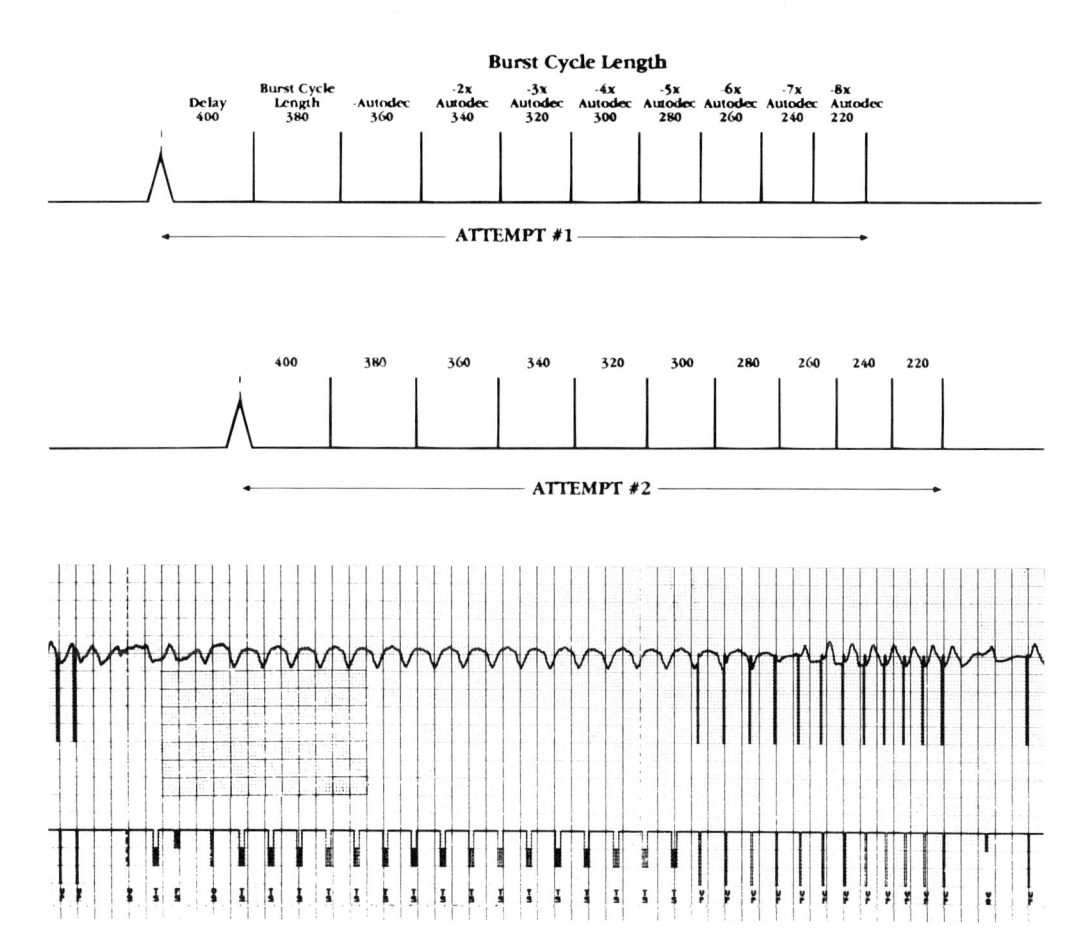

Figure 10. Top: Schematic representation of autodecremental burst pacing. (Reproduced with permission from *Clinical Manual of Electrophysiology*. Edited by I Singer, J Kupersmith. Baltimore, MD: Williams and Wilkins Medical Publishers; 1993, p. 389. **Bottom**: Noninvasive programmed stimulation. Monomorphic ventricular tachycardia is terminated by autodecremental burst pacing (PCD™ 7217 B, Medtronic, Minneapolis, MN). VP: ventricular paced beat; VS: ventricular sensed beat; TS: tachycardia sensed beat; PS: pace/sense beat; VR: ventricular refractoriness.

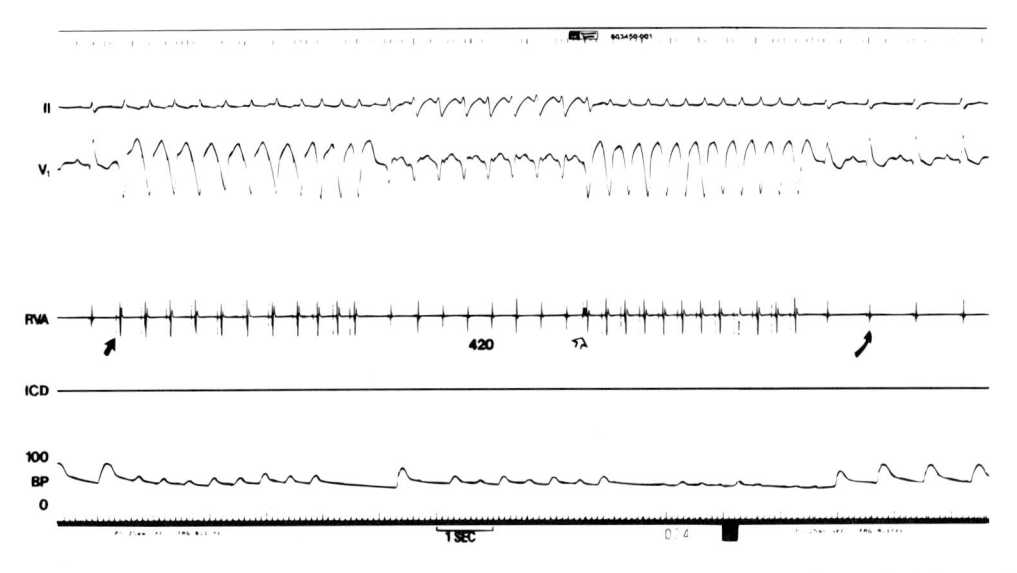

Figure 11. Ventricular tachycardia initiated by noninvasive programmed stimulation (solid arrow) terminated by ventricular burst stimulation (VB) (open arrow) with resumption of normal sinus rhythm (solid curved arrow). (Reproduced with permission from *Clinical Manual of Electrophysiology*. Edited by I Singer, J Kupersmith. Baltimore, MD: Williams and Wilkins Medical Publishers; 1993, p. 397.)

tolerated well hemodynamically. We rarely use the scanning techniques with individual extrastimuli. Antitachycardia pacing is effective in most patients with stable ventricular tachycardias and is reported to terminate 50% to 92.4% of ventricular tachycardia episodes.[27-35]

The effect of ATP therapy, as well as the effects of ventricular tachycardia on perfusion, should be assessed during electrophysiologic study.[25,26] Termination of ventricular tachycardia is an insufficient therapeutic goal, since syncope may occur even with successful ventricular tachycardia termination. Antitachycardia pacing therapy may be potentially hazardous if used inappropriately. Prolonged ATP routines may result in cardiac ischemia, hemodynamic collapse, or cerebral hypoperfusion. A delay in arrhythmia termination may increase DFTs and result in ineffective cardioversion or defibrillation. Ideally, a hemodynamic sensor could be used to assess ICD efficacy. However, current ICDs do not have hemodynamic sensors.

Another way to deal with this issue is to limit the duration of ATP therapy by programming the maximum time beyond which the therapy cannot be extended (eg, 20 seconds), after which the device proceeds to the most aggressive therapy. If ventricular tachycardia is not terminated within the specified time period, cardioversion/defibrillation shock is administered.

Finally, ATP therapy must be demonstrated to be effective. Multiple inductions and successful ventricular tachycardia terminations are necessary to ensure that the programmed therapy is effective and appropriate.

The limitations of electrophysiologic testing should also be recognized. The testing conditions in the electrophysiology laboratory are not analogous to real-life circumstances. Patients are often sedated and tested in the supine position only. The influence of autonomic nervous system cannot be adequately assessed in this setting. Serum levels of antiarrhythmic drugs may fluctuate over time. However, serum and tissue concentrations of drugs may influence ventricular tachycardia characteristics. Effects of ischemia, exercise, vascular tone or other physiologic variables cannot be adequately tested in the setting of the electrophysiology laboratory. Therefore, it must be anticipated that outcomes may differ from day-to-day. These limitations notwithstanding, electrophysiologic testing still provides the only available means to test ICD therapy.

Ventricular Fibrillation Induction

Defibrillation threshold testing is a vital component of intraoperative ICD testing. Adequate DFTs and safety margins must be ensured. Further, it is crucial to ensure that sensing during ventricular tachycardia and ventricular fibrillation are appropriate. Oversensing might lead to inappropriate shocks and undersensing of ventricular fibrillation may be fatal (Figure 12).

It is our current practice to induce at least one ventricular fibrillation during routine predischarge electrophysiology study. Inappropriate ICD function may result

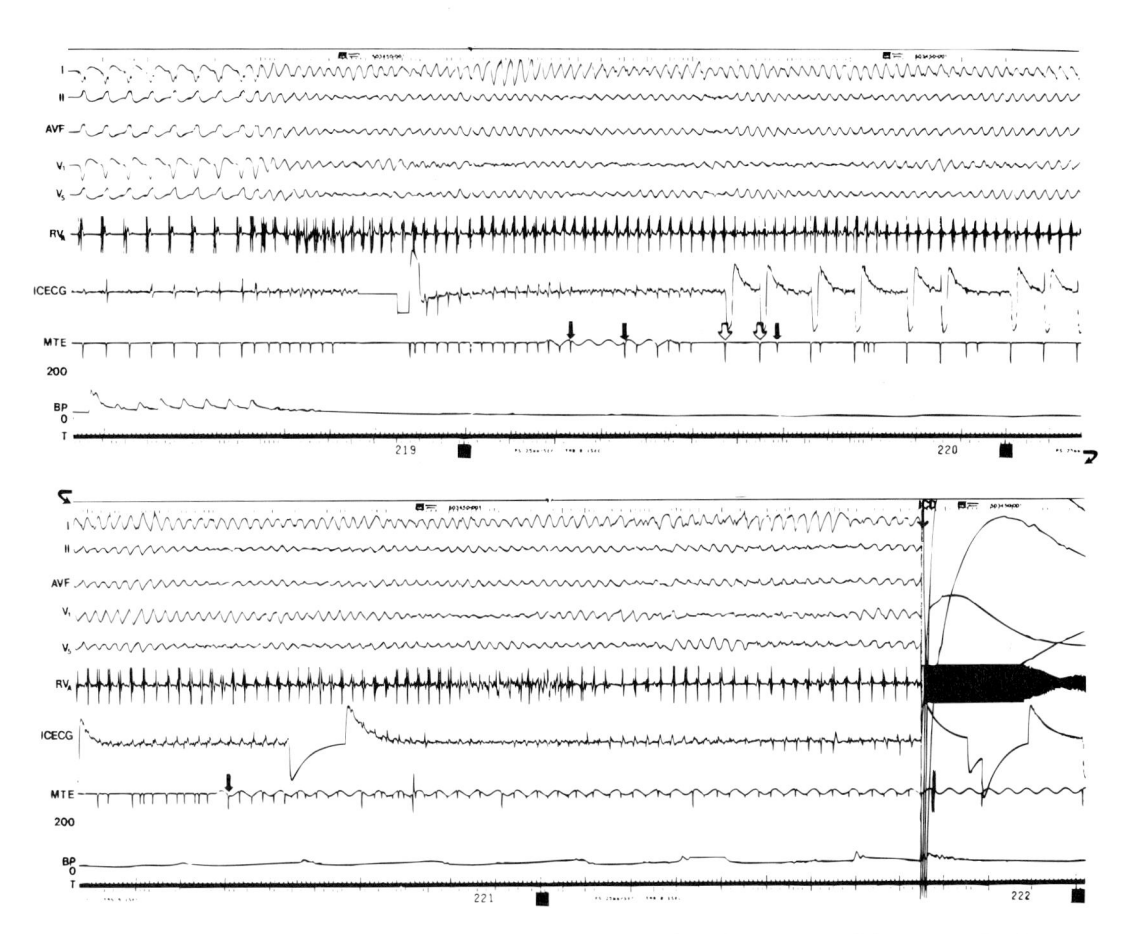

Figure 12. Undersensing during ventricular fibrillation (Guardian™ ATP 4210, Telectronics, Englewood, CO). The device is programmed to the maximum sensitivity of 1 mV. Intermittent undersensing with signal dropout (solid arrows) during ventricular fibrillation and inappropriate pacing (open arrows) are seen. Ventricular fibrillation is eventually redetected with implantable cardioverter-defibrillator (ICD) shock. This device has fixed gain sensitivity that halves (to 0.5 mV, in this case) when ventricular fibrillation is detected. Top and bottom strips are continuous: surface leads I, II, aVF, V_1, V_5, intracardial electrograms (ICECG), main timing events (MTE), blood pressure (BP), time lines (T). (Reproduced with permission from Singer I, et al: *PACE*, 16(5):1070, 1993 and Singer I, Kupersmith J, eds. *Clinical Manual of Electrophysiology*. Baltimore, MD: Williams and Wilkins Medical Publishers; 1993, p. 396.)

from: 1) endocardial rate sensing lead displacement; 2) patch displacement or crimping; 3) increase in DFTs due to antiarrhythmic drugs (eg, amiodarone); 4) pericardial effusion resulting in increased DFT; and 5) unsuspected lead fracture or loose lead-connector screw.

Third-generation devices permit induction of ventricular fibrillation by ventricular burst stimulation or T wave shock (Jewel™, Medtronic, Minneapolis, MN). Second-generation devices (Ventak), require placement of an endocardial electrode to induce ventricular fibrillation by burst pacing or alternating current.

Short-acting intravenous sedative (eg, midazolam) is given prior to ventricular fibrillation induction in combination with a narcotic analgesic (morphine sulphate or equivalent). The patient is oxygenated prior to the ventricular fibrillation induction. A standby external defibrillator must be available with a back-up defibrillator.[36] Failure of ICD to defibrillate is followed by external defibrillation. Resuscitative equipment and trained personnel must be readily available. With adequate monitoring, ventricular fibrillation induction in the electrophysiology laboratory is safe.[36]

Testing may uncover potential problems, including increased DFTs, lead-related problems (lead displacement), sensing problems (undersensing or oversensing), inappropriate programming, and so on. Therefore, unless specific contraindications exist, we recommend that all patients undergo at least one ventricular fibrillation induction at predischarge electrophysiologic study.

Follow-Up

The follow-up period begins with preimplant assessment and continues after hospital discharge. The fundamental objective of follow-up is continuous life-long patient care that should be distinguished from device surveillance alone. This process extends from the preoperative patient and family education to the full scope of postoperative surveillance. The specific clinical goals are listed in Table 1.

Table 1
Clinical Goals of ICD Patient Follow-Up

- Monitoring of ICD generator and lead performance
- Optimizing clinical effectiveness of ICD by making suitable programming adjustments
- Maximizing ICD pulse-generator longevity and performance
- Minimizing ICD-related symptoms and complications
- Anticipating the need for elective ICD pulse generator replacement
- Addressing clinical problems as they arise
- Dealing with device recalls and advisories
- Patient and family education

Methods

Unlike pacemaker follow-up, transtelephonic monitoring currently has no role in ICD follow-up. The basic method for ICD patient follow-up is direct (hands-on) examination. Follow-up visits provide an opportunity for: 1) assessment of symptoms; 2) physical evaluation of the ICD generator site; 3) assessment of lead integrity, ICD generator function, and pacing and sensing thresholds (third-generation ICDs); 4) detection and evaluation of clinical problems unrelated to ICD function; and 5) continuing psychological support for the patient and family.

Instrumentation

Instrumentation for direct evaluation includes: 1) at least one ICD programming device suitable for each ICD generator followed; 2) an electrocardiographic (ECG) display monitor; 3) an ECG strip-chart recorder; 4) a doughnut magnet; 5) 12-lead ECG recorder; and 6) a crash cart equipped with an external defibrillator. Optional facilities include: 1) facilities for ambulatory echocardiographic examination; 2) exercise test facilities; 3) access to radiological and fluoroscopic examination; 4) transient arrhythmia recorders (event monitors); 5) availability of transesophageal echocardiography and Doppler facilities; and 6) computerized database.

Personnel

A qualified staff capable of providing the full scope of clinical and administrative services must be available. At a minimum, this should include a trained electrophysiologist experienced in all aspects of ICD therapy and arrhythmia management, trained cardiovascular nurse, and technical support staff. Care should be available 24 hours a day. Detailed and separate administrative records that keep track of patients, manage device recalls and advisories as needed, perform troubleshooting, and provide a quick access to data are also essential.

Current Practice

Frequency of Follow-Up

Presently there is no consensus on what constitutes optimal follow-up frequency for ICD patients. Therefore, current practice is individualized by physicians to best accommodate the device type and patient's requirements. The frequency of follow-up is dictated by the need for capacitor reformation (Ventak, at 2-month intervals) and protocol needs for investigational devices (generally 3-month intervals). For example, a need for therapy adjustment due to appropriate or inappropriate ICD therapy, frequent shocks, or suspected device or antiarrhythmic drug complications dictate more frequent or immediate assessment. Symptoms unrelated to the device per se may initiate a follow-up visit by the patient, eg, recurrent angina, heart failure symptoms, syncope, and so on.

In the absence of complications, the usual routine is to see patients within the first 2 weeks postimplant to assess the incision site, check antiarrhythmic drug levels, and assess pacing and sensing function of the ICD. Thereafter, visits are scheduled at 2-month intervals to reform capacitors (eg, Ventak) or at 3- to 6-month intervals with devices that have automatic capacitor reforming capabilities (eg, Cadence). The role of follow-up electrophysiologic testing to assess sensing and therapy prescriptions for third-generation devices is not clearly established. Current "routines" are to some extent dictated by the investigational protocol requirements. It should however, be acknowledged that optimal frequency of visits and electrophysiologic evaluations have not been established.

Assessment of Battery Integrity and Capacitor Charge Times

First-generation (AID™, AICD™, Intec, Pittsburgh, PA) and second-generation devices (Ventak) require manual capacitor reformation. Battery charge and capacitor reformation times are elicited by using an external programmer. The usual charge times for Ventak are 6.5–8.5 seconds. These charge times are compared to the beginning-of-life and anticipated elective replacement indicator supplied by the manufacturer (Figure 13).

Some third-generation devices (eg, Guardian ATP 4211, and Cadence) perform capacitor reformation automatically on a periodic basis. Battery voltage may also be elicited by interrogation of some devices.

Assessment of Implantable Cardioverter-Defibrillator Sensing

Appropriate sensing is crucial for proper device function. Oversensing and undersensing may occur under certain circumstances (Figure 14). The causes of un-

```
****************
   VENTAK P
   MODEL 1600
  PULSE GENERATOR
****************
PRESENT PARAMETERS
_____

MODE        ACTIVE
RATE        175 BPM
PDF         OFF
DELAY
  1ST         5 SEC
  2-5       2.5 SEC
SHOCK ENERGY
  1ST       30 JOULES
  2-5       30 JOULES

_____

CHARGE TIME
              6.6 SEC
LEAD IMPEDANCE
              TEST OHMS
PG BATTERY STATUS
          EVALUATE ERI
CAPACITOR FORM
             33.0 SEC
COUNT
  1ST SHOCK        7
  2-5 SHOCK        7
  TOTAL PATIENT   14
  TEST SHOCK      18

****************
```

Figure 13. Ventak P™ (CPI, St. Paul, MN) interrogation with printout of programmed parameters, charge, and capacitor reformation times. Datalog provides only limited information including the number of shocks delivered for first, subsequent shocks and battery testing (test shocks).

dersensing and oversensing are discussed in detail in Chapters 4 and 21.

First- and second-generation devices provided limited information in this regard. AID, AICD, and Ventak provided no direct information. Placement of a doughnut magnet over the device elicited audible tone signals synchronous with QRS detections. Double, triple, or multiple sensing could be detected by phonocardiographic recordings of audible beeps if signals other than ventricular depolarizations were sensed (Figure 14).

Some third-generation ICDs provide real-time electrograms for analysis (eg, Cadence, Ventak P-2, Guardian ATP 4210 and 4211) (Figure 15). Therefore, sensing function of these ICDs may be assessed directly. Other third-generation ICD devices provide R-R interval logs that give indirect information about device sensing.

We routinely assess sensing during spontaneous rhythm (with strip chart recording) and if necessary, with provocative maneuvers (change in posture, arm and shoulder abduction, device and lead manipulation). It should be emphasized, however, that appropriate sensing during sinus rhythm does not guarantee proper sensing during arrhythmias (ventricular tachycardia or ventricular fibrillation). If inappropriate sensing is suspected (eg, spurious shocks), then electrophysiologic testing with assessment of sensing during ventricular tachycardia and ventricular fibrillation may be required to troubleshoot a suspected problem (see Chapter 21).

Pacing Thresholds and Lead Impedance

Third-generation devices provide facilities to test pacing thresholds and lead impedance. With some devices, this function may be performed automatically (eg, Guardian ATP 4210 and 4211; Figure 8). Lead impedance may also be telemetered. Lead integrity and position will affect pacing thresholds and lead impedance providing further diagnostic clues useful in troubleshooting suspected lead or lead-device system malfunctions.

Datalog Analysis

Third-generation devices provide extensive datalogs with summary of diagnostic information, including the date and the

AICD DOUBLE COUNT

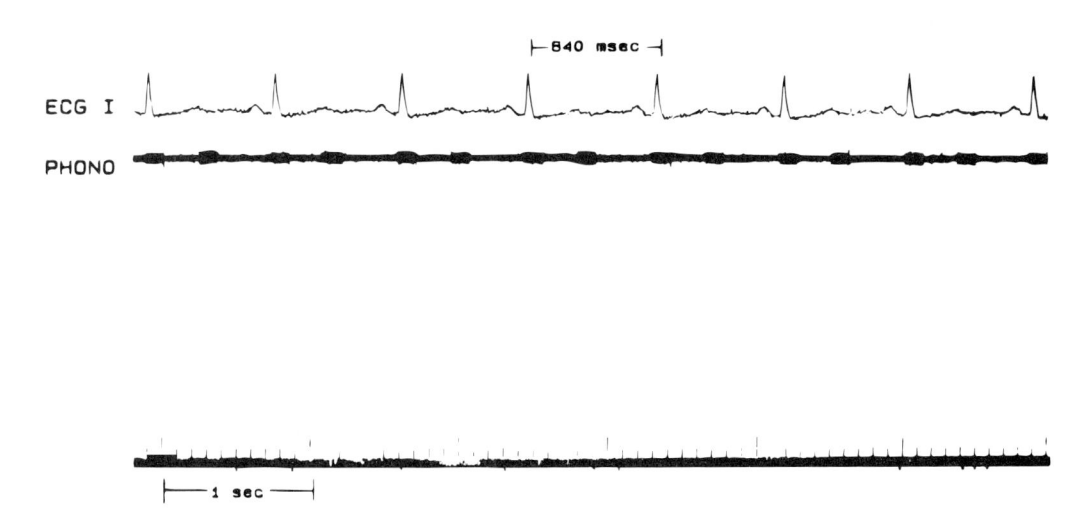

Figure 14. Double counting of AICD™ (Intec, Pittsburgh, PA) due to T wave sensing. Phonocardiographic recording demonstrates QRS and T wave detections with audible tones synchronous with electrogram detection.

time of recorded tachyarrhythmia episodes, episode details, details of administered therapy and outcome of therapy. Some devices provide analog signals (eg, Cadence, Ventak P-2) while others provide more limited information, such as R-R interval log (eg, Guardian ATP 4210 and 4211; PCD, Medtronic, Minneapolis, MN). Limited "peaks" at electrogram prior to and post-therapy ("snapshots") are a feature of Guardian ATP 4210 and 4211 devices (Figures 15, 16, and 17).

Datalogs enable the physician to more accurately assess: 1) arrhythmia frequency; 2) sensing; 3) efficacy of ICD and antiarrhythmic drug therapy; and 4) to troubleshoot suspected device, lead or lead-device problems. For further discussion see also Chapters 21 and 22.

Assessment of Implantable Cardioverter-Defibrillator Discharges

Prodrome of near syncope or syncope and/or palpitations followed by shock may on occasion be elicited from patients. More commonly, however, shocks are not preceded by symptoms. The absence of clearly defined symptoms does not mean that ICD shocks are inappropriate. Analysis of diagnostic datalogs clarifies the diagnosis in most instances. If still in doubt, transient event recorders or continuous recorders (Holter monitor) may be used to supplant datalogs and confirm the diagnosis.

Inappropriate shocks should be suspected when frequent or unexpected shocks occur at rest or during a specific postural maneuver (eg, bending, arm movement) in absence of symptoms suggestive of clinical tachycardia. These historical clues suggest oversensing, or "noise" detections (Figure 16) that may be due to lead fracture, lead connector "noise" (due to a loose pin or connector fracture) (Figure 17), or far field or myopotential sensing (see Chapter 21).

Inappropriate ICD discharges may also occur in the absence of ICD lead system malfunction when rhythms other than the clinical ventricular tachycardia are fre-

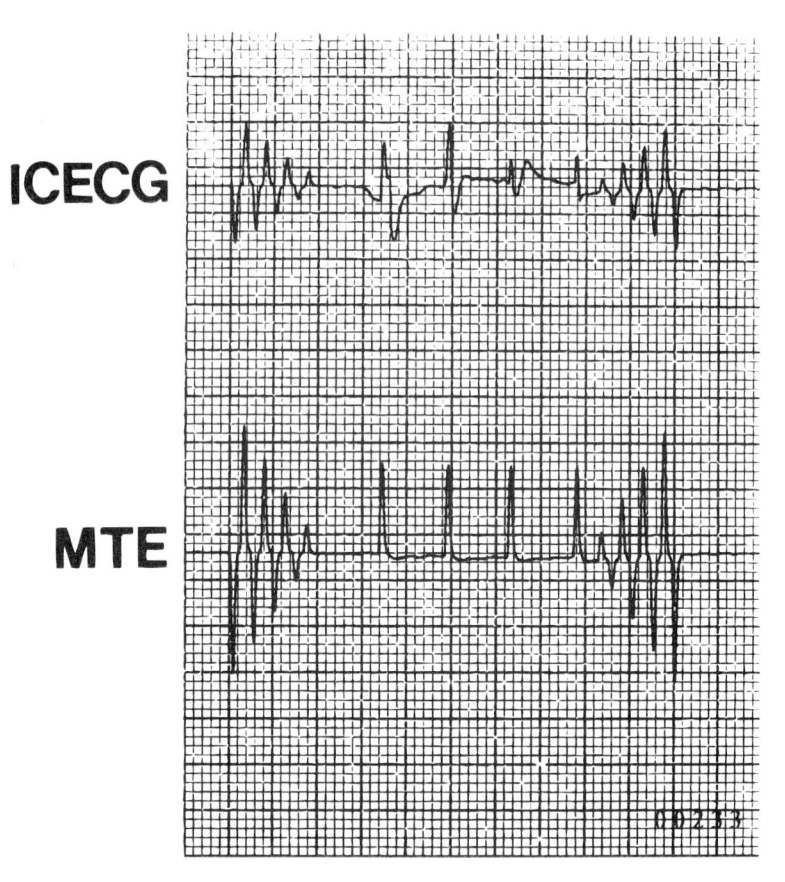

Figure 15. "Snapshot" of polymorphous ventricular tachycardia (Guardian™ ATP 4210, Telectronics, Englewood, CO). ICECG: intracardiac electrogram; MTE: main timing events.

quent. For example, atrial fibrillation with rapid ventricular response may result in ICD shocks if the rate exceeds the programmed ventricular tachycardia detection rate (Figure 1). If nonsustained episodes of ventricular tachycardia occur long enough to meet the detection criteria, shocks may occur in sinus rhythm despite arrhythmia termination if the device is "committed." If, however, the device is "noncommitted," frequent internal shock "dumps" may result in premature battery depletion. Presence of atrial fibrillation that meets the ventricular tachycardia detection criteria should prompt administration of digitalis, β- or calcium-channel blocking drugs to slow AV node conduction. Similarly, frequent nonsustained ventricular tachycardia detections may require antiarrhythmic drug therapy administration to suppress or abolish frequent ventricular tachycardia episodes.

Psychiatric and Social Issues

Preimplant Period

Before implant patients face potentially fatal tachyarrhythmias. During electrophysiologic studies the patients may experience fear and discomfort of external cardioversion/defibrillation. Patients may also experience side effects of treatment with antiarrhythmic medications. If these medications have not controlled the arrhythmia occurrences, a disappointed patient may internalize a sense of personal failure or guilt. This entire experience may cultivate a feeling of helplessness and powerlessness.

A

MAR 24, 1991
10:54 AM

GUARDIAN ATP4210
SN A02226678 ON

08:26 AM 24MAR91
    TCL170ms SPONT*
08:26 AM 24MAR91
    TCL310ms SPONT*
08:10 AM 24MAR91
    TCL 185ms SPONT*
08:10 AM 24MAR91
    TCL 275ms SPONT*
07:47 AM 25MAR91
    TCL 75ms SPONT*
01:43 AM 24MAR91
    TCL 315ms SPONT*
08:28 PM 23MAR91
    TCL 70ms SPONT*
08:20 PM 23MAR91
    TCL 100ms SPONT*
08:08 PM 23MAR91
    TCL 210ms SPONT*
05:38 PM 23MAR91
    TCL 65 ms SPONT*

05:36 PM 23MAR91
    TCL 80ms SPONT*05:33
PM 23MAR91
    TCL 70ms LATE*
05:05 PM 23MAR91
    TCL 90ms SPONT*
04:09 PM 23MAR91
    TCL 100ms SPONT*
01:42 PM 23MAR91
    TCL 170ms SPONT*
12:44 PM 23MAR91
    TCL 75ms SPONT*
12:20 PM 23MAR91
    TCL 95ms SPONT*
10:51 AM 23MAR91
    TCL 100ms SPONT*
10:44 AM 23MAR91
    TCL 70ms SPONT*
08:08 AM 23MAR91
    TCL 105ms SPONT*
08:08 AM 23MAR91
    TCL 80ms LATE*
05:37 AM 23MAR91
    TCL 80ms SPONT*

B

0 seconds
    Tachy detection
    TCL 310ms (194PPM)

0 seconds
    Sense History (ms)
    65   650   65
    655 65   655
    65   660   65
    660 65   665
    65   660   65
    660 65   655
    65   655 65
    655 65   660
    65   435   375
    325 295   320
    270 360
    Detection

3 seconds
    Sense History (ms)
    380 420   360
    350 305   300
    Confirmation

3 seconds
    Tachy still present
    TCL 330ms (183PPM)

7 seconds
    Sense History (ms)
    305 120   200
    135 265   175
    225 180   230
    270
    Confirmation

7 seconds
    Tachy still present
    TCL 225ms (269PPM)

19 seconds
    Sense History (ms)
    330 150   170
    325 150   175
    310 345   250
    135 260   385
    250 150   135
    345 350   325

    340 320   330
    330 270   160
    215 345   335
    330 330   330
    330 285
    Confirmation

19 seconds
    Tachy still present
    TCL 315ms (190PPM)
    Defib (25 J)
        delvrd 29.2 Joules
        impedance 36 ohms

23 seconds
    Sense History (ms)
    390 655   850
    690
    Reversion

Figure 16. Oversensing leading to shock (Guardian® ATP 4210, Telectronics, Englewood, CO). **A**: Datalog display demonstrates multiple "tachyarrhythmia detections" with "spontaneous" or "late" reversions. Note that the "tachycardia" cycle lengths are unphysiologically short (< 100 msec). **B**: Analysis of a single episode demonstrates long-short intervals typical of noise detections. Same patient as Figure 12.

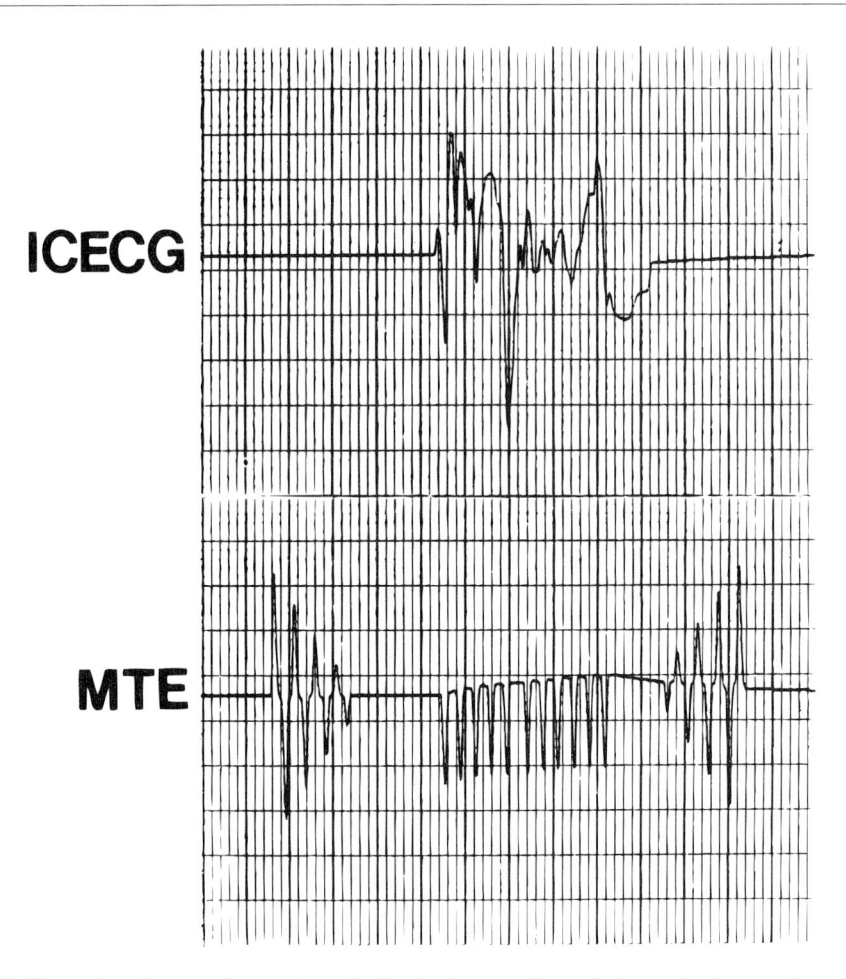

Figure 17. "Snapshots" preceding tachyarrhythmia therapy. Snapshot clearly demonstrates "noise" with multiple spontaneous detections. This patient had a connector fracture, leading to multiple "tachyarrhythmia" detections and inappropriate shocks (Guardian™ ATP 4210, Telectronics). ICECG: intracardiac electrograms; MTE: main timing events.

Fricchione and Vlay[37,38] suggested four critical components to deal with anxieties experienced by patients with life-threatening arrhythmias. They include the cardiologist, a consulting psychiatrist, anxiolytic medication if indicated, and behavioral intervention techniques. The cardiologist should provide information and education about the treatment procedures in terms that are understandable to the patient and family. It is advisable for the cardiologist to address hopeful solutions and potential frustrations. Hopefulness and knowledge of potential benefit from the treatment facilitate a reaction of confidence and decreased apprehension from the unknown. A consulting psychiatrist or specially trained nursing professional can provide supportive therapy that encourages patients to verbalize their perceptions and concerns while identifying therapeutic coping skills. Adaptive approaches initiated by the patient should not be discouraged unless maladaptive denial begins to obstruct compliance with therapy. Maladaptive denial should be addressed and altered to develop a more therapeutic coping behavior.

Postimplant Period

Immediately after the implant, the pain and discomfort from surgery confront the patient. The protrusion of the device may evoke emotions related to the patient's change in body image. The patient may feel a loss of independence and capability, and may question ability to function in the accustomed roles. This may result in anxiety and depression. Of those patients who have completed the Minnesota Multiphasic Personality Inventory (MMPI) and the California Personality Inventory after implant, "moderate levels of self-doubt, depression, helplessness, and high levels of emotional upset and distress" were revealed.[39] The early postoperative phase requires continued psychological support, active listening, and empathy. Positive adaptive skills should be acknowledged and reinforced, allowing identification of aspects of care about which the patient will decide and manage. Plans for greater autonomy should be acknowledged, involving the patient in the planning.

Morris et. al.[40] observed a 50% occurrence of adjustment disorders and depression in patients who had received a cardioverter/defibrillator in the past 3 to 21 months. This occurrence is similar to that documented for other medically ill patients. The recovery from the surgical implantation may be more rapid than the recovery from the depressive state that can occur as a complication. These patients may continue to be adapting to a perceived loss of control and independence associated with the sick role. A more elementary and less therapeutic level of adaptation may be observed if the patient manifests illness regression. Patients may report insomnia, fears, depression, and emotional instability. Increased sympathetic tone may accompany anxiety, contributing to the patient's risk of arrhythmias. This provides an additional reason to modify the patient's anxiety. Severity of illness, functional level and the ability to work influence depressive mood changes. This psychopathology may be a reactive adjustment disorder that is usually transient, decreasing or resolving when a more therapeutic level of adaptation is reached. Therefore, intervention aimed to help patients regain their previous functional activities and productivity is helpful. Previous expectations must be balanced by the perception of benefit from the device. If expectations were unrealistic, disappointment, frustration and anger may result. A reminder that ICD is an effective protection from sudden cardiac death can reinforce positive adaptation, particularly in patients who are self-limiting and overlook their productive and active roles.

A common concern of patients is the ability to resume employment and personal roles and responsibilities. From a small patient population, Vlay[38] reported that all patients with an ICD returned to an active lifestyle. Kalbfleisch et al.[41] found that 62% of patients returned to work after implantation of a cardioverter/defibrillator. This is comparable to the reemployment rate of patients with coronary artery disease after medical and surgical treatment. A major determinant of the ability to return to work is the patient's level of education. As these patients attempt to resume normal daily activities and employment, fears from the inability to predict the occurrence of an arrhythmic episode and shocks may inhibit adaptation. Those patients who feel forced into retirement may become despondent.

Most patients voice economic concerns from the impact of illness combined with treatment by ICD. Because an ICD does not prevent most patients from returning to work, the economic impact is not considered as significant as debilitating illnesses that may require repeated hospitalizations resulting in limitations in activity and employment. The cost of the device and implant hospitalization may be a burden for some, however, research in cost analysis will objectively clarify the future economic impact from treatment with the ICD (see Chapter 27).

Some patients may experience anxiety from the realization that not all physicians are familiar with the device. Patients may feel reluctant to travel, resulting in further loss of independence. In some states, patients may no longer be permitted to hold a driver's license. Medication, follow-up visits, fears of additional electrophysiologic studies, device failure, and the need to replace the ICD generator periodically are particular concerns to some patients.

Changes in sexual activity and performance may be self-imposed by the patient or their sexual partner. Changes in body-image present another adjustment. In terms that are understandable, education about the device and the patient's medical condition is vital for therapeutic adjustment. Health care professionals can encourage the patient to be creative and flexible with this information to resolve concerns and independence needs. Interdisciplinary teams composed of a social worker, financial counselor, cardiac nurse, and/or a psychiatric nurse can be particularly effective in assisting the patient with these varied concerns as the patient and the family attempt to return to normal living patterns.

Family and Support Systems

The patient's family or support system shares the concerns experienced by the patient. Anxiety and depression can be manifested by family members, creating an adaptational maladjustment on a group level. Anxiety and feelings of guilt may motivate the family to direct anger at the patient. Shifts in power and roles may occur within the family creating independence-dependence conflicts. Families can impose overprotective attitudes on the patients, forcing the patients to function in a more restricted, dependent manner. The degree of social support perceived by the patient may determine the reaction to stressful life events.

It cannot be assumed that a physical illness or life-threatening event will mobilize the patient's support system. The patient's condition may prove to be an overwhelming anxiety and emotional distress on the family, paralyzing therapeutic adaptation. The patient's presentation to the hospital may have followed resuscitation by a family member. This family member may place guilt upon themselves if they feel that they did not adequately assist the patient. Often families live far away from their homes and familiar community. The relationship between the patient's psychiatric morbidity and social support may require that health care professionals direct assessment and intervention toward the support system if the patient's psychological status and coping skills regress. Supportive individual and family counseling that encourages healthy family interaction, role adjustments, and long-term patterns of adaptation may be helpful.

Support Groups

The group process has been used by some to provide therapeutic intervention for specific patient populations.[42,43] Information can be shared, hopefulness inspired, isolation relinquished, and interpersonal learning can be fostered by the support group. A support group is a practical and effective method to provide physical and psychosocial well being for ICD patients and their families. Consistent issues observed in groups for postcardiac patients include: fear of death, depression secondary to helplessness and lack of accomplishment, and the feeling of abandonment when caregivers are not present. In a supportive environment, patients have shown positive responses to the group experience. The environment can encourage the patient to draw on available resources to resolve issues. The patient can observe and learn from those who have healthy, adaptive coping styles. The group experience provides a supportive structural environment where confrontation is of value. Maladaptive perspectives, adaptations and defenses are difficult to maintain when challenged by the group and the therapist. Patient feelings and perspectives about their condition can be verbalized, allowing one to move beyond individual concerns. The group experience provides for the ventilation of feelings and frustrations, with a collective response of reassurance, confrontation, and problem solving. A support group can afford the opportunity to provide formal education and confidence to patients and their support system. Accurate information can dispel any misconceptions that may interfere with optimal social participation by the patient.

Quality of Life and Coping Mechanisms

Depending on the patient's health experience before the implant of an ICD, the device may pose either a threat to or restoration of roles and freedoms important to the individual. Implantable cardioverter-defibrillators may restore freedom and productivity in patients who have undergone previous antiarrhythmic drug therapy. This is particularly true for patients who have experienced uncomfortable side effects or in whom drug therapy did not control the arrhythmias. Fear of arrhythmia reoccurrence resulting in ICD shocks may cause the patient to fear uncontrolled environments and reinforce social isolation. For the patient who lacked previous symptoms before an emergent sudden cardiac death event, the ICD may be implanted during a stage when the person is still in the process of accepting the diagnosed condition. In this case, an ICD may be a reminder of the condition the patient wishes to deny. Therefore, the patient may not immediately perceive the benefit of the ICD and may require a longer adjustment period to realize the positive aspects of the device.

The coping style will determine the depth of information a patient can use positively. Coping is effective when the person's integrity, functional ability, social interaction, productivity, and level of self-esteem are maintained.

For the patient who lives with the threat of sudden cardiac death, the ICD can provide more effective treatment than antiarrhythmic drug therapy. This technology has the potential to allow greater control and freedom from the disruption of the patient's normal way of life. To integrate this technology with optimum psychosocial adaptation, the health care team must strive to nurture positive self-esteem and inspire hope in this unique group of patients.

Conclusion

The integrated team approach to the follow-up of patients with ventricular tachyarrhythmias includes the electrophysiologist, referring physician, cardiac surgeon, cardiovascular nurse, psychologist, and social worker. The goal of follow-up is to optimize therapy, minimize discomfort, provide positive feedback and encouragement, and return the patient to productive work, to his or her family and social environment.

References

1. Saksena S, Tullo NG, Krol RB, et al: Initial clinical experience with endocardial defibrillation using an implantable cardioverter/defibrillator with a triple-electrode system. *Arch Intern Med* 149:2333, 1989.
2. Paul VE, Anderson M, Jones S, et al: Cardiologist implanted cardioverter defibrillators: early experience of three systems. *Eur J Cardiac Pacing Electrophysiol* 1:21, 1991.
3. Goldman L, Caldera DL, Nussbaum SR, et al: Multifactorial index of cardiac risk in noncardiac surgical procedures. *N Engl J Med* 297:845, 1977.
4. Winkle RA, Mead RH, Ruder MA, et al: Long-term outcome with the automatic implantable cardioverter-defibrillator. *J Am Coll Cardiol* 13:1353, 1989.
5. Edel TB, Maloney JD, Moore S, et al: Six-year clinical experience with the automatic implantable cardioverter defibrillator. *PACE* 14(Part II):1850, 1991.
6. Mosteller RD, Lehmann MH, Thomas AC, et al: Participating Investigators. Operative mortality with implantation of the automatic cardioverter-defibrillator. *Am J Cardiol* 68:1340, 1991.
7. Akhtar M, Avitall B, Jazayeri M, et al: Role of implantable cardioverter defibrillator therapy in the management of high-risk patients. *Circulation* 85(Suppl I):I-131, 1992.
8. Lehmann MH, Mitchell LB, Saksena S, et al: Worldwide PCD Investigators. Operative (30-day) mortality with transvenous vs. epicardial ICD implantation: an intention-to-treat analysis (abstract). *Circulation* 86:I-656, 1992.

9. Kelly PA, Cannom DS, Garan H, et al: The automatic implantable cardioverter-defibrillator: efficacy complications and survival in patients with malignant ventricular arrhythmias. *J Am Coll Cardiol* 11:1278, 1988.
10. Kim SG, Fisher JD, Choue CW, et al: Influence of left ventricular function on outcome of patients treated with implantable defibrillators. *Circulation* 85:1304, 1992.
11. Levine JH, Mellits ED, Baumgardner RA, et al: Predictors of first discharge and subsequent survival in patients with automatic implantable cardioverter-defibrillators. *Circulation* 84:558, 1991.
12. Epstein A, Ellenbogen K, Kirk K, et al: Clinical characteristics and outcome of patients with high defibrillation thresholds: a multicenter study. *Circulation* 86:1206, 1992.
13. Kay GN, Epstein AE, Kirklin JK, et al: Fatal postoperative amiodarone pulmonary toxicity. *Am J Cardiol* 62:490, 1988.
14. Nalos PC, Kass RM, Gang ES, et al: Life-threatening postoperative pulmonary complications in patients with previous amiodarone pulmonary toxicity undergoing cardiothoracic operations. *J Thorac Cardiovasc Surg* 93:904, 1987.
15. Watkins L Jr, Mirowski M, Mower MM, et al: Implantation of the automatic defibrillator: the subxyphoid approach. *Ann Thorac Surg* 34:515, 1982.
16. Lawrie G, Griffin JC, Wyndham C: Epicardial implantation of the automatic implantable defibrillator by left subcostal thoracotomy. *PACE* 7(Part II):1370, 1984.
17. Joye JD, Paulowski JJ, Fogoros RN, et al: Perioperative morbidity and mortality after ICD implantation in 150 consecutive patients (abstract). *Circulation* 84(Suppl II):II-608, 1991.
18. Gartman DM, Bardy GH, Allen MD, et al: Short-term morbidity and mortality of implantation of automatic implantable cardioverter-defibrillator. *J Thorac Cardiovasc Surg* 100:353, 1990.
19. Bardy GH, Troutman C, Poole JE, et al: Clinical experience with a tiered-therapy multiprogrammable arrhythmia device. *Circulation* 85:1689, 1992.
20. Cardiac Pacemakers, Inc.: Endotak™ lead system clinical report, premarket approval application to the Food and Drug Administration, December 1991.
21. Block M, Hammel D, Isbruch F, et al: Results and realistic expectations with transvenous lead systems. *PACE* 15(Part III):665, 1992.
22. Singer I, Guernieri T, Kupersmith J: Implanted automatic defibrillators: effects of drugs and pacemakers. *PACE* 11:2250, 1988.
23. Marchlinski FE, Flores B, Miller JM, et al: Relation of the intraoperative defibrillation threshold to successful postoperative defibrillation with an automatic implantable cardioverter defibrillator. *Am J Cardiol* 62:393, 1988.
24. Schamp DJ, Langberg JJ, Lesh MD, et al: Post-implant/pre- discharge automatic implantable defibrillator testing. Is it mandatory (abstract)? *PACE* 10:510, 1990.
25. Singer I, van der Laken J, Edmonds HL Jr, et al: Is defibrillation threshold testing safe? *Proceedings of IXth World Symposium on Cardiac Pacing and Electrophysiology.* PACE 14(11):1899, 1991.
26. Singer I, Rodriguez R, Edmonds HL Jr: Can cerebral perfusion predict appropriateness of implantable cardioverter-defibrillator therapy? *PACE* 16(5):1160, 1993.
27. Greve H, Koch T, Gulker H, et al: Termination of malignant ventricular tachycardias by use of an automatic defibrillator (AICD) in combination with an antitachycardial pacemaker. *PACE* 11:2040, 1988.
28. Newman DM, Lee MA, Herre JM, et al: Permanent antitachycardia pacemaker therapy for ventricular tachycardia. *PACE* 12:1387, 1989.
29. Bonnet CA, Fogoros RN, Elson JJ, et al: Long-term efficacy of an antitachycardia pacemaker and implantable defibrillator combination. *PACE* 14:814, 1991.
30. Fromer M, Schlapfer J, Fischer A, et al: Experience with a new implantable pacer-, cardioverter-defibrillator for the therapy of recurrent sustained ventricular tachyarrhythmias: a step toward a universal ventricular tachyarrhythmia control device. *PACE* 14:1288, 1991.
31. Luderitz B: The impact of antitachycardia pacing with defibrillation. *PACE* 14:312, 1991.
32. Saksena S, Mehta D, Krol RB, et al: Experience with a third- generation implantable cardioverter-defibrillator. *Am J Cardiol* 67:1375, 1991.
33. Singer I, Austin E, Nash W, et al: The initial clinical experience with an implantable cardioverter defibrillator/antitachycardia pacemaker. *PACE* 14:1119, 1991.
34. Block M, Borggrefe M, Hammel D, et al: Pacer-cardioverter- defibrillator (PCD): utilization, efficacy and complications of antitachycardia pacing (abstract). *J Am Coll Cardiol* 17:54A, 1991.
35. Ellenbogen K, Welch W, Luceri R, et al: Clinical evaluation of the Guardian ATP 4210 implantable pacemaker/defibrillator: worldwide experience (abstract). *PACE* 14:623, 1991.
36. Singer I: Approach to resuscitation in the electrophysiologic laboratory. In: *Clinical*

Manual of Electrophysiology. Edited by I Singer, J Kupersmith. Baltimore, MD: Williams and Wilkins Medical Publishers; 1993, p. 437.
37. Fricchione GL, Vlay SC: Psychiatric aspects of patients with malignant ventricular arrhythmias. *Am J Psych* 143:1518, 1986.
38. Vlay SC: The automatic internal cardioverter defibrillator: comprehensive clinical follow-up, economic and social impact: the Stony Brook experience. *Am Heart J* 112:189, 1986.
39. Pycha C, Gulledge AD, Jutzler J, et al: Psychological responses to the implantable defibrillator: preliminary observations. *Psychosomatics* 27(12):841, 1986.
40. Morris PL, Badger J, Chmielewski C, et al: Psychiatric morbidity following implantation of the automatic cardioverter defibrillator. *Psychosomatics* 32(1):58, 1991.
41. Kalbfleisch KR, Lehmann MH, Steinman RT, et al: Reemployment following implantation of the automatic cardioverter defibrillator. *Am J Cardiol* 64:199, 1989.
42. Badger JM, Morris PLP. Observations of a support group for automatic implantable cardioverter-defibrillator recipients and their spouses. *Heart & Lung* 18(3):238, 1989.
43. Teplitz L, Egenes KJ, Brask L. Life after sudden death: the development of a support group for automatic implantable cardioverter-defibrillator patients. *J Cardiovasc Nurs* 4(2):20, 1990.

Chapter 20

Complications of Implantable Cardioverter-Defibrillator Surgery: Diagnosis and Management

Igor Singer

Complications associated with implantable cardioverter-defibrillator (ICD) therapy may be considered under two categories: 1) operative complications and 2) complications due to ICD system malfunction. An extensive discussion of complications related to ICD system malfunction is found in Chapter 21; surgical complications are considered in this chapter.

Operative Complications (Table 1)

The incidence of cardiac complications related to the ICD implantation per se is difficult to assess because thoracotomy lead systems are frequently implanted during combined surgical interventions, such as coronary revascularization or valvular surgery. Prior to the availability of nonthoracotomy lead systems, a variety of thoracotomy approaches were used to implant the ICD system (see Chapter 15). The frequency of anticipated complications varied depending on the patient-related variables (eg, left ventricular [LV] function), the operative approach, and the surgical experience of the implanting team.

Arrhythmias

Arrhythmic complications after ICD implantation can be expected to reflect the underlying arrhythmogenic substrate of the implantees. Sustained ventricular arrhythmias occur relatively frequently in the postoperative period, and have been reported to occur in up to 17% of patients.[1-4] These arrhythmias may represent exacerbation of the arrhythmogenic substrate by a variety of operative and postoperative factors including fluid and electrolyte shifts, fluctuations in antiarrhythmic drug concentrations, exacerbation of ischemia, myocardial stunning due to defibrillation threshold (DFT) testing, or they may arise de novo.[5] However, the arrhythmogenic effect of epicardial patches cannot be entirely discounted. In the absence of a control group (no prospective clinical trials have been reported to date), it is difficult to separate the role of surgical intervention per se from a direct effect of the epicardial patch placement on the heart. Results of the ongoing CABG Patch trial, where patients with LV dysfunction (left ventricular ejection fraction [LVEF] $\leq$ 0.35) positive signal-averaged electrocardiogram (ECG) and surgi-

From Singer I, (ed.) Implantable Cardioverter-Defibrillator. Armonk, NY: Futura Publishing Company, Inc.; © 1994.

Table 1

Operative Complictions
Systemic
Cardiac
- Arrhythmias
  - atrial fibrillation
  - VT/VF exacerbation
- Myocardial infarction

Pulmonary
- Pleural effusion
- Atelectasis
- Pneumonia
- ARDS
- Embolism
- Pneumothorax

Pericardial
- Pericarditis
- Tamponade

Noncardiac
- Infection
- Cerebrovascular accident

Surgical Complications Related to the Leads and ICD Pulse Generator
- Hemorrhage (hematoma)
  - pocket hematoma
  - pocket seroma
- Erosion
- Injury to vagus nerve
- Lead dislodgement
- Lead perforation
- Air embolism
- Loose set screw
- Failure to insulate set screw
- Subclavian stick technique
- Microdislocation
- Active fixation lead malfunction
- Malposition
- Phrenic nerve stimulation
- Diaphragmatic stimulation
- Exit block
- Wire fracture
- Insulation fracture
- Venous thrombosis
- Embolism

cally correctable coronary artery disease are randomized to coronary revascularization (coronary artery bypass grafting [CABG]) or CABG and ICD implantation, may shed some light on this important question.[6]

Atrial fibrillation has been reported as occurring in up to 19% of cases.[1,4] Some caveats apply to its incidence. The effect of pericardiotomy is difficult to separate from the patch-related mechanical irritation and inflammatory reaction. In this authors opinion, patch lead placement does increase the frequency of atrial fibrillation postoperatively independent of the thoracotomy and the pericardiotomy effects.

Myocardial Infarction

Myocardial infarction is an infrequent complication of ICD surgery. It has been reported in 1% of cases.[1,7,8] Careful intraoperative hemodynamic and electrocardiographic monitoring helps limit the incidence of this complication. Revascularization (transluminal coronary angioplasty or coronary artery revascularization) should precede ICD implantation whenever coronary perfusion is compromised.

Heart failure may follow ICD surgery, in absence of myocardial infarction. On occasion, this complication may be precipitated by aggressive DFT testing protocols resulting in transient myocardial stunning.

Pulmonary Complications

Pulmonary complications are not infrequent following thoracotomy lead systems implantation.[1,2,7-10] These complications may be expected with thoracotomy per se, however, the presence of intrapericardial and/or extrapericardial patch leads may further exacerbate them by causing pain and pleuropericarditis. The incidence of pleural effusions, atelectasis, and postoperative pneumonia has been variously reported to occur in 3% to 27% of patients postthoracotomy ICD placement.[1,2,7-10]

The wide differences reported in the clinical series are likely related to the frequency and the extent of the concomitant cardiac surgery. Effects of ICD patch lead implantation are difficult to separate from the effects of additional cardiac surgery, in the absence of a true control group (ICD only). Most reported series have not separated the effect of ICD surgery from those associated with cardiac surgery, eg, coronary artery bypass, valvular surgery, etc.

The effect of the ICD patch leads as a causative factor unrelated to the effects of other cardiac surgery will likely emerge from the prospective data currently accumulated in the CABG Patch trial.[6] However, even this trial will only provide data relative to coronary revascularization.

Many factors may impact upon the frequency of pulmonary complications. These include the age of the patient, preoperative pulmonary status, duration of anesthesia, the length of time the patient requires ventilator support postoperatively, the surgical approach (eg, median sternotomy versus subxiphoid approach), cardiac status, and whether the patient is exposed to amiodarone preoperatively.[11-17] Adult respiratory distress syndrome after ICD surgery has been associated with long-term amiodarone therapy.[12] This adverse effect is not peculiar to the ICD patients and has also been reported in transplantation patients who have received amiodarone.[17]

The impact of various surgical approaches on the incidence of postoperative pulmonary complications has not been studied systematically. However, surgical approaches designed to minimize the "invasiveness" such as subxiphoid[18] and thoracoscopic approach[19] are likely to be associated with reduced incidence of perioperative complications. The advantage of reduced invasiveness, however, must be balanced against the relatively limited operative surgical exposure.

The management of pulmonary complications arising from ICD surgery is not unlike the management of these complications postthoracotomy in the absence of an implanted ICD. We encourage rapid weaning from the ventilator and extubation, vigorous chest physiotherapy, and generous analgesia. Postoperative pneumonia management should be directed at the etiologic organism, with appropriate cultures of sputum, pleural fluid, and blood preceding antibiotic therapy.

The management of postoperative effusions with conventional chest tube drainage does not differ from the management of postoperative effusions of any cause. It is worth mentioning that small postoperative effusions are commonly associated with patch leads, and the temptation to aspirate the fluid by percutaneous pleurocentesis should be avoided at all costs, unless the fluid accumulation is substantial and interferes with lung expansion. The danger of introducing organisms by external puncture in an environment where a foreign body (the leads) is present is fraught with risk, and should be avoided. In most patients the pleural fluid reabsorbs spontaneously.

Pulmonary Embolism

The incidence of pulmonary embolism post-ICD implantation is difficult to assess accurately. It is probable that pulmonary emboli occur more commonly than clinically recognized. They are more likely to occur with nonthoracotomy lead systems due to the presence of intravascular electrodes. It is, however, difficult to separate other contributing factors (low ejection fraction, atrial fibrillation, congestive heart failure) from ICD lead system effects. Embolisms have been reported in up to 3% of patients.[1,2,7-10]

Pulmonary emboli should be suspected in patients with unexplained right heart failure, episodic dyspnea with minimal signs of congestive heart failure, new chest x-ray infiltrates in the absence of demonstrable infection as well as with more classic presentations such as a new onset pleuritic pain, dyspnea, or hemoptysis.

With nonthoracotomy lead systems transthoracic or transesophageal echocardiography may reveal a lead associated thrombus. Conventional therapy with systemic heparin, followed by oral anticoagulation is indicated. The risk of bleeding in the immediate postoperative period may be minimized by careful titration of therapy and frequent monitoring of activated partial thromboplastin time. Oral anticoagulation should be administered for a minimum of

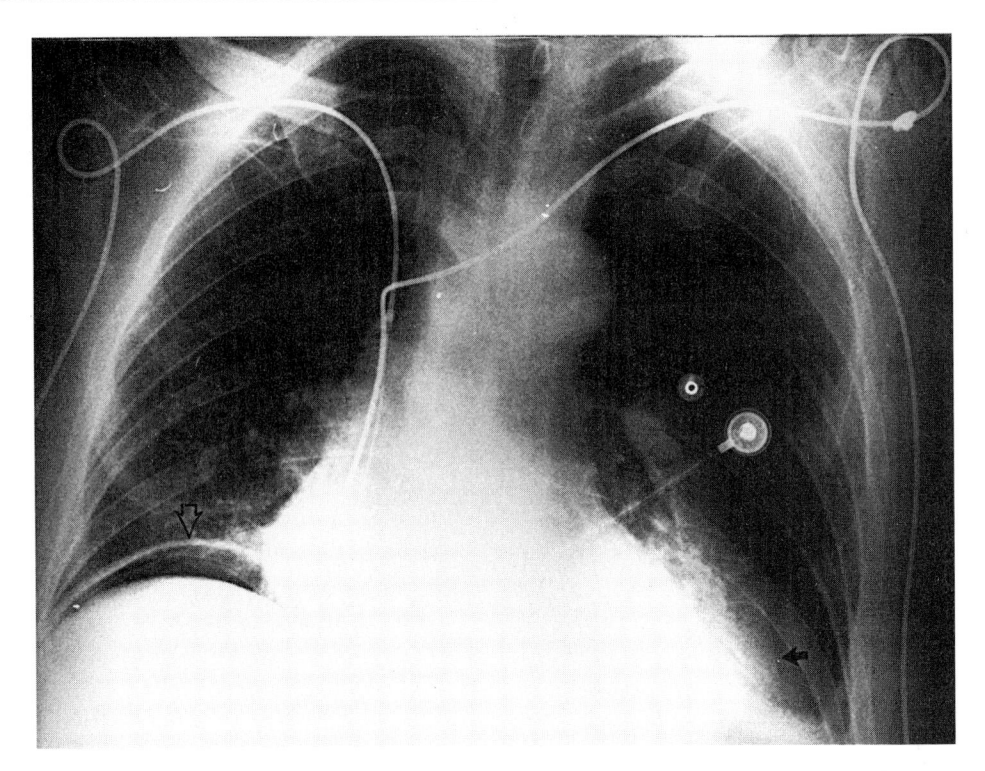

Figure 1. Chest x-ray demonstrating a pneumothorax (right), dark arrow after a nonthoracotomy (NTL) lead placement due to inadvertent lung puncture during left subclavian stick (EnGuard™ lead system, Telectronics, Englewood, CO). A pneumoperitoneum is also noted (left), open arrow.

6 weeks, or indefinitely in patients at high risk of recurrence (patients with dilated cardiomyopathy and LVEF < 20%).

Pneumothorax

Pneumothorax is most frequently associated with subclavian stick technique used for nonthoracotomy lead placement and is estimated to occur in 1% of patients.[1,2,7–9,20] However, a transvenous endocardial rate sensing lead is frequently used for thoracotomy ICD systems. If the pneumothorax is small, it may require no specific treatment. However, if the pneumothorax is large or if it is associated with tension, chest tube drainage is required (Figure 1). The incidence of pneumothorax may be minimized by the use of cephalic cutdown and by careful attention to the subclavian stick technique.

Pericarditis

Postoperative pericarditis after pericardiotomy and patch lead placement is almost a universal finding. However, its manifestations are often nonspecific. It may be associated with postoperative pain, pericardial or pleuropericardial rubs, and fever, but usually requires no specific therapy. Anti-inflammatory drugs may be helpful when pericarditis is persistent and causes clinically significant pericardial effusion. Symptomatic clinical pericarditis has been estimated to occur in 3% to 4% of patients and significant pericardial effusion has been reported in 2% to 3% of patients.[1,2,8]

Infection

Infectious complications may be considered as either ICD or non-ICD related.

Infective complications unrelated to the device include pneumonia and incision site infections. The incidence of nondevice-related infections is similar to postoperative infections associated with thoracotomy. The source of infection may be from intravascular catheters used for perioperative monitoring or postoperative intravenous catheter placement, or related to the surgical incisions. The management of these infections does not differ from the conventional management of postsurgical infections of any cause.

Device-related infections range from 1% to 7% in various series.[1,3,7,9,21] Device infections are more common with device replacements. The most frequent organism causing device and lead infection is *Staphylococcus aureus*, although *Staphylococcus epidermis*, diphteroids, and occasionally gram-negative organisms have been implicated as well. The incidence of infections is to a large extent related to the surgical technique, but other patient-related factors, such as depressed immunity, diabetes, and age of the patient may play a role. The role of prophylactic antibiotic therapy is unclear, although we routinely administer preoperative antistaphylococcal antibiotic prophylaxis (usually vancomycin) and continue antibiotics 48–72 hours postoperatively. Routinely, we also irrigate the pocket with Bacitracin or equivalent solution. These prophylactic measures do not substitute for good aseptic surgical technique. Therefore, all efforts should be made to enforce the aseptic technique.

In the presence of a superficial infection it is possible to achieve a cure with parenteral antibiotics (eg, vancomycin in the case of a staphylococcal infection), but in the presence of a deep pocket infection it is necessary to explant the ICD and the lead system.

The development of bacterial endocarditis is a serious and a potentially fatal complication when associated with transvenous leads.[22] Endocarditis involving the tricuspid valve is best diagnosed by the transesophageal echocardiography. With implanted pacemakers, recovery has been reported with antibiotic therapy,[23] but usually a complete removal of the entire system is required, whether endocardial or epicardial.[24–26]

The incidence of infections may be minimized by careful surgical technique and possibly by local and systemic antibiotic prophylaxis.

Cerebrovascular Accident

Cerebrovascular accidents have been reported in 1% to 2% of patients implanted with thoracotomy lead systems.[3,7,9,10,21] Preoperative evaluation of the cerebrovascular status by noninvasive and invasive techniques is indicated in high-risk patients, particularly in the presence of carotid bruits or a prior history of strokes or transient ischemic attacks.

Intraoperative monitoring with quantitative electroencephalogram (QEEG) and transcranial Doppler techniques[27] may minimize the operative risk of patients at high risk of strokes (those patients with preexisting cerebrovascular disease). In the high-risk patients, the DFT testing should be minimized and confined to proving the safety margins, rather than determining the actual DFT (see Chapters 10 and 15) (Figures 2 and 3).

Surgical Complications Related to the Leads and Implantable Cardioverter-Defibrillator Pulse Generator

Erosion

In our experience, the incidence of pulse generator erosion is rare. Erosion of the pulse generator or lead through the skin may occur at any time postimplantation. In some cases this may be related to incorrect location of the pulse generator or the leads. If the generators are placed subcutaneously, the blood supply to the skin may be im-

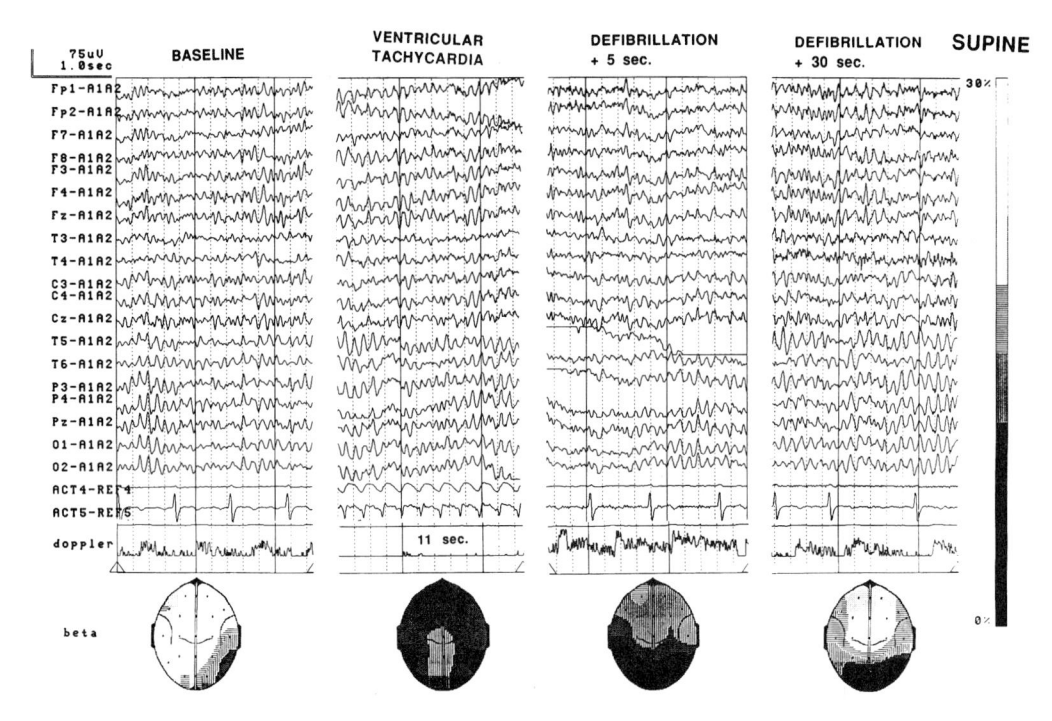

Figure 2. Quantitative electroencephalogram (EEG) during ICD testing in the electrophysiology laboratory. Note beta activity (normal) at baseline with loss of beta activity during ventricular tachycardia and fibrillation, followed by a residual effect seen in the occipital area at 30 seconds postdefibrillation indicating cerebral ischemia. **Top**: analog signals; **bottom**: schematized head views from above: nose in front, occiput behind.

paired leading to erosion. Contributing factors may include thin patients, and the bulk or shape of the pulse generator (sharp corners and edges). We generally prefer the submuscular generator placement for that reason. A more rounded design of the pulse generator may eliminate most cases of pulse generator erosion.

The surgical management of pulse generator erosion depends on the clinical stage. In early cases where skin thinning and erythema are present, but without the actual breach in the skin integrity, the pocket is still sterile and surgical relocation of the generator to a submuscular plane is indicated. If the pulse generator has eroded through the skin and there is communication between the pocket and the outside environment, one must assume that the system is contaminated. It is unlikely that under these circumstances the system can be salvaged.

Pocket Hematoma

Hematoma involving the generator pocket is seen only occasionally. Most frequently, it occurs in anticoagulated patients, eg, postcardiopulmonary bypass, or patients on oral anticoagulants in whom the anticoagulation either cannot be completely reversed for ICD surgery or discontinued in the most immediate perioperative period (eg, patients with prosthetic valves). Management of pocket hematoma should be conservative, unless massive or expanding, in which case surgical reexploration is recommended in a scrupulously sterile environment such as the operating room. Surgical reexploration is also indicated if the suture lines are bulging or a threatened wound dehiscence seems imminent.

A hematoma involving the generator pocket predisposes to secondary bacterial infection. Therefore, every caution must be

VENTRICULAR TACHYCARDIA
13 sec

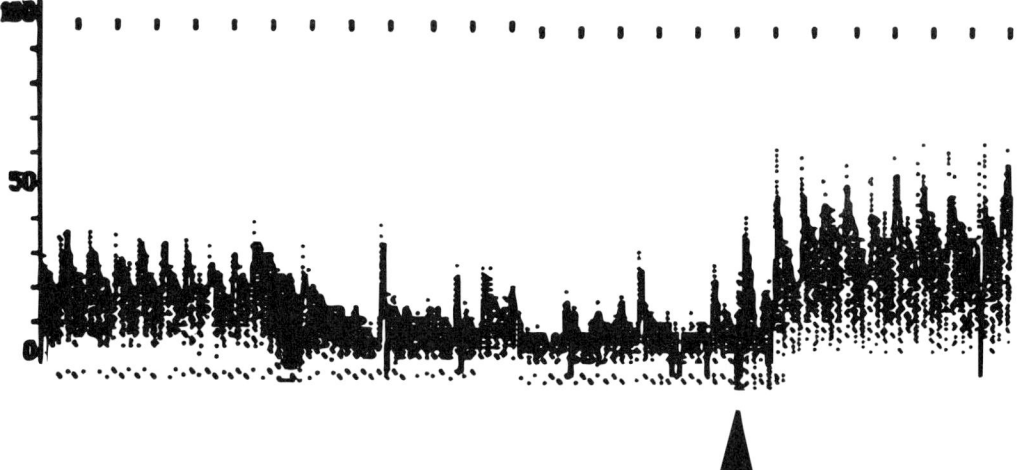

Figure 3. Transcranial Doppler during ventricular tachycardia in another patient, demonstrating a profound impairment in cerebral perfusion during tachycardia, and a hyperemic response postdefibrillation. Prolonged hyperemia is associated with cerebral hypoxia.

exercised during the operation to ligate all bleeding vessels and to scrupulously "dry" the pocket prior to wound closure. Immediate anticoagulation post-ICD surgery, if required, should be carefully monitored with the activated thromboplastin times kept at the lower range of therapeutic (1.5 × control) in the immediate postoperative period (48–72 hours).

Pocket Seroma

Pocket seroma is defined as a sterile effusion of the generator pocket that causes pocket fluctuance, but without inflammatory changes (fever, erythema, purulent discharge). Pocket seromas are a relatively frequent and benign occurrence. They may follow pocket hematomas and are especially frequent after generator change. This is particularly prone to occur when the replacement generator is smaller than the original ICD generator, thus resulting in a potential free space, which encourages seromatous fluid accumulation. The main significance of seromas is to distinguish them from frank pocket infections. The main distinguishing signs are absence of inflammatory reaction, fever, and leukocytosis. The temptation to aspirate the fluid percutaneously should be strenuously discouraged and avoided because exogenous invasion of the fluid by bacterial contamination is a disastrous complication that can result in ICD system infection and a need to explant the ICD system. Management of pocket seromas should, therefore, be expectant and reassurance to the patient is usually all that is required.

Lead Dislodgment

Dislodgment usually occurs within 24–48 hours postoperatively, but it may occur up to several weeks postimplantation. It is usually accompanied by the loss of sensing and capture (ICDs with pacing capabilities), oversensing and/or undersensing that may result in inappropriate shocks, or inability to properly detect ventricular tachycardia and fibrillation. Displacement of the rate sensing ventricular endocardial lead to the atrium or atrioventricular junction may result in detection of atrial as well as ventricular electrograms, resulting in double counting and inappropriate shocks. When gross, lead displacement may be readily recognized by radiographic means. Immediate repositioning of the lead is indicated (Figure 4).

Nonthoracotomy leads have defibrillation coils incorporated in the lead (Endotak™, CPI, St. Paul, MN; or Transvene™, Medtronic, Minneapolis, MN). Displacement of the defibrillation coil may be anticipated to change the DFTs and hence may result in ineffective defibrillation.

Lead Perforation

In our experience, lead perforation with nonthoracotomy leads is a rare occurrence. Clues to lead perforation are loss of ventricular capture and sensing, which may be associated with diaphragmatic pacing (ICDs with pacing capabilities). Occasionally, perforation may be confirmed radiographically by an unusual lead position, but more frequently the chest x-ray is unrevealing.

If right ventricular perforation is suspected, the lead should be gently withdrawn and repositioned using fluoroscopic guidance. Cardiac tamponade usually does not occur unless the patient is anticoagulated.

Perforation can be avoided by careful lead positioning and by ensuring that the lead stylet is partially withdrawn prior to positioning of the tip of the lead in the right ventricular apex. Appropriate lead curvature should be ensured in the right atrium. Too loose a loop may potentiate a tendency for the lead migration, but a short loop may predispose to a lead dislocation.

Superior Vena Caval Lead Migration

Migration of superior vena caval (SVC) lead has been reported in up to 6% of patients.[28] This complication is also more likely with nonthoracotomy leads that do not have a distal anchoring mechanism (eg, SVC spring electrode, Transvene electrode). When the anchoring sutures on the lead sleeve are not tight enough, the lead may migrate to the right atrial-inferior vena caval junction, or into the inferior vena cava, resulting in ineffective defibrillation. With two lead nonthoracotomy systems, anchoring of the SVC electrode (eg, EnGuard™, Telectronics, Englewood, CO) may help minimize the incidence of this complication (Figure 5). Appropriate anchoring of the lead with firm suturing to the pectoral muscle may help to minimize the incidence of this complication.

Loose Set Screw

This complication is probably very rare and is easily preventable. It may manifest as oversensing, resulting in spurious shocks or failure to pace with increase in lead impedance, or both. If the set screws are not tightened properly with the patch leads, energy shunting may occur, resulting in inadequate energy output and failure to defibrillate.

The surgeon should always tug on the leads to ensure that the set screws are tightened properly. It is also recommended that noninvasive measurements of lead impedance and electrogram characteristics be obtained prior to the pocket closure where noninvasive telemetry facilities exist (third-generation ICDs).

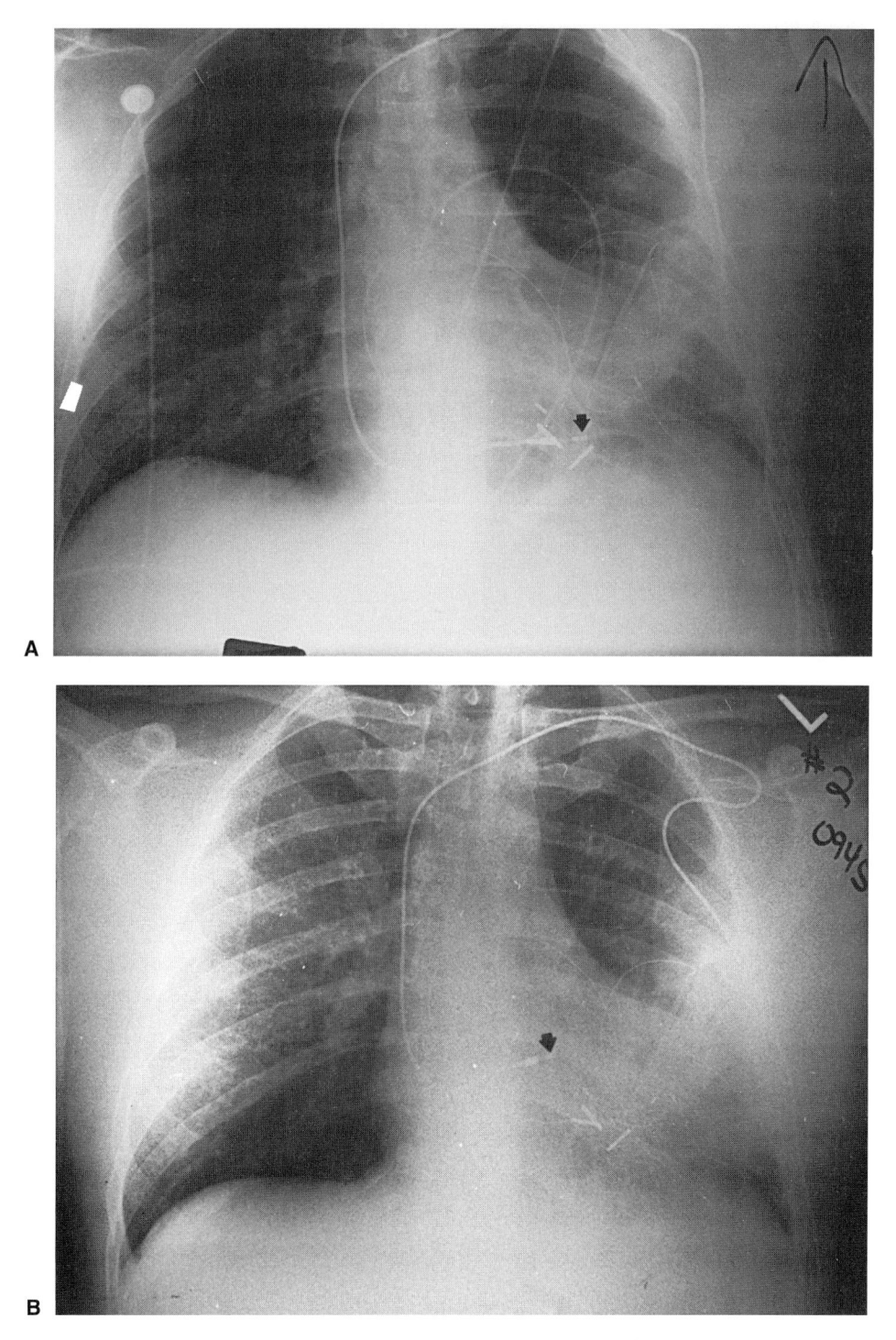

Figure 4. Endocardial pace/sense lead displacement. **A:** position of the lead tip (dark arrow) after the implant. **B:** displacement of the endocardial lead to the atrioventricular junction. *(continues)*

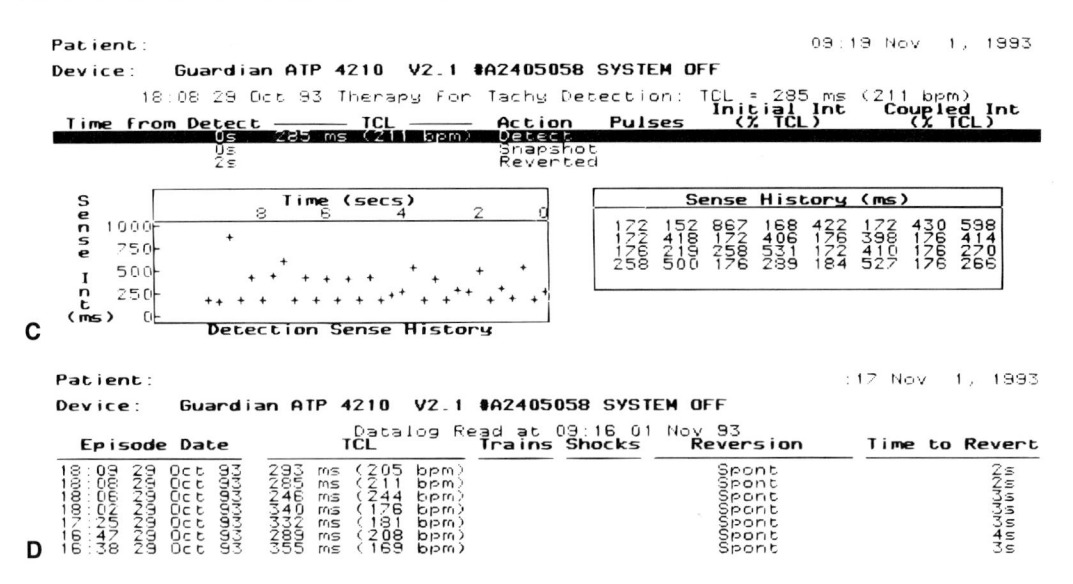

Figure 4. *(Continued)* **C:** sensing of both atrial and ventricular electrograms due to the lead displacement, resulting in **(D)** multiple spurious arrhythmia detections.

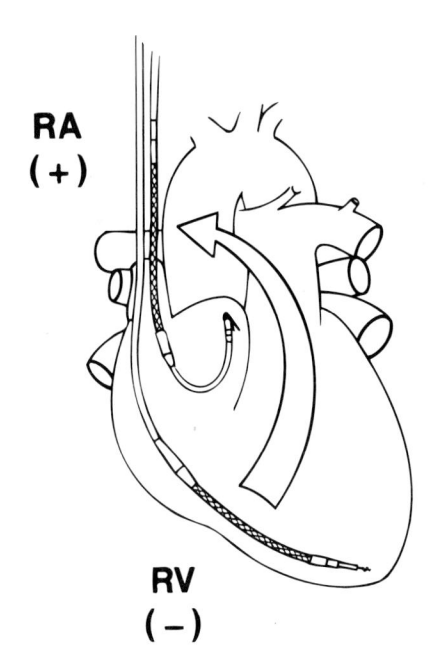

Figure 5. EnGuard™ (Telectronics, Englewood, CO) transvenous endocardial lead system demonstrating the atrial anchoring mechanism, with a J-shaped atrial lead.

Failure to Insulate the Set Screws

Some pulse generators have self-sealing insulation allowing introduction of the Allen wrench through the insulation to tighten the screw. Some, however, have a silastic button that has to be screwed on after the set screws are tightened (eg, Cadence™, Ventritex, Sunnyvale, CA; Res-Q™, Intermedics, Angleton, TX). Failure to place the silastic buttons may result in premature battery depletion, shock shunting, and ineffective defibrillation and local muscle stimulation during pacing. Therefore, meticulous surgical technique and attention to detail are important to avoid these preventable complications.

Complications Resulting from the Subclavian Stick Technique

Since its introduction, the subclavian stick technique has largely replaced the cephalic cutdown as the preferred approach because of its simplicity.[29,30] While this technique is generally associated with minimal complications in experienced hands, this technique does have some potential risks.

Pneumothorax

The incidence of pneumothorax may be minimized by a careful subclavian stick technique, the use of deep Trendelenburg position during the stick, and avoidance of repeated attempts to stick the vein in difficult cases and shift to alternative approaches. Pneumothorax is occasionally a benign complication and may resolve without further intervention. However, it may also be associated with lung collapse and tension, resulting in hemodynamic compromise. In that event, apical chest tube should be placed with suction to reexpand the lung. Postoperative chest x-ray is mandatory to screen for this complication whenever the subclavian stick technique is used.

Hemothorax

Hemothorax is a rare complication, but may occur when blood vessel is injured and a simultaneous pneumothorax occurs. In the absence of a concomitant pneumothorax, the blood is usually tamponaded by the lung pressure. If, however, the lung has collapsed, blood escapes into the thorax and may lead to a fatal hemorrhage. This complication has been reported in the pacemaker literature,[31,32] but is clearly not unique to the pacemakers and may occur whenever the subclavian stick technique is used, whether for ICD or pacemaker lead placement. The management of this complication is surgical with exploratory thoracotomy, surgical blood vessel repair, and chest tube drainage.

Subclavian Artery Puncture

Subclavian artery puncture is not uncommon when subclavian vein stick technique is used. Recognition of an arterial puncture is generally straightforward, with pulsatile flow of blood being easily recognized. On occasion, when the needle is not completely intraluminal, it is not possible to be sure that the blood is arterial. Passage of the guidewire to the inferior vena cava under fluoroscopy, which can be identified by the medial position of the guidewire to the right side of the spinal column, is reassuring to the operator. If the guidewire does not take this typical course, or if there is difficulty in advancing the guidewire, the needle and the guidewire must be withdrawn and pressure applied for approximately 10 minutes at the site of the needle puncture. Generally, when recognized, subclavian artery puncture is a benign complication, unless it is also associated with pneumothorax.

Air Embolism

Air embolism is somewhat more likely to occur with nonthoracotomy lead ICD systems than with pacemakers whenever a subclavian stick technique is used. This is related to the size of the lead and the necessity of using larger introducers (12F to 14F), depending on the lead system. The incidence of this potentially fatal complication may be minimized by the use of a deep Trendelenburg position during the stick, and by pinching the sheath between the thumb and the index finger prior to the introduction of the endocardial lead(s), with a rapid lead passage. Unless massive, air embolism is usually not fatal, but may be associated with transient or permanent neurological sequelae. It must be emphasized that in experienced hands this complication is exceedingly rare.

Bleeding

Continued bleeding may occasionally occur with the subclavian stick method. This problem may be eliminated by placement of purse-string suture in the pectoralis major muscle and the puncture site. Bleeding may also arise from the subcutaneous or muscular arteries. Therefore, a careful search and cautery of bleeding vessels is required prior to the wound closure.

Hemoptysis

Hemoptysis may occur if the lung is punctured during the subclavian vein puncture. It is usually associated with pneumothorax. Hemoptysis is usually self-limiting and does not require surgical intervention.

Brachial Plexus Injury

Brachial plexus is located close to the site of the subclavian vein puncture. Therefore, it is possible to injure the brachial plexus with the needle stick. This complication should be suspected if the patient complains of paresthesia or pain in the arm after the lead placement. This complication is rare, and can be avoided by careful technique.

Subclavian Arteriovenous Fistula

If the posterior wall of the artery is punctured and the vein encountered during the stick, it is possible to cause arteriovenous fistula to develop. Correction of the fistula requires surgical repair. Again and fortunately, this complication is extremely uncommon.

Lead-Related Complications

Microdislocation

Endocardial electrodes are frequently used for sensing with transthoracic patch lead placement because the long-term performance of endocardial leads with respect to pacing and sensing is superior to epicardial leads. With nonthoracotomy lead systems, pacing and sensing are accomplished between the tip of the lead (cathode) and the shocking coil (anode). Gross lead dislodgment has already been discussed. However, microdislodgment may occur as with pacing leads. In this complication, the lead is in the anatomically correct position, but the tip of the lead and the endocardium are not in good contact. The chest x-ray demonstrates no change in the lead position, however, pacing thresholds are high and failure to capture occurs. Sensing however, may be adequate. Microdislodgment requires repositioning of the lead, particularly if bradycardia or antitachycardia pacing functions are absolutely required. In general, the lead should be replaced by an active fixation lead.

Malposition

Lead malposition may occur inadvertently. The most common site is the coronary sinus when the right ventricular outflow is sought. Malposition may be detected by lateral fluoroscopy if available, with the lead noted to take a posterior course. Failure to pace the ventricle, with atrial capture may be noted with the coronary sinus malposition. Other diagnostic clues are failure of the lead to move synchronously with the ventricular systole, lack of premature ventricular contractions as the lead is advanced, and atrial and ventricular electrogram recordings from the lead.

Another potential site for lead malposition may be passage of the lead via a patent foramen ovale into the left ventricle. This would make the tip of the lead flush with the apex of the LV silhouette. This is likely to result in systemic emboli and therefore, the lead should be withdrawn and repositioned.

Diaphragmatic Stimulation

Diaphragmatic pacing may occur with right ventricular perforation with the lead and is usually accompanied by the loss of capture. It may also occur with active fixation electrode, when the screw penetrates the thin right ventricular wall. This complication is routinely tested for in our laboratory by pacing at a high output (10 V, pulse width 1–1.5 msec). If diaphragmatic pacing is noted, regardless of the acceptability of other parameters, the lead is repositioned. If the phenomenon appears postoperatively, reduction in output is attempted, if unsatisfactory, the lead may have to be repositioned.

Exit Block

Exit block occurs when excessive scar tissue forms around the pace/sense electrode resulting in inability to capture at high output. This complication occurs late (several weeks to months), distinguishing it from microdislodgment.

Sensing is often well preserved, and usually there is no significant change in the lead impedance. If the threshold is so high that the increase in thresholds cannot be compensated for by increasing the generator pacing output, then the lead needs to be replaced. If the pacing function of the ICD is not absolutely required, and sensing remains adequate, then the lead may be retained.

The use of steroid eluting electrodes is likely to make this problem infrequent. Occasionally, a short course of oral steroids has been described as useful in lowering the pacing thresholds.[33]

Lead Wire Fractures

Conductor fracture usually occurs at the point where the lead enters the venous system, at the point of fixation, or in the ICD pocket. Excessive angulation and pinching of the lead between the clavicle and the first rib may cause wire fracture. Fracture of the conductor may occur at other sites less commonly, primarily due to the metal fatigue. Superior vena caval spring lead fractures were reported in up to 9% of patients in one large series.[28] This high incidence was associated with earlier silver tinsel design, which is now no longer used. Patch lead fractures are rare and are reported to occur in approximately 1% of cases.[27] Transvenous pace/sense lead fractures occur in approximately 1% to 2% of cases.[28]

The presence of conductor fracture is rarely obvious on chest x-ray. If it is obvious, ie, if complete distraction of the fractured ends occurs in a pace/sense lead, a complete loss of sensing and pacing will be noted with high lead impedance ($> 1,500$ Ω). More commonly, however, partial fracture occurs, where the fractured ends are intermittently in contact with each other. In this situation, pacing may be intermittent and contact of wire ends may result in electrical interference leading to spurious ventricular fibrillation detections and inappropriate ICD shocks. Fractures may also occur in the lead connector when transvenous electrodes are used (Figure 6). In the case of defibrillator coil or wire fracture, inadequate defibrillation will result with potentially disastrous consequences. Inadequate energy delivery, shunting of the current and high impedance are noted (Figures 7 and 8).

When the conductor fracture is suspected, reoperation is mandatory. Direct lead recordings using the pacing analyzer are necessary. The surgeon should tug on the pace/sense lead while pacing. Intermittent loss of capture is noted with possible fluctuating impedance.

Repair of electrodes is not recommended with ICDs. Removal of the offending lead or capping of the lead and positioning of another lead is recommended.

Insulation Break

Insulation break may occur due to inadvertent placement of a suture around the lead body without a protective sleeve, accidental cut with a sharp instrument during surgery, or due to the material fatigue. Insulation break leads to the battery current drain. If the leakage occurs close to the pectoral muscle, pectoral pacing may be noted (pacing ICDs). Measurement of impedance

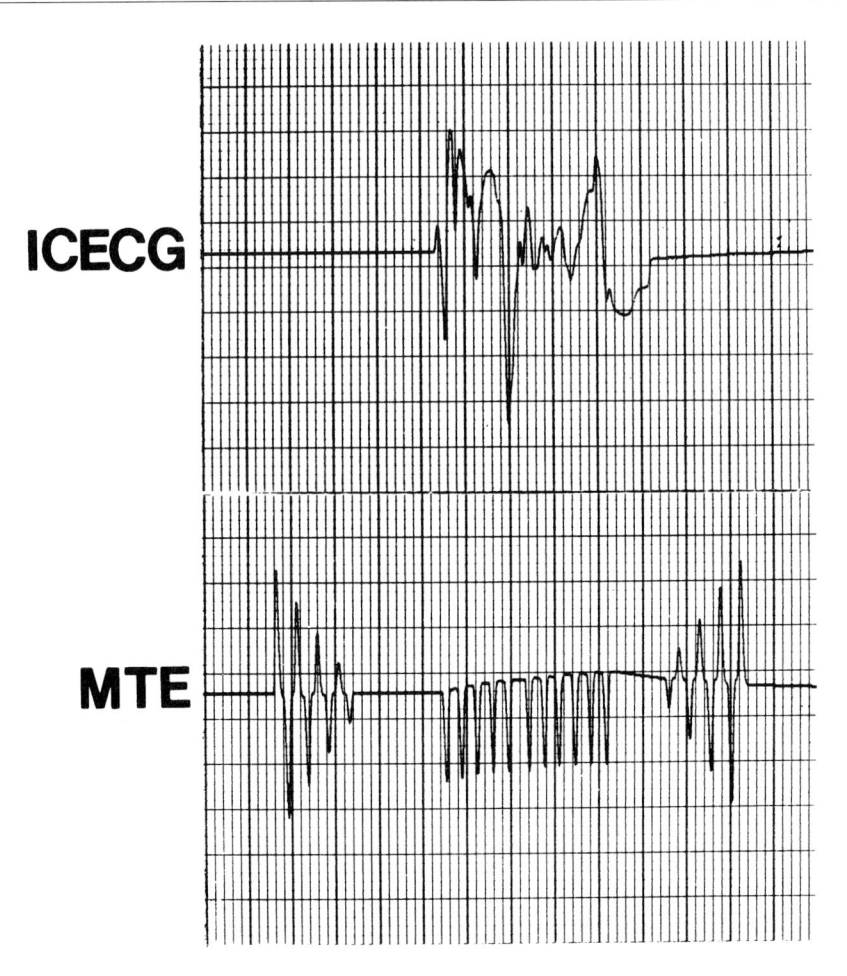

Figure 6. Lead connector fracture (Guardian ATP™ 4210, Telectronics, Englewood, CO) resulting in lead connector noise. **Top**: intracardiac electrocardiogram (ICECG); **Bottom**: main timing events (MTE). Note multiple spurious signals that may trigger inappropriate implantable cardioverter-defibrillator (ICD) shocks.

will generally show a decrease. If insulation break occurs with the high-voltage (shocking) leads, current shunting with inability to defibrillate may be found. Integrity of the high-voltage leads may be tested by giving a low-energy shock in sinus rhythm (with a backup defibrillator available) and measuring the lead impedance and energy delivered. Decrease in impedance suggests insulation break, with less energy delivered to the patient. If insulation break occurs in the shocking leads, the lead(s) must be replaced.

Venous Thrombosis

Thrombosis of subclavian and axillary veins has been reported in association with the permanent pacing leads.[33-36] Although reported in < 1% of ICD cases[28] it is likely that clinically insignificant subclavian thrombosis may occur in greater number of patients.[37] Clinically significant thrombosis presents as unilateral arm swelling, but if it involves the SVC it may give rise to the SVC syndrome.[38,39]

Treatment is usually effective with arm elevation and systemic, followed by oral an-

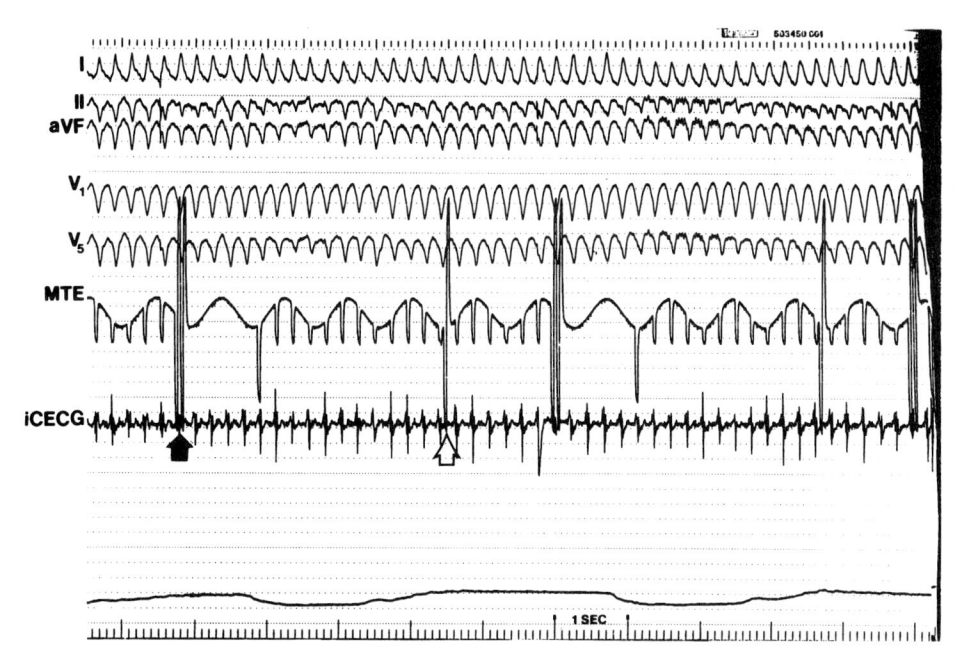

Figure 7. Failure of multiple shocks to terminate ventricular fibrillation due to endocardial defibrillation lead fracture (Accufix DF™ lead; Telectronics, Englewood, CO). From top to bottom: surface leads I, II, aVF, V_1, V_6, main timing events (MTE), intracardiac electrocardiogram (iCECG), blood pressure (BP), and time lines (T). Dark arrow denotes an unsuccessful shock, open arrow, charging of the capacitors.

ticoagulation. Conservative management usually results in resolution of symptoms and development of collateral circulation.

Embolism

Embolic complications have been reported in approximately 1% to 3% of patients with implanted pacemaker electrodes. The incidence of emboli with non-thoracotomy lead systems is currently unknown, but it is likely that it may be higher than reported for a variety of reasons.[1,2,7,10] The leads have an exposed defibrillation coil that may be thrombogenic. The leads are bulkier and present a greater surface area for clot formation. Patient-related factors such as poor LV function, atrial fibrillation, or other dysrhythmias may further predispose to thrombotic complications.

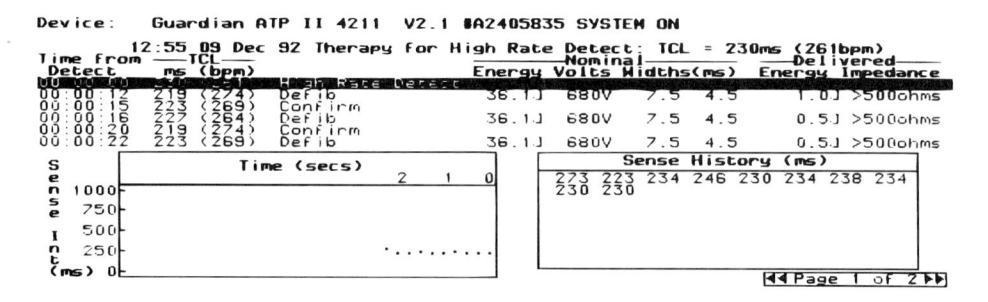

Figure 8. Telemetry of the recorded event (Figure 7). Note appropriate detection, followed by the ICD shock delivery of 36.1 J (three times) with an actual delivery of 1.0, 0.5, and 0.5 J and lead impedance > 1,500 Ω, indicative of a defibrillation lead fracture.

Currently, there are no clear guidelines as to whether to routinely anticoagulate these patients. It is our current practice to anticoagulate if the benefits of anticoagulation are not outweighed by the risks. In patients with suspected thrombi involving the endocardial leads, the transesophageal echocardiography may be a useful diagnostic tool.

Subcutaneous Patch Hematoma

Nonthoracotomy lead systems require the use of a subcutaneous patch electrode in approximately 20% to 30% of patients to achieve acceptable DFTs (see Chapters 23 and 24).[40,41] Although placement of subcutaneous patch leads is usually associated with less trauma than thoracotomy, persistent pain and discomfort related to the patch have been reported.

We have seen a case where the subcutaneous patch caused late erosion of an artery, causing a large hematoma requiring reexploration. Less commonly, smaller patch-related hematomas and seromas have been observed. Small hematoma or seroma is managed conservatively, through a frank arterial or venous bleed requires reexploration to control the bleeding.

Patch crimping and folding has also been noted. Proper fixation may minimize the incidence of this complication. It is not yet clear whether the use of SQ-array™ (CPI, St. Paul, MN) is associated with fewer undesirable complications than the subcutaneous patch lead placement.

Summary

Complications associated with ICD surgery occur infrequently in experienced clinical centers. A learning curve, as with any other surgical or medical technique, is operative with less complications occurring in the experienced, high-volume clinical centers. While the data with transvenous ICDs are still preliminary, it is certain that the postoperative mortality and morbidity are likely to be decreased with this less invasive approach. The early data suggest a perioperative mortality of < 2% overall.[40,41] It is likely, however, that lead-related complications (lead displacement, fractures, and so on) may occur more frequently with this surgical approach. A longer follow-up (5–10 years) is required to enable a meaningful comparison of the thoracotomy and the nonthoracotomy lead systems. However, it is likely that nonthoractomy lead systems will replace the thoracotomy lead systems as the surgical approach of choice in most cases, except where concomitant cardial surgery is contemplated, where high DFTs are encountered, or when other special situations exist requiring an alternative surgical approach.

References

1. Saksena S, Tullo NG, Krol RB, et al: Initial clinical experience with endocardial defibrillation using an implantable cardioverter/defibrillator with a triple-electrode system. *Arch Intern Med* 149:2333, 1989.
2. Manolis AS, Tan-DeGuzman W, Lee MA, et al: Clinical experience in seventy-seven patients with the automatic implantable cardioverter defibrillator. *Am Heart J* 118:445, 1989.
3. Edel TB, Maloney JD, Moore S, et al: Six-year clinical experience with the automatic implantable cardioverter defibrillator. *PACE* 14(Part II):1850, 1991.
4. Kim SG, Fisher JD, Choue CW, et al: Influence of left ventricular function on outcome of patients treated with implantable defibrillators. *Circulation* 85:1304, 1992.
5. Kim SG, Fisher JD, Furman S, et al: Exacerbation of ventricular arrhythmias during the postoperative period after implantation of an automatic defibrillator. *J Am Coll Cardiol* 18:1200, 1991.
6. The CABG Patch Trial Investigators and Coordinators: The CABG Patch Trial. *Prog Cardiovasc Dis* 36(2):97, 1993.
7. Gartman DM, Bardy GH, Allen MD, et al: Short-term morbidity and mortality of implantation of automatic implantable cardioverter-defibrillator. *J Thorac Cardiovasc Surg* 100:353, 1990.

8. Cohen TJ, Reid PR, Mower MM, et al: The automatic implantable cardioverter-defibrillator. *Arch Intern Med* 152:65, 1992.
9. Joye JD, Paulowski JJ, Fogoros RN, et al: Perioperative morbidity and mortality after ICD implantation in 150 consecutive patients (abstract). *Circulation* 84(Suppl II):II-608, 1991.
10. Gohn D, Edel T, Pollard C, et al: Determinants of operative mortality in implantable cardioverter defibrillators (abstract). *J Am Coll Cardiol* 17:86A, 1991.
11. Epstein A, Ellenbogen K, Kirk K, et al: Clinical characteristics and outcome of patients with high defibrillation thresholds: a multicenter study. *Circulation* 86:1206, 1992.
12. Greenspan AJ, Kidwell GA, Hurley W, et al: Amiodarone-related postoperative adult respiratory distress syndrome. *Circulation* 84(Suppl III):III-407, 1991.
13. Mullen GM, O'Sullivan EJ, Liao Y, et al: Amiodarone increases respiratory complications after cardiac transplantation (abstract). *Circulation* 84(Suppl II):II-489, 1991.
14. Kay GN, Epstein AE, Kirklin JK, et al: Fatal postoperative amiodarone pulmonary toxicity. *Am J Cardiol* 62:490, 1988.
15. Nalos PC, Kass RM, Gang ES, et al: Life-threatening postoperative pulmonary complications in patients with previous amiodarone pulmonary toxicity undergoing cardiothoracic operations. *J Thorac Cardiovasc Surg* 93:904, 1987.
16. Tuczu M, Maloney JD, Sangani F, et al: Cardiopulmonary effects of chronic amiodarone therapy in the early postoperative course of cardiac surgery patients. *Cleve Clin J Med* 54:491, 1987.
17. Amirana O, Klevan LR, Baker LD, et al: Effect of long-term preoperative amiodarone on mortality of implantable cardioverter defibrillator placement (abstract). *PACE* 15(Part II):544, 1992.
18. Watkins L Jr, Mirowski M, Mower MM, et al: Implantation of the automatic defibrillator: the subxiphoid approach. *Ann Thorac Surg* 34:515, 1982.
19. Gershman A, Reznik G, Grundfest WS: Percutaneous endoscopic implantation of automatic implantable cardioverter/defibrillator (AICD). *Circulation* 84(Suppl II):II-609, 1991.
20. Marchlinski FE, Flores BT, Buxton AE, et al: The automatic implantable cardioverter-defibrillator: efficacy, complications, and device failures. *Ann Intern Med* 104:481, 1986.
21. Kelley PA, Cannom DS, Garan H, et al: The automatic implantable cardioverter-defibrillator: efficacy, complications and survival of patients with severely depressed left ventricular function associated with coronary artery disease. *Am J Cardiol* 67:812, 1991.
22. Schwartz ES, Pervez N: Bacterial endocarditis associated with a permanent transvenous cardiac pacemaker. *JAMA* 218:736, 1971.
23. Ward C, Naik DR, Johnstone MC: Tricuspid endocarditis complicating pacemaker implantation demonstrated by echocardiography. *Br J Radiol* 52:501, 1979.
24. Furman S, Escher DJW: *Principles and Techniques of Cardiac Pacing*. First edition. New York, NY: Harper and Row; 1970, p. 91.
25. Choo MH, Holmes DR, Gersh BJ, et al: Permanent pacemaker infections: characterization and management. *Am J Cardiol* 48:559, 1981.
26. Choo MH, Holmes DR, Gersh BJ, et al: Infected epicardial pacemaker systems-partial versus total removal. *J Thorac Cardiovasc Surg* 82:794, 1981.
27. Singer I, Edmonds H Jr: Changes in cerebral perfusion during third generation ICD testing. Proceedings of the International Symposium on Electrical Device Therapy (Bonn/Koniqswinter, GERMANY). *Am Heart J* 127(4 Part 2):1052, 1994.
28. Winkle RA, Mead RH, Ruder MA, et al: Long-term outcome with the automatic implantable cardioverter-defibrillator. *J Am Coll Cardiol* 13:1353, 1989.
29. Littleford PO, Spector SD: Device for the rapid insertion of a permanent endocardial pacing electrode through the subclavian vein: preliminary report. *Ann Thorac Surg* 27:265, 1979.
30. Littleford PO, Parsonnet V, Spector SD: Method for the rapid and atraumatic insertion of permanent endocardial pacemaker electrodes through the subclavian vein. *Am J Cardiol* 43:980, 1979.
31. Rao G: Subclavian puncture for dual-chamber pacing (letter to the editor). *Ann Thorac Surg* 33(5):528, 1982.
32. Kessinger JM, Holter AR, Geha AS: Implantation of permanent transvenous pacemaker via subclavian vein. *Arch Surg* 117:1105, 1982.
33. Smyth NPD, Millette ML: The isotopic cardiac pacer: a ten-year experience. *PACE* 7:82, 1984.
34. Kenney EL, Allen RP, Weidner WA, et al: Recurrent pulmonary emboli secondary to right atrial thrombus around a permanent pacing catheter: a case report and review of the literature. *PACE* 2:196, 1979.
35. Krug H, Zerbe F: Major venous thrombosis: a complication of transvenous pacemaker electrodes. *Br Heart J* 44:158, 1980.
36. Lee ME, Chaux A: Unusual complications of endocardial pacing. *J Thorac Cardiovasc Surg* 80:934, 1980.
37. Stoney WS, Addlestone RB, Alford WC, et

problems, which are quite normal for a therapy that started just 13 years ago. All aspects of the entire implantation procedure (see Chapters 14 and 15), as it relates to the specific patient in question need to be discussed and agreed upon by the entire implant team prior to beginning the procedure. The role of each member, the exact sequence to follow, and a precise plan for managing specific complications should be clarified. The need to perform concomitant bypass or other cardiac surgery, the existence of previous coronary artery bypass grafts, prosthetic heart valves, or pacemakers all impact greatly on the surgical aspects, device testing, and postoperative care of such patients. One of the most devastating complications of ICD therapy is infection ranging in incidence from 0% to 7%[2] and nearly always require removal of the entire system.[3] Prophylactic antibiotics, special draping, and other precautions have been advocated by various groups as means of preventing or at least minimizing infection.[4] Defibrillation threshold (DFT) testing and other procedures that influence the length of the intervention may also influence the incidence of infections. Diabetic patients and those undergoing kidney dialysis are known to be particularly prone to infection, and therefore warrant special precautions.[5]

Another major area where prevention is the best cure relates to interoperative testing of the ICD lead system. High DFTs and/or the absence of adequate DFT testing have been directly implicated in a significant number of the 1% to 2% of sudden deaths that have occurred in ICD patients.[6] As DFT testing is covered in detail in Chapters 10 and 15, we would simply remind all that adequate testing—to the extent permitted by the patient's hemodynamics—remains an important prerequisite to optimal long-term results.

Troubleshooting Methodology

The sequence we follow and advocate to others is:

Problem → Possible causes → Methodology for identifying root causes

We will troubleshoot four distinct categories of ICD-related problems: 1) Suspected inappropriate shocks or antitachycardia pacing (ATP); 2) Failure to deliver therapy; 3) Ineffective shocks or ATP; and 4) Device deactivated. There are a host of medical complications including infections, pulmonary complications, pericarditis, etc., that are not unique to ICD therapy, which we will not cover; diagnosis of these problems is in the realm of current medical practice, not requiring the specialized troubleshooting methodology on which we have focused. Table 1 provides an overview of troubleshooting these four categories of problems in the absence of electrocardiographic documentation.

Troubleshooting is of course, much easier—often immediate and self evident—when the event(s) are documented via electrocardiogram (ECG) monitoring (Holter, event recorders, or in-hospital monitors) or via stored electrograms (EGMs) from the ICD. For each of the four categories of problems, we describe how to troubleshoot with and in the absence of documentation.

Suspected Inappropriate Shocks or Antitachycardia Pacing

The most frequent complications associated with ICD therapy fall in this category. Before doing anything else, one has to verify, by interrogating the device, whether in fact therapy has been delivered. There have been cases of ICD patients imagining or dreaming of shocks that never took place![7] Once it is clear that shocks (or ATP) have occurred, we need to determine their etiology. Table 1 lists 10 possible causes.

In the Absence of Documentation

Asymptomatic, but Appropriate Therapy

To start, seek specific evidence that the therapy was indeed inappropriate. (The fact that a patient was asymptomatic at the time of shock delivery is by no means proof that the shock was inappropriate.[8-10]) What were the circumstances leading up to the ICD discharges? The telemetry for most current ICDs provides detailed information on the detected R-R intervals preceding the shock (Figure 1). These are helpful in ascertaining whether sinus tachycardia or supraventricular tachycardia could have provoked the ICD discharges. Of additional use in the diagnosis is whether the patient received isolated discharges versus a "cluster" of shocks (or ATP) over a few hours.

Table 1
Troubleshooting[a] ICDs

Problem	Possible Causes	Means of Identifying the Source of the Problem
A. (Suspected) inappropriate therapy (Tx) shocks or ATP[b]	1. Asymptomatic, but appropriate, ie, sustained VT > R[c]	1.1 Check circumstances leading to Tx 1.2 Analyze device's "therapy history", esp. R-R intervals, vs. settings 1.3 If cause 1 is eliminated, investigate causes 2–10
	2. Sinus tachycardia	2.1 Can pt[d] under exercise and/or stress exceed R? 2.2 If yes, do 1.2. If no, consider causes 3–10
	3. SVT[e] (atrial fibrillation, atrial flutter, SVT), with rapid ventricular conduction	3.1 Is Pt. susceptible to SVT? 3.2 If yes, is resulting ventricular rate >R? 3.3 If both 3.1 and 3.2 are yes, check steps 1.1 and 1.2 3.4 If still unclear, do rapid atrial pacing, utilizing "beep-o-grams" and/or marker channels to check ICD detection 3.5 If either 3.1 or 3.2 are no, consider causes 4–10
	4. NSVT[f] (nonsustained VT)	4.1 Is there evidence (past history or via ECG monitoring) of NSVT? 4.2 If yes, is ICD a "committed" device (or prog'd to "comm.")? 4.3 If 4.1 and 4.2, yes, do 1.2; check in particular whether programmed "detection delay" exceeds length of NSVT episode 4.4 If cause 4 (and 1–3) can be ruled out, consider causes 5–10
	5. T wave or P wave oversensing	5.1 Check "beep-o-gram" and/or marker channels 5.2 Do 1.2 5.3 Check for position/dislodgment of ICD sensing leads 5.4 In devices without AGC[g], check if sensitivity the cause
	6. Pacemaker "spikes" or evoked potentials	6.1 Same as 5.1. If necessary, repeat with increased pacer output 6.2 Same as 1.2
	7. Lead fracture, insulation break, loose set screws, dislodgement, etc.	7.1 Same as 5.1. Do if necessary, during upper body exercise and/or manipulation near ICD connectors 7.2 Do 1.2 7.3 Check lead impedance values (also, during body exercise) 7.4 Check X-rays for lead or insulation breaks, dislodgements, etc.
	8. Outside sources (EMI, MRI, electrocautery)[h]	8.1 Same as 1.1 8.2 Do 5.1
	9. "Device Proarrythmia"	9.1 Same as 1.1 9.2 Same as 1.2
	10. Faulty detection algorithm	10.1 Same as 1.1 10.2 Same as 1.2 10.3 Same as 5.1 10.4 Analyze whether detection algorithm may have been set too sensitive

(continued)

Table 1 *(continued)*
Troubleshooting[a] ICDs

B. Failure to deliver Tx (In case Tx delivered but ineffective, see C)	1. Sensitivity problems	1.1 Same as B5.1
		1.2 In devices without AGC[g], check whether programmed sensitivity may be responsible for undersensing of R-waves (see text for explanation)
		1.3 Check A2. 1–2 with VT induced
	2. Lead problems	2.1 Same as A-7
	3. Post shock signal attenuation and undersensing	3.1 Same as A5. 1–3
		3.2 Verify whether amplitude of R-waves are sufficient for good sensing pre- and post-shock (within 5–10 seconds)
	4. Separate pacemaker[i]	4.1 Same as A5.1–2
	5. Faulty sensing algorithm or programming	5.1 Same as A1.1–2, 5.3
		5.2 Analyze whether detection algorithm set too sensitive: i.e., determine whether detection enhancements[j] might be inhibiting Tx
	6. Antiarrythmic drugs	6.1 Determine effect of change in antiarrythmic drugs on pt's rate and morphology vis-a-vis R and the det. enhancements
	7. Outside interference	7.1 Same as A8. 1–2
C. Ineffective Tx (shocks and/or ATP ineffective)	1. Inadequate shock output or programming	1.1 Retest DFT (problem not simply due to "probabilistic nature" of defibrillation?)
		1.2 Verify that the energy levels set for VF/PMVT are at maximum
	2. Rise in DFT due to impedance changes	2.1 Check (from device telemetry) impedance of the shocking leads
		2.2 If increased, check if device's delivered energy still ample
		2.3 Check for causes of impedance rise (see A7)
	3. Influence of drugs on DFT	3.1 Re-test DFT, following changes in antiarrythmic drug administration, especially amiodarone
	4. Lead problems (incl. "patch crumpling")	4.1 Same troubleshooting techniques as used in A7 (but concentrate on both shocking and pacing leads)
	5. Exacerbated CHF or degradation of LVF	5.1 Re-test DFTs, and if marginal, revise the shocking lead system
	6. Failed ATP modes	6.1 Same as A1. 1–2
		6.2 Retest ATP modes. Have substrate changes altered previous success?
	7. Inadequate pacing output ("exit block")	7.1 Retest pacing thresholds, including post-shock
		7.2 Same as A7. 3–4
D. Device deactivated	1. Inadvertently (via magnet or programmer)	1.1 Check on possibility that hospital staff inadvertently turned off device
		1.2 Similarly, with pt., his/her family, local physician
	2. Outside interference (EMI)	2.1 Check (by listening for audio tones from the implanted or equivalent device) whether pt.'s environment (home, work, hobbies) had EMI
	3. Battery depletion or circuit failure	3.1 Test device's battery status
		3.2 Interrogate ICD to determine its functional status
	4. "Shut-down" mode	4.1 Interrogate ICD to determine its functional status

[a] When no Documentation (ECG strips, Holter ECG, "event recorders" ECG, ICD electrogram (EGM)) available
[b] Tx = Therapy (shocks or ATP)
[c] R = ICD programmed "cutoff rate"
[d] Pt. = ICD patient
[e] SVT = Supraventricular tachycardia
[f] NSVT defined ... arbitrarily as runs of 5+ consecutive ventricular extrasystoles, at rates > R, and, self-terminating within 30 seconds.
[g] AGC = "Automatic Gain Control" (Automatic Sensitivity)
[h] Note: except for electrocautery, these sources have almost never been implicated as causes of inappropriate Tx.
[i] Note: unipolar pacing generally contraindicated in combination with ICD
[j] Sudden onset, stability, "PDF on", "noncommitted", "reconfirmation"

```
LAST EPISODE DETECTION SEQUENCE:
 -19. R-R INTERVAL- 430 MS
 -18. R-R INTERVAL- 430 MS
 -17. R-R INTERVAL- 290 MS
 -16. R-R INTERVAL- 300 MS
 -15. R-R INTERVAL- 290 MS
 -14. R-R INTERVAL- 280 MS
 -13. R-R INTERVAL- 290 MS
 -12. R-R INTERVAL- 290 MS
 -11. R-R INTERVAL- 290 MS
 -10. R-R INTERVAL- 290 MS
  -9. R-R INTERVAL- 290 MS
  -8. R-R INTERVAL- 300 MS
  -7. R-R INTERVAL- 300 MS
  -6. R-R INTERVAL- 300 MS
  -5. R-R INTERVAL- 300 MS
  -4. R-R INTERVAL- 290 MS
  -3. R-R INTERVAL- 300 MS
  -2. R-R INTERVAL- 300 MS
  -1. R-R INTERVAL- 300 MS
  -0. R-R INTERVAL- 300 MS
  -0. VF DETECTED

EVENTS AFTER LAST THERAPY:
  +0. VF THERAPY #1 DELIVERED
  +1. R-R INTERVAL- 950 MS
  +2. R-R INTERVAL- 650 MS
  +3. R-R INTERVAL- 490 MS
  +4. R-R INTERVAL- 480 MS
  +5. R-R INTERVAL- 390 MS
  +6. R-R INTERVAL- 820 MS
  +7. R-R INTERVAL- 370 MS
  +8. R-R INTERVAL- 500 MS
  +9. R-R INTERVAL- 420 MS
 +10. R-R INTERVAL- 420 MS
 +10. THERAPY WAS SUCCESSFUL
```

Figure 1. Telemetry from the PCD™ (Medtronic, Minneapolis, MN) reveals the last 20 intervals prior to delivery of therapy, and the 10 R-R intervals after the delivery of therapy. The R-R intervals shown strongly suggest that the arrhythmia treated was ventricular tachycardia with a relatively stable cycle length (290–300 msec), which persisted for 18 cycles prior to delivery of therapy.

The former is typical of ICD discharges for ventricular tachycardia (VT), whereas repetitive shocks usually point to inappropriate shocks for one of the causes (Table 1), or exacerbated heart failure or ischemia.[11] On the basis of this information and what you know about the patient's history and electrophysiology, you can establish with near certainty whether the therapy was appropriate or not.

Sinus Tachycardia

If sinus tachycardia is suspected, the ICD telemetry usually provides the needed evidence. It may be necessary to have the patient undergo exercise testing to assure that his/her maximum exercise rate remains below the ICDs programmed cutoff rate.

Supraventricular Tachyarrhythmias

Once it has been established that the shocks or ATP were in fact inappropriately delivered, ie, for rhythms other than sustained ventricular tachycardia/fibrillation (VT/VF) exceeding the programmed cutoff rates, the most frequent cause is usually supraventricular tachycardia with rapid conduction to the ventricles. Data supporting these diagnoses comes first and foremost from knowledge or investigation of the patients' susceptibility to such rhythms, and whether their resulting ventricular rates could "trigger" the ICD. As stated, the devices' stored R-R intervals information is also very helpful. Many of the ICDs now available or undergoing clinical trials have marker channels similar to those used with pacemakers. Examining the markers related to detection, concurrently with the patient's ECG, provides information on what signals the device is sensing as R waves. Figure 2 shows an example of how marker channels in combination with a surface ECG help in diagnosing the source of ICD shocks. If these sources still do not clarify the root cause, 24-hour Holter monitoring plus exercise testing may be required. Some investigators have reported on the utility of event

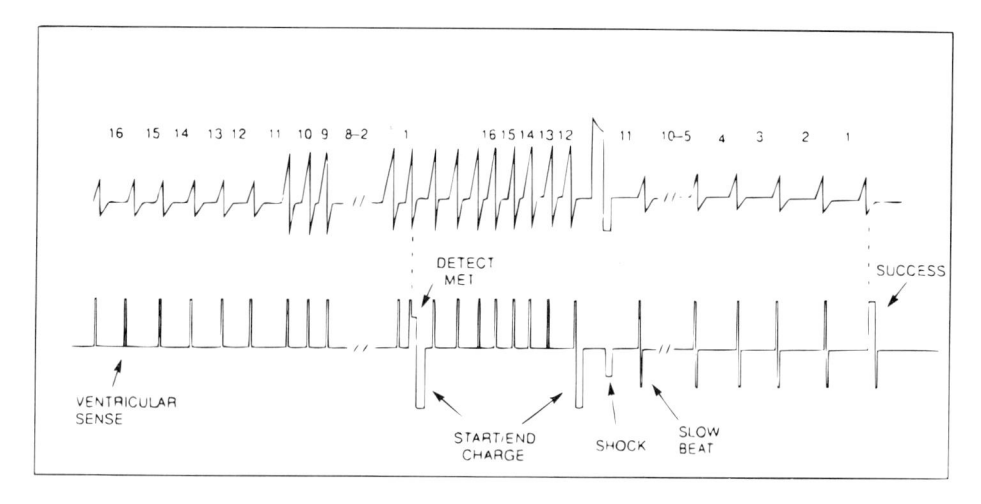

Figure 2. An ECG strip and corresponding event markers from a PRx-1™ (CPI, St. Paul, MN) illustrate how the R-R intervals are counted for pre- and postepisode history storage.

recorder with a memory loop, capable of capturing ECG tracings immediately preceding ICD discharges.[12]

Nonsustained Supraventricular Tachycardia

The cause may be nonsustained ventricular tachycardia (NSVT), ie, VT that terminates spontaneously prior to ICD discharge. The latter problem, although significantly diminished by the use of programmable detection delays and noncommitted devices (requiring a reconfirmation of a detected VT before giving shocks), still occurs.[13] These same techniques provide valuable data on NSVT episodes that the patient is subject to, particularly indicating whether their rate and duration might be sufficient to trigger the ICD.

T Wave or P Wave Oversensing

This methodology should permit you to ascertain or eliminate the first four causes listed in Table 1 as potential sources of the problem. Identification of one of the next four listed causes (in the absence of documentation accompanying ICD discharges) is greatly facilitated by the "beep-o-gram" technique.[14] All Cardiac Pacemakers, Inc. (CPI, St. Paul, MN) devices emit audible tones synchronous with sensed signals when a magnet is held over them in the "EP Test mode".[15] Figure 3 illustrates several examples of how the "beep-o-gram" identified doublecounting of P waves or T waves, or artifacts due to lead fractures. For other manufacturers' devices, the use of the marker channels and/or Holter monitoring as described should hopefully uncover the source of the problem. In trying to troubleshoot problems possibly due to oversensing of P or T waves, one needs to be particularly vigilant with devices using a programmable but fixed sensitivity. To prevent missing detection of fine fibrillation, possibly as low as 1 mV or lower, it may be necessary to program such a device to its maximum sensitivity, which in turn makes it susceptible to picking up P or T waves.[16-18] To minimize this problem, most ICDs currently in use utilize some type of automatic gain control (see Chapter 4).[19]

Pacemakers

Patients with a separate pacemaker in addition to their ICD are subject to large pacemaker spikes inhibiting the ICDs recognition of much smaller VT/VF signals, or ICD oversensing (ie, doublecounting) of pacemaker spikes and evoked R waves, and postshock. (It is for these reasons that uni-

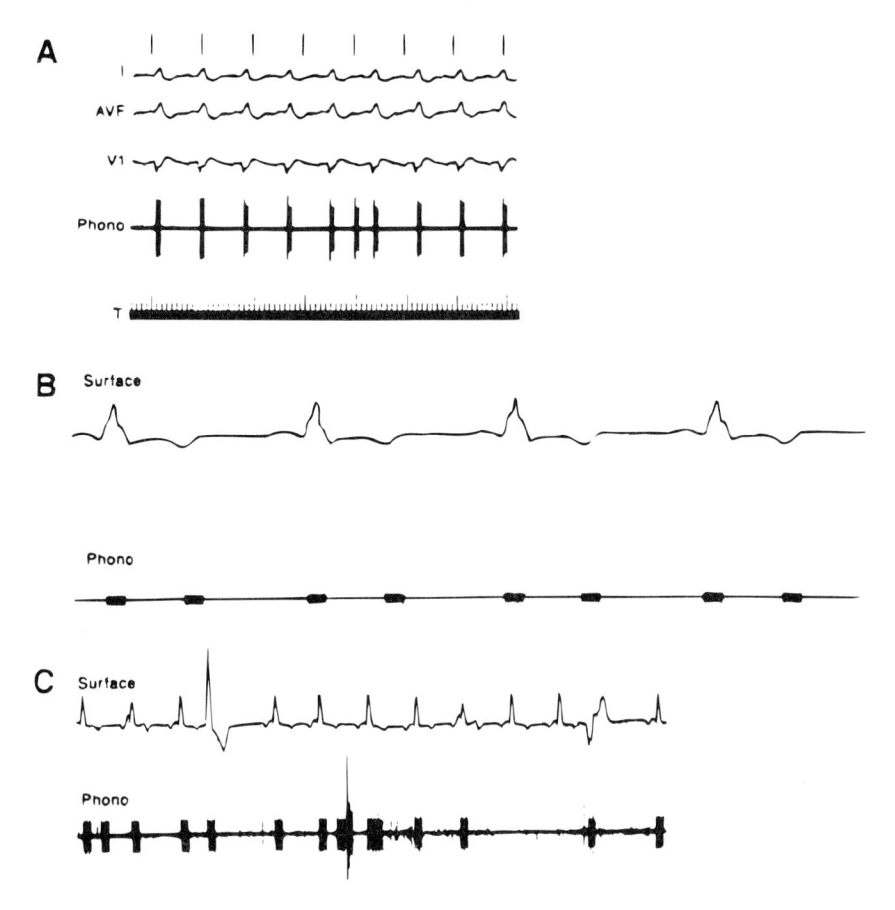

Figure 3. Examples of use of phonocardiogram to help in evaluating shocks (for CPI devices). **A**: Intermittent sensing of atrial pacing spikes (courtesy of Peter D. Chapman, MD). **B**: T wave sensing: beeping tone evaluation reveals T wave sensing. Poststellate block QT, 342 msec (courtesy of Robert G. Hauser, MD). **C**: Abnormal beeping tones during upper extremity exercise. Normal beeping tones are obtained while patient is at rest. Note: AICD™ (CPI, St. Paul, MN) under and oversensing during upper extremity exercise (courtesy of Jay W. Mason, MD). (Reproduced with permission from Alt F, Klein H, Griffith J, eds: *The Implantable Cardioverter/Defibrillator*. Springer-Verlag; 1992, p. 283.)

polar pacemakers are strictly contraindicated in conjunction with the ICD.) Troubleshooting involves, once again, use of the devices' therapy history as well as "beep-o-grams" and/or marker channels to see whether the ICD is 1) picking up signals from the pacemaker or 2) being inhibited from appropriate VT/VF detection.

Lead Related

Problems can be caused by lead discontinuities and position/disdodgment. Complementary to the methods described for *Pacemakers*, you may have to resort to chest x-rays to assess the integrity of the lead system. In addition, just as with cardiac pacemakers, measurement of lead impedance can be very helpful in uncovering lead problems. On some present and probably all future ICDs, lead impedance values can be obtained noninvasively. Infinite lead impedance—at least intermittently—is indicative of a lead fracture, whereas insulation breaks will be associated with abnormally low impedance. X-rays are of course very helpful in ascertaining whether the ICD leads are properly positioned and whether displacement has occurred.

Outside Sources

In order to be complete, we have included outside sources such as electromagnetic interference (EMI), magnetic resonance imaging (MRI), etc., as there is at least a theoretical possibility that these could trigger device discharges under certain circumstances. In fact the devices' circuit designs have effectively shielded them, so that as of this date, we are unaware of any such reports. Troubleshooting involves a careful analysis of the circumstances that led to the discharges, and the use of "beep-o-grams" or marker channels in the presence of these suspected sources.

Device Proarrhythmia

Implantable cardioverter-defibrillator iatrogenic proarrhythmia has been reported.[20] The devices' stored therapy history logs indicate failed therapy or acceleration, also providing pre- and posttherapy R-R intervals and rate, which generally suffice to make this diagnosis. Be aware that in the early postoperative period, high ventricular irritability commonly occurs, especially with epicardial leads.

Faulty Algorithms

The detection algorithms themselves and how they are programmed can lead to inappropriate shocks or ATP.[21] The self-incriminating evidence for these occurrences is usually available by interrogation of the device. The useful recent feature known as reconfirmation successfully "aborts" most of the shocks that would have been given for inappropriate detections.[22] The diagnosis of these remains important, since even the aborted shocks can reduce battery life considerably. In an attempt to assure essentially 100% sensitivity for detection of dangerous arrhythmias, the person performing the ICD implantation may inadvertently tune the device's programmable detection parameters too sensitively. He or she can retune on the basis of data available from the stored therapy history, marker channels, etc.

With Documentation

Troubleshooting the source of shocks or ATP is usually straightforward and simple when you have ECG documentation of the suspected inappropriate events. Occasionally, the EGMs provided by the ICD are not conclusive, and must be complemented by additional techniques in order to complete the diagnosis.[23,24] It has also been demonstrated that "tachycardias, which cannot be identified solely on the basis of their cycle length as being of ventricular or supraventricular origin, are more easily discriminated using EGMs from defibrillation electrodes than EGMs of sensing electrodes."[25]

In Figure 4 an example of a patient hospitalized to evaluate the occurrence of asymptomatic shocks is shown, with ECG evidence that the ICD provided a legitimate, life-saving shock, although the patient was free of symptoms. Figures 5 and 6 show examples of how EGMs from implanted devices facilitated the diagnosis of atrial flutter with rapid ventricular conduction and nonsustained VT, respectfully. Figure 7 illustrates the use of device EGM to establish a lead fracture as the cause of inappropriate shocks.

Use of Far-Field Electrograms in Implantable Cardioverter-Defibrillators

As has been demonstrated, the availability of stored intracardiac EGMs can make troubleshooting ICDs a relatively straightforward task in many cases. The Cadence™ (Ventritex, Sunnyvale, CA) stores EGMs recorded from the sensing electrodes. Generally, these EGMs yield bipolar signals that are similar to signals recorded in the electrophysiology laboratory from bipolar electrode catheters.

Another alternative, used in the P2™ and PRx-2™ (CPI, St. Paul, MN), records EGMs from the shocking electrodes. These electrodes cover a much larger surface area, and the signals resemble a far-field surface

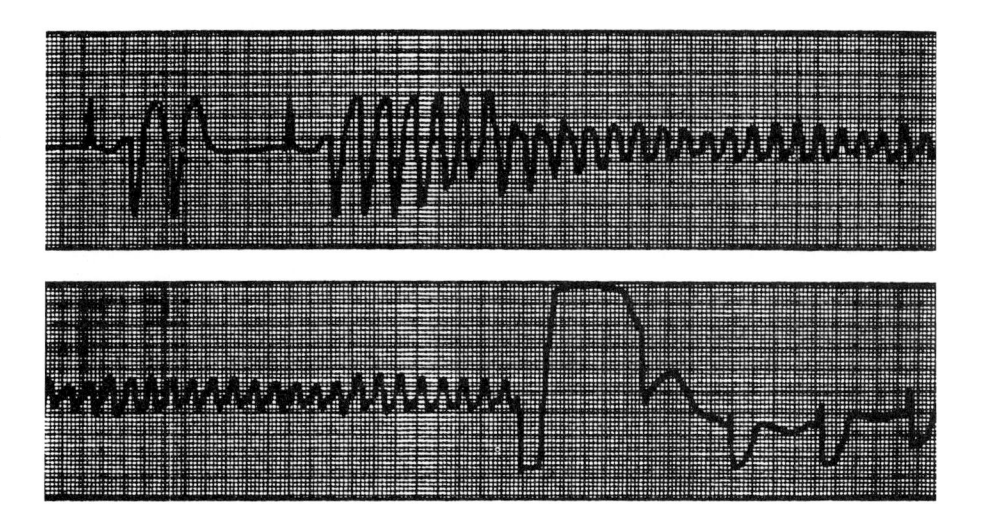

Figure 4. Cardiac rhythm during an asymptomatic run of rapid ventricular tachycardia terminated by device discharge. This patient was sitting in bed watching television when he developed ventricular tachycardia. The patient was asymptomatic until the time of device discharge. This example shows that device response can be quick enough that even with rapid ventricular tachycardias, patients may be asymptomatic at the time of cardioversion. (Reproduced with permission from Tchou P, et al: *Ann Intern Med* 109:529, 1988.)

ECG more than an intracardiac bipolar signal, as shown in Figure 8.

In many cases, the far-field signals yield valuable information otherwise not available. In Figure 9, monomorphic VT has occurred at a cycle length of 300 msec. The EGM from the sensing leads shows a rapid, regular tachycardia, but does not clearly allow differentiation from supraventricular tachycardia. Inspection of the EGM from the shocking electrodes, however, reveals that "p" waves are clearly visible in a 2:1 pattern, and that the patient is therefore in VT with 2:1 retrograde conduction. In Figure 10, the EGMs recorded from the sensing leads in sinus rhythm (left panel) and in VT (right panel) show similar morphologies. During VT, therefore, the EGM does not allow clear differentiation between ventricular and supraventricular tachycardias here. However, the EGM recorded from the shocking electrodes clearly shows a significant morphological change, with a much wider QRS complex, during VT.

Thus, far-field EGMs may yield better diagnostic information regarding arrhythmias than closely spaced bipolar EGMs. Quite possibly, future external cardioverter-defibrillators (ECDs) may allow the option of storing EGMs from the shocking leads instead of from the sensing leads.

Failure to Deliver Therapy

The lives of patients with ICDs literally depend on their receiving shocks and/or ATP to terminate the ventricular tachyarrhythmias to which they are susceptible. Therefore, the failure to deliver effective therapy is an extremely serious problem demanding immediate diagnosis and resolution. The problem of shocks or ATP that were delivered, but for some reason ineffective in terminating VT is treated later in this chapter. In this section we concentrate on troubleshooting the nondelivery of electrical therapy. It is important to remember that an ICD will only deliver therapy after having sensed tachyarrhythmias. Therefore, the starting point in troubleshooting this category of problems is the sensing system (device and leads).

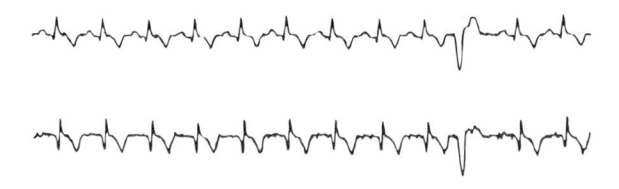

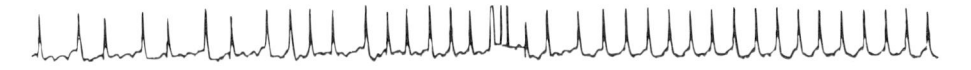

Figure 5. Demonstration of electrogram recording from endocardial shocking leads from Ventak P2™ ICD device (CPI, St. Paul, MN) showing shock for probable atrial fibrillation/flutter. In the top panel, ECG lead II and recordings from the endocardial shocking lead are shown during a simultaneous recording in sinus rhythm. Of note, there is a suggestion of atrial activity documented in the sinus rhythm recording from the endocardial shocking leads. In the bottom panel there is irregular ventricular activity leading to ICD shock. There is also suggestion of atrial activity consistent with atrial fibrillation/flutter preceding the ICD shock therapy. The wide bipolar endocardial recordings permits the detection of atrial activity on the recording in some patients, allowing for the appropriate identification of the relationship between atrial and ventricular activation. (Reproduced with permission from Reference 24.)

In the Absence of Documentation (Table 1)

Sensitivity

The "beep-o-gram" technique and the use of marker channels may help establish problems related to a device's sensitivity. If these methods show no evidence of missed beats during sinus rhythm, you may well have to repeat them during induced VT episodes because the magnitude (also morphology, slew rate, etc.) of the ventricular signal may change—be reduced—during episodes of VT/VF. As explained previously, you may need to be particularly attentive in those patients having ICDs with fixed sensitivity; Figure 11 illustrates this problem. These VT/VF signals may be considerably smaller than during sinus rhythm.

Lead Problems

Nondetection and subsequent nondelivery of therapy, may also be due to a lead problem or nonsecure connection to the ICD pulse generator. Troubleshooting for problems due to these causes may be made difficult by the fact that these lead discontinuities are often intermittent and only discernible during certain body movements. Lead disdodgment can be a calamitous complication for ICDs, because both detection and therapy delivery can be interrupted. In contrast to pacing where nonsensing simply leads to asynchronous pacing, in an ICD, generally no therapy would be delivered. The other aspect that makes lead disdodgment far more ominous with an ICD than with a pacemaker is that the problem may only manifest itself at precisely the moment when the patient needs therapy. For lead problems the techniques described ("beep-o-grams," marker channels, chest x-rays, and lead impedance measurements) will help establish the source of the problem. Lead-related sensing problems generally manifest themselves during sinus rhythm, obviating the need to induce the patient's arrhythmia.

Postshock Sensing

Transient sensing problems due to postshock attenuation of the sensed signals

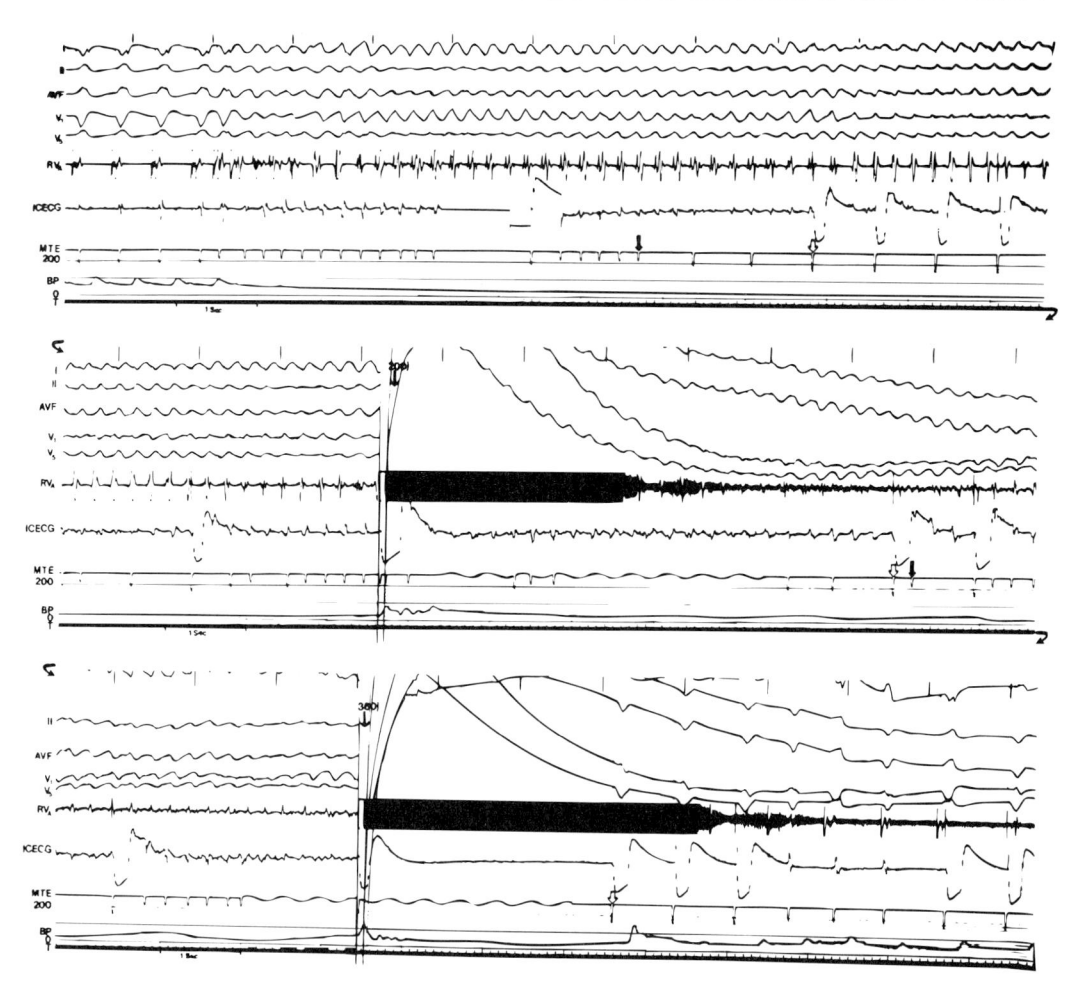

Figure 11. Failure of Guardian ATP™ 4210 (Telectronics, Englewood, CO) to sense ventricular fibrillation in the electrophysiology laboratory. Programmed sensitivity 1 mV (that doubles during ventricular tachycardia detection). Black arrow indicates undersensing, white arrow shows pacing in ventricular fibrillation. Rescue, after 37.5 seconds by external shock. From top to bottom: Surface leads I, II, aVF, V, and V_5; intracardiac ECG (IECG); main timing events (MTE); blood pressure (BP); and time lines (T). The ECGs are continuous. (Figure courtesy of Dr. Igor Singer, Louisville, KY.)

trying to trace the source of DFT-related difficulties, it is important to remember that the energies required for converting VF or polymorphic VT are generally much higher than those needed for monomorphic VT.[38] The problem may be as simple as having programmed the energy too low, ie, an inadequate safety margin, in which case the solution is simple and immediate.

Impedance Changes

More troublesome are cases in which the DFT has changed as a function of impedance variations in the defibrillating electrode-heart interface (see also Chapters 5 and 10).[19,39] Simply stated, the energy required for defibrillation will change as impedance increases and decreases.[40] It is precisely this phenomenon that accounts for the well-known differences between stored and delivered defibrillation energy. Implantable cardioverter-defibrillators using fixed pulse width will deliver a different, ie, lower energy if the impedance increases, for instance, from 50 J–75 J. (CPI devices use a design, whereby the pulse

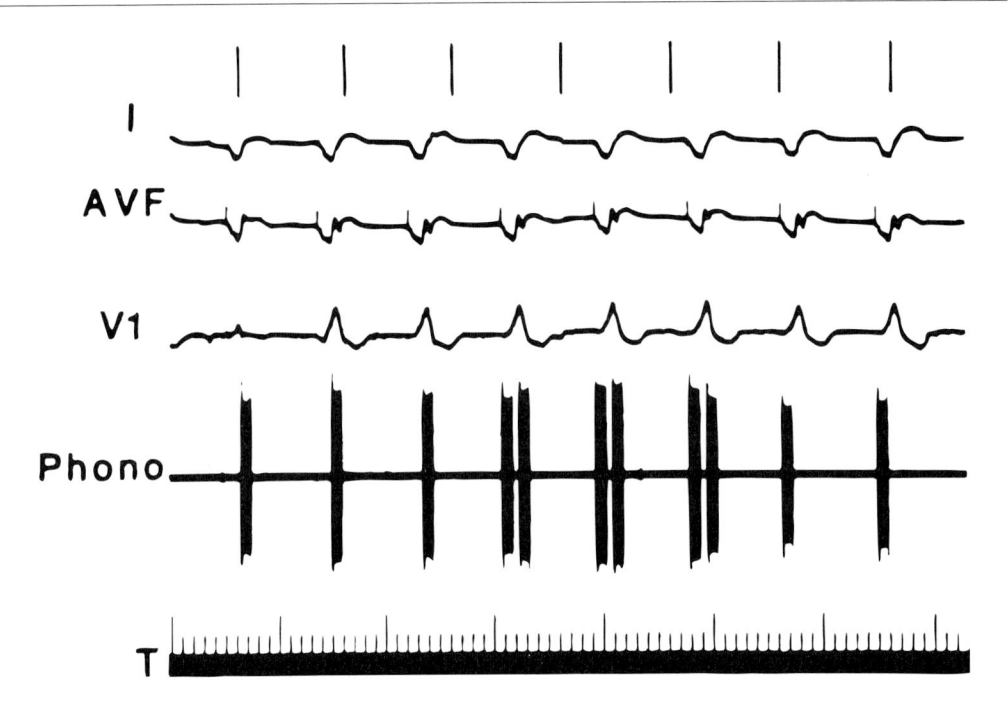

Figure 12. Phonocardiogram (Phono) druing VVI pacing (pulse width 0.5 msec, amplitude 5.0 V). Intermittent sensing of both the ventricular pacemaker stimulus and the evoked QRS complex is demonstrated with occasional double counting (fourth through sixth QRS complex from left). Paper speed 25 mm/sec. Time lines (T) are also shown (interval between the longer lines is 1 second). (Reproduced with permission from Reference 14.)

width automatically changes as a function of impedance variations, so as to assure constant energy delivery.[41]) This information may appear overly technical, but for someone troubleshooting an exhibited DFT problem with fixed pulse width devices, it may be important to know whether its source was an impedance rise opposed to other factors.

Antiarrhythmic Drugs

There are multiple reports on the influence of antiarrhythmic drugs (especially amiodarone) on DFT.[42-46] From a troubleshooting aspect, it suffices that one is aware that a change in the patient's drug regimen may have caused the DFT problem.

Lead Complications

Lead fractures, insulation breaks, loose set screws, crumpled patches, etc., as well as lead disdodgments, can all interrupt the ICD-heart circuit, resulting in ineffective shocks or ATP. Troubleshooting problems emanating from these causes, is quite similar to the techniques previously described.

Degraded Substrate

There have been some isolated cases where exacerbation of a patient's heart failure or ongoing degradation of left ventricular function was felt to have caused elevations in defibrillation energy requirements.[47,48] The awareness of this possibility may prevent the physician from losing time exploring other causes.

Antitachycardia Pacing Modes

Any and all modes of ATP may fail to convert a given VT, depending on the patient, his/her VT, and other circumstances. All ICDs with integrated ATP functions log the successes and failures of the ATP attempts, thereby facilitating the troubleshooting. For example, the Guardian™ (Telectronics, Englewood, CO) device provides a 1-second "snapshot" in addition to a summary log of sensed events (Figure 13). Anti-

SENSE HISTORY AND SNAPSHOTS

SINGLE VT EPISODE TERMINATED BY ATP

DURING VT

IECG

MARK

REVERSION

IECG

MARK

SENSE HISTORY

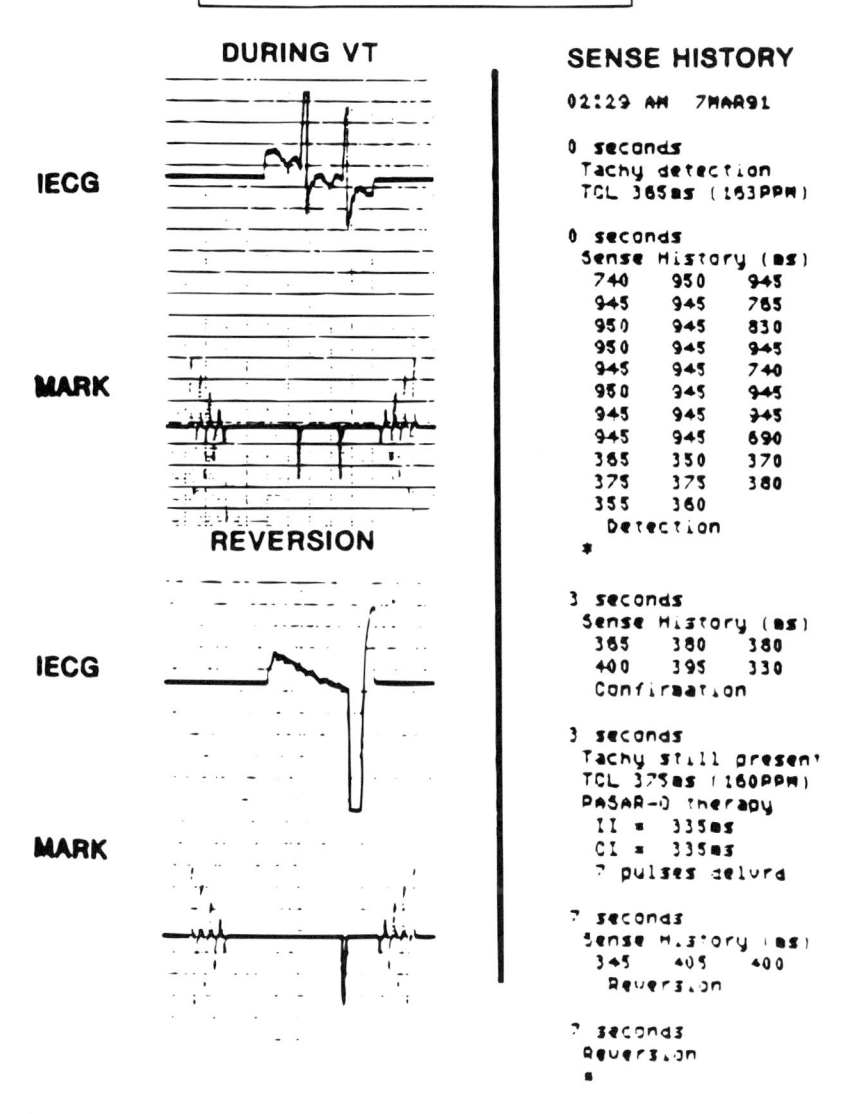

02:29 AM 7MAR91

0 seconds
Tachy detection
TCL 365ms (163PPM)

0 seconds
Sense History (ms)
740	950	945
945	945	765
950	945	830
950	945	945
945	945	740
950	945	945
945	945	945
945	945	690
365	350	370
375	375	380
355	360	
Detection
*

3 seconds
Sense History (ms)
| 365 | 380 | 380 |
| 400 | 395 | 330 |
Confirmation

3 seconds
Tachy still present
TCL 375ms (160PPM)
PASAR-0 therapy
II = 335ms
CI = 335ms
7 pulses delivd

7 seconds
Sense History (ms)
| 345 | 405 | 400 |
Reversion

7 seconds
Reversion
■

Figure 13. Sense history and electrcardiogram (ECG) snapshots from a single episode of spontaneous ventricular tachycardia (VT) terminated by antitachycardia pacing (ATP) by Guardian™ 4210 (Telectronics, Englewood, CO). **Left**: intracardiac electrograms (IECG) and markers. **Right**: sense history printout from programmer. Tachycardia was detected and terminated by a single burst of ATP (seven pulses); reversion is documented by a snapshot (*). (Reproduced with permission from Luceri R, Puchferran RL, Brownstein SL, et al: Improved patient surveillance and data acquisition with a third generation implantable cardioverter defibrillator. *PACE* 14:1870, 1991.)

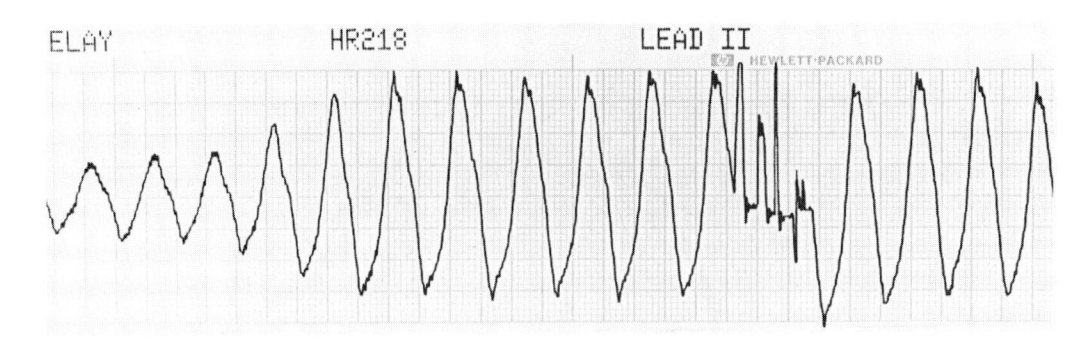

Figure 14. A stored electrogram from a patient with a P2™ (CPI, St. Paul, MN), in whom increased defibrillation thresholds resulted in high-energy shocks failing to terminate ventricular tachycardia. The "marker" for the delivery of the shock is indicated by the rapid, sharp deflections appearing beneath the words "Lead II."

tachycardia pacing failure (non-VT termination or even acceleration) often leads to syncope or presyncope, followed by ICD shocks. Information from the patient and/or witnesses, together with the device's therapy history permits further investigation in the electrophysiology laboratory.

Exit block

If pacing spikes are seen to be ineffective, one usually suspects either a rise in pacing threshold (exit block) or lead disdodgment. Another problem demanding vigilance is the loss of effective pacing (usually only for a few seconds) after an ICD shock.[29,41] In order to minimize this eventuality, some of the ICDs that have integrated pacing functions automatically increase the pacing amplitude postshock.

With Documentation

The diagnosis of failed ICD shocks or ATP is, of course, greatly facilitated when ECG tracings or EGMs from the implanted device are available. Figure 14 illustrates an EGM from a patient with a Ventak P2™ (CPI, St. Paul, MN), showing a failed ICD shock due to rise in DFT. Figure 15 is a Holter tracing from a patient with a PCD™ (Medtronic, Minneapolis, MN), document-

ing first atrial fibrillation causing VT and VF, followed very unfortunately by unsuccessful ATP and shock therapy. Figures 16 and 17 are examples of successful and non-successful inappropriate ATP attempts, respectively.

Device Deactivated

Inadvertent deactivation of an ICD is, of course, a serious problem. Indeed a fair number of the reported sudden deaths were in patients whose ICDs were turned off, intentionally or not.[6] There is relatively little that can be said regarding troubleshooting for this problem. It is generally discovered during routine patient check-ups: a magnet evoking audible tones and/or a designated programmer readily verifies the "ON/OFF" status. The real diagnostic task is to uncover how and why a device became deactivated.

Inadvertent Deactivation

The design of all available ICDs is such that the operator must go through a deliberate, unmistakable procedure to turn active device off. For example, the Cadence has an "All Functions Off" mode, which must be programmed by its programmer.[50] CPI devices (which can also be turned off by a pro-

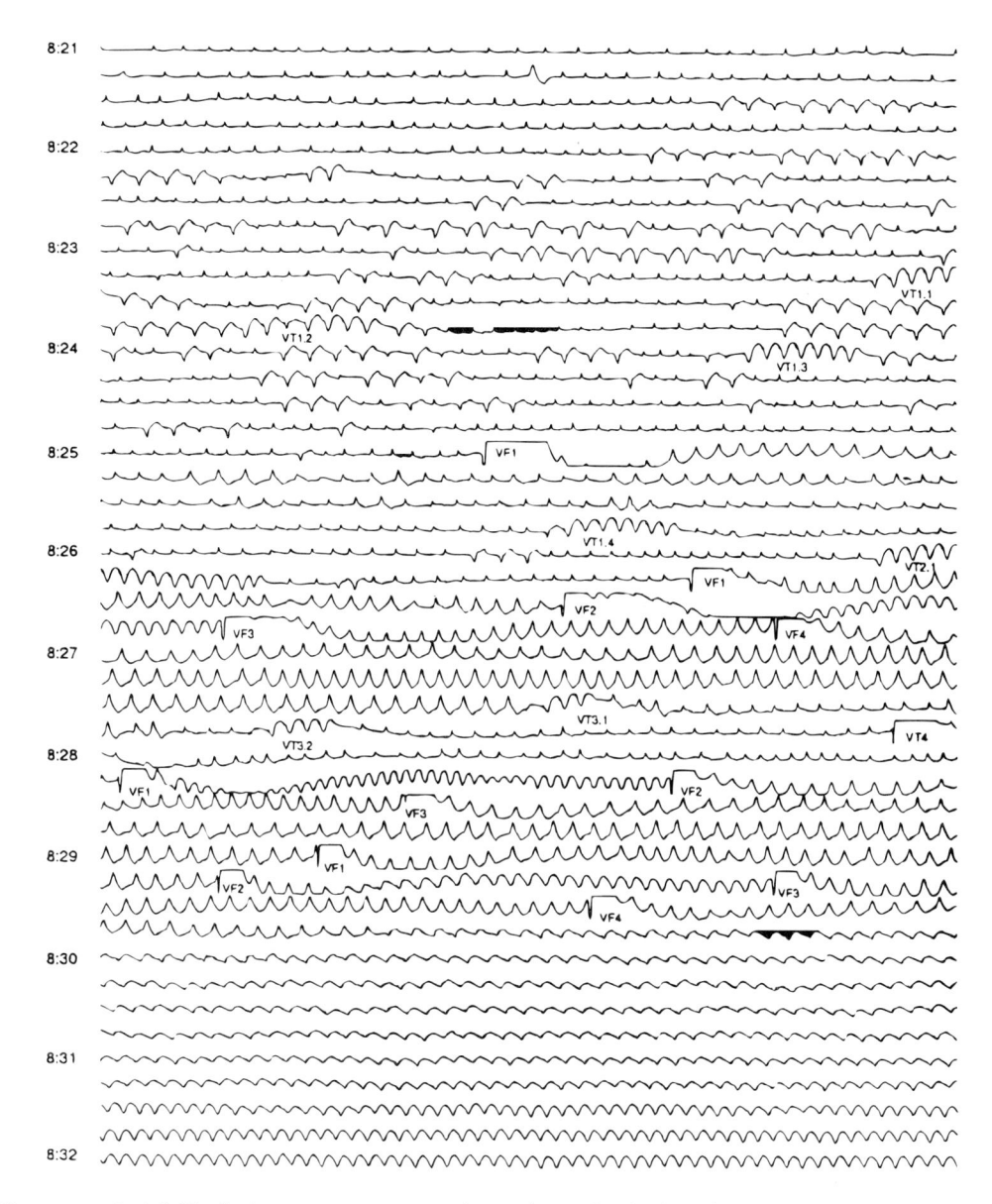

Troubleshooting Implantable Cardioverter-Defibrillators • 451

Figure 15. Atrial fibrillation causing ventricular tachycardia (VT) and ventricular fibrillation (VF) detection and therapy during the terminal episode. The PCD™ (Medtronic, Minneapolis, MN) delivered antitachyardia pacing (ATP) bursts at VT 1:1–1:3, and a 34-J shock (VF 1 at 8:25 AM). A fourth sequence of ATP was delivered (VT 1:4), causing acceleration and resulting in VT therapy 2 (VT 2: 1), then followed by four defibrillation shocks (VF 1–4). Two further ATP bursts (VT 3: 1–2) and one shock (VT 4) were followed by three VF shocks (3 VF 1–3), somewhat reducing the rate temporarily, which the device therefore considered as successful termination. A renewed final sequence of VF therapy (VF 1–4) remained unsuccessful. (Reproduced with permission from Birgersdotter-Green U, Rosenqvist M Lindemans FW, et al: Holter documented sudden death in a patient with an implanted defibrillator. *PACE* 15:1008. 1992.)

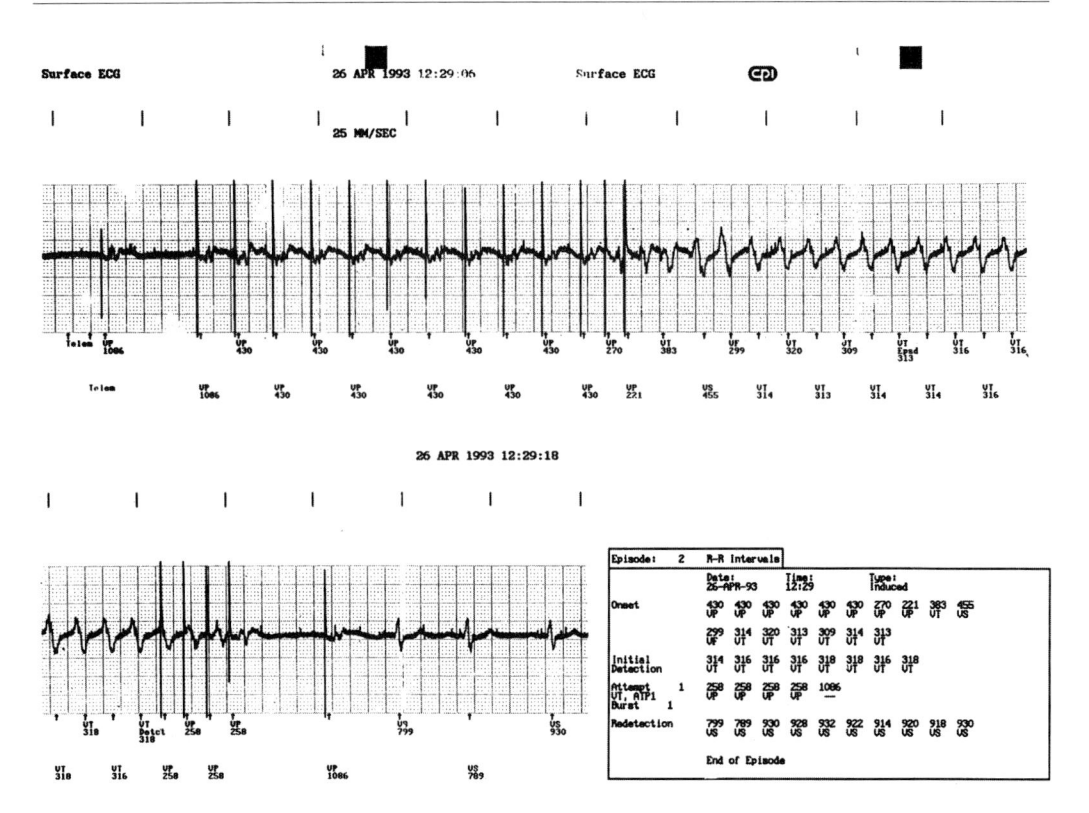

Figure 16. Ventricular tachycardia (VT) induced, then terminated by antitachycardia pacing (ATP). This strip, from a patient with a Ventak PRx2™ (CPI, St. Paul, MN), shows how marker channels and the corresponding "episode report" supplement the surface electrocardiogram (ECG). After ventricular pacing (cycle length = 1086), rapid pacing induces VT (cycle length ≈ 310). The markers show the intervals, the moment when the "VT episode is declared, subsequent reconfirmation ("VT detect"), immediately followed by a four-beat ATP burst, which interrupts the VT and results in sinus rhythm (cycle length ≈ 930 msec). The episode report, printed out after the episode, provides a quick resume. The printout of the real-time permits correlating the arrhythmia episode to the patient's activity. VP: ventricular pace; VS: ventricular sense; Telem: telemetry retrieved from implanted device.

grammer) can additionally be deactivated by a lengthy (> 30 second), uninterrupted placement of a very strong magnet directly over the pulse generator. Thus, the first step in tracing how deactivation occurred is to interrogate any and all hospital personnel, and then the patient and his or her family.

Outside Interference

Once the possibility of inadvertent or deliberate human deactivation has been eliminated, it will then be necessary to investigate whether some other type of strong outside EMI could have turned the device off, eg, MRI, arc welders, powerful radio and TV transmitters or antennas, poorly shielded electrical motors, or ignition systems. One patient's device was turned off for several minutes by proximity to a bingo wand![51] There is no industrially available measurement device as capable of checking on this problem as an active ICD itself: audible tones emanate from CPI devices if and when the strength, proximity, and orientation of a magnetic field are sufficient.

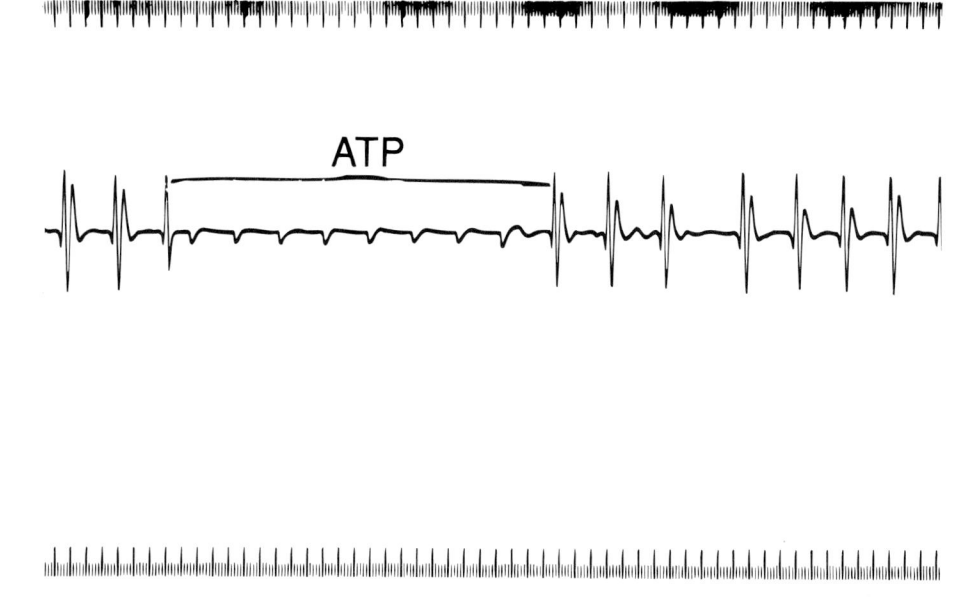

Figure 17. A stored electrogram from a patient with a Cadence™ (Ventritex, Sunnyvale, CA), in whom antitachycardia pacing (ATP) failed to terminate an episode of ventricular tachycardia. Irregular R-R intervals after ATP suggests atrial fibrillation, explaining the lack of termination of tachycardia by ATP.

Battery Depletion

Of course, a device will be off if its batteries are depleted or by a circuit fault. The elective replacement indicators for these devices generally provide ample time to replace them, but premature battery exhaustion as well as a barrage of shocks can accelerate the process.

Shut-Down Mode

Certain tiered-therapy devices inactivate the device when a fault is detected with the logic or operation of the system, such that delivery of therapy cannot be guaranteed to be safe or reliable.[52] This may be caused by a random bit-flip in the computer memory of the device, or a fault determined through self-checking routines of the device. In that case, the device may enter shut-down mode, where no therapies would be delivered. Only interrogation of the device will show that shut-down mode is operational.

Summary

Systematic troubleshooting of ICDs involves categorizing the observed (or suspected) problems, and then using available methods to identify the root causes responsible. Electrocardiogram documentation of the problem episode(s) makes troubleshooting straightforward. The major problem lies in uncovering the problem source in the absence of ECG documentation. In the latter case, a given device's telemetry and printouts, together with its markers, and the use of "beep-o-grams" provides a useful complement to the clinical evidence associated with the episode(s).

References

1. Joyce J, Paulowski J, Fogoros R: Perioperative morbidity and mortality after ICD implantation in 150 consecutive patients (abstract). *Circulation* 84:608, 1991.
2. Troup P, Nisam S: Complications associated with the automatic implantable cardioverter defibrillator. In: *The Implantable Cardioverter Defibrillator*. Edited by E Alt, H Klein, J Griffin. Berlin/Heidelberg/New York/: Springer-Verlag; 1992, p. 253.
3. Almassi G, Olinger G, Troup P, et al: Delayed infection of the automatic implantable cardioverter-defibrillator: current recognition and management. *J Thorac Cardiovasc Surg* 95:908, 1988.
4. Bakker A, Hauer W, Wever D: Infections involving implanted cardioverter defibrillator devices. *PACE* 15:654, 1992.
5. Christensen D, Baddour M, Hasty L, et al: Microbial and foreign body factors in the pathogenesis of medical device infections. In: *Infections Associated with Indwelling Medical Devices*. Edited by A Bisno, F Waldvogel. Washington DC: American Society for Microbiology; 1989, p. 27.
6. Mosteller D, Lehmann H, Thomas C, et al: Operative mortality with implantation of the automatic cardioverter-defibrillator. *Am J Cardiol* 68:1340, 1991.
7. Kowey P, Marinchak R, Rial S: Things that go bang in the night. *N Engl J Med* 327:1884, 1992.
8. Grimm W, Flores B, Marchlinski E: Symptoms and electrocardiographically documented rhythm preceding spontaneous shocks in patients with implantable cardioverter-defibrillator. *Am J Cardiol* 71:1415, 1993.
9. Maloney J, Masterson M, Khoury D, et al: Clinical performance of the implantable cardioverter defibrillator: electrocardiographic documentation of 101 spontaneous discharges. *PACE* 14:280, 1991.
10. Mehta D, Saksena S, Krol B, et al: Diagnostic use of significant symptoms underestimates appropriate ventricular tachyarrhythmia reversions by programmable pacemaker defibrillators (abstract). *PACE* 15:231, 1992.
11. Fogoros R, Elson J, Bonnet C: Actuarial incidence and pattern of occurrence of shocks following implantation of the automatic implantable cardioverter defibrillator. *PACE* 12:1465, 1989.
12. Luceri R, Habal S, Castellanos A, et al: Mechanism of death in patients with the AICD. *PACE* 11:2014, 1988.
13. Strambler B, Wood M, Feller C, et al: Limitations of tachycardia confirmation algorithms of a third generation implantable cardioverter defibrillator (ICD): is it truly a noncommitted device (abstract)? *Circulation* 86(4):I-59, 1992.
14. Chapman P, Troup P: The automatic implantable cardioverter defibrillator: evaluating suspected inappropriate shocks. *J Am Coll Cardiol* 7:1075, 1986.
15. *CPI Physicians Manual*. St. Paul, MN: CPI; 1991.
16. Ellenbogen K, Wood M, Stambler B, et al: Measurement of ventricular electrogram amplitude during intraoperative induction of ventricular tachyarrhythmias. *Am J Cardiol* 70:1017, 1992.
17. Wilber D, Poczobutl-Johanos M: Time-dependent sensing alterations in implantable defibrillators: lessons from the Telectronics Guardian 4202/4203 (abstract). *PACE* 14:624, 1991.
18. Singer I, Adams L, Austin E: Potential hazards of fixed gain sensing and arrhythmia reconfirmation for implantable cardioverter defibrillators. *PACE* 16:1070, 1993.
19. Troup P: Implantable cardioverters and defibrillators. In: *Current Problems in Cardiology*. Edited by R O'Rourke, M Crawford, F Beller, et al. Chicago, IL: Yearbook Medical Publishers; 1989, p. 724.
20. Cohen T, Chien W, Lurie K, et al: Implantable cardioverter defibrillator proarrhythmia: case report and review of the literature. *PACE* 14:1326, 1991.
21. Johnson N, Marchlinski F: Arrhythmias induced by device antitachycardia therapy due to diagnostic nonspecificity. *J Am Coll Cardiol* 18:1418, 1991.
22. Luceri R, Habal S, David I, et al: Changing trends in therapy delivery with a third generation noncommitted implantable defibrillator: results of a large single center clinical trial. *PACE* 16:159, 1993.
23. Callans D, Hook B, Marchlinski F: Use of bipolar recordings from patch-patch and rate sensing leads to distinguish ventricular tachycardia from supraventricular rhythms in patients with implantable cardioverter defibrillators. *PACE* 14(II):1917, 1991.
24. Marchlinski F, Gottlieb C, Sarter B, et al: ICD data storage: value in arryhthmia management. *PACE* 16:527, 1993.
25. Block M, Isbruch F, Clerc G, et al: ECGs of defibrillation electrodes yield more information than ECG's of sensing electrodes (abstract). *Eur J Cardiac Pacing Electrophysiol* (2):A122, 1992.

26. Isbruch F, Clock M, Hammel D, et al: Influence of defibrillation shocks on the endocardial sensing signal of an integrated sense/pace/defibrillation lead (abstract). Eur Heart J 12:363, 1991.
27. Jung W, Manz M, Moosdorf R, et al: Failure of an implantable cardioverter-defibrillator to redetect ventricular fibrillation in patients with a nonthoracotomy lead system. Circulation 86:1217, 1992.
28. Ellis J, Martin D, John R: Failed defibrillation shocks have no effect on ventricular fibrillation redetection time in the Endotak transvenous lead system (abstract). PACE 16:897, 1993.
29. Calkins H, Brinker J, Veltri E, et al: Clinical interactions between pacemakers and automatic implantable cardioverter-defibrillators. J Am Coll Cardiol 16:666, 1990.
30. Callans D, Hook B, Kleiman R, et al: Signal oversensing and undersensing in 4th generation implantable cardioverter-defibrillators (abstract). Circulation 84:II-428, 1991.
31. Sperry R, Ellenbogen K, Wood M, et al: Failure of a second and third generation implantable cardioverter defibrillator to sense ventricular tachycardia: implications for fixed gain sensing devices. PACE 15:749, 1992.
32. Singer I, Austin E, Nash W, et al: Initial clinical experience with an implantable cardioverter defibrillator/antitachycardia pacemaker. PACE 14:1119, 1991.
33. Davy J, Fain E, Dorian P, et al: The relationship between successful defibrillation and delivered energy in open-chest dogs: reappraisal of the "defibrillation threshold" concept. Am Heart J 113:77, 1987.
34. Singer I, Lang D: Defibrillation threshold: clinical utility and therapeutic implications. PACE 15:932, 1992.
35. Wetherbee J, Chapman P, Troup P, et al: Long-term internal cardiac defibrillation threshold stability. PACE 12:443, 1989.
36. Vester E, Kuhls S, Perings C, et al: Efficacy and long-term stability of a single endocardial lead configuration for permanent implantation of cardioverter/defibrillators (abstract). PACE 16:875, 1993.
37. Norenberg M, Sakun V, Roberts D, et al: Long-term clinical experience with PCD Transvene system: worldwide experience (abstract). PACE 16:874, 1993.
38. Winkle R, Stinson E, Bach S, et al: Cardioversion/defibrillation thresholds in man using a truncated exponential waveform and an apical patch-SVC spring electrode configuration. Circulation 69:766, 1984.
39. Chapman P, Wetherbee J, Vetter J, et al: Strength-duration curves of fixed pulse width variable tilt truncated exponential waveforms for nonthoracotomy internal defibrillation in dogs. PACE 11:1045, 1988.
40. Lade K: Clinical implications of changes in AICD defibrillation lead impedance (abstract). PACE 14:722, 1991.
41. CPI Concept Paper: *The Clinical Importance of Constant Energy Delivery*. 1992; p. 7855. Physician's Manuals for all CPI automatic implantable cardioverter defibrillators.
42. Jung W, Manz M, Pfeifer D, et al: Effects of antiarrhythmic drugs on epicardial defibrillation energy requirements and the rate of defibrillator discharges. PACE 16:198, 1993.
43. Epstein A, Ellenbogen K, Kirk K, et al: Clinical characteristics and outcome of patients with high defibrillation thresholds. Circulation 86:1206, 1992.
44. Fogoros R: Amiodarone-induced refractoriness to cardioversion. Ann Intern Med 100: 699, 1984.
45. Haberman R, Veltri E, Mower M: The effect of amiodarone on defibrillation threshold. J Electrophysiol 2:415, 1988.
46. Echt D, Black J, Barbey J, et al: Evaluation of antiarrhythmic drugs on defibrillation energy requirements in dogs: sodium channel block and action potential prolongation. Circulation 79:1106, 1979.
47. Lucy S, Jones D, Klein G: Increased defibrillation threshold and cardiac hypertrophy in a rapid pacing model of congestive heart failure in the dog (abstract). J Am Coll Cardiol 13:67A, 1989.
48. Neuzner J, Pitschner H: Personal communication. Kerckhoff Klinik, Bad Nauheim, Germany.
49. Khastgir T, Lattuca J, Aarons D, et al: Ventricular pacing threshold and time to capture postdefibrillation in patients undergoing implantable cardioverter-defibrillator implantation. PACE 14:768, 1991.
50. *Ventritex Cadence Physician's Manual*. 1990.
51. Ferrick K, Johnston D, Kim S, et al: Inadvertent AICD inactivation while playing bingo. Am Heart J 206, 1991.
52. Crosby P, Singer I: Letter-to-the-Editor. PACE 14:1554, 1991.

namic tolerance of these in addition to the underlying heart disease. For example, a patient presenting with syncope who is found to be easily induced into monomorphic VT at relatively low rates that are well tolerated for 30 seconds or more before hemodynamic symptoms appear and that are repetitively converted with some mode of antitachycardia pacing (ATP), should receive a tiered-therapy device, capable of ATP as well as low- and high-energy cardioversion. A patient who has been resuscitated from cardiac arrest, however, and who is noninducible in the electrophysiology laboratory is not likely to benefit from ATP, and therefore would be a better candidate for a simpler, cheaper device that does not necessarily offer ATP. Whether or not a patient will be amenable to various ATP modes is generally established prior to implant, then "fine tuned" during predischarge testing.

For those patients who are able to be induced, it is well known that the probability of reliably terminating their VT with ATP diminishes at higher VT rates.[1-3] Further complicating the problem with ATP therapy is the fact that, in general, the higher the patient's VT rate, the poorer his or her overall hemodynamic tolerance. For the patients who do respond to ATP, there is little doubt that this is the preferred treatment; we and others have had many patients with multiple successful conversions, rarely even perceptible to the patients. There is also an intermediate group of patients whose VTs respond rarely or not at all to ATP, but do respond reliably to low-energy cardioversion of approximately ≤ 10 J, and often as low as 1–2 J.[4,5] We must add that some of the above considerations may be significantly modified by antiarrhythmic drugs. For example, many ICD patients who were originally nonresponsive to ATP therapy respond well to ATP after the administration of various antiarrhythmic drugs.[2,6]

Detection Enhancements

Much of the time involved and expertise required for programming ICDs is aimed at optimizing VT detection. As emphasized earlier, inappropriate detection (leading to inappropriate therapy or no therapy) remains the primary cause of ICD complications. Current and future devices provide a large choice of detection enhancements, which are parameters that permit fine tuning for detection of tachyarrhythmias (see also Chapter 4).[7,8] Nearly all of these programmable detection parameters are based on RR intervals: rate, sudden onset, stability, acceleration, sustained rate duration (SRD), also called extended high rate (EHR). In one device (PRx-1™, CPI, St. Paul, MN), there is also an R wave morphology criterion, somewhat analogous to the probability density function (PDF) available in earlier devices. Figure 1 illustrates the detection criteria for a PRx device configured as a three-zone device. These criteria apply for the initial detection of an episode of VT/VF. Some of these criteria may be applied again before therapy is delivered during reconfirmation that the same episode is ongoing or sustained. Some may again apply during redetection or posttherapy detection, to test whether the programmed therapy did in fact convert the episode. More detailed explanations of these detection enhancements are provided. However, they vary considerably from one manufacturer's device(s) to another, so that reference to the pertinent physician manual will obviously remain a prerequisite to programming these parameters.

Rate Cutoff

The programming of the rate cutoff, which is the most fundamental and far reaching of the detection criteria, simply sets up a specific minimum RR interval (sometimes also referred to as tachycardia detection interval [TDI]), with which every RR interval is compared. The algorithms by which an ICD establishes that VT is present differ between models from the various manufacturers. Most devices require the

Detection Criteria for a Three-Zone Configuration

Parameter	Zone One Values	Zone Two Values	Zone Three Values
Rate Criterion[1]	90–200 bpm in 5-bpm increments, 210 bpm, and 220 bpm (nominal = 125 bpm)	Same as Zone One (nominal = 145)	Same as Zone One (nominal=165)
Duration[1]	8–30 cardiac cycles in 1-cycle increments, 30–50 cardiac cycles in 5-cycle increments, 50–100 cardiac cycles in 10-cycle increments, 100–250 cardiac cycles in 50-cycle increments (nominal = 10 cycles)	Same as Zone One	Same as Zone One
Sustained Rate Duration[1]	OFF, 1–5 sec in 1-sec increments, 5–45 sec in 5-sec increment, 1–2 min in 10-sec increments, 2–5 min in 30-sec increments, 5–10 min in 1-min increments, 15, 20, 25, 30, 45, 60 min (nominal = OFF)	Not available	Not available
TPM[1,3]	ON, OFF (nominal = OFF)	Same as Zone One	Not available
Onset[3,4]	OFF, 9–15%, 19–34%, or 38–50% in 3%-increments (nominal = OFF)	Not available	Not available
Stability[1,3]	OFF, 8, 16, 23, 31, 39, 47, or 55 ms (nominal = OFF)	Not available	Not available

1. Tolerance is + 8 ms.
2. The rate criterion for Zone One must be less than the rate criterion for Zone Two. Likewise, the rate criteria for Zone Two must be less than the rate criteria for Zone Three. (Zone Two minimum = Zone one rate plus 10 bpm. Zone Three minimum = Zone Two rate plus 10 bpm.)
3. If TPM is ON in Zone One, Onset and Stability must be OFF in Zone One and vice versa
4. Percentage calculation tolerance is + 16 ms.

Figure 1. Programmable detection criteria and restrictions for setting up a PRx-1™ (CPI, St. Paul, MN) to operate as a three-VT/VF zone device. TPM: turning point morphology (see text). (Reproduced with permission from Reference 12.)

fulfillment of two criteria, ie, the programmed *rate* criterion must be exceeded for a programmed *number* of intervals (duration). The Guardian™ (Teletronics, Englewood, CO) uses an X-of-Y detection algorithm that requires, for example, 8 out of 10 intervals to be shorter or equal to TDI. The PCD™ (Medtronic, Minneapolis, MN) detects fibrillation when 75% of the programmed number of intervals are shorter than the programmed fibrillation detection interval (FDI). In essence, all of these techniques represent some type of running average of the VT rate.

Rate Zones

Most current ICDs can be configured as single or multiple zone devices: bradycardia zone, lower tachycardia zones, medium VT zone, and high-rate VT/VF zone. Programming involves setting the "ceilings" or boundaries of these zones.

Sudden Onset

Sudden onset measures the abruptness (in percentage or in milliseconds) of the onset of a tachycardia in an attempt to discriminate between a sinus tachycardia, which begins gradually, and a pathological VT, which generally begins abruptly. Figure 2 demonstrates the use of sudden onset in the PCD device. The actual algorithms differ between different manufacturer's models, but the common thread is that this criterion is only calculated once a VT has begun. The function of sudden onset is to suppress delivery of the therapy until the programmed sudden onset is satisfied; hence, as a precaution, it is generally recommended to limit the time needed to satisfy the sudden onset criterion.

Stability

Stability measures the degree (percentage) of fluctuation between VT RR intervals.

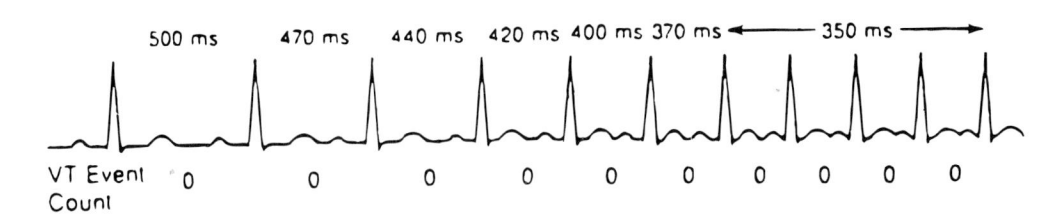

Figure 2. Example of onset criterion unfulfilled. Illustrates a sinus rhythm with a gradually accelerating rate. No interval is < 81% of the average of the four previous intervals. Thus, this rhythm would not be detected by the PCD™ (Medtronic, Minneapolis, MN) device as a ventricular tachycardia (VT). This example demonstrates how the onset criterion may be used to help differentiate between a sinus tachycardia (possibly exercise induced) and a pathological VT. (Reprinted with permission from *PCD Model 7217A Physicians' Manual*. Medtronic, Minneapolis, MN.)

In principle, a true VT is distinguished by relatively stable tachycardia intervals, whereas fast venticular rates resulting from supraventricular tachycardias, eg, atrial fibrillation, are usually unstable. As with sudden onset, this enhancement also serves to suppress programmed therapy, until it is satisfied or a programmed safety time-out is reached.

Sustained Rate Duration or Extended High Rate

Sustained rate duration (SRD) or extended high rate (EHR) is essentially a safety feature, a timer, that ensures that the programmed therapy will be delivered for a VT sustained beyond the SRD or EHR, regardless of whether the sudden onset and/or stability criterion are satisfied. To use this feature, it needs to be programmed "ON" and the time in seconds selected.

Acceleration

This feature checks the average rate posttherapy, whether ATP or cardioversion shock(s), for acceleration of the rate; it is programmed as a percentage. Safety is the main purpose of this feature. For instance, in the PRx device, if the algorithm deems that acceleration has occurred, the ongoing therapy (eg, ATP) is immediately superseded, and defibrillation shocks delivered.

Morphology

This parameter, denoted in the PRx device as turning point morphology (TPM), is somewhat similar to PDF, which was available (or programmable) in previous devices and is the only parameter not based on RR intervals. While the algorithms differ, both PDF and TPM attempt to minimize the relative time the sensed electrograms spend on or away from the isoelectric line. This feature is intended to help discriminate between narrow QRS tachycardias versus wide pathological VTs. If PDF is turned on, therapy will be inhibited until PDF is satisfied; if TPM is programmed on, therapy (shocks) will be accelerated whenever the TPM criterion is met. Siemens, Telectronics, and probably other manufacturers envision the possibility of including morphology criteria in their future ICDs.[9-11]

Noncommitted

Following detection of VT, after charging but just before delivery of therapy, it is often desirable to "look again" to see if the VT is still present. Several devices offer the possibility of programming to "Noncommitted," which means that the programmed therapy will only be delivered if the "relook" confirms that the VT is sustained.

Antitachycardia Pacing Time-Out

This safety feature limits the time a patient continues receiving ATP schemes. The implanter, aware of how well and how long a patient can tolerate a given VT, programs EHR or "ATP time-out" to the time that he/she feels ATP can continue without compromising the patient's safety. At the end of the time-out, the device delivers defibrillation shocks.

Posttherapy Confirmation

It is well known that ATP schemes often fail to terminate a VT and even cardioversion/defibrillation shocks may occasionally fail, or even accelerate a VT. With this in mind, all ICDs have been designed to reexamine the arrhythmia within seconds of the delivered therapy. The algorithms for postherapy detection are similar, but not always identical to those involved in the initial VT detection. The primary difference, in recognition of the fact that the situation is now much more urgent, is that the VT specificity enhancements (eg, sudden onset, rate stability, TPM) are disabled, in most devices leading to fast decisions and rapid delivery of aggressive therapy, usually defibrillation.

Rules of Arbitration

With the number of permutations possible in these devices' attempts to properly identify and discriminate arrhythmias, the process can become extremely complex. Thus, decision making in these devices often requires resolution in case rate and/or other criteria overlap. An example, taken from the *PRx Physicians' Manual*,[12] illustrates the necessity and complexity of this issue (Figure 3):

(During post-shock monitoring), If the maximum number of intervals following a shock is reached without the most recent four falling within one tachyarrhythmia zone or below the lowest tachyarrhythmia zone, then a "voting" scheme is used as follows:

1. If three of the four intervals fall below the lowest tachyarrhythmia rate zone boundary, the episode is declared successfully ended (detection reset).

2. If three of the four intervals fall above the lowest tachyarrhythmia rate zone boundary, the episode is declared not ended.

3. If two of the last four intervals fall below the lowest rate zone, then the last four-interval average is used to determine whether the arrhythmia is terminated. If the four-interval average falls above the lowest rate zone boundary, the episode is declared not ended. If the four-interval average falls below the lowest rate zone boundary, the episode is declared successfully ended.

If the tachycardia episode is not ended, then in all cases the average of the four intervals is used to decide which therapy to use next.

Other devices incorporate various "voting" schemes, so the reader will have to examine the pertinent physician manual.

Potential Dangers of Using Detection Enhancements

The main point that the clinician must keep in mind when deciding whether to use detection enhancement such as sudden onset and rate stability is that these enhancements have the effect of delaying or withholding antitachycardia therapy. If these detection enhancements are programmed appropriately, they can be beneficial in helping to withhold inappropriate therapy. However, if they are programmed suboptimally, they can result in the inappropriate withholding of therapy in pa-

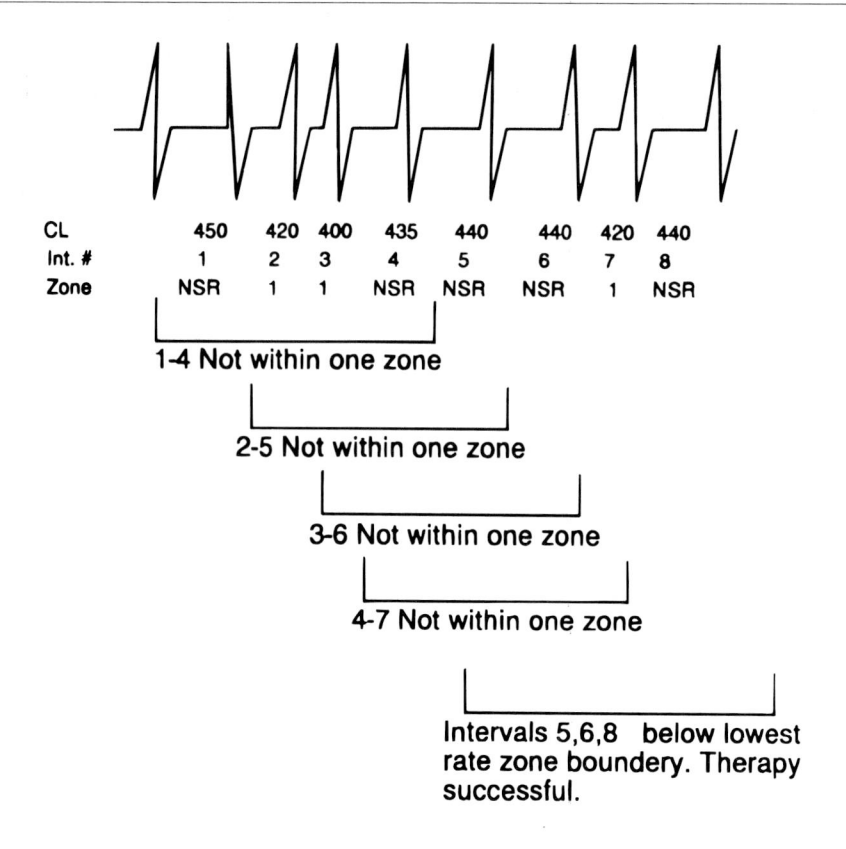

```
CL     450  420  400  435  440  440  420  440
Int. #  1    2    3    4    5    6    7    8
Zone   NSR   1    1   NSR  NSR  NSR   1   NSR
```

1-4 Not within one zone

2-5 Not within one zone

3-6 Not within one zone

4-7 Not within one zone

Intervals 5,6,8 below lowest rate zone boundery. Therapy successful.

A

Figure 3A. The postshock delay for the PRx™ (CPI, St. Paul, MN) is met for zone 1 at interval 30. Since the first four intervals are not all within zone 1 or below the rate boundary, the window begins sliding. In this case four intervals are not found and the device reaches the maximum detect delay at interval 35 where a decision must be made.

tients with potentially lethal arrhythmias. Because inappropriate shocks are merely painful while withholding appropriate shocks may be lethal, the clinician who elects to use these detection enhancements is obligated to take every precaution to prevent this latter eventuality. As a general rule, detection criteria should be limited to rate cutoff only, unless there is a compelling reason to choose otherwise.

If it is necessary to use rate stability criteria to avoid inappropriate therapy during atrial fibrillation, then the clinician is obligated to document that the patient's VT will be detected without delay when rate stability is programmed "ON," and also, whenever possible, to document that rate stability will result in the withholding of therapy during rapid atrial fibrillation.

The sudden onset criterion is used to help distinguish sinus tachycardia from VT. Unfortunately, with the sudden onset parameter, no provocative testing of VT (to make sure the tachycardia will be detected appropriately) is possible. The clinicians should probably not consider using the sudden onset parameter unless at least one episode of the patient's spontaneous ventricular arrhythmia has been documented and the change in heart rate as VT begins is indeed "sudden" (ie, there is no significant "warm up" as tachycardia begins).

The morphology parameter (PDF), used in some devices from CPI, was another feature designed to withhold ICD therapy unless the QRS complex was wide enough. In practice, PDF has not proven to be very useful, and since it was not programmable

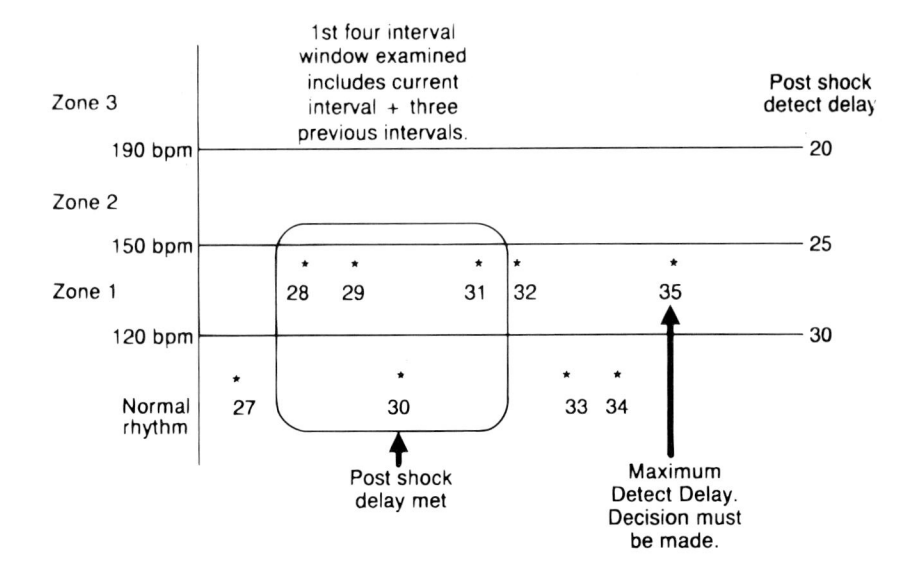

Programming of Implantable Cardioverter-Defibrillators • 463

Figure 3B. Basic redetection algorithm in action. Each interval is classified into a zone, since four consecutive intervals are not located in the same zone, at the end of eight cycles the device uses a voting scheme to make a decision.

(except for "on" or "off"), the presence of PDF made troubleshooting relatively difficult in those cases in which a shock was apparently withheld inappropriately. Most clinicians have chosen not to use PDF. The newer morphology detector (TPM) is designed, in contrast to PDF, to accelerate a shock if appropriate criteria are met. Very little clinical data exists on the benefits of using TPM.

In summary, when using detection enhancements the clinician must weigh the potential benefits against the potential risks. Since the risk (for most detection enhancements) is withholding life-saving therapy, detection enhancements should be used with great caution, if at all.

Multizone Sequenced Tiered Therapy

The whole objective of detection of a VT and assigning it to a specific zone is obviously to provide electrical therapy, programmed as most applicable to the identified VT. This concept is based on the established principles that the most dangerous arrhythmia—VF and sustained polymorphic VT—require the most aggressive therapy, high-energy defibrillation shocks[13]; well-organized, monomorphic relatively lower rate VT often responds to the least aggressive therapy (ATP) certainly least perceptible for the patient[1-3]; between these two extremes, there will be patients with VTs amenable to low-energy conversion and/or more aggressive ATP modes.[4,5] In programming an ICD within this hierarchy of therapies, the probability of successful conversion is obviously the dominant factor. Unfortunately, there are concurrent, competing risks that need to be considered, according to each patient's electrophysiologic and hemodynamic tolerance: VT acceleration to polymorphous VT and/or VF; the effect of prolonged therapy, eg, multiple and lengthy ATP schemes on the patient's hemodynamic and cerebral status[14]; and the possibility that delaying shocks may increase ischemia and raise the DFT, thereby increasing the risk of them no longer being successful.[15,16]

Several tachycardia therapy options

are programmable in some, but not all ICDs: waveform (biphasic or monophasic), shock polarity, and committed versus noncommitted. The remainder of the programming options depend on the selected hierarchy of therapies, and are covered individually below.

Low- and High-Energy Cardioversion

For the reasons indicated previously, a physician may for selected patients opt for devices offering these modes of therapy, or configure tiered ICDs to provide only low-energy cardioversion and defibrillation. Such devices can be programmed with single- or double-tachycardia zone detection and therapy. In a single-zone configuration, the level of the energy for the first, and if needed, subsequent shocks is programmable. In a two-zone configuration, differential detection and therapy can be independently programmed in each zone: low-energy shocks, for the lower rate tachycardias, and high-energy shocks for VF or rapid VTs.

Antitachycardia Pacing

For those patients amenable to ATP therapy, an ICD is usually configured as a two- or three-tachycardia zone device. The possibility does exist, although physicians use it infrequently, to program ATP in a single-zone configuration. The device can then deliver the programmed ATP scheme, which if unsuccessful is followed by low-energy cardioversion, then defibrillation, or defibrillation directly. In a device configured to operate with a "Tach A" and "Tach B" zone, different programmed detection criteria have to be fulfilled for each zone, whereupon the therapy programmed for that zone is delivered. Figure 4 shows an example of the Cadence™ (Ventritex, Sunnyvale, CA) programmed as a two-zone device. Typically, the lower zone would be programmed for single or multiple modes of ATP, and up to two or three cardioversion shocks, and the second zone would permit a programmed, limited number of low-energy conversion shocks, with high-energy defibrillation mandatory (not programmable), should the lower hierarchy

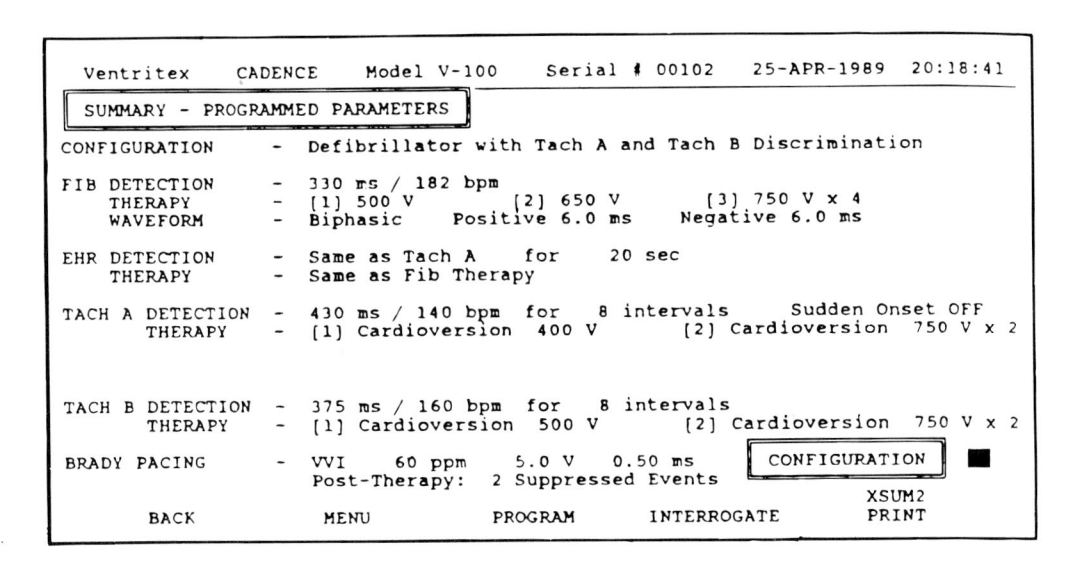

```
Ventritex      CADENCE      Model V-100      Serial # 00102      25-APR-1989  20:18:41
 ┌─────────────────────────────────────┐
 │ SUMMARY - PROGRAMMED PARAMETERS     │
 └─────────────────────────────────────┘
   CONFIGURATION       -  Defibrillator with Tach A and Tach B Discrimination

   FIB DETECTION       -  330 ms / 182 bpm
         THERAPY       -  [1] 500 V         [2] 650 V         [3] 750 V x 4
         WAVEFORM      -  Biphasic    Positive 6.0 ms    Negative 6.0 ms

   EHR DETECTION       -  Same as Tach A    for    20 sec
         THERAPY       -  Same as Fib Therapy

   TACH A DETECTION    -  430 ms / 140 bpm  for   8 intervals    Sudden Onset OFF
          THERAPY      -  [1] Cardioversion  400 V       [2] Cardioversion  750 V x 2


   TACH B DETECTION    -  375 ms / 160 bpm  for   8 intervals
          THERAPY      -  [1] Cardioversion  500 V       [2] Cardioversion  750 V x 2

   BRADY PACING        -  VVI   60 ppm    5.0 V    0.50 ms    ┌─────────────┐ ■
                          Post-Therapy:  2 Suppressed Events  │CONFIGURATION│
                                                              └─────────────┘
                                                                    XSUM2
              BACK           MENU            PROGRAM      INTERROGATE    PRINT
```

Figure 4. Summary screen for Cadence™ ICD (Ventritex, Sunnyvale, CA) with tachycardia response (Tach A and Tach B discrimination, nominal values). (Reprinted with permission from *Cadence V-100 Physicians' Manual*. Ventritex, Sunnyvale, CA.)

therapies fail to terminate the VT/VF. Some devices offer a third or even fourth VT zone, but the concept is the same: ATP alone and/or low-energy conversion in the lowest VT rate zone, more aggressive ATP modes and/or low-energy conversion in the intermediate zone(s), and defibrillation (sometimes preceded by low-engery conversion) in the highest zone, which is also referred to as the "V-Fib" zone.

Some devices offer physicians the option to use the lower zone of a three-zone device as a monitor-only, no-therapy zone. This permits a physician to program his/her device to capture in memory and retrieve by telemetry arrhythmias below a rate for which the given patient requires therapy.

There is, of course, the possibility of a tachycardia moving from one zone to another, spontaneously or as a result of ICD therapy. All these devices have fairly complex algorithms for dealing with VTs that accelerate or decelerate, but remain nonconverted. For details on how this works for any given model, it will be necessary to examine the physician's manual and/or contact the company's technical support staff. As a general rule, however, most devices deal with acceleration, ie, movement from one VT zone to a higher zone, by mandating aggressive therapy, usually defibrillation. In some devices, acceleration calls for the next programmed therapy and defibrillation is mandated only if the rate has crossed the fibrillation boundary, ie, the RR intervals have dropped below the FDI.

Diagnostics

The programming related to setting up the devices to provide diagnostic information is very device- and manufacturer-specific, and is not covered here. In essence, the major programmable aspects cover the type of diagnostic data desired, the sampling period, the form of visual display, etc.

Case Reports

Eight selected cases illustrating important aspects of programming follow. For each case, the rationale guiding the programming of the detection enhancements and of the therapy options is explained.

Case 1: Patient with well-tolerated ventricular tachycardia at a rate slower than peak sinus rate

Case: A 58-year-old man with prior inferior wall myocardial infarction, well-preserved left ventricular function (ejection fraction = 0.45), who presented with sustained VT at a rate of 180 beats per minute and presyncope. During drug testing, procainamide was found to slow VT to 130–140 beats per minute, which made the VT well tolerated, and made it amenable to termination with ATP. Peak sinus rate during treadmill testing is 150 beats per minute.

Detection considerations: Since ICD must detect VT with rates as low as 130 beats per minute, yet avoid delivering inappropriate therapy during sinus tachycardia, a device with the detection parameter of sudden onset should be used. The sudden onset parameter should reduce the risk of treating sinus tachycardia inappropriately.

Treatment considerations: A) Since on procainamide the VT is well tolerated and terminable by ATP, a tiered-therapy device should be used, and multiple episodes of ATP should be attempted before defaulting to a shock (unless acceleration occurs). B) Sustained rate duration should be programmed "OFF," or programmed to a long period of time to reduce the chances of shocks being delivered inappropriately for sinus tachycardia. C) The use of β blockers should be strongly considered to reduce the peak sinus rate.

Case 2: Patient with rapid VT causing hemodynamic collapse

Case: A 65-year-old female with prior myocardial infarction presents with cardiac arrest. After recovery, electrophysiologic evaluation reveals that she has inducible VT, rate of 180 beats per minute, which is terminable by pacing but that causes collapse within 15–20 seconds of onset. The patient's peak sinus rate was 150 beats per minute.

Detection considerations: Because VT is much faster than peak sinus rate, we can use rate-only detection.

Treatment considerations: A shock-only device would be quite appropriate in this patient. A tiered-therapy device could be considered, since the VT can be terminated by pacing. However, if ATP is to be used, only a brief attempt at ATP (one or two pacing sequences) is warranted before defaulting to shocks, because hemodynamic collapse is quick.

Case 3: Cardiac arrest survivor with no inducible VT

Case: A 70-year-old man with a prior myocardial infarction, left ventricular ejection fraction of 0.35, resuscitated from a cardiac arrest. The patient has no inducible arrhythmias. Peak sinus rate is 130 beats per minute.

Detection considerations: Detection should be using rate criteria only, at a relatively high rate cutoff (at least 170 beats per minute).

Treatment considerations: A simple shock-only ICD should be used.

Case 4: Patient with long runs of nonsustained VT

Case: A 55-year-old man with idiopathic cardiomyopathy, left ventricular ejection fraction of 0.40, presenting with cardiac arrest. Subsequent evaluation shows that he has inducible VT at rates of 170–200 beats per minute of multiple morphologies. Clinically, the patient has relatively long runs of nonsustained VT, with rates of 170–220 beats per minute; peak sinus rate is 160 beats per minute.

Detection considerations: Since peak sinus rate is slower than rate of VT, a rate-only detection scheme should be used.

Treatment considerations: To avoid inappropriate shocks for nonsustained VT, one or more of these strategies might be used: A) A noncommitted device (a device that checks to see if VT is still present just before delivering shock) can be used. The potential disadvantage is that numerous charging cycles can be wasted if frequency of nonsustained VT is high, thus reducing the longevity of the device. B) A device with a programmable detection delay (in some, committed/noncommitted is programmable) can be used, so that charging does not begin until the VT has been sustained for a programmable length of time. The potential disadvantage is that postponing a shock for up to 10 extra seconds might result in loss of consciousness before shock is finally delivered. C) Aggressive use of antiarrhythmic drugs might be used to reduce frequency of nonsustained VT. Ideally, antiarrhythmic drug regimen should be determined before ICD implantation, so that defibrillation thresholds are determined on the patient's long-term regimen.

Case 5: Patient with paroxysmal atrial fibrillation

Case: A 68-year-old female with prior myocardial infarction, left ventricular ejection fraction of 0.25, presents with sustained monomorphic VT at a rate of 150 beats per minute and presyncope. The VT is readily inducible, and moderately terminable with ATP, but the patient became very symptomatic from VT within 10–15 seconds. The patient also has a history of paroxysmal atrial fibrillation once or twice per month, lasting 15–20 minutes, with rates of 140–160 beats per minute. Antiarrhythmic drugs have been ineffective in controlling atrial fibrillation.

Detection considerations: Use of rate stability criteria should be considered, to avoid delivering treatment during atrial fibrillation.

Treatment considerations: The problem here is to deliver therapy quickly (because VT produces hemodynamic compromise), while trying to avoid inappropriate therapy for atrial fibrillation. Since VT is moderately responsive to ATP, one might consider a "quick burst" of ATP (with a tiered-therapy device) before defaulting to a shock. To avoid delivering an inappropriate shock for atrial fibrillation, there is some chance that the rate will transiently fall below detection parameters during the "second look." Aggressive usage of atrioventricular nodal blocking drugs, or even atrioventricular nodal ablation, should be considered.

Case 6: Patient with multiple VTs

Case: A 69-year-old man with prior myocardial infarction, left ventricular ejection fraction of 0.30, presents with sustained VT at a rate of 170 beats per minute that is poorly tolerated. During electrophysiologic testing, clinical VT is inducible, and while it responds reasonably well to ATP, the VT is poorly tolerated. In addition, a second VT is occasionally inducible. This second VT is slower (130 beats per minute), well tolerated, and terminable with ATP, but usually only after multiple attempts. The peak sinus rate is 140 beats per minute.

Detection considerations: To avoid inappropriate therapy for sinus tachycardia, using the sudden onset parameter should be considered.

Treatment considerations: This patient would seem to be a candidate for a tiered-therapy device that can be set up with three different zones of therapy. Zone 1 would be for the slower VT and would utilize multiple attempts at ATP. (It is in zone 1 that sudden onset should be considered as a detection enhancement). Zone 2 would be for the faster VT, and therapy might consist of a "quick burst" of ATP, and then defaulting immediately to shocks. Zone 3, of course, is the VF zone.

Case 7: Patient with poor tolerance of ATP

Case: A 73-year-old female with prior myocardial infarction, left ventricular ejection fraction 0.25, presenting with well-tolerated sustained VT at rates of 130–140 beats per minute. Peak sinus rate is 120 beats per minute. During preoperative testing, the patient's VT was virtually always terminable by ATP, but several attempts were often required, and terminating the VT required relatively long bursts (15–20 beats) at relatively rapid rates (> 200 beats per minute). During the bursts themselves, the patient became symptomatic from hypotension.

Detection considerations: Since the peak sinus rate is slower than the VT, rate-only detection should be used (see below).

Treatment considerations: This case presents a rare instance in which redetection of VT between episodes of VT becomes important. In this patient, the VT itself was well tolerated, but ATP produced hemodynamic compromise. Antitachycardia pacing delivered in rapid succession might cause serious hemodynamic compromise, even while the rate of the VT is unchanged. Some tiered-therapy devices (PRx and Cadence) have a fixed (nonprogrammable) redetection interval that in patients such as this, might present a significant problem. With some other tiered-therapy devices (PCD), redetection is indirectly programmable, in that the criteria for redetection are the same as for initial detection. Thus, redetection of VT can be delayed by setting the device up to require a large number of intervals above the rate cutoff before diagnosing VT (thus also increasing the amount of time between bursts of ATP). In this patient, selecting the appropriate tiered-therapy device is critical.

Case 8: Frequent sustained VT

Case: A 50-year-old man with prior aortic valve replacement and moderate left ventricular dysfunction (ejection fraction = 0.38), presents with frequent sustained VT (at least daily episodes of VT lasting up to 15 minutes), with rates of 200 beats per minute, causing significant light-headedness, but no loss of consciousness. Ventricular tachycardia persists despite therapy with high-dose amiodarone in combination with several other drugs. The VT is moderately amenable to ATP. Peak sinus rate 160 beats per minute.

Detection considerations: Rate-only criteria should be used.

Treatment considerations: In general, unless an ATP scheme can be found which almost always (> 90%) terminates VT, or unless extremely low-energy shocks can be shown to terminate the VT painlessly and reliably, then some therapy other than ICD therapy (such as surgical or catheter ablation) should be strenuously sought in this patient. In this patient an ICD will almost certainly result in frequent shocks that are likely to be entirely intolerable. This case is an illustration of the fact that there are some patients in whom ICD therapy is simply inappropriate.

Summary

As is evident from the foregoing explanations and these illustrative cases, programming ICDs can, for some patients, represent a formidable challenge. Once it has been determined whether a patient requires a shock-only device or one offering multiple therapies, the detection enhancements must be selected with great care to assure above all that no VT/VF episodes are missed or detected late. At the same time, to maximize patient comfort (and preserve device longevity), the detection enhancements should be fine-tuned to minimize inappropriate detections, in particular for atrial fibrillation with rapid ventricular conduction. The concomitant use of antiarrhythmic drugs and/or β blockers can facilitate the programming of the detection parameters, but can also complicate the process; therefore, retesting after any changes in drugs is highly recommended. Once VT/VF sensing is adequately programmed, the task of programming therapy is somewhat easier. The latter depends primarily on the patient's observed response to the therapy options ATP and/or low-energy cardioversion. In cases where there is no response (or patient is noninducible, making testing of ATP impossible), the patient will generally be better off with shocks only, or at most brief attempts at ATP/low-energy cardioversion quickly defaulting to shocks. For those patients responding to ATP and/or low-energy cardioversion, the critical question is their hemodynamic tolerance, which in turn determines how aggressive and how long these "painless" therapies can be attempted before reversion once again to defibrillation shocks.

References

1. Ip J, Winters S, Schweitzer P, et al: Determinants of pace-terminable ventricular tachycardia: implications for implantable antitachycardia devices. *PACE* 14:1777, 1991.
2. Naccarelli G, Zipes D, Rahilly G, et al: Influence of tachycardia cycle length and antiarrhythmic drugs on pacing termination and acceleration of ventricular tachycardia. *Am Heart J* 105:1, 1983.
3. Roy D, Waxman H, Buxton A, et al: Termination of ventricular tachycardia: role of tachycardia cycle length. *Am J Cardiol* 50:1346, 1982.
4. Gottlieb C, Powers M, Kay H, et al: Efficacy and safety of the implantable defibrillator's programmable functions (abstract). *PACE* 13:518, 1990.
5. McVeigh K, Mower M, Nisam S, et al: Clinical efficacy of low-energy cardioversion in automatic implantable cardioverter defibrillator patients. *PACE* 14(II):1846, 1991.
6. Prystowsky E: Antiarrhythmic drug therapy as an adjunct or alternative to an implantable cardioverter defibrillator. *PACE* 15:678, 1992.
7. Wietholt D, Block M, Isbruch F, et al: Clinical experience with antitachycardia pacing and improved detection algorithms in a new implantable cardioverter/defibrillator. *J Am Coll Cardiol* 21(4):885, 1993.
8. Sowton E, Sulke N: Clinical experience with

the Siemens Pacesetter Siecure. *J Cardiovasc Electrophysiol* 3:515, 1992.
9. Davies W. Personal communication. St. Mary's Hospital, London, UK.
10. Farrugia S, Yee H, Nickolls P: Implantable cardioverter defibrillator electrogram recognition with a multilayer perceptron. *PACE* 16:228, 1993.
11. Chiang C-M, Jenkins J, DiCarlo L, et al: Real-time arrhythmia identification from automated analysis of intraatrial and intraventricular electrograms. *PACE* 16:223, 1993.
12. *PRx Physicians' Manual*. Cardiac Pacemakers, Inc., St. Paul, MN, 1991.
13. Winkle R, Stinson E, Bach S, et al: Cardioversion/defibrillation thresholds in man using a truncated exponential waveform and an apical patch-SVC spring electrode configuration. *Circulation* 69:766, 1984.
14. Singer I, van der Laken, Edmonds H, et al: Is defibrillation testing safe? In: Proceeding of IXth World Symposium on Cardiac Pacing and Electrophysiology. *PACE* 14(11):1899, 1991.
15. Echt D, Barbey J, Black J: Influence of ventricular fibrillation duration on defibrillation energy in dogs using bidirectional pulse discharges. *PACE* 11:1315, 1988.
16. Winkle R, Mead R, Ruder M, et al: Effect of duration of ventricular fibrillation on defibrillation efficacy in humans. *Circulation* 81:1477, 1990.

Chapter 23

Clinical Results: An Overview

Igor Singer

Since the introduction of the implantable cardioverter-defibrillator (ICD) to clinical practice in February 1980, many important advances in technology have occurred at a breathtaking pace. The original device (AID™, Intec, Pittsburgh, PA), a nonprogrammable defibrillator designed to treat ventricular fibrillation (VF) and sinusoidal ventricular tachycardia (VT), evolved into a nonprogrammable device capable of treating VT and VF (AID B™ and AID C™) with additional rate sensing electrode(s) added for improved detection and discrimination of VT. The initial clinical performance of these devices, despite their nonprogrammability was impressive.[1] The device manufacturing techniques have also evolved. Integrated circuit technology has replaced the individual component manufacture, and nonprogrammable devices were superseded by ICDs with limited programming capabilities (Ventak™ 1550, 1555, 1600, CPI, St. Paul, MN).

As other manufacturers entered ICD research and development, the pace of technological advances quickened. Recognition of the effectiveness of antitachycardia pacing (ATP) for termination of monomorphic stable VT led to incorporation of ATP and bradycardia pacing capabilities into the next generation of devices, with the emergence of tiered-therapy strategies (Cadence™, Ventritex, Sunnyvale, CA; PCD™, Medtronic, Minneapolis, MN; and other devices still undergoing clinical trials). It was also recognized that multiprogrammability of detection and therapy algorithms is essential to optimize and individualize therapy. Equally important was the ability to acquire data about arrhythmia history and efficacy of therapy, so that the therapy could be individualized and enhanced and the troubleshooting of problems simplified. Consequently, the so-called third-generation devices now incorporate these capabilities to a greater or a lesser extent (see also Chapters 9, 12, and 22).

Another evolution paralleled the advances in technology and therapy. Mirowski's original concept was to have an implantable device with a transvenous catheter capable of treating VT and VF. Although the original design envisioned a transvenous catheter coupled to the ICD, its development was delayed by technical and clinical issues. Nevertheless, a totally implantable system is now a reality and a transvenous lead system (Endotak™, CPI, St. Paul, MN) has been approved by the Food and Drug Administration (FDA) for clinical use. More recently, the Transvene™ lead system (Medtronic, Minneapolis, MN) was also approved for clinical use in the United States. Other transvenous lead systems may follow in the near future.

From Singer I, (ed.) Implantable Cardioverter-Defibrillator. Armonk, NY: Futura Publishing Company, Inc.; © 1994.

With advances in technology and implantation techniques, the acceptance of the ICD and the enthusiasm for its use have grown. The indications for ICD use have expanded from the original, deliberately chosen stringent requirements, where the device was used as the last resort, to the point where its use is contemplated early in the therapeutic cascade. Indeed, the ICD has become the gold standard for therapy of aborted sudden cardiac death against which other therapies are now compared.[2] The use of the ICD for primary prevention of sudden cardiac death is seriously contemplated[3] and a number of prospective clinical trials are in progress to evaluate this application (see Chapter 26).[4]

Although a variety of devices are currently in use, some commercially available, others investigational, the largest available clinical database comes from a single clinical manufacturer database, CPI, St. Paul, MN. As of the last published report (June 2, 1992) more than 25,000 patients have been entered into the database. These data were summarized and presented by Nisam et al.[5] As of the time of this writing, although the absolute number of implants have increased, the data regarding ICD results have remained substantially unchanged and are consistent with those previously reported.[6] Although these data have been criticized by skeptics as incomplete or possibly biased, the data are in remarkable agreement with the largest published clinical databases from independent clinical investigators, substantiating its overall accuracy and objectivity.[7,8]

The clinical results are reviewed in light of the available data and with regard to the improvements in the device and leads technology.

Results With Thoracotomy Lead Systems

With expanding indications for ICD use, it is important to examine whether the patient populations treated with ICD therapy has changed. Table 1, adapted from Nisam et al.[5] provides an overview of the characteristics of patients who underwent the implantation of ICD from some of the largest series reported in the literature.[7-19] As Nisam et al.[5] points out, despite a substantial institutional differences in treatment strategy, there is a remarkable lack of divergence between the earlier and the more recent data. A single exception to this conclusion is the overall difference in the patient selection with respect to the primary presentation. More recent implantees are older than in the earlier series, with less prevalence of aborted sudden cardiac death as the primary indication. The availability of tiered therapy and ATP has probably contributed to the earlier use of the ICD for patients presenting with pace-terminable monomorphic VTs.

Figure 1 shows the survival of patients with three generations of devices. The actuarial 1-year freedom from all cause mortality was 92.8%, 92.9% and 90.7%, respectively, for the Ventak, Ventak-P, and PRx™ (CPI, St. Paul, MN) series of devices.[5] Since all of these devices were implanted by thoracotomy, it is reasonable to assume that with the endocardial leads (nonthoracotomy lead systems), the causes of mortality may improve even further, due to a reduction in the perioperative morbidity and mortality. Figure 2 shows the actuarial patient survival for 22,798 patients with implanted CPI ICDs. Results from two of the largest reported clinical series are plotted on the same graph.[7,20] Although there is minor divergence in the results (from years 2–5) between the reported series and the CPI database, the results of these independent series are very similar. The somewhat larger number of deaths in the two clinical series compared to the CPI database is likely due to the underreporting of the late deaths to the manufacturer. Nevertheless, the survival from all cause mortality at 5 years in the clinically reported series is approximately 75%.

While the reported results are impres-

Table 1*
Patient Characteristics from Major ICD Series

	1988 or Earlier							1989–1992				
Author	Mirowski[9]	AID™/B/BR[10]	Echt[11]	Tchou[12]	Thomas[12]	Kelly[14]	Winkle[7]	Klein[15]	Ventak P™[16]	Nisam[17]	Akhtar[8]	Ventak™/PRx™[18]
N (Patients)	52	323	70	70	3610	94	270	120	292	9807	300	372
Year Published	1983	1985	1985	1988	1988	1988	1989	1990	1990	1991	1992	1992
% Males	71.2	80.8	78.6	72.9	80.4	76.6	80.4	90.9	78.8	80.7	80.0	86.0
Mean Age (Years)	52.0	66.0	54.0	59.7	59.0	58.6	58.2	57.0	61.5	60.9	61.9	63.6
% Mean EF	33.7	33.0		36.7	32.8	33.0	34.0	29.0	34.0	33.0	34.3	31.5
% Cad	67.3	74.6	68.6	76.0	76.7	64.9	78.2	72.5	78.4	75.3	79.0	78.2
% Concomitant AARx	—	—	68.6	59.4	64.0	49.0	68.9	61.0	66.4	55.1	44.0	61.6
% Concomitant Surgery (most often CABG)	28.8	—	25.7	22.9	18.8	11.7	30.0	25.0	16.0	20.3	—	13.2
VF or VT/VF (%)	100.0	—	54.3	77.0	64.7	54.3	80	59.2	41.4	—	—	17.2
Average No. Cardiac Arrests	3.9	—	1.9	—	—	—	1.5	115 had previous CA	168 had previous CA	—	—	—
Mean No. of Drug Failures	—	—	4.0	3.1	—	—	3.4	3.4	—	—	2.6	—

— Taken from earlier series (N = 200) from same authors.

EF: left ventricular ejection fraction; CAD: coronary artery disease; AARx: antiarrhythmic drug therapy; CABG: coronary artery bypass graft; VF: ventricular fibrillation; VT: ventricular tachycardia.

(* Reproduced with permission from Reference 5.)

sive, it must be acknowledged that these results cannot be compared to a control group treated by the available alternative therapeutic modalities, for example, antiarrhythmic drugs. In fact, a large number of patients with implanted ICDs are also concurrently treated with antiarrhythmic drugs, a trend that is likely to continue. While most independent observers and investigators acknowledge the ICD effectiveness in reducing sudden cardiac death rates, in most clinical studies to less than 3% to 8% at 1 and 3 years, respectively,[1,7,12,21–23] skeptics have questioned the magnitude of the ICDs contribution to the overall survival.[24–26] Randomized controlled studies comparing

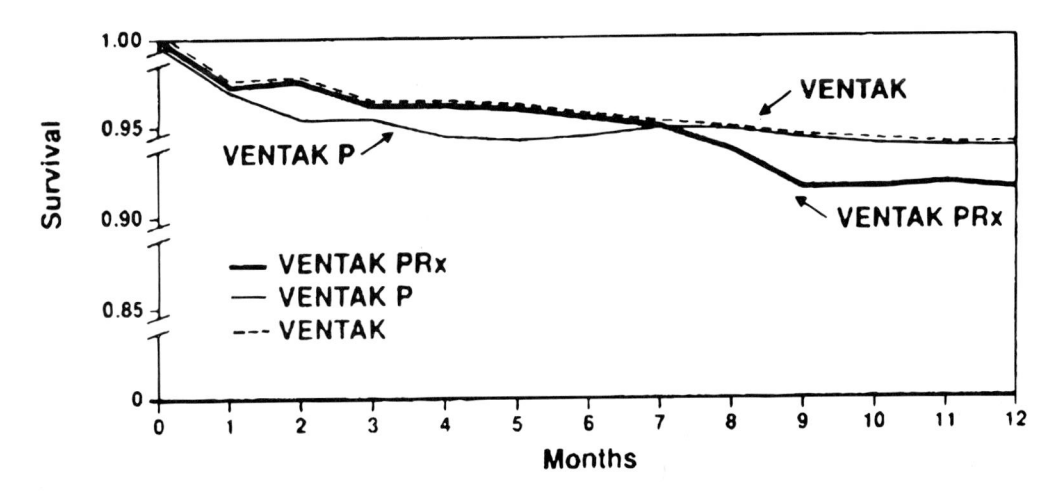

Figure 1. Survival of patients with three generations of devices. (Reprinted with permission from Reference 5.)

AICD SURVIVAL
Freedom From All Causes of Mortality

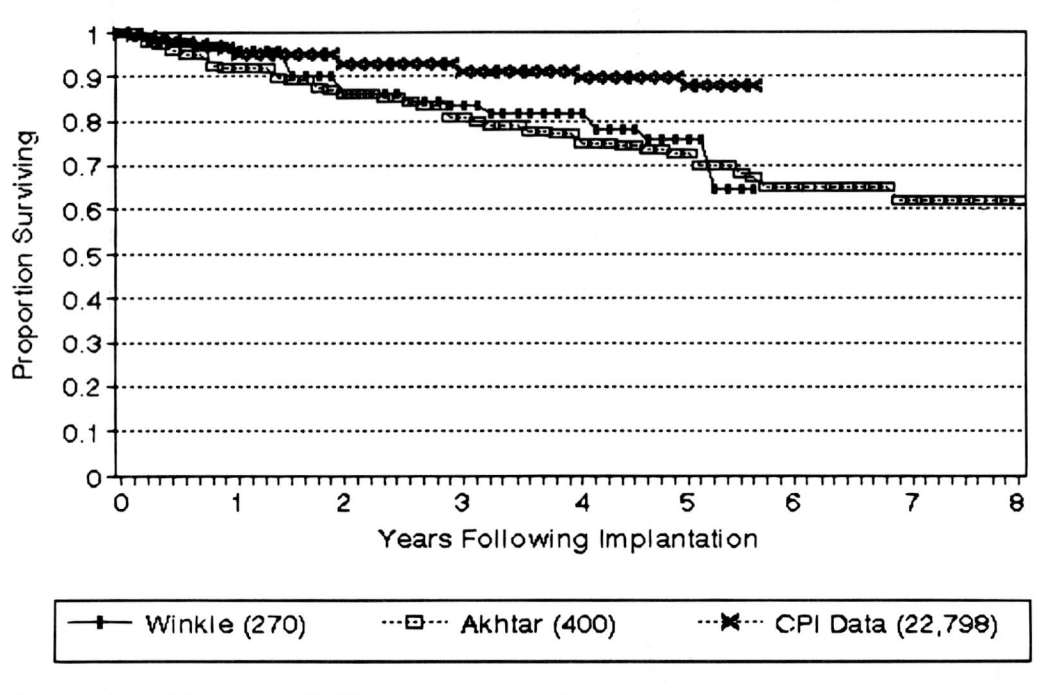

Figure 2. Actuarial survival of 22,798 patients with implanted CPI (St. Paul, MN) implantable cardioverter defibrillators (ICDs) compared to two of the largest reported series in the literature. (Reprinted with permission from Reference 5.)

the ICD to other therapies were not done because in the early days of ICD development, even the concept itself was called into question, precluding a fair and unbiased comparison of this, then a revolutionary concept, and the accepted therapeutic norms. A number of such clinical trials are currently ongoing in an attempt to address this important question (see Chapter 26).

Despite the controversy regarding the magnitude of reduction in mortality due to the therapeutic benefits of the device, the efficacy of the ICD in terminating VT and VF is unquestioned. Although it should be obvious that despite near-elimination of sudden death by implantation of ICDs the mortality benefit will be limited by the concurrent competing cardiac risks such as the extent of the left ventricular dysfunction, persistent unrelieved ischemia, and other cardiovascular and noncardiovascular pathologies, some skeptics continue to question the relative value of the ICD in reduction of overall mortality.

In the absence of randomized studies, the influence of ICD therapy on survival has been examined by direct mortality comparisons between patients who received ICDs and a control population who did not, or by inferred benefit based on the "appropriate" ICD shock, presumed to have been the lifesaving shock. There are potential methodological pitfalls with both methods. The first is handicapped by the definition of a control group, which must be defined retrospectively, and the second is handicapped by the presumption that the shocks are in fact "appropriate," because the earlier devices lacked the documentation of the causative arrhythmia. The second assumption, that had the shock not been delivered the patient would have died, is also inappropriate. We know that not all ventricular tachyarrhythmias result in death, and a number of VT episodes terminate spontaneously or are aborted by medical or other therapeutic intervention. Nevertheless, it is instructive to review the published series that have attempted to separate the ICD survival benefit to an alternative therapy, by comparing the ICD-treated patients to a comparable control group.

Three published series have compared survival of patients with implanted ICDs and a control population. Fogoros et al.[21] compared the survival of 21 patients with drug-refractory symptomatic VT who presented with cardiac arrest or syncope and received ICD and amiodarone with 29 patients treated with amiodarone alone (due to the unavailability of devices), and a group of 28 patients with less symptomatic VT (no syncope) also treated with amiodarone. There were no significant differences between these groups for age, mean left ventricular ejection fraction, gender, the baseline electrophysiologic characteristics (except for the shorter VT cycle length for the first two groups), or arrhythmia recurrence during follow-up. After 2-years follow-up, the sudden cardiac death and total mortality rates were 0% and 5% for the ICD patients compared with 24% and 37% for the non-ICD treated patients. The results for the patients who did not present with syncope or aborted sudden death and were treated with amiodarone were somewhat better than the former amiodarone-treated group; 4% and 19% for sudden and overall mortality, respectively.

Newman et al.[27] used a carefully matched retrospectively defined control group from the same institution to compare a population of patients who presented with aborted sudden cardiac death or with sustained VT. Sixty patients who received ICDs were matched to two historical control patients each, a total of 120 patients. The variables matched were age, type of underlying cardiac disease, ejection fraction, and antiarrhythmic drug therapy (amiodarone). Survival estimates were matched from the time that the ICD was implanted (the study group), to the hypothetical time that the device would have been implanted in the control group (arrhythmia recurrence or discontinuation of amiodarone therapy due to serious side effects or toxicity). The analysis included the operative mortality in the ICD group. Actuarial survival demonstrated a survival benefit for the ICD group (89% compared to 72% for the first year, and 65% versus 49% the third year). Total sudden deaths were reduced 50% and the third-year mortality was reduced 31% with the ICD therapy. The conferred survival advantage disappeared over time as the two survival curves converged by 40 months. This convergence in the survival may be explained by the emergence of the nonsudden deaths in the ICD-treated group over time, ie, that when there are two concurrent competing risks, arrhythmia and heart failure, the overall benefit of arrhythmic survival will eventually be overshadowed by the heart failure risk. This is entirely to be expected and does not invalidate the early survival benefit conferred by ICD therapy.

A more recent study has retrospectively compared the long-term outcomes of ICD therapy versus electrophysiologically guided antiarrhythmic drug therapy in 331 survivors of out-of-hospital cardiac arrest.[28] One hundred and fifty patients were treated with an ICD and 181 patients with drug therapy. The two groups were dissimilar with respect to the left ventricular ejection fraction (ICD group: 35% versus non-ICD group: 45%) and the lower revascularization rates for the ICD group (22% versus 37%). A multivariate analysis identified absence of ICD as a significant predictor of cardiac mortality (a relative mortality risk of 2.7) and a marginally significant predictor of overall mortality (relative risk of 2.27). Implantable cardioverter-defibrillators conferred a survival benefit in patients with ejection fractions of > 39% at 5 years (96% compared to 82%), but not at 1 or 3 years. For patients with ejection fraction of < 40%, treatment with ICDs conferred a survival benefit at 1 (94% versus 86%) and 5 (64% versus 43%) years, compared to the patients with drug suppressible arrhythmias not treated with an ICD. Patients with inducible arrhythmias not suppressed by antiarrhythmic therapy who did not receive an ICD did worse than the patients with ICD or the patients with drug suppressible arrhythmias, irrespective of the ejection fraction.

Several studies have attempted to measure the survival benefit of the ICD by comparing the presumed survival benefit based upon a true positive shock, which otherwise might have resulted in the patients death from VT or VF. This approach has several limitations that have already been discussed. For example, Fogoros et al.[22] analyzed the survival of 119 patients with drug-refractory VT or VF who had ICDs implanted. Eighteen percent of patients (7 of 40) with ejection fractions < 30% had at least one appropriate shock and died a mean of 11 months after the shock, compared to patients with ejection fractions > 29%, 4% (3 of 79) of whom died a mean of 42 months after the initial shock.

Bocker et al.[28] analyzed the survival of 107 patients treated with third-generation ICDs capable of storing intracardiac electrograms or tachycardia cycle lengths prior to therapy. Thus, this analysis restricts the estimation of the survival benefit to documented fast tachycardia. These investigators estimated the survival benefit from the difference between total mortality and the fast VT (> 240 beats per minute) that most likely would have been fatal without the ICD intervention. Actuarial survival rate at 6, 12, and 18 months was 100% for sudden death, and 97% for nonsudden arrhythmia-related death. In contrast, the actuarial survival rate for fast VT at 6, 12, and 18 months was 83%, 74%, and 69%, respectively. Therefore, the estimated survival benefit was 14%, 23%, and 28% at 6, 12, and 18 months.

The most powerful predictor of survival is the left ventricular ejection fraction, independent of whether the ICD shocks were received by the patient.[29–31] The true measure of the survival benefit resulting from a lifesaving shock for VT or VF is difficult to measure accurately with these historically and methodologically handicapped studies. Inclusion of patients at high risk of nonsudden cardiac death (for example advanced heart failure or incomplete revascularization) will dilute the survival benefit of the ICD due to the competing risk of heart failure or ischemia. For ICD benefit to be assessed appropriately, the nonsudden risk must be reasonable, and the duration of follow-up sufficient to measure the benefit. Prospective randomized trials underway, may shed further light on this otherwise waxing intellectual dilemma.

Clinical Results With Endocardial Lead Systems

The clinical efficacy of thoracotomy lead systems has been established in the clinical trials over the past decade. The controversy regarding the overall impact of ICD therapy on survival notwithstanding, the success in terminating VF and VT by the implanted ICDs is unquestioned. The new generation of lead systems are designed to be implanted transvenously, as originally conceived by Mirowski, thus precluding the requirement for thoracotomy. The first such system approved for the clinical use is the Endotak lead system. The Endotak lead is a 100-cm long, tined endocardial lead that combines bipolar rate sensing and defibrillation in a single lead. A porous tip functions as the rate-sensing cathode; a right ventricular spring electrode serves as both the shocking cathode and the rate-sensing anode; and a superior vena cava spring electrode serves as a defibrillation anode. The endocardial lead may be combined with a subcutaneous patch electrode, by using a Y connector to provide additional lead configurations and to provide improvements in the defibrillation efficacy.

Prior to the FDA submission of the therapeutic efficacy of this lead system,

1,652 patients were tested, and of these, 1,393 patients were implanted with the Endotak lead system in one of four standard configurations. For the latter part of the study, 91.2% of patients were implanted with this lead system.[32] At implant, 48.2% of patients received concomitant antiarrhythmic therapy. The profile of the patient population with respect to the clinical variables such as age, gender, underlying cardiac disease, and left ventricular function was otherwise similar to the previous thoracotomy lead system ICD series. The defibrillation threshold (DFT) protocol used for testing is shown in Figure 3. Long-term implantation of the lead system was permitted only for patients who met the protocol DFT requirements. The four lead configurations tested are shown in Figure 4. Figure 5 summarizes the DFT testing performed in each of the Endotak lead configurations for all patients tested. Figure 6 summarizes the overall efficacy of the four lead configurations.

The sudden cardiac death actuarial survival rate at 12 months is presented in Table 2. The survival of the Endotak population is compared to patients implanted during the clinical investigation of CPI Ventak P model 1600 AICD™ (CPI, St. Paul, MN)

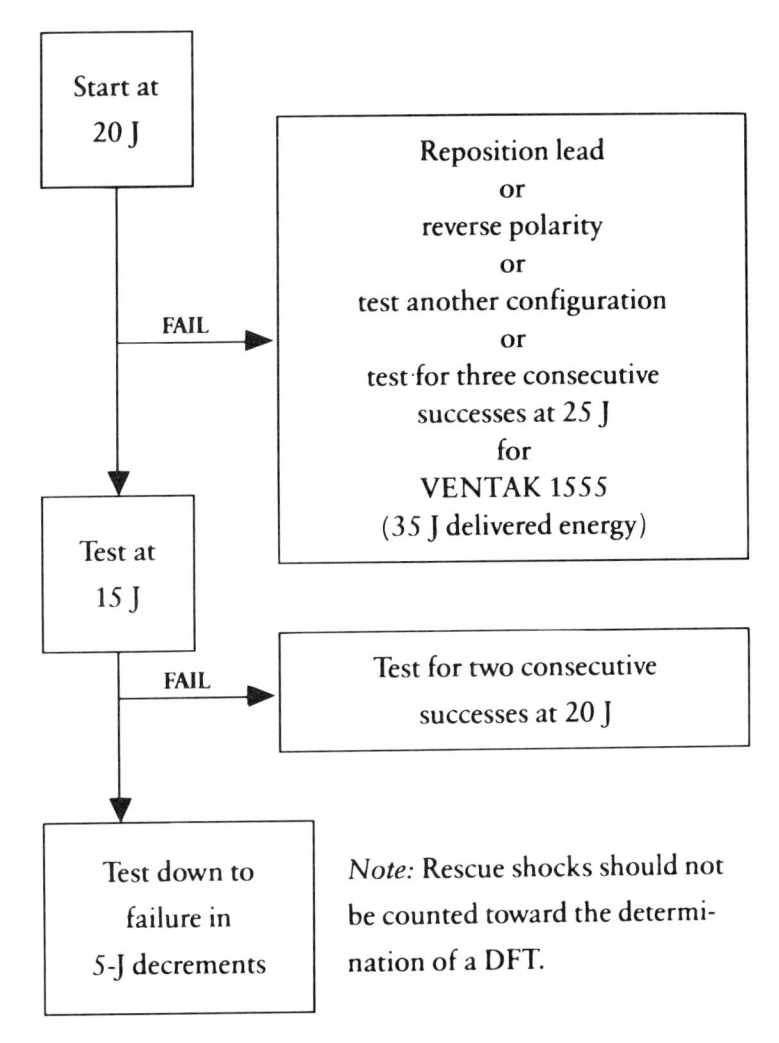

Figure 3. Protocol defibrillation threshold (DFT) testing flow chart. (Reprinted with permission from Reference 32.)

A

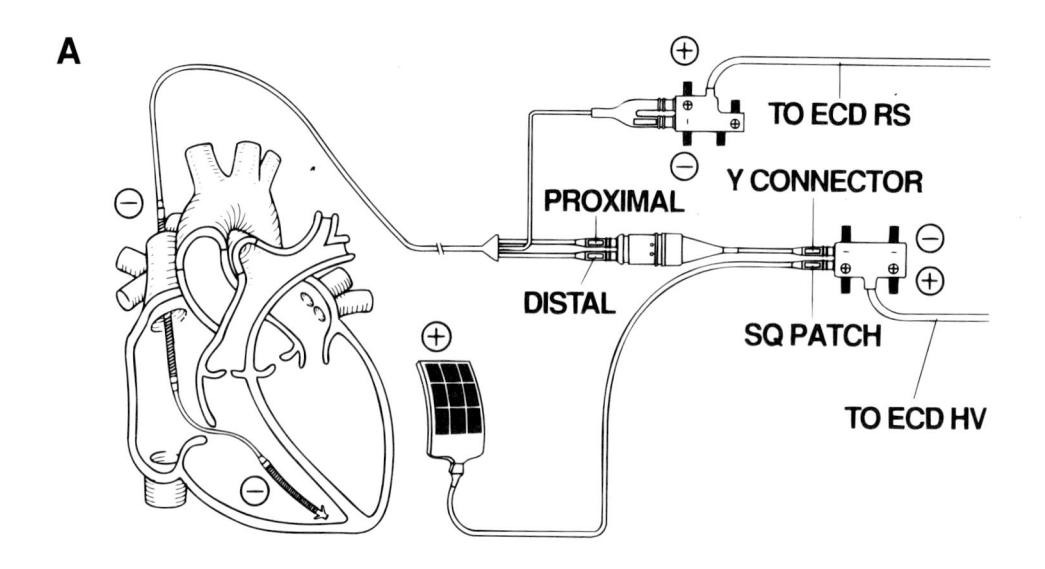

Horizontal (Configuration 1)

ENDOTAK C proximal and distal spring electrode connected together as cathode (−) to the ENDOTAK SQ patch as anode (+)

Orthogonal (Configuration 2)

ENDOTAK C distal electrode as cathode (−) to ENDOTAK C proximal spring electrode and ENDOTAK SQ connected together as anode (+)

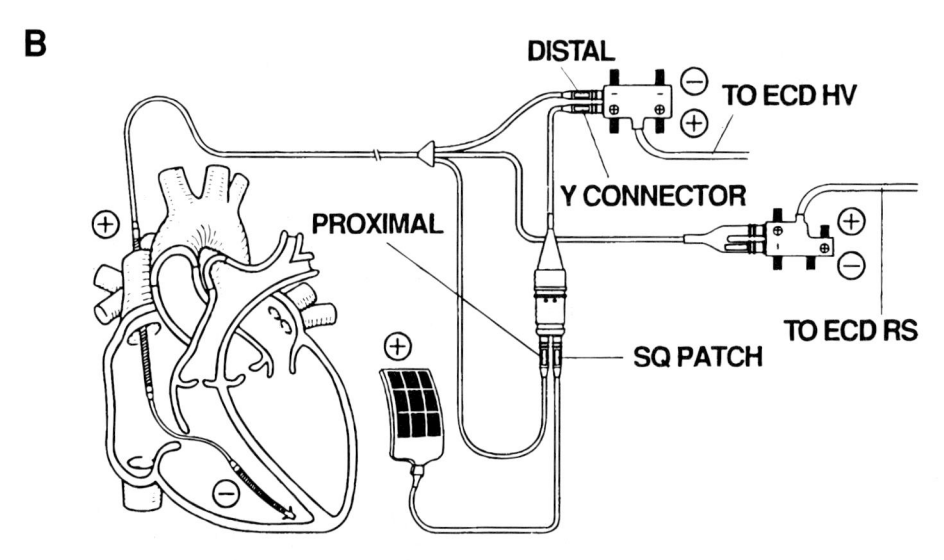

B

Figure 4. The Endotak™ (CPI, St. Paul, MN) lead configurations (panels A to D). (Reprinted with permission from Reference 32.)

C Lead Only (Configuration 3)

ENDOTAK C alone, distal spring as cathode (−), proximal spring as anode (+)

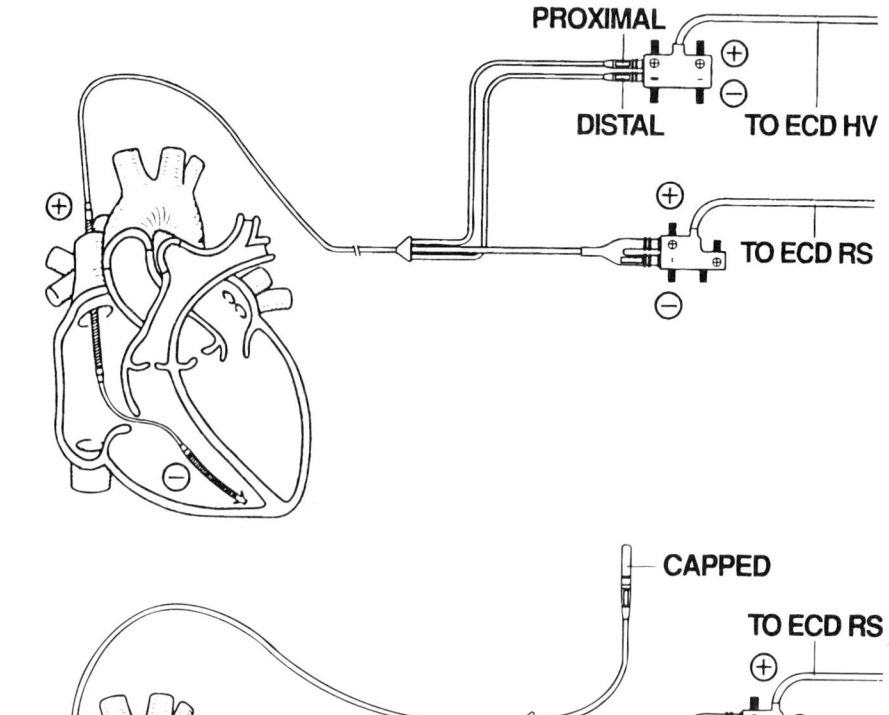

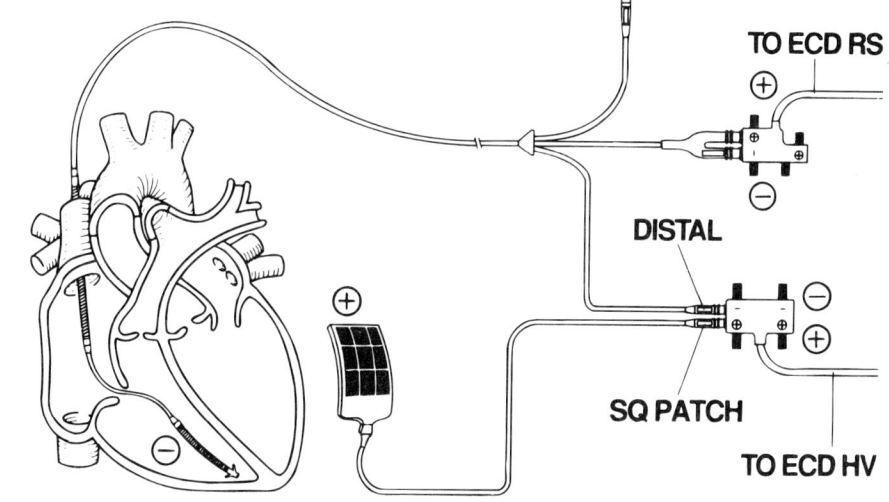

D

Parallel (Configuration 4)

ENDOTAK C distal spring electrode as cathode (−) to ENDOTAK SQ as anode (+)

Figure 4. *(Continued)*

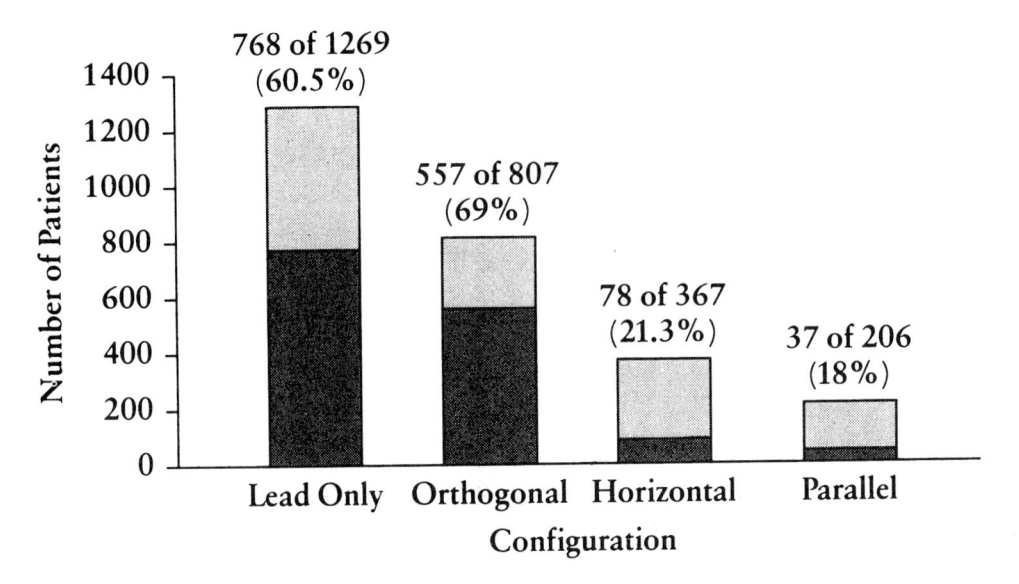

Figure 5. Defibrillation threshold testing by configuration. (Reprinted with permission from Reference 32.)

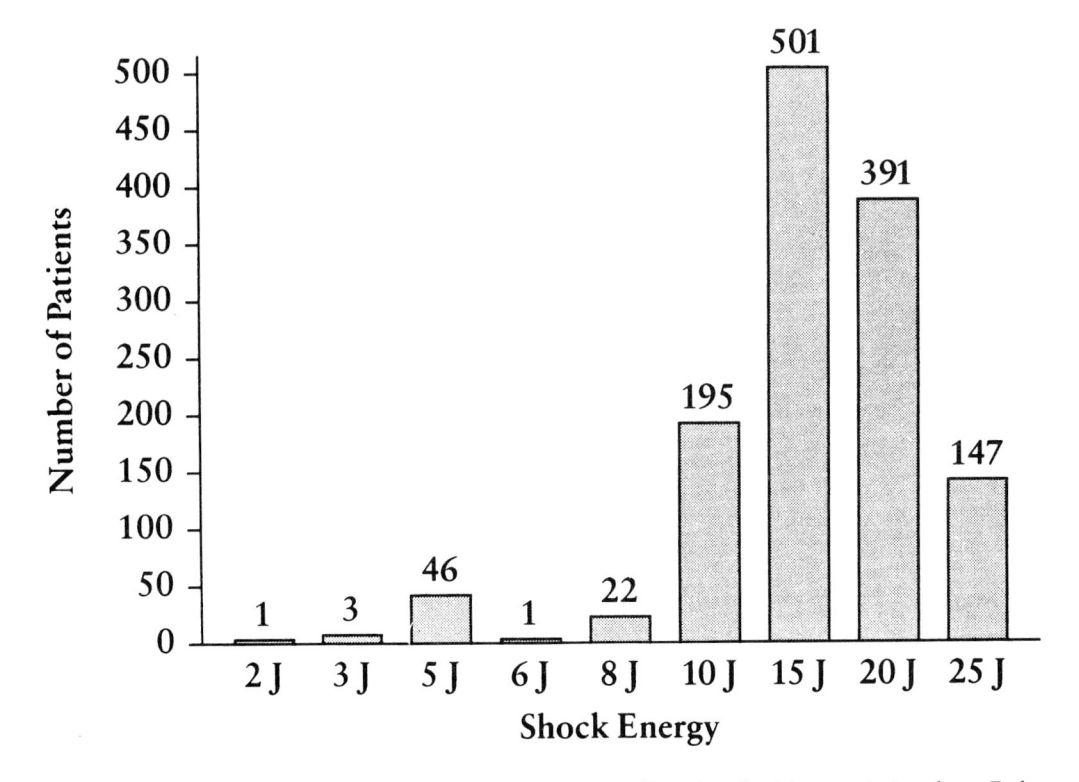

Figure 6. Lowest defibrillation energy, any configuration. (Reprinted with permission from Reference 32.)

Table 2
Patient Survival at 12 Months*

Patient Survival	Endotak™ Population	Comparison Group
Sudden cardiac death survival	98.7%	98.6%
Non sudden cardiac death survival	96.8%	96.7%
Total cardiac death survival	95.5%	95.3%
Total death survival	93/9%	90.7%

(* Reproduced with permission from Reference 32.)

Table 3*
Clinical Observations Related to Morbidity
(N = 1393)

Observation	Number	Implants (%)
Infection	28	2.0
Hematoma	6	0.4
Fluid accumulation	4	0.3
AICD™ pocket erosion	2	0.1
Cerebral vascular accident	2	0.1
Postshock asystole	2	0.1
Syncope	1	0.07
Muscle tear	1	0.07
Pneumothorax	1	0.07
Psychological problems	1	0.07
Pulmonary embolus	1	0.07
RV perforation	1	0.07
Increased ectopy	1	0.07
Left subclavian vein thrombosis	1	0.07
Swelling in area of SQ patch	1	0.07
Transient ischemic attacks	1	0.07
Endotak C™ lead inadvertently in the coronary sinus	1	0.07
Poor pocket healing	1	0.07
SQ patch erosion/torn patch	1	0.07
SQ patch folded	1	0.07
SQ patch crinkled	1	0.07
Blurring of left eye	1	0.07
Pressure of superficial skin from excess C lead (no strain relief loop)	1	0.07
Total observations	62	4.5

(* Reproduced with permission from Reference 32.)

pulse generator with epicardial patches (n = 292). There were no significant differences in either sudden or total cardiac survival between the two groups.

The operative mortality for the Endotak population was found to be 1% compared to that observed for the comparison group, which was 2.7%. The incidence of morbidity related to the Endotak was also significantly lower than the morbidity for the Ventak P 1600 control population with epicardial patches, which was 7.8%.[32] The observed morbidity is summarized in Table 3.

Another transvenous lead system, Transvene, has undergone extensive clinical trials and has received FDA approval for clinical use in the United States. As of June 11, 1993, 757 patients received the Transvene lead system. The patient profile in most respects was similar to the patient population implanted with the Ventak 1600 devices (the retrospective control group).[33] The lead system differs from the Endotak lead in that the cathodal and the anodal defibrillation coils are located on two separate leads, the superior vena caval lead and the right ventricular (RV) endocardial lead. The RV also has the sensing bipolar electrodes located at its distal end. The sensing is accomplished from the bipolar distal lead, and is therefore truly bipolar, while the pacing is accomplished between the cathodal tip and the common electrode. The presence of two endocardial electrodes provides a greater flexibility in lead location. For example, the RV electrode might be positioned in the outflow tract or in a less typical right ventricular location, as dictated by the clinical needs. Similarly, the second electrode is positioned in the superior vena cava and a third electrode may be positioned in the coronary sinus. An additional subcutaneous patch electrode may be used with this lead system. The frequency with which the various lead configurations were used during the clinical trials and the relative defibrillation thresholds (DFTs) achieved are presented in Table 4.

The overall efficacy for treating sponta-

Table 4*

PCD™ Transvene System Mean LED and DFT Values

Lead System	Implant Frequency	Mean LED	Implant Frequency	Mean DFT
Total Systems	702	16.0 J	316	14.8 J
RV-SVC-SQ	455	16.7 J	187	15.8 J
RV-CS-SQ	210	14.6 J	110	12.8 J
RV-CS-SVC	37	37	19	16.0 J

LED: lowest energy defibrillation; DFT: defibrillation threshold.
(* Reproduced with permission from Reference 33.)

neous VT/VF episodes was 98.4% in over 10,000 documented episodes. The perioperative mortality was 0.7% (5 of 757 patients) compared to 5.3% mortality for the epicardial leads patients with PCD (39 of 742).[33] One-year actuarial survival for all causes is summarized in Table 5.

The comparison of the Transvene data to a reference Ventak epicardial system patient population presented in the PMA summary to the FDA on May 2, 1991 is presented in Table 5.[33] The Transvene patient population did not differ significantly in the baseline patient characteristics from the Ventak patient population. The sudden cardiac death survival and the overall survival are summarized in Table 6. The PCD Transvene system sudden cardiac death survival of 99.7% was comparable to that of Ventak at 1 year, and the actuarial survival

Table 5*

PCD™ Transvene System One Year Actuarial Survival

	Received a Transvene System (N = 757)	Screened for a Transvene™ System (N = 854)
Sudden Cardiac Death	99.5%	99.4%
Nonsudden Cardiac	96.2%	96.6%
All Cardiac	95.8%	96.1%
Noncardiac	98.1%	98.3%
Perioperative	0.7%	1.6%
Overall	93.3%	92.9%

(* Reproduced with permission from Reference 33.)

Table 6*

PCD™ Transvenous System Survival Comparison PCD versus Ventak-P™

	PCD™ Transvenous System	Ventak-P™ Epicardial System
Sudden Cardiac	99.7%	98.6%
Overall	94.2%	90.8%

(* Reproduced with permission from Reference 33.)

Table 7*

PCD™ Transvene System Reported Complications./Observations By Category—U.S. and International

Category	Complications Num (% of Pts) U.S.	Complications Num (% of Pts) Int'l	Observations Num (% of Pts) U.S.	Observations Num (% of Pts) Int'l
Increased defibrillation requirements	6(1.4%)	3(1.0%)	4(0.9%)	4(1.3%)
Inappropriate ventricular fibrillation therapy delivery	—	—	3(0.7%)	11(3.5%)
Inappropriate ventricular tachycardia therapy delivery	—	—	19(4.3%)	38(12.1%)
Loss of capture	4(0.9%)	2(0.6%)	4(0.9%)	9(2.9%)
Oversensing	—	—	31(7.0%)	21(6.7%)
Undersensing	—	—	—	—
Skin erosion	1(0.2%)	4(1.3%)	1(0.2%)	—
Pocket infection	12(2.7%)	12(3.8%)	7(1.6%)	3(1.0%)
Seroma	4(0.9%)	2(0.6%)	1(0.2%)	13(4.1%)
Hematoma	4(0.9%)	2(0.6%)	6(1.4%)	11(3.5%)
Pneumothorax	1(0.2%)	1(0.3%)	1(0.2%)	—
Pacemaker syndrome	—	—	2(0.5%)	—
Perforation	4(0.9%)	2(0.6%)	—	—
Subclavian vein thrombosis	1(0.2%)	—	2(0.5%)	1(0.3%)
Lead fracture	5(1.1%)	4(1.3%)	—	—
Subcutaneous patch crinkling	—	7(2.2%)	3(0.7%)	2(0.6%)
Early device explant	4(0.9%)	—	—	—
Total lead dislodgement	53(12.0%)	33(10.5%)	6(1.4%)	6(1.9%)
Total	99	72	90	119

(* Reproduced with permission from Reference 33.)

for all cause mortality was 94.2% compared to 90.8% for the Ventak series.[33]

Complications were reported in 19.4% of patients and were comparable to other market-released AICD systems in the categories of ineffective VT/VF therapy, pocket infection, and pocket erosion. The complications are summarized in Table 7.

These data indicate that the transvenous leads systems are associated with less perioperative morbidity and mortality, while the clinical efficacy is not compromised. Endocardial lead systems, therefore, lend themselves to implantation in patients who may otherwise be considered relatively poor candidates for thoracotomy. An additional benefit may be derived from earlier postoperative recovery period, lessened discomfort to the patient and earlier postsurgical discharge. These factors make the endocardial transvenous systems the first choice for most patients.

Conclusions

Implantable cardioverter-defibrillator therapy has evolved over a relatively short period of time from a relatively simple device to a considerably more complex system capable of dealing with a variety of arrhythmias. Furthermore, with the development of nonthoracotomy leads, the overall morbidity and mortality has been significantly reduced, to the point where these devices may be considered early in the therapeutic cascade for therapy of malignant ventricular tachycardia. The desirable object of any therapy is primary prevention. Similarly, the use of ICDs for primary prevention of sudden cardiac death should also be considered strongly. This application awaits the completion of the ongoing clinical trials comparing the ICD to no therapy in high-risk patients, or to another currently recognized alternative therapeutic modality.

References

1. Mirowski M, Reid P, Watkins L, et al: Clinical treatment of life-threatening ventricular tachyarrhythmias with the automatic implantable defibrillator. *Am Heart J* 102:265, 1981.
2. Lehmann M, Steinman R, Schuger C, et al: The automatic implantable cardioverter defibrillator as antiarrhythmic treatment modality of choice for survivors of cardiac arrest unrelated to acute myocardial infarction. *Am J Cardiol* 62:803, 1988.
3. Bigger JT: Should defibrillators be implanted in high-risk patients without a previous sustained ventricular tachyarrhythmia? In: *Implantable Cardioverter-Defibrillators*. Edited by G Naccarelli, E Veltri. Boston, MA: Blackwell Medical Publishers; 1993, p. 284.
4. Klein H, Troster J, Haverich A: AICD as a bridge to transplant (abstract). *Rev Eur Technol Biomed* 12:110, 1990.
5. Nisam S, Mower M, Thomas A, et al: Patient survival comparison in three generations of automatic implantable cardioverter defibrillators: review of 12 years, 25,000 patients. *PACE* 16(1):174, 1993.
6. MADIT Executive Committee: Multicenter Automatic Defibrillator Implantation Trial (MADIT): design and clinical protocol. *PACE* 14:920, 1991.
7. Winkle R, Mead R, Ruder M, et al: Long-term outcome with the automatic implantable cardioverter defibrillator. *J Am Coll Cardiol* 13:1353, 1989.
8. Akhtar M, Avitall B, Jazayeri M, et al: Role of implantable cardioverter defibrillator therapy in the management of high-risk patients. *Circulation* 85(1):I-131, 1992.
9. Mirowski M, Reid P, Winkle R, et al: Mortality in patients with implanted automatic defibrillators. *Ann Intern Med* 98:585, 1983.
10. *AID B/BR Clinical Report*. CPI Medical Records. St. Paul, MN. 1985.
11. Echt D, Armstrong K, Schmidt P, et al: Clinical experience, complications and survival in 70 patients with the automatic implantable cardioverter/defibrillator. *Circulation* 71:289, 1985.
12. Tchou P, Kadri N, Anderson J, et al: Automatic implantable cardioverter defibrillators and survival of patients with left ventricular dysfunction and malignant ventricular arrhythmias. *Ann Intern Med* 109:529, 1988.
13. Thomas A, Moser S, Smutka M, et al: Implantable defibrillation: eight years clinical experience. *PACE* 11(II):2053, 1988.
14. Kelly P, Canom D, Garan H, et al: The automatic implantable cardioverter defibrillator: efficacy, complications and survival in patients with malignant ventricular arrhythmias. *J Am Coll Cardiol* 11:1278, 1988.
15. Klein H, Troster J, Treppe H, et al: Derimplantierbare automatische Kardioverter-Defibrillator (AICD). *Herz Kardiovaskulare Erkrankungen* 15:111, 1990.
16. *Ventak P Clinical Report*. CPI Medical Records. St. Paul, MN. 1990.
17. Nisam S, Mower M, Moser S: ICD clinical update: first decade, initial 10,000 patients. *PACE* 14(II):255, 1991.
18. *Ventak PRx Clinical Report*. CPI Medical Records. St. Paul, MN. 1992.
19. Axtell K, Tchou P, Akhtar M: Survival in patients with depressed left ventricular function treated by automatic implantable cardioverter defibrillator. *PACE* 14:291, 1991.
20. Masood A: Personal communication. June 1992.
21. Fogoros RN, Fiedler SB, Elson JJ: The automatic implantable cardioverter-defibrillator in drug-refractory ventricular tachyarrhythmias. *Ann Intern Med* 107:635, 1987.
22. Fogoros RN, Elson JJ, Bonnet CA, et al: Efficacy of the automatic implantable cardioverter-defibrillator in prolonging survival in patients with severe underlying cardiac disease. *J Am Coll Cardiol* 16:381, 1990.
23. Kim SG, Fisher JD, Furman S, et al: Benefits of implantable defibrillators are overestimated by sudden death rates and better represented by the total arrhythmic death rate. *J Am Coll Cardiol* 17:1587, 1991.
24. Furman S: AICD benefit. *PACE* 12:399, 1989.
25. Connolly SJ, Yusuf S: Evaluation of the implantable cardioverter-defibrillator in survivors of cardiac arrest: the need for randomized trials. *Am J Cardiol* 69:959, 1992.
26. Kim SG: Implantable defibrillator therapy: does it really prolong life? How can we prove it? *Am J Cardiol* 71:1213, 1993.
27. Newman D, Suave MJ, Herre J, et al: Survival

after implantation of the cardioverter defibrillator. *Am J Cardiol* 69:899, 1992.
28. Bocker D, Block M, Isbruch F, et al: Do patients with implantable defibrillators live longer? *J Am Coll Cardiol* 21:1638, 1993.
29. Levine JH, Mellits ED, Baumgardner RA, et al: Predictors of first discharge and subsequent survival in patients with automatic implantable cardioverter-defibrillators. *Circulation* 84:558, 1991.
30. Mehta D, Saksena A, Krol R: Survival of implantable cardioverter-defibrillator recipients: role of left ventricular function and its relationship to device use. *Am Heart J* 124:1608, 1992.
31. Grimm W, Flores BT, Marchlinski FE: Shock occurrence and survival in 241 patients with implantable cardioverter-defibrillator therapy. *Circulation* 87:1880, 1993.
32. *Endotak Clinical Summary Report*. CPI, St. Paul, MN. August 1993.
33. Medtronic PCD™ Transvene™. FDA PMA Application P920015, 1993.

Chapter 24

Clinical Results With Implantable Cardioverter-Defibrillator Therapy

Hans-Joachim Trappe and Helmut Klein

Introduction

Sudden cardiac death is a major health problem in the western world. In the majority of patients, it is caused by ventricular tachyarrhythmias.[1-3] Recently, controlled clinical trials with antiarrhythmic drugs have raised serious questions regarding the long-term benefit and efficacy of pharmacological therapy for ventricular arrhythmias.[4,5] Therefore, nonpharmacological alternatives (map guided surgery, transcatheter ablation, and automatic implantable cardioverter-defibrillator [ICD] therapy) have been regarded as the more attractive alternatives.[6,7] Clinical experience to date suggests that no other therapeutic approach is more effective for prevention of sudden cardiac death than ICD therapy. The growing acceptance and increased use of this therapy is reflective of this view. More than 40,000 cardioverter defibrillators have been implanted worldwide to date.[8,9] Our experience with ICD therapy within the last 10 years is described here.

Historical Background

The concept of an ICD was developed by Michel Mirowski between 1966 and 1967.[10] The first human implant was performed in 1980.[11] Since then, significant interest and enthusiasm has developed for ICD use for patients with life-threatening ventricular tachyarrhythmias. First- and second-generation devices had defibrillation capabilities only, whereas the recently developed third-generation devices combine antitachycardia pacing (ATP), low-energy cardioversion, defibrillation, and back-up bradycardia pacing.[12-14] Until 1989, epicardial defibrillation leads were implanted by the thoracotomy approach. More recently, the nonthoracotomy lead (NTL) systems have become the method of choice. This partially explains the fact that NTL system implantation is associated with lower perioperative mortality and morbidity than the epicardial approach.[15,16]

Device Implantation

In all patients the ICD and leads were implanted under general anesthesia. During the first 5 years, an epicardial defibrillation lead system was used and leads were implanted via a median sternotomy or left anterior thoracotomy (Figure 1).[15] The epicardial lead system consists of two defibrillation patch electrodes and two myocardial

---

From Singer I, (ed.) Implantable Cardioverter-Defibrillator. Armonk, NY: Futura Publishing Company, Inc.; © 1994.

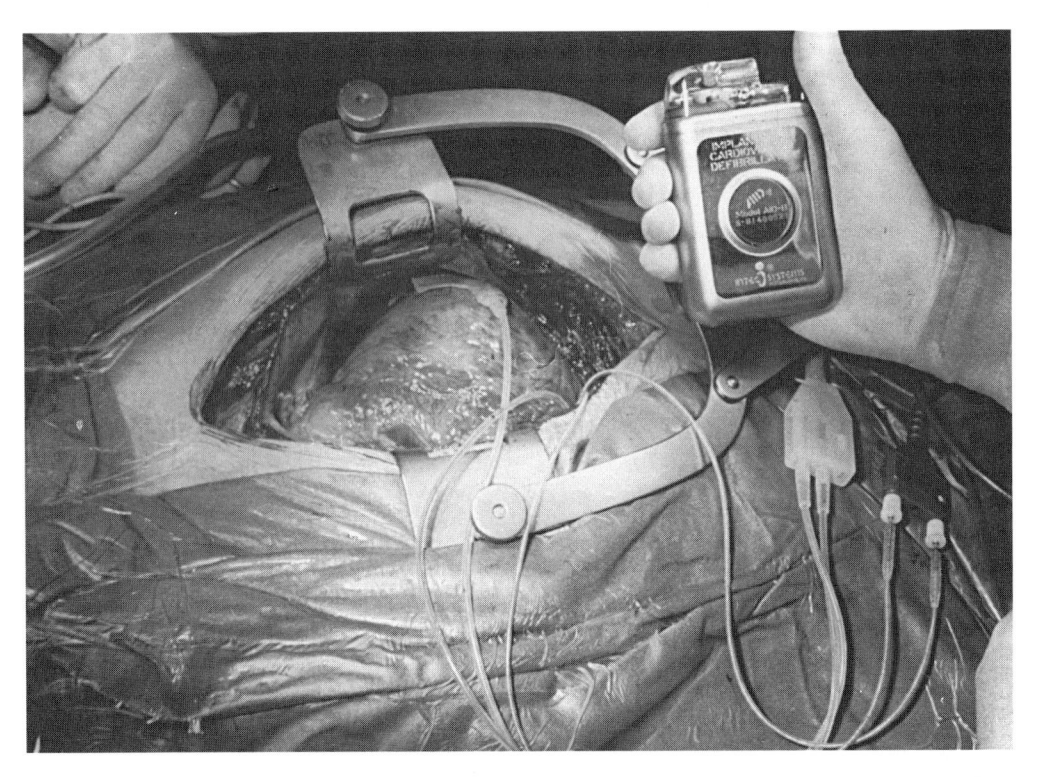

Figure 1. Implantation of the cardioverter defibrillator system through median sternotomy. The chest and the pericardium are opened and two screw-in and two patch lead electrodes are visible, connected to an external cardioverter-defibrillator (ECD™, CPI, St. Paul, MN.)

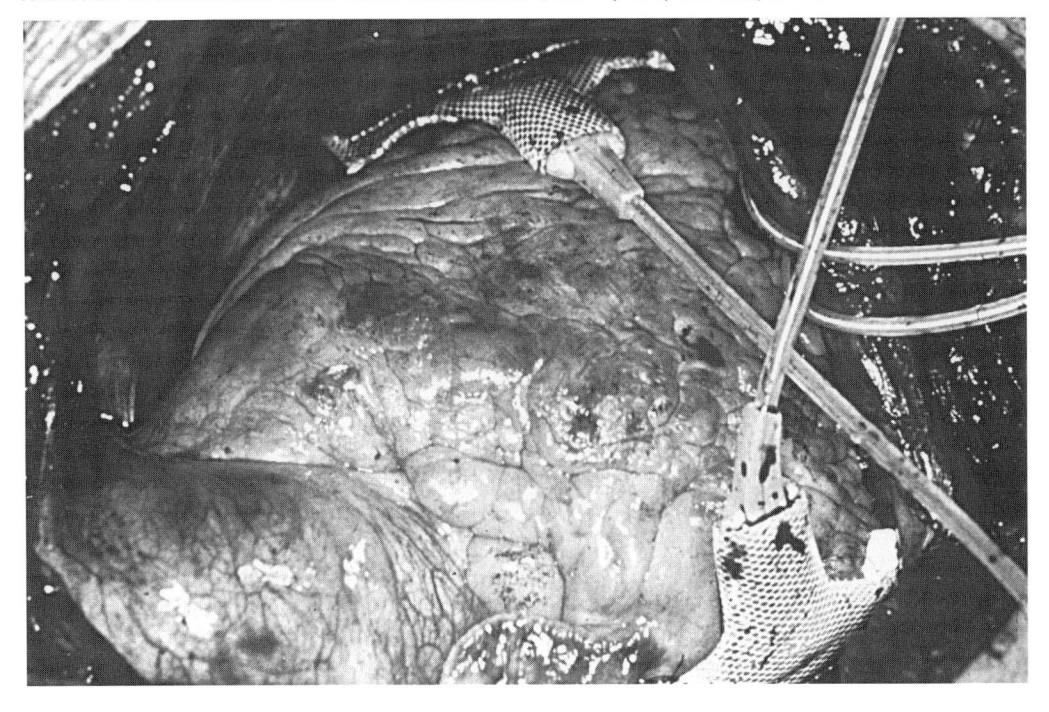

Figure 2. Intraoperative view of a patient with epicardial patch implantation. Two epicardial screw-in leads and two patch electrodes are clearly visible.

screw-in leads that are used for sensing and pacing (Figure 2). The NTL used almost exclusively at our institutions for the past 3 years has been the Endotak™ lead (CPI, St. Paul, MN).

The operative techniques used for lead insertion are discussed in Chapters 15, 16, and 17. The lead is advanced via the subclavian or the cephalic vein to the right atrium and then to the right ventricle. The distal tip

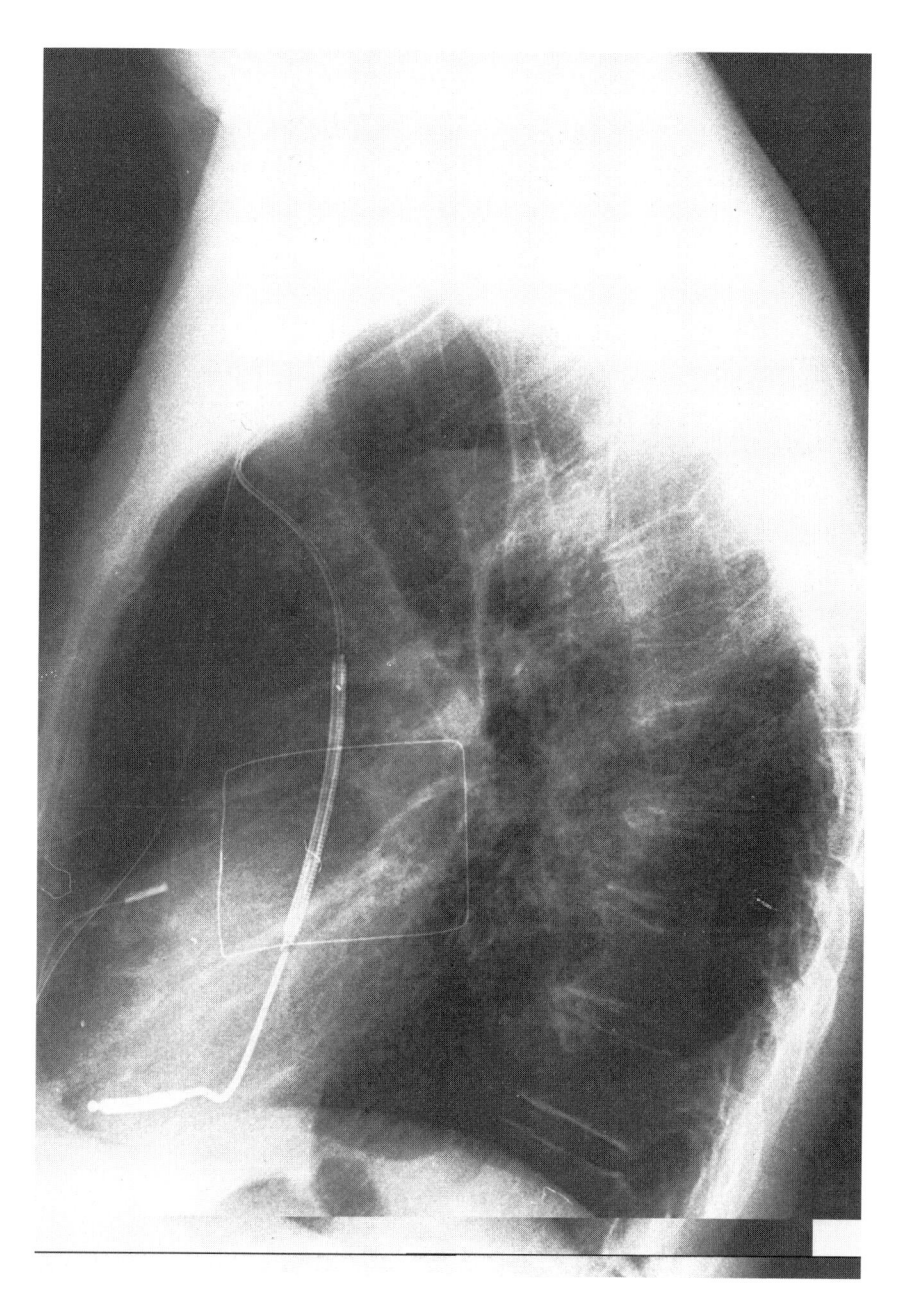

Figure 3. Chest x-ray of an implanted nonthoracotomy lead system (Endotak™ lead system, CPI, St. Paul, MN) combined with a subcutaneous patch electrode (lateral view). One electrode for sensing, pacing, and defibrillation is placed in the right ventricular apex, a subcutaneous patch electrode for defibrillation is placed subcutaneously.

of the lead is lodged in the right ventricular apex. The distal defibrillation coil is positioned in the right ventricular cavity below the tricuspid valve, with the proximal coil located in the right atrium, close to the superior vena caval junction (Figures 3 and 4). Recently, we used a new transvenous lead system (TVL™) (Ventritex Inc., Sunnyvale, CA) that consists of two electrodes, one positioned in the right ventricular apex, the other above the junction of the superior vena cava and the right atrium (Figure 5 and 6). The leads are then tunneled to the abdominal pocket subcutaneously and attached to the pulse generator, which is placed subcutaneously or submuscularly

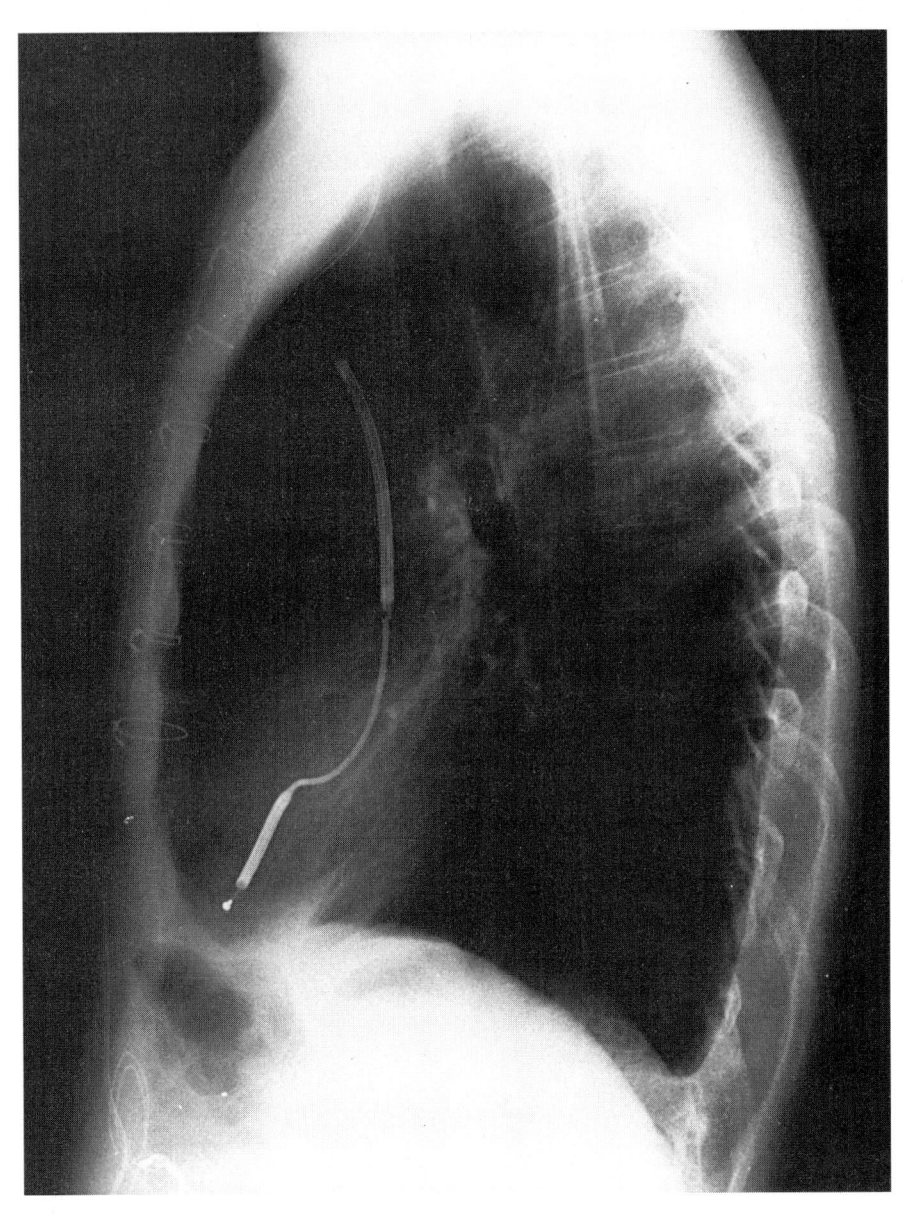

Figure 4. Chest roentgenogram of the implantaed nonthoracotomy lead system (Endotak™ lead system, CPI, St. Paul, MN) without an additional subcutaneous patch in a patient with previous aortocoronary bypass grafting.

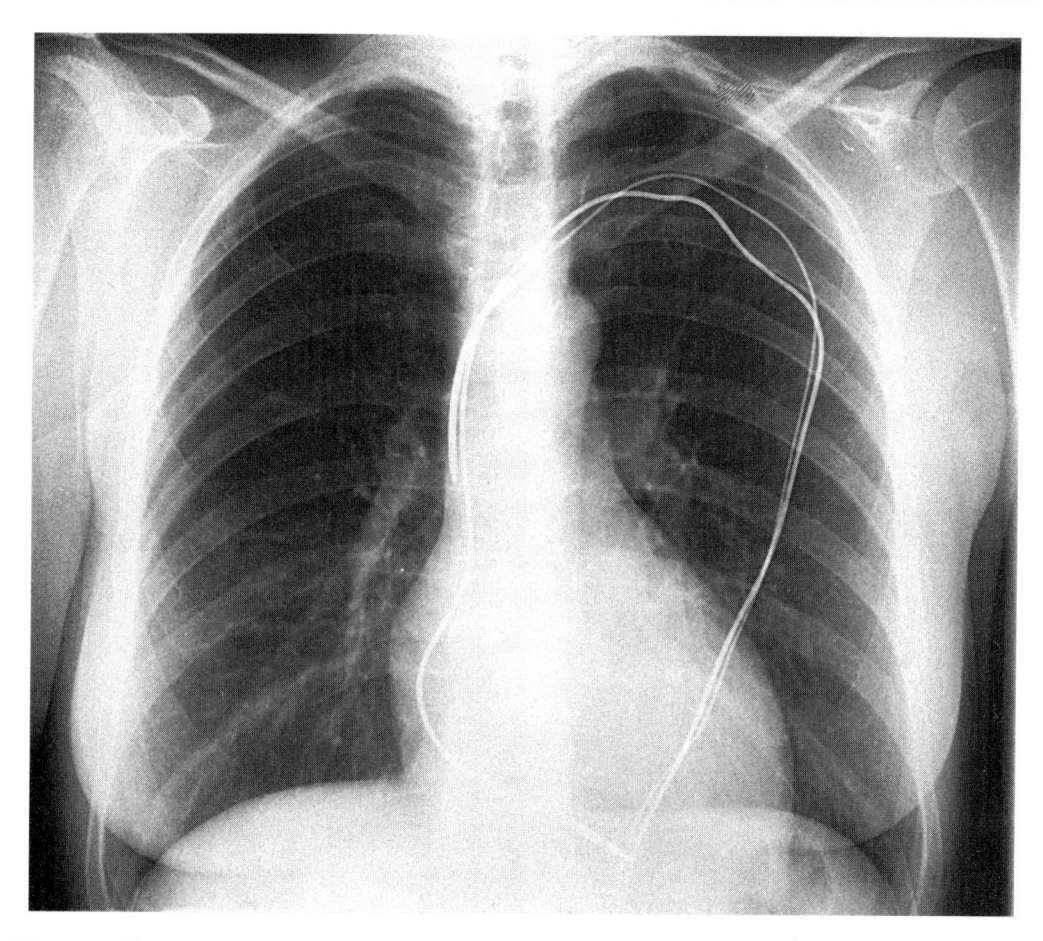

Figure 5. Chest roentgenogram of an implanted nonthoracotomy lead system with transvenous electrodes (TVL™ lead system, Ventritex Inc., Sunnyvale, CA). One electrode for sensing, pacing, and defibrillation is placed in the right ventricular apex, another electrode for defibrillation is placed at the right atrium-superior vena cava junction (posteroanterior view).

(see Chapter 15) (Figure 7). Intraoperative leads and device testing are described extensively in Chapters 10 and 15, and are not discussed here.

Patient Characteristics

The first cardioverter defibrillator was implanted in January 1984, more than 3 years after Mirowski's first implant. Our ICD experience now extends for a period of approximately 10 years. Within this time period 342 patients (308 males, 34 females), mean age of 57 ± 11 years (range 10–78 years) underwent ICD implantation. The majority (246 patients or 71%) had coronary artery disease with a prior history of myocardial infarction. Fifty-one patients (15%) had dilated cardiomyopathy, 5 patients (1%) had hypertrophic cardiomyopathy, and 18 patients (5%) ventricular tachycardia (VT) associated with right and/or left ventricular dysplasia. Twelve patients (3%) had valvular heart disease; a variety of different pathologies were present in the remaining 14 patients (myocarditis, tetralogy of Fallot, and primary electrical disease).

Life-threatening ventricular tachyarrhythmias (sustained monomorphic or polymorphic VT and ventricular fibrillation [VF]) were documented in 328 patients

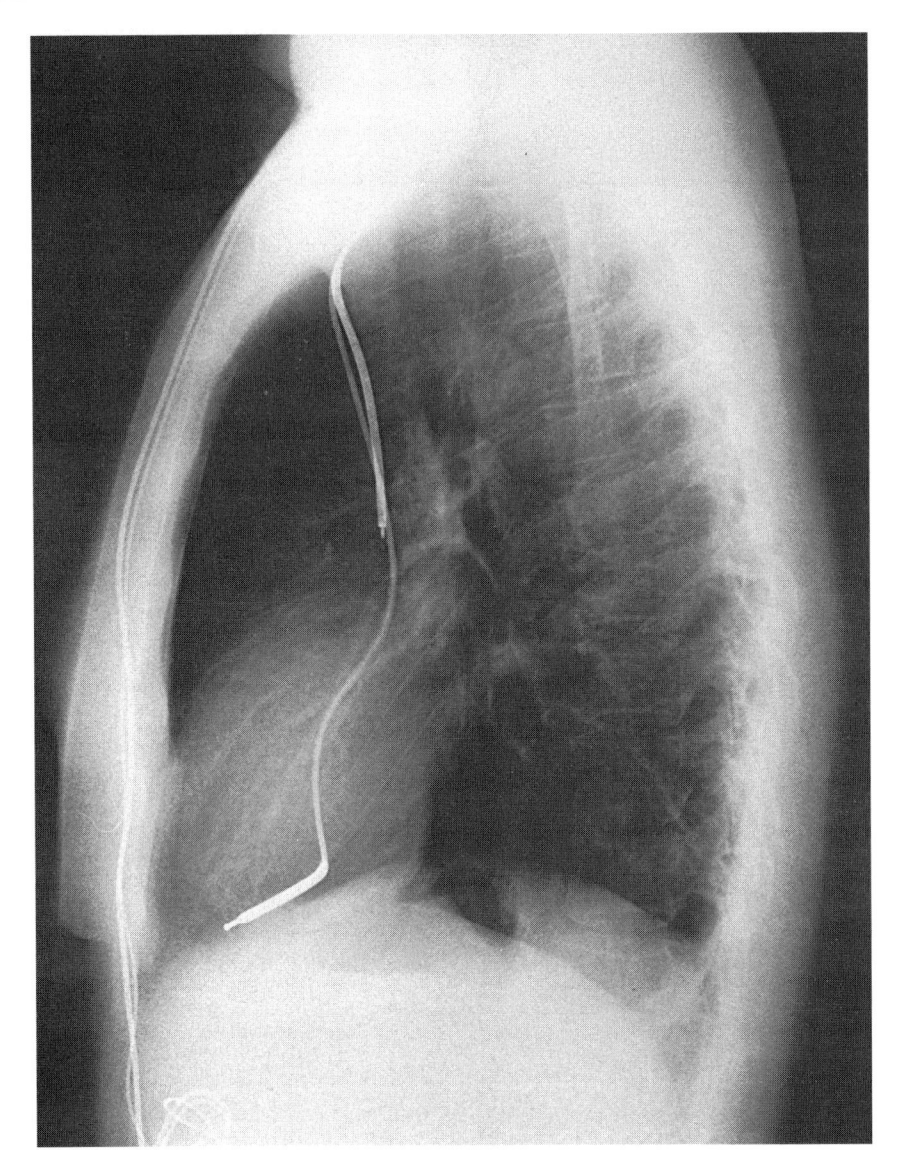

Figure 6. Chest x-ray of an implanted nonthoracotomy lead system with transvenous electrodes (TVL™ lead system, Ventritex Inc., Sunnyvale, CA). One electrode for sensing, pacing, and defibrillation is placed in the right ventricular apex, another electrode for defibrillation is placed above the right atrial-superior vena cava junction.

(95%), while the remaining 17 patients (5%) underwent cardioverter defibrillator implantation for prophylactic use as part of the MADIT[17] and CAT study protocols.[18] A history of recurrent episodes of sustained VT was present in 112 patients (32%), VF or cardiac arrest caused by ventricular tachyarrhythmias occurred in 213 patients (63%).

All patients had complete hemodynamic evaluation with left ventriculography, coronary angiography, and electrophysiologic study prior to ICD implantation. The mean left ventricular ejection fraction was 34% ± 13% (range 12% to 85%) indicating poor ventricular function in the majority of cases. Coronary angiography

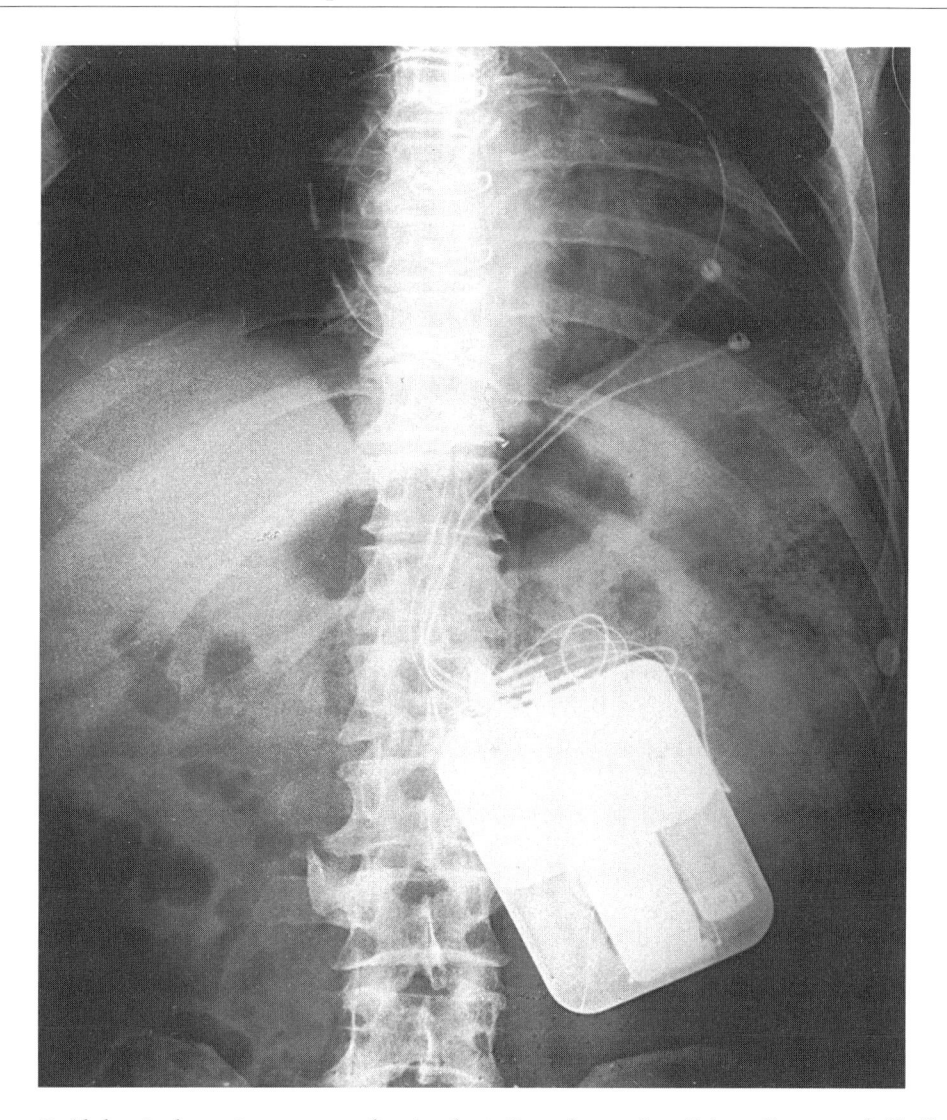

Figure 7. Abdominal roentgenogram after implantation of an epicardial cardioverter defibrillator lead system. Two screw-in leads and two patch electrodes are visible and connected to a pulse generator that is implanted in a left abdominal pocket.

identified coronary artery disease in 246 patients. Patients with other pathologies had either normal or minimal lesions on angiography.

Electrophysiologic study prior to ICD implantation induced sustained VT (mean tachycardia rate 180 ± 40, range 140–210 beats per minute) or VF in 310 patients (90%). Unsustained VT or no tachycardia were observed in 35 patients, despite spontaneous clinical episodes of life-threatening ventricular tachyarrhythmias.

Device Implantation

In 207 patients, epicardial approach was used. The mean R wave amplitude of the myocardial screw-in pace/sense leads was 12 ± 6 mV (range 6–25 mV). The pacing threshold at pulse width of 0.5 msec was 0.8 ± 0.5 V (range 0.2–1.5 V) with a mean lead impedance of 573 ± 210 Ω (range 220–980 Ω). The mean defibrillation threshold (DFT) was 16 ± 10 J (range 5–40 J).

For NTL systems, the R wave amplitude was 9 ± 2 mV (range 6–25 mV) and the pacing threshold at 0.5-msec pulse width was 0.5 ± 0.2 V (range 0.1–1.3 V) with a lead impedance of 470 ± 75 Ω (range 280–610 Ω). Defibrillation threshold for the endocardial lead system patients was 15 ± 9 J (range 5–30 J).

Results

Operative Mortality

Epicardial leads were implanted in 207 (60%) of patients, while 138 patients (40%) underwent NTL system implantation. Concomitant cardiac surgery was performed in 77 (22%) patients, including aortocoronary bypass grafting in 64, left ventricular aneurysmectomy in 4, cryoablation in 3, and valvular replacement in the remaining 6 patients.

Operative mortality (defined as death occurring within 30 days of ICD implantation) was 3%. One of 12 patients died intraoperatively after induction of VF that could not be terminated. The cause of death was fatal rupture of the right ventricle. This patient had prior coronary bypass grafting and was on amiodarone at the time of ICD implantation. Ten of the 12 patients who died had coronary artery disease. Operative mortality proved to be significantly higher in patients with epicardial leads (5%) compared with the NTL implants (< 1%; $P < 0.01$). Eight of the 12 patients who died during the perioperative period had concomitant cardiac surgery, whereas 4 of 345 patients (< 1%) died secondary to the ICD-only surgery.

Long-Term Mortality

A total of 333 patients were followed for a mean of 26 ± 23 (range < 1–112) months. During this time period, 63 patients (19%) died. The cause of death in 8 patients was sudden arrhythmic death. Another 6 patients died suddenly, but no ICD discharges were documented at the time of death. The cause of death in these patients remains unclear.

Thirty-six patients (11%) died from cardiac nonarrhythmic causes (congestive heart failure or myocardial reinfarction) and 13 patients (4%) died of noncardiac causes. The Kaplan-Meier survival curves demonstrated 1-year, 3-year, and 5-year survival of 90%, 75%, and 62%, respectively. Sudden arrhythmic death occurred in approximately 2% of patients per year, with a 1-year, 3-year, and 5-year survival of 99%, 94%, and 91%, respectively. Cardiac mortality was 19%, with survival of 96%, 87%, and 78% at 1, 3, and 5 years, respectively (Figure 8).

Implantable Cardioverter-Defibrillator Discharges

During the follow-up period, 235 patients (68%) had ICD discharges with a mean of 22 ± 44 (range 0–628) shocks. Implantable cardioverter defibrillator shocks occurred more frequently in patients with dilated cardiomyopathy (78%) than in patients with coronary disease (65%) or other cardiac pathologies (75%). The incidence of ICD discharges was higher in patients with dilated cardiomyopathy (26 ± 12 shocks) compared to patients with coronary disease (16 ± 10 shocks) or other underlying cardiac pathologies (21 ± 12 shocks). The time interval from the device implantation to the first shock was 10 ± 11 (range 1–76) months (Figure 9).

Nonthoracotomy Defibrillation Lead Systems

After the introduction of NTL systems, the epicardial approach was almost completely abandoned at our center. Because NTL systems can be implanted with low morbidity and mortality, they became the method of choice for most patients.[19,20] Long-term results have to demonstrate,

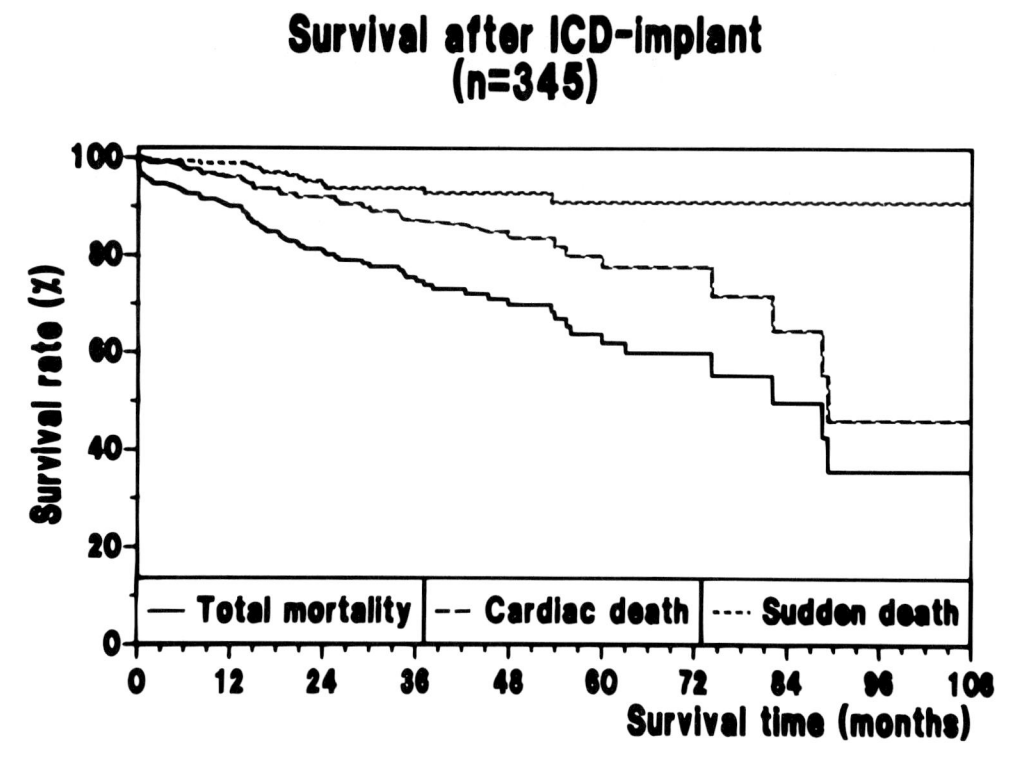

Figure 8. Kaplan-Meier survival curves in patients after cardioverter defibrillator implantation.

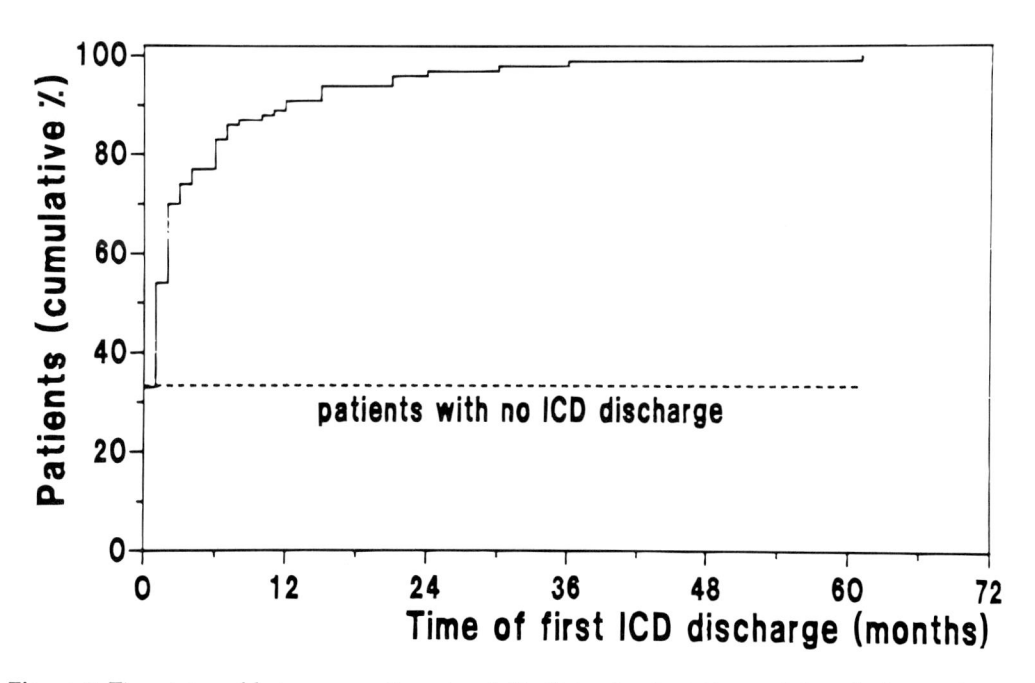

Figure 9. Time interval between cardioverter defibrillator implantation and first device stock.

however, that the nonthoracotomy approach is as safe and effective as the use of the well-established epicardial defibrillation leads.[21]

At our institution, 138 patients (126 males, 12 females), mean age of 57 ± 11 years underwent NTL system implantation. This approach was attempted in 144 patients and was successfully performed in 138 patients (96%). In 3 patients, due to high DFTs (> 25 J) and in 3 other patients because of technical considerations, we were unable to find stable endocardial lead electrode positions or sufficiently low DFTs. Therefore, these 6 patients received epicardial patch lead implantation. These were the only patients who received epicardial patch leads after introduction of the NTL systems.

For the first 46 patients with endocardial leads we purposely implanted an additional subcutaneous patch as part of the protocol (Figure 3). Later, having observed sufficiently low DFTs and reliable arrhythmia terminations with stable lead position, we continued to implant a single lead Endotak electrode without the subcutaneous patch (Figure 4). In 106 patients, the single lead approach was attempted and successfully performed in 92 patients (87%). In 14 patients (13%), no acceptable DFTs (≤ 20 J) could be achieved, and therefore, an additional subcutaneous patch was used.

The first 78 patients (57%) underwent NTL and cardioverter defibrillator implantation in the operating room. However, ICD implantation was performed in 60 patients (43%) in the cardiac catherization laboratory. No perioperative death was observed with NTL system implantation. During the mean follow-up of 13 ± 10 months (range < 1 to 42) months, 6 of 138 patients died (4%); 1 patient (< 1%) died from sudden arrhythmic death; 1 patient (< 1%) most likely died suddenly from pulmonary embolism. Three patients (2%) died from congestive heart failure and another patient (< 1%) died from a fatal cerebrovascular accident.

During the follow-up period, arrhythmic episodes occurred in 90 (65%) patients with a mean incidence of 8 ± 5 shocks (range 0–45) per patient.

Third-Generation Devices

The main advantage of third-generation ICDs is availability of antitachycardia and back-up bradycardia pacing capabilities. Holter monitoring has shown that most episodes of VF are preceded by VT.[22,23] Timely termination of VT by ATP could, therefore, reduce frequent and unpleasant ICD shocks. Because ATP may also accelerate VT to VF, there is a potential for ATP to lead to unnecesary ICD shocks.[14,24]

Another important advance is the availability of biphasic shocks in the newer devices. In general, biphasic shocks are more effective because they decrease the DFTs and reduce the energy requirements. The reduction in the energy requirements permit implantation of NTL systems in a greater number of patients and allow for a smaller device size, due to the reduction in the capacitor size.

At our institution, 154 patients (140 males, 14 females) with a mean age of 58 ± 12 years (range 10–78) received third-generation devices. Ninety patients received a third-generation device to take advantage of the tiered therapy, whereas 64 patients received devices to take advantage of biphasic shocks for documented high DFTs.

Further discussion here will therefore focus on the results of 90 patients with a demonstrable need for tiered therapy. All patients had at least one episode of spontaneous sustained monomorphic VT. During a preoperative electrophysiologic study, three ATP modes were tested by an external version of the Ventak™ PRx (CPI, St. Paul, MN) programmer. Predischarge testing was performed applying the most effective pacing mode demonstrated preoperatively.[25] Patients were discharged with the most appriopriate and reliable ATP mode tested during the predischarge electrophysiologic study.

```
38  01   TEL 13  26 JAN 96   0112 ***VE_TACHY
```

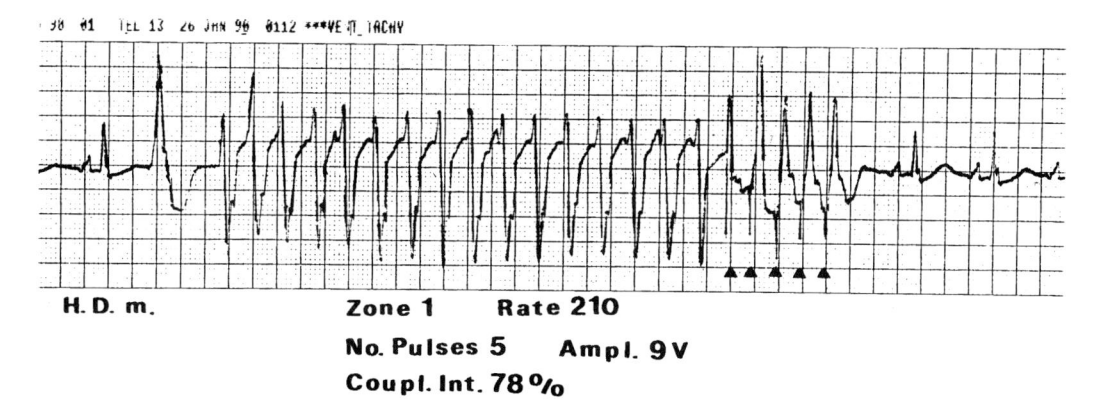

H. D. m.   Zone 1   Rate 210
                No. Pulses 5   Ampl. 9 V
                Coupl. Int. 78 %

Figure 10. Noninvasive testing of the Ventak™ PRx II (CPI, St. Paul, CA). Ventricular tachycardia (VT) (rate 200 beats per minute) is induced and is correctly detected. After first stimulation attempt (burst coupling interval 81%) with four stimuli, VT is terminated. ATP: antitachycardia pacing; M: marker channel; I, II, III: limb leads.

After hospital discharge, all patients were closely monitored and all arrhythmia episodes evaluated using stored electrograms. During a mean follow-up of 12 ± 9 months (range < 1–49), 3,542 arrhythmia episodes occurred. Fast VT rates (> 220 beats per minute) were observed in 778 episodes (22%) and these episodes were appropriately terminated by biphasic shocks. Antitachycardia pacing was attempted in 2,764 arrhythmic episodes (78%) and succesfully terminated in 2,484 episodes (90%) (Figures 10 and 11). Acceleration of VT to VF occurred in 83 episodes (3%); however, these episodes were successfully terminated by ICD shock (Figure 12). Antitachycardia pacing was unsuccessful in 197 episodes (7%) requiring subsequent ICD shocks (Figure

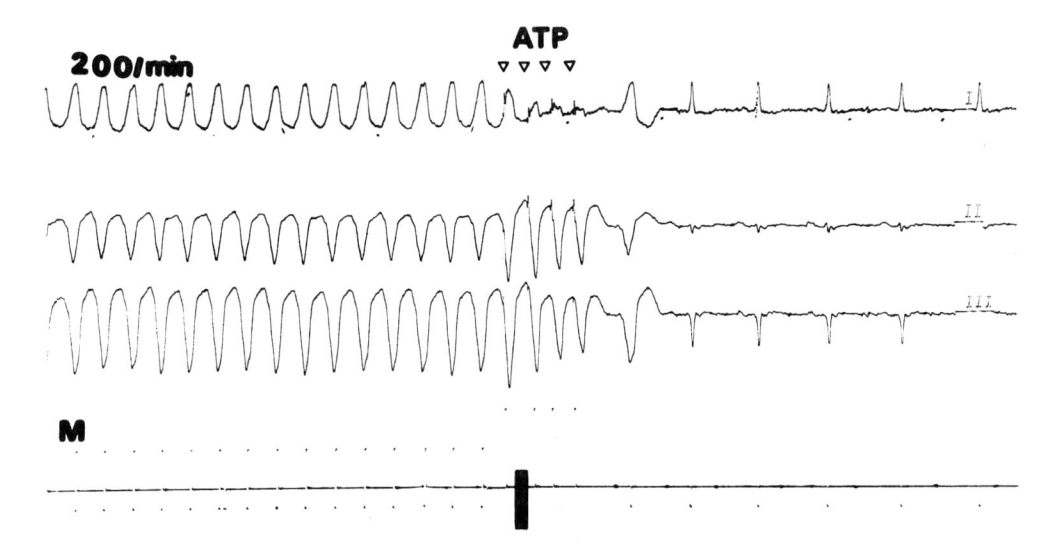

200/min   ATP
               ▽ ▽ ▽ ▽

Figure 11. Holter recording in a patient after implantation of the Ventak™ PRx I (CPI, St. Paul, MN). Ventricular tachycardia (rate 210 beats per minute) is visible, correctly detected and after first stimulation attempt (zone 1 with a burst coupling interval of 78%) with five extrastimuli terminated.

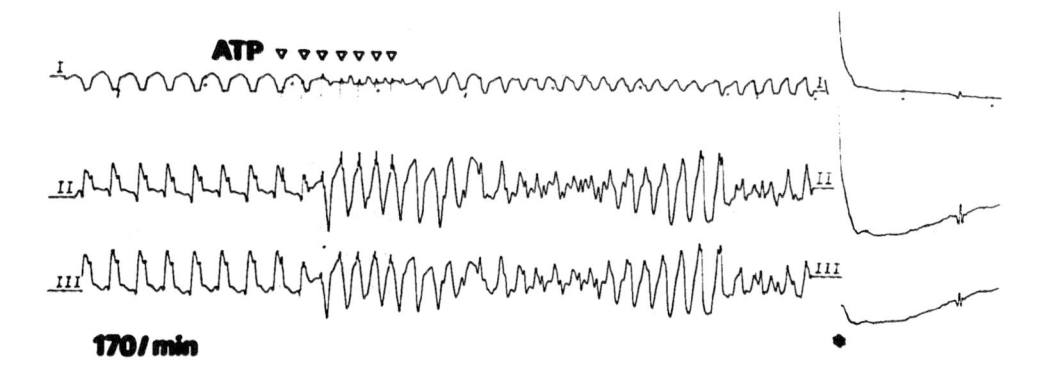

Figure 12. Noninvasive testing of the Ventak™ PRx 1700 (CPI, St. Paul, MN). Ventricular tachycardia (rate 170 beats per minute) is correctly detected. The first pacing attempt (coupling interval 75%) with seven extrastimuli is ineffective, acceleration into ventricular fibrillation is visible, and the arrhythmia is terminated by a 20-J shock (star). I, II, III: limb leads.

13). Despite the high success rates for ATP, the number of patients who used ATP exclusively for VT termination was low (8%) in contrast to the majority of patients (82%) who used both ATP and ICD shocks.

During the follow-up period, reprogramming of the ATP was necessary in 15% of patients, mainly due to ineffectiveness of the ATP, or because of acceleration of VTs.

Problems and Complications

Implantable cardioverter defibrillator therapy, although extremely effective for therapy of VT and VF, may be associated with problems and potential complications.[26–28] The undoubted benefit has to be considered and balanced against any possible complications.[29] Perioperative mortality with the first- and second-generation devices using the epicardial approach is reported to be 5% to 8%.[27] These mortality figures, however, have to be taken within the context of combined surgical procedures that undoubtedly account, for the most part, for these relatively high mortality statistics. It has been shown that operative mortality could be reduced significantly by NTL systems, with perioperative mortality below 1%.[30,31]

Operative mortality with epicardial approaches was mainly influenced by concomitant surgical procedures.[32,33] Currently, in patients who need concomitant surgical interventions a two-step procedure is recommended.

Another serious complication is infection of the implanted system, which was seen in 4% to 5% of our patients over the total follow-up period.[34,35] An infected ICD system is most often associated with serious morbidity, prolonged hospitalization, and higher mortality.[36] Once infection of the generator pocket has occurred, explantation of the entire system is usually necessary, because control of the infection with conservative management is ineffective.[7]

Infection occurred in 12 patients (3%), more frequently in patients with epicardial (11 of 207 patients, 5%) than in those with NTL systems (1 of 138 patients, < 1%) ($P < 0.01$). Infections occurred more frequently after pulse generator replacement (7 of 12 patients) than after initial ICD implantation. In all patients, explantation of the entire system (lead system and pulse generator) was finally necessary, although we initially tried to leave the electrodes in place. During follow-up, 7 patients died, 6 from congestive heart failure, and 1 patient from myocardial infarction after the device was removed. Reimplantation of a new device was performed in 4 patients with a mean interval

```
Episode - 43        Date : 01/19/1990

  Defibrillation occurred in this episode

    The Pre-shock R-R intervals in milliseconds were:
      266,281,258,258,266,281,281,273,281,281,281,273,289,281,281,289 msec.

    The Post-episode R-R intervals in milliseconds were:
      1992,1055,586,578,883,664,680,617,1070,750,922,859,578,680,570,648 msec.

Attempt - 1
  Time of detection        - 06:11:37
  Duration of therapy      - 00:00:02
  Pre-attempt R-R mean     - 281 msec./213 BPM
  Detection criteria met   - Rate only
  Zone of Therapy          - 1
  Therapy used             - Anti-Tachy Pace#1  ←
  Conversion successful    - No
  Therapy aborted          - No
  Arrhythmia accelerated   - No
  Post-attemp monitoring-  6 cycles
  Post-attempt R-R mean    - 227 msec./265 BPM

Attempt - 2
  Time of detection        - 06:11:39
  Duration of therapy      - 00:00:22
  Pre-attempt R-R mean     - 227 msec./265 BPM
  Detection criteria met   - Duration
  Zone of Therapy          - 2
  Therapy used             - Defib @27.3 joules  ←
  Conversion successful    - Yes
  Therapy aborted          - No
  Arrhythmia accelerated   - No
  Post-attempt monitoring- 16 cycles
  Post-attempt R-R mean    - 617 msec./ 97 BPM
```

Figure 13. Printout of therapy history during follow-up visit of a patient with Ventak™ PRx 1700 (CPI, St. Paul, MN) device. Note that with attempt 1 (arrow) antitachycardia pacing was unsuccessful within zone 1 but accelerated ventricular tachycardia (cycle length 227 msec). In zone 2 defibrillation was mandatory and terminated ventricular tachycardia successfully (arrow).

of 2.8 ± 1.3 (range 2–4 months) months after ICD explantation. Two patients remained without devices. One patient is still alive, the other died 2 years later, due to sudden arrhythmic death.

Complications with electrode lead systems have been reported in 5% to 10% of patients.[37,38] These are due to lead dislocation, lead connector problems, insulation defects, or lead fractures. The majority of patients with lead complications experience inappropriate ICD shocks. However, lead problems may also result in inappropriate sensing of ventricular tachyarrhythmia leading to a fatal outcome.[39,40]

In our own series, dislocation of the Endotak electrode was observed in 3 of 138 patients (2%), leading to frequent inappropriate ICD shocks. Three patients (2%) had inappropriate ATP therapy due to T wave oversensing after bradycardia pacing. Noise sensing resulted in inappropriately aborted therapy and inappropriate delivery of therapy in three patients (3%) with NTL systems. This was caused by adapter connector failure of the Endotak lead system to the Cadence™ V-100 (Ventritex, Sunnyvale, CA) pulse generator. Insulation defects of the Endotak electrode occurred in 8 patients (6%) due to mechanical problems produced by suboptimal surgical fixation of the lead.

Inappropriate shocks due to sinus

tachycardia, atrial fibrillation, or flutter with fast atrioventricular (AV) conduction, has been reported to account for as many as 30% of ICD shocks.[41] Antiarrhythmic therapy may be required to suppress unsustained VT and to avoid unpleasant and unnecessary ICD shocks. At our center, supraventricular tachyarrhythmias with inappropriate ICD discharges occurred in 52 patients (15%), more frequently in patients with epicardial lead systems (18%) compared to those with NTL systems (10%). Interruption or slowing of AV conduction by digitalis or verapamil to limit the ventricular response during atrial fibrillation episodes was necessary in 35 patients (67%), and reprogramming of the ATP therapy in 15 patients (29%). In two patients (4%), transvenous catheter ablation of the AV conduction system was necessary to interrupt rapid ventricular rates during atrial fibrillation. Availability of stored data is extremely helpful for recognizing and managing supraventricular tachycardias and VT.[42,43]

Discussion

The availability of cardioverter defibrillator therapy has provided the physician with an enormous improvement in therapy for patients with life-threatening ventricular tachyarrhythmias.[44–46] It has been shown that no other therapeutic approach is more capable of preventing or reducing sudden cardiac death.[47–50] Tiered therapy has expanded the current indications for ICD therapy.[51–53]

Mortality

Various studies have demonstrated that the annual rate of sudden cardiac death in patients with ICDs is < 2%.[54–58] Other than a reduction in actual arrhythmic deaths and subsequent overall cardiac mortality, ICD therapy is likely to prolong life in patients who ultimately would have died.[59,60] The most common cause of death in patients who have received an ICD is congestive heart failure.[48,61,62] Survival is mainly influenced by the underlying cardiac disease and the degree of systolic left ventricular dysfunction, which is assessed by the left ventricular ejection fraction and the functional class of heart failure.[63,64] It has been reported that patients with life-threatening ventricular tachyarrhythmias with implanted ICD and poor left ventricular function show lower sudden death rates and better actuarial survival than patients treated with antiarrhythmic drugs, even when serial drug testing is performed.[65] It is difficult, however, to compare these two therapeutic alternatives directly, because no randomized controlled data are currently available.

Nonthoracotomy Lead Systems

It has been shown that operative mortality is < 1% using the NTL approach.[21,29,39,55,61,66,67] Our own data confirmed the benefit of the endocardial lead systems. The presented data from our institution demonstrated operative mortality to decrease significantly, from 5% with epicardial to < 1% with the nonthoracotomy approach. However, experience with endocardial lead systems is still too short to assess whether this approach is as safe as the epicardial lead systems longer term.[68] Our own results are in agreement with other reports comparing epicardial with endocardial leads.[19,69,70]

Third-Generation Implantable Cardioverter-Defibrillators

More than two decades ago it was demonstrated that VT can be prevented by pacing at physiological rates.[71–73] Antitachycardia pacing using various pacing algorithms has been recommended to interrupt sustained VTs.[14] We and others have previously used two separate devices to achieve the benefits embodied in the third-generation defibrillators.[25] In this report we were able to demonstrate that ATP incorportated into an ICD is capable of terminating VT effectively in most patients with stable monomorphic VT. Antitachycardia pacing was effective for termination of spontaneously occurring VT in up to 90% of episodes. This is similar to the data reported by other authors, with success rates of > 75%.[74-76] Despite the promising results with ATP for VT, patients who exclusively benefit from ATP are rarely found.[60,77] Our own data concur with these findings.

Several ATP modalities have been used for VT termination. The most effective ATP mode is still unclear.[78,79] It has been recommended that a pacing mode using an automatically increasing number of stimuli with adaptive coupling intervals is the most effective mode that is associated with low incidence of VT acceleration.[80] However, we have found that there is no significant superiority of one or the other mode when randomly tested in a prospective fashion.[25] We believe that at the present time there is no ideal pacing mode that allows reliable pace-termination to be predicted by predischarge electrophysiologic testing.

The least desired complication of ATP is acceleration of a well-tolerated VT to VF.[81] In our patient population an acceleration was observed in 3% of patients. This has also been shown by others, with acceleration rates of 3% to 11% reported by various authors.[82,83] We have found that acceleration is independent of the adaptive coupling intervals, with similar acceleration rates with coupling intervals of 69%, 75%, and 81%, both during preoperative and at predischarge electrophysiologic studies.[25] This was not confirmed by other observers, showing higher acceleration rates with shorter coupling intervals, particularly with adaptive bursts of < 75% of the tachycardia cycle length.[51,79] We and others have noted that acceleration rates were more frequent during pre- and postoperative electrophysiologic studies compared to the observations during follow-up.[25] This might be due to the effects of sympathetic tone, anesthesia, or other factors.

Clincial Implications

Without a doubt, ICD therapy has had an enormous impact on the safer management of patients with life-threatening ventricular tachyarrhythmias. Although there are other therapeutic options available, the ICD provides benefits to patients at high risk of sudden arrhythmic death that no other therapeutic approach has demonstrated so far. The endocardial approach has almost completely replaced the epicardial implantation techniques. Endocardial lead systems are not only easier to implant but are also associated with a lower operative mortality and similar efficacy to the epicardial leads. Nonthoracotomy defibrillation lead systems are preferred for the vast majority of patients.

Third-generation ICDs allow individualized therapy prescription for the majority of VTs. Biphasic shock waveforms decrease DFTs significantly. Despite the excellent results with ATP, the number of patients who benefit exclusively from ATP is small. Bradycardia pacing back-up has further improved ICD therapy. Availability of electrogram storage and retrieval has provided further insight into mechanisms of life-threatening VTs. Electrogram storage has proven to be most useful for detection of inappropriate defibrillator discharges.

There is a growing interest in primary prevention of sudden death with prophylactic treatment with ICDs for patient populations that can be identified at high risk for cardiac arrest. Ongoing prospective randomized trials will demonstrate if the most effective treatment of patients identified as being at high risk is prophylactic ICD implantation. Devices appropriate for such indications need to be simple, reliable, and have better generator longevity, with smaller size suitable for pectoral implantation.

References

1. Trappe HJ, Klein H, Lichtlen PR: Ursachen des akuten Herz-Kreislauf-Stillstandes. *Internist* 33:289, 1992.
2. Horowitz LN: The automatic implantable cardioverter defibrillator: review of clinical results, 1980–1990. *PACE* 15:604, 1992.
3. Wellens HJJ, Brugada P: Sudden cardiac death: a multifactorial problem. In: *Cardiac Arrhythmias. Where To Go From Here?* Edited by P Brugada, HJJ Wellens. Mount Kisco, NY: Futura Publishing Company; 1987, p. 391.
4. The Cardiac Arrhythmia Suppression Trial (CAST) Investigators: Preliminary report: effect of encainide and flecainide on mortality in a randomized trial of arrhythmia suppression after myocardial infarction. *N Engl J Med* 321:406, 1989.
5. The Cardiac Arrhythmia Suppression Trial II Investigators: Effect of the antiarrhythmic agent morizicine on survival after myocardial infarction. *N Engl J Med* 327:227, 1992.
6. Breithardt G, Borggrefe M, Wietholt D, et al: Role of ventricular tachycardia surgery and catheter ablation as complements or alternatives to the implantable cardioverter defibrillator in the 1990s. *PACE* 15:681, 1992.
7. Trappe HJ, Klein H, Frank G, et al: Nonpharmacological treatment of ventricular tachycardia. In: *Sudden Cardiac Death*. Edited by A Bayes de Luna, P Brugada, J Cosin Aguilar, F Navarro-Lopez. Dordrecht: Kluwer Academic Publishers; 1991, p. 147.
8. Klein H, Trappe HJ: Implantierbare Defibrillatoren. *Z gesamte Inn Med* 47:209, 1992.
9. Nisam S, Mower MM, Thomas A, et al: Patient survival comparison in three generations of automatic implantable cardioverter defibrillators: review of 12 years, 25000 patients. *PACE* 16:174, 1993.
10. Mirowski M, Mower MM, Staewen WS, et al: Standby automatic defibrillator: an approach to prevention of sudden coronary death. *Arch Intern Med* 126:158, 1970.
11. Mirowski M, Reid PR, Mower MM, et al: Termination of malignant ventricular arrhythmias with an implanted automatic defibrillator in human beings. *N Engl J Med* 303:322, 1980.
12. Saksena S: Recent advances in implantable cardioverter- defibrillator therapy. In: *Interventional Electrophysiology*. Edited by S Saksena, B Lüderitz. Mount Kisco, NY: Futura Publishing Company, Inc.; 1991, p. 395.
13. Akhtar M, Jazayeri MR, Sra JS, et al: Implantable cardioverter defibrillator therapy for prevention of sudden cardiac death. In: *Cardiology Clinics*. Edited by M Akhtar. Philadelphia, PA: WB Saunders Company; 1993, p. 97.
14. Fisher JD, Furman S, Kim SG, et al: Antitachycardia pacing, cardioversion, and defibrillation: from the past to the future. In: *The Implantable Cardioverter/Defibrillator*. Edited by E Alt, H Klein, JC Griffin. Berlin/Heidelberg/New York: Springer-Verlag; 1992, p. 157.
15. Frank G, Lowes D: Implantable cardioverter defibrillators: surgical considerations. *PACE* 15:631, 1992.
16. Trappe HJ, Fieguth HG, Weber-Conrad O, et al: Results and experience with transvenous cardioverter defibrillator therapy. *Med Klinik* 87:615, 1992.
17. Moss AJ: Prospective antiarrhythmic studies assessing prophylactic pharmacological and device therapy in high risk coronary patients. *PACE* 15:694, 1992.
18. The Cardiomyopathy Trial Investigators: Cardiomyopathy trial. *PACE* 16:576, 1993.
19. Block M, Hammel D, Isbruch F, et al: Results and realistic expectations with transvenous lead systems. *PACE* 15:665, 1992.
20. Saksena S, DeGroot P, Krol RB, et al: Low energy endocardial defibrillation using an axillary or a pectoral thoracic electrode location. *Circulation* 88:2655, 1993.
21. Brooks R, Garan H, Torchiana D, et al: Determinants of successful nonthoracotomy cardioverter-defibrillator implantation: experience in 101 patients using two different lead systems. *J Am Coll Cardiol* 22:1835, 1993.
22. Bayes de Luna A, Coumel P, Lerclerq JF: Ambulatory sudden death: mechanisms of production of fatal arrhythmia on the basis of data from 157 cases. *Am Heart J* 117:151, 1989.
23. Olshausen VK, Witt T, Pop T, et al: Sudden cardiac death with wearing a Holter monitoring. *Am J Cardiol* 67:381, 1991.
24. Leitch JW, Gillis AM, Wyse DG, et al: Reduction in defibrillator shocks with an implantable device combining antitachycardia pacing and shock therapy. *J Am Coll Cardiol* 18:145, 1991.
25. Trappe HJ, Klein H, Kielblock B: Role of antitachycardia pacing in patients with third generation cardioverter defibrillators. *PACE* (in press).
26. Trappe HJ, Klein H, Fieguth HG, et al: Problems and complications after cardioverter-defibrillator implantation. *Med Klinik* 88:619, 1993.
27. Troup PJ, Nisam S: Complications associated with the automatic implantable cardioverter

defibrillator. In: *The Implantable Cardioverter/Defibrillator*. Edited by E Alt, H Klein, JC Griffin. Berlin/Heidelberg/New York: Springer Verlag; 1993, p. 253.
28. Meesmann M: Factors associated with implantation-related complications. *PACE* 15:649, 1992.
29. Kelly PA, Cannom DS, Garan H, et al: The automatic implantable cardioverter-defibrillator: efficacy, complications and survival in patients with malignant ventricular arrhythmias. *J Am Coll Cardiol* 11:1278, 1988.
30. Grimm W, Flores BF, Marchlinski FE, et al: Complications of implantable cardioverter defibrillator therapy: follow-up of 241 patients. *PACE* 16:218, 1993.
31. Trappe HJ, Klein H, Fieguth HG, et al: Initial experience with a new transvenous defibrillation system. *PACE* 16:134, 1993.
32. Alfieri O, Benedini G, Caradonna E, et al: The implantable cardioverter defibrillator and concomitant coronary artery bypass grafting: special considerations. *PACE* 15:642, 1992.
33. Trappe HJ, Klein H, Wahlers T, et al: Risk and benefit of additional aortocoronary bypass grafting in patients undergoing cardioverter-defibrillator implantation. *Am Heart J* 127:75, 1994.
34. Trappe HJ, Fieguth HG, Kielblock B, et al: Infections after cardioverter defibrillator implantation (abstract). *Eur Heart J* 14:411, 1993.
35. Bakker PFA, Hauer RNW, Wever EFD, et al: Infections involving implanted cardioverter defibrillator devices. *PACE* 15:654, 1992.
36. Siclari F, Klein H, Tröster J, et al: Infectious complications after AICD implantation (abstract). *PACE* 13:547, 1990.
37. Frame R, Brodman R, Gross J, et al: Initial experience with transvenous implantable cardioverter defibrillator lead systems: operative morbidity and mortality. *PACE* 16:149, 1993.
38. Yee R, Klein GJ, Leitch JW, et al: A permanent transvenous lead system for an implantable pacemaker cardioverter- defibrillator. Nonthoracotomy approach in implantation. *Circulation* 85:196, 1992.
39. Gabry MD, Brodman R, Johnston D, et al: Automatic implantable cardioverter defibrillator: patient survival, battery longevity, and shock delivery analysis. *J Am Coll Cardiol* 9:1349, 1987.
40. Josephson ME: Evaluation of electrical therapy for arrhythmias. In: *Clinical Cardiac Electrophysiology*. Edited by ME Josephson. Philadelphia, PA: Lea and Febiger; 1993, p. 683.
41. Marchlinski FE, Buxton AE, Flores BF: The automatic implantable cardioverter defibrillator: follow-up and complications. In: *Cardiac Pacing and Electrophysiology*. Edited by N El-Sherif, P Samet P. Orlando, FL: Grune and Stratton; 1990, p. 743.
42. Hook BG, Perlman RL, Johnson NJ, et al: Value of stored electrograms and programmable sensing criteria in optimizing management of patients receiving pacing and shocks for asymptomatic arrhythmias (abstract). *J Am Coll Cardiol* 17:85A, 1991.
43. Wilkoff BL, Igel DA, Pinski L, et al: Ventricular arrhythmia identification by electrogram pattern analysis (abstract). *J Am Coll Cardiol* 21:127A, 1993.
44. Kim YH, O'Nunian S, Ruskin JN, et al: Nonpharmacological therapies in patients with ventricular tachyarrhythmias. In: *Cardiology Clinics*. Edited by M Akhtar. Philadelphia, PA: WB Saunders Company; 1993, p. 85.
45. Cannom DS, Winkle RA: Implantation of the automatic implantable cardioverter defibrillator (AICD): practical aspects. *PACE* 9:793, 1986.
46. DiMarco JP: Nonpharmacological therapy of ventricular arrhythmias. *PACE* 13:1527, 1990.
47. Fisher JD, Kim SG, Roth JA, et al: Ventricular tachycardia/fibrillation: therapeutic alternatives. *PACE* 14:370, 1991.
48. Winkle RA, Mead AH, Ruder MA, et al: Long-term outcome with the automatic implantable cardioverter-defibrillator. *J Am Coll Cardiol* 13:1353, 1989.
49. Akhtar M, Garan H, Lehmann MH, et al: Sudden cardiac death: management of high risk patients. *Ann Intern Med* 114:499, 1991.
50. Klein H, Trappe HJ: Treatment algorithm for patients with life-threatening ventricular tachyarrhythmias. In: *The Implantable Cardioverter/Defibrillator*. Edited by E Alt, H Klein, JC Griffin. Berlin/Heidelberg/New York: Springer-Verlag; 1992, p. 203.
51. Almendral J, Arenal A, Villacastin JP, et al: The importance of antitachycardia pacing for patients presenting with ventricular tachycardia. *PACE* 16:535, 1993.
52. Fogoros RN: The effect of the implantable cardioverter defibrillator on sudden death and on total survival. *PACE* 16:506, 1993.
53. Akhtar M, Jazayeri M, Sra J, et al: Implantable cardioverter defibrillator for prevention of sudden cardiac death in patients with ventricular tachycardia and ventricular fibrillation: ICD therapy in sudden cardiac death. *PACE* 16:511, 1993.
54. Borbola J, Denes P, Ezri MD, et al: The automatic implantable cardioverter-defibrillator: clinical experience, complications, and follow-up in 25 patients. *Arch Intern Med* 148:70, 1988.
55. Veltri EP, Mower MM, Mirowski M, et al:

Follow-up of patients with ventricular tachyarrhythmias treated with the automatic implantable cardioverter defibrillator: programmed electrical stimulation results do not predict clinical outcome. *J Electrophysiol* 3:467, 1989.
56. Manolis AS, Tan-DeGuzman W, Lee MA, et al: Clinical experience in seventy-seven patients with the automatic implantable cardioverter defibrillator. *Am Heart J* 118:445, 1989.
57. Cappucci A, Boriani G: Drugs, surgery, cardioverter defibrillator. A decision based on the clinical problem. *PACE* 16:519, 1993.
58. Furman S, Kim SG, Brodman R, et al: Statistical analysis of ICD data. In: *Interventional Electrophysiology*. Edited by S Saksena, B Lüderitz. Mount Kisco, NY: Futura Publishing Company; 1991, p. 455.
59. Akhtar M, Jazayeri M, Sra J, et al: Implantable cardioverter defibrillator for prevention of sudden cardiac death in patients with ventricular tachycardia or ventricular fibrillation: ICD therapy in sudden cardiac death. *PACE* 16:511, 1993.
60. Böcker D, Block M, Isbruch F, et al: Do patients with implantable defibrillator live longer? *J Am Coll Cardiol* 21:1638, 1993.
61. Tchou PJ, Kadri N, Anderson J, et al: Automatic implantable cardioverter defibrillators and survival of patients with left ventricular dysfunction and malignant ventricular arrhythmias. *Ann Intern Med* 109:529, 1988.
62. Luceri RM, Habal SM, Castellanos A, et al: Mechanism of death in patients with the automatic implantable cardioverter defibrillator. *PACE* 11:2015, 1988.
63. Myerburg RJ, Luceri RM, Thurer R, et al: Time to first shock and clinical outcome in patients receiving an automatic implantable cardioverter defibrillator. *J Am Coll Cardiol* 14:508, 1989.
64. Mehta D, Saksena S, Krol RB, et al: Device use pattern and clinical outcome of implantable cardioverter defibrillator patients with moderate and severe impaired left ventricular function. *PACE* 16:179, 1993.
65. Swerdlow CD, Winkle RA, Mason JW, et al: Determinants of survival in patients with ventricular tachyarrhythmias. *N Engl J Med* 308:1436, 1983.
66. Reid PR, Griffith LSC, Platia EV, et al: The automatic implantable cardioverter-defibrillator. Five-year clinical results. In: *Nonpharmacological Therapy of Tachyarrhythmias*. Edited by G Breithardt, M Borggrefe, DP Zipes. Mount Kisco, NY: Futura Publishing Company; 1987, p. 477.
67. Hauser RG, Nisam S, McVeigh KC, et al: World-wide experience with the Endotak transvenous defibrillation lead. *New Trends Arrhythmias* 8:69, 1992.
68. Saksena S, Parsonnet V: Implantation of a cardioverter defibrillator without thoracotomy using a triple electrode system. *JAMA* 259:66, 1988.
69. McGowan R, Maloney J, Wilkoff B, et al: Automatic implantable cardioverter-defibrillator implantation without thoracotomy using an endocardial and submuscular patch system. *J Am Coll Cardiol* 17:415, 1991.
70. Hauser RG, Kuraschinski DT, McVeigh K, et al: Clinical results with nonthoracotomy ICD systems. *PACE* 16:141, 1993.
71. Escher DJW: The treatment of tachyarrhythmias by artificial pacing. *Am Heart J* 78:829, 1969.
72. Heiman DF, Helwig J Jr: Suppression of ventricular arrhythmias by transvenous intracardiac pacing. *JAMA* 195:172, 1966.
73. Lew HT, March HW: Control of recurrent ventricular fibrillation by transvenous pacing in the absence of heart block. *Am Heart J* 73:794, 1967.
74. Fromer M, Brachmann J, Block M, et al: Efficacy of automatic multimodel device therapy for ventricular tachyarrhythmias as delivered by a new implantable pacer-, cardioverter- defibrillator. Results of a European multicenter study incorporating 102 implants. *Circulation* 86:363, 1992.
75. Saksena S, Mehra D, Krol RB, et al: Experience with a third- generation implantable cardioverter-defibrillator. *Am J Cardiol* 67:1375, 1991.
76. Leitch JW, Gillis AM, Wyse G, et al: Reduction in defibrillation shocks with an implantable device combining antitachycardia pacing and shock therapy. *J Am Coll Cardiol* 18:145, 1991.
77. Trappe HJ, Klein H: Is antitachycardia pacing really an advantage in patients with cardioverter defibrillators (abstract)? *J Am Coll Cardiol* 205A, 1994.
78. Klein LS, Miles WM, Zipes DP: Antitachycardia devices: realities and promises. *J Am Coll Cardiol* 18:1349, 1991.
79. Porterfield JG, Porterfield LM, Bray L: Ninety-six episodes of spontaneous ventricular tachycardia in 1 week: success of ramp pacing by pacer-cardioverter-defibrillator. *PACE* 14:1440, 1991.
80. Charos GS, Haffajee GI, Gold RL, et al: A theoretically and practically more effective method for interruption of ventricular tachycardia: self adapting auto decremental overdrive pacing. *Circulation* 73:309, 1986.
81. Fisher JD, Kim SG, Waspe LE, et al: Mechanisms for the success and failure of pacing

for termination of ventricular tachycardia: clinical and hypothetical considerations. *PACE* 6:1094, 1983.
82. Fromer M, Schläpfer J, Fischer A, et al: A new comprehensive ventricular tachyarrhythmia control device: efficacy of hierachial therapy (abstract). *J Am Coll Cardiol* 17:87A, 1991.
83. Siebels J, Geiger M, Schneider MAE, et al: The automatic implantable cardioverter defibrillator: does low energy cardioversion offer any advantage over antitachycardia pacing in patients with ventriculasr tachycardia (abstract)? *J Am Coll Cardiol* 17:129A, 1991.

Chapter 25

Clinical Results With Nonthoracotomy Lead Systems and Implications for Implantable Cardioverter-Defibrillator Practice:
The European Experience

Samuel Lévy, Philippe Ricard, and Eric Dolla

Introduction

The implantable cardioverter defibrillator (ICD) is a major therapeutic tool for the management of patients at high risk of sudden death. When it was introduced by Mirowski et al. in 1980,[1] the electrodes were placed on the epicardium via a median thoracotomy, a lateral thoracotomy, or a subxiphoid approach. However, since 1971, Mirowski et al.[2] thought that an intravascular catheter approach could be a solution. However, technical problems and the lack of support have probably delayed the early use of such an approach. As the ICD was demonstrated as effective for the treatment of malignant arrhythmias, the cardiologists, influenced by the widespread use of antibradycardia pacemakers have expressed the need for a transvenous approach for ICD implantation. The first reports date back to 1988,[3–6] but a reliable lead system was not available until 1991 (Endotak™, CPI, St. Paul, MN).

In this chapter, the results and advantages of transvenous techniques as well as the desirable future improvements are discussed. This new approach represents a major breakthrough in the management of patients with malignant ventricular arrhythmias.

Available Transvenous Lead Systems

The first electrode lead system used was a single lead (Endotak). This 12F lead comprises of two defibrillation electrodes and is introduced typically through the left subclavian vein and the tip positioned at the apex of the right ventricle (Figure 1). If the defibrillation threshold (DFT) is too high to implant the lead only, a subcutaneous patch (SQ) or more recently a lead array may be positioned subcutaneously to encompass the left ventricle in the defibrillation field. The bipolar electrodes used for sensing and pacing are connected to the generator after subcutaneous tunneling to the ICD abdominal pocket.

The transvenous lead system Transvene™, provided by Medtronic Inc. (Minneapolis, MN) consists of two or three leads. A 10.5F right ventricular (RV) lead is used

---

From Singer I, (ed.) Implantable Cardioverter-Defibrillator. Armonk, NY: Futura Publishing Company, Inc.; © 1994.

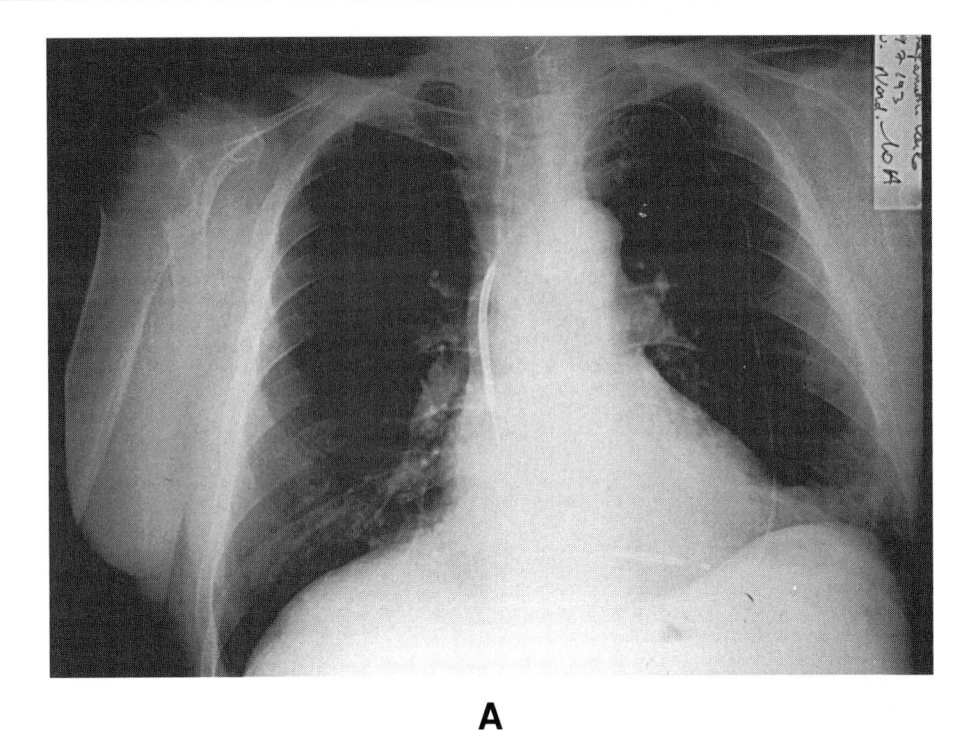

Figure 1. Various available lead systems for nonthoracotomy implantation of cardioverter defibrillators. **A:** Radiographs of the chest showing single lead system (Endotak™, CPI, St. Paul, MN). **B:** Transvene™ system (Medtronic, Minneapolis, MN) using a superior vena cava coil (SVC) electrode, an electrode positioned at the apex of the right ventricle, and a subcutaneous patch. **C:** EnGuard™ system (Telectronics, Englewood, CO) using an electrode in the right atrium and an electrode in the right ventricle (see text).

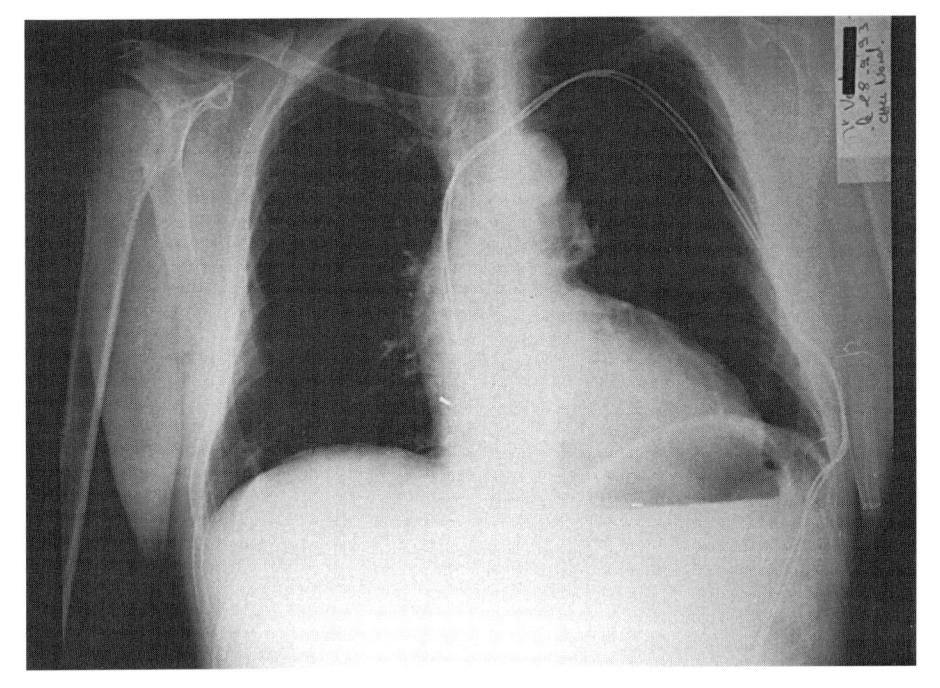

C

Figure 1. *(Continued)*

for defibrillation, pacing, and bipolar sensing. This lead has an active fixation mechanism. Another catheter (6.5F) with a coil electrode is positioned in the majority of patients in the high superior vena cava (SVC) or in some cases in the coronary sinus (CS). A SQ electrode may be used if the DFTs are too high with the endocardial electrode system.[7,8]

The third nonthoracotomy lead (NTL)

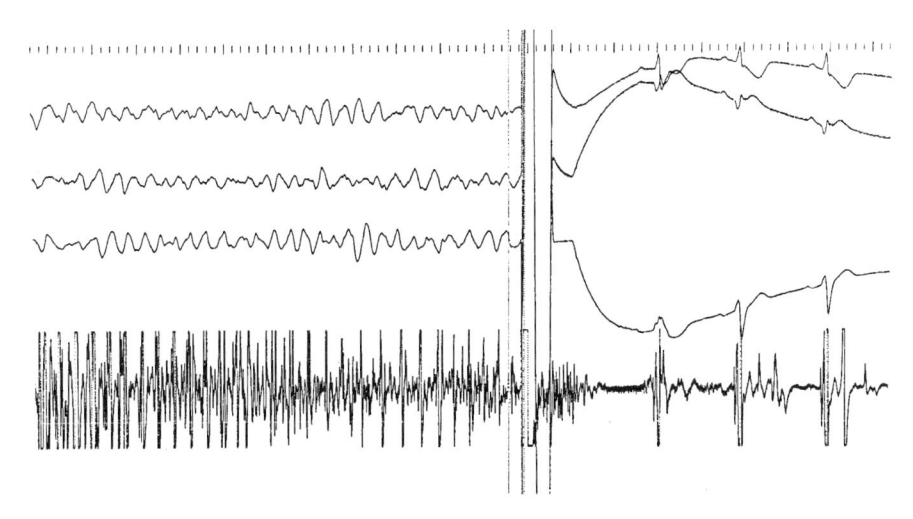

Figure 2. Defibrillation threshold testing after induction of ventricular fibrillation. A 25-J shock was found to reproducibly convert ventricular fibrillation to sinus (from top to bottom ECG leads I, II, and V_1 and right ventricular electrocardiogram).

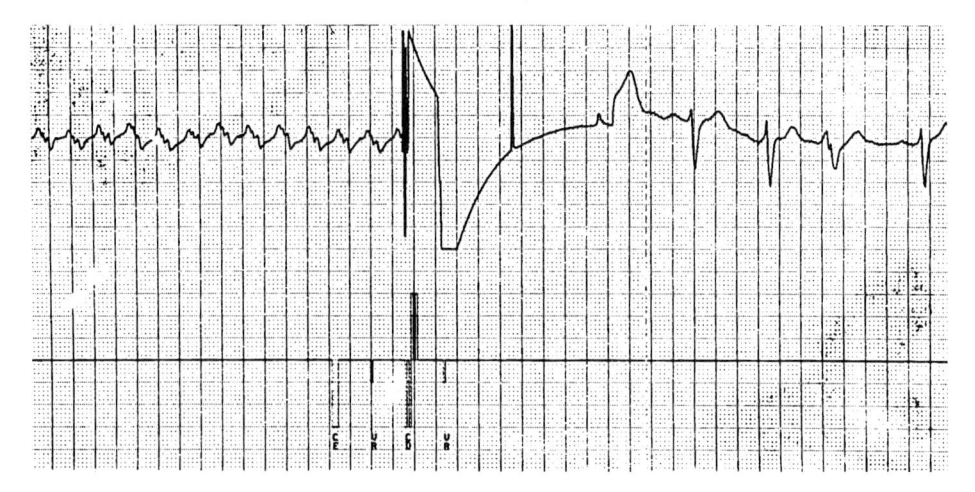

Figure 3. Termination of rapid ventricular tachycardia with cardioversion. **Top:** recorded surface ECG. **Bottom:** marker channel (PCD™, Medtronic, Minneapolis, MN).

system available in Europe is EnGuard™ (Telectronics, Denver, CO). This system consists of two endocardial leads. A pace/sense and defibrillation lead in the right ventricle with active, or more recently passive fixation mechanism, combined with a passive tined J-shaped defibrillation lead placed in the right atrial appendage, with the more proximal defibrillation coil in the SVC. As with other systems, an SQ electrode may be combined with the endocardial leads if the results of DFT testing are unsatisfactory with the two endocardial leads. Currently, two other transvenous lead systems and third-generation ICDs (Siecure™, Siemens Pacesetter, Sylmar, CA)[9] and NTL system designed by Intermedics Inc. (Angleton, TX) with Res-Q™ ICD are undergoing clinical trials.

The techniques used for the implantation of the leads are described in Chapters 15, 16, and 17. Examples of DFT (Figure 2) and ICD testing are shown (Figure 3).

Results of the Nonthoracotomy Lead System

Personal Experience

We attempted this technique in 33 patients. For 22 patients, a mean follow-up of 11 months was available (from February 2, 1991–November 9, 1992). The mean age was 58 years (range 29–74). Coronary artery disease was the underlying etiology in the majority of patients (17 patients). Ventricular fibrillation was the presenting rhythm in 6 patients. The mean left ventricular ejection fraction was 0.28 (range 0.10–0.70). An acceptable DFT, defined as DFT < 25 J, was documented in 16 patients (72.7%). There were no operative or perioperative deaths.

With a mean follow-up of 11 months (range 3–22 months) there were 3 deaths. The cause of death was congestive heart failure in 2 patients at 3 months (following incessant ventricular tachycardia [VT]), and at 6 months due to pulmonary edema after implantation of the ICDs, and a sudden cardiac death at 7 months in 1 patient. In this patient, late displacement of the SVC lead was noted, and death occurred before the electrode could be repositioned. An infection that required explantation of the defibrillation system occurred in 1 patient (4.5%).

With a mean follow-up of 11 months, 5 patients experienced ventricular fibrillation that was successfully treated by shock; 6 patients had VT that was successfully treated in 4 of these patients by antitachycardia pacing (ATP) and in 2 of these patients by defibrillation after unsuccessful ATP. In 9 patients (56%), no ICD intervention or tachyarrhythmias were detected. Analysis of factors that were predictive of success or failure of ICD therapy showed that the only factor that tended to predict failure was antiarrhythmic therapy, particularly amiodarone at the time of the ICD implant.

This experience is consistent with that of a collaborative French study that also includes this patient group. In the collaborative study, the transvenous approach could be applied to 62 of 77 patients (80%) and the perioperative mortality was 1.6%.

Review of the Literature

Several groups have reported their NTL system experience. Yee et al.[7] reported on 14 patients in whom the transvenous implant technique was attempted and found feasible in 11 of these 14 patients using the CS, an RV, and an SVC lead in 7 patients, and an SQ in the remaining 4 patients. No operative deaths were reported.

The European PCD™ (Medtronic, Minneapolis, MN) study includes 103 of 162 patients[10] in whom the Transvene system was attempted (87.6%). The mean age of the patients was 55 years. Predominant male gender (86%) was observed, comparable to other reported ICD series. The mean left ventricular ejection fraction was 38%. This patient population was compared to a retrospective control group of patients with implanted epicardial leads. The 1-year survival was better for the Transvene patients (96.4% versus 86.3%), mainly due to a decrease in perioperative mortality. Reporting on the worldwide experience of 757 patients with the Transvene NTL leads, Norenberg et al.[11] found a perioperative mortality of 0.7% and an overall 1-year survival rate of 95.3% for this patient population. Considering the sudden and the nonsudden cardiac deaths, the survival was 99.8% and 96.8%, respectively. The lead configurations used were RV-SVC-SQ in 65.6%; RV-CS-SQ in 29.3%; and RV-CS-SVC in 5.1% of patients.

Bocker et al.[12] reported on the Münster NTL experience. The operative mortality was 1%. The ICDs used were Ventak™ PRx and Ventak™ P2 (CPI, St. Paul, MN) in combination with the Endotak lead, and PCD combined with the Transvene leads. During the follow-up period of 12 ± 8 months, the actuarial survival was 100% for sudden cardiac and 95% for total cardiac deaths. Considering the arrhythmic survival based on the documented shocks for rapid ventricular arrhythmia (> 240 beats per minute) by the device telemetry, which the authors assumed would have resulted in certain death without the shock, they estimated that the ICD survival benefit to be 30% at 18 months. The arrhythmic death mortality was not significantly different in the group with an ejection fraction below 30% compared to the group of patients with an ejection fraction above 30%.

Hauser et al.[13] reviewed the results of 414 patients from a multicenter Endotak clinical trial and compared these results to a retrospective control group of 292 patients who received epicardial leads with Ventak ICDs. The two groups were comparable with respect to age, gender, underlying heart disease, and documented clinical arrhythmias. The operative mortality was lower for the transvenous (1.3%) compared to the epicardial group (2.7%). The complications rates were reportedly similar for both groups. Considering total cardiac mortality, sudden and nonsudden, the survival rate was high for both groups. At 12 months it was 93.1% for the NTL and 88.3% for the epicardial group. If only sudden cardiac deaths were taken into account, 98.8% and 98.6% were alive in the two groups, respectively.

Frame et al.[14] reported their experience with 34 patients. A successful implantation was achieved in 30 patients (88.2%) with the transvenous lead system. Although there were no deaths in the perioperative period, three patients developed pulmonary edema and low cardiac output that responded to therapy. Three additional patients developed electromechanical dissociation during

DFT testing. These complications were ascribed to prolonged anesthesia and DFT testing. In fact, one patient received up to 35 shocks in their series.

The experience of Trappe et al.[15] with 13 patients using the Endotak system also confirmed the feasibility of the endocardial approach. An operative death due to cardiac rupture occurred in 1 patient.

Advantages of the Transvenous Approach

Feasibility

It is clear from the review of the literature and from our own experience that the transvenous approach is feasible for most patients. The transvenous approach obviates the need for thoracotomy and its inherent complications. The hospital stay is shortened, making this technique more cost effective. Although in most institutions this technique is performed by a thoracic or cardiovascular surgeon in the operative suite, in our institution the last 21 implants were performed in the electrophysiology laboratory by appropriately trained cardiologists without the help of a surgeon. Our experience is similar to that of Gross et al.[16] It is important to emphasize that the electrophysiology laboratory should fulfill the requirements of an operating room in most respects, including equipment, dimension standards, and aseptic technique. The operative mortality with the NTL approach is reduced, compared to the epicardial approach, from 3% to 4% to approximately 1%. Furthermore, this technique may be applied to patients with poor left ventricular function (ejection fraction < 0.20) in whom thoracotomy may otherwise be contraindicated due to a higher operative risk.

Efficacy

The transvenous approach appears to be as effective as the epicardial approach in the short term. The NTL systems combined with third-generation cardioverter defibrillators capable of ATP with burst or ramp (autodecremental) pacing have success rates for termination of VT approaching 90% (Figures 4 and 5).[15] Therefore, for the majority of patients, the need for ICD shocks is reduced, as well as the associated discomfort. The battery life of the ICD may therefore be enhanced, which is likely to improve the cost effectiveness of ICD therapy.

For all these reasons, the transvenous approach is the first-line approach for ICD implantation. If a DFT with a satisfactory safety margin cannot be achieved even after an SQ has been placed, the epicardial approach is then considered.

Future Developments

Infection remains a potential problem with ICD use, however, rigorous asepsis,

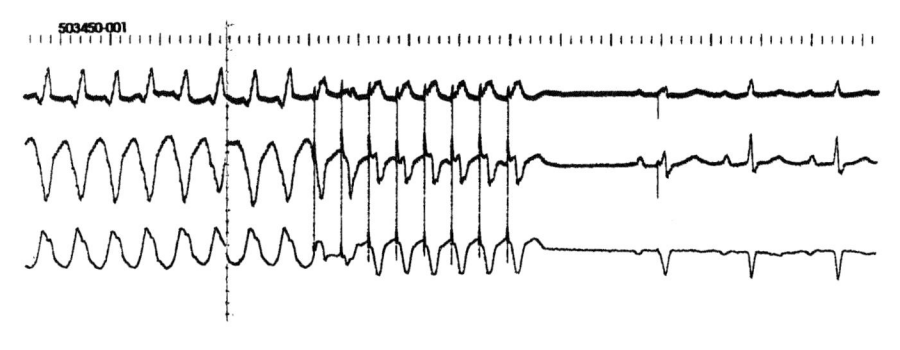

Figure 4. Termination of ventricular tachycardia with burst pacing.

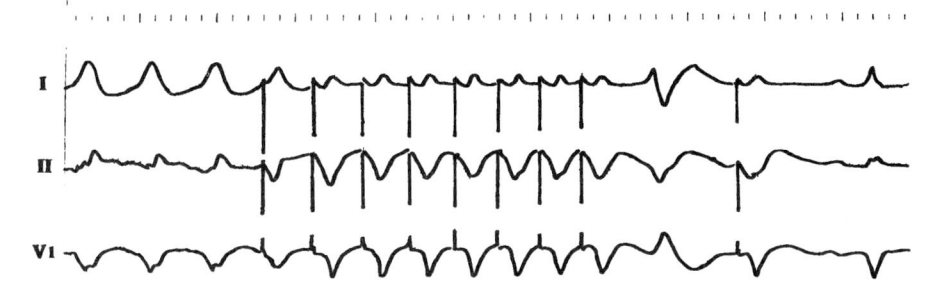

Figure 5. Termination of ventricular tachycardia with autodecremental pacing. From top to bottom: surface leads I, II, and V_1. Arrhythmia conversion is followed by a single paced beat.

prophylactic antibiotic therapy, and careful patient selection and preparation (which include tooth extraction and treatment of other potential infection), comparable to that of patients undergoing valvular surgery may help minimize the infection potential.

Lead displacement is another potential complication of the transvenous approach. Displacement of the SVC lead particularly requires attention. It is possible that the single lead systems, with or without an SQ, may supersede two- and three-lead systems. It appears that passive or active fixation of leads is feasible.

Although the current generation of ICDs have data logging capabilities designed to detect ventricular electrograms, analog ECG tracing may be needed to clarify the diagnosis. Dual-chamber pacing and sensing would be another useful addition to the ICD therapy, providing physiological pacing and the ability to analyze atrial electrograms, which could improve the specificity for VT recognition (see Chapter 34).

Biphasic shocks lower DFTs and enable implantation of transvenous ICDs in a greater number of patients. Significantly lower DFTs are likely to result in reduction of the generator size, as the need for high-output devices is reduced, thus permitting the use of the transvenous subpectoral ICDs for most patients.

References

1. Mirowski M, Reid P, Mower M, et al: Termination of malignant ventricular arrhythmias with an implanted automatic defibrillator in human beings. *N Engl J Med* 303:322, 1980.
2. Mirowski M, Mower MM, Staewen WS, et al: The development of the transvenous automatic defibrillator. *Arch Intern Med* 129:773, 1972.
3. Saksena S, Parsonnet V: Implantation of a cardioverter defibrillator without thoracotomy using a triple electrode system. *JAMA* 259:69, 1988.
4. Winkle RA, Bach SM Jr, Mead RH et al: Comparison of defibrillation efficacy in humans using a new catheter and superior vena cava spring left ventricular patch electrode. *J Am Coll Cardiol* 11:365, 1988.
5. Bach S, Barstadt J, Harper N, et al: Initial clinical experience. Endotak™ implantable transvenous system (abstract). *J Am Coll Cardiol* 13:65A, 1989.
6. Nisam S, Barold S: Historical evolution of the automatic implantable cardioverter defibrillator in the treatment of malignant ventricular arrhythmias. In: *The Implantable Cardioverter-Defibrillator*. Edited by E Alt, H Klein, JC Griffin. Berlin: Springer-Verlag; 1993, p. 3.
7. Yee R, Klein GJ, Leitch JW, et al: A permanent transvenous lead system for an implantable pacemaker cardioverter-defibrillator: nonthoracotomy approach to implantation. *Circulation* 85:196, 1992.
8. Bardy GH, Hofer B, Johnson G, et al: Implantable transvenous cardioverter-defibrillators. *Circulation* 87:1152, 1993.
9. Weismuller P, Hemmer W, Wiecha J, et al: Initial clinical experience with the new ICD Siecure (abstract). *PACE* 16(Part II):874, 1993.

10. *European PCD Study. Patients with Transvene Lead System.* Maastricht: Medtronic Bakken Research Center Report. November 1991.
11. Norenberg MS, Sakun V, Roberts D, et al: Long-term clinical experience with PCD Transvene system: worldwide experience (abstract). PACE 16(Part II):874, 1993.
12. Bocker D, Block M, Isbruch F, et al: Do patients with an implantable defibrillator live longer? *J Am Coll Cardiol* 21:1638, 1993.
13. Hauser RG, Kurschinski DT, McVeigh K, et al: Clinical results with nonthoracotomy ICD systems. PACE 16:141, 1993.
14. Frame R, Brodman R, Gross J, et al: Initial experience with transvenous implantable cardioverter defibrillator lead systems: operative morbidity and mortality. PACE 16:149, 1993.
15. Trappe JH, Klein H, Fieguth HG, et al: Clinical efficacy and safety of the new cardioverter defibrillator systems. PACE 16:153, 1993.
16. Gross JN, Ben-Zur UM, Furman S, et al: Transvenous ICD implantation: feasibility of implantation by cardiologists in a catheterization laboratory environment (abstract). PACE 16:902A, 1993.

Chapter 26

Primary Prevention of Sudden Cardiac Death Using Implantable Cardioverter-Defibrillators

J. Thomas Bigger, Jr.

Although the efficacy of implantable cardioverter-defibrillators (ICDs) is established for termination of sustained ventricular tachycardia (VT) and ventricular fibrillation (VF), the benefit in terms of overall survival has not been demonstrated. Implantable cardioverter-defibrillator therapy became available in 1985, well after electrophysiologically guided antiarrhythmic drug therapy was established as a standard of practice. Therefore, no randomized controlled study of ICD therapy versus no therapy was ever done in patients with malignant ventricular arrhythmias. No trials comparing ICD therapy with drug therapy in patients with malignant ventricular arrhythmias have been completed as yet either, but several are ongoing and we discuss these briefly in this chapter.

There is no randomized, controlled clinical trial yet completed that justifies primary prevention (prophylaxis) of sudden cardiac death with ICDs. Currently, most of the effort is directed at secondary prevention of sudden cardiac death, ie, treatment is directed at survivors of cardiac arrest. The limited success of this approach has sparked interest in primary prevention. In this chapter, we discuss the prospects for primary prevention of sudden cardiac death using ICD prophylaxis and describe some of the ongoing studies that are evaluating this approach.

The Case for Primary Prevention of Sudden Cardiac Death

There are good arguments for primary prevention of sudden cardiac death. Each year, 400,000 or more sudden cardiac deaths occur in the United States, almost 1 per minute.[1,2] A similar number die each year in western Europe. Fewer than 5% of cardiac arrest victims are resuscitated and leave the hospital alive. A few well-organized communities, eg, Seattle, have higher salvage rates, but even in these communities, more than three fourths of the cardiac arrest victims die. The survivors of cardiac arrest are

---

Supported in part by NIH Grants HL-48159 and HL-48120 from the National Heart, Lung, and Blood Institute, Bethesda, MD and RR-00645 from the Research Resources Administration, NIH; and by funds from Cardiac Pacemakers, Inc., The Bugher Foundation, The Dover Foundation, and Mrs. Adelaide Segerman, New York, NY.

From Singer I, (ed.) Implantable Cardioverter-Defibrillator. Armonk, NY: Futura Publishing Company, Inc.; © 1994.

treated vigorously, usually with electrophysiologically guided drug therapy or with ICDs. However, the success of this approach is limited by the very small fraction of patients who survive a cardiac arrest to take advantage of modern treatment. The poor salvage rate for patients experiencing cardiac arrest provides strong motivation for prophylaxis. A significant fraction of deaths due to cardiac arrest cannot be addressed by prophylaxis, because sudden cardiac death is the first and last manifestation of coronary heart disease for many individuals. Many of the deaths of patients who were previously asymptomatic probably have an ischemic mechanism.[3-5] However, about three fourths of sudden cardiac deaths occur in patients with previously recognized heart disease, quite often severe heart disease. Arrhythmias account for a significant fraction of deaths in patients with advanced heart disease and congestive heart failure. Large numbers of patients with previously recognized heart disease are available for screening, risk stratification, and prophylaxis.[6,7] If those patients with heart disease who will experience cardiac arrest can be identified, preventive measures could have a substantially larger impact on the sudden cardiac death problem than is currently achieved with the salvage and treat strategy.

The Case Against Primary Prevention of Sudden Cardiac Death

A strategy of prediction and prevention of high-risk patients requires that the tests to detect high-risk patients be accurate and that the treatments be effective. The tests currently available to identify patients for ICD prophylaxis are not ideal. Tests that predict cardiac mortality and sudden cardiac death include left ventricular ejection fraction (LVEF), spontaneous, unsustained ventricular arrhythmias quantified in 24-hour continuous electrocardiographic (ECG) recordings, RR variability over a 24-hour or shorter interval, signal-averaged ECG, and electrophysiologic studies. These tests have high negative predictive accuracy, ie, > 90% of the patients with a negative test will remain free of arrhythmic events during follow-up. Thus, the tests do an admirable job of identifying low-risk groups. Unfortunately, however, these tests have low positive predictive accuracy, about 15% to 30%.[8-19] This means that at least 70% of the patients in the high-risk group will not have a cardiac arrest during a 2- to 3-year period of follow-up. If the high-risk group is treated, then 70% will be exposed to the risk, inconvenience, and expense of treatment even though they would not have had an event if left untreated. The more dangerous, inconvenient, and costly a treatment is, the less appealing it is when the screening tests have low to moderate positive predictive accuracy.

There is encouraging preliminary data to suggest that recently evaluated risk predictors, eg, signal-averaged ECG, cardiac electrophysiologic studies, and RR variability can be combined with more established risk predictors, eg, LVEF or ventricular ectopy, to obtain positive predictive accuracies > 50%.[20,21] This level of predictive accuracy may warrant prophylaxis, even with a treatment that has significant mortality and morbidity. However, these findings are preliminary and require additional studies.

Drug Prophylaxis to Prevent Sudden Cardiac Death

β-Adrenergic Blocking Drugs, Aspirin, and Converting Enzyme Inhibitors

Drug prophylaxis for sudden cardiac death has not proved very effective. The only class of antiarrhythmic drugs shown to be effective against sudden cardiac death to a greater extent than for all-cause mortality or cardiac death is β-adrenergic blocking drugs and their benefit is modest.[22-25] It is not clear whether the beneficial effect of β-adrenergic blocking drugs on postinfarction survival is an antiarrhythmic action, an anti-ischemic action, or both. The suppression of ventricular arrhythmia by most β-adrenergic blocking drugs is modest. Many patients who are at high risk for sudden cardiac death have severe left ventricular dysfunction (LVEF < 0.36) or a clinical heart failure syndrome (New York Heart Association [NYHA] functional Class II-IV), groups that physicians are reluctant to treat with β-adrenergic blocking drugs.[26] In controlled clinical trials, two other drug classes have been proven to improve survival in patients with coronary heart disease: aspirin and converting enzyme inhibitors.[27-33] However, both of these have relatively modest effects on mortality and seem to have less effect on sudden cardiac death than on all-cause mortality or cardiac death. Some studies have even suggested that aspirin may increase sudden cardiac death even though it has an overall beneficial effect on mortality.[34]

Drugs With Class I Antiarrhythmic Action

Until recently, it was hoped that drugs that suppressed prognostically significant ventricular arrhythmias would improve survival. The Cardiac Arrhythmia Suppression Trial (CAST) disproved this hypothesis for Class I drugs. Encainide and flecainide treatment was associated with a 2.5-fold increase in the mortality rate, even though they substantially suppressed prognostically significant ventricular arrhythmias.[35,36] Moricizine was not significantly different from placebo, ie, even when moricizine substantially reduced ventricular arrhythmias, it did not improve survival.[37] Also, moricizine seemed to increase mortality during the dose finding phase of the study (before randomization). The pooled experience from additional small studies of drugs with Class I antiarrhythmic action is also discouraging.[38-42]

Drugs With Class III Antiarrhythmic Action

Currently, drugs with Class III antiarrhythmic action are regarded as most effective for treatment of malignant ventricular arrhythmias. This view has significant support, but the data are not definitive. In 1991, Yusuf and Teo[43] published an overview of randomized clinical trials of antiarrhythmic drug therapy. In the four trials that compared amiodarone with a control group, there were 55 deaths among 577 patients treated with amiodarone compared to 73 deaths among 575 controls. These trials showed a nonsignificant trend toward benefit. The odds of dying while on amiodarone therapy were 0.71 that of the control groups (95% confidence interval for the odds ratio was 0.48–1.03). None of these trials recruited patients with malignant ventricular arrhythmias.

The Basel Antiarrhythmic Study of Infarct Survival

The Basel Antiarrhythmic Study of Infarct Survival (BASIS) was among those included in Yusuf and Teo's overview.[44] Between 1981 and 1987, BASIS randomized 312 patients who had complex ventricular arrhythmias at the time of discharge after acute myocardial infarction: 100 were randomized to individualized therapy with Class I antiarrhythmic drugs, 98 to amiodarone, and 114 to no antiarrhythmic drugs. The average LVEF for the three groups was: 0.41 in the Class I antiarrhythmic drug group, 0.46 in the amiodarone group, and 0.42 in the control group. Drugs were chosen in the individualized antiarrhythmic therapy group by demonstrating suppression of the arrhythmia by Holter ECG assessment. Amiodarone was given empirically, 1,000 mg/day for 5 days, followed by a daily dose of 200 mg/day. BASIS was not a blinded study. During 12 months of follow-up, there were 30 deaths: 10 in the Class I antiarrhythmic drug group, 5 in the amiodarone group, and 15 in the control group. This borderline result may be attributed, in part, to the LVEF advantage had by the amiodarone group.

Polish Postinfarction Amiodarone Study

In 1992, Ceremuzynski et al.[45] published the results of a pilot study of amiodarone prophylaxis after acute myocardial infarction that was conducted between 1986 and 1989. Patients < 75 years of age with myocardial infarction and a contraindication for therapy with β-adrenergic blocking drugs were recruited (heart failure, bronchial asthma, treated diabetes, or peripheral artery disease with claudication); 308 were randomized to placebo and 305 to amiodarone. During 1 year of follow-up, there were 33 deaths (10.7%) in the placebo group compared with 21 deaths (6.9%) in the amiodarone group (odds ratio 0.62, 95% confidence interval 0.35–1.08, $P = 0.095$). This is a borderline result.

Ongoing Trials With Amiodarone

There are three large trials currently underway that compare amiodarone to placebo: the Canadian Myocardial Infarction Amiodarone Trial (CAMIAT), the European Myocardial Infarction Amiodarone Trial (EMIAT), and the Veterans Administration Study of Amiodarone in Heart Failure. CAMIAT recruits patients with prognostically significant, unsustained ventricular arrhythmias after acute myocardial infarction without any LVEF requirement. EMIAT recruits patients with LVEF < 0.40 after myocardial infarction regardless of their ventricular arrhythmias. The Veterans Administration study recruited patients with significant left ventricular dysfunction and unsustained ventricular arrhythmias. CAMIAT and EMIAT are actively recruiting and together plan to randomize more than 3,000 patients. The Veterans Administration study has completed recruiting approximately 700 patients and is following its sample. These studies, together with the small number of already completed studies should clarify the benefit and risk of amiodarone therapy after myocardial infarction. These studies will not clarify the efficacy and safety of amiodarone for patients with malignant ventricular arrhythmias. At the moment, the evidence for the efficacy of amiodarone to prevent malignant ventricular arrhythmias in high-risk patients is inadequate to support a definite recommendation for prophylaxis.

Implantable Cardioverter-Defibrillator Therapy for Secondary Prevention of Sudden Cardiac Death

Uncontrolled Studies Indicate Efficacy of Implantable Cardioverter-Defibrillator Therapy for Sudden Death

Perhaps the most important argument against ICD prophylaxis is the lack of any evidence from a randomized, controlled trial to indicate an increased survival attributable to ICD treatment in the patients who currently have indications for treatment, ie, patients with sustained VT or VF. Uncontrolled studies have reported that ICD treatment reduces the sudden cardiac death rate to < 2% per year.[46-48]

Possible Biases in Uncontrolled Studies of Implantable Cardioverter-Defibrillator Therapy

Recently, such optimistic results have been questioned.[49] First, sudden cardiac death is a judgmental diagnosis, ie, a man-made assignment of cause of death and is thus subject to unconscious bias in assignment. Second, the nonsudden death rates are low in ICD follow-up studies that show low sudden cardiac death rates. This could indicate a benefit of ICD treatment on nonarrhythmic death, but this possibility seems unlikely because ICD therapy should uniquely affect arrhythmic mortality. More likely, low nonsudden death rates in ICD-treated patients are due to patient selection, to concomitant therapy, and to a long interval between the presenting arrhythmia and initiation of treatment. Until recently, ICD treatment was used as a last resort, usually a long time after the presenting event, eg, cardiac arrest or sustained VT. As a result of delay, the sickest patients may die, making the mortality rate for ICD therapy lower than for historical controls who were started on alternate treatments with less delay. Aspirin and converting enzyme inhibitors are used much more frequently since the advent of ICD therapy and may account for some of the apparent benefit when ICD treatment is compared with historical controls.

Biases due to patient selection, longer time to treatment, and use of sudden cardiac death as an end point affect all available studies. Despite this, sudden cardiac death rates of 5% to 8% at 5 years are so low that it seems likely that ICD treatment does provide protection against sudden cardiac death. However, even if sudden death were totally eliminated by ICD treatment, it might not have much impact on the occurrence of death of all causes. Patients dying of malignant ventricular arrhythmias usually have other risks as well as arrhythmic risk, eg, chronic multivessel coronary disease and left ventricular dysfunction. Implantable cardioverter-defibrillator treatment might not prolong survival very much because death from ischemia or pump failure may nullify the potential benefit of eliminating arrhythmic deaths.

Connolly and Yusuf[49] argue that the reduction in all-cause mortality could not be larger than 33%. They point out that < 50% of deaths are sudden, some of the sudden deaths are not tachyarrhythmic (eg, cardiac rupture, cerebral hemorrhage, bradyarrhythmias), some tachyarrhythmic deaths are not prevented by ICD treatment, and that the operative mortality of an ICD implant via thoracotomy averages about 3%.

Does Implantable Cardioverter-Defibrillator Therapy Reduce Overall Mortality?

By 1985, when ICD therapy arrived on the scene, electrophysiologically guided antiarrhythmic drug therapy was well established as a standard of practice. Although the efficacy of electrophysiologically guided antiarrhythmic drug therapy was never established in controlled trials either, physicians were not willing to randomize patients with malignant ventricular arrhythmias to no therapy. We probably will never see a large-scale, randomized clinical trial that compares ICD treatment with no therapy in patients who have survived an episode of cardiac arrest or sustained VT. Thus, the magnitude of the improvement in overall survival by ICD therapy for patients with malignant ventricular arrhythmias will always remain unknown.

Is Implantable Cardioverter-Defibrillator Therapy Better Than Antiarrhythmic Drug Therapy?

We are fortunate that at least three studies will compare ICD therapy to drug therapy in patients with malignant ventricular arrhythmias: the Canadian Implantable Defibrillator Study (CIDS), the Cardiac Arrest Study of Hamburg (CASH), and the Antiarrhythmics Versus Implantable defibrillators (AVID) trial.

The Canadian Implantable Defibrillator Study

CIDS began enrollment early in 1991. CIDS is recruiting patients who have had VF without myocardial infarction, VT with syncope, and VT with presyncope and an LVEF < 0.36. Patients who enroll are randomized in equal proportions to amiodarone or to ICD treatment. Patients who are randomized to amiodarone are given 1,200 mg or more per day for at least a week, 400 mg or more per day for 10 weeks, and, then given 300 mg or more per day until the end of the trial. It is recommended that amiodarone not be used in the ICD group to treat patients with atrial fibrillation. Patients who are randomized to ICD therapy can be treated with any available ICD system. The primary end point is arrhythmic death as defined by Hinkle and Thaler.[50] During the planning of CIDS, a 15% 3-year mortality rate was assumed for the group assigned to amiodarone. CIDS has 80% power to detect a 58% difference between the two treatment assignments. CIDS originally planned to randomize 400 patients and follow them an average of 3 years; recently the sample size was increased to 500. At the end of April 1993, 205 patients had been randomized in CIDS. In the group assigned to ICD treatment, 22% are taking amiodarone; in the group assigned to amiodarone treatment, 5.3% have had ICDs implanted.

The Cardiac Arrest Study of Hamburg

CASH began in 1987 and is nearing completion of its enrollment phase. CASH is testing the hypothesis that ICD therapy is better than drug therapy. When planning the trial, it was assumed that 50% of the patients who survived the index cardiac arrest would die within 2 years without treatment and that the 2-year death rate would be reduced to 31% in the group assigned to ICD therapy. The target randomization number was 400, 100 to each of four treatments. Patients who had cardiac arrest and inducible VT or VF were randomized to ICD treatment or one of three drug treatments each with a different mechanism of action: propafenone (IC), metoprolol (II), or amiodarone (III).[51]

Details of Treatment

A loading dose of 1,000 mg of amiodarone per day was given for 7 days followed by a dose of 400–600 mg per day starting on day 8.[52] Metoprolol was started at a low initial dose of 12.5–25 mg per day and increased to the maximum tolerated dose or 300 mg per day over 2 weeks. Propafenone was started at 450 mg per day and increased to the maximum tolerated dose or 900 mg per day over 2 weeks. A variety of ICDs manufactured by Cardiac Pacemakers Inc. (St. Paul, MN) were implanted in the CASH study: AID-B™, Ventak™ 1500 and 1520, Ventak 1600, and Ventak 1700 and 1705. In the programmable ICDs, the rate cutoff was programmed between 170 and 200 per minute. The primary therapy was a high-energy discharge in all cases.

When repeated episodes of documented VT occurred, investigators were permitted to activate antitachycardiac pacing (ATP) if the patient had a device with this capability. Many patients who had recurrences of sustained, but nonfatal ventricular tachyarrhythmias during long-term drug therapy crossed over to ICD therapy.[52]

Patient Sample

The average age of the patients in the CASH study was 57 years; 80% were male. Seventy-nine percent had coronary heart disease and a surprising 19% had no heart disease. The average LVEF was relatively high, ie, 0.42, for a group of cardiac arrest survivors. Patients with ischemic ST depression during an exercise test or a positive thallium scan were revascularized (angioplasty or coronary artery bypass graft [CABG] surgery) prior to randomization. Following this policy, about 20% of the patients in CASH were revascularized. The primary end point for CASH was all-cause mortality for the ICD limb and all-cause mortality or recurrence of nonfatal cardiac arrest in the three drug limbs.

In March 1992, after 229 patients were randomized, enrollment was stopped in the propafenone limb because of an excess of events.[52] Eighteen percent of the patients in the propafenone group experienced sudden cardiac death compared with none in the ICD group.[53] All-cause mortality was 34% in the propafenone group compared with 17% in the ICD group. All-cause mortality or cardiac arrest occurred in 44% of the propafenone group compared with 18% of the ICD group. The results of electrophysiologic testing (positive or negative) had no predictive value for death or nonfatal arrhythmic events during follow-up on propafenone therapy. This finding led the CASH investigators to conclude that propafenone treatment cannot be recommended in survivors of cardiac arrest even when the drug converts inducible VT to not inducible.[52] Randomization continues in the other three limbs. By the end of April 1993, 298 patients had been randomized in the CASH study.[53] Stopping recruitment early for the propafenone group will complicate the primary analysis, which should have been a comparison of the ICD group with the three drug groups combined. CASH also has been compromised by a series of interim reports of outcome data.

Antiarrhythmics Versus Implantable Defibrillators

The National Heart, Lung, and Blood Institute (NHLBI) is conducting a trial to determine whether there is a significant difference in efficacy, safety, quality of life, and cost between ICD therapy and drug treatment with either amiodarone or sotalol. The NHLBI trial is called Antiarrhythmics Versus Implantable Defibrillators (AVID). The 1-year pilot phase began in June 1993 in 20 clinical centers in the United States. The purpose of the pilot study is to evaluate feasibility, safety, and procedures for a full-scale trial. The full-scale trial will test the hypothesis that the policy of implanting an ICD in patients who survive cardiac arrest or sustained VT will improve survival compared with treatment with amiodarone or sotalol (Figure 1). AVID is enrolling patients who were defibrillated for cardiac arrest due to VF, or experienced syncope due to documented sustained VT. For these two groups, there is no LVEF criterion to qualify. Patients who have hemodynamically compromising sustained VT without syncope are eligible, but must have an LVEF < 0.41. There are no age restrictions for enrollment. Patients who qualify and lack exclusions (Table 1) are randomized with equal probability to ICD treatment or drug treat-

The AVID Trial

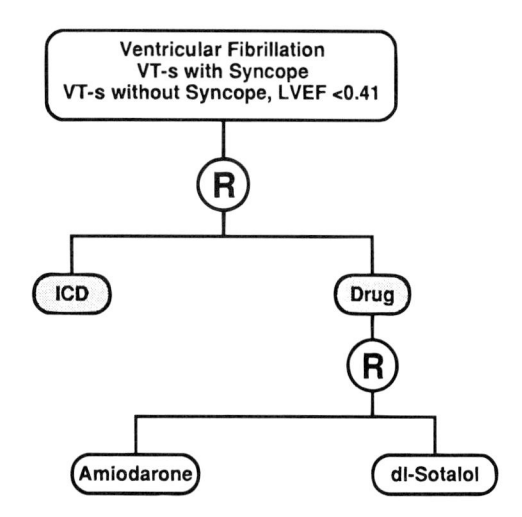

Figure 1. Flow diagram for the Antiarrhythmics Versus Implantable Defibrillators (AVID) trial pilot study. The R in the circle indicate the points of randomization. The shaded boxes indicate the main comparison for the trial. ICD: implantable cardioverter-defibrillator; LVEF: left ventricular ejection fraction; VT-s: sustained ventricular tachycardia.

ment. Those assigned to drug treatment will be randomized to start treatment with amiodarone or with sotalol (Figure 1). In AVID, amiodarone therapy is empiric, but dl-sotalol therapy can be guided either by Holter assessment or electrophysiologic studies. Patients who are randomized to drug therapy, but cannot be assessed by either Holter recordings or electrophysiologic studies (< 30 ventricular premature complexes and uninducible), will be treated empirically with amiodarone.

Baseline Studies

Clinically indicated baseline tests to define the type and extent of disease and the need for revascularization (CABG surgery or percutaneous transluminal coronary agnioplasty [PTCA]), eg, coronary angiography, radionuclide ventriculogram, exercise tests, are done before randomization. Deci-

Table 1
Exclusion Criteria for the AVID Trial Pilot Study

1. Transient or correctable cause of the index arrhythmic event
2. Index arrhythmic event occurred while on amiodarone
3. CABG surgery performed since index arrhythmic event
4. Revascularization (CABG or PTCA) is planned and LVEF is >0.40
5. Inability to undergo thoracotomy or have an ICD implanted
6. Contraindications to amiodarone
7. More than 6 weeks exposure to amiodarone in the last 6 months or maximum plasma level of amiodarone of 0.2 mcg/mL
8. Supraventricular arrhythmia requiring Class I or III antiarrhythmic drug
9. Less than age of consent
10. Long QT syndrome
11. Index event within 7 days of revascularization (either CABG or PTCA)
12. Mechanical device or inotropic drug (excluding digitalis) required for hemodynamic support
13. NYHA Class IV heart failure
14. On a heart transplant waiting list
15. Life expectancy <1 year
16. Chronic serious bacterial infection
17. Unable to give informed consent
18. Psychiatric condition likely to limit cooperation
19. Geographically inaccessible for follow-up
20. Concurrent use of an investigational antiarrhythmic drug or device

CABG: coronary artery bypass graft; PTCA: percutaneous transluminal coronary angioplasty; LVEF: left ventricular ejection fraction; ICD: implantable cardioverter-defibrillator.

sions about the use of β blockers, angiotensin converting enzyme inhibitors, and aspirin therapy are made before randomization. Holter recordings and electrophysiologic studies are not required at baseline, but are utilized as needed to establish a diagnosis of the index rhythm or characterize the disease.

Enrollment Cascade

It is anticipated that about 50% of the patients presenting with malignant ventricular arrhythmias will be eligible for the trial and that about 50% of the eligible patients will be willing to enroll.

Design Features and Sample Size

AVID is designed as a fixed sample size, randomized clinical trial with group sequential monitoring for safety. Like all of the other ICD trials, AVID is not blinded. Patients who agree to join the study are randomized 50:50 to ICD or drug therapy. This primary randomization to ICD or drug therapy is stratified on clinical center and primary rhythm disorder (VF versus sustained VT). The primary end point for the study is all-cause mortality. The primary hypothesis will be tested using the intention to treat principle; data will be analyzed by the Cox regression model and the significance of differences between groups will be tested with the log rank test. The alpha error is set at 0.05 (two tailed) and the power between 0.85 and 0.90. The drop-in rate (crossover from drug therapy to ICD therapy) was estimated at 20% and the dropout rate at 0%. For the sample size calculation, the 2.5-year primary event rate in the group assigned to drug therapy was assumed to be 35% and ICD therapy was assumed to reduce this rate by 30%, ie, to 24.5%. These parameters yield a sample size of about 1,000 patients, 500 in each group.

Implantable Cardioverter-Defibrillator Therapy

AVID attempts to implant ICDs using nonthoracotomy lead systems wherever possible. Pulse generators with tiered therapy, including ATP and antibradycardia pacing, were chosen for the pilot study. No ICD systems that include both tiered-therapy devices and nonthoracotomy leads were marketed in June 1993 so AVID is implanting ICD systems under the control of an Investigational Device Exemption from the Food and Drug Administration. Nonthoracotomy leads are tried first unless the patient is undergoing thoracotomy for revascularization or valvular surgery. If a

10-J safety margin for defibrillation thresholds cannot be obtained on nonthoracotomy leads, an ICD system is implanted via thoracotomy. Patients who are undergoing CABG surgery have an ICD system with epicardial leads implanted during the operation. Devices are turned on in the operating room at the time of implant with a VF detection criterion of ≥ 200 per minute and with VF therapy activated. Before discharge, the final settings are programmed and tested; at least one test of the device against induced VF is recommended. For patients who qualified with sustained VT, ATP is programmed and tested. To the extent possible, arrhythmias that occur after ICD implantation are managed by ICD reprogramming alone. Addition of antiarrhythmic drug therapy in the group assigned to ICD therapy is discouraged.

Drug Therapy

Patients assigned to the drug limb are randomized to start sotalol or amiodarone first. Patients assigned to amiodarone are not required to have electrophysiologic or Holter assessment. Loading doses of 800–1,600 mg/day are given for 1–3 weeks. Then, doses of 400–800 mg/day are given for 4 weeks. Thereafter, a maintenance dose is given, usually 400 mg/day; the minimum acceptable maintenance dose is 200 mg, 5 days a week. It is recommended that a loading dose of 10 gm be achieved before discharge. Sotalol is started at a dose of 80 mg twice a day. The dose is advanced every 2–3 days to a maximum of 320 mg twice a day. Sotalol therapy is guided by Holter recordings or electrophysiologic studies, chosen by the investigator. For Holter assessment, a baseline 24-hour recording is done. A Holter done on sotalol must show a $\geq 75\%$ suppression of ventricular premature complexes and $> 90\%$ suppression of couplets and unsustained VT. For electrophysiologic assessment, at least two sites of stimulation and two pacing cycle lengths (one of which must be 400 msec) are used. Double and triple premature stimuli must be used, both for drug-free, baseline study and for drug assessment. To be evaluated with electrophysiologic studies, patients with sustained VT as their qualifying clinical event must have inducible sustained (uniform) VT. Patients with VF as their clinical event must have inducible sustained (uniform or multiform) VT, sustained ventricular flutter, or sustained VF. Drug success is defined as inability to induce > 15 complexes of unsustained VT. If the first drug tried is not effective or not tolerated, the patient may be crossed over to the other, ie, sotalol to amiodarone or vice versa. If neither drug is effective/tolerated, investigators can choose another antiarrhythmic regimen.

Events During Follow-Up

The primary end point for AVID is death of any cause; nonfatal cardiac arrest is not a primary end point. The mode of death will be classified using the CAST definitions.[35,36] Deaths will be classified as noncardiac or cardiac, and cardiac deaths will be subclassified as arrhythmic or nonarrhythmic. Treatments will be assessed for effect on quality of life and cost effectiveness. Patients who experience nonfatal cardiac arrest or a recurrence of sustained VT in the drug limb can be managed using conventional standards of care. Investigators are asked to consider whether the patient can be managed by increasing drug doses, by changing the drug, or by adding a drug.

What Will We Learn from AVID?

We will learn how ICD therapy and therapy with Class III antiarrhythmic drugs compare with respect to survival, arrhythmia recurrences, quality of life, and cost effectiveness. The results of AVID combined with those from CIDS should give a definitive evaluation of the relative merits of amiodarone and ICD therapy for malignant ventricular arrhythmias.

What Will We Learn from Trials That Compare Implantable Cardioverter-Defibrillator and Drug Therapy?

CIDS, CASH, and AVID cannot accurately estimate the magnitude of ICD benefit because each has a positive control group, ie, ICD treatment is being compared to drug therapy. For example, in CIDS, no difference between ICD and amiodarone therapy could result if both treatments have little effect, or if both have beneficial or harmful effects of similar magnitude. A large difference in favor of ICD treatment could indicate a substantial benefit of ICD therapy or a modest benefit combined with a harmful effect of amiodarone or another comparison drug. A difference in favor of amiodarone could occur because of benefits unrelated to an antiarrhythmic action, eg, an anti-ischemic action or a vasodilator action. Similarly, the apparent advantage of ICD treatment over propafenone found in CASH could represent no benefit from ICD treatment combined with substantial harm from propafenone. It would not be surprising if propafenone doubled the all-cause mortality rate in patients with malignant ventricular arrhythmias since this was the magnitude of the adverse effect on mortality seen with encainide and flecainide in CAST. If this is so, then the results indicate no benefit of ICD therapy on all-cause mortality. However, there could be modest benefit in the ICD group and modest harm in the propafenone group. It should be recognized that antiarrhythmic drug treatment is mostly empiric in all three of these trials so they will not answer how well electrophysiologically guided antiarrhythmic drug therapy would compare with ICD therapy. Regardless of the difficulty of interpreting the ICD trials that have positive control groups, if any of these trials shows a substantially better outcome for patients assigned to ICD treatment, it will create additional interest in ICD prophylaxis. Given our current state of knowledge, however, ICD prophylaxis is not warranted until controlled data is available to support this approach.

Randomized Controlled Clinical Trials of Implantable Cardioverter-Defibrillator Prophylaxis

Definitive data are not available to support the prophylactic use of ICD therapy. Nevertheless, one study is attempting to evaluate the role of the ICD in electrophysiologically guided therapy of patients with unsustained VT. Two randomized, controlled clinical trials are exploring ICD treatment in patients who are at high risk to arrhythmic death but have not yet experienced a sustained arrhythmia. The Multicenter UnSustained Tachycardia Trial (MUSTT) aims to determine whether electrophysiologically guided treatment, including drugs and ICD, will improve survival without arrhythmic events. The Multicenter Automatic Defibrillator Implantation Trial (MADIT) is comparing ICD prophylaxis with conventional treatment for patients who have left ventricular dysfunction and unsustained VT. The CABG Patch Trial is comparing ICD therapy with no therapy for high-risk patients undergoing CABG surgery. In addition to these, there are two ICD trials being planned for patients with heart failure and ventricular arrhythmias: the Dilated Cardiomyopathy Trial and Defibrillator Implantation As a Bridge to Later Transplantation.

The Rationale for Prophylactic Treatment of Patients With Unsustained Ventricular Tachycardia

Two of the trials that we discuss, MUSTT and MADIT, are evaluating ICD prophylaxis for coronary heart disease patients who have left ventricular dysfunction and unsustained VT. Unsustained VT is an excellent predictor of death after myocardial infarction and has an association with death comparable to that of LVEF < 0.40.[54] A number of studies have been done to determine whether programmed ventricular stimulation can stratify the risk of patients with coronary heart disease and unsustained VT.

Inducible Ventricular Arrhythmias and Arrhythmic Events in Patients With Unsustained Ventricular Tachycardia

Recently, a meta-analysis was done with 12 studies that reported the results of programmed ventricular stimulation in patients with coronary heart disease and unsustained VT and also reported arrhythmic events during follow-up.[55] The number of patients in the 12 studies totaled 926. The mean age was 61 years, 80% were male, 88% had coronary heart disease, and 72% had previous myocardial infarction. One third ($n = 302$) of the patients had sustained ventricular arrhythmias induced by programmed ventricular stimulation and 251 (83%) of the inducible patients were treated with antiarrhythmic drugs. The studies that limited programmed ventricular stimulation to patients with LVEF < 0.40 had higher percentages of positive tests, about 45%. During an average follow-up of 19.4 months, 100 arrhythmic events occurred: 60 sudden cardiac deaths, 39 episodes of spontaneous, sustained VT, and 1 episode of syncope attributed to VT. The arrhythmic event rate was 17.9% for the inducible patients and 7.4% for noninducible patients, a relative risk of 2.4 (Figure 2). The prevalence of long-term antiarrhythmic drug use was high (> 80%) even when no drug was found that rendered the patient uninducible or

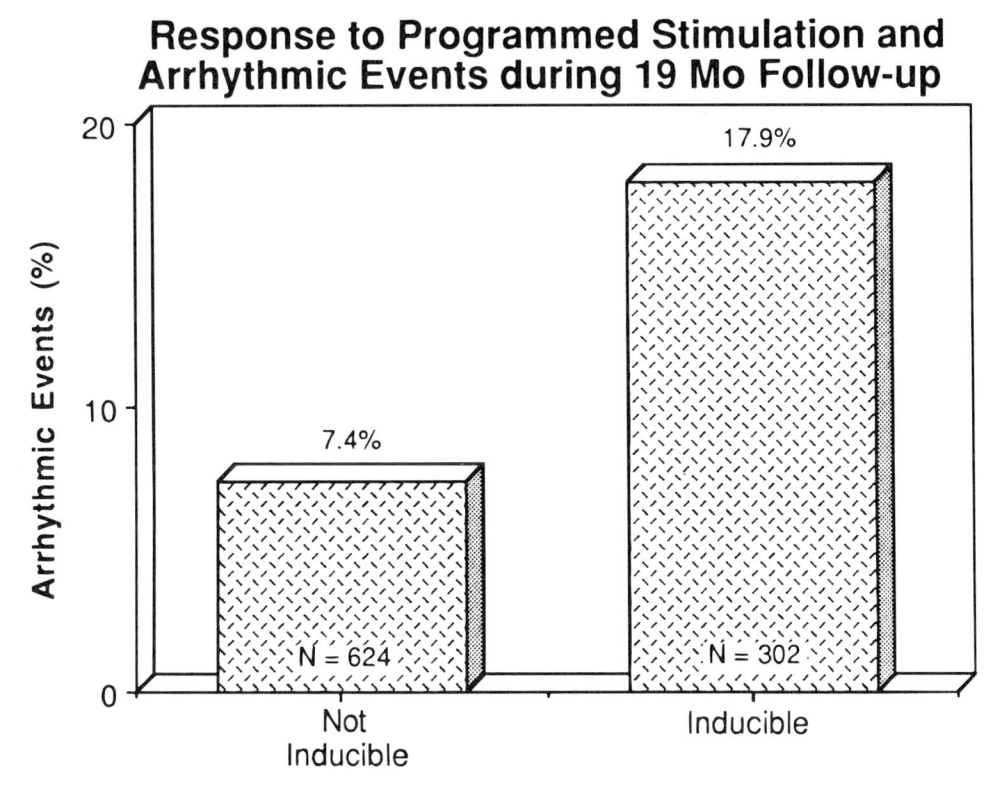

Response to Programmed Stimulation and Arrhythmic Events during 19 Mo Follow-up

Figure 2. Results of meta-analysis to determine the significance of unsustained ventricular tachycardia (VT). Patients with inducible sustained VT had a 2.4 times greater chance of experiencing sudden cardiac death or spontaneous, sustained VT during 19.4 months of follow-up. The high prevalence of antiarrhythmic drug use in the inducible group complicates the interpretation of these data. (Reproduced with permission from Reference 55.)

slowed the tachycardia enough to make it hemodynamically stable. The frequent use of antiarrhythmic drugs makes it impossible to determine the natural history of unsustained VT. During follow-up, arrhythmic events were common in the inducible patients despite or because of the high prevalence of antiarrhythmic drug use in this group. The characteristics of programmed ventricular stimulation as a test to predict risk were: sensitivity, 54%; specificity, 70%; positive predictive accuracy, 18%; and negative predictive accuracy, 93%. Taken together, these studies show that programmed ventricular stimulation has considerable merit to identify the patients at low risk to arrhythmic events during follow-up and, to a lesser extent, to identify the patients at high risk.

The Predictive Value of Inducible Ventricular Tachycardia for Arrhythmic Events

Overall, uncontrolled data from the pooled studies does not suggest that selecting drug therapy by programmed ventricular stimulation identified drugs that prevent arrhythmic events in patients with unsustained VT and inducible sustained VT. The study by Wilber et al.[56,57] is the only one that suggested that programmed ventricular stimulation has merit for evaluating drug therapy. In this study, 100 patients with coronary heart disease, LVEF < 0.40, and unsustained VT were evaluated with programmed ventricular stimulation. In 57 patients, no sustained ventricular arrhythmia was induced; these were discharged on no therapy. Of the remainder, 40 had serial drug evaluation using programmed ventricular stimulation; 20 were suppressed (ie, not inducible) on a drug and were discharged on the drug predicted to be efficacious. Twenty were not suppressed but were discharged on a drug that increased the cycle length of the induced VT by ≥ 100 msec and made the tachycardia hemodynamically well tolerated. Sudden death or cardiac arrest, during an average of 16.7 months of follow-up, were the end points of the study. The 2-year actuarial rates of sudden death or cardiac arrest at 2 years of follow-up were: not inducible, 6%; inducible but suppressed, 11%; and inducible but not suppressed, 50% (Figure 3). Wilber et al.[56] concluded that only 50% of patients with left ventricular dysfunction and inducible sustained VT responded to drug therapy and that the partial responders remained at high risk. In 1991, the authors updated their results after 32.1 months average follow-up.[57] The 2-year actuarial rates of arrhythmic events were: not inducible, 6%; inducible but suppressed, 28%; and inducible but not suppressed, 50%. Independent predictors of sudden death or cardiac arrest were: inducible VT at baseline, inducible VT at discharge, and LVEF < 0.30 (all but one of the patients who experienced an end point had an ejection fraction < 0.30). The authors concluded that electrophysiologically guided antiarrhythmic drug treatment may have limited efficacy in this population whether or not induced arrhythmias are suppressed.[57] This study suggested that electrophysiologic testing is excellent for predicting risk, but has limited value for predicting drug efficacy in patients who have unsustained VT.

At this time, there is no clear indication that antiarrhythmic drug therapy guided by results of programmed ventricular stimulation should be employed in patients with left ventricular dysfunction and unsustained VT. However, the high risk of this group for arrhythmic events makes it a prime target for studies aimed at preventing lethal or morbid outcomes. The poor prognosis of patients with unsustained VT also provides a rationale for randomized controlled trials to evaluate treatment effects on survival.

The Multicenter UnSustained Tachycardia Trial

MUSTT will test the hypothesis that electrophysiologically guided antiarrhyth-

Response to Serial EP Drug Testing and Arrhythmic Events during 32-Mo Follow-up

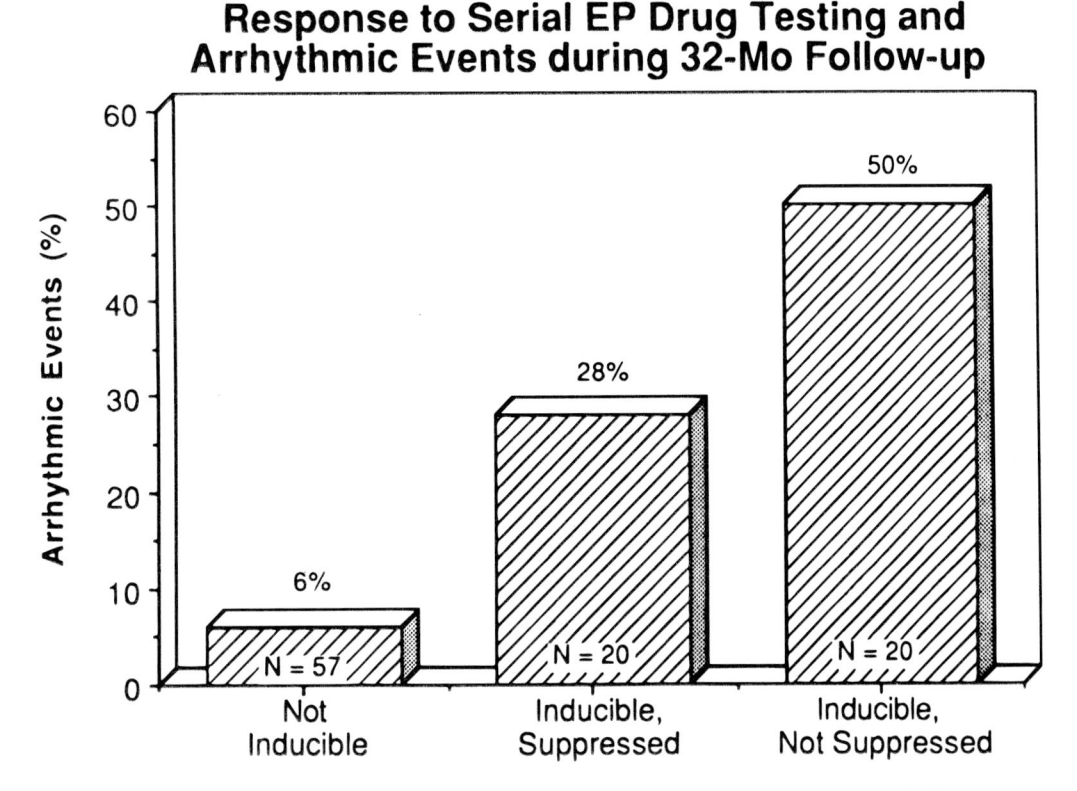

Figure 3. Results of the study of unsustained ventricular tachycardia by Wilber et al.[56,57] The study included 100 patients followed an average of 32.1 months. The 57 patients who were not inducible were not treated with antiarrhythmic drugs and had a 6% rate of mortality or nonfatal sustained ventricular arrhythmia. Of the 20 patients who completed serial drug testing and were suppressed, 28% had arrhythmic events during follow-up. Of the 20 patients who were not suppressed, 50% had arrhythmic events during follow-up. (Reproduced with permission from References 56 and 57.)

mic therapy will reduce the risk of arrhythmic death or cardiac arrest in patients with unsustained VT and left ventricular dysfunction (Table 2). MUSTT started in October 1991 with 25 clinical centers in North America participating. MUSTT is enrolling patients with coronary heart disease who are < 80 years of age, have an LVEF < 0.41, and have asymptomatic, or minimally symptomatic, unsustained VT. Patients who qualify and lack exclusions (Table 3) are asked to have an electrophysiologic study. Patients who have qualifying sustained ventricular arrhythmias induced by programmed ventricular stimulation and who consent are randomized to be followed on no antiarrhythmic treatment or to have antiarrhythmic treatment guided by serial electrophysiologic studies (Figure 4).

Baseline Studies

Coronary heart disease must be documented by coronary angiography or by previous myocardial infarction. When it began, MUSTT excluded patients whose most recent infarct occurred within 4 weeks of enrollment. This exclusion criterion was changed to 4 days during the second year of enrollment. Patients must have had LVEF quantified within 1 year of enrollment by left ventriculogram, radionuclide angiography, or echocardiogram. Unsustained VT (duration, 3 complexes to 30 seconds, rate,

Table 2
Design Features of ICD Prophylaxis Trials in Patients with Coronary Heart Disease

	MUSTT	MADIT	CABG Patch II
Design	Fixed sample size	Sequential	Fixed sample size
Stratification variable(s)	Center	Center	Center
		Time after MI	LV ejection fraction
Eligibility criteria	Coronary heart disease	Q-wave MI	CABG surgery
	Age <80	Age <75	Age <80
	LVEF <0.41	LVEF <0.36	LVEF <0.36
	Unsustained VT	Unsustained VT	SAECG positive
	Inducible VT	Inducible VT, fail procainamide	
Primary Endpoint	Sudden death, cardiac arrest	Death of any cause	Death of any cause
Minimum follow-up (months)	24	6	24
Average follow-up (months)	36	26	40
Event Rate			
Control group	15.0% (24 mos.)	30.0% (26 mos.)	36.5% (40 mos.)
ICD group	10.0% (24 mos.)	16.3% (26 mos.)	27.0% (40 mos.)
Percent reduction	33.3%	46.0%	26.0%
Alpha	5.0%	5.0%	5.0%
Power (1-beta)	80.0%	85.0%	85.0%
Drop-in rate	not estimated	<5.0%	11.0%
Dropout rate	not estimated	<5.0%	6.0%
Sample size (each group)	450	140	400

VT: ventricular tachycardia; LVEF: left ventricular ejection fraction; SAECG: signal averaged electrocardiogram; MI: myocardial infarction.

Table 3
Exclusion Criteria for The Multicenter Unsustained Tachycardia Trial

1. Previous syncope, sustained ventricular tachycardia or fibrillation
2. Unsustained ventricular tachycardia due to long QT syndrome, acute ischemia, acute metabolic disorder, or drug toxicity
3. Unsustained ventricular tachycardia symptomatic enough to need treatment
4. CABG surgery or coronary angioplasty in the previous month
5. Myocardial infarction in the previous month
6. Left ventricular ejection fraction >0.40
7. Patients likely to undergo CABG or valve surgery during the study
8. History of noncompliance
9. Patients with uncontrolled congestive heart failure
10. Non-cardiac disease with likelihood of <2 years survival
12. Patients who live too far for follow-up visits

CABG: coronary artery bypass graft.

≥ 100 per minute) must be documented electrocardiographically and must be associated with no symptoms or minimal symptoms. Patients must complete a symptom limited exercise test within a 6-month interval prior to enrollment, usually combined with thallium. If the exercise test indicates ischemia, coronary angiography is performed prior to enrollment. Patients who are anticipated to need CABG surgery or angioplasty are not enrolled. A signal-averaged ECG is obtained to determine its prognostic value. A baseline electrophysiologic study is done to determine which patients are inducible. Two pacing cycle lengths are used, 600 and 400 msec. Single and double premature stimuli are performed at both the right ventricular apex and outflow tract before burst pacing or triple premature stimuli are used. Patients who have sustained, uniform VT induced by ≤ 3 premature stimuli or sustained, multiform VT or VF induced

MUSTT

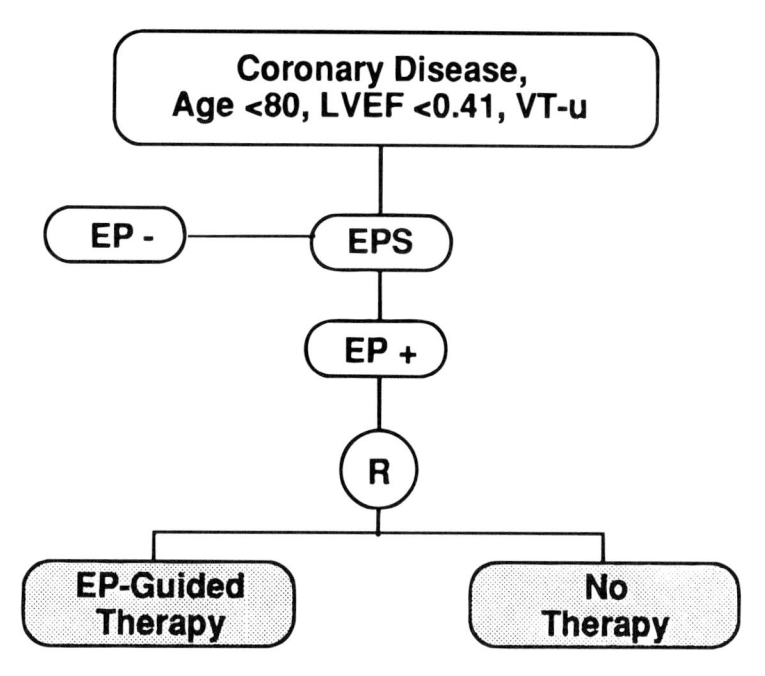

Figure 4. Flow diagram for the Multicenter Unsustained Tachycardia Trial (MUSTT). The R in the circle indicates the point of randomization. The shaded boxes indicate the main comparison for the trial. EPS: electrophysiologic study; LVEF: left ventricular ejection fraction; VT-u: unsustained ventricular tachycardia. (Reproduced with permission from Bigger JT Jr: Should defibrillators be implanted in high-risk patients without a previous sustained ventricular tachyarrhythmia? In: *Implantable Cardioverter-Defibrillators*. Edited by GV Naccarelli, EP Veltri. Boston, MA: Blackwell Scientific Publications, Inc.; 1993, p. 284.)

by ≤ 2 premature stimuli are eligible to be randomized to antiarrhythmic therapy. Ventricular tachycardia with a cycle length ≤ 220 msec or VF induced with triple premature stimuli does not qualify a patient for enrollment.

Enrollment Cascade

When planning MUSTT, it was expected that about half of the qualified patients would agree to have an electrophysiologic study, about 40% would be inducible, and about 50% of the inducible patients would agree to be randomized. A 70% success rate (VT not inducible or slowed) was expected for those randomized to electrophysiologically guided antiarrhythmic therapy and the 30% drug failures would be treated with ICDs. Between October 1991 and May 1993, about 600 patients were enrolled into MUSTT and 205 (33%) had inducible ventricular arrhythmias that qualified them for randomization; half of the qualifying ventricular arrhythmias were induced with three premature stimuli. Of the eligible patients, 189 (92%) were randomized. Ninety-four percent of the randomized patients were male and their average LVEF was 29%. Of patients who completed serial electrophysiologic testing, about 40% were offered ICD therapy, but only about half of these actually underwent implantation. From these preliminary results, it seems that one third of the patients with LVEF < 0.41 and unsustained VT will be inducible and that most will consent to serial electrophysiologic testing. Also, it appears that a smaller fraction than expected will be controlled by drug therapy, resulting in a larger fraction being offered ICD therapy.

Design Features and Sample Size

MUSTT is designed as a fixed sample size randomized clinical trial with group sequential monitoring for safety. Qualified patients who have inducible, sustained ventricular arrhythmias are randomized 50:50 to be followed 2–5 years without any antiarrhythmic treatment or to be followed on antiarrhythmic treatment guided by the results of electrophysiologic studies. Randomization is stratified only by clinical center. The primary end point for the study is arrhythmic death (definition still under discussion) and nonfatal cardiac arrest (causing loss of consciousness and requiring cardioversion). The primary hypothesis will be tested using the intention to treat principle, ie, patients will be grouped for analysis by their assignment at the time of randomization. The alpha error (ie, chance of declaring a significant difference when none exists) is set at 0.05 (two sided) and the power (the chance of finding a difference when there is one) is about 0.80. No specific estimates were made of the drop-in and dropout rates but, given the primary end point being used, these rates are likely to be small and accounted for in the conservative estimates of sample size. For the sample size calculation, the 2-year primary event rate was assumed to be 15% and treatment was assumed to reduce this rate by 33%, ie, to 10%. Using these parameters, the sample calculates to be 814 patients for a power of 0.80; the target sample size for MUSTT is rounded up to 900, 450 in each group. If all else were equal, but the 2-year primary event rate were 25%, the total sample size required would be only 460.

Antiarrhythmic Drug Therapy in MUSTT

Seven antiarrhythmic drugs are authorized for use in MUSTT (Table 4). The se-

Table 4
Drugs Used in The Multicenter Unsustained Tachycardia Trial

Drug	Recommended Dose	Target Plasma Concentration
Procainamide	—	8–10 μg/mL
Quinidine	—	3.5–5 μg/mL
Disopyramide	—	3.5 μg/mL
Mexiletine	150–200 mg q 8 h	—
Propafenone	200–300 mg TID	—
Acebutalol	200 mg BID for 2 days, 400 mg BID if tolerated	—
Amiodarone	1,000–2,000 mg/day for 1 week, 400 mg/day maintenance	—

quence of drug therapy is governed by a strategy of rounds (Figure 5). In Round A, any tolerated drug with Class IA action can be given or, alternatively, the drug with Class IC action, propafenone, can be given. If Round A is unsuccessful, patients continue to Round B as shown in Figure 3. At least two drug trials must be attempted before amiodarone is given. After three or more unsuccessful drug trials, an ICD can be implanted. Each drug will be evaluated with programmed ventricular stimulation. To declare a drug successful, the stimulation protocol, including triple premature stimuli, must be completed with < 15 consecutive VPC being induced.

What Will We Learn from MUSTT?

MUSTT should tell us whether high-risk patients with unsustained VT are significantly benefited by prophylactic antiarrhythmic treatment guided by electrophysiologic studies. The chance of finding significant benefit for electrophysiologically guided therapy will be reduced by patients in the treatment group who refuse ICD im-

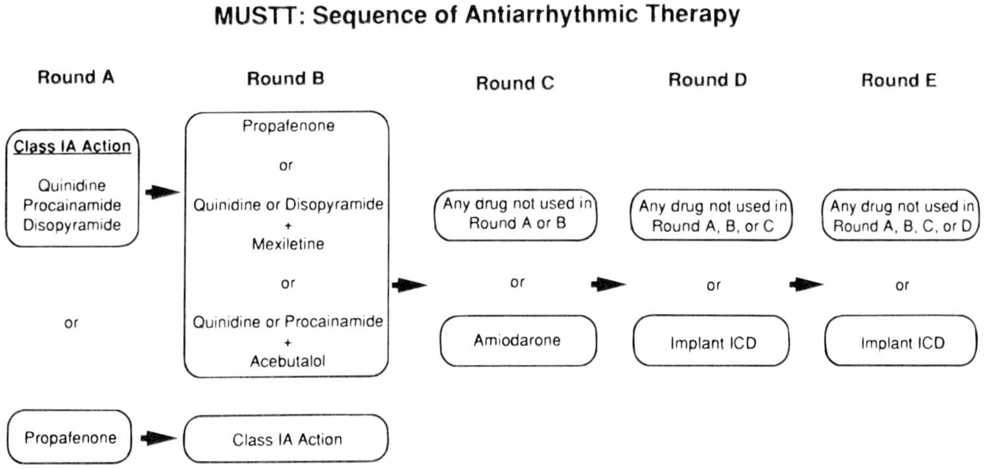

MUSTT: Sequence of Antiarrhythmic Therapy

Figure 5. The sequence of antiarrhythmic drug treatment in MUSTT. (Reproduced with permission from Bigger JT Jr. Should defibrillators be implanted in high-risk patients without a previous sustained ventricular tachyarrhythmia? In: *Implantable Cardioverter-Defibrillators.* Edited by GV Naccarelli, EP Veltri. Boston, MA: Blackwell Scientific Publications, Inc.; 1993, p. 284.)

plantation when no effective drug is found. Early experience suggests that about half of the patients who are offered ICD implantation refuse. A larger percentage may accept ICD implantation now that nonthoracotomy lead systems are on the market. MUSTT will not give a definitive answer about which drugs are more efficacious, better tolerated, or safer, although we may see trends. Similarly, we won't be able to estimate definitively the benefit of ICD therapy relative to no treatment or drug treatment, but trends may suggest relative efficacy and safety for this mode of therapy. For example, ICD therapy is likely to be used in the sickest patients, ie, those not responding to drugs. If patients treated with ICD therapy survive better than drug treated patients, we can infer that the ICD is more effective since the comparison is biased against ICD therapy. From MUSTT, we should learn how good electrophysiologic testing is for assessing risk and, for the first time, be able to compare the outcome of uninducible and inducible patients without the confounding effects of antiarrhythmic drug treatment. We should learn how the results of electrophysiology studies correlate with signal-averaged ECG results and determine the relative predictive accuracy of these two tests for arrhythmic events. These data should suggest how the two tests should be used in risk stratification of patients with left ventricular dysfunction and unsustained VT. It may be that one test or the other dominates for prediction of arrhythmic events. Or, if patients with positive electrophysiologic studies prove to be a subset of the patients with a positive signal-averaged ECG, then the signal-averaged ECG can be used effectively to screen for patients who should have electrophysiologic studies.

The Multicenter Automatic Defibrillator Implantation Trial

MADIT is testing the hypothesis that implantation of an ICD in patients with coronary heart disease, left ventricular dysfunction, and unsustained VT will result in a significant reduction in all-cause mortality when compared to "conventional therapy" (Table 2). MADIT began enrolling in the fall of 1990 in 24 hospitals in the United States and Europe. MADIT is enrolling patients who have had a Q wave myocardial infarc-

Table 5
Exclusion Criteria for The Multicenter Automatic Defibrillator Implantation Trial

1. Previous cardiac arrest or syncopal ventricular tachycardia
2. New York Heart Association functional Class IV
3. CABG surgery or coronary angioplasty in the previous 6 months
4. Myocardial infarction in the previous month
5. Left ventricular ejection fraction >0.35%.
6. Patients likely to undergo CABG surgery during the study
7. Patients with severe cerebral vascular disease
8. Women with childbearing potential
9. Non-cardiac disease with likelihood of <2 years survival
10. Patients participating in other clinical trials
11. Patients who live too far for follow-up visits
12. Patients unwilling or unable to cooperate with the study

CABG: coronary artery bypass graft.

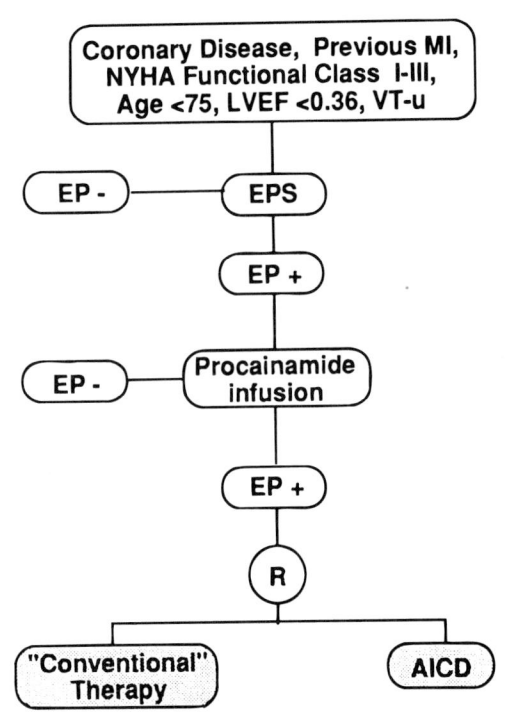

Figure 6. Flow diagram for Multicenter Automatic Defibrillator Implantation Trial. The R in the circle indicates the point of randomization. The shaded boxes indicate the main comparison for the trial. EPS: electrophysiologic study; LVEF: left ventricular ejection fraction; NYHA: New York Heart Association; MI: myocardial infarction; VT-u: unsustained ventricular tachycardia. (Reproduced with permission from Bigger JT Jr: Should defibrillators be implanted in high-risk patients without a previous sustained ventricular tachyarrhythmia? In: *Implantable Cardioverter-Defibrillators*. Edited by GV Naccarelli, EP Veltri. Boston, MA: Blackwell Scientific Publications, Inc.; 1993, p. 284.)

tion, are < 75 years of age, have an LVEF < 0.36, and have asymptomatic, unsustained VT (3 to 30 consecutive complexes, rate ≥ 120 per minute).[58] Patients who qualify and who lack exclusions (Table 5) are asked to have an electrophysiologic study. Patients who have sustained, inducible ventricular arrhythmias that do not respond to an intravenous procainamide infusion and who consent are randomized to conventional pharmacological therapy or to ICD implantation (Figure 6).

Baseline Studies

To be eligible for MADIT, patients must have had a previous Q wave myocardial infarction with the most recent occurring ≥ 4 weeks prior to enrollment. Unsustained VT must be documented by 12-lead ECG, telemetry, Holter recording, or an exercise ECG. The VT must be associated with no or minimal symptoms. The ejection fraction must be < 0.36 and the patient must be in NYHA functional Class I–III.[58] Within the 3 months prior to enrollment, patients must have been evaluated for ischemia with an exercise test, exercise thallium study, or coronary angiography and should not be candidates for CABG surgery. A baseline electrophysiologic study is done to determine which patients are inducible. The protocol involves two pacing cycle lengths, 600 and 400 msec, and three premature stimuli. Inducible sustained VT is defined as a ventricular rhythm with cycle length ≤ 350 msec that lasts 30 seconds or longer. To qualify a patient for randomization in MADIT, uniform VT with a cycle length ≤ 230 msec, multiform VT, or VF must be induced with single or double premature stimuli. The induced ventricular arrhythmia must be reproducible, ie, induced at least twice. Inducible patients are given a loading dose of 15 mg/kg of procainamide intravenously at a rate of 50 mg/min, then given a maintenance infusion of 4 mg/min. Programmed ventricular stimulation is repeated and patients who remain inducible during procainamide infusion are eligible for randomization.[59,60]

Enrollment Cascade

When planning MADIT, it was expected that about half of the patients who qualified would agree to have an electrophysiologic study, 40% would be inducible, and 80% of these would not be suppressed by intravenous procainamide infusion.[40,41] About 50% of the patients who are fully eligible were expected to consent to be randomized. As of the end of April 1993, about 90 patients had been randomized. The average age for the enrolled sample was 61 years; 93% of them were male. The average LVEF was 0.26 and 43% had had previous CABG surgery. The enrollment rate for MADIT should increase significantly now that nonthoracotomy lead systems are available.

Design Features and Sample Size

Randomization is stratified by clinical center and the time between the most recent myocardial infarction and randomization (< 6 months versus ≥ 6 months). The primary hypothesis will be tested using the intention to treat principle. The primary end point for the study is all-cause mortality. To calculate sample size for MADIT, the 2-year cumulative mortality rate was assumed to be 30% (20% arrhythmic death and 10% nonarrhythmic death) and treatment was assumed to reduce this rate by 46%, ie, to 16.3% (4.4% arrhythmic death, 10.4% nonarrhythmic death, and 1.5% operative mortality associated with ICD implantation). The alpha error is set at 0.05 (two sided) and the power at 0.85. The drop-in and dropout rates are estimated to be < 5%. Using these parameters, it was calculated that about 280 patients are needed, 140 in each group. MADIT has a sequential design, and the end points are examined monthly. MADIT will be stopped when the difference in all-cause mortality between the two groups crosses a boundary indicating that the ICD group is significantly better than conventional therapy or a boundary indicating that the trial is unlikely to show benefit for ICD treatment.

Treatment in the Control Group

Patients randomized to the control group will be treated with "conventional therapy." This varies from no treatment at all to amiodarone therapy. Many patients in the control group are being treated with amiodarone. Evaluation of the efficacy and safety of drug therapy also is at the discretion of the local investigator.

What Will We Learn from MADIT?

MADIT should clarify whether prophylactic treatment with an ICD significantly improves survival in patients with left ventricular dysfunction, unsustained VT, and inducible, sustained VT. This information will clarify the choice and sequence of therapy in this high-risk group. The chance of finding a significant difference between the two approaches will be reduced by patients assigned to conventional therapy who experience syncope or cardiac arrest during follow-up and have ICD therapy as a result. Crossover from the control group to ICD therapy may increase now that nonthoracotomy leads are available. MADIT won't be able to estimate definitively the benefit of ICD therapy relative to no treatment or any particular drug therapy. Some of the patients in the control group will not be treated at all while many will be treated with drugs, including amiodarone. If ICD therapy is associated with better survival than drug-treated patients, we won't know how much benefit is due to ICD therapy and how much is due to harmful effects of drugs. Also, if no difference is found between ICD treatment and conventional therapy, we won't know whether either treatment was harmful, beneficial, or had little effect on outcome.

The CABG Patch Trial II

The CABG Patch Trial II will test the hypothesis that implantation of an ICD in patients with coronary heart disease, left ventricular dysfunction, and a positive signal-averaged ECG will reduce the risk of death from all causes. In September 1990, the CABG Patch Trial started a pilot study in 5 North American clinical centers. In January 1992, enrollment was extended to 13 hospitals in North America and Europe and, in February 1993, the CABG Patch Trial became a cooperative study with the NHLBI and enrollment was extended to 28 clinical centers. The CABG Patch Trial is enrolling patients with coronary heart disease who are having elective CABG surgery, are < 80 years of age, have an LVEF < 0.36, and have a positive signal-averaged ECG. Patients with these qualifying characteristics, lack exclusions (Table 6), and signed consent are randomized to ICD therapy or to a control group that receives no therapy in addition to their routine CABG surgery (Figure 7).

The CABG Patch Trial

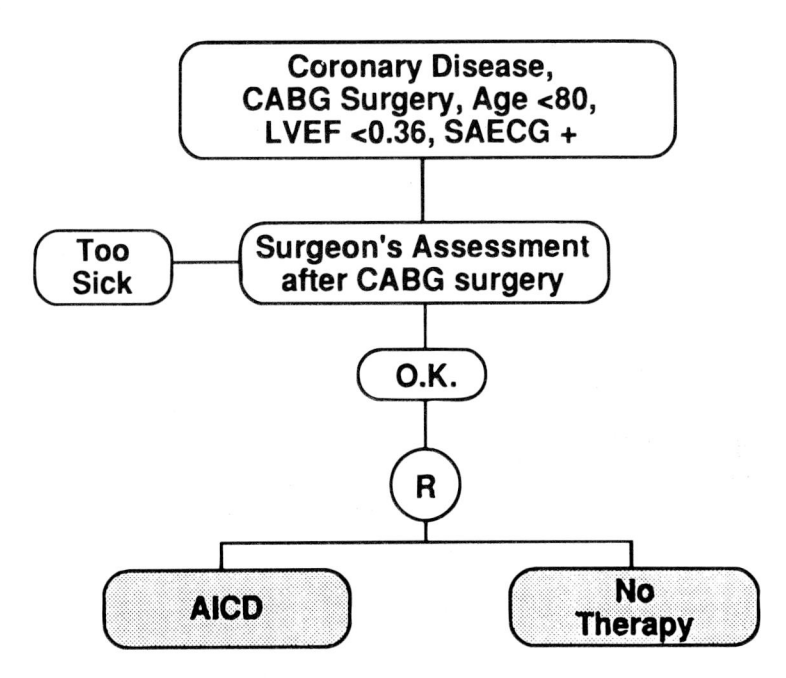

Figure 7. Flow diagram for the CABG Patch Trial. The R in the circle indicates the point of randomization. The shaded boxes indicate the main comparison for the trial. CABG: coronary artery bypass graft; LVEF: left ventricular ejection fraction; SAECG: signal-averaged ECG. (Reproduced with permission from Bigger JT Jr: Should defibrillators be implanted in high-risk patients without a previous sustained ventricular tachyarrhythmia? In: *Implantable Cardioverter-Defibrillators*. Edited by GV Naccarelli, EP Veltri. Boston, MA: Blackwell Scientific Publications, Inc.; 1993, p. 284.)

Table 6
Exclusion Criteria for The CABG Patch Trial

1. History of sustained VT, VF, or cardiac arrest with inducible VT
2. Renal dysfunction (creatinine >3 mg/dl)
3. Insulin dependent diabetes mellitus with significant vascular complications or history of poor control and recurrent infections
4. Unipolar pacemakers
5. Previous or concomitant aortic or mitral valve surgery
6. Concomitant cerebrovascular surgery
7. Emergency CABG surgery
8. Thrombolysis in the 7 days prior to CABG surgery
9. Concomitant arrhythmia surgery or aneurysmectomy
10. Comorbidity associated with expected survival less than two years
11. Lives too far away to return for follow-up visits
12. Inadequate time to obtain informed consent
13. Enrolled in another randomized controlled clinical trial
14. Physician, surgeon, or patient refusal

VT: ventricular tachycardia; VF: ventricular fibrillation; CABG: coronary artery bypass graft.

The Rationale for Prophylactic Implantable Cardioverter-Defibrillator Treatment With Coronary Heart Disease, Treatment of High-Risk CABG Surgery Patients

The planning effort that led to the CABG Patch Trial began in 1988. The planning group realized that there was a potential scientific problem with conducting a randomized controlled trial of ICD prophylaxis using a transthoracic approach for implantation of epicardial patch leads. This approach is likely to produce greater use of diagnostic coronary angiography and revascularization procedures, ie, PTCA or CABG surgery, in patients randomized to receive ICD therapy. A systematically greater use of revascularization in the ICD group would confound the interpretation of results in the following way. In the group assigned to ICD therapy, benefit due to ICD therapy could not be distinguished from that due to revascularization. Also, therapy for the control group was a troublesome issue. The CABG Patch Trial investigators thought that the striking contrast between no therapy and ICD implantation via thoracotomy would have a large negative impact on recruitment in a randomized trial. The investigators also realized that, aside from β blockers,[22–25] no antiarrhythmic drug therapy could be recommended. To the contrary, most clinical trials suggested that antiarrhythmic drugs with Class I action had a substantial harmful effect.[35–42] After discussing several groups that might benefit from ICD prophylaxis, the planning group finally selected patients at high risk for arrhythmic death who were having CABG surgery as the study group. Thus, all patients in the experiment are revascularized; this approach avoids confounding by differences in the use of revascularization in the randomized groups. A policy of no treatment in the comparison group overcame the problems anticipated for the use of antiarrhythmic drugs.

High-Mortality Rates in Patients Who Have CABG Surgery and Left Ventricular Dysfunction

Patients with two- or three-vessel coronary artery disease and reduced LVEF show better long-term survival with surgical treatment than with medical treatment.[61–63] However, after CABG surgery, mortality rates are high for patients with poor left ventricular function. Alderman et al.[64] compared the long-term survival of 231 patients in the Coronary Artery Surgery Study Registry (CASS) registry with LVEF < 0.36 who had CABG surgery between 1975 and 1979 with 420 medically treated CASS registry patients who had LVEF < 0.36. The average LVEF was 0.30 in both the medical and surgical groups. The 3-year cumulative mortality rate was 23% for surgically treated patients and 34% for medically treated patients.

Hochberg et al.[65] reported the surgical mortality and long-term survival of 466 patients with LVEF < 0.40 undergoing CABG surgery between 1976 and 1982. All of the patients had previous myocardial infarction and 36% had congestive heart failure. There were 425 patients with LVEF 0.20–0.39 and 41 patients with LVEF 0.10–0.19 in their study. In the group with LVEF of 0.20–0.39, surgical mortality was 11% and the 3-year mortality rate was 40%. In the group with LVEF 0.10–0.19, surgical mortality was 27% and the 3-year mortality rate was 85%. The patients were divided into six groups based on LVEF, each with a five-point range. The groups with LVEF 0.10–0.14, and 0.15–0.19 had an similar survival experience and the groups with LVEF 0.20–0.24, 0.25–0.29, and 0.30–0.34 had a similar survival experience that was substantially better than the groups with LVEF 0.10–0.19 and substantially worse than the group with LVEF 0.35–0.39. This study provides the rationale for stratification at an LVEF of 0.20 for randomization in the CABG Patch Trial.

Recently, Christakis et al.[66] presented a large experience with death attending CABG surgery and related operative deaths to preoperative LVEF. Between January 1982 and December 1990, 12,471 patients had CABG surgery at the University of Toronto. For 9,445 patients with LVEF > 0.40, the operative mortality rate was 2.3%; for 2,539 patients with LVEF between 0.20 and 0.40, the operative mortality rate was 4.8%; and for 487 patients with LVEF < 0.20, the operative mortality rate was 9.8%. No information was provided on long-term mortality rates or on the causes of these operative deaths.

Coronary Artery Bypass Graft Surgery Does Not Decrease the Prevalence of Ventricular Arrhythmias

In the CASS registry study reported by Alderman et al.,[64] rehospitalization for arrhythmias occurred in 21.2% of the surgical group and in 17.9% of the medical group. This study suggests that CABG surgery does not substantially reduce arrhythmic risk.

Arrhythmic Deaths are Common After Coronary Artery Bypass Graft Surgery

There is not much information on the causes of death during long-term follow-up after CABG surgery. Holmes et al.[67,68] reported the mortality experience during 5 years of follow-up in 11,843 medically treated patients and 8,103 surgically treated patients in the CASS registry. In the surgically treated patients, death was sudden in 204 patients (25%), not sudden but cardiac in 390 (47%), and not cardiac in 230 (28%).[67] There were no baseline variables in the CASS database that predicted sudden death better than nonsudden cardiac death after CABG surgery. This study confirmed a previous report by the same authors that CABG surgery reduced sudden cardiac death in the highest risk patients, but that substantial numbers of sudden deaths continue to occur after surgical treatment.[68] Bolooki[69] reported a 35% sudden death mortality after CABG surgery during a follow-up period of 50 months in a relatively small group of patients. Tresch et al.[70] reported the long-term follow-up of 49 patients who had CABG surgery after cardiac arrest. The mean LVEF for the group was 45%. Seven (16%) of the 45 patients discharged alive died during an average follow-up of 55 months. Five of the seven deaths were due to recurrent VF and two were due to congestive heart failure. This study suggests that CABG surgery alone does not eliminate arrhythmic risk.

Arrhythmic Death After Coronary Artery Bypass Graft Surgery

The summarized studies and others indicate that the reported operative mortality for CABG surgery in patients with LVEF < 0.36 ranges from 4% to 24%, 3-year all-cause mortality after CABG surgery in patients with LVEF < 0.36 ranges from 24% to 50%, and the percentage of all deaths after CABG surgery that are sudden ranges from 25% to 50%.

The Coronary Artery Bypass Graft Surgery Survey

Because there is so much variability among the reports in the literature and because most of the relevant studies are 10–20 years old, 7 of the 8 investigators in the CABG Patch Trial planning group performed a survey of CABG surgery in their institutions to determine the percentage of patients having CABG surgery during 1986 who were < 80 years of age and had LVEF < 0.36 and to determine the survival experience of this high-risk subset. The number of CABG operations done in the participating hospitals ranged from 289–794 and totaled 3,217. The percentage of patients who were < 80 years of age and had LVEF < 0.36 averaged 17%.[71] The crude mortality rate between CABG surgery and discharge from hospital for patients with LVEF < 0.36 averaged 11.6%. The overall 2-year actuarial mortality rate was 28%. A substantial number of nonfatal cardiac arrests occurred in patients with LVEF < 0.36, but the data were too incomplete to permit precise estimates of rates for nonfatal cardiac arrests. The CABG surgery survey results encouraged the investigators to proceed with planning a randomized controlled clinical trial in high-risk CABG surgery patients.

The CABG Patch Trial Pilot Study

A 1-year pilot study was undertaken between September 1, 1990 and August 31, 1991 to obtain information needed to plan a full-scale trial.[71] The major objectives of the pilot study were to determine: 1) whether the signal-averaged ECG was a worthwhile arrhythmia qualifier; 2) the percentage of CABG surgery patients who were fully eligible for the trial; 3) the percentage of fully eligible patients who would consent to the study; and 4) the percentage of enrolled patients who could be randomized. The investigators wanted a marker that would permit them to enroll patients at high risk for arrhythmic events during follow-up. Three arrhythmia markers were considered: 1) signal-averaged ECG, 2) ventricular arrhythmias in 24-hour Holter ECG recordings, and 3) electrophysiologic studies. The signal-averaged ECG was chosen based on its practicality and its predictive value for arrhythmic events shown in previous studies. Most patients are admitted < 24 hours before their CABG surgery, making 24-hour ECG recordings or electrophysiologic studies less practical than the signal-averaged ECG that only takes 15–30 minutes to complete. Also, in previous studies, the signal-averaged ECG has performed very consistently for identifying patients at high risk for arrhythmic events (sudden cardiac death or nonfatal cardiac arrest) after myocardial infarction; the average relative risk for a positive signal-averaged ECG is 6 to 8.[14,72] The investigators thought that a positive signal-averaged ECG must have a relative risk of at least 2.0 to be worth using in the full-scale trial. During the 1-year pilot study, 2,508 patients were screened and 18% of them were < 80 years of age and had an LVEF < 0.36; these percentages are remarkably similar to those found previously in the survey of CABG surgery.[71] Overall, 3.3% of the screened patients were fully eligible and 68% of the eligible patients signed a consent form. Of those who signed a consent form, 80% were randomized. About 65% of the otherwise eligible patients had a positive signal-averaged ECG and the relative risk of patients with positive versus negative tests for death of any cause or a nonfatal arrhythmic event was > 3.0.

The Full-Scale CABG Patch Trial—CABG Patch II

Since the pilot study showed that the signal-averaged ECG performed well and enrollment was feasible, the trial was extended to 13 clinical centers on January 1, 1992 and an NIH grant application was submitted for a full-scale trial (CABG Patch I). The joint end point proposed for CABG Patch I was all-cause mortality or nonfatal cardiac arrest whichever came first. During the review of the grant application for the CABG Patch Trial, the NHLBI recommended that all-cause mortality be used as the primary end point rather than all-cause mortality or cardiac arrest. This recommendation was accepted by the investigators and a second grant application was submitted to NHLBI. The change in end point increased the sample size from 320 to about 800 and necessitated an increase in the number of clinical centers from 13 to 28. A grant was awarded by NHLBI for a full-scale trial using all-cause mortality as the primary end point; CABG Patch II and began in February 1993.

Baseline Studies

Patients with coronary artery disease who are scheduled for elective CABG surgery are screened at the CABG Patch Trial clinical centers. All patients have had coronary angiography and measurement of LVEF within a year, most within a month of the CABG surgery. The coronary angiograms are reviewed and the left ventriculograms are quantified for ejection fraction. Ejection fraction also can be quantified using radionuclide angiography or two-dimensional echocardiography, but > 85% are determined from a left ventriculogram. A 12-lead ECG, signal-averaged ECG, and Holter recording are obtained at baseline. The criteria for a positive signal-averaged ECG are any one of the following: 1) a filtered QRS duration of $\geq$ 114 msec; 2) a root mean square voltage < 20 μV in the terminal 40 msec of the filtered QRS duration; or 3) duration of the terminal filtered QRS complex of > 38 msec after the QRS voltage falls below 40 μV. These criteria were selected to exclude low-risk patients while qualifying more high-risk patients than conventional criteria would. Many of the Holter ECG recordings are substantially shorter than 24 hours because of the short time between admission and surgery. Holter information is used to characterize patients at baseline, but there are no Holter requirements to qualify for the study.

Enrollment Cascade

It was shown in the CABG surgery survey that 95% of patients scheduled for elective CABG surgery were < 80 years of age and that about 18% of age-eligible patients had an LVEF < 0.36. The pilot study showed that about 40% of otherwise eligible patients have a negative signal-averaged ECG and other exclusion criteria are present in about half of the patients with LVEF < 0.36. Patients who are fully eligible and sign consent forms proceed to CABG surgery. After the bypass grafts are done, the surgeon makes the judgment whether the patient is stable enough to implant an ICD and, if so, the patient is randomized. Randomization takes place in the operating room after the coronary artery bypass grafts are completed, usually while patients are on partial cardiopulmonary circulatory assistance. Eighty percent of patients who sign a consent form are randomized. For patients randomized to ICD treatment, patch electrodes are sutured to the pericardium and the pulse generator is connected, implanted, and tested before the patient leaves the operating room. At the end of April 1993, about 20,000 patients had been screened and 246 had been randomized in the CABG Patch Trial. Also, about 350 patients had been enrolled in the substudy to determine the value of the signal-averaged ECG for predicting death or nonfatal arrhythmic events after CABG surgery.

Design Features and Sample Size

The CABG Patch Trial is designed as a fixed sample size, randomized clinical trial with group sequential monitoring for safety.[71] Qualified patients who have positive signal-averaged ECGs are randomized 50:50 to be followed 2–5 years without any antiarrhythmic treatment or with ICD therapy. The average follow-up is expected to be 40 months. Randomization is stratified by clinical center and LVEF (≤ 0.20 versus 0.21–0.35). The primary end point for the study is all-cause mortality. The primary hypothesis will be tested using the intention to treat principle; data will be analyzed using the Cox regression model; the significance of differences between groups will be tested with the log rank test. The alpha error is set at 0.05 (two tailed) and the power at about 0.85. The drop-in rate was estimated at 11% and the dropout rate at 6%. For the sample size calculation, the 40-month primary event rate was assumed to be 36.5% and treatment was assumed to reduce this rate by 26%, ie, to 27.0%. Using these parameters, the sample size required for the trial is calculated to be about 800 patients, 400 in each group.

Treatment in the Control Group

No systematic antiarrhythmic treatment is given in the control group. Both groups are recommended to take aspirin prophylaxis and there is a policy that patients are not to be treated with antiarrhythmic drugs in either group for asymptomatic or minimally symptomatic ventricular arrhythmias. About 15% of the patients in both groups are treated with antiarrhythmic drugs, mostly for atrial fibrillation.

What Will We Learn from the CABG Patch Trial?

The CABG Patch Trial will determine whether ICD prophylaxis will improve survival of high-risk patients having CABG surgery. This is the only randomized controlled trial of ICD therapy in which the control group is not given antiarrhythmic treatment. Thus, the CABG Patch Trial will be the only trial able to estimate the magnitude of the effect of ICD therapy on survival and on cardiac arrest. The CABG Patch Trial also will determine the surgical mortality rates of high-risk patients managed with modern surgical techniques and will detect any adverse effect of ICD implantation on surgical mortality. The predictive accuracy of the signal-averaged ECG for death or cardiac arrest in high-risk CABG surgery patients will be determined. The CABG Patch Trial will not be confounded by the effects of thoracotomy or by ischemic events since both the ICD-treated group and the control group have thoracotomy and complete surgical revascularization. Since both randomly assigned groups have a thoracotomy, the effect of thoracotomy can be factored out and the results should apply to future ICD systems that use nonthoracotomy leads. Since the treatment used in the CABG Patch Trial only addresses tachyarrhythmic deaths and the control group gets no treatment that could cloud the issue, the trial should estimate the percentage of deaths after CABG surgery that are arrhythmic with better precision than ever before. The trial also will validate or call into question current criteria used to classify deaths as sudden or arrhythmic. The CABG Patch Trial II overcomes a major weakness of the CABG Patch Trial I—the joint end point (death or nonfatal cardiac arrest). The joint end point could not determine how much ICD treatment increases overall survival. Implantable cardioverter-defibrillator treatment could prevent cardiac arrest (a primary end point proposed for CABG Patch Trial I) only to have patients die of heart failure or noncardiac deaths shortly thereafter. If a large fraction of the primary end point events were nonfatal cardiac arrests, the effects of ICD therapy on all-cause mortality would not be clarified using the joint end point, death or nonfatal cardiac arrest. This would be an unfortunate outcome because the effect of ICD therapy on all-cause mortality is a burning issue. Broadening the indications for ICD therapy and obtaining reimbursement for broader indications depend critically on knowing how much ICD therapy prolongs life and on knowing the cost effectiveness of ICD and alternate therapies. Such considerations prompted the CABG Patch Trial investigators to conduct a larger study using all-cause mortality as the primary end point (CABG Patch Trial II).

Trials of Implantable Cardioverter-Defibrillator Therapy in Heart Failure

Two studies are being planned to evaluate ICD therapy in patients with congestive heart failure, the Dilated CArdiomyopathy Trial (CAT) and Defibrillator Implantation as Bridge to Later Transplantation (DEFIBRILAT).

The Rationale for Implantable Cardioverter-Defibrillator Prophylaxis in Patients With Heart Failure

Patients with heart failure classified as NYHA functional Class III or IV have a very high mortality rate, eg, 40% to 50% during 2 years of follow-up and about 40% of this mortality is sudden, presumably arrhythmic, death.[73–76] A higher percentage of the deaths are sudden in Class II or III patients than in Class IV patients.[76]

Heart Failure Patients Might Benefit from Implantable Cardioverter-Defibrillator Prophylaxis

Treatment with an ICD has been suggested as a bridge to heart transplantation, ie, as therapy for patients who are accepted for heart transplantation, but who are waiting for a donor heart. About half of the patients on a heart transplant waiting list die before they get their transplant.[77,78] Two preliminary studies[79,80] have shown that patients on the heart transplant waiting list with LVEF < 0.20 tolerated thoracotomy and ICD implantation very well (no operative mortality in 20 patients). Nineteen of 20 patients survived to transplant; 95% used their ICD during the first year after implant. About half of the patients used their ICD > 10 times. There was no increase in difficulty of the subsequent transplant operation due to previous ICD implantation. Patients who are evaluated for heart transplantation and not accepted also have a very high mortality rate and ICD treatment could be helpful in this group as well.[81] Klein et al.[82] studied 81 patients referred for heart transplantation but considered too well for an immediate transplant; 60 had cardiomyopathy and 21 had coronary heart disease. During a mean follow-up of 20 months, 38 patients (47%) died; 45% of the deaths ($n = 17$) were sudden. In the subgroup of 39 patients selected by presence of spontaneous, complex ventricular arrhythmias, 21 were treated with antiarrhythmic drugs and 18 with ICDs. There were 8 (38%) sudden deaths in the drug-treated patients and none in ICD-treated patients; 94% of the ICD pulse generators discharged during follow-up (an average of 4 ICD discharges per patient). These investigators concluded that drug therapy was unreliable and that ICD treatment was advisable to prevent sudden death in patients with congestive heart failure and complex unsustained ventricular arrhythmias.

The prophylactic use of ICD treatment in heart failure patients should be subjected to randomized controlled clinical trials before this approach is accepted because effectively treating arrhythmic risk might not increase survival very much in heart failure patients due to other lethal mechanisms, eg, pump failure and myocardial ischemia/infarction.

The Dilated Cardiomyopathy Trial

CAT addresses the hypothesis that implantation of an ICD in patients with dilated cardiomyopathy and severe left ventricular dysfunction will reduce the mortality rate.[83,84] CAT started randomizing patients in a pilot study on July 1, 1991 with 9 German centers participating. Patients with dilated cardiomyopathy are eligible if their LVEF is ≤ 0.30 and they are in NYHA functional Class II or III. The following conditions exclude patients from CAT: 1) history of sustained VT or cardiac arrest; 2) coronary atherosclerosis with > 70% stenosis of a coronary artery; 3) valvular heart disease; 4) likely to undergo cardiac transplantation within 6 months after enrollment; and 5) dilated cardiomyopathy present longer than 9 months. Patients who qualify and consent to join the study are randomized to ICD therapy or a control group that receives no formal alternate therapy. A registry is being kept on patients with dilated cardiomyopathy who have LVEF > 0.30 or a history of cardiomyopathy for longer than 9 months.

Baseline Studies

A large battery of baseline tests is performed in CAT, ie, bicycle exercise testing, 24-hour continuous ECG recording, signal-averaged ECG, coronary angiography, and programmed ventricular stimulation, but none of them are used to qualify or to stratify randomization.

Enrollment Cascade

Many of the percentages needed to design CAT are not available. Accordingly, the CAT investigators are conducting a pilot study to enroll 100 patients so they can estimate the critical parameters for the trial. Between May 15, 1991 and the end of March 1992, 42 patients were randomized. The major obstacle to enrollment in the early months of the study was the requirement that the dilated cardiomyopathy be diagnosed within the 6 months prior to enrollment. The interval was changed to 9 months during the course of the pilot study.[84]

Design Features and Sample Size

The design for CAT will not be finalized until after the pilot study, but it is anticipated that CAT will be a fixed sample size, randomized clinical trial. In the pilot study, the only stratifying variable for randomization is clinical center. The alpha error is set at 0.05 and the power at 0.80. The CAT investigators expect a 1-year mortality rate (deaths of all causes) of 30%; 60% of the deaths to be due to heart failure and 40% due to sudden cardiac death. Implantable cardioverter-defibrillator therapy is expected to reduce the 1-year mortality rate to 24% (a reduction of 20%). Originally, the CAT investigators estimated the perioperative mortality to be 5%, but the experience so far is substantially less. The lower operative mortality is attributed to implantation of nonthoracotomy lead systems (Endotak™, CPI, St. Paul, MN) with a pulse generator that provides a biphasic defibrillating pulse (Ventak P2).[84] When 100 patients have been recruited, the final design, sample size, and feasibility of CAT will be assessed and the decision made whether a full-scale trial will be conducted.

Therapy in the Control Group

The use of β-adrenergic blocking and calcium channel blocking drugs is not controlled by the protocol. CAT has a policy against using antiarrhythmic drugs in the control group.

What Will We Learn from CAT?

The primary information that will come from the pilot study is whether it is feasible to conduct a full-scale trial. The exclusion for longstanding cardiomyopathy has caused a problem already and will be examined closely. Perhaps, the time between documentation of cardiomyopathy and enrollment in CAT will be used to stratify randomization rather than excluding patients. If it turns out not to be feasible to do a full-scale trial in this patient group, some controlled information on the safety of implantation of nonthoracotomy ICD systems will be developed. Information on the frequency of ICD firing in patients with NYHA Class II and III heart failure will be determined. With 100 patients in the pilot sample, it is unlikely that any useful information will be acquired related to the potential of ICD therapy to reduce mortality. Hopefully, a full-scale trial will be conducted to provide definitive information on the magnitude of the reduction of mortality by ICD treatment in patients with Class II and III heart failure.

DEFIBRILAT as a Bridge to Later Transplantation

Planning for DEFIBRILAT has been underway for more than 2 years. The DEFIBRILAT investigators plan to test the hypothesis that prophylactic use of ICD therapy will reduce all-cause mortality in patients with heart failure (NYHA Class III) due to coronary heart disease who have been accepted for cardiac transplantation. DEFIBRILAT will enroll patients on transplant waiting lists who are < 65 years of age, have coronary heart disease, LVEF < 0.30, NYHA Class III heart failure, and unsustained VT in a 24-hour ECG recording. Patients who qualify and lack exclusions will be asked to have an electrophysiologic study. Patients who have a sustained ventricular arrhythmia induced and sign a consent form will be randomized to ICD therapy or to no antiarrhythmic therapy. The initial attempt will be to implant a nonthoracotomy system; if thresholds are above 20 J, a thoracotomy will be done to implant patch electrodes on the heart.

Baseline Studies

Baseline studies will include measurement of functional capacity, Holter recording, and electrophysiologic study.

Enrollment Cascade

It is expected that about half of otherwise eligible patients will have unsustained VT during a 24-hour ECG recording and that about half of these patients will consent to an electrophysiologic study. About 40% of the patients evaluated with programmed ventricular stimulation are expected to respond with sustained VT and 65% of these to agree to be randomized in DEFIBRILAT. Thus, about 4,500 patients will need to be screened with Holter recordings to enroll 300 patients. Nonthoracotomy lead systems will be implanted whenever possible. If the defibrillation threshold is ≥ 20 J, a thoracotomy will be done and patches will be sewn directly on the pericardium.

Design Features and Sample Size

DEFIBRILAT is considering a sequential design using all-cause mortality as the primary end point. The alpha error is set at 0.05 (two sided) and the power at 0.85. For the sample size size computation, the 1-year cumulative mortality rate was assumed to be about 45% in the control group and 22% in the group assigned to ICD therapy. The preliminary calculations lead to an estimate of sample size of about 300 patients, 150 per group. Details, like the drop-in and dropout rates, and complexities, like how to deal with the very large censoring rates due to transplantation, are still under discussion.

What Will We Learn from DEFIBRILAT?

We should learn valuable information about the causes of death in patients who are waiting for cardiac transplantation. We will have a good estimate of the morbidity and mortality rates for ICD implantation in this high-risk group. We will learn how often a nonthoracotomy lead system will have an adequate defibrillation threshold (≤ 20 J) in patients with severe heart failure. Most importantly, we will learn whether ICD therapy can substantially increase survival to the time of cardiac transplantation for patients on transplant waiting lists. The requirement for inducible sustained VT is likely to qualify substantially more patients with coronary heart disease relative to patients with cardiomyopathy. Thus, the results may not be relevant to patients with cardiomyopathy. Using conventional ICDs available today, there is likely to be a serious cost-effectiveness problem for the approach being evaluated in this trial because the ICDs implanted in this trial are likely to be removed for transplantation long before the device is expended. A less expensive ICD designed specifically for prophylactic use could overcome this problem, not just for DEFIBRILAT, but for prophylactic use in other settings as well.[85]

Conclusions

At the present time, the pitifully small salvage rate after cardiac arrest motivates the exploration of primary prevention for sudden cardiac death. However, before primary prevention is adopted, its efficacy, safety, and cost effectiveness must be demonstrated in controlled clinical trials. Some clinical trials to evaluate primary prevention have begun and others are sure to follow.

References

1. National Center for Health Statistics: *Advance Report, Final Mortality Statistics, 1981.* Monthly Vital Statistics, Vol. 33(Suppl 3): DHHS Pub. No.(PHS)84–1120, p. 4.
2. Weaver WD, Cobb LA, Hallstrom AP, et al: Factors influencing survival after out-of-hospital cardiac arrest. *J Am Coll Cardiol* 7:752, 1986.
3. Davies MJ, Thomas A: Thrombosis and acute coronary artery lesions in sudden cardiac ischemic death. *N Engl J Med* 310:1137, 1984.
4. Marshall JC, Waxman HL, Sauerwein A, et al: Frequency of low-grade residual coronary stenosis after thrombolysis during acute myocardial infarction. *Am J Cardiol* 66:773, 1990.
5. Fuster V, Badimon L, Badimon JJ, et al: The pathogenesis of coronary artery disease and the acute coronary syndromes. *N Engl J Med* 326:242, 1992.
6. Gordon T, Kannel WB: Premature mortality from coronary heart disease. The Framingham Study. *JAMA* 215:1617, 1971.
7. Lown B: Sudden cardiac death: the major challenge confronting contemporary cardiology. *Am J Cardiol* 43:313, 1979.
8. Bigger JT Jr, Fleiss JL, Kleiger R, et al: The relationships among ventricular arrhythmias, left ventricular dysfunction and mortality in the 2 years after myocardial infarction. *Circulation* 69:250, 1984.
9. Cripps TR, Bennett ED, Camm AJ, et al: High gain signal averaged electrocardiogram combined with 24-hour monitoring in patients early after myocardial infarction for bedside prediction of arrhythmic events. *Br Heart J* 60:181, 1988.
10. Kuchar DL, Thorburn CW, Sammet NL: Late potentials detected after myocardial infarction: natural history and prognostic significance. *Circulation* 74:1280, 1986.
11. Gomes JA, Winters SL, Stewart D, et al: A new noninvasive index to predict sustained ventricular tachycardia and sudden death in the first year after myocardial infarction: based on signal-averaged electrocardiogram, radionuclide ejection fraction and Holter monitoring. *J Am Coll Cardiol* 10:349, 1987.
12. Breithardt G, Borggrefe M: Recent advances in the identification of patients at risk of ventricular tachyarrhythmias: role of ventricular late potentials. *Circulation* 75:1091, 1987.
13. Simson MB: Noninvasive identification of patients at high risk for sudden cardiac death. Signal averaged electrocardiography. *Circulation* 85:I-145, 1992.
14. Steinberg JS, Regan A, Sciacca RR, et al: Predicting arrhythmic events after myocardial infarction: results of a prospective study and a meta-analysis using the signal-averaged electrocardiogram. *Am J Cardiol* 69:13, 1992.
15. Richards DA, Cody DV, Denniss AR, et al: Ventricular electrical instability: a predictor of death after myocardial infarction. *Am J Cardiol* 51:75, 1983.
16. Breithardt G, Borggrefe M, Haerten K: Role of programmed ventricular stimulation and noninvasive recording of ventricular late potentials for the identification of patients at risk of ventricular tachyarrhythmias after acute myocardial infarction. In: *Cardiac Electrophysiology and Arrhythmias.* Edited by DP Zipes, J Jalife. New York, NY: Grune & Stratton, Inc.; 1985, p. 553.
17. Roy D, Marchand E, Theroux P, et al: Programmed ventricular stimulation in survivors of an acute myocardial infarction. *Circulation* 72:487, 1985.
18. Denniss AR, Richards DA, Cody DV, et al: Prognostic significance of ventricular tachy-

cardia and fibrillation induced at programmed stimulation and delayed potentials detected on the signal-averaged electrocardiograms of survivors of acute myocardial infarction. *Circulation* 74:731, 1986.
19. Bourke JP, Richards DAB, Ross DL, et al: Routine programmed electrical stimulation in survivors of acute myocardial infarction for prediction of spontaneous ventricular tachyarrhythmias during follow-up: results, optimal stimulation protocol, and cost-effective screening. *J Am Coll Cardiol* 18:780, 1991.
20. Bigger JT Jr, Fleiss JL, Steinman RC, et al: Frequency domain measures of heart period variability and mortality after myocardial infarction. *Circulation* 85:164, 1992.
21. Farrell TG, Bashir Y, Paul V, et al: Risk stratification for arrhythmic events in postinfarction patients based on heart rate variability, ambulatory electrocardiographic variables, and the signal-averaged electrocardiogram. *J Am Coll Cardiol* 18:687, 1991.
22. Hjalmarson A, Elmfeldt D, Herlitz J, et al: Effect on mortality of metoprolol in acute myocardial infarction. A double-blind randomized trial. *Lancet* IV:823, 1981.
23. Norwegian Multicenter Study Group: Timolol-induced reduction in mortality and reinfarction in patients surviving acute myocardial infarction. *N Engl J Med* 304:801, 1981.
24. Beta-Blocker Heart Attack Trial Research Group: A randomized trial of propranolol in patients with acute myocardial infarction. I. Mortality results. *JAMA* 247:1707, 1982.
25. Yusuf S, Peto R, Lewis J, et al: Beta blockade during and after myocardial infarction: an overview of the randomized trials. *Prog Cardiovasc Dis* 27:335, 1985.
26. Lichstein E, Hager D, Gregory J, et al: The relationship between beta blocker use, various measures of left ventricular function and the chance of developing congestive heart failure. *J Am Coll Cardiol* 16:1327, 1990.
27. ISIS-2 (Second International Study of Infarct Survival) Collaborative Group: Randomized trial of intravenous streptokinase, oral aspirin, both or neither among 17,187 cases of suspected acute myocardial infarction. *Lancet* 2:349, 1988.
28. Hennekens CH, Buring JE, Sandercock P, et al: Aspirin and other antiplatelet agents in the secondary and primary prevention of cardiovascular disease. *Circulation* 80:749, 1989.
29. The CONSENSUS Trial Study Group: Effects of enalapril on mortality in severe congestive heart failure: results of the Cooperative North Scandanavian Enalapril Survival Study (CONSENSUS). *N Engl J Med* 316:1429, 1987.
30. The SOLVD Investigators: Effect of enalapril on survival in patients with reduced left ventricular ejection fractions and congestive heart failure. *N Engl J Med* 325:293, 1991.
31. Pfeffer MA, Braunwald E, Moye LA, et al: Effect of captopril on mortality and morbidity in patients with left ventricular dysfunction after myocardial infarction. *N Engl J Med* 327:669, 1992.
32. Swedberg K, Held P, Kjekshus J, et al: Effect of the early administration of enalapril on mortality in patients with acute myocardial infarction—results of the Cooperative New Scandinavian Enalapril Survival Study II (CONSENSUS II). *N Engl J Med* 327:678, 1992.
33. The SOLVD Investigators: Effect of enalapril on mortality and the development of heart failure in asymptomatic patients with reduced left ventricular ejection fractions. *N Engl J Med* 327:685, 1992.
34. Oates JA: Aspirin increases the sudden death rate (personal communication).
35. The Cardiac Arrhythmia Suppression Trial (CAST) Investigators: Effect of encainide and flecainide on mortality in a randomized trial of arrhythmia suppression after myocardial infarction. *N Engl J Med* 321:406, 1989.
36. Echt DS, Liebson PR, Mitchell LB, et al: Mortality and morbidity in patients randomized to receive encainide, flecainide, or placebo in the Cardiac Arrhythmia Suppression Trial. *N Engl J Med* 324:781, 1991.
37. The Cardiac Arrhythmia Suppression Trial II Investigators: Effect of the antiarrhythmic agent moricizine on survival after myocardial infarction. *N Engl J Med* 327:227, 1992.
38. May GS, Eberlein KA, Furberg CD, et al: Secondary prevention after myocardial infarction: a review of long-term trials. *Prog Cardiovasc Dis* 24:331, 1982.
39. Furberg CD: Effect of antiarrhythmic drugs on mortality after myocardial infarction. *Am J Cardiol* 52:32C, 1983.
40. Hine L, Laird N, Hewitt P, et al: Meta-analysis of empiric chronic antiarrhythmic therapy after myocardial infarction. *JAMA* 262:3037, 1989.
41. Coplen SE, Antman EM, Berlin JA, et al: Efficacy and safety of quinidine therapy for maintenance of sinus rhythm after cardioversion. A meta-analysis of randomized control trials. *Circulation* 82:1106, 1990.
42. Morganroth J, Goin JE: Clinical investigation: quinidine-related mortality in the short-to-medium-term treatment of ventricular arrhythmias: a meta-analysis. *Circulation* 84:1977, 1991.

43. Yusuf S, Teo KK: Approaches to prevention of sudden death: need for fundamental re-evaluation. *J Cardiovasc Electrophysiol* 2:S233, 1991.
44. Burkart F, Pfisterer M, Kiowski W, et al: Effect of antiarrhythmic therapy on mortality in survivors of myocardial infarction with asymptomatic complex ventricular arrhythmis: Basel Antiarrhythmic Study of Infarct Survival (BASIS). *J Am Coll Cardiol* 16:1711, 1990.
45. Ceremuzynski L, Kleczar E, Krzeminska-Pakula M, et al: Effect of amiodarone on mortality after myocardial infarction: a double-blind, placebo-controlled, pilot study. *J Am Coll Cardiol* 20:1056, 1992.
46. Mirowski M, Reid PR, Winkle RA, et al: Mortality in patients with implanted automatic defibrillators. *Ann Intern Med* 98:585, 1983.
47. Winkle RA, Mead RH, Ruder MA, et al: Long-term outcome with the automatic implantable cardioverter-defibrillator. *J Am Coll Cardiol* 13:1353, 1989.
48. Tchou PJ, Kadri N, Anderson J, et al: Automatic implantable cardioverter defibrillators and survival of patients with left ventricular dysfunction and malignant ventricular arrhythmias. *Ann Intern Med* 109:529, 1988.
49. Connolly SJ, Yusuf S: Evaluation of the implantable cardioverter defibrillator in survivors of cardiac arrest: the need for randomized trials. *Am J Cardiol* 69:959, 1992.
50. Hinkle LE Jr, Thaler HT: Clinical classification of cardiac deaths. *Circulation* 65:457, 1982.
51. Kuck HK, Siebels J, Schneider M, et al: Preliminary results of a randomized trial, AICD versus drugs (abstract). *Rev Eur Technol Biomed* 12:110, 1990.
52. Siebels J, Cappato R, Ruppel R, et al: ICD versus drugs in cardiac arrest survivors: preliminary results of the Cardiac Arrest Study Hamburg. *PACE* 16:552, 1993.
53. Kuck K-H: *Update on the Cardiac Arrest Study Hamburg*. Presented at NASPE, May 8, 1993.
54. Bigger JT Jr, Fleiss JL, Rolnitzky LM, et al: Prevalence, characteristics and significance of ventricular tachycardia detected by 24-hour continuous electrocardiographic recordings in the late hospital phase of acute myocardial infarction. *Am J Cardiol* 58:1151, 1986.
55. Kowey PR, Taylor JE, Marinchak RA, et al: Does programmed stimulation really help in the evaluation of patients with nonsustained ventricular tachycardia? Results of a meta-analysis. *Am Heart J* 123:481, 1992.
56. Wilber DJ, Olshansky B, Moran JF, et al: Electrophysiologic testing and nonsustained ventricular tachycardia: use and limitations in patients with coronary artery disease and impaired ventricular function. *Circulation* 82:350, 1990.
57. Wilber D, Olshansky B, Moran J, et al: Electrophysiological testing and nonsustained ventricular tachycardia. *Circulation* 84:II-21, 1991.
58. MADIT Executive Committee: Multicenter Automatic Defibrillator Implantation Trial (MADIT): design and clinical protocol. *PACE* 14:920, 1991.
59. Waxman HL, Buxton AE, Sadowski LM, et al: The response to procainamide during electrophysiologic study for sustained ventricular tachyarrhythmias predicts the response to other medications. *Circulation* 67:30, 1983.
60. Kuchar DL, Rottman JN, Berger RE, et al: Prediction of successful suppression of sustained ventricular tachyarrhythmias by serial drug testing from data derived at the initial electrophysiologic study. *J Am Coll Cardiol* 12:982, 1988.
61. Read RC, Murphy ML, Hultgren HN, et al: Survival of men treated for chronic stable angina pectoris: a cooperative randomized study. *J Thorac Cardiovasc Surg* 75:1, 1978.
62. European Coronary Surgery Study Group: Long-term results of prospective randomized study of coronary artery bypass surgery in stable angina pectoris. *Lancet* 2:1173, 1982.
63. CASS Principal Investigators and Their Associates: Coronary Artery Surgery Study (CASS): a randomized trial of coronary artery bypass surgery: survival data. *Circulation* 68:939, 1983.
64. Alderman EL, Fisher LD, Litwin P, et al: Results of coronary artery surgery in patients with poor left ventricular function (CASS). *Circulation* 68:785, 1983.
65. Hochberg MS, Parsonnet V, Gielchinsky I, et al: Coronary artery bypass grafting in patients with ejection fractions below forty percent. Early and late results in 466 patients. *J Thorac Cardiovasc Surg* 86:519, 1983.
66. Christakis GT, Weisel RD, Fremes SE, et al: Coronary artery bypass grafting in patients with poor left ventricular function. *J Thorac Cardiovasc Surg* 103:1083, 1992.
67. Holmes DR, David K, Gersh BJ, et al: Risk factor profiles of patients with sudden cardiac death and death from other cardiac causes: a report from the Coronary Artery Surgery Study (CASS). *J Am Coll Cardiol* 13:524, 1989.
68. Holmes DR Jr, Davis KB, Mock MB, et al: The effect of medical and surgical treatment on subsequent sudden cardiac death in patients with coronary artery disease: a report

from the Coronary Artery Surgery Study. *Circulation* 73:1254, 1986.
69. Bolooki H: Discussion of Hochberg MS, Parsonnet V, Gielchinsky I, et al: Coronary artery bypass grafting in patients with ejection fractions below forty percent. Early and late results in 466 patients. J Thorac Cardiovasc Surg 86:519, 1983. *J Thorac Cardiovasc Surg* 86:526, 1983.
70. Tresch DD, Wetherbee JN, Siegel R, et al: Long-term follow-up of survivors of prehospital sudden cardiac death treated with coronary bypass surgery. *Am Heart J* 110:1139, 1985.
71. The CABG Patch Trial Investigators and Coordinators: The CABG Patch Trial. *Prog Cardiovas Dis* 36(2):97, 1993.
72. Cripps TR, Bennett ED, Camm AJ, et al: High gain signal averaged electrocardiogram combined with 24-hour monitoring in patients early after myocardial infarction for bedside prediction of arrhythmic events. *Br Heart J* 60:181, 1988.
73. Bigger JT Jr: Why patients with congestive heart failure die: arrhythmias and sudden cardiac death. *Circulation* 75(suppl IV):28, 1987.
74. Packer M: Sudden unexpected death in patients with congestive heart failure: a second frontier. *Circulation* 72:681, 1985.
75. Francis G: Should asymptomatic ventricular arrhythmias in patients with congestive heart failure be treated with antiarrhythmic drugs? *J Am Coll Cardiol* 12:274, 1988.
76. Kjekshus J: Arrhythmias and mortality in congestive heart failure. *Am J Cardiol* 65:42I, 1990.
77. DEFIBRILAT Study Group: Actuarial risk of sudden death while awaiting cardiac transplantation in patients with atherosclerotic heart disease. *Am J Cardiol* 68:545, 1991.
78. Stevenson L, Chelimsky-Fallick C, Tillisch J, et al: Unacceptable risk of sudden death without transplantation if low ejection fraction is due to coronary artery disease (abstract). *J Am Coll Cardiol* 15:222A, 1990.
79. Bolling S, Deeb M, Morady F, et al: AICD: a new "bridge" to transplantation (abstract). *J Am Coll Cardiol* 15:223A, 1990.
80. Jeevanandam V, Bielefeld MR, Auteri JS, et al: The implantable defibrillator: an electronic bridge to cardiac transplantation. *Circulation* 86:II-276, 1992.
81. Stevenson L, Fowler M, Schroeder J, et al: Poor survival of patients with idiopathic cardiomyopathy considered too well for transplantation. *Am J Med* 83:871, 1987.
82. Klein H, Troster J, Haverich A: AICD as a bridge to transplant (abstract). *Rev Eur Technol Biomed* 12:110, 1990.
83. The German Dilated Cardiomyopathy Study Investigators: Prospective studies assessing prophylactic therapy in high risk opatients: the German Dilated Cardiomyopathy Study (GDCMS)—study design. *PACE* 15:697, 1992.
84. The Cardiomyopathy Trial Investigators: Cardiomyopathy trial. *PACE* 16:576, 1993.
85. Hauser RG: Attributes of a prophylactic implantable cardioverter defibrillator: how close are we? *PACE* 16:582, 1993.

Chapter 27

The Implantable Cardioverter-Defibrillator: Economic Issues

Mark H. Anderson and A. John Camm

Introduction

The development and rapid expansion of usage of the implantable cardioverter-defibrillator (ICD) is just one example of the dramatic innovation that has occurred in cardiological medicine in the last 40 years. New surgical techniques, transplantation, transluminal procedures, and a wide range of drugs have been added to our armamentarium. Many of these developments demonstrably improve prognosis, and all offer symptomatic relief. However, most of these advances produce a substantial requirement for additional resources. In countries with relatively centralized provision of health care, such as the United Kingdom, this had already resulted in conflicts over resource allocation by the early 1980s. In the United States, where health care spending has traditionally accounted for a higher proportion of gross domestic product, this conflict has been relatively delayed, despite marked inequities in the delivery of care. However, even in the United States the cost of funding Medicaid and Medicare programs has resulted in a review of service provision and an attempt to rank the priority of provision of different medical therapies based on assessment of their cost-efficacy.[1] The Department of Health Agency for Health Care Policy and Research created a Center for Medical Effectiveness Research, which gave rise to the Patient Outcome Research Teams (PORTs) program, designed to assess treatment efficacy, patient benefit, and cost. While some physicians feel that economic factors have no part to play in the provision of medical resources, they may overlook the inequities in the provision of health care that have arisen from the classical politico-vocal mechanism of distributing resources "he who shouts loudest gets most."[2] It is becoming increasingly clear that even in the most affluent of western countries the cost of medical technology may be outstripping our ability to pay for it.

Thus, the development of the ICD has coincided with a period of earnest debate on the cost of provision of health services. For this reason, and because of the relatively high initial cost of the device, the use of the ICD has been subjected to more intense economic scrutiny earlier in its development than have other cardiological treatments. In this chapter we consider the concept of cost-efficacy, its applications to the ICD, the impact of technical and medical developments, and possible national resource implications of adopting various strategies of ICD use.

From Singer I, (ed.) Implantable Cardioverter-Defibrillator. Armonk, NY: Futura Publishing Company, Inc.; © 1994.

How Much Does the Implantable Cardioverter-Defibrillator Cost?

The pricing of medical hardware in the early stages of its development tends to bear little relationship to the actual cost of its manufacture, as manufacturers need to recoup their very substantial research and development costs. Although the ICD market was initially supplied by a single manufacturer, the rapid entry of five other manufacturers into the field in the late 1980s has ensured the prospect of an active competitive market in the future. The majority of devices currently produced are not market released and competition in the field of "off-the-shelf" defibrillators remains limited. However, the majority of large implanting centers are involved in investigational studies of new devices and have taken the opportunity to obtain their devices from more than one manufacturer, to broaden their experience with the device, to improve their access to new technology, and to reduce their exposure to technical problems affecting the products from a single manufacturer. An approximate price range for ICD generators of $15,000 to $30,000 (£10,000–£20,000) has developed with the newest, most sophisticated models at the top of this range, while older, less sophisticated devices are at the bottom. Nearly obsolete devices may sometimes be obtained somewhat cheaper! The current market life of any single ICD generator appears to be about 3–4 years with the full development cycle extending over a decade. In addition to the cost of the generator itself it is necessary to add the cost of the defibrillation lead system (and separate pace-sense electrodes in the case of epicardial leads) that currently costs around $3,000 to $5,000 depending on the choice of transvenous electrodes or epicardial patches and the number of electrodes required.

The relatively high initial capital cost of the ICD and its electrodes may be one reason why it has been perceived as an expensive therapy while other therapies may have equivalent in-hospital costs, but these may be less obvious as the cost may be divided between a number of items such as staff costs, equipment costs, and a prolonged hospital stay. To answer this possible criticism it is necessary to consider the cost-efficacy of the ICD and to compare this with other accepted medical therapies.

Cost-Efficacy: What Is It and Why Measure It?

Cost-efficacy (also known as cost-benefit) is simply a measure of the amount of expenditure required to obtain a given degree of medical benefit. In its simplest form, when used to examine a lifesaving therapy, the benefit may be expressed as years of patients' life gained per currency unit or, more commonly, as currency units spent to obtain 1 extra year of life (life-year). Provided that accurate costs are used and that reliable data is available on patient survival with different therapies such cost per life-year figures provide a means of comparing the cost-efficacy of different medical strategies. Such comparisons are complicated when therapies that have benefits other than prevention of death are considered. Some operations, such as hip replacement, may have little impact on overall survival but may result in a dramatic improvement in the quality of life. This observation has lead to the development of the quality adjusted life-year (QALY). A medical intervention that saves the life of one patient with a subsequent life-expectancy of 10 years whose quality of life was 100% prior to the intervention and returns to 100% afterwards produces a gain of 10 QALYs. Another medical intervention that improves the quality of life of a patient with a life expectancy of 20 years from 50% to 100% without affecting their life expectancy produces an identical gain in QALYs. The major problem with this approach is that while cost and improved survival are objective variables and can be quantified (albeit with some difficulty), quality of life is essentially a subjective concept. A number of different approaches have been adopted to assess quality of life including the Rosser-Watts classification that scores on two scales of disability and distress[3] and the quality of well being (QWB) scale that assesses functional and psychological well being.[4] Unfortunately many different quality of life assessment techniques have been used in different studies requiring cumbersome conversion to allow comparison between them.[5] The pitfalls associated with these techniques have been strikingly illustrated by the outcry that followed the draft publication by the state of Oregon of a list of priorities for the provision of health care to Medicaid recipients that was based on an analysis of cost effectiveness. Many of the rankings in the list appeared counterintuitive. For example, surgery for ectopic pregnancy was assigned a similar priority to dental caps for pulp exposure. This led some authors to question the value of cost effectiveness as a means of prioritizing therapies.[6] However, there were startling inaccuracies in the cost data (an identical cost of $98.51 was assigned to such diverse procedures as medical treatment of tinea pedis and urgent coronary angioplasty for myocardial infarction) used for some computations and problems with the definition of the QWB values used in this study[7] that did not consider societal perceptions of the value of therapies. Society has a preference for interventions that provide benefits to people alive now, rather than to people who may be alive in the future and a preference for technically impressive therapies (the so-called Rule of Rescue). The delivery of therapy itself, therefore, has a perceived value over and above any benefit from the therapy itself. These factors must all be taken into account if the values produced by QALYs or QWBs are not to appear counterintuitive. In an attempt to take these societal perceptions into account the Saved Young Life Equivalent (SAVE) has been developed. It uses society's appreciation of one particular health care outcome—saving a young life—as a unit of value, but it has yet to be widely applied in studies of cost effectiveness.[8]

While these limitations of cost-efficacy analysis must be kept in mind, there are two potentially important applications to the ICD. First, it may be used to compare the cost-efficacy of conventional patterns of ICD use with other accepted therapies. Second, the cost-efficacy of a variety of possible future applications of the ICD may be calculated to examine priorities in the development of prospective trials and to highlight ways in which the cost-efficacy of ICD therapy may be improved.

How Can the Cost-Efficacy of the Implantable Defibrillator be Measured?

The primary outcome measure of ICD use is prolonged survival and the primary costs include purchase of the device and electrodes, implantation surgery, clinical follow-up, and device replacement. It is a relatively simple matter to measure the primary outcome and primary costs. However, there are secondary outcome measures (which may have an important impact on quality of life) and secondary cost factors that may also be of considerable importance. These are summarized in Table 1. Measurement or estimation of these secondary outcome measures is more difficult because of their complex interrelationship. Data on quality of life in ICD recipients are available only from a limited number of very small studies[9-11] and no published cost analysis of the ICD has included assessment of quality of life. Although this is to be regretted, it must be remembered that the primary aim of ICD therapy is to improve survival and therefore analyses that restrict themselves to considering this measure of outcome are probably valid.

Because ICD therapy is usually compared with conventional antiarrhythmic drug therapy rather than with no therapy at all, it is common to consider the marginal

Table 1
Secondary Outcome Measures and Costs of Implantable Cardioverter-Defibrillator Therapy

Secondary Outcome Measures	Secondary Cost Factors
Quality of Life —Return to work —Psychosocial adjustment	Cost of adverse effects of the ICD (displaced leads, infection, etc.)
Avoidance of adverse reactions to antiarrhythmic drugs	Cost of alternative (drug) therapies and their associated adverse effects
Incidence of rehospitalisation	Cost of time off work (reduced tax paid and increased benefits claimed)
Ability to cope with therapies from ICD	Cost of support of patient (pensions, etc.) Cost of support for dependents if patient dies Training costs for physicians providing therapy

ICD: implantable cardioverter-defibrillator.

cost-efficacy of ICD therapy. This represents the cost-efficacy of the ICD when it is used in place of the conventional therapy and is not the same as the true cost-efficacy of the device.

The best way of collecting data on cost and quality of life in ICD patients would be to do so in parallel with prospective studies of the efficacy of the device. A number of studies of this type are in progress, but have yet to be published. Therefore all existing estimates of ICD cost-efficacy are retrospective in nature and based on modeling techniques using costs derived from a variety of sources and efficacy data pooled from a number of published studies.

Retrospective Assessment of Cost-Efficacy

Three groups have published major analyses of the cost-efficacy of the ICD, two in the United States and one in the United Kingdom. For ease of comparison, the data from the United Kingdom has been converted to United States dollars using an exchange rate of $1.50 = £1.00, this being the approximate exchange rate at the time of writing. The first study was that of Kupperman and colleagues[12]. The aim of this study was to calculate the marginal cost-efficacy of the ICD when compared to conventional electrophysiologically-guided antiarrhythmic drug therapy. Survival data for patients with the ICD were derived from a number of published studies[13-17] and compared with that for antiarrhythmic drug therapy.[18-24]

A variety of sources were used for estimating resource use including data from the Health Care Financing Administration, the 1984 Medicare Provider Analysis and Review (MEDPAR), and a panel of expert physicians. Using these data they calculated a marginal cost effectiveness versus conventional antiarrhythmic drug therapy at 1986 prices of $17,400 per life-year saved by the ICD. Because of the large number of assumptions involved in this study sensitivity analyses showed a wide range of values for this cost-efficacy figure from $2,000 to $30,000 per life-year. Assuming an extension of ICD generator life to 5 years and assuming the adoption of nonthoracotomy implantation, they predicted the cost-efficacy would improve to $7,400 per life-year by 1991.

This elegant study was a major advance in the assessment of ICD cost-efficacy, but its design illustrates the problems associated with retrospective studies. The ICD survival data was pooled from several studies. Given the similarity of sudden death-free survival reported in these studies this is adequate, but the similarly pooled data for survival on antiarrhythmic drugs displayed a wide range of survival figures and the validity of the pooled data is unclear. Much of the data on which this study was founded were collected 10 or more years ago and in the postthrombolysis era they may not satisfactorily reflect current patient outcome.

In the United Kingdom, O'Brien and co-workers[25] have used a similarly complex model to assess the cost-efficacy of the ICD in comparison with long-term amiodarone therapy. Their model studied a 20-year period using extrapolated survival data from the ICD survival study of Winkle et al.[26] and the amiodarone study of Herre et al.[27] Cost data was derived from known National Health Service drug costs, a study of costs of cardiac surgery[28] and physician interviews. The marginal cost-efficacy of the ICD versus therapy with amiodarone ranged from $12,300 to $21,300 per life-year depending on the assumed rate of nonsudden death in the two populations. They estimated that developments in devices (primarily extended ICD generator life) and transvenous implant techniques could improve cost-efficacy to $9,000 per life-year.

The most recent and most sophisticated attempt to measure the cost-efficacy of the ICD versus that of amiodarone and conventional antiarrhythmic drug therapy is that of Larsen and colleagues.[29] They used a Markov or state transition decision model to compare the ICD, amiodarone, and conventional drug therapy in three cohorts of patients assumed to be identical except for their treatment for ventricular arrhythmia. In such a model, an individual patient occupies a single health state (eg, ICD implanted well) at any one time with a range of probabilities governing their likelihood of leaving this state and passing to another (eg, ICD battery depletion, surgery). Costs are defined for each associated health state and a computer models the passage of time and the transition of patients in the population between various health states. The decision model with its multiplicity of health states used by Larsen et al.[29] is shown in Figure 1.

The costs used in this model were derived from the New England Medical Center's accounting system for real ICD patients. The probabilities of passing from one health state to another were again based on published data for ICD recipient survival,[30-32] amiodarone-treated survival,[33-35] conventional antiarrhythmic drug survival,[21,22] and complications. Using this model and assuming an ICD generator life of 2 years, the authors calculated that amiodarone produced a marginal gain in life expectancy of 1.31 years over conventional antiarrhythmic drug therapy and the ICD produced a further 2.22-year gain over and above amiodarone therapy. The marginal cost-efficacy of the ICD over amiodarone therapy was $29,200 per life-year while that of amiodarone therapy over conventional drug therapy was $6,600 per life-year. These figures were calculated for a patient aged 55 years and the cost per life-year became marginally higher for older patients. Sensitivity analysis showed that prolonging generator life from 2 years to 4 years would cause a marked improvement in cost-efficacy from $29,200 per life-year to around $19,000 per life-year. The authors also considered the impact of altered quality of life in either the drug- or ICD-treated groups on cost-efficacy (Figure 2). Even quite small reductions in quality of life from 100% with ICD therapy greatly impair its cost-efficacy, whereas the reductions in quality of life on amiodarone therapy improve the relative cost effectiveness of ICDs, but less dramatically so.

These three studies have made a substantial contribution to our knowledge of the cost-efficacy of current and past patterns of ICD usage. Table 2 shows a comparison of these cost-efficacy values with those for other therapies derived from a variety of sources[12,25,29,36,37] converted (where necessary) to United States dollars and corrected for inflation to 1991. There is a two- to threefold difference in the cost-efficacy estimates for some procedures between the United States and the United Kingdom, but such variation is likely to be accounted for by uncertainties in the costing process and differ-

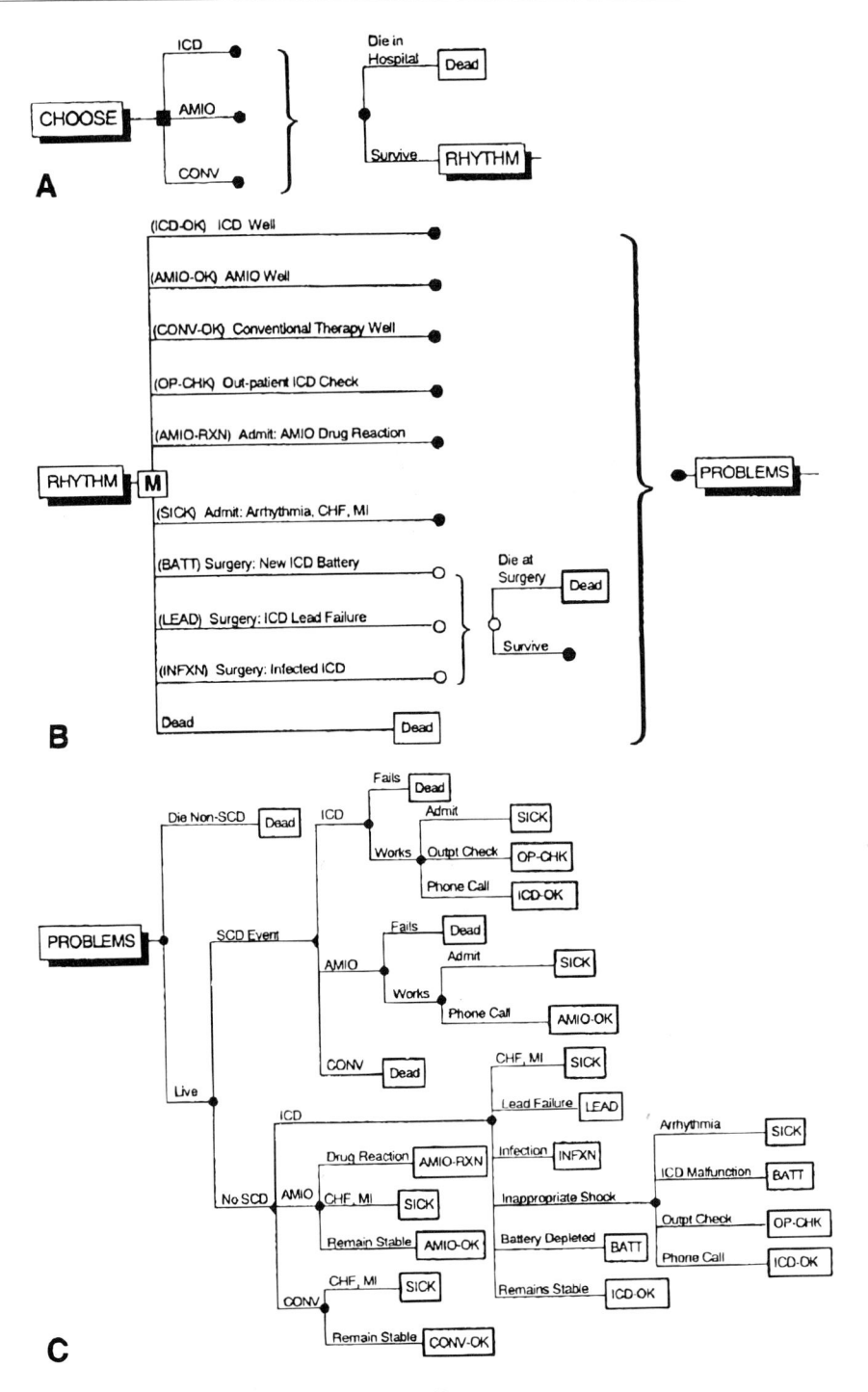

Figure 1. The Markov model used by Larsen et al.[29] At any one time an individual patient may be in any one of the health states shown. Their passage to other health states is governed by predetermined probabilities and the costs of being in each health state is known. (Reproduced with permission from Reference 29.)

COST-EFFICACY OF ICD US$,000/LIFE-YEAR

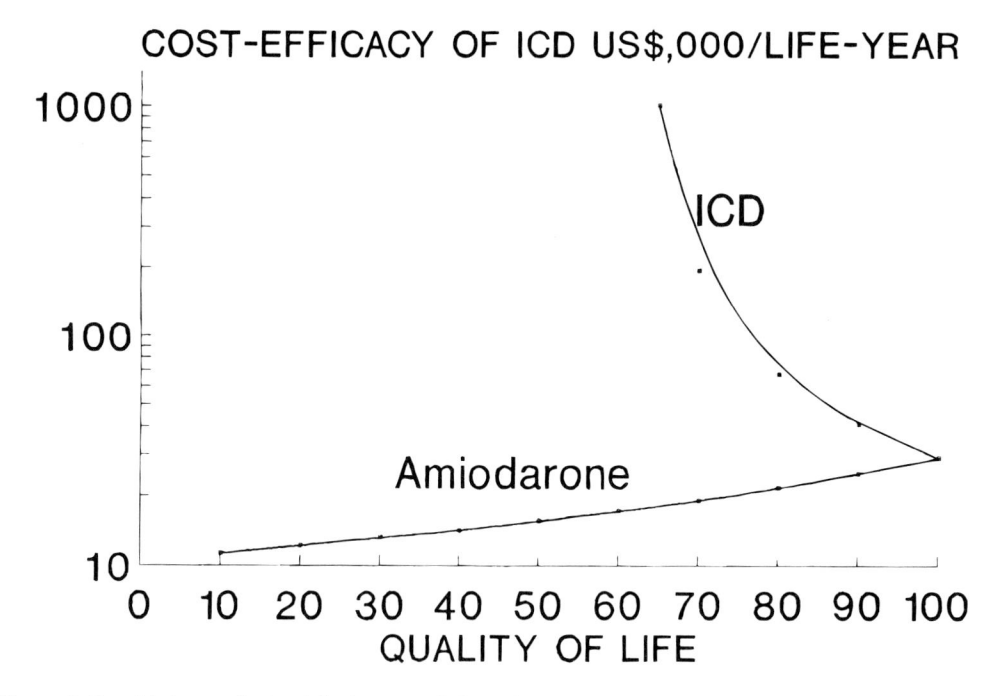

Figure 2. Sensitivity analysis of the impact of altered quality of life on the cost-efficacy of implantable cardioverter-defibrillator (ICD) use. The ICD line (ICD) shows the dramatic fall in cost-efficacy of the ICD that occurs if ICD recipients suffer quite small reductions in quality of life. The amiodarone line (Amiodarone) shows the improvement on ICD cost-efficacy that occurs if long-term amiodarone therapy is associated with impaired quality of life. (Modified with permission from Reference 29.)

ence in medical costs between the United States and United Kingdom. The similarity of the three different figures for cost-efficacy of ICD use is striking, particularly as they originate from different countries at different times. The table suggests that the cost of ICD therapy lies within the broad scope defined by other invasive medical and cardiovascular therapies.

Limitations of These Retrospective Studies of Implantable Cardioverter-Defibrillator Cost-Efficacy

The three studies of cost-efficacy described above use models of progressively increasing complexity to quantify the cost-efficacy of ICD use. The major limitations of all three of these studies is that they use survival data from relatively early published series of survival with the ICD in which the features of the patients included were often not clearly defined. So while considerable effort has gone into ensuring the accuracy of the figures produced by these studies these figures essentially tell us about past practice. The complexity of the models used in these studies limits their easy application to current and possible future uses of the ICD.

Application of a Simple, Flexible Model to the Assessment of Implantable Cardioverter-Defibrillator Cost-Efficacy

At St. George's Hospital in London, England, we[38] have developed a simple flexible model of the cost-efficacy of the ICD and applied it using a wide variety of data

Table 2
Cost per Year of Life Saved for Various Therapies

Procedure (Reference Source)	Cost-Efficacy: $,000/Life-Year (1991)
Pacemaker for complete heart block[36]	1.4
Aortic valve replacement for aortic stenosis[36]	2.2
Neonatal intensive care (babies 1,000–1,499 g)[12]	7.4
Coronary artery bypass grafting–three-vessel disease[36]	8.0
Coronary artery bypass grafting–three-vessel disease[12]	9.6
Heart transplantation[36]	*12.0*
Treatment of severe hypertension (diastolic 105 mm Hg) in men aged 40 years[12]	14.9
Lovastatin therapy for cholesterol >250 mg/dL (6.47 mmol/L) in men aged 55–64[37]	19.1
PTCA for single-vessel disease[36]	25.7
ICD versus conventional drug therapy[12]§	23.3
ICD versus amiodarone[25]§	*23.8*
ICD versus amiodarone[29]§	29.2
Treatment of mild hypertension (diastolic 95–104 mm Hg) in men aged 40 years[12]	31.1
Hospital hemodialysis[36]	*33.6*
Heart transplantation[12]§	36.0
Coronary artery bypass grafting at single-vessel disease[12]	59.2
Chronic ambulatory peritoneal dialysis[12]	76.8
Hospital hemodialysis[12]	79.7

All figures refer to quality-adjusted life-years except those marked §.
All costs have been converted to United States dollars and corrected for inflation to 1991 prices.
Figures in italics derived from United Kingdom, all others for United States.
ICD: implantable cardioverter-defibrillator; PTCA: percutaneous transluminal angioplasty.

from published studies to assess the cost-efficacy of ICD use in a variety of circumstances. Because of the limited availability of long-term survival data for ICD recipients, a fixed time period of 3 years has been used in this model. In calculating the total cost of ICD use they take the cost of identifying the patient at risk (screening tests), the cost of the hospital stay required for ICD implantation, the cost of the implantation surgery, the cost of the ICD generator and leads, and the cost of follow-up over the life of the generator. These costs are written off over the 3-year period of the study. Subsequent generator replacement costs are ignored by the model as are any benefits accruing from the initial ICD therapy after the initial 3-year period is completed.

To calculate the gain in years of life accruing from the use of the ICD in any particular population, a simple calculation is performed. Figure 3 shows the survival curve for a hypothetical population of 100 subjects in which the sudden death mortality is 16% in the first year, 8% in the second year, and 4% in the third year. If the ICD prevents all the sudden deaths over the 3-year predicted ICD generator life, then 16 patients who would have died during the first year will gain a mean additional survival of 2.5 years (assuming sudden deaths are evenly distributed through the year) giving a total gain of 40 life-years. A similar calculation can be performed for the second and third years. However, patients who die as a result of ICD implantation actually lose life-years and this must also be taken into account. Their deaths also reduce the number of life-years gained by the rest of the population. Knowing the cost for a defibrillator implant and follow-up over the 3-year period and the net gain in life-years accruing from each

Calculation of Gain in Life-Years from Survival Curve

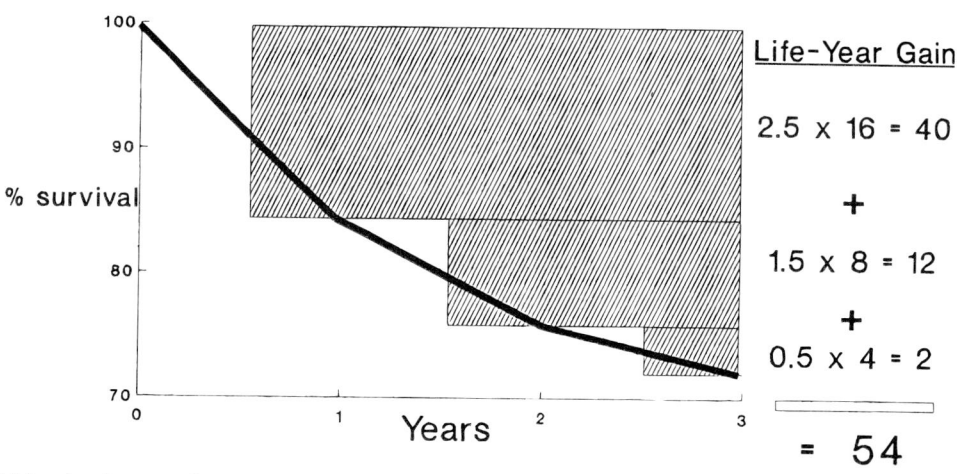

Life-Year Gain

2.5 x 16 = 40

+

1.5 x 8 = 12

+

0.5 x 4 = 2

= 54

If implant mortality is 3% only 97% of population stand to benefit. and 3% of population have lost 3 years of life.

FINAL GAIN = (54 X 0.97) - (3 X 3) = 43.4 LIFE-YEARS/100 patients

Figure 3. Method of calculation of gain in life-years. The dark line shows the untreated survival free of sudden death in a hypothetical population of 100 patients. The shaded boxes represent the gain in life-years accruing if the implantable cardioverter-defibrillator (ICD) prevents all sudden deaths. The total gain of 54 life-years calculated is reduced to 52.4 years (54 × 100 − 3/100) as the 3% of the population who die gain no benefit from the ICD. In addition the three patients each lose a potential 3 life-years (totaling 9 life-years) so the final gain from the strategy is 43.4 life-years.

implant the cost per life-year can be calculated.

The cost assumptions that have been used in the St. George's model are shown in Table 3. These are based on 1991 prices and have been derived from a number of sources. The single most expensive item at any ICD implant is the ICD generator itself. The figure of $15,000 that was used in the St. George's model allows the purchase of a modern device without antitachycardia pacing but with data logging/Holter functions. Pace/sense electrodes and epicardial patches (two or three) or a transvenous electrode(s) with or without an axillary patch electrode are also required. Although the costs of individual components of these systems vary quite markedly between manufacturers, the total cost of a complete lead system is remarkably similar. The figure of

Table 3
The Costing Assumptions Used in the
St. George's Costing Model (1991 figures)

Item	Cost ($)
Screening tests	
Echocardiogram	82
Signal-averaged ECG	75
Holter recording and analysis	150
Limited electrophysiological study (VT stimulation)	750
Repeat VT stimulation study	225
ICD generator	15,000
ICD leads (including patches and pace/sense leads)	2,470
ICD implantation surgery cost[25]	4,800
Additional hospital stay (day charge)	400
Follow-up visit (6 in first year and 4 in subsequent years)	150

ICD: implantable cardioverter-defibrillator; VT: ventricular tachycardia.

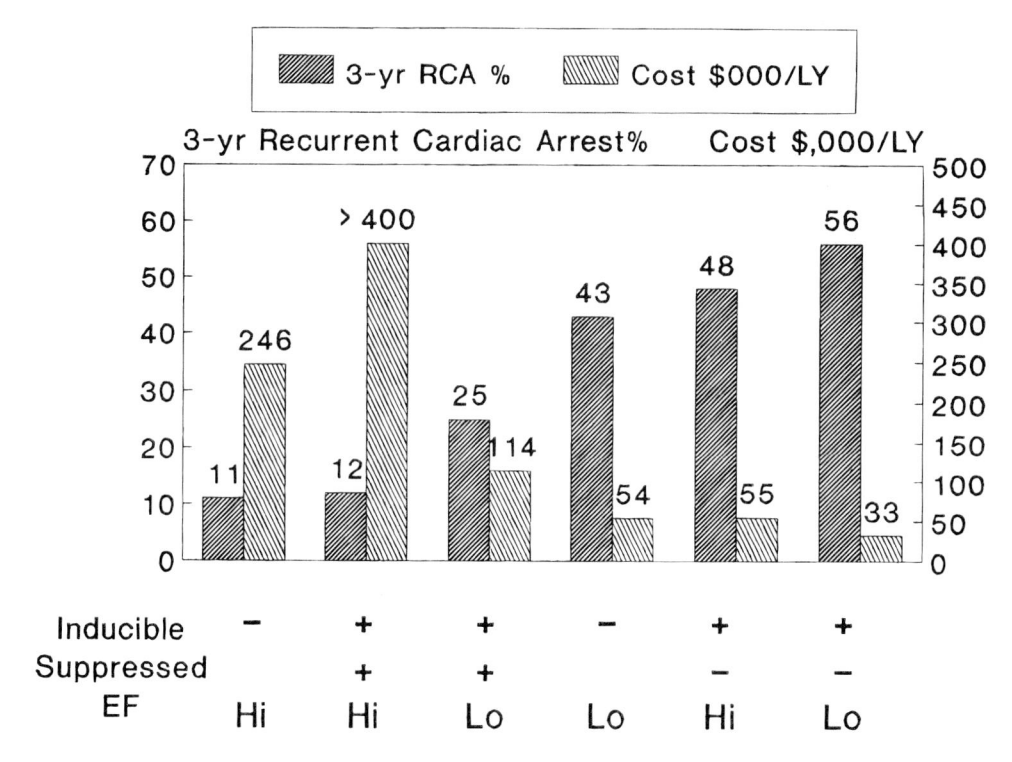

Figure 5. Three-year recurrent cardiac arrest (RCA) incidence and cost of implantable cardioverter-defibrillator (ICD) use in thousand dollars per life-year in the six groups shown in Figure 4.

physiologically guided investigation (Figure 6). A strategy of early implantation in all patients appeared to cost $40,400 versus $48,900 for a strategy of electrophysiologically guided evaluation with ICD implantation only in patients in whom an effective pharmacological agent could not be found. In light of this, we have applied the model to assess the cost-efficacy of a more simple approach to selection of patients for ICD implantation using either baseline inducibility at a single electrophysiologic study or ejection fraction alone. A single electrophysiologic study costs $750 and may involve 1 or 2 extra days in-hospital. In Wilber et al.'s group[22], 79% of patients had an inducible arrhythmia and 86.2% of recurrent cardiac arrests occur in this group. However, because of the cost of using an electrophysiologic study to identify this large group at relatively low risk of sudden death, the cost per life-year of this strategy is $85,500. This is identical to that of using no screening test at all and appears to offer no advantage over such a policy. In contrast, measurement of ejection fraction is cheap and involves no extra hospital stay. The low ejection fraction subgroup comprises 33% of the population and 52% of recurrent cardiac arrests occur in this subgroup. The cost-efficacy of ICD use in this subgroup alone is $38,250 per life-year that is a considerable improvement when compared to ICD use in the whole population ($85,500 per life-year). However, despite the shorter hospital stay this approach is less cost effective than use of the ICD in the combined high-risk group ($38,250 versus $35,400) as described and would prevent a smaller proportion (52% versus 56%) of the total number of sudden deaths.

The St. George's costing model suggests that generalized use of the ICD in all cardiac arrest survivors is an expensive strategy. The cost-efficacy may be improved by restricting ICD use to subgroups at

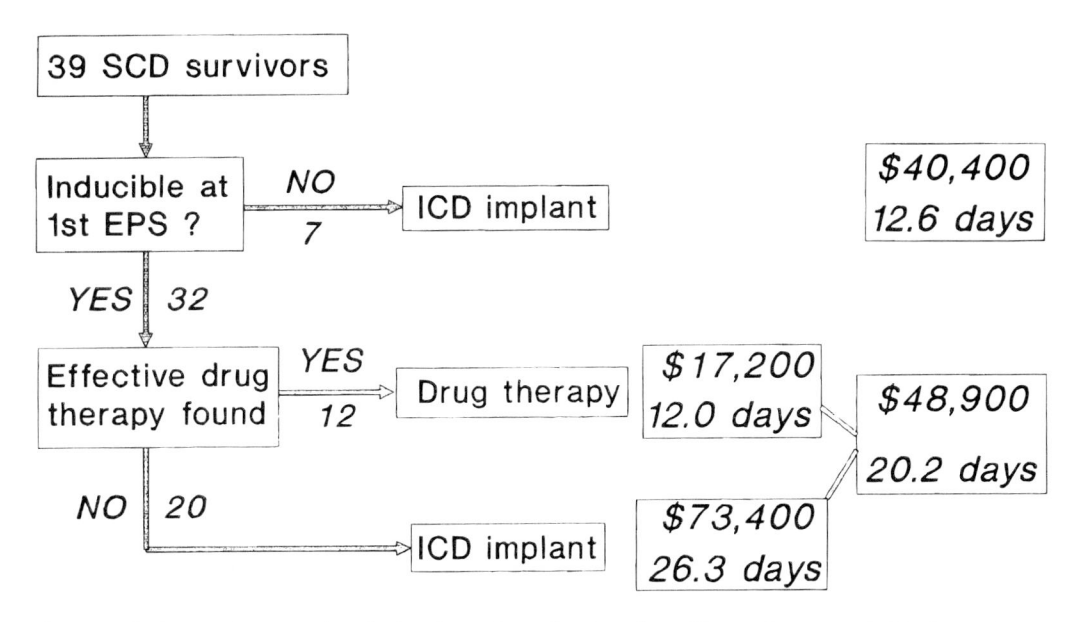

Figure 6. In-hospital costs of early implantation of an implantable cardioverter-defibrillator (ICD) versus full electrophysiologic investigation with late ICD implantation if no effective drug therapy is found. (Data from Reference 39.)

higher risk of sudden death. The model suggests that a combination of ejection fraction measurement and electrophysiologic assessment is superior in identifying a cost-effective high-risk subgroup than either of these investigations alone. The dichotomization of the ejection fraction as performed by Wilber et al.[22] may overlook additional information that may be obtained by retaining it as a continuous variable. Some studies have suggested that much of the apparent value of the electrophysiologic study as a predictive investigation is accounted for by difference in the values of ejection fraction between the inducible and noninducible groups.[40]

The relationship between cost-efficacy and yield of sudden death prevention for various strategies outlined above is illustrated in Figure 7. A number of studies are in progress to compare ICD use in cardiac arrest survivors with conventional electrophysiologically guided drug therapy and many of these studies are aiming to collect cost data in parallel with evidence of efficacy. The Dutch Prospective Study[41] is specifically addressing the issue of cost-efficacy. The results of these studies should enable a more accurate assessment of the cost-efficacy of ICD use in these patients that may provide a guide to the rational use of the ICD in these patients.

Costing Future Applications of the Implantable Cardioverter-Defibrillator

A number of controlled trials of the ICD are currently planned or underway (Table 4). Among these trials are a number that aim to evaluate ICD implantation in novel risk groups.[42,43] These include patients with nonsustained ventricular tachycardia (VT), high-risk patients after myocardial infarction, patients undergoing coronary artery bypass grafting, and patients with severe dilated cardiomyopathy awaiting cardiac transplantation. As described, the simple costing model has been applied to assess the cost-efficacy of the strategies proposed by these trials using published survival data for the various groups at risk.

% of total sudden deaths preventable

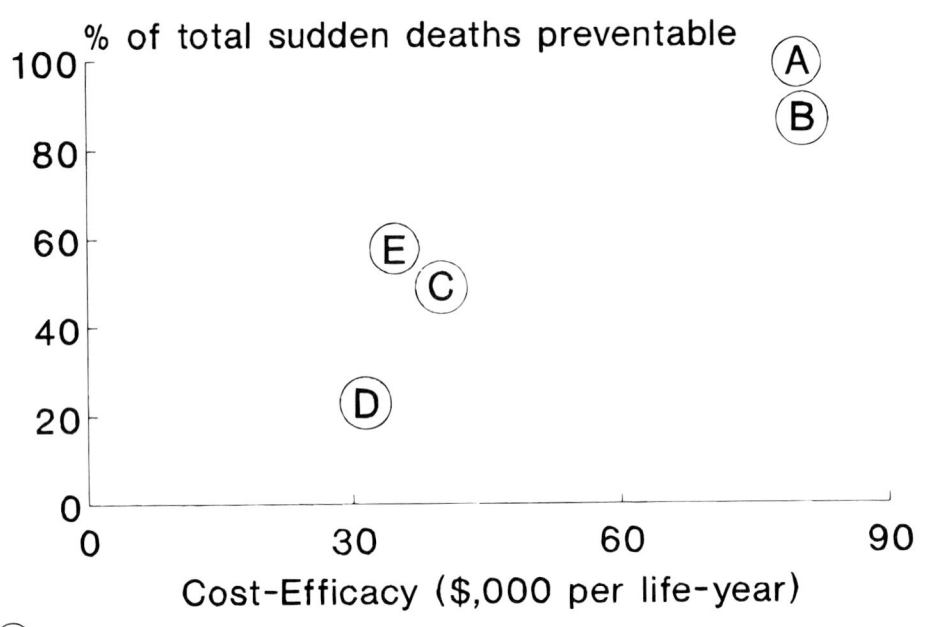

Ⓐ - ICD in all cardiac arrest survivors
Ⓑ - ICD in pts with inducible arrhythmias only
Ⓒ - ICD in patients with Low EF only
Ⓓ - ICD in highest risk gp (Lo EF, inducible, non-suppressed)
Ⓔ - ICD in the 3 highest risk groups combined

Figure 7. Relationship between cost-efficacy and yield of prevention of sudden death for a variety of selection strategies.

Table 4
Some of the Current Trials of Novel Applications of the Implantable-Cardioverter Defibrillator

Risk Group	Trial
Nonsustained ventricular tachycardia	Multicenter Automatic Defibrillator Implantation Trial (MADIT)
	Multicenter Unsustained Tachycardia Trial (MUSTT)
High-risk patients postmyocardial infarction	Australasian Clinical Trial of the Automatic Implantable Defibrillator (ACTAID)
Patients undergoing coronary artery bypass grafting with impaired left ventricular function and positive signal-average ECG.	CABG-Patch Trial
Dilated cardiomyopathy (Bridge to transplant)	CAT (The Cardiomyopathy Trial) DEFIBRLAT

Implantable Cardioverter-Defibrillator Cost-Efficacy in Patients With Nonsustained Ventricular Tachycardia

Three separate trials of the use of the ICD in patients with nonsustained VT and known coronary artery disease, but without a history of sustained VT or ventricular fibrillation (VF) are in progress. The Multicenter Automatic Defibrillator Implantation Trial (MADIT) study that recruits patients with nonsustained VT who have inducible arrhythmias at baseline electrophysiologic study that remain inducible on procainamide.[44] These patients are randomized to ICD or conventional drug therapy. Multicenter Unsustained Tachycardia Trial (MUSTT) compares electrophysiologically-guided drug therapy with placebo for patients with inducible arrhythmia. In the electrophysiologically-guided patients, the ICD is used for patients who remain inducible despite drug therapy. The rationale for these studies is that the presence of inducible arrhythmias at electrophysiologic study correlates closely with subsequent VT or VF[45,46] and that patients with nonsustained VT have a high incidence of inducible arrhythmias and these patients in turn have a high incidence of sudden death.[47,48]

Wilber et al.[47] have published data on survival free of cardiac arrest for patients with coronary artery disease, left ventricular ejection fraction < 40%, and nonsustained VT. They have stratified this population by inducibility of sustained VT at electrophysiologic study and whether such tachycardias could be suppressed by antiarrhythmic drug therapy. The results of this stratification are shown in Figure 8. Using these data and the simple model, the strategy of ICD use proposed by the MADIT trial costs $63,900 per life-year and the strategy of the MUSTT trial costs $35,200 per life-year. This cost-efficacy is similar to that gained by using the ICD in cardiac arrest

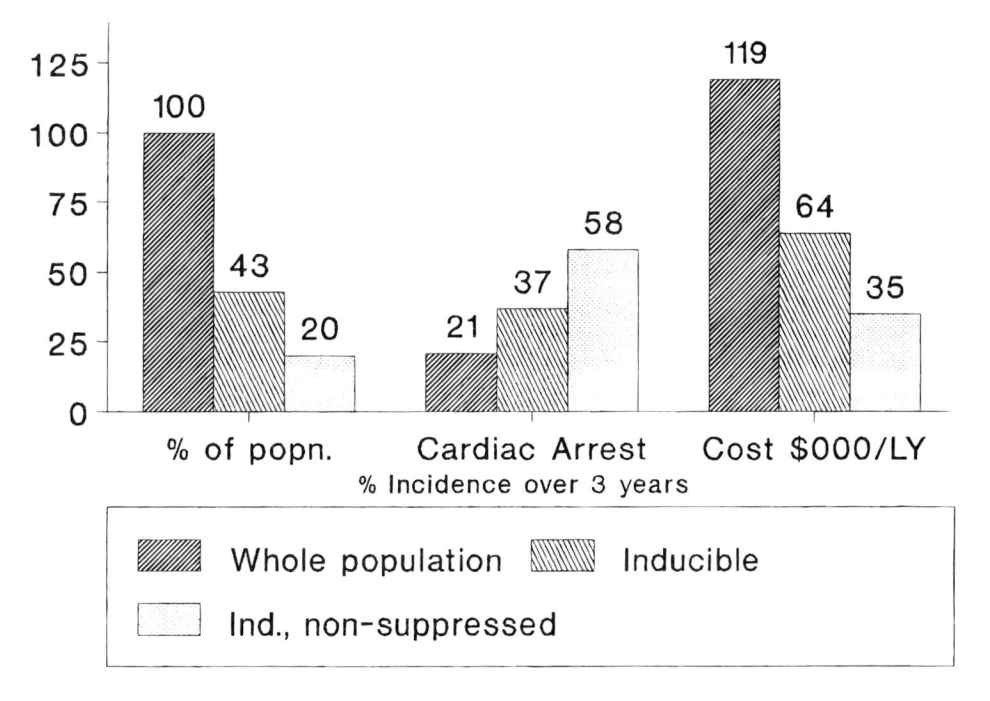

Figure 8. Stratification of patients with nonsustained ventricular tachycardia (VT) using electrophysiologic studies. The costing model has been used to calculate the cost-efficacy of ICD use in each group. (Survival data from Reference 47.)

survivors. However, difficulty with recruitment for the MADIT trial suggest that the prevalence of inducible arrhythmias noted in the Wilber et al.[47] study (43%) may not be representative of this group as a whole. This would increase the number of patients who need to be screened to find one patient at risk and reduce the cost-efficacy of this strategy.

Implantable Cardioverter-Defibrillator Cost-Efficacy in Patients at High Risk After Myocardial Infarction

Survivors of myocardial infarction represent a large population who are known to be at increased risk of sudden cardiac death. Much interest has centered on the identification of subgroups of this population who are at particularly high risk. Although electrophysiologic studies have been reported to be effective at identifying patients with a high risk of recurrent cardiac events[49] most interest has focused on the use of noninvasive screening tests. At St. George's Hospital, we have a large database of myocardial infarction survivors. Over 500 patients have now been followed for 3 years or more and the population has been studied for predictors of sudden death. Currently the best group of tests to identify patients at high risk appear to be the combination of reduced heart rate variability, more than 10 ventricular ectopic beats per hour, and a positive signal-averaged ECG.[50] At 3 years this population has a sudden death mortality of 29.9% in comparison with 4.5% for the population as a whole, and 7.5% for those patients with an ejection fraction < 40% (Figure 9).

The cost of ICD use in this high-risk population with a 29.9% 3-year sudden death rate is $54,700 per life-year, which is less than twice that of using the device in

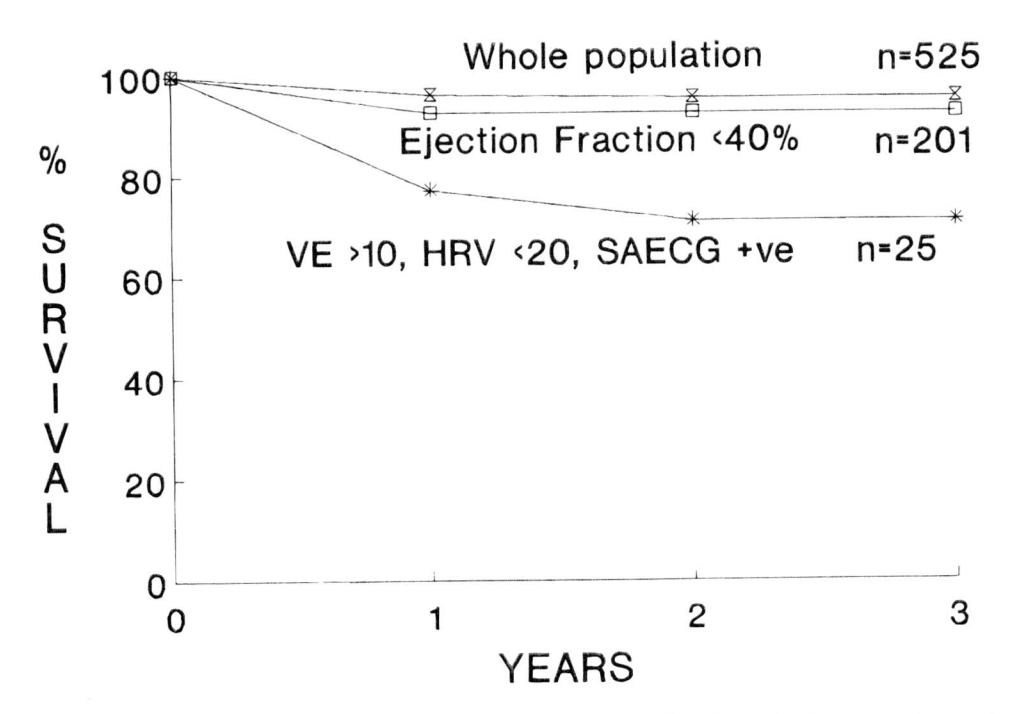

Figure 9. Stratification of myocardial infarction survivors using data from the St. George's Hospital database. A high-risk group of patients with frequent ventricular extrasystoles, reduced heart rate variability, and positive signal-averaged ECG have a 29.9% 3-year mortality from sudden death.

highest risk subgroup of cardiac arrest survivors. However, while this group may be approaching an acceptable level of cost effectiveness, it includes only 26% of the patients who will die suddenly in this period and this represents only 10.5% of the total deaths. Extending the use of the ICD to the larger group with an ejection fraction of < 40% (which contains 38% of the population) increases the cost nearly fivefold to $255,000 per life-year. The overall impact of ICD use on postinfarction mortality is likely to remain small unless the sensitivity and specificity of screening tests for patients at risk of sudden death improves. The Australasian Clinical Trial of the Automatic Implantable Defibrillator (ACTAID) study, which evaluates the implantation of the ICD in patients with inducible arrhythmias postinfarction, is in the early stages of recruitment and should provide valuable data on the role of the ICD in survivors of myocardial infarction.

Implantable Cardioverter-Defibrillator Cost-Efficacy in Patients with Low Ejection Fraction and Positive Signal-Averaged ECG

The CABG Patch study is already in progress,[43] recruiting patients already destined for coronary artery bypass grafting with impaired left ventricular function (ejection fraction < 36%) and a positive signal-averaged ECG. Patients are randomized to coronary artery bypass grafting or to coronary artery bypass grafting plus ICD. Insertion of the ICD at the same time as coronary artery bypass grafting surgery saves on both surgical and bed stay costs for implantation.

There are no published survival data for an identical group, but the study is apparently based on a retrospective study of these patients by the investigators[42] that showed an unexpectedly high mortality. Data is available for a similar group of patients with a positive signal-averaged ECG and ejection fraction of < 40%.[51] The 1-year mortality in this group appears to be about 12% to 14%. Extrapolation is required to produce a 3-year sudden death mortality of 21% so that the costing figure of $66,000 per life-year is subject to wide confidence limits. Using data from the postinfarction database at St. George's Hospital suggests that patients with an ejection fraction < 36% and a positive signal-average ECG have a 3-year sudden death rate of just 4.2%. This produces a very high cost of $855,000 per life-year. However, the patients in the St. George's database do not necessarily require coronary artery bypass grafting and might therefore be presumed to be at lower risk of sudden death than those entering the CABG Patch study. Clearly it is not possible to make any definitive conclusions about the strategy proposed by this trial pending the availability of survival data from the trial itself.

Implantable Cardioverter-Defibrillator Cost-Efficacy in Patients Awaiting Cardiac Transplantation

About 40% of deaths from congestive heart failure are thought to be of an arrhythmic nature[52,53] and patients with dilated cardiomyopathy awaiting cardiac transplantation appear to be at particularly high risk of sudden death.[54] This has given rise to the suggested use of the ICD as a bridge to transplantation (DEFIBRLAT = Defibrillator Implantation as Bridge to Later Transplantation[55]) although the protocol of this study has yet to be published. Stevenson et al.[54] found a 34% 1-year sudden death mortality in the group with an ejection fraction < 25% and the mortality rose to 57% in those patients with a stroke volume of < 40 mL. In these patients the costing model was adjusted to assume a 1-year wait to transplantation with a 50% 5-year survival rate after transplantation. Because of the high mortality and short follow-up period in this group, the defibrillator appears highly cost effective ($24,000 per life-year in the whole group and $13,900 per life-year in the high-risk group). However, it must be remembered that these costs are additional to the cost per life-year of the transplant itself.

Expenditure Implications of the Strategies Proposed by the Current Generation of Controlled Implantable Cardioverter-Defibrillator Trials

Application of the St. George's model suggests that the cost-efficacy of the various proposed applications of the ICD varies markedly. By calculating the approximate number of patients in the various risk groups we can calculate the expenditure implications for the United States of adopting the strategies proposed by these trials (Table 5). The current population of the United States is 251,000,000 and nearly 1,500,000 patients suffer from myocardial infarction annually.[56] The case-fatality rate has fallen dramatically over the last 40 years such that it is now < 10% and we can safely assume there will be 1,300,000 infarct survivors annually. Even if only half of these are first infarctions, there will be 650,000 new myocardial infarction survivors per annum. The basic cost of each ICD implant alone (without any allowance for screening test or follow-up costs) is $25,070. If ICD use is restricted to just those patients with reduced heart rate variability, a positive signal-averaged ECG and increased ventricular ectopic beats, 30,800 ICD implants would be needed annually at a cost of $775,000,000 per annum or 0.013% of gross domestic product.

The approximate number of cardiac arrest survivors per annum can be estimated from the results of community based interventions for out-of-hospital cardiac arrest. Early schemes for out-of-hospital resuscitation in urban areas achieved survival figures to hospital discharge of 10% to 15%[57,58] improving in the 1980s to about 25%.[59] In rural populations the figures are likely to be lower due to longer response times and the figure of 12.5% in the Heartstart Scotland study[60] may be more representative. This is equivalent to 6 cardiac arrest survivors per 100,000 population per annum and similar

Table 5
Annual Expenditure Implications for the United Kingdom of Adopting the Strategies Proposed by the Various Controlled Trials of the Implantable Cardioverter-Defibrillator

Risk Group	Number of Patients	Annual Cost $
Cardiac Arrest Survivors		
All patients	17,600	441 × 10⁶
Low EF	5,900	147 × 10⁶
Inducible, nonsuppressed, low EF	2,060	52 × 10⁶
Nonsustained VT		
ie, MADIT	14,000	350 × 10⁶
ie, MUSTT and SDPS	6,500	163 × 10⁶
SAECG positive + low EF (ie, CABG Patch)	15,500	390 × 10⁶
Dilated Cardiomyopathy awaiting transplant (ie, DEFIBRLAT)	650	16 × 10⁶
ICD use postmyocardial infarction (high-risk group)	30,800	775 × 10⁶

EF: ejection fraction; MADIT: Multicenter Automatic Defibrillator Implantation Trial; VT: ventricular tachycardia; SAECG: signal-average ECG; MUSTT: Multicenter Unsustained Tachycardia Trial; SDPS: Sudden Death Prevention Study; DEFIBRLAT: Defibrillator Implantation as Bridge to Later Transplantation.

to the 8.3 per 100,000 population per annum from a study in rural Iowa.[61] Assuming a figure of 7 per 100,000 per annum to be representative, this would give a figure of 17,600 resuscitated cardiac arrest survivors for the United States. Assuming all these patients receive an ICD the total annual expenditure would be $441,000,000. If ICD implantation is restricted to those with a low ejection fraction, then this figure falls to $147,000,000 per annum and use of the ICD only in the highest risk group with inducible nonsuppressed arrhythmias reduces expenditure to $52,000,000 per annum.

In patients with nonsustained VT we can assume that these are selected from the 650,000 first myocardial infarction survivors per annum. In the St. George's study group 5% of such patients had nonsustained VT on Holter monitoring. If we restrict ICD use to the highest risk group with inducible tachycardias (like the MUSTT trial) not suppressed by conventional antiarrhythmic drug therapy, the annual cost would be $163,000,000 per annum. If we adopt the broader strategy of device use in all patients with an ejection fraction below 40% and inducible ventricular arrhythmias (like the MADIT trial) the cost rises to $350,000,000 per annum.

In 1990, approximately 1,080 coronary artery bypass operations were performed per million population in the United States[62] giving a total of 272,000 procedures. In the St. George's database, 5.7% of patients had a positive signal-averaged ECG and reduced ejection fraction that would qualify them for the CABG Patch trial. This extrapolates to 15,500 ICD implants per annum in the United States at a cost of $390,000,000 per annum.

Approximately 2,000 heart transplants were performed in the United States in 1990.[63] If ICD use were restricted to the group at highest risk of sudden death (ejection fraction < 25% and stroke volume < 40 mL) the number of ICD implants required would be 650 and the cost would be just $16,000,000 per annum.

Future Technical Developments in the Implantable Cardioverter-Defibrillator and Screening Tests

The considered costing scenarios above have been based on a number of assumptions that are likely to change over the next few years. Using the simple costing model, we can assess the impact of these developments in our high-risk postmyocardial infarction group where the cost per life-year is currently $54,700. Use of the ICD in this group currently appears relatively expensive when compared to other accepted medical therapies.

Increased Generator Life

If we assume an increase in generator life to 5 years and that the sudden deaths are distributed so that two thirds of them occur in the first 3 years after ICD implantation, the cost of ICD use in the high-risk postinfarction group falls to $37,500 per life-year. The relationship between generator life and cost-efficacy is illustrated in Figure 10. Further extensions of generator life beyond 5 years will have relatively small impact on ICD cost-efficacy.

Generator Price Reduced

Assuming a 50% reduction in the real cost of a simple defibrillator, the cost of ICD use in the high-risk postinfarction group falls to $42,000 per life-year. The relationship between generator price and cost-efficacy is shown in Figure 11. It is interesting to note that even if the ICD generator was free, the cost of this strategy would still be $29,200 per life-year.

Transvenous Implantation

Transvenous implantation is likely to be associated with shorter hospital stay and reduced cost of implantation surgery. How-

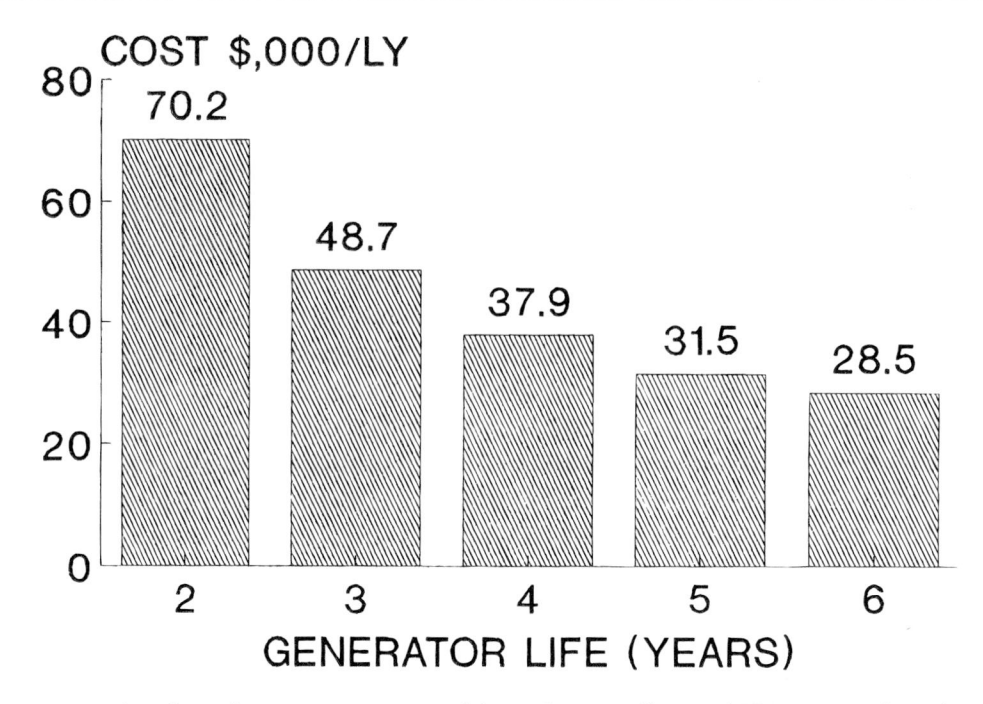

Figure 10. The effect of increasing generator life on the cost-efficacy of ICD use in a hypothetical population with a 3-year sudden mortality of 28%.

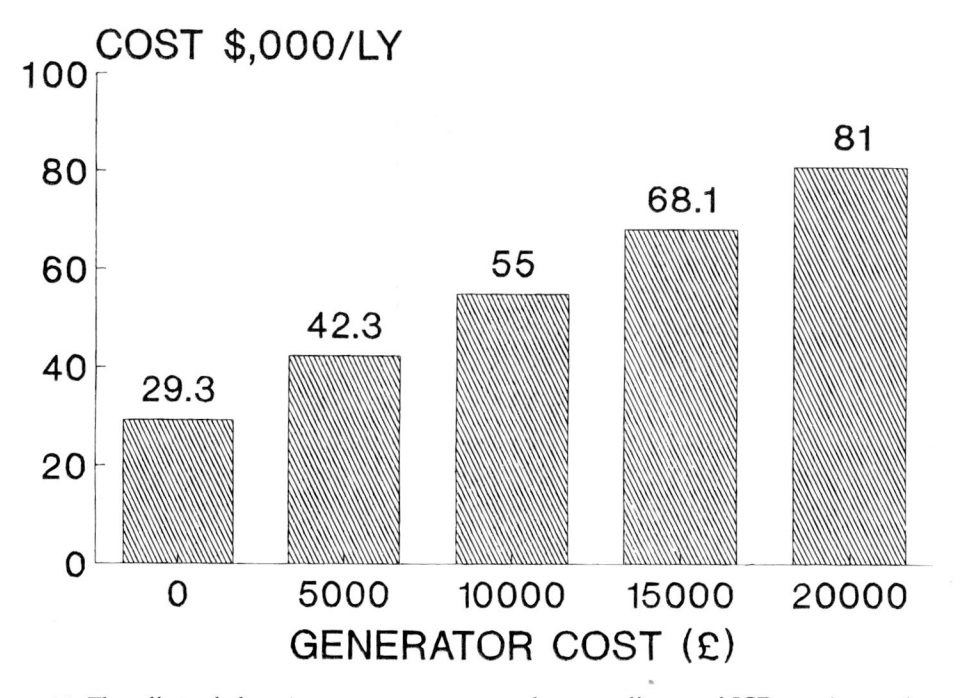

Figure 11. The effect of changing generator cost on the cost-efficacy of ICD use in survivors of myocardial infarction at high risk of sudden cardiac death.

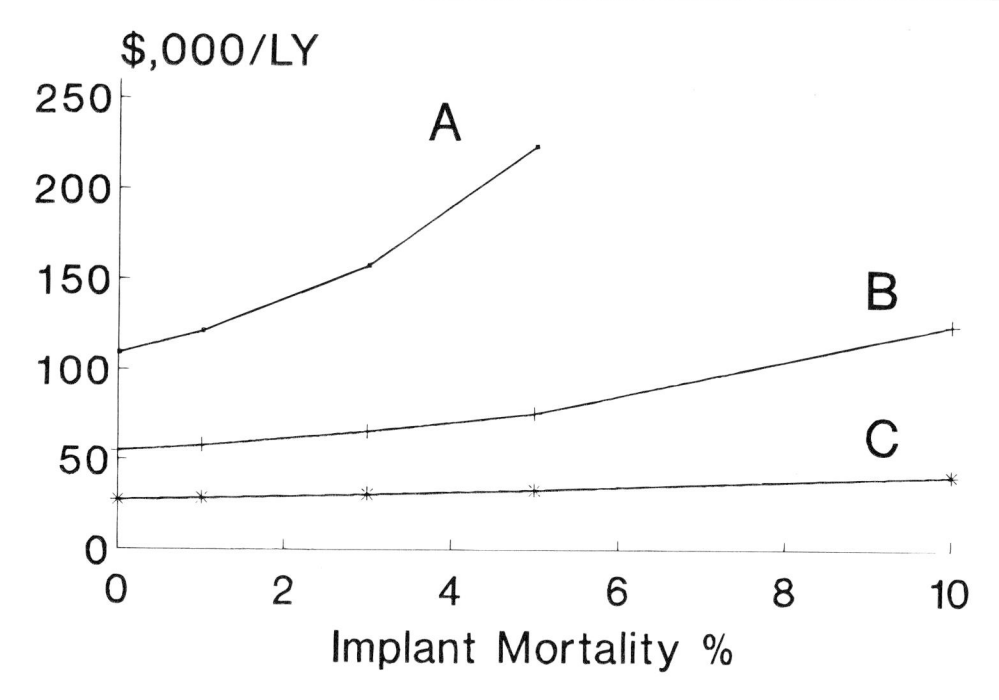

Figure 12. The effect of altering implant mortality on the cost-efficacy of ICD use is illustrated in three populations with differing 3-year sudden death rates: A: 14%; B: 28%; C: 56%. The improvement in cost-efficacy from improved implant-related mortality is greatest where the use of the implantable cardioverter-defibrillator (ICD) is marginal, ie, where sudden death mortality is low.

ever, the cost of the defibrillator is unchanged and most transvenous lead systems are marginally more expensive than their epicardial counterparts. Calculation of cost-efficacy on this basis alone produces only a marginal improvement in cost-efficacy to $48,000 per life-year. A more important means by which transvenous implantation may improve cost-efficacy is by reducing the mortality associated with ICD implantation. The exact scale of this reduction remains to be determined but the study of Lehmann et al.[64] suggested a reduction from 4.7% to 1.6%. The potential improvement in cost-efficacy that could result if implant mortality is reduced, particularly in groups whose annual sudden death mortality is relatively small, is graphically illustrated in Figure 12.

Screening Tests

Despite considerable effort, improvements in screening tests to identify patients at high risk of sudden death have been slow and not always reproducible in different centers. However, the interest in screening test improvement is understandable when the economic effects are considered. A screening test able to detect a group with a 3-year sudden death rate of 60% would improve cost-efficacy to $27,000 per life-year. However, any new screening test must be relatively cheap as well as being sensitive and specific. Figure 13 shows the relationship between screening test cost and the size of the population at risk identified by the test. For a population such as the postinfarction high-risk group, where the group at risk represents approximately 5% of the population screened the total screening test cost should be below $375 per patient if it is not to adversely affect overall cost-efficacy.

Combined Future Scenario

A combined future scenario with a halved generator cost, 5-year generator life,

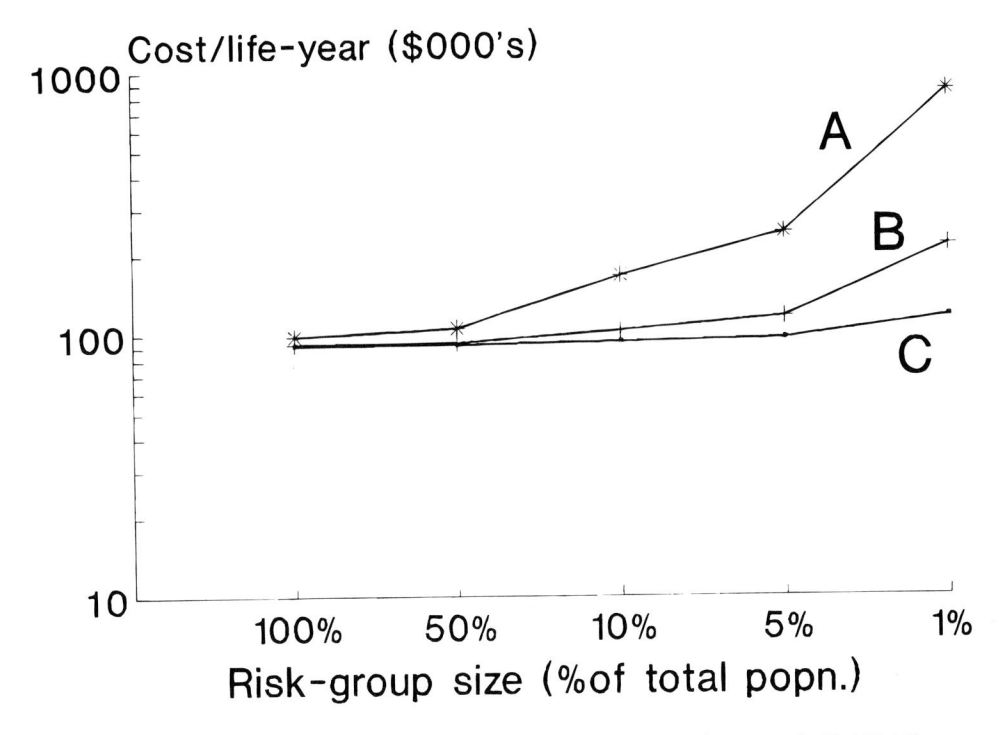

Figure 13. The effect of different screening test costs (A: $75.00; B: $375.00; C: $2,250.00) on cost-efficacy in relation to the size of the group selected by the test. The smaller the high-risk group selected, the more sensitive it is to screening test cost.

transvenous implantation with 1.5% implant mortality, and improved screening test would improve the cost-efficacy to $11,500 per life-year, a reduction of over 75% of the current cost. Changes of this magnitude would have a dramatic effect on the perception of the ICD as an expensive therapy.

Other Factors of Importance in the Assessment of Cost-Efficacy

Nonsudden and Noncardiac death

Patients remain at risk of death from nonarrhythmic mechanisms even after implantation of an ICD. The rate of nonarrhythmic death may have an important influence on the cost-efficacy of the implantable defibrillator. It is clear from large series[65] of ICD patients that the nonsudden death rate considerably exceeds that due to sudden cardiac death and this reflects the efficacy of the ICD in preventing sudden cardiac death. The nonsudden death rate appears to be between 6% and 14% per annum[66-69] and there has been much interest in identifying factors that predict a higher risk of death. Underlying cardiac function, expressed as left ventricular function is clearly important. Some authors[66] have found that concurrent coronary artery bypass graft surgery reduces subsequent mortality, while others[70] have not. Similarly, it remains unclear whether ICD shock delivery itself is an independent predictor of subsequent mortality.

The St. George's model has also been used to examine the effect of varying levels of nonsudden mortality and the hypothesis that ICD shock delivery is associated with patients at increased risk of nonsudden death on the overall cost-efficacy of the ICD in two hypothetical populations (Figure 14).

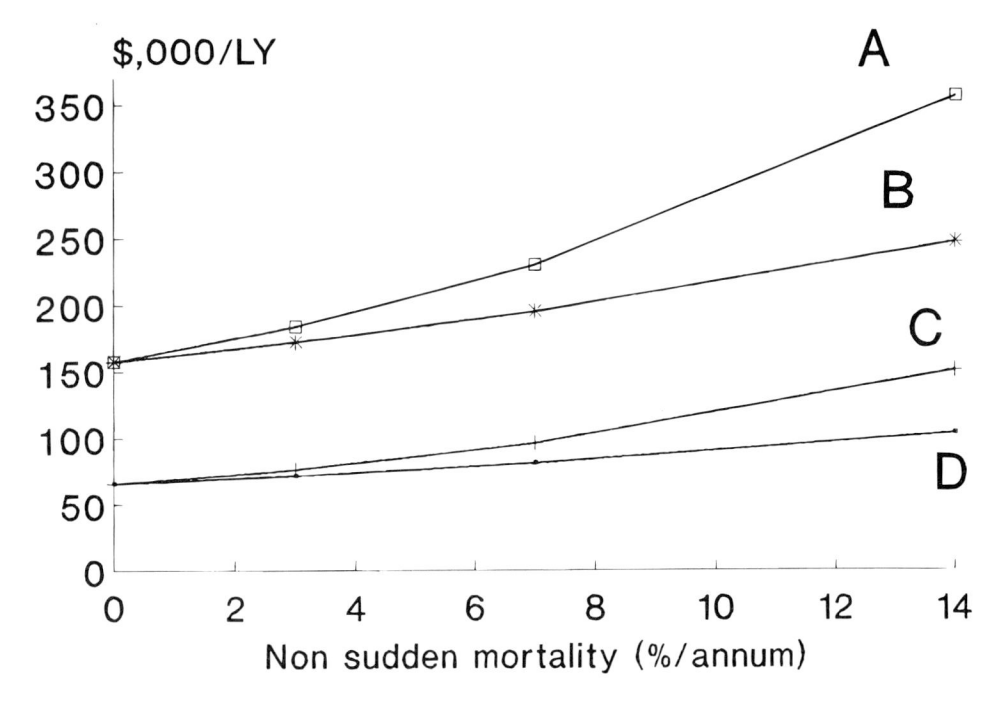

Figure 14. The impact of nonsudden mortality on cost-efficacy. Lines B and D show the impact of altering nonsudden mortality in implantable cardioverter-defibrillator (ICD) patients with a 14% and 28% 3-year sudden death mortality. Lines A and C show the impact of the same nonsudden mortality with the assumption that patients who receive ICD therapy have a doubled risk of subsequent nonsudden mortality.

Efficacy of the Implantable Cardioverter-Defibrillator in Preventing Sudden Cardiac Death

It is clear that the ICD will not prevent every sudden arrhythmic death, as there will be a small number of device or lead failures or devices that are inactive. Most studies[26,71,72] have reported an annual incidence of sudden arrhythmic death of around 2% in patients with the ICD, but Gross et al.[73] studied 56 ICD patients and found that the cumulative survivals free of sudden death was 93% at 1 year, 89% at 3 years, and 75% at 5 years suggesting the figure is closer to 7% to 8% per annum. A reduction in device efficacy has a predictable effect on cost-efficacy. A reduction of device efficacy to 50% doubles the cost per life-year saved. Even assuming that the figures of Gross et al.[73] are more representative than those of the other studies, then the error in the cost-efficacies calculated using the St. George's model, which assumes 100% efficacy in prevention of sudden death, would still be < 10%.

Implications of Economic Issues for the Pattern of Use and Potential Impact of the Implantable Cardioverter-Defibrillator on Sudden Cardiac Death

Sudden cardiac death remains a public health problem of massive proportion in the western world and despite a slow but steady decline in incidence, there were over 300 sudden deaths per 100,000 men per annum in the United States in 1985 and around one third this rate in women.[74] Despite the availability in some communities of cardiopulmonary resuscitation by bystanders and out-of-hospital defibrillation, < 1 in 3 patients suffering a cardiac arrest are resuscitated and survive to hospital discharge.[75] About two thirds of cardiac arrest victims have some form of cardiac disease recognized before the terminal event and the potential exists to identify those at risk of sudden cardiac death in advance. However, until the development of the ICD there was little incentive to do so. The dramatic increase in the frequency of implantation of the ICD illustrates the perception of the need for such a device. Initial retrospective studies have suggested that the device is efficacious in preventing sudden cardiac death.[32,65,72] The relative expense of ICD therapy has however lead to close scrutiny of its cost-efficacy as a means of preventing sudden death.

The basic concept of cost-efficacy is quite simple, but the determination of numerical values for cost-efficacy, particularly when considering quality of life issues, is complex and can be controversial. Nonetheless, because the primary outcome measure of ICD therapy is the prevention of sudden cardiac death, three studies have attempted to quantify the cost effectiveness of conventional ICD use[12,25,29] as it has been. Remarkably, considering their different provenance, the three studies produced very similar figures for cost-efficacy of about $25,000 per life-year. This reflects the cost of the current pattern of usage of the ICD, which is similar to that in the guidelines for ICD implantation recently defined by several national and international cardiological bodies.[76-78] While this is very expensive compared with some cardiovascular therapies such as pacing for complete heart block, it is comparable with other invasive therapies such as heart transplantation, coronary angioplasty, and hemodialysis.

By using a relatively simple model of cost-efficacy it is possible to examine a policy of stratified application of the ICD in groups of cardiac arrest survivors at differing levels of risk of recurrence. Not surprisingly those patients at highest risk of recurrence have the best cost-efficacy figures, although a variety of other factors such as the cost of screening tests and the incidence of nonsudden mortality can modify this relationship.

It is particularly clear from the application of the St. George's model that the best way to optimize the cost-efficacy of the ICD is to implant the device in patients at high risk of sudden cardiac death and at low risk of death from other causes. At least some of the strategies proposed by the current generation of controlled trials approach this target. However, it is also clear that the current generation of screening tests have relatively poor sensitivity and specificity and that improved screening tests for patients at risk of sudden death could substantially improve the cost-efficacy of the ICD. Whether this improvement can be achieved by the development of new screening tests or whether there is a fundamentally random component to the occurrence of fatal arrhythmias that may prevent it remains to be seen. With current levels of sensitivity and specificity of screening tests, acceptable levels of cost-efficacy can only be achieved by accepting very low levels of sensitivity, which means that the yield of sudden death prevention due to ICD use will be small. Nonetheless some of the proposed strategies for ICD implantation in the current generation of prospective studies of the ICD have very significant implications for national health care expenditure requiring up to 0.1% additional spending on health care.

Along with improved screening tests, sensitivity analysis with the St. George's model suggest that technical developments and alterations in the true cost of the device may allow a substantial improvement in the cost-efficacy. In combination with improvements in screening tests, a greater than fourfold improvement in cost-efficacy is feasible.

Conclusion

The capital cost of the ICD generator and its leads are considerable. Application of cost analysis to ICD implantation suggests that the ICD is a relatively expensive therapy, although comparable in cost with other accepted medical and surgical therapies. The limitations of currently available screening tests means that the overall impact of the ICD on the population burden of sudden cardiac death will be small, even if ICD use is extended to the populations proposed by some of the current generation of controlled trials of the device. However, developments in screening tests and technical and economic development of the ICD could easily lead to a fourfold improvement in cost-efficacy of ICD therapy. Controversial analysis of the cost-efficacy of new therapies is helpful in enabling their most appropriate use and in guiding research into new applications.

References

1. Klevit HD, Bates AC, Castanares T, et al: Prioritization of health care services. A progress report by the Oregon Health Services Commission. *Arch Intern Med* 151:912, 1991.
2. Chamberlain D, Alderslade R: Can rationing of cardiological services be rational? *Br Heart J* 64:219, 1990.
3. Rosser R, Watts V: The measurement of hospital output. *Int J Epidemiol* 1:361, 1972.
4. Kaplan R, Anderson J: A general health policy model: update and applications. *Health Serv Res* 23:203, 1988.
5. Carr-Hill RA, Morris J: Current practice in obtaining the "Q" in QALYs: a cautionary note. *Br Med J* 303:699, 1991.
6. Hadorn DC: Setting health care priorities in Oregon: cost-effectiveness meets the Rule of Rescue. *JAMA* 265:2218, 1991.
7. Eddy DM: Oregon's methods. Did cost-effectiveness analysis fail? *JAMA* 266:2135, 1991.
8. Nord E: An alternative to QALYs: the saved young life equivalent (SAVE). *Br Med J* 305:875, 1992.
9. Vlay SC, Olson LC, Fricchione GL, et al: Anxiety and anger in patients with ventricular tachyarrhythmias. Responses after automatic implantable internal cardioverter defibrillator implantation. *PACE* 12:366, 1989.
10. Keren R, Aarons D, Veltri EP: Anxiety and depression in patients with life-threatening ventricular arrhythmias: impact of the implantable cardioverter-defibrillator. *PACE* 14:181, 1991.
11. Kalbfleisch KR, Lehmann MH, Steinman RT, et al: Reemployment following implantation of the implantable cardioverter defibrillator. *Am J Cardiol* 64:199, 1989.
12. Kupperman M, Luce BR, McGovern B, et al: An analysis of the cost effectiveness of the implantable defibrillator. *Circulation* 81:91, 1990.
13. Echt DS, Armstrong K, Schmidt P, et al: Clinical experience, complications and survival in 70 patients with the automatic implantable cardioverter/defibrillator. *Circulation* 71:289, 1985.
14. Mirowski M, Reid PR, Winkle RA, et al: Mortality in patients with implanted automatic defibrillators. *Ann Intern Med* 98:585, 1983.
15. Reid PR, Griffith LSC, Platia EV, et al: The automatic implantable cardioverter defibrillator: five-year clinical results. In: *Nonpharmacological Therapy of Tachyarrhythmias*. Edited by G Breithardt, M Borggrefe, DP Zipes. Mt. Kisco, NY: Futura Publishing Company, Inc.; 1987, p. 477.
16. Kelly PA, Cannom DS, Garan H, et al: The automatic implantable defibrillator (AICD): efficacy, complications and survival of patients with left ventricular dysfunction and malignant ventricular arrhythmias. *J Am Coll Cardiol* 11:1278, 1988.
17. Tchou PJ, Kadri N, Anderson J, et al: Automatic implantable cardioverter-defibrillators and survival of patients with left ventricular dysfunction and malignant ventricular arrhythmias. *Ann Intern Med* 109:529, 1988.
18. Graboys TB, Lown B, Podrid PJ, et al: Long-term survival of patients with malignant ventricular arrhythmia treated with antiarrhythmic drugs. *Am J Cardiol* 50:437, 1982.
19. Roy D, Waxman HL, Kienzle MG, et al: Clinical characteristics and long-term follow-up in 119 survivors of cardiac arrest: relation to inducibility at electrophysiologic testing. *Am J Cardiol* 52:969, 1982.
20. Stein J, Podrid PF, Lampert S, et al: Long-term mexiletine for ventricular arrhythmia. *Am Heart J* 107:1091, 1984.
21. Swerdlow CD, Winkle RA, Mason JW: Determinants of survival with ventricular arrhythmia. *Am Heart J* 107:1091, 1984.
22. Wilber DJ, Garan H, Finkelstein D, et al: Out-of hospital cardiac arrest. Use of electrophysiological testing in the prediction of long-term survival. *N Engl J Med* 318:19, 1988.
23. Hohnloser SH, Garan H, Raeder EA, et al:

Short- and long-term therapy with tocainide for malignant ventricular tachyarrhythmias. *Circulation* 75(Suppl III):146, 1987.
24. Tordjman T, Podrid PJ, Raeder E, et al: Safety and efficacy of encainide for malignant ventricular arrhythmias. *Am J Cardiol* 58:87C, 1986.
25. O'Brien B, Buxton MJ, Rushby JA: Cost effectiveness of the implantable cardioverter defibrillator: a preliminary analysis. *Br Heart J* 68:241, 1992.
26. Winkle RA, Mead H, Ruder MA, et al: Long-term outcome with the automatic implantable cardioverter-defibrillator. *J Am Coll Cardiol* 13:1353, 1989.
27. Herre JM, Sauve MJ, Malone P, et al: Long-term results of amiodarone therapy in patients with recurrent sustained ventricular tachycardia or ventricular fibrillation. *J Am Coll Cardiol* 13:442, 1989.
28. Price Waterhouse: *Cardiothoracic Costing Study*. Sheffield: Trent Regional Health Authority; 1988.
29. Larsen GC, Manolis AS, Sonnenberg FA, et al: Cost-effectiveness of the implantable cardioverter-defibrillator: effect of improved battery life and comparison with amiodarone therapy. *J Am Coll Cardiol* 119:1323, 1992.
30. Winkle RA, Mead RH, Ruder MA, et al: Long-term outcome with the automatic implantable cardioverter-defibrillator. *J Am Coll Cardiol* 13:1353, 1989.
31. Manolis AS, Tand-DeGuzman W, Lee MA, et al: Clinical experience in seventy-seven patients with the automatic implantable cardioverter defibrillator. *Am Heart J* 118:445, 1989.
32. Mirowski M, Reid PR, Winkle RA, et al: Mortality in patients with implanted automatic defibrillators. *Ann Intern Med* 98:585, 1983.
33. Manolis AS, Uricchio F, Estes NAM: Prognostic value of early electrophysiologic studies for ventricular tachycardia recurrence in patients with coronary artery disease treated with amiodarone. *Am J Cardiol* 63:1052, 1989.
34. Horowitz LN, Greenspan AM, Spielman SR, et al: Usefulness of electrophysiologic testing in evaluation of amiodarone therapy for sustained ventricular tachyarrhythmias associated with coronary artery disease. *Am J Cardiol* 55:367, 1985.
35. Yazaki Y, Haffajee CI, Gold RL, et al: Electrophysiologic predictors of long-term clinical outcome with amiodarone for refractory ventricular tachycardia secondary to coronary artery disease. *Am J Cardiol* 60:293, 1987.
36. Williams A: Economics of coronary artery bypass grafting. *Br Med J* 291:326, 1985.
37. Goldman L, Weinstein MC, Goldman PA, et al: Cost-effectiveness of HMG-CoA reductase inhibition for primary and secondary prevention of coronary heart disease. *JAMA* 265:1145, 1991.
38. Anderson MH, Camm AJ: Implications for present and future applications of the implantable cardioverter-defibrillator resulting from the use of a simple model of cost-efficacy. *Br Heart J* 69:83, 1993.
39. O'Donoghue S, Platia EV, Brooks-Robinson S, et al: Automatic implantable cardioverter-defibrillator: is early implantation cost-effective? *J Am Coll Cardiol* 16:1258, 1990.
40. Anderson M, Poloniecki J, Jones S, et al: Ejection fraction alone predicts recurrence of arrhythmias in implantable cardioverter defibrillator patients (abstract). *Eur Heart J* (in press).
41. Wever EFD, Hauer RNW: Cost-effectiveness considerations: the Dutch prospective study of the automatic implantable cardioverter defibrillator as first-choice therapy. *PACE* 15: 690, 1992.
42. Nisam S, Thomas A, Mower M, et al: Identifying patients for prophylactic implantable cardioverter defibrillator therapy: status of prospective studies. *Am Heart J* 122:607, 1991.
43. Bigger JT: Prophylactic use of implantable cardioverter defibrillators: medical, technical, economic considerations. *PACE* 14:376, 1991.
44. MADIT Executive Committee: Multicenter automatic defibrillator implantation trial (MADIT): design and clinical protocol. *PACE* 14:920, 1991.
45. Denniss AR, Richards DA, Cody DV, et al: Prognostic significance of ventricular tachycardia and fibrillation induced at programmed stimulation and delayed potentials detectable on the signal-averaged electrocardiograms of survivors of acute myocardial infarction. *Circulation* 69:731, 1986.
46. Richards D, Taylor A, Fahey P, et al: Identification of patients at risk of sudden death after myocardial infarction: the continued Australian experience. In: *Cardiac Arrhythmias: Where to Go From Here?* Edited by P Brugada, HJJ Wellens. Mount Kisco, NY: Futura Publishing Company; 1987, p. 329.
47. Wilber DJ, Olshansky B, Moran JF, et al: Electrophysiological testing and nonsustained ventricular tachycardia. *Circulation* 82:350, 1990.
48. Kadish A, Schmaltz S, Calkins H, et al: Outcome of patients undergoing electrophysiological testing for nonsustained ventricular tachycardia (abstract). *Circulation* 82:III-82, 1990.
49. Richards DAB, Byth K, Ross DL, et al: What is the best predictor of spontaneous ventricu-

lar tachycardia and sudden death after myocardial infarction. *Circulation* 83:756, 1991.
50. Farrell TG, Bashir Y, Cripps T, et al: Risk stratification for arrhythmic events in postinfarction patients based on heart rate variability, ambulatory electrocardiographic variables and the signal-averaged electrocardiogram. *J Am Coll Cardiol* 18:687, 1991.
51. Gomes JA, Winters SL, Stewart D, et al: A new noninvasive index to predict sustained ventricular tachycardia and sudden death in the first year after myocardial infarction: based on signal-averaged electrocardiogram, radionuclide ejection fraction and Holter monitoring. *J Am Coll Cardiol* 10:349, 1987.
52. Packer M: Sudden unexpected death in patients with congestive heart failure: a second frontier. *Circulation* 72:681, 1985.
53. Francis G: Should asymptomatic ventricular arrhythmias in patients with congestive heart failure be treated with antiarrhythmic drugs? *J Am Coll Cardiol* 12:274, 1988.
54. Stevenson LW, Fowler MB, Schroeder JS, et al: Poor survival of patients considered too well for cardiac transplantation. *Am J Med* 83:871, 1987.
55. Bolling S, Deeb M, Mired F: AICD: a new "bridge" to transplantation (abstract). *J Am Coll Cardiol* 15:223A, 1990.
56. American Heart Association: *1990 Heart Facts*. Dallas, TX: American Heart Association National Center, 1990, p. 1.
57. Baum RS, Alvarez H, Cobb LA: Survival after resuscitation from out-of-hospital ventricular fibrillation. *Circulation* 50:1231, 1974.
58. Liberthson RR, Nagel EL, Hirschman JC, et al: Pathophysiological observations in prehospital ventricular fibrillation and sudden cardiac death. *Circulation* 49:790, 1974.
59. Myerburg RJ, Conde CA, Sung RJ, et al: Clinical, electrophysiologic and hemodynamic profile of patients resuscitated from prehospital cardiac arrest. *Am J Med* 68:568, 1980.
60. Cobbe SM, Redmond MJ, Watson JM, et al: "Heartstart Scotland"—initial experience of a national scheme for out-of-hospital defibrillation. *Br Med J* 302:1517, 1991.
61. Stults KR, Brown DD, Schug VL, et al: Prehospital defibrillation performed by emergency medical technicians in rural communities. *N Engl J Med* 310:219, 1984.
62. Unger F: European survey on open heart surgery. *Ann Acad Sci Artium Eur* 2:3, 1991.
63. *UNOS Update*. 1991; 7(Oct-Nov):(1O).
64. Lehmann MH, Mitchell LB, Saksena S, et al: Operative (30-day) mortality with transvenous vs. epicardial ICD implantation: an intention-to-treat analysis (abstract). *Circulation* 86:I-656, 1992.
65. Nisam S, Mower M, Moser S: ICD clinical update: first decade, initial 10,000 patients. *PACE* 14:255, 1991.
66. Levine JH, Mellits D, Baumgardner RA, et al: Predictors of first discharge and subsequent survival in patients with automatic implantable cardioverter-defibrillators. *Circulation* 84:558, 1991.
67. Zilo P, Gross JN, Benedek M, et al: Occurrence of ICD shocks and patient survival. *PACE* 14:273, 1991.
68. Axtell K, Tchou P, Akhtar M: Survival in patients with depressed left ventricular function treated by implantable cardioverter defibrillator. *PACE* 14:291, 1991.
69. Palatianos GM, Thurer RJ, Cooper DC, et al: The implantable cardioverter-defibrillator: clinical results. *PACE* 14:297, 1991.
70. Klein H, Tröjster HJ, Trappe F, et al: Outcome after defibrillator implantation with or without concomitant coronary artery bypass grafting (abstract). *Eur Heart J* 12:365, 1991.
71. Winkle RA, Mead RH, Ruder MA, et al: Ten year experience with implantable defibrillators (abstract). *Circulation* 84:II-426, 1991.
72. Fogoros RN, Fielder SB, Elson JJ: The automatic implantable cardioverter-defibrillator in drug-refractory ventricular tachyarrhythmias. *Ann Intern Med* 107:635, 1987.
73. Gross J, Zilo P, Ferrick K, et al: Sudden death mortality in implantable cardioverter defibrillator patients. *PACE* 14:250, 1991.
74. Gillum RF: Sudden coronary death in the United States 1980–1985. *Circulation* 79:756, 1989.
75. Weaver WD, Cobb LA, Hallstrom AP, et al: Factors influencing survival after out-of-hospital cardiac arrest. *J Am Coll Cardiol* 7:752, 1986.
76. Dreifus LS, Gillette PC, Fisch C, et al: Guidelines for implantation of cardiac pacemakers and antiarrhythmia devices. *J Am Coll Cardiol* 18:1, 1991.
77. Task Force of the Working Groups on Cardiac Arrhythmias and Cardiac Pacing of the European Society of Cardiology: Guidelines for the use of implantable cardioverter defibrillators. *Eur Heart J* 13:1304, 1992.
78. Lehman MH, Saksena S: Implantable cardioverter defibrillators in cardiovascular practice: report of the Policy Conference of the North American Society of Pacing and Electrophysiology. *PACE* 14:969, 1991.

Part 4

Alternative Approaches to Implantable Cardioverter-Defibrillator Therapy

Chapter 28

Pharmacological Therapy

L. Brent Mitchell

Introduction

Patients who have experienced an episode of spontaneous ventricular tachycardia (VT) or ventricular fibrillation (VF) in the absence of a reversible cause are at significant risk of both future episodes of arrhythmia recurrence and sudden death. Accordingly, for the past 50 years, a variety of therapeutic approaches to the prevention of arrhythmia recurrence and sudden death for patients with VT/VF have been under evaluation. This chapter summarizes and compares the efficacies of approaches that use antiarrhythmic drug therapies. Given the paucity of published randomized clinical trial data comparing the efficacies of various therapeutic approaches to either no treatment or to one another, the comparative statements made here must be considered to be speculative. Of course, within one therapeutic approach, a wide divergence of results might be expected as a result of application of the approach with varying methodological details and as a result of application of the approach to VT/VF populations with varying prognostic characteristics. Potential inaccuracies in reaching a summary statement regarding the efficacies of each approach can only be magnified by subsequent comparisons of the relative efficacies of differing approaches. Nevertheless, until properly controlled randomized trial results are available such comparisons are necessary to guide our choice of therapeutic alternatives. Furthermore, the summary statements made for the published efficacies of each approach may serve as average "expectations" for the success of each approach to allow interpretation of the results of randomized approach comparisons when they ultimately became available.

Natural History of Ventricular Tachycardia/ Ventricular Fibrillation

Ethical considerations have precluded determination of the contemporary natural history of untreated VT/VF. Reports that appeared in the mid-1970s describing the follow-up of patients resuscitated from out-of-hospital cardiac arrest[1-4] are frequently cited when quoting the natural history of VF recurrence even though these studies are clearly dated and even though some of the patients in each of these reports received empiric antiarrhythmic therapy.

The report of Liberthson et al.[1] examined the natural history of 42 patients who survived to be discharged after resuscitation from out-of-hospital VF (29 of whom were receiving empiric standard antiarrhythmic drug therapy). After discharge, 12

From Singer I, (ed.) Implantable Cardioverter-Defibrillator. Armonk, NY: Futura Publishing Company, Inc.; © 1994.

of the 42 patients (28%) died suddenly during a mean follow-up period of 1 year. The early Seattle experience reported by Baum et al.[2] demonstrating the high-risk state of the patient surviving out-of-hospital VF in the absence of a new Q wave myocardial infarction, was subsequently extended by Schaffer and Cobb[3] and Cobb et al.[4] The former report[3] described an arrhythmia recurrence/sudden death rate for patients successfully resuscitated from an initial episode of out-of-hospital VF of 31% (57 of 183 patients) over a 1.2-year follow-up. Over 70% of the patients experiencing recurrent arrhythmic events in this study were receiving empiric antiarrhythmic drug therapy. The report of Cobb et al.[4] described the Seattle study population when it reached 200 patients. By actuarial analysis the 2-year probability of death or cardiac arrest recurrence in this population was 47% (Figure 1).

Estimation of the recurrence probability for untreated patients with spontaneous episodes of VT is even more difficult as the natural history data is even more dated.[5-11] Nevertheless, the data of Trevor Cooke and White[8] was presented in a format that permits determination of actuarial death/arrhythmia recurrence probabilities after exclusion of the many patients with VT secondary to digitalis intoxication. Follow-up of the remaining patients suggested that the

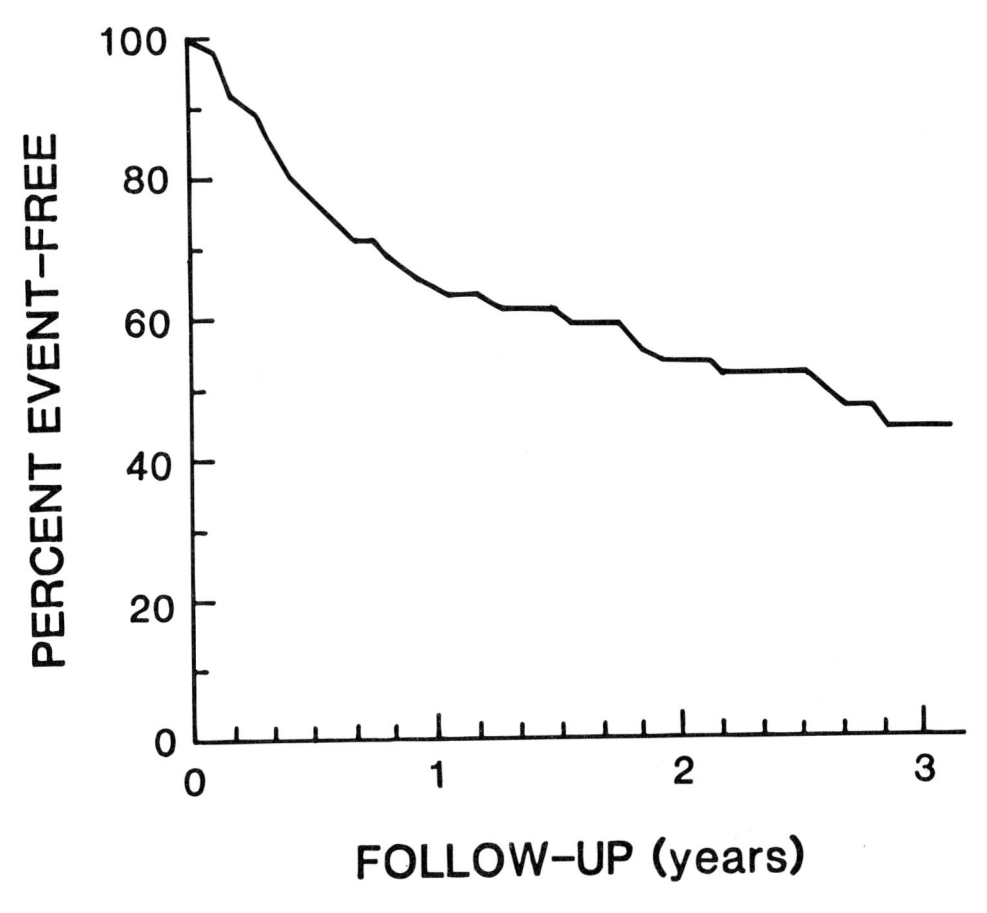

Figure 1. Cumulative probabilities of survival (%) over 3 years of follow-up in patients experiencing an out-of-hospital ventricular fibrillation (VF) arrest in the absence of a new Q wave myocardial infarction who were treated with no antiarrhythmic drug therapy or with empiric standard antiarrhythmic drug therapy. (Redrawn with permission from Figure 6, Reference 4.)

2-year probability of arrhythmia recurrence or death may be as high as 90% for patients with VT in the absence of a reversible cause. These data are consistent with prevalent opinion that the arrhythmia recurrence rates of patients with VT are higher than are those of patients with VF.

A newer patient population appropriate for determination of the natural history of arrhythmia recurrence in the absence of preventative drug therapy is the population of patients with VT/VF that have had an automatic implantable cardioverter-defibrillator (ICD) implanted as primary therapy and have not been prescribed antiarrhythmic drug therapy. In the randomized Cardiac Arrest Study Hamburg (CASH),[12] patients presenting after an out-of-hospital VT/VF cardiac arrest have a 2-year actuarial probability of receiving an appropriate ICD shock (during syncope or documented VF) of 23%. This probability is likely an underestimate of the arrhythmia recurrence risk as many individuals experiencing VT/VF that is terminated by an ICD do not experience syncope.[13] Other reported ICD populations have not utilized the device exclusively as the first and only antiarrhythmic therapy. Nevertheless, reports of experiences that have minimized the use of concomitant antiarrhythmic drug therapy provide ICD utilization rates that support the arrhythmia recurrence constructs of the older data. Bardy et al.[14] described a population of 55 VF and 25 VT patients who received a tranvenous ICD system of whom only 4 patients (5%) received postimplantation antiarrhythmic drugs prior to demonstration of unacceptable postoperative VT/VF frequency. The arrhythmia recurrence rate in these 80 patients over a 1-year follow-up period was 39% (31 of 80). In support of the concept that arrhythmia recurrence rates are higher for VT patients than for VF patients, Leitch et al.[13] described a 54% (25 of 46 patients) arrhythmia recurrence rate during a 6-month follow-up of 38 VT patients and 8 VF patients whose primary antiarrhythmic therapy was an ICD. However, 29% of the patients described in that report received postimplantation antiarrhythmic drugs prior to a postoperative episode of VT/VF.

Recognizing the hazards of historical controls, the published evidence that is available suggests that the probability of arrhythmia recurrence/sudden death for patients who have survived out-of-hospital VF in the absence of a reversible cause is 30% to 36% over the first year and 10% to 15% during the second year,[15] for a 2-year arrhythmia recurrence/sudden death probability of 40% to 50%. To the extent that patients with VT tend to have more frequent recurrences, the arrhythmia recurrence/sudden death probability for untreated VT patients is expected to be somewhat greater than that of untreated VF patients. Although it is likely that recent advances in both medical and surgical approaches to the treatment of coronary artery disease and advances in the medical treatment of ventricular contractile dysfunction have improved the untreated natural history of patients with VT/VF compared to historical controls, contemporary primary ICD data argue in favor of a recurrence rate not substantially different from that suggested by Figure 1. Therefore, for the purposes of subsequent argument, the untreated, natural history 2-year arrhythmia recurrence/sudden death probability of an average VT/VF patient population will be taken to be 45%.

Empiric Standard Antiarrhythmic Drug Therapy

No study reported to date has examined the efficacy of any therapeutic intervention for VT/VF in a randomized, placebo controlled fashion. Accordingly, we still lack conclusive evidence that any therapeutic modality improves the outcome of patients with VT/VF. However, most potential therapeutic approaches to these patients have been reported to favorably influence recurrence and sudden death rates at least when compared to historical controls.

The one exception to this trend has been the use of empiric antiarrhythmic drugs from Vaughan Williams Class I (referred to as standard antiarrhythmic drugs). Even uncontrolled comparisons of standard antiarrhythmic drug therapy for VT/VF have suggested that the empiric use of these agents is no better than no treatment[16–18] and may be worse than no treatment.[1,19,20] Myerburg et al.[16] reported the outcomes of empiric standard antiarrhythmic drug therapy in 16 patients resuscitated from out-of-hospital VF who were then treated with empiric Class I antiarrhythmic drug therapy (procainamide or quinidine). After a minimum event-free follow-up period of 1 year the sudden death/arrhythmia recurrence rate was 50% (8 of 16 patients)—no better than the expected untreated natural history of such patients. The data of this report suggested that the outcome of patients treated with empiric Class I antiarrhythmic therapy was better if the plasma level of the empiric agent was maintained in the therapeutic "target" range. In a later report of 61 similar patients, Myerberg et al.[17] assessed this hypothesis by noting that 14 of 16 victims of recurrent arrest (87%) had plasma antiarrhythmic drug concentrations below the target range while only 10 of 34 (29%) matched samples from long-term survivors were below the target range. In this report, the 2-year actuarial probability of recurrent cardiac arrest was only 15%. The authors attributed the improvement, in part, to their plasma level-guided dosing protocol. Nevertheless, other investigators had much less success with empiric standard antiarrhythmic drug therapy. Vlay et al.[18] reported a 40% arrhythmia recurrence/sudden death rate and a 34% sudden death rate over 16 months of follow-up in 80 patients resuscitated from out-of-hospital cardiac arrests who were then treated with empiric investigational antiarrhythmic drugs. More recently two other groups have reported outcome data relevant to the use of empiric standard antiarrhythmic drug therapy.[19–21] Moosvi et al.[19] described the outcome of 209 patients resuscitated from out-of-hospital VF between 1975 and 1982. Among these patients, 116 patients received no antiarrhythmic drug therapy and had a follow-up 2-year actuarial sudden death probability of 11% while 93 patients received empiric procainamide or quinidine therapy and had a 2-year sudden death probability of 31% ($P < 0.01$). Extension of the follow-up of these patients has been provided by Goldstein et al.[20] That report included a multivariate analysis of potential predictors of subsequent sudden death, the 2-year actuarial probability of which was 19%. The factors independently related to follow-up sudden death were the use of empiric quinidine therapy and the presence of ventricular premature beats (VPB) pairs on a postdischarge ambulatory ECG monitoring examination. However, in these reports the treatment allocations were neither random nor even described. Considering that 40% of these patients had an acute myocardial infarction at the time of their index VT/VF, the study population included a readily identifiable low-risk subpopulation that was likely over-represented in the patient group that did not receive antiarrhythmic drug therapy. The large contribution from this low-risk group is also the most likely explanation for the apparent improvement over the expected untreated natural history risk. In support of the contention that empiric standard antiarrhythmic drug therapy may be harmful, Leclercq et al.[21] evaluated empiric antiarrhythmic drug therapy in 295 patients with sustained monomorphic VT. The treatments included empiric standard antiarrhythmic agent therapy, empiric β-adrenergic blocking agent therapy, and empiric amiodarone therapy. Patients receiving empiric standard antiarrhythmic drug therapy had a higher 2-year actuarial probability of death (58%) than did those receiving other therapies (13%). Again, empiric standard antiarrhythmic drug therapy appears to produce an outcome that is no better than, and is possibly worse than, the expected untreated natural history of VT/VF patients. Finally, Willems et al.[22] have reported outcome data on 268 patients with sustained

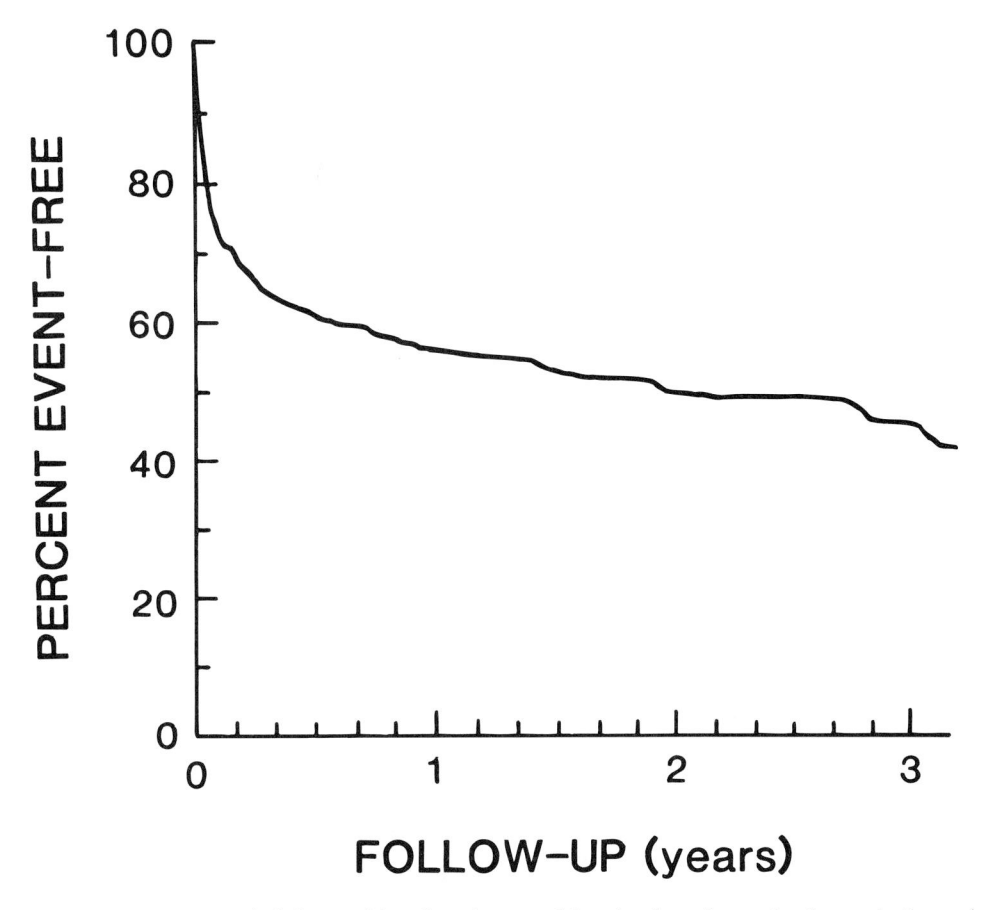

Figure 2. Cumulative probabilities of freedom from sudden death and sustained ventricular tachycardia/ventricular fibrillation (VT/VF) (%) over 3 years of follow-up in patients with sustained VT/VF primarily treated with empiric standard antiarrhythmic drug therapy. (Redrawn with permission from Figure 2, Reference 22.)

VT and 122 patients with VF occurring late (> 48 hours) after myocardial infarction. Of these 390 patients, 75% were treated with empiric antiarrhythmic drugs alone. The 2-year arrhythmia recurrence/sudden death probability for the entire group was 49% (Figure 2) and the 2-year sudden cardiac death probability was 18%.

Thus, we can conclude that the average patient who presents with VT/VF in the absence of a reversible cause has a 2-year probability of VT/VF recurrence of approximately 45% if left untreated or if prescribed empiric standard antiarrhythmic drug therapy. For patients with VF, the majority of recurrences are expected to result in sudden death (a 2-year sudden death probability of approximately 30%).[23] For patients with VT the minority of recurrences are expected to result in sudden death (a 2-year sudden death probability of approximately 20%—estimated from the data of Leclercq et al.[21]).

Individualized Standard Antiarrhythmic Drug Therapy

Recognizing the inefficacy of the empiric use of standard antiarrhythmic drug therapies in patients with a demonstrated propensity to VT/VF, two approaches have been developed to predict the long-term efficacy of a specific antiarrhythmic drug therapy in a specific patient during a short-term trial of that therapy. Each of the approaches identifies an index of ventricular electrical instability in an antiarrhythmic drug-free state and then assess the ability of specific antiarrhythmic drug therapies to suppress the index of electrical instability. The noninvasive approach[24-46] uses spontaneous VPBs and nonsustained runs of VT as the baseline index of ventricular electrical instability, while the invasive approach[32,36-40,43-98] uses VT/VF induced by the techniques of programmed stimulation as the baseline index of electrical instability. Antiarrhythmic drug therapy is then individualized for a specific patient by demonstration of its ability to suppress one or the other of these instability indices.

The Noninvasive Approach

The noninvasive approach to individualized antiarrhythmic drug therapy for VT/VF, popularized by Lown and co-workers[25,28,29,30,33,34,42,44] begins with an antiarrhythmic drug-free 24-hour ambulatory ECG examination and exercise tolerance test. To be useful in guiding subsequent antiarrhythmic drug therapy these baseline studies must disclose spontaneous ventricular arrhythmia. Early in the history of use of the noninvasive approach, the mere presence of complex forms of VBPs (couplets or nonsustained VT) on an ambulatory monitoring examination was considered an adequate index to guide the noninvasive approach.[24,26,32,35,37,40] Subsequently, more experience with the noninvasive approach led Lown and co-workers to the following definition of the minimum frequency and complexity of spontaneous ventricular arrhythmia adequate to guide the approach: at least 30 VPBs per hour for at least 50% of monitored hours and at least 3 hours containing one or more ≥ 3-beat runs of VT during 24 hours of ambulatory monitoring (which they usually repeated twice).[44] Nevertheless, most investigators have used the simpler definition of a mean of ≥ 30 VPBs per hour averaged over a 24-hour recording.[27,31,38,39,41,43] A baseline exercise tolerance test is considered to have sufficient arrhythmia to guide the noninvasive approach if it reproducibly produces VT or VF.[43] When these baseline spontaneous ventricular arrhythmia requirements are applied, the reported percentages of patients with sufficient spontaneous ventricular arrhythmia to guide the noninvasive approach ranges from 31% when spontaneous ventricular triplets or longer repetitive forms were required[40] to 89% when a mean hourly VPB frequency of only 10 per hour is considered acceptable.[45] When more standard minimum spontaneous ventricular arrhythmia criteria are applied the percentage of patients with VT/VF who are appropriate candidates for application of the noninvasive approach is approximately 60%.[33,38,42-44] The demographic and clinical characteristics (if any) that distinguish VT/VF patients who have sufficient spontaneous ventricular arrhythmia to guide the noninvasive approach from those who do not have not been determined.

Once the frequency and complexity of a patient's spontaneous ventricular arrhythmia has been determined in an antiarrhythmic drug-free state, antiarrhythmic agents or combinations of antiarrhythmic agents are then prescribed until a therapy is identified that is associated with suppression of the spontaneous ventricular arrhythmia. Recognizing the day-to-day spontaneous variability in spontaneous ventricular arrhythmia frequency, marked suppression of ventricular arrhythmia is required before the suppression can be reasonably ascribed to effective antiarrhythmic drug therapy.[27] Nevertheless, there is no general agreement as to the degree of spontaneous arrhythmia suppression necessary to suggest long-term efficacy of antiarrhythmic drug therapy. Typical recommendations for the degree of suppression of isolated VPB frequency required range from ≥ 50%[25,28,30,33,34,39,41,42] to ≥ 80%.[43] However, most investigators agree that ventricular couplets should be suppressed by ≥ 90% and ventricular triplets and longer repetitive forms should be eliminated from both the treatment 24-hour ambulatory ECG monitoring examination and the treatment exercise tolerance test.[25,26,28,30,32-35,37,39-44]

Isolated use of the noninvasive approach to individualizing antiarrhythmic drug therapy for patients with VT/VF has been reported to identify a therapy that is predicted to be effective for between 73%[24] and 100%[40,43] of patients with VT/VF. Combining the published studies reporting such data[24,25,28,30,37,40,43-45] suggests that the percentage of VT/VF patients for whom predicted effective therapy will be found by a noninvasive approach is approximately 80%. The demographic and clinical correlates of finding a therapy that the noninvasive approach predicts will be effective in long-term use include better left ventricular function and fewer monitoring hours with ventricular triplets or longer repetitive forms.[44,45]

Lown and Graboys[25] have compared the relative, follow-up antiarrhythmic efficacy of therapy predicted to be effective by the noninvasive approach to that of the (then) standard of empiric antiarrhythmic drug therapy. The study group consisted of 43 patients of whom 33 had been resuscitated from VF. Of this group, 26 received therapy selected by the noninvasive approach and 17 received empiric standard antiarrhythmic drug therapy. Unfortunately, the group assignments were not randomized but, instead, "clinical factors were decisive in determining a therapeutic strategy." Thus, comparison of the outcomes of the two groups is suspect. Nevertheless, the sudden death rate over a 20-month follow-up period of patients treated with empiric standard antiarrhythmic drugs was 41% while the sudden death rate over a 17-month follow-up period of patients treated with agents selected by the noninvasive approach was 8%. The noninvasive approach to individualizing antiarrhythmic drug therapy for patients with VT/VF appeared to represent a therapeutic advance.

Several reports have compared the follow-up antiarrhythmic efficacy of therapy predicted to be effective by the noninvasive approach to that predicted to be ineffective by the noninvasive approach.[24,28,30,32,35-37,44] In this regard, two general study formats have been followed. The first study design is to examine the predictive values of negative and positive results of a noninvasive evaluation of the final antiarrhythmic drug therapy chosen, by some other approach, for a group of patients with VT/VF.[32,35-37] As this design is likely to be lacking baseline antiarrhythmic drug-free ambulatory ECG monitoring data, studies of this sort commonly define their efficacy prediction by virtue of the elimination of repetitive ventricular beats on a treatment ambulatory ECG monitoring examination without quantitative reference to a baseline ambulatory ECG examination. The study of Vlay at al.[35] demonstrates this study design and its results. Fifty-nine survivors of symptomatic VT or VF who had failed empiric treatment with standard antiarrhythmic drugs and had ventricular triplets or longer repetitive forms during baseline monitoring received empiric therapy with investigational antiarrhythmic agents. Therapy was chosen empirically. Thereafter, the predictive values of elimination of ventricular triplets or longer repetitive forms on a treatment ambulatory ECG were determined. The observed 2-year actuarial probability of arrhythmia recurrence or death in the 26 patients receiving therapy predicted to be effective by the noninvasive approach was 18% while that of the 18 patients receiving therapy predicted to be ineffective was 42% ($P < 0.002$). Similar results have been described from similar studies.[36,37] The second general study design comparing the follow-up efficacy of therapy predicted to be effective by the noninvasive approach to that predicted to be ineffective by the noninvasive approach prospectively identifies patients who can and who cannot have predicted effective therapy identified by the noninvasive approach and then compares their follow-up outcomes.[24,28,30,44]

This study design and its results are well illustrated by the report of Graboys et al.[30] These investigators described results of the application of the noninvasive approach to individualized antiarrhythmic drug therapy in 56 patients with hypotensive VT and 67 patients with VF. All had required at least one resuscitation or emergency cardioversion for treatment of their ventricular tachyarrhythmia. Of these 123 patients, application of the noninvasive approach indentified 98 patients (80%) for whom a drug therapy was predicted to be effective (> 50% suppression of VPBs, > 90% suppression of ventricular couplets, elimination of ventricular triplets and longer repetitive forms, and elimination of R-on-T VPBs on both ambulatory ECG monitoring and exercise tolerance testing) and 25 patients (20%) for whom these goals could not be acheived. The latter group received drug therapy that was, therefore, predicted to be ineffective. On follow-up the 2-year actuarial probability of sudden death for the predicted effective therapy group (approximately 8%) was lower than that of the predicted ineffective therapy group (approximately 52%) (Figure 3). Other studies of this type[24,28,44] have shown similar results.

Thus, application of the noninvasive approach separates patients into a group with a 2-year actuarial follow-up sudden

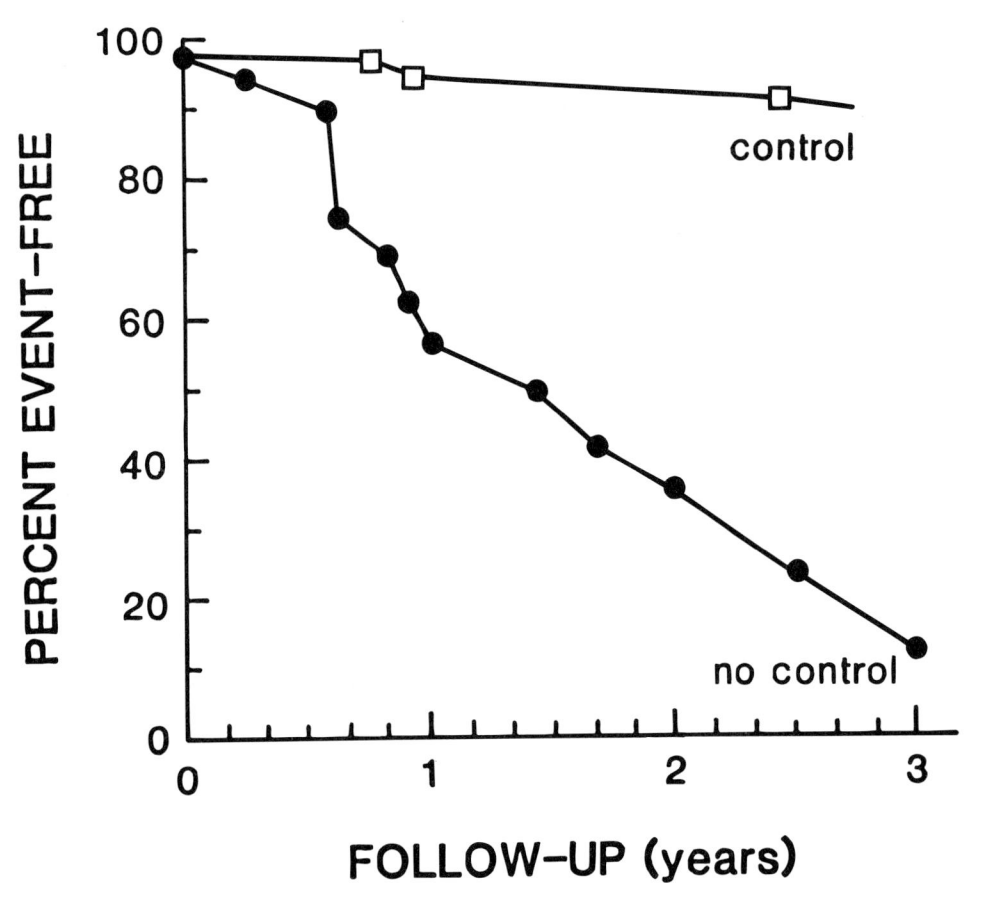

Figure 3. Cumulative probabilities of freedom from sudden death (%) over 3 years of follow-up in patients with hemodynamically compromising VT/VF treated with antiarrhythmic drugs predicted to be effective by the noninvasive approach (☐, control) or predicted to be ineffective by the noninvasive approach (●, no control). (Redrawn with permission from Figure 2, Reference 30.)

death probability substantially better than and a group with a 2-year probability of sudden death substantially worse than the expected untreated natural history sudden death probability of a 50:50 VT:VF study population of 25%.

The efficacy of therapy for the prevention of VT/VF individualized by the noninvasive approach may be estimated from those studies reporting actuarial follow-up data.[30,34,35,41,43] The size of each study population was used as a weighting factor in the calculation of an overall mean result. Calculated in this way, the estimated 2-year actuarial sudden death probability of patients receiving therapy predicted to be effective by the noninvasive approach is 10% and the estimated 2-year actuarial arrhythmia recurrence/sudden death probability of such patients is 25%. Demographic and clinical factors associated with freedom from sudden death/arrhythmia recurrence on follow-up include better left ventricular function and satisfactory spontaneous ventricular arrhythmia suppression with more than 50% of the antiarrhythmic agents tested.[44] These values contrast with those of the untreated natural history and empiric standard antiarrhythmic drug arguments presented, suggesting a potential role for the noninvasive approach in the treatment of patients with VT/VF.

The Invasive Approach

Shortly after the work of Wellens et al.[47,48,50] and Denes et al.[49] demonstrated that the techniques of programmed ventricular stimulation were capable of inducing a clinically relevant VT in susceptible individuals, reports[51-55] began to appear describing the use of programmed stimulation for the prediction of antiarrhythmic drug efficacy in such patients. These initial reports formed the groundwork for the development of the invasive approach to individualizing antiarrhythmic drug therapy for patients with VT/VF. The invasive approach begins with an antiarrhythmic drug-free transvenous catheter electrophysiologic study. To be useful in guiding subsequent antiarrhythmic drug therapy the baseline programmed stimulation study must reproducibly induce the patient's ventricular tachyarrhythmia. Recognizing the nonspecific nature of the induction of VF,[79] the baseline induction of VF is generally considered a positive result only in patients who have experienced spontaneous VF. The process of selection of antiarrhythmic drug therapy by the invasive approach has been validated best when the induced ventricular arrhythmia to be used as the index of electrical instability is sustained monomorphic VT. Sustained in this context has been defined as that which lasts at least 30 seconds or requires termination prior to that time secondary to hemodynamic collapse.[99] Nevertheless, some investigators have used reproducibly inducible nonsustained VT to guide the approach.[43,60,73,76,89,90,95,100,101]

Application of the techniques of programmed stimulation in the invasive approach to therapy selection has been less well standardized than has application of the techniques of spontaneous arrhythmia monitoring in the noninvasive approach to therapy selection. The initial programmed stimulation protocols used consisted of up to two programmed ventricular extrastimuli delivered during a variety of basic drive cycle lengths at the right ventricular apex.[52,54,59,60,63,64] Data supporting the use of stimuli with a 2-msec duration and an intensity twice the late diastolic capture threshold have been published.[102] When the yield of inducible sustained VT/VF using such stimulation protocols was found to be low the aggressiveness of stimulation was increased by stimulation at a second right ventricular site,[76] by stimulation at one or more left ventricular sites,[82,103] by stimulation after the administration of isoproterenol,[104] and by the use of up to 3,[80,82] 4,[75] or 5[105] programmed ventricular extrastimuli. Of these maneuvers, use of more than two programmed extrastimuli appears to provide the greatest increment in clinical VT inducibility. However, the use of more than two programmed extrastimuli also has the greatest potential to permit the induction of nonclinical (and presumably irrelevant) polymorphic VT/VF. Most investigators have settled upon a programmed stimulation protocol that concludes after the delivery of three programmed ventricular extrastimuli at three basic ventricular cycle lengths from two right ventricular sites. The time required to maximize clinical VT/VF induction probability is shortened by the addition of the third extrastimulus prior to stimulation at a second site. However, the probability of induction of nonclinical polymorphic VT/VF is minimized by stimulation with two extrastimuli at two sites prior to the addition of the third extrastimulus. Most investigators are adopting the latter approach. When this stimulation protocol fails to reproduce a patient's clinical VT/VF, and reproduction of the patient's VT/VF is a clinical imperative, consideration can then be given to further right ventricular stimulation after isoproterenol administration, left ventricular stimulation, or use of more than three programmed ventricular extrastimuli. Use of a programmed stimulation protocol limited to three programmed ventricular extrastimuli will reproduce clinical sustained VT in approximately 80% of a general population of VT patients[38,53,74,76,80,82,83] with spontaneous sustained VT. However, in patients who have experienced an out-of-hospital cardiac arrest the induction of clinical VT/VF is less common—approximately 60%.[15,40,73,74,77,80,83,88–91,95,96,98] In addition to whether the presenting arrhythmia was VT or VF,[15,74,85,88,91] other clinical and demographic factors have been associated with a greater probability of VT/VF induction by programmed stimulation. The most consistently reported correlates of inducible VT/VF are male gender,[85,91] the presence of structural heart disease (especially coronary artery disease, previous myocardial infarction, left ventricular aneurysm),[15,74,77,85,88–91,93] and depressed left ventricular ejection fraction.[15,77,88,90,91,93]

After demonstration of reproducibility, induction of the patient's (preferably) sustained VT/VF in an antiarrhythmic drug-free state by programmed stimulation, antiarrhythmic agents or combinations of antiarrhythmic agents are then prescribed until a therapy is identified that is associated with the inability of programmed stimulation to induce VT/VF at a subsequent treatment electrophysiologic study. Unfortunately, there is also a great deal of variability in the aggressiveness of the programmed stimulation protocol used at drug assessment electrophysiologic studies. Typically, the maximum stimulation stress applied includes the number of extrastimuli that would have been used in a negative baseline study delivered to the pacing site that permitted reproducible VT/VF induction at the patient's drug-free study. Isoproterenol is most commonly administered during a drug assessment electrophysiologic study only if it had been required for induction at the baseline study. Nevertheless, drug assessment induction stresses both less and more stringent than this standard have been suggested. More stringent drug assessments include delivery of the full stimulation protocol at at least two right ventricular sites,[68,86] delivery of the full stimulation protocol at both right and left ventricular sites,[73,89] and delivery of the full stimulation protocol during isoproterenol administration[106] before accepting a drug efficacy prediction regardless of the absence of a need for such ancillary stresses for VT/VF induction at the baseline study. Less stringent drug assessments include limiting the number of applied ventricular extrastimuli at the treatment study to the number that permitted reproducible VT/VF induction at the baseline study[92] and avoidance of triple extrastimuli unless their use had been required at the baseline study.[44,45] The rationale for the latter process is based entirely upon a small, retrospective study by Swerdlow et al.[107] that found no differences between the the follow-up arrhythmia recurrence probability of one group of 14 patients with VT induced at a baseline study with one or two extrastimuli who then received antiarrhythmic drug therapy predicted to be effective at a treatment study that included only two extrastimuli and the follow-up arrhythmia recurrence probability of another group of 19 patients with VT induced at a baseline study with one or two extrastimuli who then received therapy predicted to be effective at a treatment study that included three extrastimuli.

A drug efficacy prediction by the invasive approach also includes a maximum acceptable patient response to the programmed stimulation protocol. Most investigators would agree that the primary goal of drug therapy assessed by the invasive approach is to render the VT/VF "noninducible." However, the definitions of noninducible vary from the absence of inducible sustained VT/VF[54,56,59,64–66,69,71,77,86,92,96] to absence of an inducible ventricular triplet.[37,40,60] There is nothing in the literature to suggest that the long-term efficacy of therapy chosen by application of these extremes in response criteria differ. Nevertheless, most laboratories use a noninducible cutoff of between 5 and 15 repetitive ventricular reponses.[32,39,43,55,62,68,70,72–74,78,81,84,85,89,90,94,95,98] Recognizing, the marked effects that antiarrhythmic therapy can have on the morphology and cycle length of VT/VF that remains inducible, most investigators do not accept the concept of the induction, on drug therapy, of a nonclinical and therefore irrelevant VT/VF. Thus, the most prevalent definition of predicted effective antiarrhythmic drug therapy for VT/VF by the invasive approach is that which, when given to a patient with inducible sustained VT (or VF if VF has been previously documented), is associated with the inability to induce more than 15 repetitive ventricular responses with a programmed stimulation protocol that includes up to three ventricular extrastimuli delivered to the site that permitted reproducible VT/VF induction at an antiarrhythmic drug-free baseline programmed stimulation study. When criteria for an efficacy prediction such as these are applied, the percentage of patients for whom a predicted effective therapy can be found is approximately 40% to 45% in populations dominated by VT patients[36,39,43,53,62,70,74,84,97] and somewhat higher (55%) in populations dominated by VF patients.[74,84,90,95,98] Several studies have examined clinical, demographic, and electrophysiologic factors associated with the ability of drug therapy to suppress inducible VT/VF.[69,70,74,85,90,92,94,108] The most consistently reported clinical correlates of inducible VT/VF suppression by drug therapy have been younger age,[69,70,94] the absence of structural heart disease (especially coronary artery disease, previous myocardial infarction, left ventricular aneurysm),[69,70,92,108] higher left ventricular ejection fraction,[69,90,92,94,108] fewer previous empiric drug trial failures,[70,74,85] and the induced (or presenting) arrhythmia—sustained VT being more difficult to suppress than VF.[74,85,92] Electrophysiologic predictors of the ability of drug therapy to suppress inducible VT/VF include the absence of an intraventricular conduction defect or HV interval prolongation,[69] induction of VT/VF with multiple rather than one extrastimuli,[69,92] and shorter baseline indices of ventricular repolarization-QTc interval and ventricular refractory periods.[108]

To my knowledge the long-term performance of therapy for VT/VF selected by the invasive approach has not been compared to that of empiric standard antiarrhythmic drug therapy or to an untreated control population. However, several groups have compared the follow-up antiarrhythmic efficacy of therapy predicted to be effective by the invasive approach to that predicted to be ineffective by the invasive approach. In this instance the vast majority of such studies are of the design that prospectively identifies patients who can and who cannot have predicted effective therapy identified by the invasive approach and then compares their follow-up outcomes. Studies of this sort have been reported for both patient populations dominated by VT patients[54–56,59,62,63,65,69,72,78,84,86,94] and for out-of-hospital cardiac arrest patients.[15,60,73,74,77,89,90,93,96,98] Such studies that refer to patients with VT are well illustrated by the report of Horowitz et al.[65] although the results are rather extreme. In this study, the invasive approach to antiarrhythmic drug treatment was applied to 111 patients with inducible sustained VT. A medical regimen predicted to be effective, by virtue of prevention of VT induction, was found for 65 patients. The remaining 46 patients were treated with regimens that were predicted to be ineffective after failure to find a predicted effective therapy. After a mean follow-up of 18 months the percentage with recurrent VT or sudden death was 6% (4 of 65) in the predicted effective therapy group and 91% (42 of 46) in the predicted ineffective therapy group. Similar, although less dramatic, results have been reported by each of the other studies of this type in VT patients.[54–56,59,62,63,69,72,78,84,86,94] The actuarial analysis of the results of the largest such study, reported by Waller et al.[86] are shown in Figure 4. Studies of this sort in patients with out-of-hospital cardiac arrest are illustrated by the report of Ruskin et al.[74] Of 69 patients surviving an out-of-hospital cardiac arrest who were found to have inducible VT/VF and underwent serial electropharmacological testing, a therapy pre-

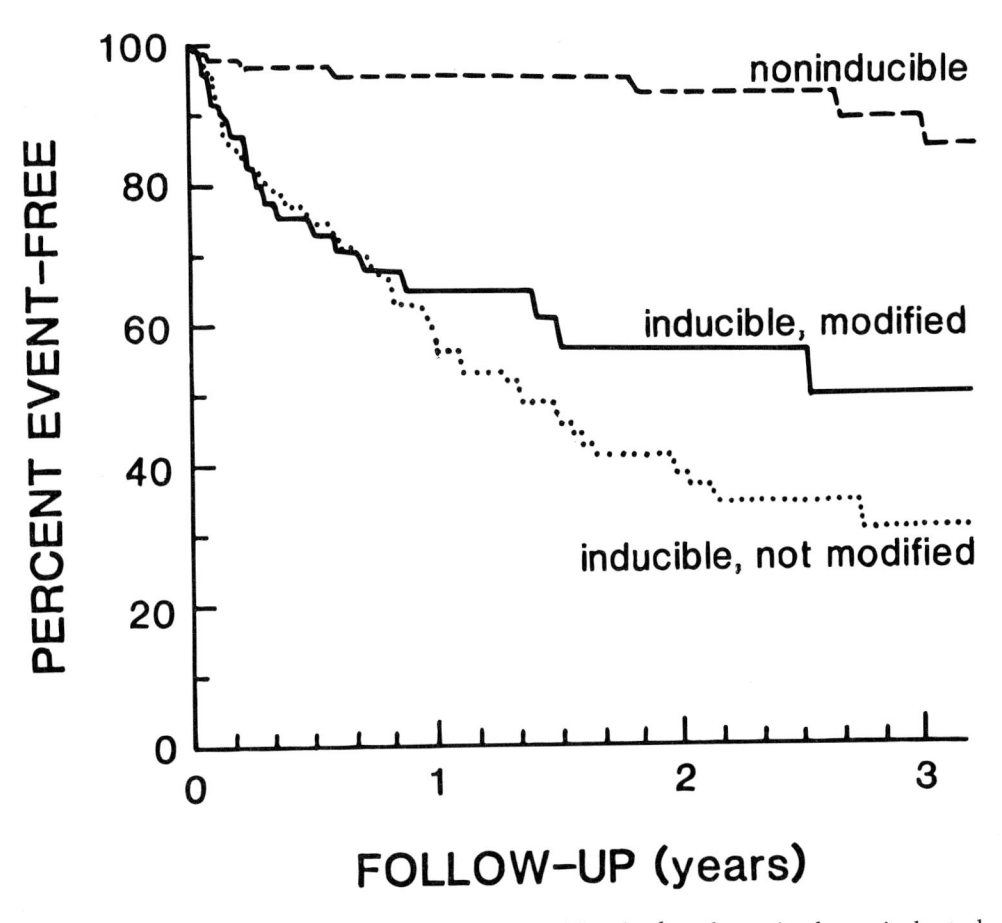

Figure 4. Cumulative probabilities of freedom from sudden death and sustained ventricular tachycardia/ventricular fibrillation (VT/VF) (%) over 3 years of follow-up in patients with inducible sustained VT/VF treated with antiarrhythmic drugs predicted to be effective by the invasive approach (dashed line, noninducible) or predicted to be ineffective by the invasive approach with modification of the inducible VT/VF (solid line, inducible, modified) or without modification of the inducible VT/VF (dotted line, inducible, not modified). (Redrawn with permission from Figure 1, Reference 86.)

dicted to be effective by the invasive approach was found for 55 patients and was not found for 14 patients. Four of the 55 patients (7%) receiving predicted effective therapy died suddenly during a mean 22-month follow-up period. However, 5 of the 14 patients (35%) who received therapy predicted to be ineffective died suddenly during follow-up. Several other investigators have reported similar results from this study design.[15,40,71,89,90,93,98] However, such studies in patients resuscitated from out-of-hospital cardiac arrests have not produced uniform results. Those studies that did not demonstrate a significant difference in the follow-up probabilities of arrhythmia recurrence and sudden death[73,77,96,98] are characterized by the frequent use of empiric amiodarone or electrosurgery in the patients for whom no predicted effective therapy could be found. In these studies, the outcomes of patients receiving predicted effective therapy was improved over that of an untreated natural history population. However, the outcome of patients treated with empiric amiodarone or electrosurgery was similarly improved.

The strength and independence of the predictive value of the invasive approach to therapy selection for patients with VT/VF have been assessed by univariate and multivariate analysis of predictors of arrhythmia recurrence and/or sudden death in large cohorts of patients.[15,72,90,94] Swerdlow et al.[72] reported such a study in a population dominated by VT patients. Of 217 patients with sustained VT and 22 patients with VF, 205 patients had inducible VT/VF at a baseline electrophysiologic study and were managed primarily by the invasive approach. Patients who were not inducible at baseline electrophysiologic study and patients for whom no drug therapy was predicted to be effective were treated with antiarrhythmic drugs that decreased the rate and duration of induced VT or rendered VT more difficult to induce, with antiarrhythmic drugs that were selected by the noninvasive approach, or with surgical approaches to arrhythmia therapy. For the whole group, the 2-year actuarial sudden death probability was identical to that of the expected untreated, natural history of a VT/VF population at 25%. However, for patients receiving treatment predicted to be effective by the invasive approach, the 2-year sudden death probability was 18% compared to a 2-year sudden death probability of 41% in patients receiving therapy predicted to be ineffective by the invasive approach. This study reports a higher 2-year sudden death probability for patients receiving therapy predicted to be effective than that reported by any other actuarial report. This may be due to the fact that at the time of sudden death, 7 of the 13 patients contributing an end point to the effective therapy group were not receiving the therapy predicted to be effective: 1 died before long-term therapy was instituted, and 6 died after a drug predicted to be effective had been discontinued or its dose had been decreased. Multivariate analysis of 34 variables describing age, gender, cardiac disease, clinical arrhythmia, and induced arrhythmia in patients who were inducible at the baseline electrophysiologic study revealed two independent predictors of sudden death—higher NYHA functional class and persistent VT/VF induciblity on the discharge treatment. Another study of this sort, reported by Borggrefe et al.[94] found the dominant predictor of recurrent VT/VF or sudden death on follow-up to be persistent inducibility of VT/VF on the discharge therapy. Patients discharged on a therapy predicted to be ineffective by the invasive approach were eight times more likely to experience an arrhythmic event during follow-up than were patients discharged on therapy predicted to be effective by the invasive approach. Similar results have been reported in the out-of-hospital cardiac arrest population.[15,90] Wilber et al.[90] described the outcomes of 166 patients with out-of-hospital cardiac arrest. Patients with inducible VT/VF who received therapy that was predicted effective by the invasive approach had a 2-year actuarial probability of recurrent cardiac arrest of approximately

5%, while those who received therapy that was predicted to be ineffective by the invasive approach had a 2-year probability of recurrent cardiac arrest of approximately 45%. By multivariate analysis the independent predictors of recurrent cardiac arrest in this population were persistent inducibility of VT/VF on the discharge therapy, left ventricular ejection fraction < 0.30, and the absence of cardiac surgery. When the analysis was limited to patients with inducible VT/VF at the baseline electrophysiologic study the only predictor of recurrent cardiac arrest by multivariate analysis was persistent inducibility of VT/VF on the discharge therapy. Patients discharged on a therapy predicted to be ineffective by the invasive approach were seven times more likely to experience a recurrent cardiac arrest during follow-up than were patients discharged on therapy predicted to be effective by the invasive approach (Figure 5).

Thus, as with the noninvasive approach, application of the invasive approach separates patients into a group with a 2-year actuarial sudden death probability substantially better than, and a group with a 2-year sudden death probability substantially worse than the expected untreated natural history sudden death probability of a 50:50 VT:VF study population of 25%. Two potential explanations exist for these

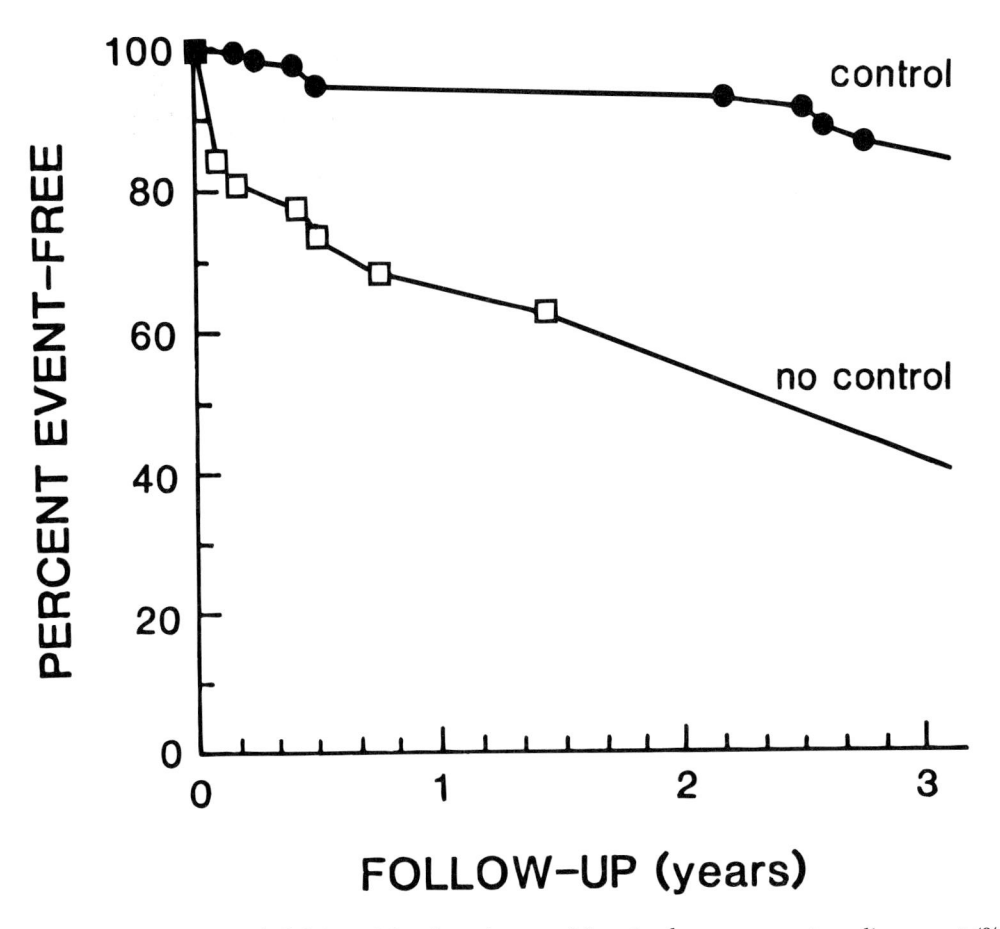

Figure 5. Cumulative probabilities of freedom from sudden death or recurrent cardiac arrest (%) over 3 years of follow-up in patients resuscitated from out-of-hospital cardiac arrest treated with antiarrhythmic drugs predicted to be effective by the invasive approach (●, control) or predicted to be ineffective by the invasive approach (□, no control). (Redrawn with permission from Figure 2, Reference 90.)

results. First, therapy predicted to be effective by these approaches may indeed be responsible for the improved outcome relative to natural history sudden cardiac death rate. If so, we must also conclude that therapy predicted to be ineffective by each approach is not only ineffective but is also harmful in that the outcome on predicted ineffective therapy is worse than the expected natural history of the arrhythmia. Second, it is also possible that the ability to satisfactorily suppress the index arrhythmia by either approach identifies a population of patients with a good prognosis irrespective of the subsequent use of the drug therapy chosen. Similarly, inability to suppress the index arrhythmia may simply identify a population of patients with a poor prognosis. In this way, the natural history of the arrhythmia may be redistributed with a lower sudden death probability in the good prognosis group and a higher sudden death probability in a poor prognosis group with the weighted average of the two remaining equivalent to the natural history sudden death probability. Which of these two possibilities is operative remains to be defined. My personal bias is that the former scenario is most probable given the frequent reporting of arrhythmia recurrence/sudden death shortly after the patient or his/her physician has discontinued antiarrhythmic drug therapy that was predicted to be effective.[25,54,64,72] Such events would be expected to be infrequent if the approach had identified a patient with an inherently good prognosis regardless of subsequent therapy.

The efficacy of therapy for patients with VT/VF individualized by the invasive approach may be estimated in a manner analogous to that described above for the noninvasive approach. The estimated 2-year actuarial sudden death probability while receiving therapy predicted to be effective by the invasive approach in populations dominated by VT patients is 8% and the estimated 2-year actuarial arrhythmia recurrence/sudden death probability of such patients is 12%.[43,62,72,78,84,86,94] Similarly, for patients with cardiac arrest the 2-year actuarial sudden death probability and 2-year arrhythmia recurrence/sudden death probability on therapy predicted to be effective by the invasive approach are estimated at 6% and 13%, respectively.[90,95,98,99] Thus, the estimated 2-year actuarial sudden death probability of an average VT/VF population treated with individualized drug therapy selected by the invasive approach is 7% and the estimated 2-year actuarial arrhythmia recurrence/sudden death probability of such patients is 12%. Again, these values contrast those of the untreated natural history and empiric standard antiarrhythmic drug arguments presented above suggesting a potential role for the invasive approach in the treatment of patients with VT/VF.

Empiric Amiodarone Therapy

Amiodarone is a benzofuran derivative orginally introduced as a coronary vasodilator and antianginal agent in the late 1960s.[109,110] Its antiarrhythmic potential was first recognized in the early 1970s[111-113] and was introduced into clinical use by investigators in Europe and South America.[114-118] Subsequently, numerous clinical studies have evaluated its safety and efficacy in patients with ventricular tachyarrhythmias.[119-173] From these studies amiodarone has acquired a reputation as an extremely effective antiarrhythmic agent, albeit one with a significant adverse effect profile in the dosages commonly used to treat life-threatening arrhythmias.[121,129,130,150,174-179] Its antiarrhythmic actions are sufficiently potent as to have prompted one investigator to refer to its effects as "arrhythmolytic."[126]

The dominant antiarrhythmic actions of amiodarone are those of Vaughan Williams Class III.[112,113] Nevertheless, the agent is also a Class I antiarrhythmic drug, a noncompetitive β-adrenergic blocker, and a calcium channel blocker.[140,180] Furthermore, it has been suggested that amiodarone exerts beneficial antiarrhythmic effects, at least in

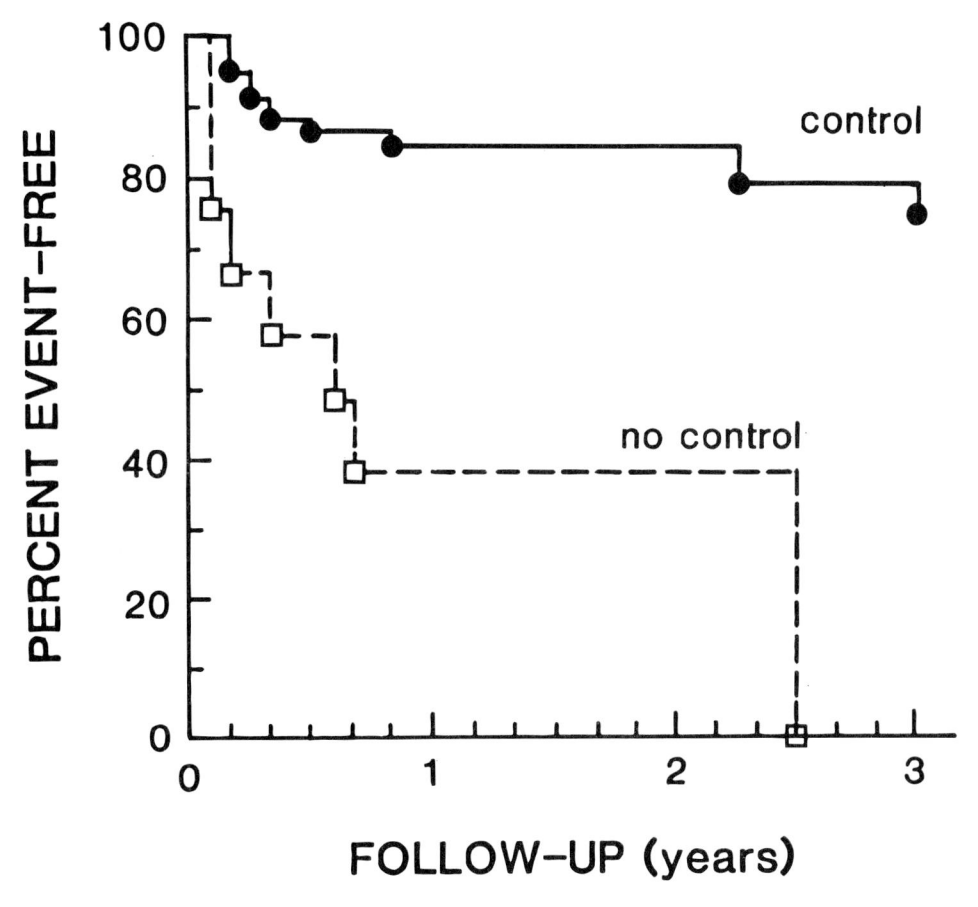

Figure 6. Cumulative probabilities of freedom from death or recurrent sustained ventricular tachycardia/ventricular fibrillation (VT/VF) (%) over 3 years of follow-up in patients with sustained VT/VF treated with amiodarone predicted to be effective by the noninvasive approach (●, control) or predicted to be ineffective by the noninvasive approach (□, no control). (Redrawn with permission from Figure 4, Reference 162.)

mean of 12 months and symptomatic VT/VF recurred in 38 of the 80 patients (48%). The 2-year arrhythmia recurrence/sudden death probability was 67% (Figure 7). Again, the predictive values of this invasive evaluation of the long-term efficacy of amiodarone do not differ substantially from those presented above for the invasive evaluation of the long-term efficacy of other antiarrhythmic agents. These observations have called into question the proported uniqueness of amiodarone as an antiarrhythmic agent in patients with VT/VF.

These observations notwithstanding, most practitioners prescribe amiodarone on an empiric basis. Over the past 4 years, three reports of the long-term antiarrhythmic efficacy of empiric amiodarone in patients with VT/VF have appeared.[170,171,173] The results of these studies were remarkably encouraging and remarkably consistent. Combined these reports describe the outcome of a total of 1,076 patients who received amiodarone after failure of standard antiarrhythmic agents for the treatment of VT/VF (of whom only 81 had nonsustained VT [8.5%]). The combined population was typical of drug resistant VT/VF patients: 793 patients (72%) had atherosclerotic heart disease; 45 patients (4%) had no evident struc-

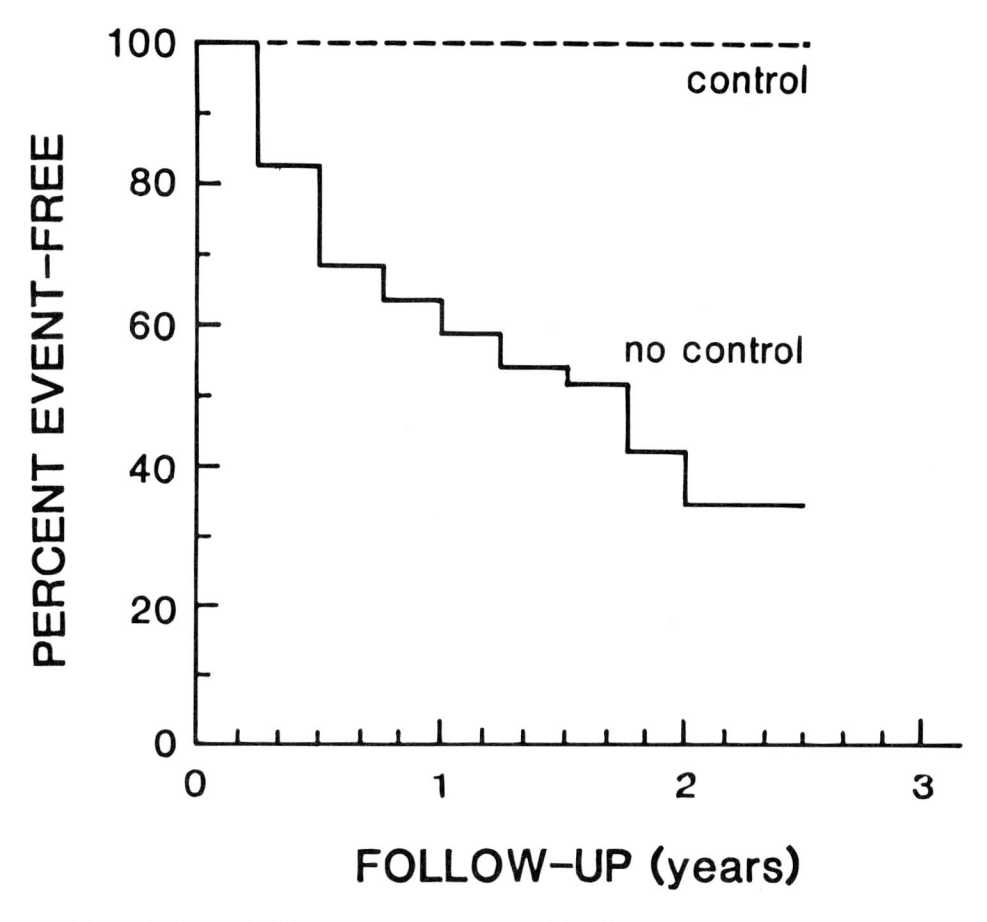

[Figure: step plot showing Percent Event-Free vs Follow-up (years); control line flat near 100%, no control line declining to ~35% by 2.5 years]

Figure 7. Cumulative probabilities of freedom from sudden death or recurrent sustained ventricular tachycardia/ventricular fibrillation (VT/VF) (%) over 3 years of follow-up in patients with sustained VT/VF treated with amiodarone predicted to be effective by the invasive approach (dashed line, control) or predicted to be ineffective by the invasive approach solid line, no control). (Redrawn with permission from Figure 1, Reference 153.)

tural heart disease; and the mean left ventricular ejection fractions in these studies ranged from 0.34–0.36. After standard, although somewhat variable, loading dosages the maintenance amiodarone dosages averaged between 350 and 450 mg/day. Two of these studies[170,173] reported 2-year actuarial probabilities of recurrent sustained VT/VF or sudden death—both 26% (Figure 8). All three studies[170,171,173] reported 2-year actuarial probabilities of sudden death. They ranged from 9% to 13% with a sample size weighted mean of 12%. Results such as these, in drug resistant patients, have reawakened interest in empiric amiodarone therapy as a primary treatment modality in patients with VT/VF. These large studies also evaluated the potential for clinical characteristics to predict arrhythmia recurrence/sudden death during empiric amiodarone treatment. Each study[170,171,173] identified a lower ejection fraction as a significant predictor of arrhythmia recurrence/sudden death. Other predictors of arrhythmia recurrence/sudden death identified by these studies included older age,[170,173] higher NYHA dyspnea functional class,[171,173] cardiac arrest with the present-

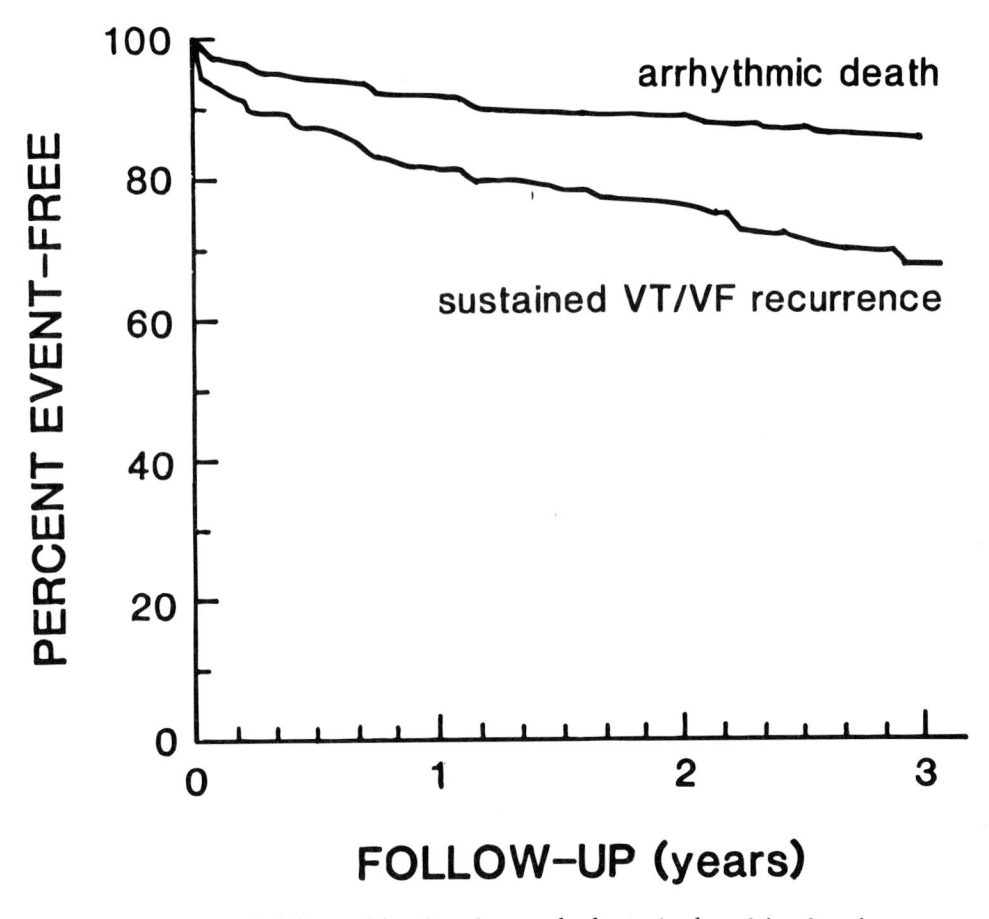

Figure 8. Cumulative probabilities of freedom from arrhythmic death and freedom from recurrent sustained ventricular tachycardia/ventricular fibrillation (VT/VF) (%) over 3 years of follow-up in patients with sustained VT/VF treated with empiric amiodarone therapy. (Redrawn with permission from Figure 2, Reference 170.)

ing arrhythmia,[170] and the presence of structural, especially atherosclerotic, heart disease.[173]

Empiric β-Adrenergic Blocking Therapy

The efficacy of β-adrenergic blocking agents for the acute and chronic management of patients with VT/VF has been under assessment since these agents were first used as antiarrhythmic drugs.[194–196] Early assessments suggested that β-adrenergic blocking drugs had specific indications, but were not a particularly potent therapy for the largest group of patients with VT/VF—those with stable atherosclerotic heart disease and remote myocardial infarction. The specific settings where β-adrenergic blocking drugs were considered indicated included VT/VF occurring in the settings of mitral valve prolapse,[197] exercise,[198–200] acute myocardial infarction,[194,196,201] the long QT interval syndromes,[202] and in the absence of identifiable structural heart disease.[199,203,204]

β-Adrenergic blocking agents have little or no measurable effects on the in vitro electrophysiology of normal ventricular myocardial or Purkinje tissue when administered acutely in concentrations matching those typically used in clinical settings. However, in intact preparations under autonomic influences and in abnormal or ischemic tissue, the acute electrophysiologic effects, β-adrenergic blocking agents become more evident. Furthermore, with long-term use some β-adrenergic blockers (propranolol, metoprolol) also prolong the rate corrected QT interval, ventricular action potential duration, and ventricular effective refractory period in humans. Finally, all β-adrenergic agents so tested have demonstrated the ability to increase the VF threshold in experimental preparations. For details of the electrophysiologic effects of β-adrenergic blocking agents as applicable to ventricular arrhythmias the reader is referred to the excellent review of Venditti et al.[205] Thus, the rationale for the use of β-adrenergic blocking agents to treat VT/VF is based upon their chronic electrophysiologic effects, their effects on abnormal or ischemic ventricular tissue, and their ability to prevent the arrhythmogenic effects of acute sympathetic stimulation.

With this rationale, β-adrenergic blocking agents have been used in patients with VT/VF as primary therapy individualized by suppression of noninvasive markers of arrhythmia propensity,[206–209] as primary therapy individualized by suppression of invasive markers of arrhythmia propensity,[208–212] as adjuvant therapy to enhance the efficacy of other antiarrhythmic agents,[213–216] and as empiric primary therapy.[12,21,217]

When solitary β-adrenergic blocking drug therapy for patients with VT/VF is evaluated by either the noninvasive or the invasive approach the results are not substantially different from those of other antiarrhythmic drugs evaluated by these approaches. The proportion of patients responding to β-adrenergic blocking therapy as assessed by the noninvasive approach has been reported to range from 33% to 75%.[206,207,209] Patients treated with β-adrenergic blocking agents whose therapy has been predicted to be effective by the noninvasive approach have reported arrhythmia/sudden death rates ranging from 0% after 14 months of follow-up[206] to 29% after 3 years of follow-up.[209] The latter study discharged patients on β-adrenergic blocking drugs regardless of the results of the noninvasive assessment of the adequacy of therapy. After 3 years of follow-up the arrhythmia recurrence/sudden death rate was 29% in patients whose therapy was predicted to be effective and 50% in patients whose therapy was predicted to be ineffective by the noninvasive approach.[209] This difference did not reach statistical significance in this small ($n = 13$) study. The proportion of patients responding to β-adrenergic blocking therapy as assessed by the invasive approach has been reported to range from 21% to 44%.[209–212] Patients treated with β-adrenergic blocking agents whose therapy had been predicted to be effective by the invasive approach have reported arrhythmia recurrence/sudden death rates ranging from 0% after 34 months of follow-up[211] to 25% after 3 years of follow-up.[209] Two of these studies discharged patients on β-adrenergic blocking drugs regardless of the results of the invasive assessment of the adequacy of therapy. Brodsky et al.[209] reported that the arrhythmia recurrence/sudden death rate after 3 years of follow-up was 25% in patients whose therapy was predicted to be effective by the invasive approach and 50% in patients whose therapy was predicted to be ineffective by the invasive approach. This difference did not reach statistical significance in this small ($n = 14$) study. Leclercq et al.[212] reported that the arrhythmia recurrence/sudden death rate was 12.5% in patients whose therapy was predicted to be effective and 60% in patients whose therapy was predicted to be ineffective by the invasive approach after 28 months of follow-up. The difference did reach statistical significance in this larger ($n = 36$) study. These two investigations also provide efficacy estimates for the empiric use of β-adrenergic blocking drug therapy in patients with VT/VF. The overall arrhythmia recurrence/sudden death rate was 25% after 3 years of follow-up in the study of Brodsky et al.[209] and 39% after 28 months of follow-up in the study of Leclercq et al.[212] These results are not particularly supportive of the concept of empiric β-adrenergic blocking therapy for patients with VT/VF.

Nevertheless, support for the use of empiric β-adrenergic blocking therapy for patients with VT/VF is provided by the numerous reports of a reduction in the probability of sudden death with empiric β-adrenergic blocking therapy in patients convalescing from an acute myocardial infarction.[218–223] Furthermore, in a retrospective evaluation of the outcomes of patients with sustained VT and left ventricular ejection fractions of < 30% treated with a variety of empiric therapies reported by Leclercq et al.,[21] patients whose therapy included β-adrenergic blocking drugs had a lower 2-year actuarial cardiac mortality probability (approximately 9%) than did those whose therapy did not include a β-adrenergic blocking drug (approximately 34%). Thus, available data do not strongly support solitary empiric β-adrenergic blocking therapy in patients with VT/VF for the purpose of preventing arrhythmia recurrence. However, the postmyocardial infarction trials and the study of Leclercq et al. raise the possibility of a more prominent role of β-adrenergic blocking therapy for the purpose of prevention of sudden death in such patients.

In this setting, Steinbeck et al.[217] recently published the results of a prospective assessment of the efficacy of empiric metoprolol therapy in 54 patients with documented, sustained VT/VF or syncope. All patients had a baseline electrophysiologic study that reproducibly induced at least 20 consecutive beats of VT or VF. These patients received metoprolol 25 mg twice a day with subsequent dose increments, as tolerated, to 100 mg twice a day. The 2-year probability of recurrent sustained VT/VF or sudden death was approximately 45% (Figure 9). The 2-year probability of sudden death was approximately 15% for these patients.

From these limited data we might conclude that the 2-year probability of arrhythmia recurrence in a patient with VT/VF in the absence of a reversible cause is not substantially altered by the use of empiric β-adrenergic blocking drug therapy. Nevertheless, the data do suggest that this approach to treatment lowers the 2-year probability of sudden death. Clearly, these data indicate the need for further evaluation of empiric β-adrenergic blocking therapy in patients with VT/VF, particularly in patients with VT/VF manifest as cardiac arrest.

Comparisons of Approaches

At present, viable approaches to the medical treatment of patients with a demonstrated propensity to VT/VF include individualized antiarrhythmic drug therapy selected by the noninvasive approach, individualized antiarrhythmic drug therapy selected by the invasive approach, empiric amiodarone therapy, and (perhaps) empiric β-adrenergic blocking therapy. Although each of these therapeutic approaches is likely "best" under specific clinical circumstances, there has been interest in determining which is "best" when more than one approach is applicable. However, opinion remains divided over how "best" in this setting should be defined. While the purest definition of "best" may be overall predictive accuracy, this measure has no meaning for empiric antiarrhythmic drug therapy and does not reflect clinical practice when individualized drug therapy is used. Currently, patients with VT/VF are not often discharged on therapy that is predicted to be ineffective. Instead, if predicted effective therapy cannot be identified for a specific patient then alternative approaches to medical therapy or nonmedical approaches to therapy are generally used. Thus, since the goal of therapy is to prevent VT/VF recurrence and sudden death, "best" will be defined as that approach that selects therapy that best prevents VT/VF recurrence and

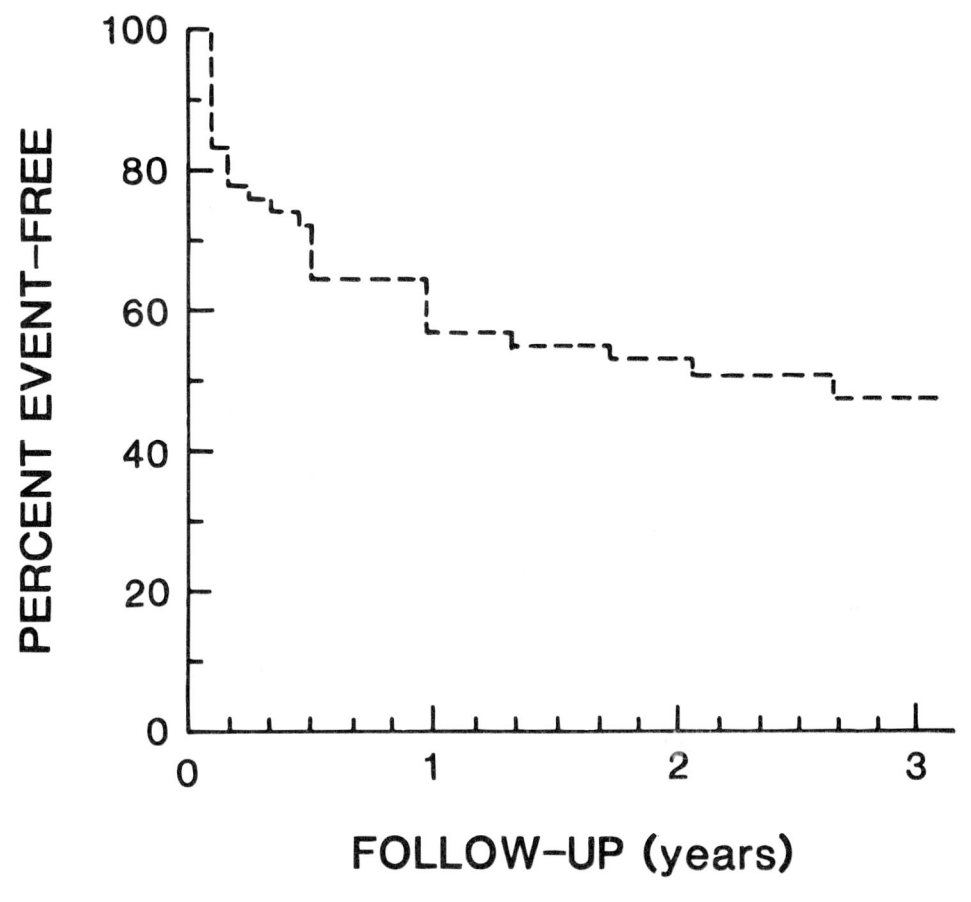

Figure 9. Cumulative probabilities of freedom from sudden death or sustained ventricular tachycardia/ventricular fibrillation (VT/VF) (%) over 3 years of follow-up in patients with sustained VT/VF or syncope with inducible VT/VF treated with empiric metoprolol therapy. (Redrawn with permission from Figure 1, Reference 217.)

sudden death in patients discharged on therapy. For the individualized therapeutic approaches this translates into the negative predictive value of the assessment (predictive value of the absence of the index of electrical instability on drug therapy for the follow-up absence of VT/VF on drug therapy). For the empiric therapy approaches this translates into the overall result of the empiric therapy. A summary of the efficacies, so defined, of each approach to therapy for an average 50:50 VT/VF population are presented in Table 1. A number of clinical trials have compared (or are in the process of comparing) the outcomes of therapy selected by these approaches.

Table 1
Estimated Two-Year Actuarial Event Rates in a 50:50 VT/VF Patient Population by Method of Treatment

	Sudden Death	Arrhythmia Events
"Natural history"	25%	45%
Empiric standard AA drugs	25%	45%
Holter-guided standard AA drugs	10%	25%
EPS-guided standard AA drugs	7%	12%
Empiric amiodarone	12%	25%
Empiric β blockade	15%	45%

AA: antiarrhythmic; arrhythmic events: sustained VT/VF recurrence plus sudden death; EPS: electrophysiologic study.

The relative efficacies of therapy selected by the two approaches to individualized antiarrhythmic drug therapy have been prospectively compared in randomized clinical trials twice with disparate results. Mitchell et al.[43] performed 24-hour ambulatory ECG monitoring, exercise tolerance testing, and programmed stimulation in 105 consecutive consenting patients surviving hypotensive VT or VF to identify 57 individuals with an index to guide either the noninvasive or the invasive approach to antiarrhythmic drug selection. These patients were randomized to have their therapy selected by either the noninvasive approach or by the invasive approach. The two populations were equivalent in all known codeterminants of long-term outcome. After a mean of 3.2 drug trials, therapy predicted to be effective by the noninvasive approach was found for each of the 29 patients randomized to that approach. After a mean of 5.5 drug trials, therapy predicted to be effective by the invasive approach was found for 15 of the 28 patients (54%) randomized to that approach. Patients for whom no predicted effective therapy could be found received empiric amiodarone therapy. The 2-year, actuarial probability of symptomatic, sustained VT/VF recurrence or sudden death was significantly lower on therapy predicted to be effective by the invasive approach (7%) than on therapy predicted to be effective by the noninvasive approach (43%) ($P < 0.04$) (Figure 10). This study did not have sufficient power to assess the statistical significance of the difference between the 2-year actuarial probabilities of sudden death on therapy predicted to be effective by the invasive approach (4%) and on therapy predicted to be effective by the noninvasive approach (7%). Nevertheless, this study indicated that therapy selected by the invasive approach prevents VT/VF recurrence better than does that selected by the noninvasive approach. Therapy predicted to be effective by the noninvasive approach failed to improve the expected natural history of untreated VT/VF patients with respect to arrhythmia recurrence. These results contrast with those of the recently completed Electrophysiologic Study Versus Electrocardiographic Monitoring (ESVEM) study.[45,45a] The design of ESVEM was not markedly different from that of Mitchell et al. although different results were obtained. In the EVSEM study, a therapy predicted to be effective by the noninvasive approach was found for 188 of the 244 patients randomized to that approach and a therapy predicted to be effective by the invasive approach was found for 108 of the 242 patients randomized to that approach. There was no significant difference between the 2-year actuarial probabilities of arrhythmia recurrence or sudden death on therapy predicted to be effective by the noninvasive approach (51%) and that on therapy predicted to be effective by the invasive approach (47%) (P = NS) (Figure 11). Thus, in the ESVEM study, neither approach selected therapy that appeared to improve the expected natural history of arrhythmia recurrence in a VT/VF population. Potential explanations for this aberrant finding include a preponderance of antiarrhythmic drug resistant patients in the study population and the use of lax criteria for the prediction of drug efficacy in the noninvasive/invasive approach limbs of the ESVEM study.[45]

Determination of the relative efficacies of individualized antiarrhythmic drug therapy and empiric amiodarone therapy in patients resuscitated from cardiac arrest was the subject of study in the Cardiac Arrest in Seattle: Conventional versus Amiodarone Drug Evaluation (CASCADE) study.[224] Patients resuscitated from a VT/VF cardiac arrest were randomized to receive individualized conventional antiarrhythmic drug therapy or empiric amiodarone. Patients randomized to the conventional therapy limb underwent electrophysiologic study. If sustained VT/VF could be induced in an antiarrhythmic drug-free state the first approach to drug therapy selection was the invasive approach. If sustained VT/VF could not be induced, or if no therapy was predicted to be effective by the invasive ap-

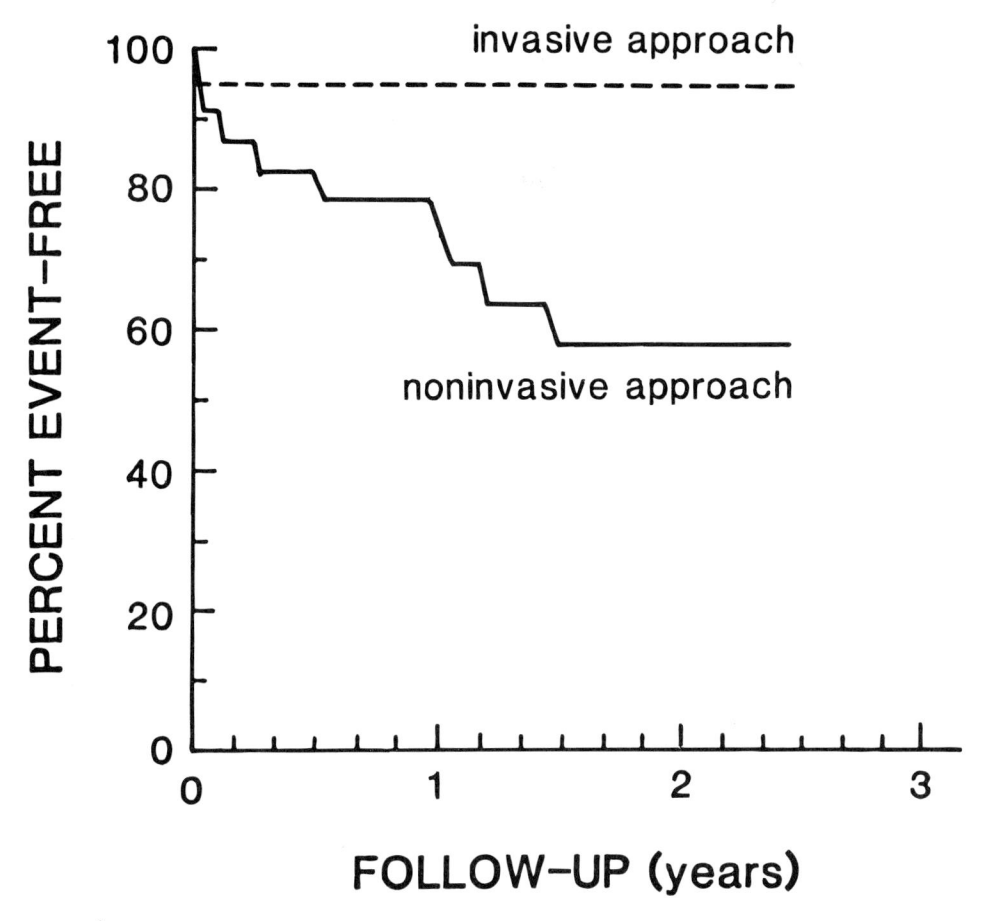

Figure 10. Cumulative probabilities of freedom from sudden death or sustained VT/VF (%) over 2.5 years of follow-up in patients with symptomatic VT/VF randomly assigned to antiarrhythmic drug treatment predicted to be effective by the invasive approach (dotted line) or to treatment predicted to be effective by the noninvasive approach (solid line). (Redrawn with permission from Figure 3, Reference 43.)

proach, drug therapy was selected by the noninvasive approach. During the conduct of this trial a higher than expected sudden death probability was noted for the whole group. Therefore, the investigators elected to implant an automatic cardioverter-defibrillator when possible in all subsequent patients. Thus, the primary outcome variable cluster was cardiac mortality, complete syncope followed by an ICD shock, or resuscitated cardiac arrest recurrence. The 2-year actuarial probability arrhythmia recurrence, so defined, was higher in patients receiving conventional antiarrhythmic drug therapy (31%) than in patients receiving empiric use of amiodarone therapy (18%) (Figure 12).[225] Thus, in a cardiac arrest population, the empiric use of amiodarone therapy appeared superior to the use of standard antiarrhythmic drug therapy individualized by the invasive approach where applicable and successful and by the noninvasive approach otherwise. To date, no data regarding the relative predictive values of the invasive and noninvasive approaches in the CASCADE study have been published. Accordingly, the results of the CASCADE study cannot be extrapolated to suggest that the empiric use of amiodarone therapy is superior to the use of standard antiarrhyth-

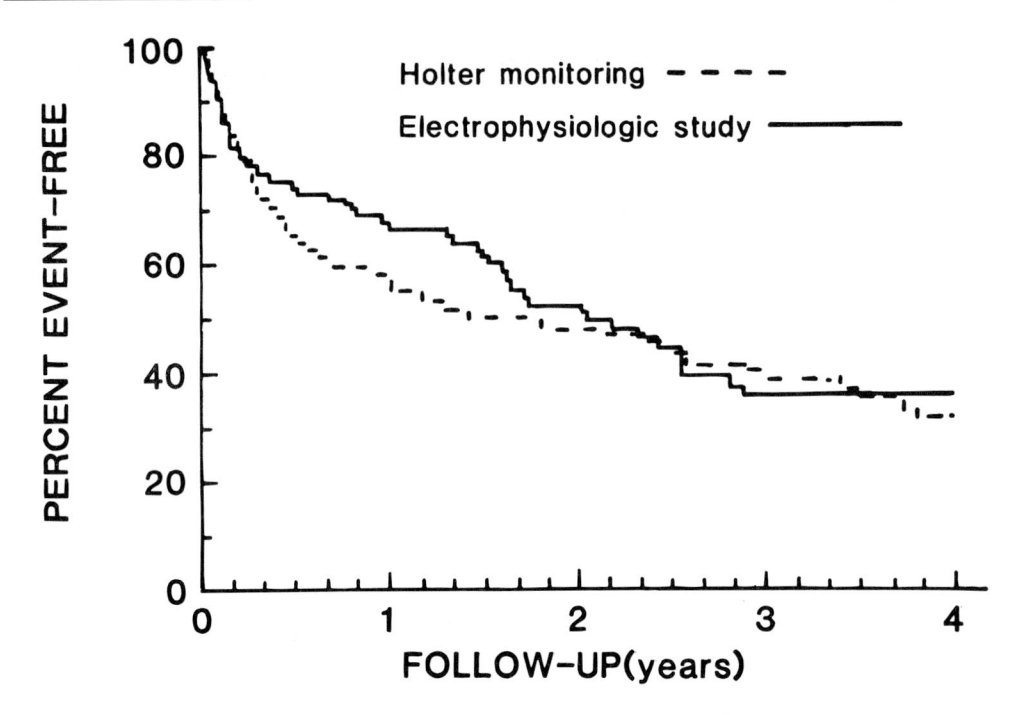

Figure 11. Cumulative probabilities of freedom from ventricular tachycardia (VT) of > 15 beats duration, ventricular fibrillation (VF), torsade de pointes, unmonitored syncope, cardiac arrest, or death caused by arrhythmia over 4 years of follow-up of VT/VF patients randomly assigned to antiarrhythmic drug treatment predicted to be effective by the invasive approach (solid line) or to treatment predicted to be effective by the noninvasive approach (dashed line). (Redrawn with permission from Figure 1, Reference 45a.)

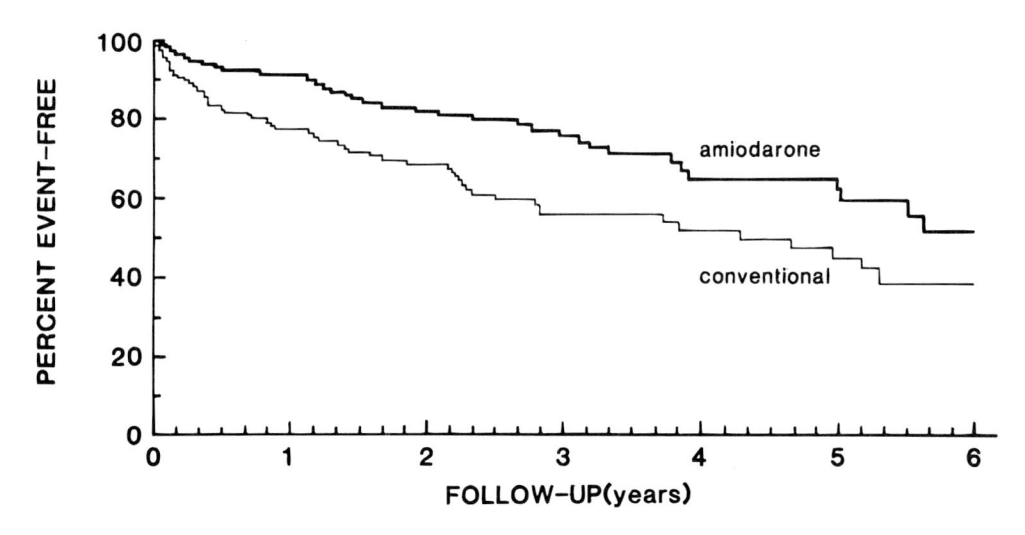

Figure 12. Cumulative probabilities of freedom from cardiac mortality, complete syncope followed by an implantable cardioverter-defibrillator (ICD) shock, or resuscitated cardiac arrest recurrence over 6 years of follow-up in patients resuscitated from cardiac arrest randomly assigned to treatment with empiric amiodarone (heavy line) or to treatment with conventional antiarrhythmic drugs individualized by the invasive approach if applicable and successful or by the noninvasive approach (solid line). (Redrawn with permission from Figure 2, Reference 225.)

mic drug therapy individualized by the invasive approach if, as suggested by Mitchell et al.[43] the invasive approach provides results that are significantly better than those of the noninvasive approach.

Steinbeck et al.[217] recently published the results of a prospective, randomized, clinical trial comparing the efficacy of antiarrhythmic therapy chosen by the invasive approach to that of empiric metoprolol therapy. Patients were included if they had documented, sustained VT/VF or syncope. Randomization to the study therapeutic approaches was dependent upon a baseline electrophysiologic study that reproducibly induced at least 20 consecutive beats of VT or VF. The baseline electrophysiologic study identified 115 patients eligible for randomization. Sixty-one patients were randomized electrophysiologically guided therapy and 54 to empiric metoprolol. The randomization process was apparently successful in distributing known codeterminants of outcome equally between the two groups. Patients randomized to the empiric metoprolol arm received metoprolol 25 mg twice a day with subsequent dose increments, as tolerated, to 100 mg twice a day. Patients randomized to electrophysiologically guided therapy underwent a mean of 2.8 electropharmacological trials to identify predicted effective therapy in 48% of the patients. The remaining patients randomized to the electrophysiologically guided therapy arm received antiarrhythmic drug therapy that was predicted to be ineffective. The outcome data were analyzed by intention-to-treat with an end point cluster of recurrent symptomatic sustained VT/VF or sudden death. The study concluded that there was no difference in the 2-year probabilities of these outcomes between patients randomized to electrophysiologically guided therapy and those randomized to empiric metoprolol therapy. Each group had a 2-year recurrence probability of approximately 45% (P = NS) (Figure 13). Analysis restricted to the 2-year probability of sudden death also revealed no difference between the two treatment groups, approximately 15% for the metoprolol group and approximately 25% for the electrophysiologically guided therapy group (P = NS). However, subgroup analysis of the patients randomized to the electrophysiologically guided therapy arm of the study showed that the 2-year recurrence probability was only 20% in those patients receiving therapy predicted to be effective while it was 70% in those patients receiving therapy that was predicted to be ineffective. Although a statistical analysis of the three-way comparison was not presented, it appears that the 2-year recurrence probability of patients receiving therapy that the electrophysiologically guided approach predicted to be effective (approximately 20%) was better than that of patients receiving empiric metoprolol therapy (approximately 45%), which in turn, was better than that of patients receiving therapy that the electrophysiologically guided approach predicted to be ineffective (approximately 70%). This assessment of the result was supported by the authors description of a multivariate regression analysis of their data which indicated that persistently inducible VT/VF despite therapy was the only independent variable associated with arrhythmia recurrence or sudden death. When the analysis is restricted to the end point of sudden death differences among the three treatment groups are less evident (2-year sudden death probabilities of approximately 15% for patients receiving predicted effective therapy, 15% for patients receiving empiric metoprolol therapy, and 35% for patients receiving predicted ineffective therapy).

Alternative approaches to the medical therapy of patients with VT/VF are also being assessed in CASH.[12] In this study, patients resuscitated from a VT/VF cardiac arrest were randomized to receive one of either empiric amiodarone therapy, empiric propafenone therapy, empiric metoprolol therapy, or an ICD with a primary outcome variable of total mortality. After 230 of the 400 patient planned enrollment had been

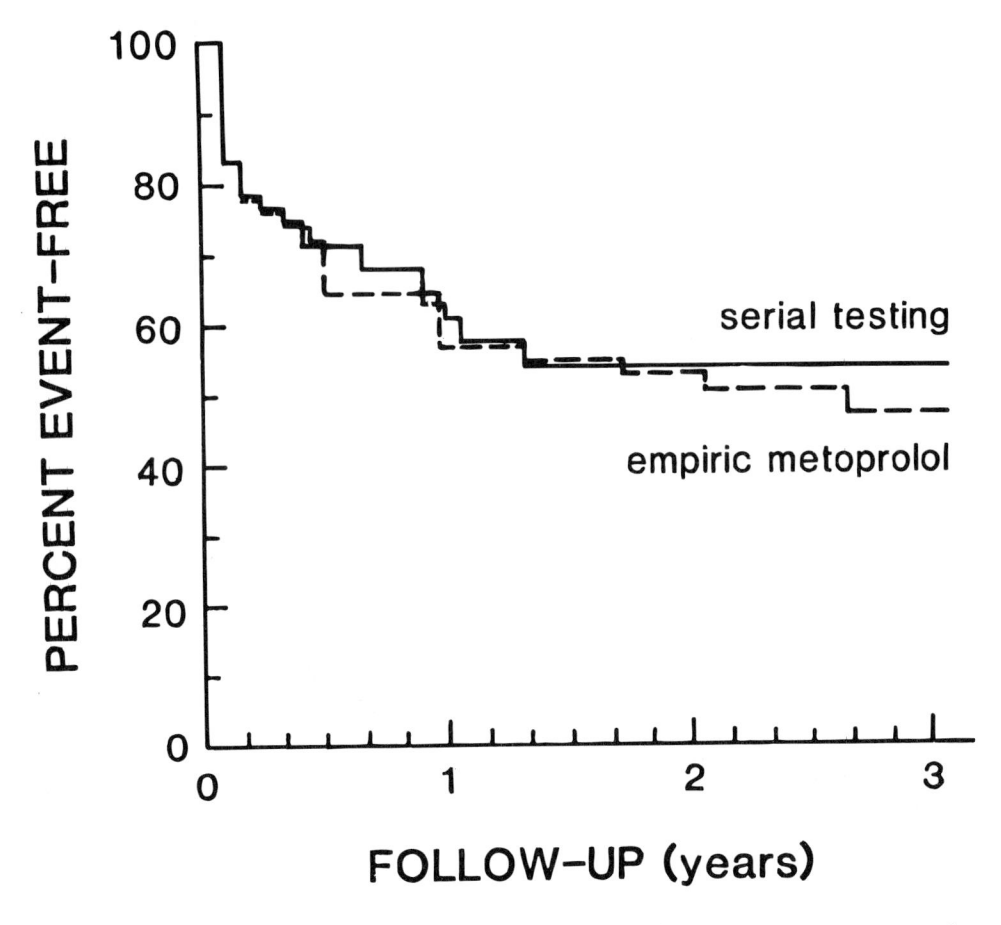

Figure 13. Cumulative probabilities of freedom from sudden death or sustained ventricular tachycardia/ventricular fibrillation (VT/VF) (%) over 3 years of follow-up in patients with sustained VT/VF or syncope with inducible VT/VF randomly assigned to antiarrhythmic drug treatment selected by the invasive approach (48% on predicted effective therapy, 52% on empiric therapy after failure to find predicted effective therapy) (solid line, serial testing) or to treatment with empiric metoprolol therapy (dotted line). (Redrawn with permission from Figure 1, Reference 217.)

completed, the Safety Monitoring Board of CASH recommended that the empiric propafenone arm be closed as the total mortality rate of patients in this arm was statistically significantly higher than in the other three treatment limbs.[12] At that time, there were no statistically significant differences comparing empiric amiodarone, empiric metoprolol, and ICD treatments.

Thus, presently available data from randomized clinical trials of various therapeutic alternatives to medical therapy for patients with VT/VF have suggested that empiric standard antiarrhythmic drug therapy is inappropriate,[12] that individualized antiarrhythmic therapy selected by the invasive approach is preferable to individualized antiarrhythmic therapy selected by the noninvasive approach,[43] that individualized antiarrhythmic therapy selected by the invasive and noninvasive approaches are equivalently ineffective,[45] in patients with demonstrated antiarrhythmic drug resistance,[45a] and that empiric amiodaone therapy is preferable to the combined use of the invasive and noninvasive approaches to individualized antiarrhythmic drug therapy.[225]

References

1. Liberthson RR, Nagel EL, Hirschman JC, et al: Prehospital ventricular fibrillation. Prognosis and follow-up course. N Engl J Med 291:317, 1974.
2. Baum RS, Alvarez H III, Cobb LA: Survival after resuscitation from out-of-hospital ventricular fibrillation. Circulation 50:1231, 1974.
3. Schaffer WA, Cobb LA: Recurrent ventricular fibrillation and modes of death in survivors of out-of-hospital ventricular fibrillation. N Engl J Med 293:259, 1975.
4. Cobb LA, Baum RS, Alvarez H III, et al: Resuscitation from out-of-hospital ventricular fibrillation: 4 years of follow-up. Circulation 52(Suppl III):III-223, 1975.
5. Strauss MB: Paroxysmal ventricular tachycardia. Am J Med Sci 179:337, 1930.
6. Lundy CJ, McLellan LL: Paroxysmal ventricular tachycardia: an etiological study with special reference to the type. Ann Intern Med 7:812, 1934.
7. Williams C, Ellis LB: Ventricular tachycardia: an analysis of thirty-six cases. Arch Intern Med 71:137, 1943.
8. Trevor Cooke W, White PD: Paroxysmal ventricular tachycardia. Br Heart J 5:33, 1943.
9. Herrmann GR, Hejtmancik MR: A clinical and electrocardiographic study of paroxysmal ventricular tachycardia and its management. Ann Intern Med 28:989, 1948.
10. Armbrust CA Jr, Levine SA: Paroxysmal ventricular tachycardia: a study of one hundred and seven cases. Circulation 1:28, 1950.
11. Herrmann GR, Park HM, Hejtmancik MR: Paroxysmal ventricular tachycardia: a clinical and electrocardiographic study. Am Heart J 57:166, 1959.
12. Siebels J, Cappato R, Ruppel R, et al: ICD versus drugs in cardiac arrest survivors: preliminary results of the Cardiac Arrest Study Hamburg. PACE 16:552, 1993.
13. Leitch JW, Gillis AM, Wyse DG, et al: Reduction in defibrillator shocks with an implantable device combining antitachycardia pacing and shock therapy. J Am Coll Cardiol 18:145, 1991.
14. Bardy GH, Hofer B, Johnson G, et al: Implantable transvenous cardioverter-defibrillators. Circulation 87:1152, 1993.
15. Furukawa T, Rozanski JJ, Nogami A, et al: Time-dependent risk of and predictors for cardiac arrest recurrence in survivors of out-of-hospital cardiac arrest with chronic coronary artery disease. Circulation 80:599, 1989.
16. Myerburg RJ, Conde C, Sheps DS, et al: Antiarrhythmic drug therapy in survivors of prehospital cardiac arrest: comparison of effects on chronic ventricular arrhythmias and recurrent cardiac arrest. Circulation 59:855, 1979.
17. Myerburg RJ, Kessler KM, Estes D, et al: Long-term survival after prehospital cardiac arrest: analysis of outcome during an 8 year study. Circulation 70:538, 1984.
18. Vlay SC, Reid PR, Griffith LSC, et al: Relationship of specific coronary lesions and regional left ventricular dysfunction to prognosis in survivors of sudden cardiac death. Am Heart J 108:1212, 1984.
19. Moosvi AR, Goldstein S, VanderBrug Medendorp S, et al: Effect of empiric antiarrhythmic therapy in resuscitated out-of-hospital cardiac arrest victims with coronary artery disease. Am J Cardiol 65:1192, 1990.
20. Goldstein S, Landis JR, Leighton R, et al: Predictive survival models for resuscitated victims of out-of-hospital cardiac arrest with coronary heart disease. Circulation 71:873, 1985.
21. Leclercq J-F, Coumel P, Denjoy I: Long-term follow-up after sustained monomorphic ventricular tachycardia: causes, pump failure, and empiric antiarrhythmic therapy that modify survival. Am Heart J 121:1685, 1991.
22. Willems AR, Tijssen JGP, van Capelle FJL, et al: Determinants of prognosis in symptomatic ventricular tachycardia or ventricular fibrillation late after myocardial infarction. J Am Coll Cardiol 16:521, 1990.
23. Goldstein S, Landis R, Leighton R, et al: Characteristics of the resuscitated out-of-hospital cardiac arrest victim with coronary artery disease. Circulation 64:977, 1981.
24. Winkle RA, Alderman EL, Fitzgerald JW, et al: Treatment of recurrent symptomatic ventricular tachycardia. Ann Intern Med 85:1, 1976.
25. Lown B, Graboys TB: Management of patients with malignant ventricular arrhythmias. Am J Cardiol 39:910, 1977.
26. Fasola AF, Noble RJ, Zipes DP: Treatment of recurrent ventricular tachycardia and fibrillation with aprindine. Am J Cardiol 39:903, 1977.
27. Morganroth J, Michelson EL, Horowitz LN, et al: Limitations of routine long-term electrocardiographic monitoring to assess

ventricular ectopic frequency. *Circulation* 58:408, 1978.
28. Lown B: Sudden cardiac death: the major challenge confronting contemporary cardiology. *Am J Cardiol* 43:313, 1979.
29. Lown B: Management of patients at high risk of sudden death. *Am Heart J* 103:689, 1982.
30. Graboys TB, Lown B, Podrid PJ, et al: Long-term survival of patients with malignant ventricular arrhythmia treated with antiarrhythmic drugs. *Am J Cardiol* 50:437, 1982.
31. The Flecainide-Quinidine Research Group: Flecainide versus quinidine for treatment of chronic ventricular arrhythmias: a multicenter clinical trial. *Circulation* 67:1117, 1983.
32. Chua W, Roth H, Summers C, et al: Programmed stimulation versus ambulatory monitoring for therapy of malignant arrhythmias (abstract). *Circulation* XX:III-55, 1983.
33. Podrid PJ, Lown B: Management of malignant ventricular arrhythmia—experience with lorcainide. *Am J Cardiol* 54:28B, 1984.
34. Stein J, Podrid PJ, Lampert S, et al: Long-term mexiletine for ventricular arrhythmia. *Am Heart J* 107:1091, 1984.
35. Vlay SC, Kallman CH, Reid PR: Prognostic assessment of survivors of ventricular tachycardia and ventricular fibrillation with ambulatory monitoring. *Am Heart J* 54: 87, 1984.
36. Ezri MD, Huang SK, Denes P: The role of Holter monitoring in patients with recurrent sustained ventricular tachycardia: an electrophysiologic correlation. *Am Heart J* 108:1229, 1984.
37. Platia EV, Reid PR: Comparison of programmed electrical stimulation and ambulatory electrocardiographic (Holter) monitoring in the management of ventricular tachycardia and ventricular fibrillation. *J Am Coll Cardiol* 4:493, 1984.
38. Swerdlow CD, Peterson J: Prospective comparison of Holter monitoring and electrophysiologic study in patients with coronary artery disease and sustained ventricular tachyarrhythmias. *Am J Cardiol* 56:577, 1985.
39. Kim SG, Seiden SW, Matos JA, et al: Discordance between ambulatory monitoring and programmed stimulation in assessing efficacy of Class Ia antiarrhythmic agents in patients with ventricular tachycardia. *J Am Coll Cardiol* 6:539, 1985.
40. Skale BT, Miles WM, Heger JJ, et al: Survivors of cardiac arrest: prevention of recurrence by drug therapy as predicted by electrophysiologic testing or electrocardiographic monitoring. *Am J Cardiol* 57:113, 1986.
41. Kim SG, Seiden SW, Felder SD, et al: Is programmed stimulation of value in predicting the long-term success of antiarrhythmic therapy for ventricular tachycardias? *N Engl J Med* 315:356, 1986.
42. Hohnloser SH, Lange HW, Raeder EA, et al: Short- and long-term therapy with tocainide for malignant ventricular tachyarrhythmias. *Circulation* 73:143, 1986.
43. Mitchell LB, Duff HJ, Manyari DE, et al: A randomized clinical trial of the noninvasive and invasive approaches to drug therapy of ventricular tachycardia. *N Engl J Med* 317: 1681, 1987.
44. Hohnloser SH, Raeder EA, Podrid PJ, et al: Predictors of antiarrhythmic drug efficacy in patients with malignant ventricular tachyarrhythmias. *Am Heart J* 114:1, 1987.
45. The ESVEM Investigators: The ESVEM trial: electrophysiologic study versus electrocardiographic monitoring for selection of antiarrhythmic therapy of ventricular tachyarrhythmias. *Circulation* 79:1354, 1989.
45a. Mason JW, Electrophysiologic Study versus Electrocardiographic Monitoring Investigators: A comparison of electrophysiologic testing with Holter monitoring to predict antiarrhythmic drug efficacy for ventricular tachyarrhythmias. *N Engl J Med* 329:445, 1993.
46. The ESVEM Investigators: Determinants of predicted efficacy of antiarrhythmic drugs in the electrophysiologic study versus electrocardiographic monitoring trial. *Circulation* 87:323, 1993.
47. Wellens HJ, Schuilenburg RM, Durrer D: Electrical stimulation of the heart in patients with ventricular tachycardia. *Circulation* 46:216, 1972.
48. Wellens HJJ, Lie KI, Durrer D: Further observations on ventricular tachycardia as studied by electrical stimulation of the heart: chronic recurrent ventricular tachycardia and ventricular tachycardia during acute myocardial infarction. *Circulation* 49: 647, 1974.
49. Denes P, Wu D, Dhingra C, et al: Electrophysiological studies in patients with chronic recurrent ventricular tachycardia. *Circulation* 54:229, 1976.
50. Wellens HJJ, Duren DR, Lie KI: Observations on mechanisms of ventricular tachycardia in man. *Circulation* 54:237, 1976.
51. Wu D, Wyndham CR, Denes P, et al: Chronic electrophysiological study in patients with recurrent paroxysmal tachycardia: a new method for developing success-

ful oral antiarrhythmic therapy. In: *Reentrant Arrhythmia: Mechanisms and Treatment.* Edited by HE Kulbertus. Lancaster, PA: MTP Press Limited; 1977, p. 294.
52. Hartzler GO, Maloney JD: Programmed ventricular stimulation in management of recurrent ventricular tachycardia. *Mayo Clin Proc* 52:731, 1977.
53. Fisher JD, Cohen HL, Mehra R, et al: Cardiac pacing and pacemakers II. Serial electrophysiologic-pharmacologic testing for control of recurrent tachyarrhythmias. *Am Heart J* 93:658, 1977.
54. Horowitz LN, Josephson ME, Farshidi A, et al: Recurrent sustained ventricular tachycardia 3. Role of the electrophysiologic study in selection of antiarrhythmic regimens. *Circulation* 58:986, 1978.
55. Mason JW, Winkle RA: Electrode-catheter arrhythmia induction in the selection and assessment of antiarrhythmic drug therapy for recurrent ventricular tachycardia. *Circulation* 58:971, 1978.
56. Josephson ME, Horowitz LN: Electrophysiologic approach to therapy of recurrent sustained ventricular tachycardia. *Am J Cardiol* 43:631, 1979.
57. Vandepol CJ, Farshidi A, Spielman SR, et al: Incidence and clinical significance of induced ventricular tachycardia. *Am J Cardiol* 45:725, 1980.
58. Josephson ME, Horowitz LN, Spielman SR, et al: Electrophysiologic and hemodynamic studies in patients resuscitated from cardiac arrest. *Am J Cardiol* 46:948, 1980.
59. Denes P, Wu D, Wyndham C, et al: Chronic longterm electrophysiologic study of paroxysmal ventricular tachycardia. *Chest* 77:478, 1980.
60. Ruskin JN, DiMarco JP, Garan H: Out-of-hospital cardiac arrest: electrophysiologic observations and selection of long-term antiarrhythmic therapy. *N Engl J Med* 303:607, 1980.
61. Myerburg RJ, Conde CA, Sung RJ, et al: Clinical, electrophysiologic and hemodynamic profile of patients resuscitated from prehospital cardiac arrest. *Am J Med* 68:568, 1980.
62. Mason JW, Winkle RA: Accuracy of the ventricular tachycardia-induction study for predicting long-term efficacy and inefficacy of antiarrhythmic drugs. *N Engl J Med* 303:1073, 1980.
63. Breithardt G, Abendroth RR, Loogen F: Serial electrophysiologic testing of antiarrhythmic drug efficacy in patients with recurrent ventricular tachycardia. *Eur Heart J* 1:11, 1980.
64. Herling IM, Horowitz LN, Josephson ME: Ventricular ectopic activity after medical and surgical treatment for recurrent sustained ventricular tachycardia. *Am J Cardiol* 45:633, 1980.
65. Horowitz LN, Spielman SR, Greenspan AM, et al: Role of programmed stimulation in assessing vulnerability to ventricular arrhythmias. *Am Heart J* 103:604, 1982.
66. Swiryn S, Bauernfeind RA, Strasberg B, et al: Prediction of response to class I antiarrhythmic drugs during electrophysiologic study of ventricular tachycardia. *Am Heart J* 104:43, 1982.
67. Livelli FD, Bigger JT Jr, Reiffel JA, et al: Response to programmed ventricular stimulation: sensitivity, specificity and relation to heart disease. *Am J Cardiol* 50:452, 1982.
68. Morady F, Hess D, Scheinman MM: Electrophysiologic drug testing in patients with malignant ventricular arrhythmias: importance of stimulation at more than one ventricular site. *Am J Cardiol* 50:1055, 1982.
69. Spielman SR, Schwartz JS, McCarthy DM, et al: Predictors of the success or failure of medical therapy in patients with chronic recurrent sustained ventricular tachycardia: a discriminant analysis.
70. Swerdlow CD, Gong G, Echt DS, et al: Clinical factors predicting successful electrophysiologic-pharmacologic study in patients with ventricular tachycardia. *J Am Coll Cardiol* 1:409, 1983.
71. Benditt DG, Benson W Jr, Klein GJ, et al: Prevention of recurrent sudden cardiac arrest: role of provocative electropharmacologic testing. *J Am Coll Cardiol* 2:418, 1983.
72. Swerdlow CD, Winkle RA, Mason JW: Determinants of survival in patients with ventricular tachyarrhythmias. *N Engl J Med* 308:1436, 1983.
73. Morady F, Scheinman MM, Hess DS, et al: Electrophysiologic testing in the management of survivors of out-of-hospital cardiac arrest. *Am J Cardiol* 51:85, 1983.
74. Ruskin JN, Schoenfeld MH, Garan H: Role of electrophysiologic techniques in the selection of antiarrhythmic drug regimens for ventricular arrhythmias. *Am J Cardiol* 52:41C, 1983.
75. Mann DE, Luck JC, Griffin JC, et al: Induction of clinical ventricular tachycardia using programmed stimulation: value of third and fourth extrastimuli. *Am J Cardiol* 52:501, 1983.
76. Doherty JU, Kienzle MG, Waxman HL, et al: Programmed ventricular stimulation at a second right ventricular site: an analysis of 100 patients, with special reference to sensitivity, specificity and characteristics of

patients with induced ventricular tachycardia. *Am J Cardiol* 52:1184, 1983.
77. Roy D, Waxman HL, Kienzle MG, et al: Clinical characteristics and long-term follow-up in 119 survivors of cardiac arrest: relation to inducibility at electrophysiologic testing. *Am J Cardiol* 52:969, 1983.
78. Mason JW, Swerdlow CD, Winkle RA, et al: Ventricular tachyarrhythmia induction for drug selection: experience with 311 patients. In: *Clinical Pharmacology of Antiarrhythmic Therapy*. Edited by BR Lucchesi, JV Dingell, RP Schwarz Jr. New York, NY: Raven Press; 1984, p. 229.
79. Brugada P, Green M, Abdollah H, et al: Significance of ventricular arrhythmia initiated by programmed ventricular stimulation: the importance of the type of ventricular arrhythmia induced and the number of premature stimuli required. *Circulation* 69:87, 1984.
80. Buxton AE, Waxman HL, Marchlinski FE, et al: Role of triple extrastimuli during electrophysiologic study of patients with documented sustained ventricular tachyarrhythmias. *Circulation* 69:532, 1984.
81. Raviele A, Di Pede F, Delise P, et al: Value of serial electropharmacological testing in managing patients resuscitated from cardiac arrest. *PACE* 7:850, 1984.
82. Morady F, DiCarlo L, Winston S, et al: A prospective comparison of triple extrastimuli and left ventricular stimulation in studies of ventricular tachycardia induction. *Circulation* 70:52, 1984.
83. Stevenson WG, Brugada P, Waldecker B, et al: Clinical, angiographic, and electrocardiographic findings in patients with aborted sudden death as compared with patients with sustained ventricular tachycardia after myocardial infarction. *Circulation* 71:1146, 1985.
84. Rae AP, Greenspan AM, Spielman SR, et al: Antiarrhythmic drug efficacy for ventricular tachyarrhythmias associated with coronary artery disease as assessed by electrophysiologic studies. *Am J Cardiol* 55:1494, 1985.
85. Shoenfeld MH, McGovern B, Garan H, et al: Determinants of the outcome of electrophysiologic study in patients with ventricular tachyarrhythmias. *J Am Coll Cardiol* 6:298, 1985.
86. Waller TJ, Kay HR, Spielman SR, et al: Reduction in sudden death and total mortality by antiarrhythmic therapy evaluated by electrophysiologic drug testing: criteria of efficacy in patients with sustained ventricular tachyarrhythmia. *J Am Coll Cardiol* 10:83, 1987.
87. Pratt CM, Thornton BC, Magro SA, et al: Spontaneous arrhythmia detected on ambulatory electrocardiographic recording lacks precision in predicting inducibility of ventricular tachycardia during electrophysiologic study. *J Am Coll Cardiol* 10:97, 1987.
88. Swerdlow CD, Bardy GH, McAnulty, et al: Determinants of induced sustained arrhythmias in survivors of out-of-hospital ventricular fibrillation. *Circulation* 76:1053, 1987.
89. Eldar M, Sauve MJ, Scheinman MM: Electrophysiologic testing and follow-up of patients with aborted sudden death. *J Am Coll Cardiol* 10:291, 1987.
90. Wilber DJ, Garan H, Finkelstein D, et al: Out-of-hospital cardiac arrest: use of electrophysiologic testing in the prediction of long-term outcome. *N Engl J Med* 318:19, 1988.
91. Freedman RA, Swerdlow CD, Soderholm-Difatte V, et al: Clinical predictors of arrhythmia inducibility in survivors of cardiac arrest: importance of gender and prior myocardial infarction. *J Am Coll Cardiol* 12:973, 1988.
92. Kuchar DL, Rottman J, Berger E, et al: Prediction of successful suppression of sustained ventricular tachyarrhythmias by serial drug testing from data derived at the initial electrophysiologic study. *J Am Coll Cardiol* 12:982, 1988.
93. Kehoe R, Tommaso C, Zheutlin T, et al: Factors determining programmed stimulation responses and long-term arrhythmic outcome in survivors of ventricular fibrillation with ischemic heart disease. *Am Heart J* 116:355, 1988.
94. Borggrefe M, Trampisch H-J, Breithardt G: Reappraisal of criteria for assessing drug efficacy in patients with ventricular tachyarrhythmias: complete versus partial suppression in inducible arrhythmias. *J Am Coll Cardiol* 12:140, 1988.
95. Hays LJ, Lerman BB, DiMarco JP: Nonventricular arrhythmias as precursors of ventricular fibrillation in patients with out-of-hospital cardiac arrest. *Am Heart J* 118:53, 1989.
96. Poole JE, Mathisen TL, Kudenchuk PJ, et al: Long-term outcome in patients who survive out of hospital ventricular fibrillation and undergo electrophysiologic studies: evaluation by electrophysiologic subgroups. *J Am Coll Cardiol* 16:657, 1990.
97. Kavanagh KM, Wyse DG, Duff HJ, et al: Drug therapy for ventricular tachyarrhythmias: how many electropharmacologic trials are appropriate? *J Am Coll Cardiol* 17:391, 1991.

98. Fogoros RN, Elson JJ, Bonnet CA, et al: Long-term outcome of survivors of cardiac arrest whose therapy is guided by electrophysiologic testing. *J Am Coll Cardiol* 19:780, 1992.
99. Waldo AL, Akhtar M, Brugada P, et al: NASPE policy statement: the minimally appropriate electrophysiologic study for the initial assessment of patients with documented sustained monomorphic ventricular tachyardia. *PACE* 8:918, 1985.
100. Podrid PJ, Schoeneberger A, Lown B, et al: Use of nonsustained ventricular tachycardia as a guide to antiarrhythmic drug therapy in patients with malignant ventricular arrhythmia. *Am Heart J* 105:181, 1983.
101. Buxton AE, Waxman HL, Marchlinski FE, et al: Electropharmacology of nonsustained ventricular tachycardia: effects of Class I antiarrhythmic agents, verapamil and propranolol. *Am J Cardiol* 53:738, 1984.
102. Mitchell LB, Wyse DG, Duff HJ: Programmed electrical stimulation studies for ventricular tachycardia in man: I. The role of functional refractoriness in tachycardia induction. *J Am Coll Cardiol* 8:567, 1986.
103. Robertson JF, Cain ME, Horowitz LN, et al: Anatomic and electrophysiologic correlates of ventricular tachycardia requiring left ventricular stimulation. *Am J Cardiol* 48:263, 1981.
104. Freedman RA, Swerdlow CD, Echt DS, et al: Facilitation of ventricular tachyarrhythmia induction by isoproterenol. *Am J Cardiol* 54:765, 1984.
105. Cooper MJ, Koo CC, Skinner MP, et al: Comparison of immediate versus day to day variability of ventricular tachycardia induction by programmed stimulation. *J Am Coll Cardiol* 13:1599, 1989.
106. Jazayeri MR, VanWyhe G, Avitall B, et al: Isoproterenol reversal of antiarrhythmic effects in patients with inducible sustained ventricular arrhythmias. *J Am Coll Cardiol* 14:705, 1989.
107. Swerdlow CD, Blum J, Winkle RA, et al: Decreased incidence of antiarrhythmic drug efficacy at electrophysiologic study associated with the use of a third extrastimulus. *Am Heart J* 104:1004, 1982.
108. Gillis AM, Wyse DG, Duff HJ, et al: Drug response at electropharmacologic study in patients with ventricular tachyarrhythmias: the importance of ventricular refractoriness. *J Am Coll Cardiol* 17:914, 1991.
109. Vastesaeger M, Guillot P, Rasson G: Etude clinique d'une nouvelle medication antiangoreuse. *Acta Cardiol (Brux)* 22:483, 1967.
110. Zelvelder WG: Investigation of the therapeutic activity of amiodarone (Cordarone) in the treatment of angina pectoris. *Eur J Clin Pharmacol* 3:158, 1971.
111. Charlier R, Delaunois G, Bauthier J, et al: Recherches dans la serie des benzofuranes. XL. Properties antiarrhythmiques de l'amiodarone. *Cardiologia* 54:82, 1969.
112. Singh BN, Vaughan Williams EM: The effect of amiodarone, a new antianginal drug, on cardiac muscle. *Br J Pharmacol* 39:657, 1970.
113. Olsson SB, Brorson L, Varnauskas E: Class 3 antiarrhythmic action in man. Observations from monophasic action potential recordings and amiodarone treatment. *Br Heart J* 35:1255, 1973.
114. Van Schepdael J, Solvay H: Etude clinique de l'amiodarone dans les troubles du rythme cardiaque. *Presse Med* 78:1849, 1970.
115. Fraquet J, Nivet M, Grosgogeat Y, et al: L'influence de l'amiodaone sur le rythme cardiaque et l'electrocardiogramme. *Therapie* 25:335, 1970.
116. Vastesaeger M, Guillot P, Van Der Straeten P: L'effet antiarythmique de l'amiodarone. *Brux Med* 51:99, 1971.
117. Coumel P, Bouvrain Y: Etude clinique des effets pharmacodynamiques et antiarythmiques de l'amiodarone. *J Agrege* 6:69, 1973.
118. Rosenbaum MB, Chiale PA, Ryba D, et al: Control of tachyarrhythmias associated with Wolff-Parkinson-White syndrome by amiodarone hydrochloride. *Am J Cardiol* 34:215, 1974.
119. Rosenbaum MB, Chiale PA, Halpern MS, et al: Clinical efficacy of amiodarone as an antiarrhythmic agent. *Am J Cardiol* 38:934, 1976.
120. Leak D, Eydt JN: Control of refractory cardiac arrhythmias with amiodarone. *Arch Intern Med* 139:425, 1979.
121. Heger JJ, Prystowski EN, Jackman WM, et al: Clinical efficacy and electrophysiology during long-term therapy for recurrent ventricular tachycardia or ventricular fibrillation. *N Engl J Med* 305:539, 1981.
122. Kaski JC, Girotti LA, Messuti H, et al: Long-term management of sustained, recurrent, symptomatic ventricular tachycardia with amiodarone. *Circulation* 64:273, 1981.
123. Hamer AW, Finerman WB Jr, Peter T: Disparity between the clinical and electrophysiologic effects of amiodarone in the treatment of recurrent ventricular tachyarrhythmias. *Am Heart J* 102:992, 1981.
124. Podrid PJ, Lown B: Amiodarone therapy in symptomatic sustained refractory atrial and ventricular tachyarrhythmias. *Am Heart J* 101:374, 1981.
125. Nademanee K, Hendrickson JA, Cannom DS, et al: Control of refractory life-threaten-

ing ventricular tachyarrhythmias by amiodarone. *Am Heart J* 101:759, 1981.
126. Nademanee K, Hendrickson J, Kannan R, et al: Antiarrhythmic efficacy and electrophysiologic actions of amiodarone in patients with life-threatening ventricular arrhythmias: potent suppression of spontaneously occurring tachyarrhythmias versus inconsistent abolition of induced ventricular tachycardia. *Am Heart J* 103:950, 1982.
127. Waxman HL, Groh WC, Marchlinski FE, et al: Amiodarone for control of sustained ventricular tachyarrhythmia: clinical and electrophysiologic effects in 51 patients. *Am J Cardiol* 50:1066, 1982.
128. Nademanee K, Singh BN, Hendrickson JA, et al: Pharmacokinetic significance of serum reverse T3 levels during amiodarone treatment: a potential method for monitoring chronic drug therapy. *Circulation* 66:202, 1982.
129. Haffajee CI, Love JC, Canada AT, et al: Clinical pharmacokinetics and efficacy of amiodarone for refractory tachyarrhythmias. *Circulation* 67:1347, 1983.
130. Fogoros RN, Anderson KP, Winkle RA, et al: Amiodarone: clinical efficacy and toxicity in 96 patients with recurrent, drug-refractory arrhythmias. *Circulation* 68:88, 1983.
131. Horowitz LN, Spielman SR, Greenspan AM, et al: Ventricular arrhythmias: use of electrophysiologic studies. *Am Heart J* 106:881, 1983.
132. Heger JJ, Prystowski EN, Zipes DP: Clinical efficacy of amiodarone in treatment of recurrent ventricular tachycardia and ventricular fibrillation. *Am Heart J* 106:887, 1983.
133. Haffajee CI, Love JC, Alpert JS: Efficacy and safety of long-term amiodarone in treatment of cardiac arrhythmias: dosage experience. *Am Heart J* 106:935, 1983.
134. Peter T, Hamer A, Mandel WJ, et al: Evaluation of amiodarone therapy in the treatment of drug-resistant cardiac arrhythmias: long-term follow-up. *Am Heart J* 106:943, 1983.
135. Greene HL, Graham EL, Werner JA, et al: Toxic and therapeutic effects of amiodarone in the treatment of cardiac arrhythmias. *J Am Coll Cardiol* 2:1114, 1983.
136. Morady F, Scheinman MM, Hess DA: Amiodarone in the management of patients with ventricular tachycardia and ventricular fibrillation. *PACE* 6:609, 1983.
137. Nademanee K, Singh BN, Hendrickson J, et al: Amiodarone in refractory life-threatening ventricular arrhythmias. *Ann Intern Med* 98:577, 1983.
138. Waxman HL: The efficacy of amiodarone for ventricular arrhythmias cannot be predicted with clinical electrophysiological studies. *Int J Cardiol* 3:76, 1983.
139. Morady F, Sauve MJ, Malone P, et al: Long-term efficacy and toxicity of high dose amiodarone therapy for ventricular tachycardia or ventricular fibrillation. *Am J Cardiol* 52:975, 1983.
140. Hamer AWF, Mandel WJ, Zaher CA, et al: The electrophysiologic basis for the use of amiodarone for treatment of cardiac arrhythmias. *PACE* 6:784, 1983.
141. Nademanee K, Singh BN, Cannom DS, et al: Control of sudden recurrent arrhythmic deaths: role of amiodarone. *Am Heart J* 106:895, 1983.
142. McGovern B, Garan H, Malacoff RF, et al: Long-term clinical outcome of ventricular tachycardia or fibrillation treated with amiodarone. *Am J Cardiol* 53:1558, 1984.
143. Saksena S, Rothbart S, Shah Y, et al: Clinical efficacy and electropharmacology of continuous intravenous amiodarone infusion and chronic oral amiodarone in refractory ventricular tachycardia. *Am J Cardiol* 54:347, 1984.
144. Reddy CP, Kuo CS, Jivrajka V: Effect of amiodarone on electric induction, morphology, and rate of ventricular tachycardia and its relation to clinical efficacy. *PACE* 7:1055, 1984.
145. Kaski JC, Girotti LA, Elizari MV, et al: Efficacy of amiodarone during long-term treatment of potentially dangerous ventricular arrhythmias in patients with chronic stable ischemic heart disease. *Am Heart J* 107:648, 1984.
146. Collaborative Group for Amiodarone Evaluation: Multicenter controlled observation of a low-dose regimen of amiodarone for treatment of severe ventricular arrhythmias. *Am J Cardiol* 53:1564, 1984.
147. McKenna WJ, Krikler DM: Clinical evaluation of the efficacy of oral amiodarone. *Br Heart J* 51:241, 1984.
148. Debbas NMG, DuCailar C, Bexton RS, et al: The QT interval: a predictor of the plasma and myocardial concentrations of amiodarone. *Br Heart J* 51:316, 1984.
149. Wellens HJJ, Brugada P, Abdollah H, et al: A comparison of the electrophysiologic effects of intravenous and oral amiodarone in the same patient. *Circulation* 69:120, 1984.
150. Sanmarti A, Permanyer-Miralda G, Castellanos JM, et al: Chronic administration of amiodarone and thyroid function: a follow-up study. *Am Heart J* 108:1262, 1984.
151. DiCarlo LA, Morady F, Sauve MJ, et al: Cardiac arrest and sudden death in patients treated with amiodarone for sustained ventricular tachycardia or ventricular fibrilla-

tion: risk stratification based on clinical variables. *Am J Cardiol* 55:372, 1985.
152. Veltri EP, Reid PR, Platia EV, et al: Results of late programmed electrical stimulation and long-term electrophysiologic effects of amiodarone therapy in patients with refractory ventricular tachycardia. *Am J Cardiol* 55:375, 1985.
153. Horowitz LN, Greenspan AM, Spielman SR, et al: Usefulness of electrophysiologic testing in evaluation of amiodarone therapy for sustained ventricular tachyarrhythmias associated with coronary heart disease. *Am J Cardiol* 55:367, 1985.
154. Veltri EP, Reid PR, Platia EV, et al: Amiodarone in the treatment of life-threatening ventricular tachycardia: role of Holter monitoring in predicting long-term clinical efficacy. *J Am Coll Cardiol* 6:806, 1985.
155. Marchlinski FE, Buxton AE, Flores BT, et al: Value of Holter monitoring in identifying risk for sustained ventricular arrhythmia recurrence on amiodarone. *Am J Cardiol* 55:709, 1985.
156. Naccarelli GV, Fineberg NS, Zipes DP, et al: Amiodarone: risk factors for recurrence of symptomatic tachycardia identified at electrophysiologic study. *J Am Coll Cardiol* 6:814, 1985.
157. Sokoloff NM, Spielman SR, Greenspan AM, et al: Utility of ambulatory electrocardiographic monitoring for predicting recurrence of sustained ventricular tachyarrhythmias in patients receiving amiodarone. *J Am Coll Cardiol* 7:938, 1986.
158. Smith WM, Lubbe WF, Whitlock RM, et al: Long-term tolerance of amiodarone treatment for cardiac arrhythmias. *Am J Cardiol* 57:1288, 1986.
159. Veltri EP, Griffith LSC, Platia EV, et al: The use of ambulatory monitoring in the prognostic evaluation of patients with sustained tachycardia treated with amiodarone. *Circulation* 74:1054, 1986.
160. Kadish AH, Marchlinski FE, Josephson ME, et al: Amiodarone: correlation of early and late electrophysiologic studies with outcome. *Am Heart J* 112:1134, 1986.
161. Lavery D, Saksena S: Management of refractory sustained ventricular tachycardia with amiodarone: a reappraisal. *Am Heart J* 113:49, 1987.
162. Kim S, Felder SD, Figure I, et al: Value of Holter monitoring in predicting long-term efficacy and inefficacy of amiodarone used alone and in combination with class Ia antiarrhythmic agents in patients with ventricular tachycardia. *J Am Coll Cardiol* 9:169, 1987.
163. DiCarlo LA, Morady F, de Buitleir M, et al: Effects of chronic amiodarone therapy on ventricular tachycardia induced by programmed ventricular stimulation. *Am Heart J* 113:57, 1987.
164. Kadish AH, Buxton AE, Waxman HL, et al: Usefulness of electrophysiologic study to determine the clinical tolerance of arrhythmia recurrences during amiodarone therapy. *J Am Coll Cardiol* 10:90, 1987.
165. Yazaki Y, Haffajee, Gold RL, et al: Electrophysiologic predictors of long-term clinical outcome with amiodarone for refractory ventricular tachycardia secondary to coronary artery disease. *Am J Cardiol* 60:293, 1987.
166. Schmitt C, Brachmann J, Waldecker B, et al: Amiodarone in patients with recurrent sustained ventricular tachyarrhythmias: results of programmed electrical stimulation and long-term clinical outcome in chronic treatment. *Am Heart J* 114:279, 1987.
167. Zhu J, Haines DE, Lerman BB, et al: Predictors of efficacy of amiodarone and characteristics of recurrence or arrhythmia in patients with sustained ventricular tachycardia and coronary artery disease. *Circulation* 76:802, 1987.
168. Greenspon AJ, Volosin KJ, Greenber RM, et al: Amiodarone therapy: role of early and late electrophysiologic studies. *J Am Coll Cardiol* 11:117, 1988.
169. Klein LS, Fineberg N, Heger JJ, et al: Prospective evaluation of a discriminant function for prediction of recurrent symptomatic ventricular tachycardia or ventricular fibrillation in coronary artery disease patients receiving amiodarone and having inducible ventricular tachycardia at electrophysiologic study. *Am J Cardiol* 61:1024, 1988.
170. Herre JM, Sauve MJ, Malone P, et al: Long-term results of amiodarone therapy in patients with recurrent sustained ventricular tachycardia or ventricular fibrillation. *J Am Coll Cardiol* 13:442, 1989.
171. Myers M, Peter T, Weiss D, et al: Benefits and risks of long-term amiodarone therapy for sustained ventricular tachycardia/fibrillation: minimum of three-year follow-up. *Am Heart J* 119:8, 1990.
172. Evans SJL, Myers M, Zaher C, et al: High dose oral amiodarone loading: electrophysiologic effects and clinical tolerance. *J Am Coll Cardiol* 19:169, 1992.
173. Weinberg BA, Miles WM, Klein LS, et al: Five-year follow-up of 589 patients treated with amiodarone. *Am Heart J* 125:109, 1993.
174. Harris L, McKenna WJ, Rowland E, et al: Side effects and possible contraindications

of amiodarone use. *Am Heart J* 106:906, 1983.
175. Rakita L, Sobol SM, Mostow N, et al: Amiodarone pulmonary toxicity. *Am Heart J* 106:906, 1983.
176. Rotmensch HH, Belhassen B, Swanson BN, et al: Steady-state serum amiodarone concentrations: relationships with antiarrhythmic efficacy and toxicity. *Ann Intern Med* 101:462, 1984.
177. Raeder EA, Podrid PJ, Lown B: Side effects and complications of amiodarone therapy. *Am Heart J* 109:975, 1985.
178. Falik R, Flores BT, Shaw L, et al: Relationship of steady-state serum concentrations of amiodarone and desethylamiodarone to therapeutic efficacy and adverse effects. *Am J Med* 82:1102, 1987.
179. Greenberg ML, Lerman BB, Shipe JR, et al: Relation between amiodarone and desethylamiodarone plasma concentrations and electrophysiologic effects, efficacy and toxicity. *J Am Coll Cardiol* 9:1148, 1987.
180. Mason JW: Amiodarone. *N Engl J Med* 316:455, 1987.
181. Singh BN, Nademanee K: Amiodarone and thyroid function: clinical implications during antiarrhythmic therapy. *Am Heart J* 106:857, 1983.
182. Kanna R, Nademanee K, Hendrickson J, et al: Amiodarone kinetics after oral dosages. *Clin Pharmacol Ther* 31:438, 1982.
183. Holt DW, Tucker GT, Jackson PR, et al: Amiodarone pharmacokinetics. *Am Heart J* 106:840, 1983.
184. Staubli M, Bircher J, Galeazzi RL, et al: Serum concentrations of amiodarone during long-term therapy: relation to dose, efficacy and toxicity. *Eur J Clin Pharmacol* 24:485, 1983.
185. Rakita L, Sobol SM: Amiodarone in the treatment of refractory ventricular arrhythmias: importance and safety of initial high-dose therapy. *JAMA* 250:1293, 1982.
186. Siddoway LA, McAllister CB, Wilkinson GR, et al: Amiodarone dosing: A proposal based on its pharmacokinetics. *Am Heart J* 106:951, 1983.
187. Connolly SJ, Gupta RN, Hoffert D, et al: Concentration response relationships of amiodarone and desethylamiodarone. *Am Heart J* 115:1208, 1988.
188. Kennedy EE, Rosenfeld LE, McPherson C, et al: Evaluation by serial electrophysiologic studies of an abbreviated oral loading regimen of amiodarone. *Am J Cardiol* 56:867, 1985.
189. Mitchell LB, Wyse DG, Gillis AM, et al: Electropharmacology of amiodarone therapy initiation: time courses of onset of electrophysiologic and antiarrhythmic effects. *Circulation* 80:34, 1989.
190. Yabek SM, Kato R, Singh BN: Effects of amiodarone and its metabolite, desethylamiodarone, on the electrophysiologic properties of isolated cardiac muscle. *J Cardiovasc Pharmacol* 8:197, 1986.
191. Nattel S: Pharmacodynamic studies of amiodarone and its active N-desethyl metabolite. *J Cardiovasc Pharmacol* 8:771, 1986.
192. Talajic M, DeRoode MR, Nattel S: Comparative electrophysiologic effects of intravenous amiodarone and desethylamiodarone in dogs: evidence for clinically relevant activity of the metabolite. *Circulation* 75:265, 1987.
193. Wilkinson PR, Rees JR, Storey GCA, et al: Amiodarone: prolonged elimination following cessation of chronic therapy. *Am Heart J* 107:787, 1984.
194. Stock JPP, Dale N: Beta-adrenergic receptor blockade in cardiac arrhythmias. *Br Med J* 2:1230, 1963.
195. Zipes DP, Festoff B, Schaal SF, et al: Treatment of ventricular arrhythmia by permanent atrial pacemaker and cardiac sympathectomy. *Ann Intern Med* 68:591, 1968.
196. Wasir HS, Mahapatra RK, Bhatia ML, et al: Metoprolol—a new cardioselective beta-adrenoceptor blocking agent for treatment of tachyarrhythmias. *Br Heart J* 39:834, 1977.
197. Winkle RA, Lopes MG, Goodman DJ, et al: Propranolol for patients with mitral valve prolapse. *Am Heart J* 93:422, 1977.
198. Wu D, Kou HC, Hung JS: Exercise-triggered paroxysmal ventricular tachycardia. *Ann Intern Med* 95:410, 1981.
199. Palileo EV, Ashley WW, Swiryn S, et al: Exercise provocable right ventricular outflow tract tachycardia. *Am Heart J* 104:185, 1982.
200. Sung RJ, Olukotun AY, Baird CL, et al: Efficacy and safety of oral nadolol for exercise-induced ventricular arrhythmias. *Am J Cardiol* 60:15D, 1987.
201. Ryden L, Ariniego R, Arnmank, et al: A double-blind trial of metoprolol in acute myocardial infarction: effects on ventricular tachyarrhythmias. *N Engl J Med* 308:614, 1983.
202. Moss AJ, Schwartz PJ, Crampton RS, et al: The long QT syndrome: a prospective international study. *Circulation* 71:17, 1985.
203. Buxton AE, Waxman HL, Marchlinski FE, et al: Right ventricular tachycardia: clinical and electrophysiologic characteristics. *Circulation* 68:917, 1983.
204. Brodsky MA, Sato DA, Allen BJ, et al: Solitary beta-blocker therapy for idiopathic life-threatening ventricular tachyarrhythmias. *Chest* 89:790, 1986.

205. Venditti FJ, Garan H, Ruskin JN: Electrophysiologic effects of beta blockers in ventricular arrhythmias. *Am J Cardiol* 60:3D, 1987.
206. Woosley RL, Kornhauser D, Smith R, et al: Suppression of chronic ventricular arrhythmias with propranolol. *Circulation* 60:819, 1979.
207. Podrid PJ, Lown B: Pindolol for ventricular arrhythmia. *Am Heart J* 104:491, 1982.
208. Brodsky MA, Allen BJ, Bessen M, et al: Beta-blocker therapy in patients with ventricular tachyarrhythmias in the setting of left ventricular dysfunction. *Am Heart J* 115:799, 1988.
209. Brodsky MA, Allen BJ, Luckett CR, et al: Antiarrhythmic efficacy of solitary beta-adrenergic blockade for patients with sustained ventricular tachyarrhythmias. *Am Heart J* 118:272, 1989.
210. Duff HJ, Mitchell LB, Wyse DG: Antiarrhythmic efficacy of propranolol: comparison of low and high serum concentrations. *J Am Coll Cardiol* 8:959, 1986.
211. Huikuri HV, Cox M, Interian A Jr, et al: Efficacy of intravenous propranolol for suppression of inducibility of ventricular tachyarrhythmias with different electrophysiologic characteristics in coronary artery disease. *Am J Cardiol* 64:1305, 1989.
212. Leclercq J-F, Leenhardt A, Lemarec H, et al: Predictive value of electrophysiologic studies during treatment of ventricular tachycardia with the beta-blocking agent nadolol. *J Am Coll Cardiol* 16:413, 1990.
213. Korte DW Jr, Nash CB: Ventricular electrophysiology of quinidine-propranolol combinations in the dog heart. *J Pharmacol Exp Ther* 197:452, 1976.
214. Leahey EB Jr, Heissenbuttel RH, Giardina EGV, et al: Combined mexiletine and propranolol treatment of refractory ventricular tachycardia. *Br Med J* 281:357, 1980.
215. Hirsowitz G, Podrid PJ, Lampert S, et al: The role of beta blocking agents as adjunct therapy to membrane stabilizing drugs in malignant ventricular arrhythmia. *Am Heart J* 111:852, 1986.
216. Deedwania PC, Olukotun AY, Kupersmith J, et al: Beta blockers in combination with Class I antiarrhythmic agents. *Am J Cardiol* 60:21D, 1987.
217. Steinbeck G, Andresen D, Bach P, et al: A comparison of electrophysiologically guided antiarrhythmic drug therapy with beta-blocker therapy in patients with symptomatic, sustained ventricular tachyarrhythmias. *N Engl J Med* 327:987, 1992.
218. Multicenter International Study: Reduction in mortality after myocardial infarction with long term beta-adrenergic receptor blockade. *Br Med J* 2:419, 1977.
219. The Norwegian Multicenter Study Group: Timolol-induced reduction in mortality and reinfarction in patients surviving acute myocardial infarction. *N Engl J Med* 304:801, 1981.
220. Hjalmarson A, Herlitz J, Malek T, et al: Effect on mortality of metoprolol in acute myocardial infarction. *Lancet* 2:823, 1981.
221. Julian DG, Prescott RJ, Jackson FS, et al: Controlled trial of sotalol for one year after myocardial infarction. *Lancet* 1:1142, 1982.
222. Beta-Blocker Heart Attack Study Group: A randomized trial of propranolol in patients with acute myocardial infarction. II. Mortality results. *JAMA* 247:1707, 1982.
223. Lichstein E, Morganroth J, Harriet R, et al: Effect of propranolol on ventricular arrhythmias. The beta-blocker heart attack trial experience. *Circulation* 67(Suppl I):5, 1983.
224. The CASCADE Investigators: Cardiac arrest in Seattle: conventional versus amiodarone drug evaluation (the CASCADE study). *Am J Cardiol* 67:578, 1991.
225. The CASCADE Investigators: Randomized antiarrhythmic drug therapy in survivors of cardiac arrest (The CASCADE Study). *Am J Cardiol* 72:280, 1993.

Chapter 29

Surgical Treatment of Ventricular Tachycardia Associated With Coronary Artery Disease

Gerard M. Guiraudon, George J. Klein, Raymond Yee, and R.K. Thakur

Ventricular arrhythmias associated with coronary artery disease are the leading cause of death in North America,[1] and extensive coronary artery disease is the most prevalent finding in patients with sudden cardiac death. Surgical treatment of ventricular tachycardias (VTs) is part of the nonpharmacological electrophysiologic intervention for ventricular arrhythmias. Electrophysiologic interventions include: antitachycardia devices and implantable cardioverter-defibrillators (ICDs),[2,3] ventricular myocardial catheter ablation,[4–6] intracoronary catheter ablation (using ethanol),[7] and surgical interventions.[8–11]

Surgical interventions are multiple and can include a direct surgical approach to the anatomical arrhythmogenic substrate,[8–11] essentially the infarct scar and adjunct revascularization (coronary artery bypass grafting).[12] Surgical therapy is defined by the way the therapy is delivered, not by the therapy itself; therefore, ICD implantation is not classified as a surgical therapy, although implantation still requires a surgical approach.

Open heart cardiac surgery is still associated with significant mortality and morbidity. Most of the surgical risk is associated with ancillary surgical techniques, ie, cardiac exposure (median sternotomy, cardiopulmonary bypass techniques, cardioplegic cardiac arrest). Each adjunct has inherent mortality and morbidity.[13] A ventriculotomy is usually required for approaching the anatomical arrhythmogenic substrate and is also associated with inherent mortality and morbidity.

Because of inherent severe side effects, the surgical treatment of VT is considered only in selected patients. Stringent criteria are applied—stringent exclusion criteria to avoid mortality as well as stringent inclusion criteria to obtain high efficacy. Successful surgical ablation can provide long-term control associated with excellent functional capacity and quality of life. Surgical ablation should be the preferred intervention when feasible.

Definition of Terms

Cardiac arrhythmias are currently classified according to the site of their arrhyth-

---

Supported by the Heart and Stroke Foundation of Ontario.

From Singer I, (ed.) Implantable Cardioverter-Defibrillator. Armonk, NY: Futura Publishing Company, Inc.; © 1994.

mogenic substrate. Accordingly, five varieties of cardiac arrhythmia are described: atrial tachycardia, atrioventricular (AV) nodal reentrant tachycardia, His bundle tachycardia, ventricular arrhythmias, and AV reentrant tachycardias (preexcitation syndrome), which requires the presence of an accessory AV connection (Kent bundle).[14]

The Anatomical Arrhythmogenic Substrate

The anatomical arrhythmogenic substrate is the anatomical site of the mechanism of the arrhythmia. It can be discrete or poorly delineated, and it can be associated or not with overt pathology. In general, the anatomical substrate is confined to the part of the myocardium that harbors the obligatory segment of the working mechanism—essentially reentry. It usually does not include the entire circuit.

Electrocardiographic Presentations

Electrocardiographic presentations of ventricular arrhythmias are protean. Premature ventricular complex (PVC) is a premature activation originating in the ventricles. Premature ventricular contractions may be single or multiple, and uniform or multiform. Ventricular tachycardia is defined as a series of three or more ventricular complexes at a rate > 100 beats per minute (cycle length 600 msec). Ventricular tachycardia can be nonsustained, lasting < 30 seconds and self-terminating, or sustained lasting > 30 seconds or requiring "immediate" cardioversion because of associated hemodynamic collapse (hemodynamically significant VTs). Ventricular complexes are generally uniform, although a single patient may have multiple bouts of uniform VT with significant differences among attacks.

Ventricular tachycardia with polymorphic complexes is associated with a faster heart rate, generally > 200 beats per minute (cycle length 300 msec). Ventricular flutter is arbitrarily defined as an uninterrupted series of QRS complexes without intercalated isoelectric segments of a rate > 250 beats per minute (cycle length 240 msec).

Ventricular fibrillation is associated with chaotic ventricular depolarization with undulating irregular recordings on the surface ECG. Ventricular fibrillation is rarely self-terminating. Ventricular fibrillation can be "primary," not preceded by or "secondary" to VT.

Torsades de pointes are a subgroup of nonsustained polymorphic VT characterized by a QRS pattern that undulates and appears to rotate (torsade) around the isoelectric line.

Clinical Presentation

Premature ventricular complexes may be associated with palpitations, skipped beats, or dyspnea. Ventricular tachycardias have sudden onset and sudden termination. Their clinical characteristics fall into two patterns: patients with sustained monomorphic VTs that are hemodynamically well tolerated or patients with syncope or cardiac arrest associated with primary or secondary ventricular fibrillation and/or sustained monomorphic or polymorphic VTs.

Mechanism of Ventricular Tachycardia

Current concepts of the mechanisms of VT include reentry, abnormal, or enhanced automaticity and triggered automaticity. Most clinical VT after myocardial infarction are inducible by programmed electrical stimulation and are due to a macroreentrant circuit. Inducible VT can be studied "reliably" and "reproducibly" in the electrophysiology laboratory and in the operating room. Noninducible VTs are elusive and difficult to assess. Surgery for VTs in the presence of coronary artery disease comprises two approaches—a direct approach to the tachycardia substrate (direct ablative surgery; Figure 1), and an indirect approach (coronary artery bypass grafting). These ap-

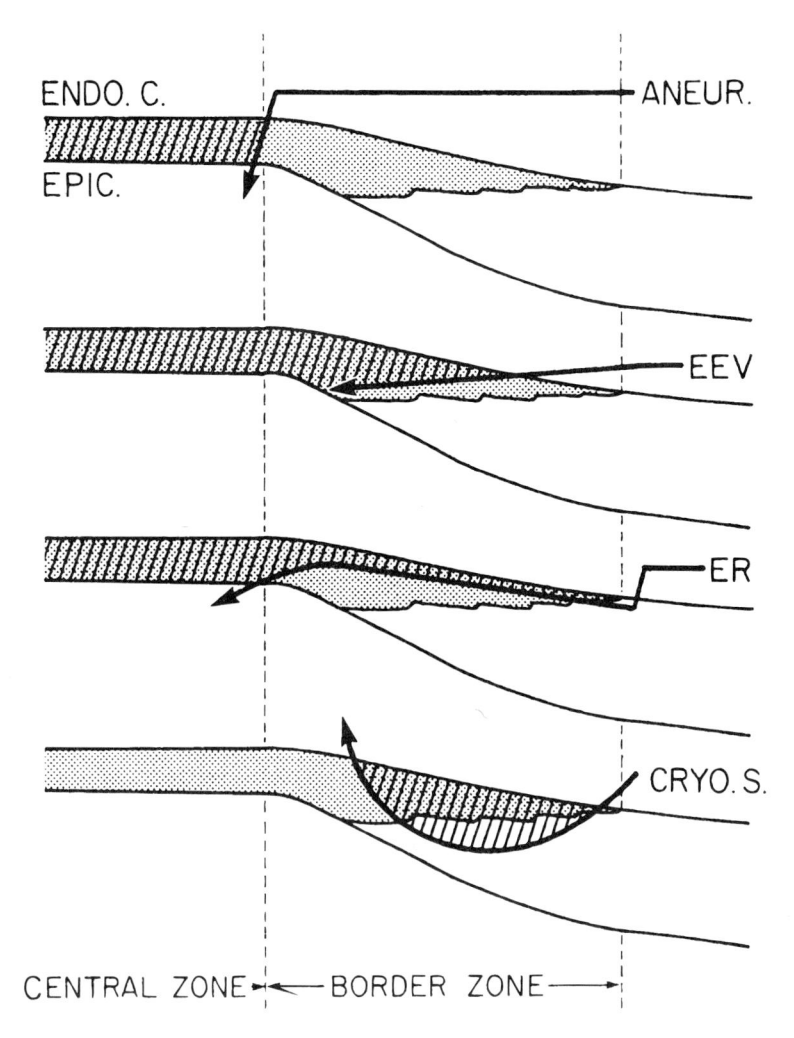

Figure 1. Schematic depiction of various surgical techniques for ventricular tachycardias. A cross section of the aneurysm shows the three segments: the central zone (the aneurysm); the border zone; and the remaining myocaridum. ANEUR: aneurysmectomy that only resects the nonarrhythmogenic central zone. EEV: the encircling endocardial ventriculotomy that "excludes" the border zone. ER: the endocardial resection that resects the arrhythmogenic subendocardium. CRYO S: cryosurgical ablation of the border zone.

proaches are not exclusive, but should be combined when feasible.

Pathophysiology

Ventricular tachycardias are associated either with acute or chronic ischemia. Acute ischemia has various clinical presentations: exercise-induced ischemia (silent or manifest), unstable angina, and the early phase of acute myocardial infarction, PVCs, polymorphic VTs, and ventricular fibrillation are the prevalent electrocardiographic presentations. Chronic ischemia is associated with 1) the infarct scar; and 2) dilated ischemic cardiomyopathy that essentially involves the "remaining" myocardium.

The infarct scar (left ventricular aneurysm or discrete segmental wall motion abnormality) develops in the chronic phase after acute myocardial infarction.[15] Typically, it comprises a central fibrotic zone, which is thin walled and was the site of transmural fibrosis. The central fibrotic zone is circumscribed by a border zone that is made of a disarray of fibrotic tissue and normal or abnormal myocardial cells. The ischemic lesions are essentially located in the subendocardium. Endocardial fibrosis develops opposite the subendocardial ischemic myocardium and constitutes a reliable anatomical landmark to delineate the extent of the infarct scar. However, rarely is the infarct scar consistent with the preceding description. The necrosis may not be manifest. The associated ischemic cardiomyopathy abolishes the discrete limits of the infarct scar (Figures 2 and 3). Large patches of chronic ischemic lesions may be present at a distance from the infarct scar.

Chronic recurrent VTs are the common presentation, the working mechanism of which is macroreentry. The arrhythmogenic anatomical substrate, ie, the anatomical and electrophysiologic milieu that allows reentry to occur and to be sustained, is usually situated in the border zone of the infarct, in the subendocardial layers. The new tissue organization, composed of surviving myocardial cells and fibrosis, is associated with a slow myocardial activation front (slow conduction and block). Slow conduction with unidirectional block is the critical pathophysiological substrate for reentry to occur.

The current accepted depiction of the reentry circuit is consistent with the figure-of-eight circuit (Figure 4).[16] The figure-of-eight circuit comprises an area of unidirectional slow conduction funneled by walls of functional block. The exit site of the slow conduction funnel enters the rest of the myocardium, and produces the QRS complex (cardiac contraction). The activation

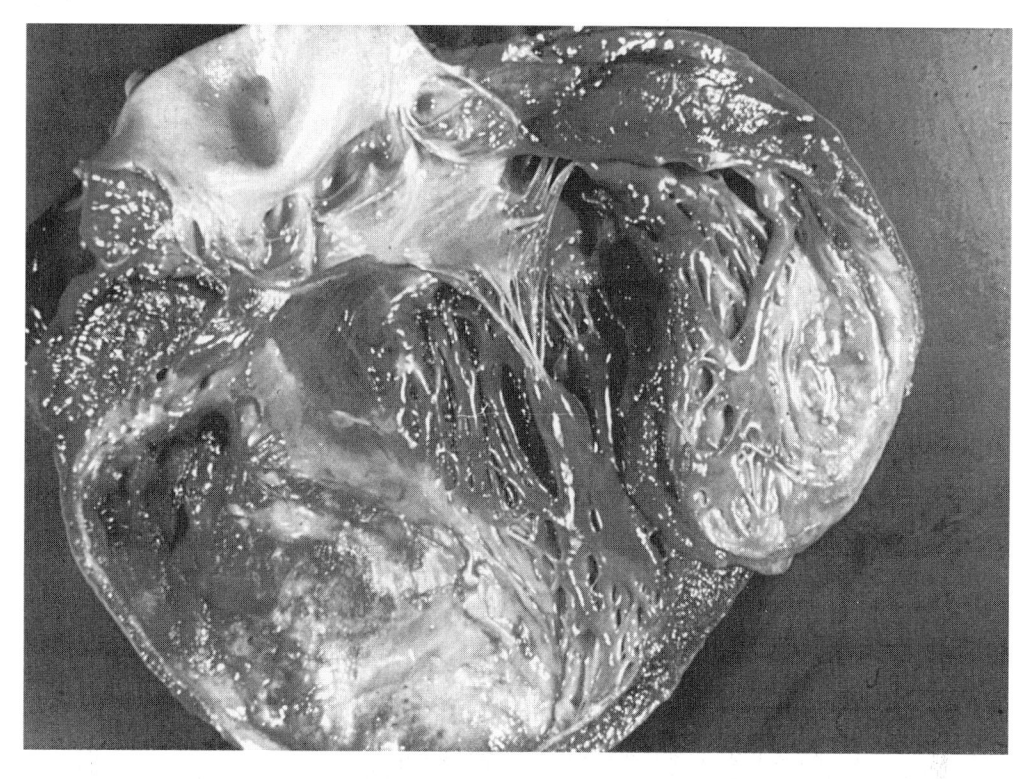

Figure 2. Pathological heart specimen that shows a typical aneurysm with the three "zones": thin-walled fibrotic central zone; border zone with endocardial fibrosis; and normal remaining myocardium.

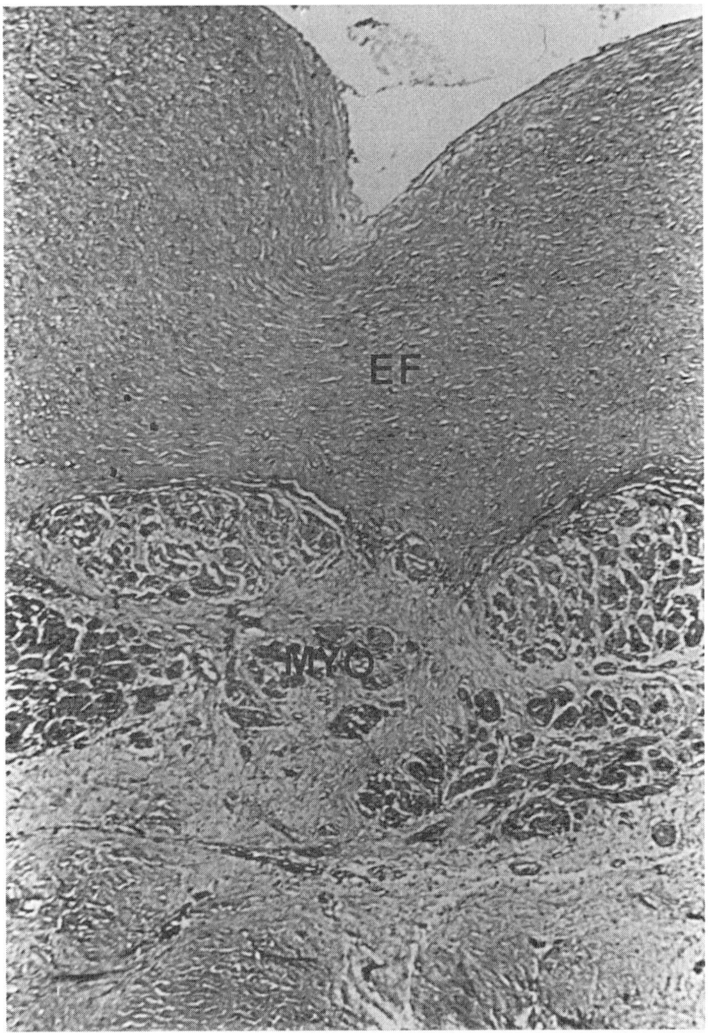

Figure 3. Histologic section of the subendocardial layers of the border zone. EF: endocardial fibrosis. MYO: subendocardium showing myocardial bundles intertwined with fibrosis.

reenters the slow conduction route at the other end. Because the arrhythmic substrate, although determined by underlying pathology, is essentially functional, its precise location and mass is poorly defined. There may be many vicarious sites. Surgical experience may have overestimated the size of anatomical substrate. Recent experience with discrete catheter ablation suggests that its volume may be small, although ablation of a large mass of tissue may decrease the risk of recurrences. The anatomical substrate may be situated within the "remaining" myocardium (ischemic cardiomyopathy).

Preoperative and intraoperative cardiac mapping allows spatial correlation of the site of the tachycardia(s) and the arrhythmogenic area(s) with the anatomical lesions. Usually a part of the lesion is documented to be arrhythmogenic. However, that does not imply that the rest of the lesion is not actually or does not have the potential to be arrhythmogenic.

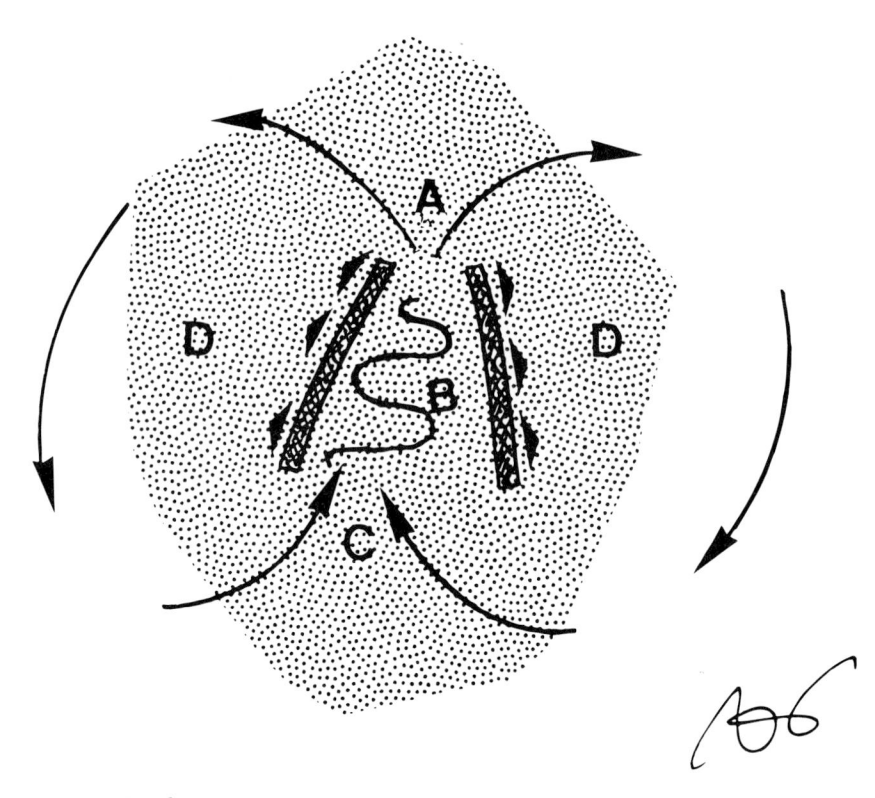

Figure 4. Figure-of-eight reentrant circuit. The entire shaded area represents the scar and is potentially arrhythmogenic. A: exit of low-conduction route corresponding to the initial activation of QRS or the origin of the tachycardia. B: slow conducting route isolated by a wall of conduction block. C: funnel of reentry. D: remaining "inactive" scar.

Intraoperative Cardiac Mapping

Cardiac mapping is a method by which the electrical activity of the heart is recorded directly from the heart and spatially depicted in an integrated manner as in a geographic map.[16-25] The site of recording can be epicardial, endocardial, or intramural. The recording mode can be unipolar or bipolar. The method of display involves activation time (isochronic map) or potential amplitude (isopotential map) or potential morphology (postexcitation map or fractionation map). Maps are obtained during sinus rhythm or induced ventricular arrhythmias.

The crucial issue is the way in which the recordings are obtained from the various cardiac sites. A unique handheld roving probe can be used. That point by point technique is feasible only if the cardiac activation is stable and each QRS complex identical to the following during the exploration. The handheld probe must be moved from one site to another after a sufficient number of complexes have been recorded at each site. The technique is time consuming, but appropriate for mapping during sinus rhythm or sustained monomorphic VT. Computerized mapping allows the simultaneous recording of a large number of sites. The epicardial electrodes may be affixed on a mesh that encompasses the heart like a sock. The endocardial electrodes array can be attached on an inflatable balloon introduced into the left ventricle via a left ventriculotomy or the aortic root or the left atrium. Epicardial and endocardial mapping can be carried out simultaneously. Computerized mapping is of particular interest when the VT are badly tolerated, and when the tachycardia are nonsustained, polymorphic, or multiple. It goes without saying that normothermic cardiopulmonary bypass is used when necessary.

Cardiac mapping provides the surgeon with two critical guides: 1) the site of origin of the arrhythmias that corresponds to the site of the earliest activation of the QRS complex during VT (exit site of figure-of-eight). In some instances the onset of the QRS can be difficult to determine, as well the activation time at various sites; and 2) the areas where abnormal electrical activity is recorded: arrhythmogenic areas where tunneled slow conduction may occur. These areas are subendocardial, or rarely, subepicardial or intramural. In a few patients, the surgeon may be provided with the actual macroreentrant circuit.

Despite the apparent precision, most of the information is crude and can be misleading even after being corroborated by thermal mapping or pace mapping. The reliability of the information depends upon the apparent site of origin (right ventricular free wall, septum, left ventricular free wall) and associated pathology. Intraoperative cardiac mapping must be also be assessed with regard to the preoperative endocardial mapping.

Preoperative Evaluation and Patient Selection

Patients with VT must be extensively investigated in terms of cardiac functional anatomy and electrophysiology. Assessment of patients with VT is documented elsewhere in this volume (see Chapter 2). Surgical indication for direct ablation is based on 1) left ventricular anatomy and function, which essentially determines the surgical risk and patient long-term prognosis[26,27]; 2) the availability of other electrophysiologic interventions; and 3) expected surgical efficacy. High efficacy is expected in patients with sustained monomorphic VT and well-identified discrete arrhythmogenic substrate. The arrhythmogenic anatomical substrate should be approachable without major impairment of the ventricular function and anatomy (coronary artery bypass is essentially an adjunct procedure in most cases). A complete plan based on all available information should be designed before surgery and should be carried out intraoperatively unless unexpected critical findings obtained from either cardiac anatomy or mapping are encountered.

Coronary Artery Bypass Grafting

Because ischemia was thought to be the main factor in initiating ventricular arrhythmia, it was anticipated that myocardial revascularization would prevent and/or interrupt ventricular arrhythmias. However, initial clinical experience with direct myocardial revascularization was disappointing.[12,28,29] Triggering factors of VTs are manifold and include exercise, acute ischemia, changes in the autonomic nervous system,[30] etc.

Ventricular arrhythmias associated with exercise testing are classified into three groups. (1) Premature ventricular complexes and nonsustained VTs are frequently induced during treadmill testing. Lown et al.[31] described a method of suppressing both spontaneous and exercise-induced ventricular arrhythmia using drug therapy guided by treadmill testing. Exercise-induced nonsustained VT, although an accurate predictor of sudden death, does not offer independent predictive value superior to those of coronary artery anatomy and left ventricular ejection fraction. The Cardiac Arrhythmias Suppression Trial (CAST)[32] documented that suppression of PVCs using drug therapy is associated with significantly higher mortality, which is probably caused by the proarrhythmic side effect of the drugs. Exercise-induced PVCs occur frequently after coronary artery bypass grafting. A recent study[33] showed that the prevalence of exercise-induced PVCs significantly increases after coronary artery bypass grafting, but is not associated with an increased risk of cardiac death. (2) Acute ischemia-induced VT can be documented in rare patients who present with exercise-induced ischemia associated with problematic sustained VT. Recently, Rasmussen et al.[34] reported on nine patients meeting these criteria who were successfully cured by coronary artery bypass grafting. These nine patients were part of a series of 400 patients consecutively undergoing coronary artery bypass grafting at the same institution. (3) Exercise-induced problematic sustained VTs are generally observed in a minority of patients with similar episodes of spontaneous VT.[35] Patients with or without exercise-induced VT do not differ significantly in history of myocardial infarction, segmental left ventricular wall motion abnormality, left ventricular function, coronary anatomy, or electrophysiologic testing. Exercise-induced VT is associated with an identical ischemic arrhythmogenic anatomical substrate with a reentry mechanism. Exertion and its multifaceted associated factors act as triggers. The most likely trigger is heart rate. Because acute ischemia is not the critical factor, coronary artery bypass grafting is not mandatory for this group of patients.

Patients With Spontaneous Recurrent Ventricular Tachycardia

Coronary artery bypass grafting, as suggested by several studies, may have a role in decreasing the incidence of arrhythmic death in patients with out-of-hospital documented cardiac arrent. Every et al.[36] showed a trend in decreasing cardiac death after coronary artery bypass grafting in such patients. Garan et al.[28] reported that 60% of patients with problematic sustained VT had negative electrophysiologic testing after coronary artery bypass grafting. In a follow-up study from the same group, Kelly et al.[29] corroborated the results obtained by coronary artery bypass grafting in patients with ischemic ventricular arrhythmia. Studying a subgroup of cardiac arrest survivors, they reported that coronary artery revascularization abolished preoperative inducible arrhythmias in a substantial number, especially when the inducible arrhythmia was ventricular fibrillation. On this basis, a good long-term prognosis may be expected. Other investigators have advocated coronary artery bypass grafting for survivors of cardiac arrest or patients with ventricular fibrillation. However, the patient selection criteria are poorly defined, as well as markers for long-term success.

Coronary artery bypass graft surgery decreases the incidence of sudden cardiac death as evidenced by the results of the CASS[26] and ECST[27] studies. Coronary artery bypass grafting may suppress sustained VTs and/or ventricular fibrillation. Coronary artery bypass grafting is most effective in the high-risk group with severe coronary artery disease and impaired ventricular function. Coronary artery bypass grafting is a critical adjunct to an electrophysiologic intervention, and should be combined whenever feasible.

Direct Surgical Approach

The direct surgical approach for VT after myocardial infarction was developed because simple aneurysmectomy proved ineffective.[37] In the late 1970s two surgical rationales were described: the encircling endocardial ventriculotomy aimed at excluding the entire arrhythmogenic border zone[10] and the endocardial resection (The Philadelphia peel)[11] aimed at resection of the arrhythmogenic segment of subendocardial tissue determined by intraoperative mapping.

Surgical Rationale

The surgical rationale is a compromise between the preservation of the cardiac function and the neutralization of the current and/or potentially arrhythmogenic lesions. It is based on two surgical concepts: 1) the concept of exclusion; and 2) the concept of ablation. The concept of exclusion is aimed at preventing the arrhythmogenic mechanism from involving the rest of the heart and producing ventricular arrhythmia. The best model of exclusion is the right ventricular free wall disconnection.[38] The concept of ablation is aimed at neutralizing the lesion(s) or a critical part (Figure 1). There are a large number of ablative techniques: transmural resection, endocardial resection, ventriculotomy, cryoablation, and laser photocoagulation.

The Surgical Implements

Surgical rationales can be implemented using various tools, eg, scalpel,[10,11] cryoablation,[39,40] lasers,[41] and chemicals such as ethanol.[7] The choice of the tool is based on the assessment of its specific advantages and disadvantages. Cryosurgery and laser photocoagulation produce well-demarcated masses of neutralized tissue that does not require further surgical intervention and do not impair normal surrounding myocardium. Cryosurgery requires concomitant cold cardiac arrest while laser photocoagulation can be used on the normothermic beating heart.

All surgical approaches are a compromise between surgical risk and efficacy. We have developed a surgical approach based on the same rationale as the encircling endocardial ventriculotomy, using cryoablation to diminish the impairment of the left ventricular function.

Encircling Endocardial Cryoablation

We recently reported our experience with 33 patients with problematic VT after myocardial infarction who underwent extensive circumferential (encircling) endocardial cryoablation of the border zone of the arrhythmogenic infarct scar,[39,40] based on the same concept as the encircling endocardial ventriculotomy.[10] The technique was designed to neutralize as much noncontractile, potentially arrhythmogenic tissue as possible without impairing the normally contracting surrounding myocardium because of the discrete fibrotic scar associated with cryolesions.

Materials and Methods

Patient Population

Thirty-three patients underwent encircling endocardial cryoablation between November 1982 and April 1993 at University Hospital in London, Ontario, Canada. There were 4 women and 29 men. Age ranged from 36–71 years (median 61). All patients had a history of acute myocardial infarction. The time interval between the myocardial infarction and the onset of ventricular arrhythmia varied from 2 weeks to 22 years with a median of 3 months. All patients had failed at least two drug trials including amiodarone in 14 patients.

Left ventricular functional anatomy was assessed using biplane left ventricular angiogram and coronary angiogram. There was a left ventricular aneurysm defined as a discrete bulging segmental wall motion abnormality in all patients. The aneurysm was anterior in 20 patients, posterior and inferior in 12 patients, and lateral (obtuse margin) in 1 patient. The remaining myocardium was graded as poor in 15 patients and good in 18. The left ventricular end-diastolic pressure ranged from 10–36 mm Hg (mean 21). The left ventricular ejection fraction ranged from 0.07–0.64 (mean 0.37). Nineteen patients presented with single vessel coronary artery disease (left anterior descending coronary artery in 13, right in 5, and obtuse marginal in 1). Eight patients had double vessel disease and five had triple vessel disease. One patient with triple vessel disease had previous coronary artery bypass graft on two vessels (LAD, OM).

Ventricular Arrhythmias

Twenty-five patients had sustained monomorphic VT with one morphology in

15, two in 8, and three in 2 patients. In 21 of the preceding 25 patients, endocardial catheter mapping localized the earliest QRS activation during VT within the aneurysm. Nonsustained monomorphic or polymorphic VTs were observed in 3 patients. In 3 patients with incessant monomorphic VT, the site of early QRS activation could not be identified and radiofrequency catheter ablation was not attempted in 2 patients. The third patient with incessant tachycardia was in circulatory collapse and was operated on an emergency basis. Two patients had primary ventricular fibrillation. One patient with one morphology of sustained VT associated with a large anterior left ventricular aneurysm had attempted intracoronary ethanol ablation via the left anterior descending coronary artery. One patient had associated Wolff-Parkinson-White syndrome with left free wall accessory pathway.

Surgical indication was empirical and did not follow a rigid algorithm. The decision was based on the presence of a discrete aneurysm, the severity of VT, and the availability or failure of other electrophysiologic interventions. The decision making evolved over time. Currently, lower risk patients as compared with our early experience are recruited. The time interval between the acute myocardial infarction and surgery varied from 3 weeks to 15 years with a mean of 7 months (mean 37 months).

Surgical Technique

The heart was exposed via a median sternotomy in all patients. A critical assessment of cardiac anatomy and function was carried out. The presence of a discrete fibrotic aneurysm allowed us to perform a satisfactory encircling endocardial cryoablation as planned. A poor remaining myocardium called for a minimal time period allocated to cardiac mapping. Four patients had unexpected pathology. Three patients had anterior myocardial dilation without fibrosis, thin wall, and endocardial fibrosis. One patient had no observable inferior aneurysm but an inferior right ventricular wall infarction.

Intraoperative Cardiac Mapping

In most patients, a roving handheld pen-like bipolar electrode was used for epicardial and/or endocardial activation mapping. A homemade epicardial multielectrode sock electrode was used when possible. Mapping was used as an adjunct when feasible or in a few cases when it was deemed necessary for critical changes or adjustment of planned surgical technique.

Either no maps or uninformative maps were obtained in 19 patients. In 2 of these 19 patients, a map was not obtained despite prolonged attempts to induce sustained VT. Mapping was deemed necessary because in one patient there was an anterior aneurysm without discrete delineation in terms of wall thickness, fibrosis, bulging, and wall motion (patient had no endocardial fibrosis at opening after attempted mapping). The second patient had emergency surgery for incessant VT associated with circulatory collapse and markedly decreased ventricular function. The VT terminated as soon as the emergency cardiopulmonary bypass was started; it could not be reinitiated. Mapping was attempted to carry out effective ablation with minimal ventricular access.

Informative mapping was obtained in 14 patients. In 12 patients the results of the mapping did not modify the planned surgical technique but did modify the surgical planning in two patients. The first patient had a dramatic discrepancy between the preoperative angiogram, which showed a discrete bulging inferior aneurysm, and the intraoperative observation, which showed a normal left ventricle with apparently a normal inferior wall thickness and contractility. The right ventricular inferior wall was akinetic and fibrotic (right ventricular myocardial infarction). Cardiac mapping documented the site of earliest QRS activation during VT over the right ventricular inferior wall scar. The second patient with a large anterior aneurysm with attempted intracoronary ethanol ablation had an earliest epicardial breakthrough of his clinical tachycardia over the inferior right ventricular wall at a distance from the septum, and suggesting a site of origin of the tachycardia outside the anatomical scar.

Cardiac mapping was carried out under normothermic cardiopulmonary bypass. Cardiac mapping was not prolonged beyond 1 hour of cardiopulmonary bypass time. Cardiopulmonary bypass time varied from 65 minutes to 4 hours, 47 minutes (mean 2 hours, 14 minutes).

Surgical Ablation

The left ventricle was entered using a ventriculotomy. Anterior aneurysms were opened using a ventriculotomy 1 cm from the septum. A segment of the fibrotic central zone was resected. The mural thrombus was carefully excised. Posterior aneurysm was approached using a posterior ventriculotomy, just along the septum and to the right of the posterior papillary muscle insertion.

Discrete endocardial fibrosis was present in 28 patients and absent in 4 patients with anterior aneurysm. The akinetic bulging part of the left ventricular wall was of normal thickness and not fibrotic. Contraction mapping was used to localize the border zone by carefully observing the limit between contracting and noncontracting myocardium on the opened normothermic beating heart.

The encircling endocardial cryoablation was carried out under cold cardioplegic arrest in 29 patients and on the normothermic fibrillating heart in 3 patients. Aortic cross-clamping time varied from 18 minutes to 94 minutes (mean 47 minutes) (Figure 5). A 15-mm probe cooled at $-60°C$ for 2 minutes was used. The probe was applied along the limits of the endocardial fibrosis, each

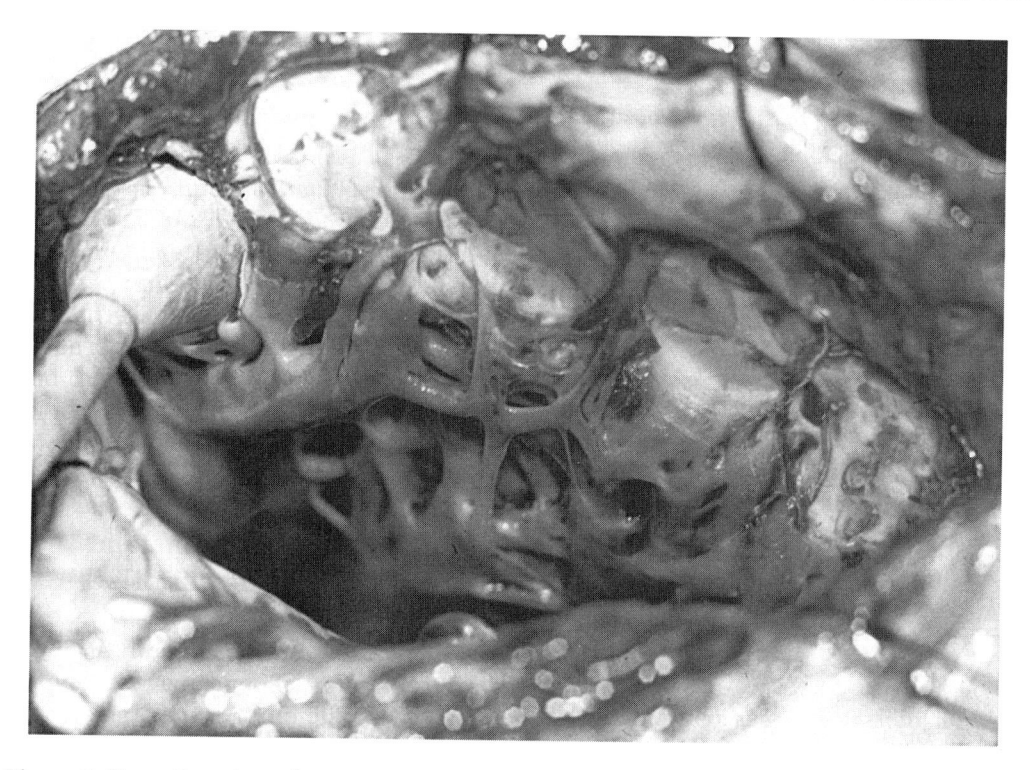

Figure 5. Operative view of an anterior aneurysm. The apical trabeculations are well seen. A 15-mm cryoprobe is applied on the border zone.

application overlapping the preceding to attain complete continuous encircling cryoablation. Two rows of cryoablation were used over the ventricular septum when anatomy permitted. In three patients transseptal cryoablation was obtained by using right ventricular septal cryoablation via a right ventriculotomy. During cryoablation, the ablated myocardium was squeezed between the large probe and a protected finger to attain deeper cryolesions. An average of 12 applications (range 5–16) were used for each patient. The left ventricle was closed using primary closure with pledgetted sutures in 24 patients. In 8 patients, a ventriculoplasty was performed using either a Dacron or pericardial patch. The patient with the clinical VT originating from the inferior wall right ventricular infarction had a partial right ventricular free wall disconnection of the right ventricular inferior wall and acute margin on the normothermic beating heart. Programmed electrical stimulation induced multiple morphologies of nonclinical VTs.

Concomitant Cardiac Procedures

Thirteen patients had concomitant coronary artery bypass grafting using a saphenous vein graft. One patient with severe congestive heart failure associated with ischemic mitral valve regurgitation had mitral valve replacement via an extended transatrial septal approach.[42] One patient with right ventricular infarction had an ICD implanted with epicardial patches and pace/sense leads. The patient with aberrant right ventricular breakthrough associated with anterior aneurysm had prophylactic patches implanted. The patient with left free wall accessory pathway had his pathway ablated using the epicardial approach.[43]

Intra-aortic balloon counterpulsation was required in 7 patients to attain adequate hemodynamics before coming off cardiopulmonary bypass. These 7 patients were all part of the 14 patients who had preoperative evidence of congestive heart failure. Before closure, pairs of temporary pacing wires were attached to the atria and ventricles for postoperative programmed electrical stimulation.

Postoperative Period

Surgical Risk

Thirty-two of 33 patients were discharged from the hospital. One patient died of uncontrolled VT 2 days after surgery. This patient had undergone surgery 1 month after an anterior myocardial infarction. At surgery, the infarct scar was still friable with a large mural thrombus. Three coronary artery bypass grafts were implanted onto the posterior descending and posterior lateral right coronary artery and the obtuse marginal coronary artery using saphenous vein grafts. Intra-aortic balloon counterpulsation was used and because of dramatically improved hemodynamics was removed the next day. However, VT associated with cardiovascular collapse reoccurred shortly thereafter. Closed chest cardiac massage was performed while the patient was taken into emergency surgery. Cryoablation of the right ventricular septum was carried out, but the patient could not be resuscitated. One patient had an early relapse. All patients had electrophysiologic testing 8–10 days after surgery using temporary epicardial pacing wires. Programmed electrical stimulation was carried out using up to two extrastimuli at right ventricular and left ventricular sites. Two patients had inducible VTs; one patient with good ventricular function and no discrete anterior aneurysm and no inducible VT refused a second operation and was discharged on amiodarone (September 1984). The other patient had an ICD implanted via a left subcostal approach (August 1989),[44] although no VTs were inducible when the ICD was tested predischarge. The patient with prophylactic ICD patches had no inducible VTs. At discharge, 29 patients (90%) were free of arrhythmia; 3 had VT, although 1 patient with ICD had no inducible VT at discharge.

Long-Term Follow-Up

The patients or their family were contacted by telephone. Their physicians, as well as the attending cardiologist, were contacted to obtain a reliable assessment of their medical condition. Four patients were lost to follow-up. The total follow-up was 134 patient years with a mean of 5 years.

Long-Term Arrhythmia

All patients who were discharged without inducible VT remained arrhythmia free. Two of the three patients with inducible arrhythmias had recurrence of VT. The patient who was discharged on amiodarone was not adequately controlled, and sustained an episode of out-of-hospital cardiac arrest. She subsequently received an ICD and has done well since then. She has not used her ICD for the last 4 years. The patient with the inferior right ventricular free wall disconnection combined with ICD implantation had frequent recurrences of ventricular arrhythmia associated with frequent ICD discharges. He refused any further interventional therapy such as heart transplant, or a more sophisticated third-generation ICD with antitachycardia pacing capabilities that might had decreased the number of shocks. The patient did not return to our institution, but requested that his ICD be deactivated and died 2 years after surgery. The third patient with an ICD, who was not inducible at discharge, had no recurrence of VT. The patient with prophylactic patches also had no VT recurrence.

Ventricular Function

Nine patients had clinical evidence of heart failure during long-term follow-up. Four patients died of heart failure 4 months, 5 months, 2 years, and 6 years, respectively, after surgery. Two patients had a heart transplantation for terminal heart failure 1 year and 6 years postoperatively.

One patient with inferior aneurysm developed a pseudoaneurysm 10 weeks after surgery. The pseudoaneurysm was not present on left ventricular angiogram at discharge. The pseudoaneurysm was repaired by closing the dehiscence of the left ventricular closure. This patient died 6 years later of cancer.

Associated Disease

Three patients died of cancer, 20 months, 30 months, and 6 years after surgery, respectively.

Cryosurgical Ablation

Cryosurgery was first used in cardiac surgery for His bundle ablation[45] and subsequently applied to the treatment of VTs.[46] The cryosurgical lesions are discrete and sharply demarcated from adjacent tissue (Figure 5). Lesions are homogeneous and nonarrhythmogenic.[47] Cryoablation induces necrosis of myocardial fibers, but spares the collagenous framework. The scar is made of dense fibrotic tissue that has no tendency to rupture or dilate. Most experiments or clinical reports deal with limited relatively discrete cryoablation. We have studied the effects of large transmural left ventricular cryoablation in dogs. We have documented that extensive cryoablation of either the posterior[48] or the anterior (unpublished data) papillary muscle in the dog is not associated with either mitral valve dysfunction or ventricular dysfunction. We have also documented that the transmural cryoablation of the left ventricular apex,[49] distal to the papillary muscle insertion, produces a thick, discrete scar without significant damage in the left ventricular anatomy and no changes in left ventricular function. Our experimental data suggests that extensive cryoablation of the infarct scar should be associated with minimum left ventricular adverse effects.

Ventricular Arrhythmia

Successful long-term ablation of ventricular arrhythmia depends on definite neutralization of the critical anatomical arrhythmogenic substrate.[10,11] More than one critical anatomical substrate may be present, especially when multiple morphologies are observed or when the tachycardia is polymorphic. Cardiac mapping may determine the location of the anatomical substrate(s). Currently, the marker of the anatomical substrate site most used is either the site of earliest activation of QRS during sustained VT[8,9,22] or the area of diastolic activation with fractionated or delayed potentials. One or both of these markers are subject to failure. Consequently, two surgical schools of thought compete: extensive surgical ablation to increase efficacy[10] or more discrete ablation.[11] We had first advocated an extensive ablation using an encircling endocardial ventriculotomy.[10] This rationale also allows surgical ablation to be carried out without relying predominantly on informative cardiac mapping. However, the adverse effect of an extensive encircling ventriculotomy on the ventricular function[50,51] prompted us to use the same principle, but a different tool. Ventricular arrhythmias have been ablated in 30 patients, while three patients had early recurrence of their arrhythmia. This accounts for an efficacy of 90%. This efficacy was not associated with significant left ventricular dysfunction.

Ventricular Function

Left ventricular dysfunction is progressive and remains the most prevalent cause of death in patients with ventricular arrhythmia. The extent of impairment of the left ventricular function is the most powerful independent risk factor for sudden cardiac death.[52,53] Fourteen patients (43%) had preoperative clinical evidence of heart failure. Seven required the assistance of intraaortic balloon counterpulsation intraoperatively. Cardiac function appeared to improve postoperatively. Only nine patients had evidence of heart failure postoperatively. There was a trend in increasing left ventricular ejection fraction postoperatively: mean 0.45 (range 0.64 to 0.31) in 16 patients where the postoperative data were available. Improvement of the left ventricular function is multifactorial, as is its aggravation. New ischemic events, progression of the coronary artery disease, or progression of cardiomyopathy are factors independent of surgical ablation and left ventricular aneurysmectomy. Our results suggest that the extensive encircling endocardial cryoablation does not impair ventricular function.

Patient Selection

Since the dramatic development of the ICD,[2,3] the role of surgical ablation has been reevaluated without definitive answers based on clinical trials. Because surgical ablation may provide the best long-term quality of life, surgery must still be considered when feasible, with low surgical risk. Ventricular score as described by van Hemel et al.[54] or other criteria as described by the Philadelphia group[55] are valuable guides, but strategies in electrophysiologic intervention for VT are still essentially empirical.[56]

Other Surgical Approaches

The University of Pennsylvania series using map-guided segmental endocardial resection with or without the adjunct of cryoablation is a monumental series that has been a model and a great reference resource for many years. All series must be compared to that standard.[57,58]

Other groups have used cryoablation,[59] or laser photocoagulation.[41,60,61] Sequential ablation based on repeat sequential mapping has been advocated.[62] Cardiac mapping has given some clues as to unexplained failure associated with inferior left ventricular aneurysm.[63] Unfortunately, there is no scientific basis to validly compare these variant approaches.[64]

Conclusion: Is There a Niche for Surgical Ablation

The sophistication of ICDs and their widespread use seems to obviate the need for direct surgery for VTs. Conference policies on indications for ICD implantation did not mention alternative surgical ablation.

Ventricular tachycardias and other ventricular arrhythmias after myocardial infarction are associated with severe prognosis. The Dutch Ventricular Tachycardia study group,[65] reported the on the outcome of 390 patients with sustained problematic ventricular arrhythmia after myocardial infarction. During follow-up (mean 1.9 years), 34% of patients died of ventricular arrhythmia and 8% of heart failure. Multivariate analysis showed that age ($\geq$ 70 years) syncopal VT, heart failure during the acute phase of infarction, anterior location infarction, and multiple infarctions were independent risk factors of mortality. One-year mortality varied from 12% to 54% in the presence of 1–5 of these factors. Other studies have emphasized poor prognosis for their patients and the determining role of ventricular function. Leclerc[66] reported a 5-year actuarial mortality of 30% when the left ventricular ejection fraction is > 30%, and a mortality of 58% when the ejection fraction is < 30%. He reported also an increase mortality in patients when patients were prescribed Class I antiarrhythmic agents.

The poor prognosis of patients with VTs after myocardial infarction is a strong incentive to use electrophysiologic interventions. However, the left ventricular function, which is the most powerful predictor of outcome, is also the main exclusion criteria for direct surgical ablation. Leclerc[66] reported no difference in outcome in patients with a left ventricular ejection fraction > 0.30, whatever the applied electrophysiologic interventions. High-risk patients with poor ventricular function are those with the greater benefit after electrophysiologic interventions[66] or coronary artery bypass grafting.[26,27]

The advantages of direct surgery are: 1) Direct surgery offers a "cure" with long-term control of the ventricular arrhythmia, with freedom from side effects of antiarrhythmic drugs, and without the dependency on the shocks and possible anxiety associated with shock anticipation with ICD use. In our experience patients do not require support after successful albative surgery and enjoy a good quality of life. Patients with ICDs may have a need for support from either social workers or psychologists. 2) Surgical ablation should be considered when it can be performed with low risk and high efficacy. 3) Efficacy is high for sustained monomorphic VT originating within a discrete infarct scar. 4) Surgical risk depends essentially on the remaining left ventricular function. Using the ventricular score that was used in the CASS study, van Hemel has recently reported 100 consecutive patients without mortality.[67] and 5) Surgical ablation is combined with coronary artery disease when indicated. Surgical ablation does not preclude the future use of antiarrhythmic drugs or an ICD.

Surgical ablation of VT should remain the first choice when technically feasible and when morality and morbidity from surgery are outweighed by the anticipated therapeutic benefits. Severe left ventricular dysfunction and heart failure, however, remain the main limitations of the primary surgical approach.

References

1. Hinkle LE, Thaler HT: Clinical classification of cardiac deaths. *Circulation* 65:457, 1982.
2. Mirowski M: The automatic implantable cardioverter-defibrillator: an overview. *J Am Coll Cardiol* 6(2):461, 1985.
3. Watkins L, Mirowski M, Mower MM, et al: Implantation of the automatic defibrillator: the subxiphoid approach. *Ann Thorac Surg* 34(5):515, 1982.
4. Fontaine G, Tonet JL, Frank R, et al: Treatment of resistant ventricular tachycardia by endocavitary fulguration associated with

antiarrhythmic therapy. In: *Ablation in Cardiac Arrhythmias*. Edited by G Fontaine, MM Scheinman. Mount Kisco, NY: Futura Publishing Company, Inc.; 1987, p. 311.
5. Schwartzman D, Jadonath RL, Preminger MW, et al: Morphology-specific radiofrequency catheter ablation of incessant ventricular tachycardia in consecutive patients with prior myocardial infarction (abstract). *PACE* 16(4):860, 1993.
6. Gonska BD, Brune S, Bethge KP, et al: Radiofrequency catheter ablation in recurrent ventricular tachycardia. *Eur Heart J* 12:1257, 1991.
7. Gursoy S, Nellens P, Guiraudon G, et al: Epicardial and subelective transcoronary chemical ablation of incessant ventricular tachycardia. *Cathet Cardiovasc Diagn* 28:323, 1993.
8. Guiraudon G, Frank R, Fontaine G: Interet des cartographies dans le traitement chirurgical des tachycardies ventriculaires rebelles recidivantes. *La Nouvelle Presse Medicale* 3(6):321, 1974.
9. Fontaine G, Guiraudon G, Frank R, et al: La cartographie epicardique et le traitement chirurgical par simple ventriculotomie de certaines tachycardies ventriculaires rebelles par reentree. *Arch Mal Coeur* 68(2):113, 1975.
10. Guiraudon G, Fontaine G, Frank R: Encircling endocardial ventriculotomy: a new surgical treatment for life-threatening ventricular tachycardias resistant to medical treatment following myocardial infarction. *Ann Thorac Surg* 26(5):438, 1978.
11. Josephson ME, Harken AH, Horowitz LN: Endocardial excision: a new surgical technique for the treatment of recurrent ventricular tachycardia. *Circulation* 60:1430, 1979.
12. Graham AF, Miller DC, Stinson EB, et al: Surgical treatment of refractory life-threatening ventricular tachycardia. *Am J Cardiol* 32:909, 1973.
13. Kirklin JW: The science of cardiac surgery. *Eur J Cardiothorac Surg* 4:63, 1990.
14. Guiraudon GM, Klein GJ, Yee R: Surgery for cardiac tachyarrhythmias. *Highlights* 6(2):5, 1990.
15. Mallory GK, White PD, Salgedo-Salgar J: The speed of healing of myocardial infarction. *Am Heart J* 18:647, 1939.
16. El-Sherif N: The figure 8 model of reentrant excitation in the canine postinfarction heart. In: *Cardiac Electrophysiology and Arrhythmias*. Edited by DP Zipes, J Jalife. Orlando, FL: Grune & Stratton, Inc.; 1985, p. 363.
17. Gallagher JJ, Kasell JH, Cox JL, et al: Techniques of intraoperative electrophysiologic mapping. *Am J Cardiol* 49:221, 1982.
18. Fontaine G, Guiraudon G, Frank R, et al: Surgical management of ventricular tachycardia not related to myocardial ischemia. In: *Tachycardias: Mechanisms, Diagnosis, Treatment*. Edited by ME Josephson, HJJ Wellens. Philadelphia: Lea & Febiger; 1984, p. 451.
19. Klein H, Karp RB, Kouchoukos NT, et al: Intraoperative electrophysiologic mapping of the ventricles during sinus rhythm in patients with a previous myocardial infarction. *Circulation* 66(4):847, 1982.
20. Durrer D, van Dam RT, Freud GE, et al: Total excitation of the isolated human heart. *Circulation* 41:899, 1970.
21. Klein GJ, Ideker RE, Smith WM, et al: Epicardial mapping of the onset of ventricular tachycardia initiated by programmed stimulation in the canine heart with chronic infarction. *Circulation* 60(6):1375, 1979.
22. de Bakker JMT, Janse MJ, Van Cappelle FJL, et al: Endocardial mapping by simultaneous recording of endocardial electrograms during cardiac surgery for ventricular aneurysm. *J Am Coll Cardiol* 2(5):947, 1983.
23. Vermeulen FEE, van Hemel NM, Guiraudon GM, et al: Cryosurgery for ventricular bigeminy using a transaortic closed ventricular approach. *Eur Heart J* 9:979, 1988.
24. Downer E, Mickleborough LL, Garris L, et al: Mapping of endocardial activation during ventricular tachycardia—a "closed heart" procedure (abstract). *J Am Coll Cardiol* 7(Suppl A):234A, 1986.
25. Downer E, Parson ID, Mickleborough LL, et al: On-line epicardial mapping of intraoperative ventricular arrhythmias: initial clinical experience. *J Am Coll Cardiol* 4(4):703, 1984.
26. Holmes DR, Davis KB, Mock MB, et al: The effect of medical and surgical treatment on subsequent sudden cardiac death in patients with coronary artery disease: a report from the Coronary Artery Surgery Study. *Circulation* 73:1254, 1986.
27. Vamauskas E, The European Coronary Surgery Study Group: Survival, myocardial infarction, and employment status in a prospective randomized study of coronary artery bypass surgery. *Circulation* 72(Suppl V):V-90, 1985.
28. Garan H, Ruskin JN, DiMarco JP, et al: Electrophysiologic studies before and after myocardial revascularization in patients with life-threatening ventricular arrhythmias. *Am J Cardiol* 51:519, 1983.
29. Kelly P, Ruskin JN, Vlahakes GJ, et al: Surgical coronary revascularization in survivors of prehospital cardiac arrest: its effect on inducible ventricular arrhythmias and long-term survival. *J Am Coll Cardiol* 15:267, 1990.
30. Coumel P: Cardiac arrhythmias and the automomic nervous system. *J Cardiovasc Electrophysiol* 4:338, 1993.

31. Lown B, Podrid PJ, DeSilva RA, et al: Sudden cardiac death: management of the patient at risk. *Curr Prob Cardiol* 4:1, 1980.
32. The Cardiac Arrhythmia Suppression Trial (CAST) Investigators: Preliminary report: effect of encainide and flecainide on mortality in a randomized trial of arrhythmia suppression after myocardial infarction. *N Engl J Med* 321:406, 1989.
33. Yli-Mayry S, Juikuri HV, Korhoenen UR, et al: Prevalence and prognostic significance of exercise-induced ventricular arrhythmias after coronary artery bypass grafting. *Am J Cardiol* 66:1451, 1990.
34. Rasmussen K, Lunde PI, Lie M: Coronary bypass surgery in exercise-induced ventricular tachycardia. *Eur Heart J* 8:444, 1978.
35. Rodriguez LM, Waleffe A, Brugada P, et al: Exercise-induced sustained symptomatic ventricular tachycardia: indicence, clinical angiographic and electrophysiologic characteristics. *Eur Heart J* 11:225, 1990.
36. Every NR, Fahrenbruch CE, Hallstrom AP, et al: Influence of coronary bypass surgery on subsequent outcome of patients resuscitation from out of hospital cardiac arrest. *J Am Coll Cardiol* 19:1435, 1992.
37. Couch OA: Cardiac aneurysm with ventricular tachycardia and subsequent excision of aneurysm. *Circulation* 20:251, 1959.
38. Guiraudon GM, Klein GJ, Gulamhusein SS, et al: Total disconnection of the right ventricular free wall: surgical treatment of right ventricular tachycardia associated with right ventricular dysplasia. *Circulation* 67(2):463, 1983.
39. Guiraudon GM, Klein GJ, Vermeulen FEE, et al: Encircling endocardial cryoablation: a technique for surgical treatment of ventricular tachycardia after myocardial infarction (abstract). *Circulation* 68:III-176, 1983.
40. Guiraudon GM, Klein GJ, Sharma AD, et al: Encircling endocardial cryoablation for ventricular arrhythmias after myocardial infarction: further experience (abstract). *Clin Invest Med* 8(Suppl B):49, 1985.
41. Svenson RH, Gallagher JJ, Selle JG, et al: Neodymium:YAG laser photocoagulation: a successful new map-guided technique for the intraoperative ablation of ventricular tachycardia. *Circulation* 76:1319, 1987.
42. Guiraudon GM, Ofiesh JG, Kaushik R: Extended vertical trans-septal approach to the mitral valve. *Ann Thorac Surg* 52:1058, 1991.
43. Guiraudon GM, Klein GJ, Sharma AD, et al: Surgery for Wolff-Parkinson-White syndrome: further experience with an epicardial approach. *Circulation* 74(3):525, 1986.
44. Guiraudon G, Klein G, Yee R: Left subdiaphragmatic implantation of the PCD defibrillator suppresses the problematic side-effects of bulky generators (abstract). *J Am Coll Cardiol* 19(3):123A, 1992.
45. Harrison L, Gallagher JJ, Kasell J, et al: Cryosurgical ablation of the AV node-His bundle: a new method for producing AV block. *Circulation* 55:463, 1977.
46. Gallagher JJ, Anderson RW, Kasell J, et al: Cryoablation of drug-resistant ventricular tachycardia in a patient with a variant of scleroderma. *Circulation* 57:190, 1978.
47. Klein GJ, Harrison L, Ideker RF, et al: Reaction of the myocardium to cryosurgery: electrophysiology and arrhythmogenic potential. *Circulation* 59:364, 1979.
48. Guiraudon GM, Guiraudon CM, McLellan DG, et al: Mitral valve function after cryoablation of the posterior papillary muscle in the dog. *Ann Thorac Surg* 47(6):872, 1989.
49. McLellan DG, Guiraudon GM, Guiraudon CM, et al: Extensive cryoablation of the left ventricular apex does not impair cardiac function (abstract). *PACE* 13(4):497, 1990.
50. Ostermeyer J, Borggrefe M, Breithardt G, et al: Direct operations for the management of life-threatening ischemic ventricular tachycardia. *J Thorac Cardiovasc Surg* 94:848, 1987.
51. Ostermeyer J, Kirklin JK, Borggrefe M, et al: Ten years electrophysiologically guided direct operations for malignant ischemic ventricular tachycardia: results. *Thorac Cardiovasc Surg* 37:20, 1989.
52. Hinkle LE, Thaler HT: Clinical classification of cardiac deaths. *Circulation* 65:457, 1982.
53. DiMarco JP, Haines DE: Sudden cardiac death. *Curr Probl Cardiol* 15:185, 1990.
54. van Hemel NM, Kingma JH, Defauw JAM, et al: Left ventricular segmental wall motion score as a criterion for selection of patients for direct surgery in the treatment of post infarction ventricular tachycardia. *Heart J* 10:304, 1989.
55. Miller JM, Kienzle MG, Harken AH, et al: Subendocardial resection for ventricular tachycardia: predictors of surgical success. *Circulation* 70:624, 1984.
56. Elefteriades JA, Biblo LA, Batsford WP, et al: Evolving patterns in the surgical treatment of malignant ventricular tachyarrhythmias. *Ann Thorac Surg* 49:94, 1990.
57. Hargrove WC, Josephson ME, Marchlinski FE, et al: Surgical decisions in the management of sudden cardiac death and malignant ventricular arrhythmias: subendocardial resection, the automatic internal defibrillator, or both. *J Thorac Cardiovasc Surg* 97:923, 1989.
58. Hargrove WC: Surgery for ischemic ventricular tachycardia—operative techniques and long-term results. *Semin Thorac Cardiovasc Surg* 1:83, 1989.

59. Caceres J, Werner P, Jazayeri M, et al: Efficacy of cryosurgery alone for refractory monomorphic sustained ventricular tachycardia due to inferior wall infarction. *J Am Coll Cardiol* 11:1254, 1988.
60. Selle JG, Svenson RH, Sealy WC, et al: Successful clinical laser ablation of ventricular tachycardia: a promising new therapeutic method. *Ann Thorac Surg* 42:380, 1986.
61. Saksena S, Hussain M, Gielchinsky I, et al: Intraoperative mapping-guided argon laser ablation of malignant ventricular tachycardia. *Am J Cardiol* 59:78, 1987.
62. Kron IL, Lerman BB, Nolan, et al: Sequential endocardial resection for the surgical treatment of refractory ventricular tachycardia. *J Thorac Cardiovasc Surg* 94:83, 1987.
63. Svenson RH, Littmann L, Gallagher JJ, et al: Termination of ventricular tachycardia with epicardial laser photocoagulation: a clinical comparison with patients undergoing successful endocardial photocoagulation alone. *J Am Coll Cardiol* 15:163, 1990.
64. Bailar JC III, Mosteller F (eds): *Medical Uses of Statistics*. Waltham, MA: NEJM Books; 1986.
65. Willems AR, Tijssen JGP, van Capelle FJL, et al: Determinants of prognosis in symptomatic ventricular tachycardia or ventricular fibrillation late after myocardial infarction. *J Am Coll Cardiol* 16:521, 1990.
66. Leclerc JF: Les tachycardies ventriculaires des cardiopathies ischemiques. *Arch Mal Coeur* 86(suppl):739, 1993.
67. van Hemel NM, Defauw JAM, Kingma JH, et al: Risk factors of map-guided surgery for post-infarction ventricular tachycardia, a multi-variate analysis (abstract). *PACE* 16(Suppl II):871, 1993.

Chapter 30

Catheter Ablation for Ventricular Tachycardia

William M. Miles and Lawrence S. Klein

Although antiarrhythmic drugs and implantable cardioverter-defibrillators (ICDs) are the most commonly used therapies for ventricular tachyarrhythmias, ablation for elimination of ventricular tachycardia (VT) has gained importance over the past few years.[1] In fact, ablation may be the therapy of first choice for selected VTs as discussed below. Although ablation for VT may be performed using either surgical or catheter techniques, the discussion in this chapter is limited to catheter ablation.

Ablation Using Direct Current Shocks

The first energy source used for catheter ablation in humans was a DC capacitor discharge, initially used for ablation of the atrioventricular (AV) junction to control the ventricular response in patients with atrial tachyarrhythmias.[2,3] In 1983, Hartzler[4] reported successful catheter ablation for VT in three patients using a DC shock. One of his patients had VT arising from the right ventricular outflow tract in a structurally normal heart, a group of patients whose VT has subsequently been reported to be particularly amenable to ablation with both DC energy[5] and radiofrequency energy.[6] The other two patients had VT postmyocardial infarction. Although these results were favorable and without complication, use of DC discharge for catheter ablation in patients with VT was slow to gain acceptance other than in patients whose VT was drug refractory, markedly symptomatic, and who were not candidates for surgical elimination of the VT.[7] Direct current ablation of VT was especially cumbersome at that time because of the lack of deflectable catheters, making precise localization of the VT origin and stable catheter contact with the endocardium difficult. The patient undergoing DC ablation requires very heavy sedation or general anesthesia during delivery of the capacitor discharge (usually 100–300 J delivered between the tip of a standard electrode catheter and a backplate using the output of a standard defibrillator). The energy delivery damages the catheter electrode, and if a second discharge needs to be delivered the catheter must be removed and

---

Supported in part by the Herman C. Krannert Fund; by grants HL-42370 and HL-07182 from the National Heart, Lung and Blood Institute of the National Institutes of Health, US Public Health Service; and the American Heart Association, Indiana Affiliate, Inc.

From Singer I, (ed.) Implantable Cardioverter-Defibrillator. Armonk, NY: Futura Publishing Company, Inc.; © 1994.

replaced with a new catheter. Discharge of DC energy within the cardiac chambers results in a pressure shock wave that may damage cardiac structures (barotrauma) and can result in cardiac perforation.[8] In addition, the lesion created by DC ablation is less homogeneous and predictable in size and location than that created by radiofrequency energy. Direct current energy delivery cannot be titrated because it is delivered over only a few milliseconds, whereas radiofrequency energy can be delivered in a more controlled fashion (ie, energy delivery may last up to 60 seconds with the ability to terminate energy delivery at any time when the desired response or an adverse response occurs). Therefore, the role of DC ablation for VT has remained limited, especially since the advent of safer forms of energy such as radiofrequency. However, using the currently available catheter designs and power availability (usually no more than 50 W), radiofrequency energy lesion size is limited; thus, in some patients in whom radiofrequency energy is unable to eliminate VT, delivery of a DC shock may create a larger and deeper lesion to ablate tachycardia in a patient whose VT was unable to be eliminated with radiofrequency energy.

Some of the difficulties involved in early ablation of VT are illustrated from the Percutaneous Mapping and Ablation Registry for VT,[9] the final report of which was published in 1988. This was a voluntary registry of patients undergoing AV junctional or VT ablation using DC energy. It was carried out before the introduction of radiofrequency energy, and therefore, most patients entered were very ill, had structural heart disease, had failed multiple drug therapies, and were not considered candidates for surgical management of the arrhythmia. There were 164 patients who underwent VT ablation with a follow-up of 12 ± 11 months. Eighteen percent of the patients had no recurrent VT and required no antiarrhythmic drug therapy and another 41% had no recurrent VT although an antiarrhythmic drug was required, for a total success (full and partial) of 59%. The other 41% of the patients had recurrent ventricular tachyarrhythmias or procedure-related death (11 patients).

Ablation Using Radiofrequency Energy

The advent of radiofrequency energy has revolutionized ablation therapy for Wolff-Parkinson-White syndrome and AV nodal reentrant tachycardia[10–12] and offered new therapeutic alternatives for VT in selected patient groups. Radiofrequency energy is alternating current with a frequency between 30 kHz and 300 MHz. For ablation purposes it is usually delivered as a continuous unmodulated sine wave with a frequency of around 500 kHz. It is the same energy used for surgical electrocautery, although the voltage used for ablation purposes is lower and it is delivered as a continuous rather than intermittent waveform, so that it heats tissue without cutting through it.[13] It is usually delivered between a 4-mm long catheter electrode and a large skin electrode, although the ideal size and shape of the catheter electrode is under investigation. It creates a lesion of approximately 5 mm in diameter and 3 mm in depth by its tissue heating effects.[14] Advantages of radiofrequency energy over DC shock include no need for anesthesia, no barotrauma, more controlled energy delivery with ability to titrate power, no catheter damage from energy delivery so that energy can be delivered multiple times without removing the catheter from the body, and a limited, discrete, homogeneous area of tissue damage. A major limitation of radiofrequency energy is the fact that a coagulum forms on the catheter tip if its temperature reaches 100°C, limiting the ability to deliver current and thus limiting lesion size.[15] This is commonly referred to as an impedance rise. If an impedance rise occurs, the catheter must be withdrawn and the coagulum removed by wiping the electrode with a damp sponge. The impedance rise may be prevented by monitoring the temperature at the tip of the catheter (using a thermister incorporated into the distal electrode) and not allowing it to exceed 100°C.[16] Contact of the catheter and tissue to be ablated is critical in radiofrequency ablation. Catheter tip temperature monitoring may also be used to verify good catheter tissue contact and may aid the operator in titrating power delivery up or down. The small volume of tissue damage by radiofrequency current may represent a disadvantage if one cannot place the catheter tip directly on the site to be ablated or if the site is deep in the myocardium. There is limited ability of radiofrequency energy to penetrate scar tissue or clot.

Feasibility of Catheter Ablation for Ventricular Tachycardia

Catheter ablation of VT uses either delivery of ablation energy to the site of origin of the VT or, in the case of bundle branch reentrant tachycardia, to the right bundle branch to eliminate one limb of the macroreentrant circuit. In the latter case the identification of the desired site for energy delivery is straightforward. However, there are several potential factors limiting the efficacy of catheter ablation for the majority of VTs. These include the presence of endocardial scar or clot limiting energy delivery to the desired site, intramyocardial or epicardial sites of VT origin, multiple morphologies or sites of origin of VT, polymorphic VT, inability to induce the VT in the electrophysiology laboratory, and induction of hemodynamically unstable VT. These limitations may be overcome to some extent in the future with multielectrode mapping catheters and computer mapping techniques. Catheter stability and tissue contact are critical but are difficult to obtain in certain areas of the ventricle using the currently available deflectable catheters. There may be difficulty identifying the site of VT origin, especially in patients with VT in the setting of coronary artery disease. In addition, new VTs may appear subsequent to ablation of the initial VT in patients who have progressive underlying structural heart disease.

Given the above factors, it is apparent that ablation is not first-line therapy in the majority of patients with VT. However, it does represent a potential first-line therapy in patients with bundle branch reentrant tachycardia and in patients with monomorphic VT associated with structurally normal hearts.

Transcoronary Chemical Ablation

An additional technique for catheter ablation of VT is transcoronary chemical ablation.[17-20] This technique was initially demonstrated to ablate aconitine-induced VT in dogs, and subsequently it has been used in limited fashion in humans (Figure 1). The general region of origin of VT is determined from the QRS morphology on 12-lead surface electrocardiography. Subsequently, coronary angiography is undertaken and the artery or arteries likely providing blood flow to the region of VT origin are cannulated with a small caliber catheter. Iced saline or lidocaine is injected directly into small branches of the arteries until the tachycardia-dependent artery is determined, ie, the injection transiently interrupts the VT. If such an artery is identified, blood flow through the artery is permanently interrupted by the injection of 1-2 cc of 95% ethanol. Although this technique may be useful for an occasional patient, it is cumbersome and the tachycardia-specific artery may either not be successfully identified or cannulated in many patients. In addition, the ultimate size of the ablation lesion is difficult to control, and inadvertent reflux of ethanol into other arterial branches may create more tissue damage than desired.

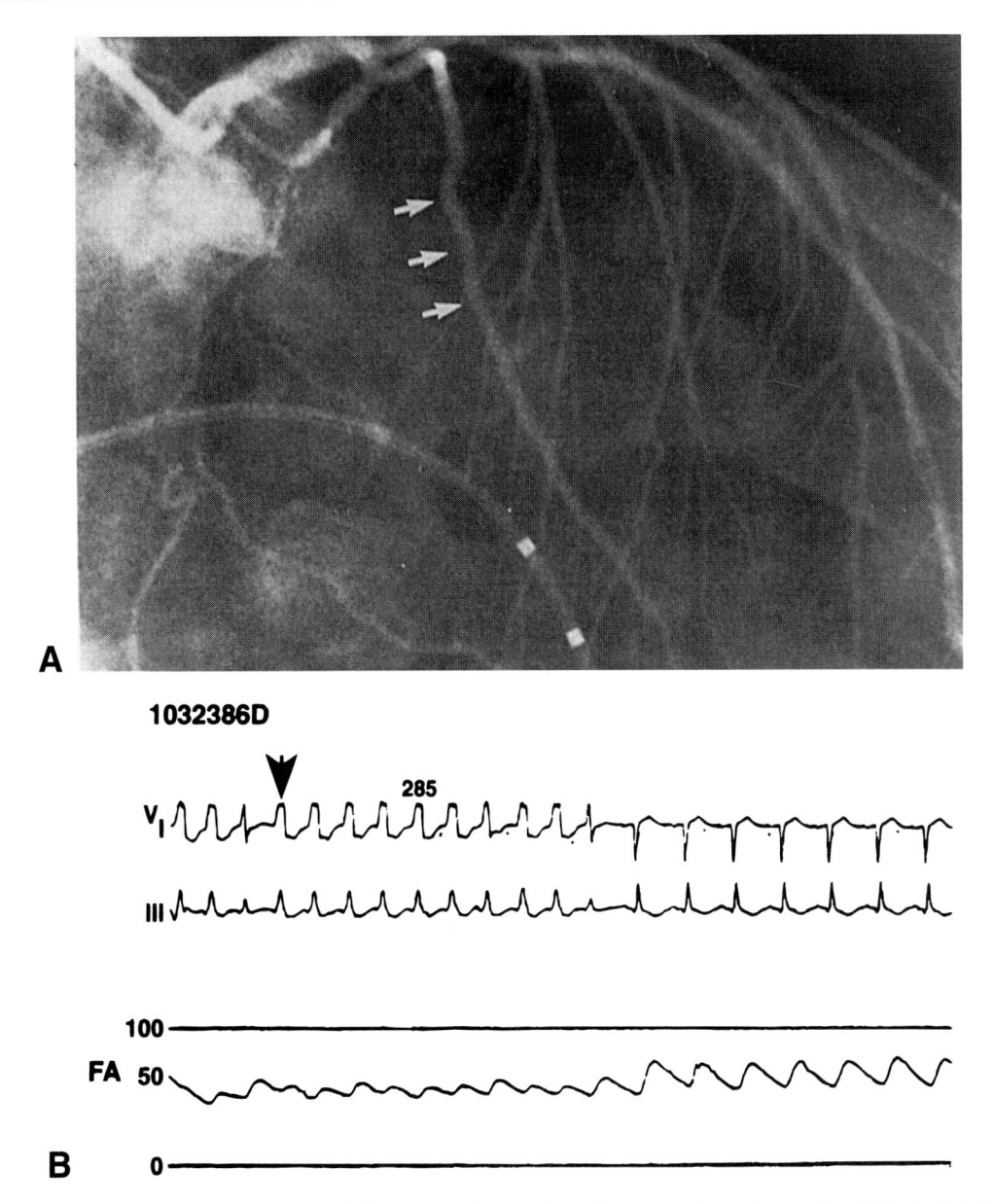

Figure 1. Transcoronary ethanol ablation for elimination of ventricular tachycardia (VT). **A:** Right oblique projection of the left coronary arteriogram. The arrows identify the coronary artery that is supplying the arrhythmic focus. **B:** Termination of VT by iced saline; arrow indicates injection.

Ablation for Elimination of Bundle Branch Reentrant Tachycardia

In normal human hearts, single induced ventricular extrasystoles commonly result in single nonstimulated bundle branch reentrant complexes.[21-23] However, in patients with prolonged His Purkinje conduction time and dilated left ventricles, a sustained VT can occur due to macroreentry within the bundle branches.[24,25] This variety of VT was initially thought to be rare, but recently it has become apparent that this mechanism is frequently responsible for VT

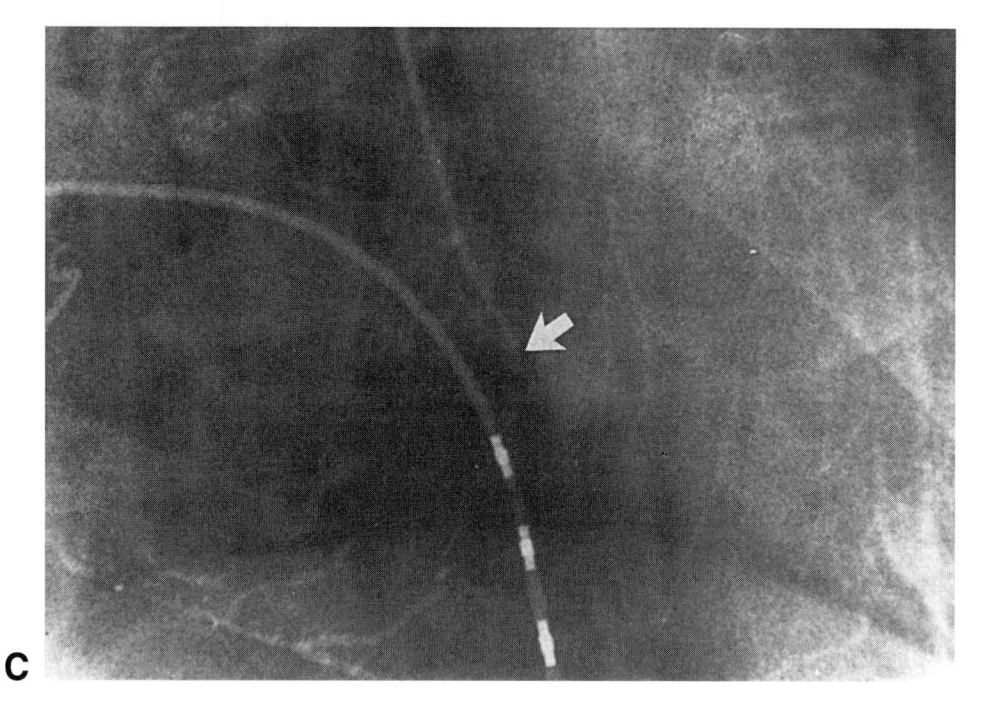

Figure 1. *(Continued)* **C**: Angiogram of left coronary artery after administration of ethanol, demonstrating occlusion (arrow) of the distal coronary artery. (Reproduced with permission from Reference 19.)

in patients with idiopathic dilated cardiomyopathy. For reentry to perpetuate within the bundle branches, there must be bundle branch conduction delay (prolonged HV interval). Ventricular dilation may also contribute to the arrhythmia by providing further prolongation of the potential tachycardia circuit. The most common form of bundle branch reentrant tachycardia has a left bundle branch block QRS morphology; its circuit consists of anterograde conduction down the right bundle branch, transseptal conduction to the left bundle branch, retrograde conduction up the left bundle branch, and subsequent reactivation of the right bundle branch anterogradely. Each QRS complex during bundle branch reentrant tachycardia is preceded by a His bundle potential with either the same HV interval as during sinus rhythm, a longer HV interval if anterograde conduction in the right bundle branch is further delayed during tachycardia, or a slightly shorter HV interval due to a proximal recording site of the His bundle potential. Recording of right or left bundle branch potentials during tachycardia may help define the tachycardia mechanism. Ventriculoatrial dissociation is usually present during tachycardia. Characteristically, any irregularity of the ventricular cycle length at the initiation of bundle branch reentry will be preceded by changes in the HH intervals, whereas in a VT with retrograde activation of the bundle branches without their integral participation in the tachycardia, HH cycle length changes would be expected to follow each respective change in the VV interval. Bundle branch reentrant tachycardia accounts for 6% of all VTs encountered in an active electrophysiology laboratory and accounts for 40% of VTs in patients with idiopathic dilated myopathy.[26] It is frequently rapid and associated with syncope and hemodynamic collapse. In an occasional patient the direction of the tachycardia circuit may be reversed, giving rise to tachycardia with a right bundle branch block QRS morphology. Even more unusual cases may involve reentry within the left anterior and left posterior fascicles (interfascicular reentry).[26]

Once the diagnosis of bundle branch reentry has been confirmed, ablation of the right bundle branch will eliminate the tachycardia (unless the tachycardia is interfascicular, in which case the right bundle branch is a bystander)[26–30] (Figure 2). To ablate the right bundle branch, an ablating electrode is positioned across the anterior leaflet of the tricuspid valve to record a typical His bundle potential. The catheter is then advanced further across the valve until a large ventricular potential is recorded, little or no atrial potential is recorded, and a right bundle branch potential is present; the interval between the right bundle branch potential and ventricular activation is at least 20 msec shorter than the HV interval

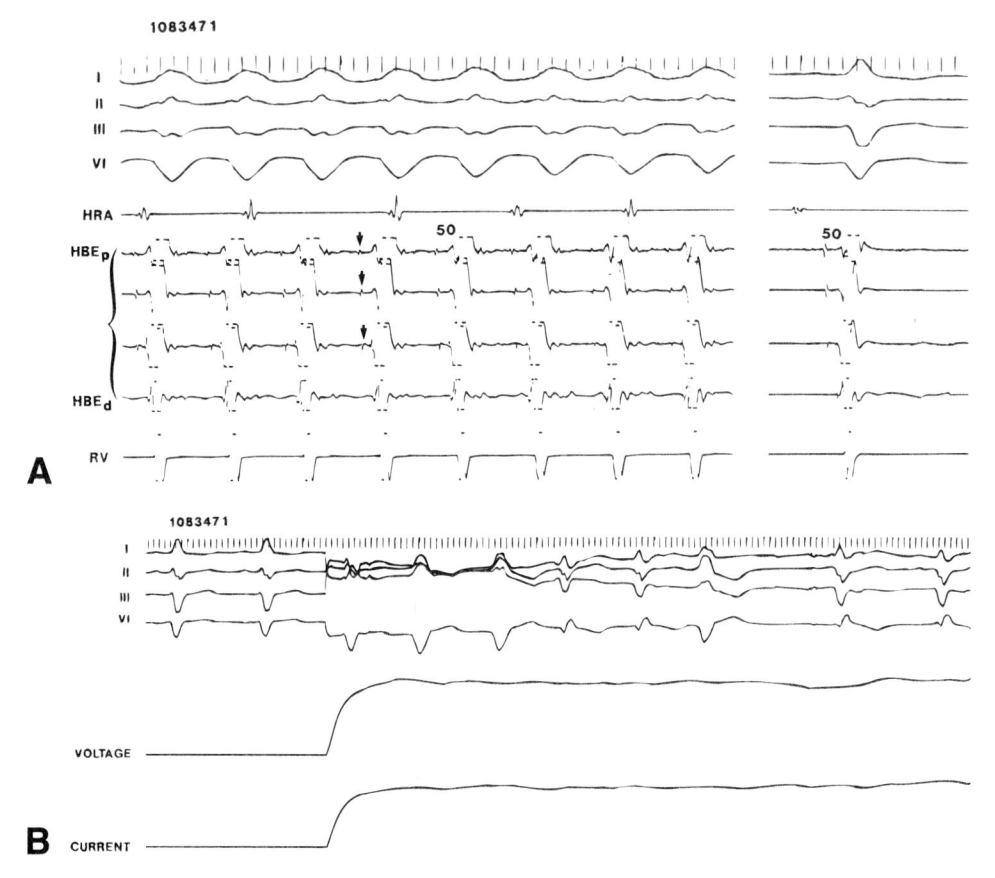

Figure 2. Ablation of bundle branch reentrant ventricular tachycardia (VT). **A:** Intracardiac recordings during bundle branch reentrant tachycardia. Surface leads I, II, III, and V_1, high right atrial (HRA), and right ventricular (RV) electrograms are shown. Four pairs of electrode catheters (indicated by the bracket) are displayed from the His bundle region, ranging from proximal (HBE_p) to distal (HBE_d). However, the His bundle catheter has been advanced so that right bundle branch potentials rather than His potentials are recorded, with a right bundle branch to ventricular interval of 50 msec (the true HV interval was 80 msec). Note that the right bundle branch to ventricular interval during bundle branch reentrant tachycardia is equal to that during sinus rhythm (right). **B:** Radiofrequency energy delivery during sinus rhythm at the HBE_d site in panel A. Ventricular ectopy occurs on introduction of energy, but complete right bundle branch block ensues as illustrated on the right of the figure. Bundle branch reentrant tachycardia was no longer inducible after the right bundle branch ablation. (Reproduced with permission from Miles et al: *Current Opinion in Cardiology* 8:75, 1993.)

measured from the distal His bundle recording electrodes. When radiofrequency energy is delivered to this area, complete right bundle branch block occurs, after which attempts at reinducing the tachycardia should be unsuccessful.

Once the diagnosis of bundle branch reentry has been verified, the right bundle branch can be ablated in virtually all patients.[26] However, patients' long-term survival may be limited by the presence of ventricular dysfunction. Although ablation of the right bundle branch eliminates the bundle branch reentrant tachycardia, these patients usually have severe underlying heart disease and may be at risk for other serious ventricular arrhythmias, which may necessitate additional antiarrhythmic drug or ICD therapy in some patients.[31] In addition, although all of these patients have prolonged HV intervals, criteria for permanent pacemaker implantation after ablation of the right bundle branch are not well defined.

Ventricular Tachycardia Ablation in Patients with Structurally Normal Hearts

Ventricular tachycardia occurring in patients with no apparent structural heart disease is often termed idiopathic VT,[32-34] accounting for up to 10% of patients referred to specialized electrophysiology centers. Related but not synonymous terms include right ventricular tachycardia, repetitive monomorphic VT, catecholamine sensitive VT, exercise-induced VT, adenosine sensitive VT, and verapamil sensitive VT. Buxton et al.[35] reported that 27% of their patients with idiopathic VT were asymptomatic, 40% presented with palpitations, 43% dizziness, and 23% syncope. Cardiac arrest has been reported, but is rare. A universally accepted classification of these tachycardias has not been developed. The VT may be classified by clinical pattern, such as repetitive monomorphic VT (multiple episodes of mostly nonsustained and self-terminating VT interrupted by occasional sinus beats) or paroxysmal sustained VT (episodes of sustained VT separated by periods of sinus rhythm). The site of VT origin can be used for classification; 70% of cases arise from the right ventricle (mostly the right ventricular outflow tract) and have a left bundle branch block QRS morphology. Tachycardia arising from the left ventricle has a right bundle branch block QRS morphology. In addition, the tachycardia may be classified by its response to pharmacological or physiological manipulations including exercise, catecholamines, verapamil, and adenosine. Potential mechanisms include reentry, abnormal automaticity, and triggered activity due to afterdepolarizations. Patient evaluation including history and physical examination, electrocardiogram, and echocardiogram are negative. In selected patients, left and right ventriculography, coronary angiography, magnetic resonance imaging scanning, and endomyocardial biopsy may be performed to exclude structural heart disease.

In the syndrome of verapamil sensitive idiopathic left VT, VT has a right bundle branch block QRS morphology with left-axis deviation. It arises from the left ventricular septum, possibly originating from the posterior fascicle.[36] It is unresponsive to β blockers, but responds to verapamil. Another unique syndrome of idiopathic VT reported by Lerman et al.[37] includes patients whose VT was initiated and terminated by programmed ventricular stimulation; VT induction was facilitated by isoproterenol; adenosine, verapamil, Valsalva, and carotid sinus massage terminated the VT; and β blockade either terminated the tachycardia or prevented its induction. These all suggest that the mechanism may be cyclic adenosine monophospate-mediated triggered activity.

In many patients with idiopathic monomorphic VT, the tachycardia cannot be initiated with programmed electrical stimulation but may occur spontaneously or be inducible during isoproterenol infusion. In addition, we have found that in some cases epinephrine but not isoproterenol may fa-

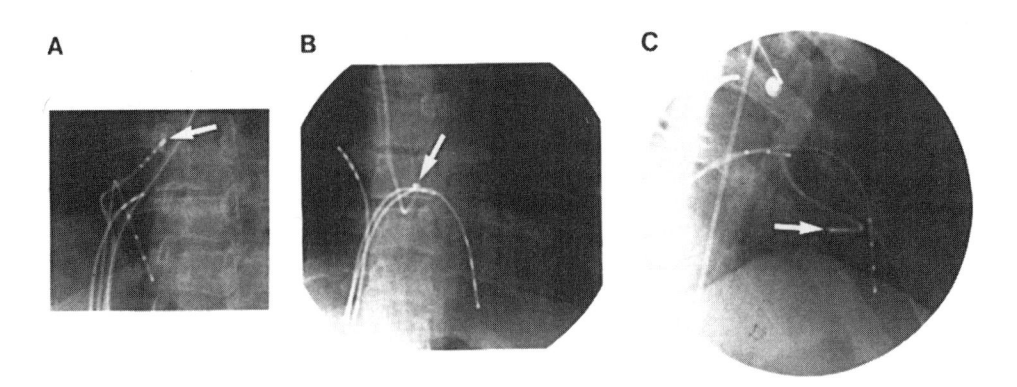

Figure 3. Catheter locations resulting in successful radiofrequency ablation of VT in patients with no structural heart disease. **A:** Left anterior oblique radiograph of a successful catheter position in a patient whose ventricular tachycardia (VT) arose from the right ventricular outflow tract. **B:** Right anterior oblique radiograph of successful catheter position in a patient whose VT arose just across the tricuspid valve near the His bundle. **C:** Right anterior oblique radiograph of successful catheter position in a patient whose VT arose from the posteroseptal region of the left ventricle. Arrows point to the electrode used for successful ablation. (Reproduced with permission from Reference 6.)

cilitate the VT, implying that α-adrenergic stimulation may be important in some patients. Idiopathic monomorphic VT may be treated chronically with β blockers, calcium blockers, or membrane active agents. Recently, however, it has become apparent that catheter ablation may be the therapy of first choice in many of these patients. These patients provide the potentially simplest substrate for VT ablation; that is, they have a monotonously monomorphic VT that is usually tolerated for periods long enough for mapping, and there is no scar, fibrosis, hypertrophy, or other abnormality of the cardiac muscle to interfere with adequate delivery of the ablation energy to the VT focus. In addition, most of these patients do not have progressive myocardial disease that would be associated with subsequent appearance of new VT foci in the future. Therefore these patients have been approached with high success using both DC energy[5] and radiofrequency energy[6,38] (Figures 3–6).

We have performed ablation in 43 such patients with a mean age of 39 years, ranging from 6–64 years.[6] Presenting symptoms were syncope in 2, presyncope in 30, palpitations in 10, and chest pain in 1. The duration of symptoms was 5.2 years, ranging from 0.1–25 years. Previous drug trials were 2.4, ranging from 0 to 10. No patient had any evidence of structural heart disease. The patients had VT induced with programmed electrical stimulation or with sympathetic stimulation using isoproterenol or epinephrine. Ablation was then carried out using a combination of activation and pace mapping. Ventricular tachycardia was eliminated in 39 of the 43 (91%) patients. Two patients required two sessions. The number of radiofrequency pulses delivered in the 39 successes were a mean of 6.8 with a range of 1–19; the median was 3 pulses with 11 patients requiring only 1 radiofrequency pulse. Ablation was never successful if there was inconsistent capture during the pace map, reflecting poor catheter tissue contact. Earliest endocardial activation during activation mapping in the 39 successes was 38 msec (range 20–80 msec) prior to onset of the VT QRS in the surface electrocardiogram, and the successful site always had the earliest endocardial activation. Over a follow-up of 14.3 months (range 1 to 37 months), there were no recurrences in the 39 successes. The sites of ventricular origin included the right ventricular out-

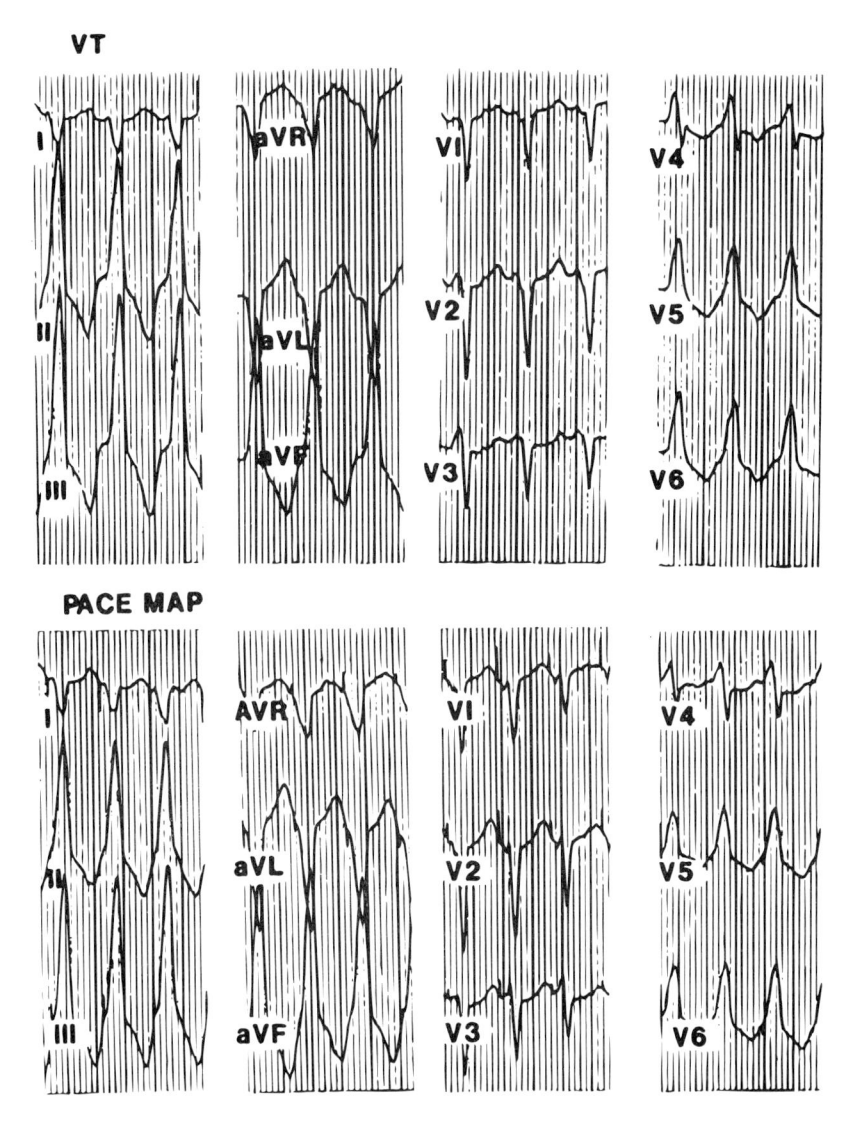

Figure 4. Electrocardiograms (ECGs) of ventricular tachycardia (top) and a pace map from the successful ablation site (bottom) in a patient with idiopathic monomorphic ventricular tachycardia arising from the right ventricular outflow tract. The site of the best pace map was the successful ablation site. This was the same site at which earliest endocardial activation was recorded during ventricular tachycardia. (Reproduced with permission from Reference 6.)

flow tract, the right ventricular septum near the His, the right ventricular free wall and the left ventricular septum, apex, or outflow tract. The success rate was 100% (27 of 27) for VT arising from the right ventricular outflow tract, but was 75% (12 of 16) for VT arising from sites other than the right ventricular outflow tract. In the patients with left VT coming from the left septum, a discrete potential preceding ventricular activation, probably Purkinje in origin, was sometimes useful for guiding ablation (Figure 7). The pace map in patients with idiopathic VT was highly reliable (in contrast to patients with coronary artery disease), and a pace map mimicking almost exactly the VT QRS morphology could usually be obtained, especially in patients with right ven-

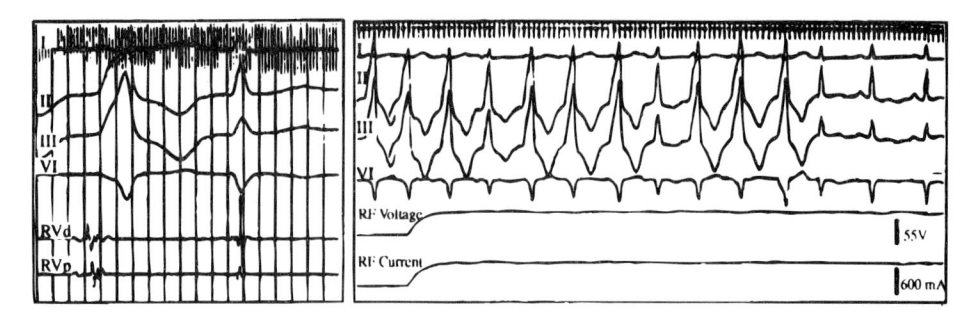

Figure 5. Radiofrequency ablation of ventricular tachycardia (VT). Left panel demonstrates recordings during ventricular bigeminy. The distal right ventricular electrogram (RVd) recorded from the right ventricular outflow tract occurred 30 msec prior to the onset of the QRS complex. The right panel demonstrates termination of the VT by radiofrequency energy. RVp: proximal right ventricular electrogram. (Reproduced with permission from Zipes DP: Management of cardiac arrhythmias: pharmacological, electrical, and surgical techniques. In: *Heart Diseases. A Textbook of Cardiovascular Medicine.* Edited by EB Braunwald. Fourth edition. Philadelphia, PA: W.B. Saunders Company; 1992.)

tricular outflow tract VT. Cardiac enzyme rise was small and follow-up Doppler echoes were normal except in two patients with cardiac perforation (one requiring catheter drainage); these were thought to have been due to right ventricular catheter manipulation rather than to the ablation itself.

Therefore, catheter ablation for elimination of monotonously monomorphic VT in patients with structurally normal hearts should be considered as a primary therapy, analogous to that in patients with Wolff-Parkinson-White syndrome or AV nodal reentrant tachycardia. It should be offered to patients on an equal basis with β blockers and calcium blockers depending on patient preference. In our opinion it is superior to

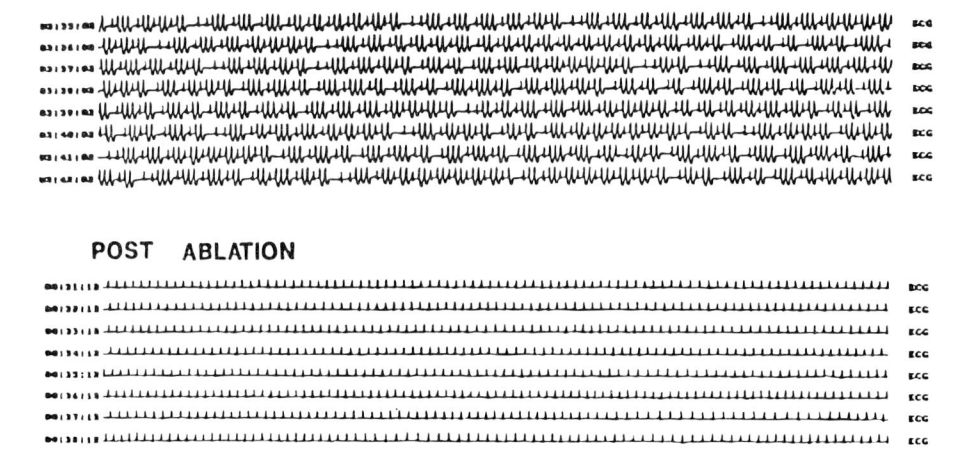

Figure 6. Tracings from a patient who presented with repetitive monomorphic ventricular tachycardia (VT). Top tracing is representative of spontaneous arrhythmia before ablation. After ablation, as displayed on the lower tracing, all spontaneous ventricular arrhythmia was eliminated. (Reproduced with permission from Reference 6.)

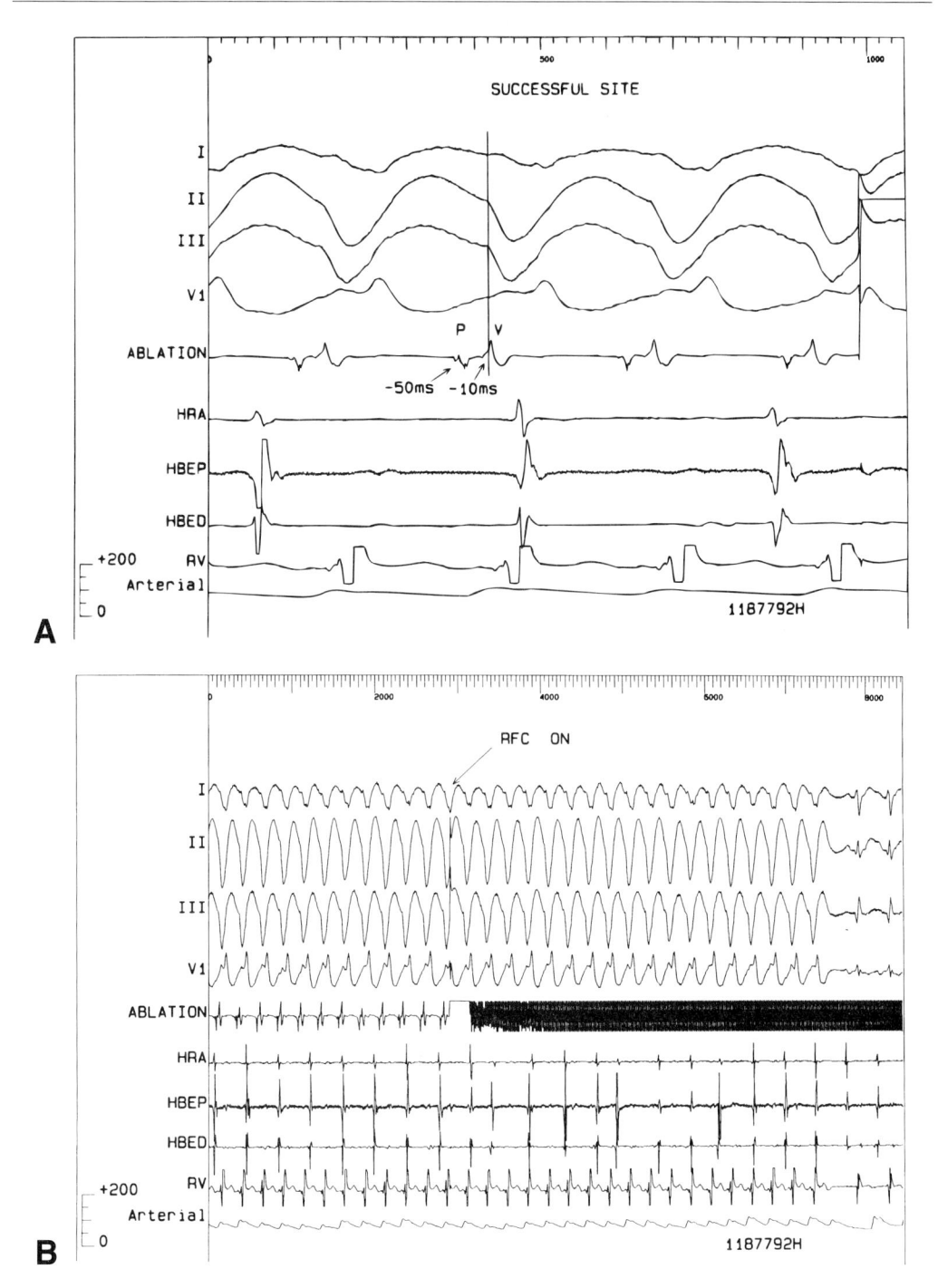

Figure 7. Verapamil sensitive ventricular tachycardia (VT) arising from the left ventricular septum. Surface leads I, II, III and V$_1$ are displayed along with a recording from the ablation electrode located in the left ventricular septal area. High right atrial (HRA), proximal and distal His bundle (HBEP and HBED) and right ventricular (RV) electrodes are displayed along with arterial pressure tracing. **A**: The electrogram from the successful site is illustrated on the ablation lead. Note that ventricular activation (V) precedes the onset of the QRS during VT by 10 msec, but a sharp potential thought to represent a Purkinje potential (P) occurs 50 msec prior to the onset of the QRS complex. **B**: VT terminates four and a half seconds after the onset of radiofrequency energy delivery (RFC ON) at the site illustrated in A. The patient had no further inducible VT.

therapy with membrane active agents, which may carry a higher risk of both nuisance and serious side effects.

Ablation of Ventricular Tachycardia in Patients With Structural Heart Disease

Ablation of VT in patients with structural heart disease is a major challenge at present, although active research may expand indications and success rates. The majority of patients with VT encountered in clinical practice have coronary artery disease. Chronic recurrent VT after myocardial infarction is likely caused by reentry involving areas of slow conduction at the border zone of infarction.[39] Mapping and ablation in these patients are complicated by all of the problems noted previously. Even when a single monomorphic VT can be reproducibly induced and targeted, ablation success is limited by difficulty in localizing the site of origin and the fact that radiofrequency energy may not penetrate scar, clot, or myocardium to sufficient depths to create lesions of sufficient size to totally eliminate the tachycardia. Pace mapping is not as reliable as it is in patients without structural heart disease,[40] probably because of myocardial fibrosis altering activation patterns and possible nonendocardial or multicentric origin of some tachycardias.

The electrogram characteristics of potential successful ablation sites are not well established.[40-45] Four major criteria have been proposed: 1) early site of activation during VT, preceding the onset of the ventricular electrogram on the surface ECG; 2) isolated mid-diastolic potentials, probably representing activation of the area of slow conduction during diastole[41] (Figure 8); 3) pace mapping, as mentioned above, may be useful but not highly reliable for guiding ablation; and 4) concealed entrainment.[44] Concealed entrainment refers to pacing from the mapping ablation catheter at the site of slow conduction, so that the tachycardia can be accelerated to the pacing rate (entrained) but the QRS morphology during concealed entrainment will be exactly the same as that during tachycardia, since exit from the site of slow conduction is identical to that during VT. None of these criteria alone have been universally successful in predicting a successful site for VT ablation. However, by using a combination of these criteria, success rates of up to 80% have been obtained at ablating the targeted VT.[40] The patients participating in such studies have been highly selected (representing < 10% of patients with coronary artery disease referred for ventricular tachyarrhythmias), not all of a given patient's VTs were able to be targeted, and the majority of patients still required antiarrhythmic drug therapy. Ablation in patients with multiple VT morphologies may be difficult; however, in some instances VT with different morphologies may use the same area of slow ventricular conduction.[46]

Indications for VT ablation in patients with coronary artery disease includes patients with incessant VT in whom implantation of an ICD is contraindicated. Candidates should have only one or two types of monomorphic VT that are inducible and hemodynamically stable enough for the mapping procedure. Patients who are not deemed surgical or ICD candidates may be candidates for an attempt at VT ablation. Ventricular tachycardia ablation may become a useful adjunct to ICD implantation; in a patient with several potential VTs, an ICD may be implanted, after which any VT leading to frequent ICD discharges may be addressed with ablation.

There is less experience in ablation of VT associated with other forms of structural heart disease. Ablation of monomorphic, inducible, hemodynamically tolerated VT in patients with dilated or hypertrophic cardiomyopathy can be attempted, although the success rate is lower than that for idiopathic VT. One must always carefully exclude bundle branch reentrant tachycardia (sometimes requiring unusual pacing methods or drug infusion for induction) in patients

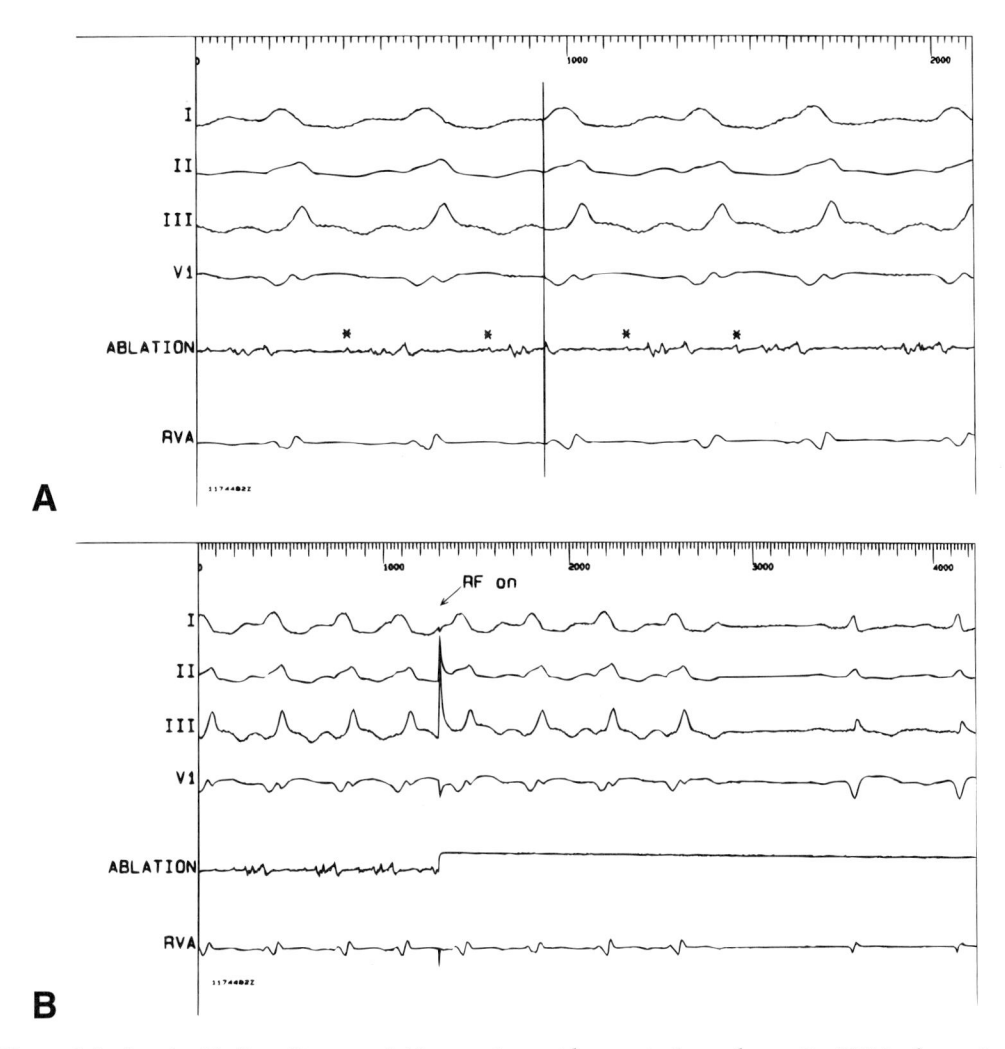

Figure 8. Isolated mid-diastolic potential in a patient with ventricular tachycardia (VT) in the setting of chronic coronary artery disease. Surface leads I, II, III, and V$_1$ are illustrated along with an ablation electrogram from the left ventricular septum and a right ventricular apical electrogram. **A**: The patient is in sustained VT. Fractionated, early ventricular activation is noted. Consistent isolated mid-diastolic activity is present (asterisks). **B**: VT terminates 1.5 seconds after onset of radiofrequency energy delivery (RF ON) at the site illustrated in A. The patient had no further inducible VT.

with idiopathic dilated cardiomyopathy if HV prolongation is present.[26]

Ablation has also been used to eliminate VT arising in arrhythmogenic right ventricular dysplasia.[47] However, it is more difficult to adequately ablate VT in these patients than in those with idiopathic monomorphic VT because multiple VT morphologies and sites of origin are usually present, and progression of the disease may result in new VTs. The risk of ventricular perforation may be increased because of the dilated and thinned right ventricular wall, and the dilated right ventricle may cause difficulty in mapping the VT and obtaining adequate contact at the ablation site. However, in patients with right ventricular dysplasia who have one predominant tachycardia morphology, ablation may be a useful option. These patients may also require antiarrhythmic medication even after the ablation procedure.

Future Directions

Investigation is ongoing to expand the indications for VT ablation. This includes improvements in tachycardia targeting; ie, new methods of identifying the correct site for delivery of ablation energy, new catheters with improved ease of manipulation, and multielectrode catheter arrays that may be introduced into the cardiac chambers for mapping of multiple sites simultaneously (aided by a computer). Intracardiac echocardiography may aid in catheter placement. In addition, improvements in energy delivery (including large-tipped catheters able to deliver higher radiofrequency power and new energy sources such as microwave, laser, and ultrasound) are being developed to provide larger and deeper lesions, lesions of varying contours, and the ability to penetrate fibrous tissue. The safety and efficacy of these energy sources have yet to be determined, but lesions larger than radiofrequency energy can currently provide are probably necessary for many cases of VT.

Conclusions

With the advent of radiofrequency energy, catheter ablation has evolved into a first-line therapy for VT due to bundle branch reentry and idiopathic monomorphic VT. It shows promise in selected patients with chronic recurrent VT associated with coronary artery disease, although new energy sources producing larger lesions and better targeting may be necessary in many of these patients. In some patients in whom catheter ablation is not satisfactory as sole therapy, it may provide useful adjunctive therapy to an ICD by eliminating recurrent VT that may be causing multiple defibrillator discharges. Ventricular tachycardia represents the next major frontier for catheter ablation.

Acknowledgment: The authors appreciate the expert secretarial assistance of Patty Owens and Robin Reid.

References

1. Zipes DP, Klein LS, Miles WM: Nonpharmacologic therapy: can it replace antiarrhythmic drug therapy? *J Cardiovasc Electrophysiol* 2:S255, 1991.
2. Gallagher JJ, Svenson RH, Kasell JH, et al: Catheter technique for closed-chest ablation of the atrioventricular conduction system. A therapeutic alternative for the treatment of refractory supraventricular tachycardia. *N Engl J Med* 306:194, 1982.
3. Scheinman MM, Morady F, Hess DS, et al: Catheter induced ablation of the atrioventricular junction to control refractory supraventricular arrhythmias. *JAMA* 248:851, 1982.
4. Hartzler GO: Electrode catheter ablation of refractory focal ventricular tachycardia. *J Am Coll Cardiol* 2:1107, 1983.
5. Morady F, Kadish AH, DiCarlo L, et al: Long-term results of catheter ablation of idiopathic right ventricular tachycardia. *Circulation* 82:2093, 1990.
6. Klein LS, Shih H-T, Hackett FK, et al: Radiofrequency catheter ablation of ventricular tachycardia in patients without structural heart disease. *Circulation* 85:1666, 1992.
7. Morady F, Scheinman MM, DiCarlo LA, et al: Catheter ablation of ventricular tachycardia with intracardiac shocks: Results in 33 patients. *Circulation* 75:1037, 1987.
8. Bardy GH, Ivey TD, Coltorti F, et al: Developments, complications, and limitations of catheter-mediated electrical ablation of posterior accessory atrioventricular pathways. *Am J Cardiol* 61:309, 1988.
9. Evans GT Jr, Scheinman MM, Zipes DP, et al: The Percutaneous Cardiac Mapping and Ablation Registry: final summary of results. *PACE* 11:1621, 1988.
10. Jackamn WM, Wang X, Friday KJ, et al: Catheter ablation of accessory atrioventricular pathways (Wolff-Parkinson-White syndrome) by radiofrequency current. *N Engl J Med* 324:1605, 1991.
11. Calkins H, Sousa J, El-Atassi R, et al: Diagnosis and cure of the Wolff-Parkinson-White syndrome or paroxysmal supraventricular tachycardias during a single electrophysiologic test. *N Engl J Med* 324:1612, 1991.
12. Jackman W, Beckman K, McClelland J, et al: Treatment of supraventricular tachycardia due to atrioventricular nodal reentry by ra-

diofrequency catheter ablation of slow-pathway conduction. *N Engl J Med* 327:313, 1992.
13. Kalbfleisch SJ, Langberg JJ: Catheter ablation with radiofrequency energy: Biophysical aspects and clinical applications. *J Cardiovasc Electrophysiol* 3:173, 1992.
14. Haines DE, Watson DD: Tissue heating during radiofrequency catheter ablation: A thermodynamic model and observations in isolated perfused and superfused canine right ventricular free wall. *PACE* 12:962, 1989.
15. Haines DE, Verow AF: Observations on electrode-tissue interface temperature and effect on electrical impedance during radiofrequency ablation of ventricular myocardium. *Circulation* 82:1034, 1990.
16. Langberg JJ, Calkins H, El-Atassi R, et al: Temperature monitoring during radiofrequency catheter ablation of accessory pathways. *Circulation* 86:1469, 1992.
17. Inoue H, Waller B, Zipes DP. Intracoronary ethyl alcohol or phenol injection ablates aconitine-induced ventricular tachycardia in dogs. *J Am Coll Cardiol* 10:1342, 1987.
18. Brugada P, de Swart H, Smeets J, et al: Transcoronary chemical ablation of ventricular tachycardia. *Circulation* 79:475, 1989.
19. Nora MO, Miles WM, Klein LS, et al: Alcohol ablation of ventricular tachycardia. *J Cardiovasc Electrophysiol* 2:456, 1991.
20. Okishige K, Friedman PL. Alcohol ablation for tachycardia therapy. *J Cardiovasc Electrophysiol* 3:354, 1992.
21. Zipes DP, de Joseph RL, Rothbaum DA. Unusual properties of accessory pathways. *Circulation* 49:1200, 1974.
22. Akhtar M, Damato AN, Batsford WP, et al: Demonstration of reentry with the His-Purkinje system in man. *Circulation* 50:1150, 1974.
23. Akhtar M, Gilbert C, Wolf FG, et al: Reentry within the His-Purkinje system: elucidation of reentrant circuit using right bundle branch and His bundle recordings. *Circulation* 58:295, 1978.
24. Lloyd EA, Zipes DP, Heger JJ, et al: Sustained ventricular tachycardia due to bundle branch reentry. *Am Heart J* 104:1095, 1982.
25. Caceres J, Jazayeri M, McKinnie J, et al: Sustained bundle branch reentry as a mechanism of clinical tachycardia. *Circulation* 79:256, 1989.
26. Blanck Z, Dhala A, Deshpande S, et al: Bundle branch reentrant ventricular tachycardia: cumulative experience in 48 patients. *J Cardiovasc Electrophysiol* 4:253, 1993.
27. Touboul P, Kirkorian G, Atallah G, et al: Bundle branch reentrant tachycardia treated by electrical ablation of the right bundle branch. *J Am Coll Cardiol* 7:1404, 1986.
28. Tchou P, Jazayeri M, Denker S, et al: Transcatheter electrical ablation of the right bundle branch: a method of treating macro-reentrant ventricular tachycardia due to bundle branch reentry. *Circulation* 78:246, 1988.
29. Langberg JJ, Desai J, Dullet N, et al: Treatment of macroreentrant ventricular tachycardia with radiofrequency ablation of the right bundle branch. *Am J Cardiol* 63:1010, 1989.
30. Cohen T, Chien W, Lurie K, et al: Radiofrequency catheter ablation for treatment of bundle branch reentrant ventricular tachycardia: results and long-term follow-up. *J Am Coll Cardiol* 18:1767, 1991.
31. Miles WM: Bundle branch reentrant tachycardia: a chance to cure? *J Cardiovasc Electrophysiol* 4:263, 1993.
32. Brooks R, Burgess JH: Idiopathic ventricular tachycardia: a review. *Medicine* 67:271, 1988.
33. Belhassen B, Viskin S: Idiopathic ventricular tachycardia and fibrillation. *J Cardiovasc Electrophysiol* 4:356, 1993.
34. Mont L, Seixas T, Brugada P, et al: The electrocardiographic, clinical, and electrophysiologic spectrum of idiopathic monomorphic ventricular tachycardia. *Am Heart J* 124:746, 1992.
35. Buxton AE, Waxman HL, Marchlinski FE, et al: Right ventricular tachycardia: clinical and electrophysiologic characteristics. *Circulation* 68:917, 1983.
36. Nakagawa H, Beckman K, McClelland J, et al: Radiofrequency ablation of idiopathic left ventricular tachycardia guided by a Purkinje potential (abstract). *PACE* 16:161, 1993.
37. Lerman BB, Belardinelli L, West A, et al: Adenosine-sensitive ventricular tachycardia: evidence suggesting cyclic AMP-mediated triggered activity. *Circulation* 74:270, 1986.
38. Wilber DJ, Baerman J, Okshansky B, et al: Adenosine-sensitive ventricular tachycardia: clinical characteristics and response to catheter ablation. *Circulation* 87:126, 1993.
39. Downar E, Harris L, Mickleborough LL, et al: Endocardial mapping of ventricular tachycardia in the intact human heart: evidence for reentrant mechanisms. *J Am Coll Cardiol* 11:783, 1988.
40. Morady F, Harvey M, Kalbfleisch SJ, et al: Radiofrequency catheter ablation of ventricular tachycardia in patients with coronary artery disease. *Circulation* 87:363, 1993.
41. Fitzgerald DM, Friday KJ, Yeung-Lai-Wah JA, et al: Electrogram patterns predicting successful catheter ablation of ventricular tachycardia. *Circulation* 77:806, 1988.
42. Morady F, Frank R, Kou WH, et al: Identification and catheter ablation of a zone of slow

conduction in the reentrant circuit of ventricular tachycardia in humans. *J Am Coll Cardiol* 11:775, 1988.
43. Stevenson WG, Weiss JN, Wiener I, et al: Slow conduction in the infarct scar: relevance to the occurrence, detection and ablation of ventricular reentry circuits resulting from myocardial infarction. *Am Heart J* 117:452, 1989.
44. Morady F, Kadish A, Rosenheck S, et al: Concealed entrainment as a guide for catheter ablation of ventricular tachycardia in patients with prior myocardial infarction. *J Am Coll Cardiol* 17:678, 1991.
45. Dubuc M, Savard P, Nadeau R: Catheter ablation of ventricular tachycardia related to coronary heart disease. *Circulation* 87:649, 1993.
46. Fitzgerald DM, Friday KJ, Yeung-Lai-Wah JA, et al: Myocardial regions of slow conduction participating in the reentrant circuit of multiple ventricular tachycardias: Report on ten patients. *J Cardiovasc Electrophysiol* 2:193, 1991.
47. Leclercq JF, Chouty F, Cauchemez B, et al: Results of electrical fulguration in arrhythmogenic right ventricular disease. *Am J Cardiol* 62:220, 1988.

Part 5

Future Perspectives

Chapter 31

Antitachycardia Pacing and Implantable Cardioverter Defibrillators for Treatment of Supraventricular Tachyarrhythmias

David G. Benditt, Stuart W. Adler, Stephen C. Remole, Scott Sakaguchi, and Keith G. Lurie

Introduction

Implanted pulse generators have been used to treat supraventricular tachycardias (SVTs) in selected patients for nearly 25 years. However, clinical acceptance has been modest and in recent years even this limited role has been largely eclipsed by improved antiarrhythmic drug management and the introduction of highly effective transcatheter ablation techniques. However, treatments for certain SVTs, particularly atrial flutter and fibrillation, remain inadequate. Potentially, the treatment of these arrhythmias may provide an arena for the application of innovative implantable devices. With the successful emergence of tiered-therapy implantable cardioverter-defibrillators (ICDs) for control of life-threatening ventricular tachyarrhythmias, there is now growing interest in the application of similar devices in the atrium.

In this chapter we examine the current status of implantable pacing systems for control of supraventricular tachyarrhythmias. Additionally, we speculate on the essential pulse generator and lead system features needed in atrial directed pacemaker cardioverter-defibrillators to assure both clinical effectiveness and physician/patient acceptance in their most important potential application—the treatment of refractory atrial fibrillation.

Implantable Pacing Techniques for Treatment and Control of Tachyarrhythmias

Evolution of Implantable Systems for Supraventricular TachycardiaControl

Tachycardia Termination

Underdrive pacing was the first method used in an implanted pulse generator for tachycardia control.[1] The technique, although not widely used at present, can still be applied with most conventional implantable pulse generators. Essentially a standard pacemaker magnet is used to convert the device temporarily from a demand pulse generator into an asynchronous pacing mode. Asynchronous underdrive pacing is maintained in the hope that fortuitous

---

From Singer I, (ed.) Implantable Cardioverter-Defibrillator. Armonk, NY: Futura Publishing Company, Inc.; © 1994.

timing of a paced beat interrupts the tachycardia. The magnet is then removed. In certain cases, devices have been developed that automatically become asynchronous when sensing a rhythm having a shorter cycle length than the programmed refractory period of the device.[2]

Currently, termination of tachycardia by underdrive pacing technique is considered to be of limited clinical utility. Essentially, underdrive pacing is only useful for interrupting relatively slow tachycardias, and even then the method may be ineffective if the pacing site is at a substantial distance from the reentry circuit making it difficult for the stimulus to interfere with rhythm. Rapid pacing methods (ie, overdrive) are usually far more effective for tachycardia termination (albeit with greater potential proarrhythmia risk).

The potential for implanted pulse generators to provide on-board electrophysiologic testing and overdrive antitachycardia capability was recognized quite early in the development of pacing systems.[3–5] At that time, it was suggested that implanted atrial pacemakers could be used in an atrial triggered mode to assess atrioventricular (AV) conduction. In the absence of telemetry control, a chest wall stimulation technique using an external adjustable pacemaker was used to trigger the device at a sufficiently rapid rate. In that circumstance, the implanted pulse generator was able to track external chest wall stimulation to rates as high as 150 beats per minute (the upper rate being limited only by the sensing refractory period of the implanted device). Ultimately, as refractory periods became shorter, even higher rates were achievable. The latter capability provided the earliest option for transcutaneous tachycardia termination by overdrive pacing technique.

Transcutaneous control of a nonpowered implantable device was perhaps the earliest implantable system designed specifically for tachycardia treatment. This system, which used an implanted antenna and a manually operated external control box (Medtronic model 5998, Minneapolis, MN) (Figure 1)[6–8] was designed primarily for atrial tachyarrhythmia conversion, and proved relatively successful in limited use. Its principal advantage was the absence of an implanted battery at a time when batteries were large and had limited longevity. As a result, the system was relatively small for its era and had indefinite longevity in the absence of electrode problems. However, the device did require both adequate positioning of a control box over the implanted antenna, and appropriate manipulation of the control box by the patient or physician. In a subsequent modification of this concept, a similar interactive system used an otherwise conventional bipolar pulse generator capable of communicating with an external patient controlled radiofrequency transmitter (Medtronic model 2331 patient programmer) (Figure 2). In a further modification the patient's transmitter was preprogrammed with information on tachycardia recognition and appropriate treatment (Medtronic SPO 500™).[9] When placed over the implanted unit, the transmitter determined whether the detected rhythm corresponded with the appropriate detection criteria, and if so, permitted the preprogrammed treatments to be delivered (Figure 3). For antitachycardia applications preprogrammed therapies were established in the electrophysiology laboratory or clinic, and were automatically delivered when the patient or operator initiated a treatment by pressing a button on the control box.

Although quite innovative and useful for their time, the limitations of interactive antitachycardia systems included the lack of automatic tachyarrhythmia detection, with the consequent possibility that patients may be unable to respond appropriately due to fear or cardiovascular incapacity. In addition, there was concern that patients may inadvertently overtreat themselves in response to nonspecific symptoms, or palpitations unrelated to a bonafide tachyarrhythmia. Finally, a new untreatable tachyarrhythmia may be induced by inappropriate device use (eg, atrial fibrillation in a patient being treated for reentrant SVT), or there may be a delay in obtaining medical

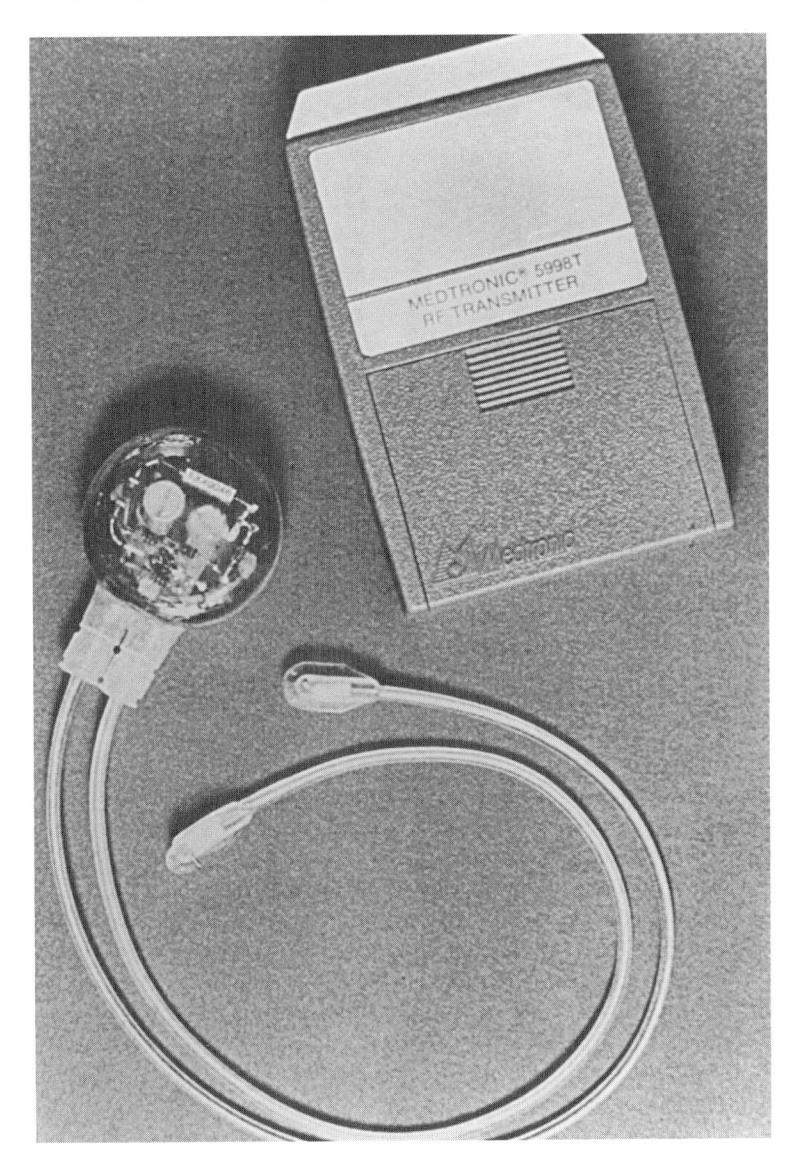

Figure 1. Photograph of a patient activated antitachycardia system (Medtronic model 5998, Minneapolis, MN) using an implantable antenna and an external radiofrequency (RF) transmitter. The implanted device was powered by the RF energy transmitted from the external unit. The RF signal was modulated to create burst pacing for treatment of atrial tachyarrhythmias. See text for details.

treatment while repeated attempts are made by the patient to interrupt a rapid rhythm that is not amenable to effective treatment by the device (eg, de novo ventricular tachycardia in a patient being treated for atrial flutter).

In the next stage of antitachycardia device development, several implantable pulse generators with burst or extrastimulus capability were made available. These pulse generators were, for the most part, dedicated to antitachycardia application with modest or no backup bradycardia function. Examples include the Cordis (Miami, FL) Orthocor™ models 234A and 239A. The Cybertach™ (Intermedics, INC., Freeport, TX) and the Medtronic model 7008 also fall into this category, but repre-

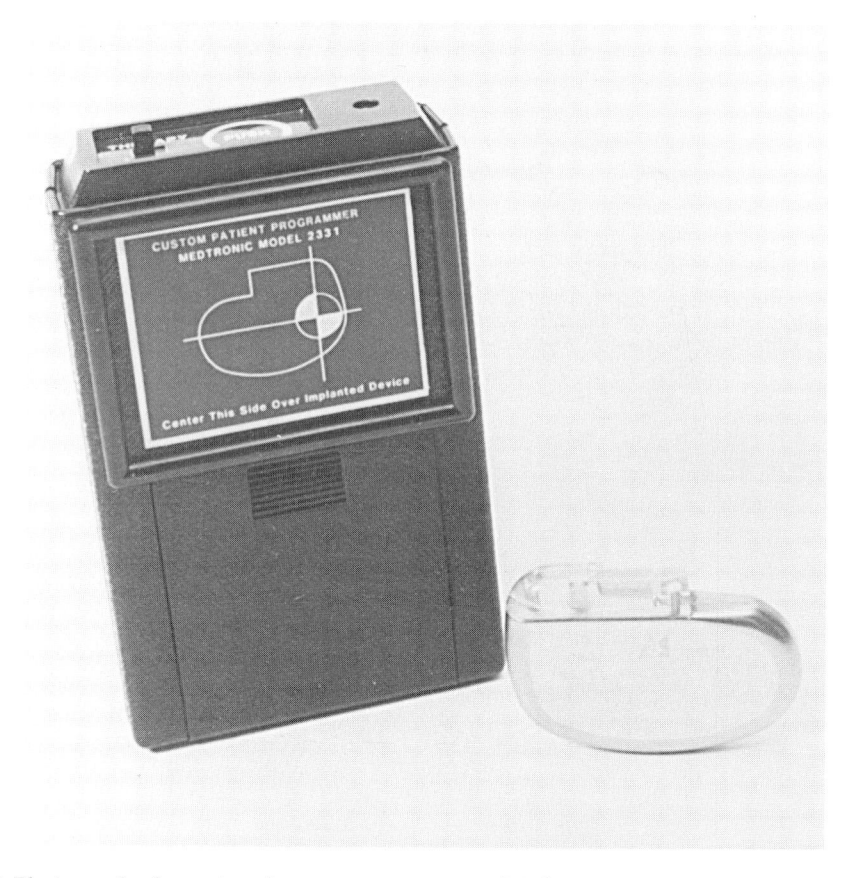

Figure 2. Photograph of an external custom programmer (Medtronic model 2331, Minneapolis, MN) used by the patient or physician to program implanted pulse generators (Spectrax models) to deliver rapid pacing bursts to terminate reentrant tachycardias.

sent important advances based on provision for both automatic tachycardia detection and variable therapy rates, as well as bradycardia backup capability. Even greater sophistication was provided by the Pasar™ family of devices (Telectronics, Inc., Englewood, CO), which provided automatic tachycardia detection (based on rate), and ultimately incorporated a variety of therapeutic stimulation capabilities including extrastimuli and scanning.

The scanning concept for antitachycardia pacing was first introduced in the mid-1970s.[10,11] This methodology appeared to provide an improvement in effectiveness over conventional burst pacing techniques and resulted in the need for fewer extrastimuli. The initial device using this concept (Pasar model 4151) was relatively effective, but experienced a number of technical problems.[12] Subsequent evolution of this early device into more recent models (Pasar model 4171) has been associated with improved success.[13,14]

The Medtronic Symbios™ model 7008[15] was the first dual-chamber pacing system to incorporate automatic antitachycardia capability. The antitachycardia features of this device were restricted to the atrial channel and incorporated the potential for delivery of up to 16 atrial extrastimuli at pacing intervals of 135–360 msec. As has been the case for most atrial antitachycardia devices, the 7008 was used in only a limited fashion and is no longer available for clinical use. In our experience in 3 patients (2 atrial flut-

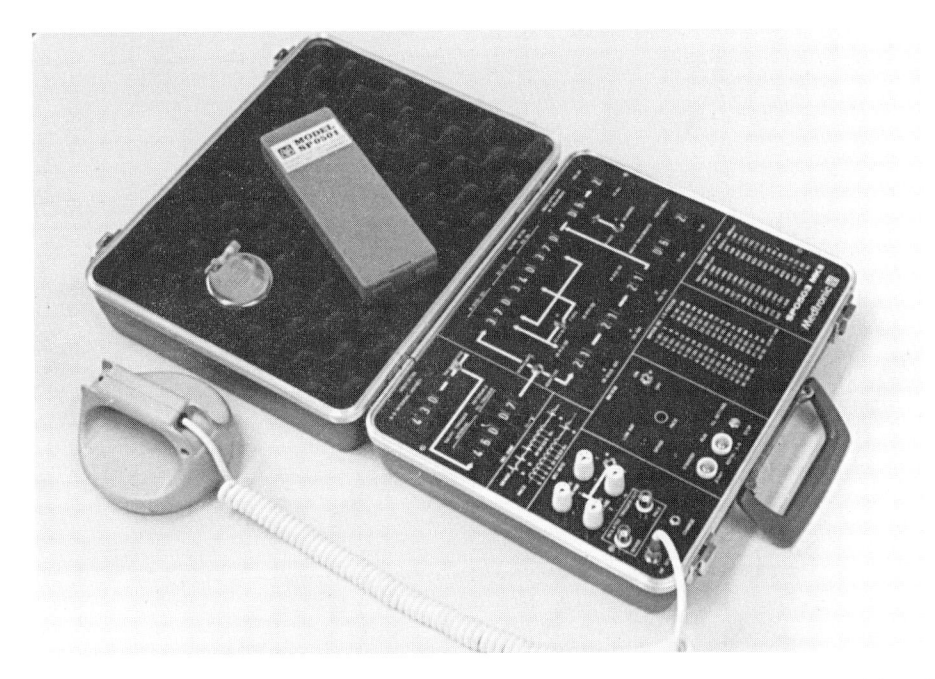

Figure 3. Photograph of a patient activated antitachycardia system (Medtronic model SPO-500, Minneapolis, MN) that was relatively advanced for its time in which tachycardia detection features and preprogrammed therapies were established by the physician for use as needed. The system was designed for both invasive and noninvasive electrophysiologic studies.

ter, 1 atrial reentry SVT) the model 7008 was associated with successful tachycardia termination in all cases during a follow-up of 2–4 years. Ultimately however, 1 patient with atrial flutter exhibited increasing frequency of atrial fibrillation (some probably device induced). The remaining 2 individuals continue to do well, although with the addition of amiodarone to their treatment regimen.

Among the implantable devices that have been specifically designed to address atrial tachyarrhythmias, only the Cybertach/Intertach family of devices remains widely available in the United States (Figure 4).[16] These pulse generators provide a relatively broad range of antitachycardia therapies with automatic arrhythmia detection. The Intertach (models 262–12 and 262–16) operates either automatically or after magnet activation. In the automatic mode, tachycardia detection is based on several possible criteria including: high rate, sudden onset, sustained high rate, and rate stability. Therapies include single or double extrastimuli, and burst stimulation up to 250 beats per minute. Initial coupling interval (delay) at onset of stimulation and subsequent stimulation cycle length are programmable, and can be fixed or set as a percentage of the tachycardia cycle length. The device can provide extrastimuli or pacing bursts in a scanning mode with programmable variables including the magnitude of the scanning step, the number of scans to be applied, and the minimum coupling interval permitted. Autodecremental stimulation is also available, with the possibility of establishing a minimum cycle length in order to prevent excessively rapid atrial pacing rates. The Intertach also includes a memory function that permits previously effective therapeutic responses to be repeated when the same tachycardia is recognized on a subsequent occasion.

Despite the sophistication of current implantable atrial antitachycardia devices, their popularity will likely remain limited

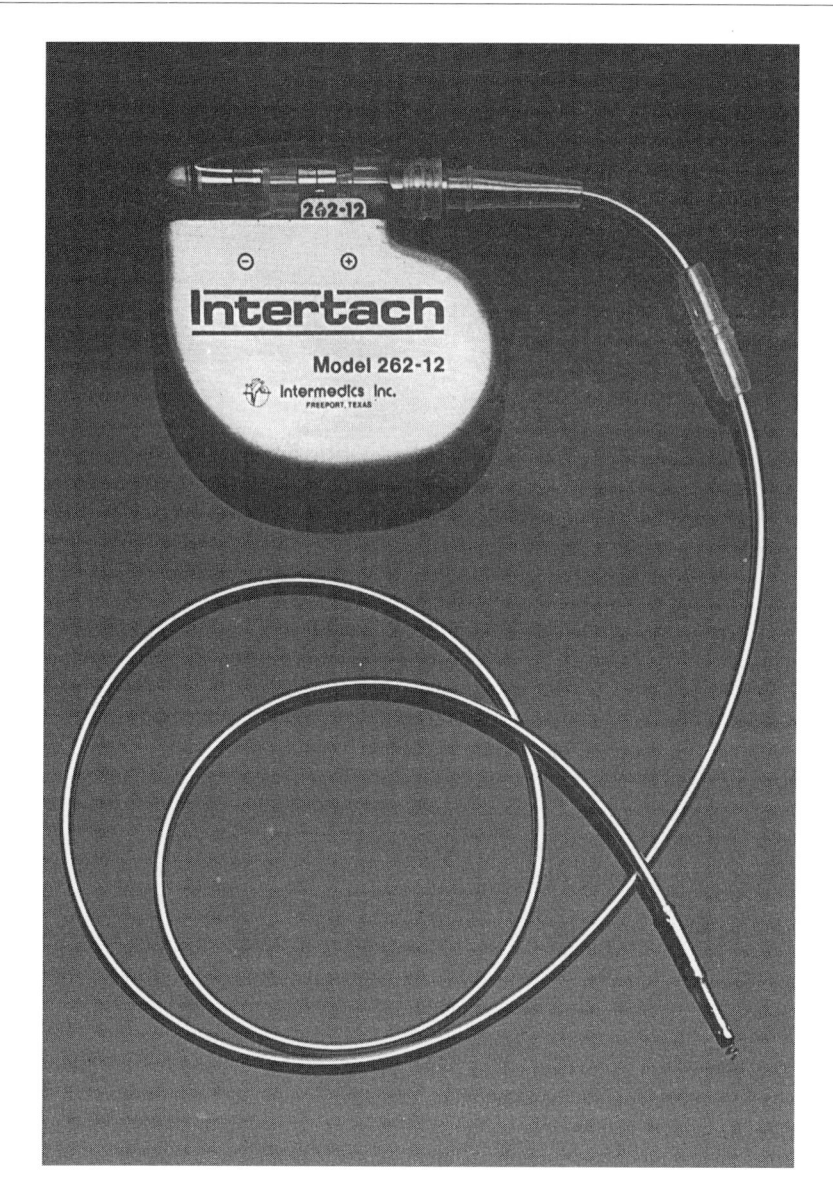

Figure 4. Photograph of the most widely available implantable pulse generator for atrial antitachycardia application in the United States. See text for description. (Intertach™, Intermedics Inc., Freeport, TX)

given the recent development of more effective antiarrhythmic drugs, and highly efficacious transcatheter ablation techniques. Perhaps their greatest advantage is in management of selected patients with the common form of recurrent atrial flutter, and some similar but relatively stable primary atrial tachycardias when they prove refractory to drugs.[17,18] Additionally, devices may be useful in a few patients with reentrant SVTs in whom drug therapy is unsuccessful and where transcatheter ablation is declined.

Tachycardia Prevention

Another approach to implantable devices for antitachycardia pacing is the use of dual-chamber pacing to prevent reentrant supraventricular tachyarrhythmias. This technique has proved useful in a few patients for control of AV nodal and AV reentry tachycardias, since synchronization of ventricular and atrial depolarization essentially prevents establishment of slow conduction through the AV node and thereby obviates the possibility of sustained reentry. Nonetheless, despite its seeming simplicity, this technique has received only limited clinical application.

Advantages and Disadvantages of Implantable Antitachycardia Systems

Fully automatic implantable antitachycardia systems offer a number of advantages[6]: 1) tachycardia treatment applied only when necessary; 2) absence of drug-related side effects; 3) freedom from drug dosing schedules; 4) appropriate treatment application in the disabled or confused patient; 5) necessity for avoidance of the potential consequences of tissue destruction by ablation (complications, proarrhythmic effects, etc.); 6) on-board antibradycardia support; 7) cost-competitive quality-of-life improvement; and 8) flexibility to pursue other therapeutic options at a later time if necessary. However, several disadvantages of the systems also bear consideration: 1) relatively high initial implantation and set-up cost; 2) device implantation risk comparable to other conventional implanted pulse generators; 3) cosmetic disadvantages; 4) imperfect diagnostic and treatment algorithms; 5) relatively frequent follow-up with testing; 6) ultimate need for pulse generator replacement; and 7) potential proarrhythmic effects (eg, induction of atrial fibrillation).

Clinical Experience With Pacing Systems for Atrioventricular Nodal and Atrioventricular Reentrant Supraventricular Tachycardias

The SVTs due to reentry within the AV node or reentry using an accessory connection are the arrhythmias most susceptible to successful treatment with pacing techniques. Although alternative treatment options have recently taken precedence, the effectiveness of antitachycardia systems in these arrhythmias has been well documented and the techniques should remain in the therapeutic armamentarium for use in selected patients.

Tachycardia Termination

A considerable body of clinical experience indicates that antitachycardia pacing techniques are effective at terminating reentrant supraventricular tachyarrhythmias. In 1986, Fisher et al.[19] provided a retrospective examination of the previous two decades of antitachycardia pacing. Their review comprised published studies using both available and custom design pulse generators. The techniques for tachycardia termination varied widely among these devices, but essentially included most of the antitachycardia modalities presently available (ie, underdrive, scanning methods, multiple premature extrastimuli, etc.). The findings from 25 papers encompassing 268 patients (average duration of follow-up approximately 12–15 months) suggested that clinical outcomes were for the most part quite satisfactory. In only 4% of cases were results considered to be poor. On average, 20% to 50% of patients were treated with concomitant antiarrhythmic drug therapy.

Currently, only fully automatic antitachycardia pacing systems with adequate bradycardia backup are appropriate for clinical use. Within such systems a variety of treatment options are programmable, with overdrive pacing at rates above the detected tachycardia rate generally being considered the most effective means of tachycardia termination. Some of the more widely used or intriguing of these overdrive modalities include (Figure 5): 1) extrastimuli alone in which single or multiple extrastimuli scan the tachycardia cycle or automatically adapt their coupling interval to

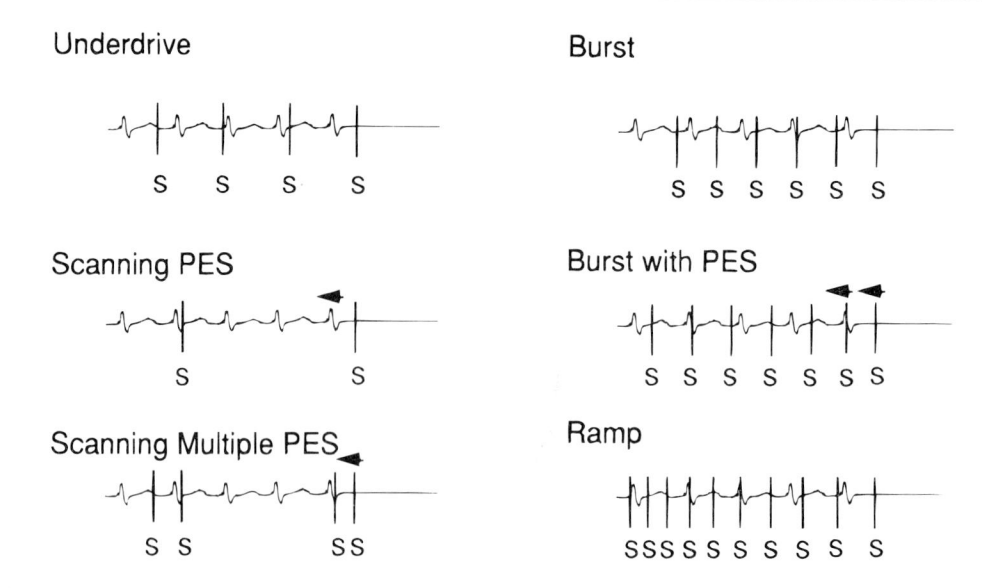

Figure 5. Simulated electrocardiograms illustrating various pacing techniques for use in atrial tachycardia termination. (Modified with permission from Reference 19.)

the tachycardia rate; 2) scanning burst in which each successive termination attempt results in reduction of the interstimulus interval by the same amount although the coupling interval of the first stimulus is usually kept constant; 3) ramp bursts in which the cycle length of the stimulation sequence gradually shortens (rate speeds up); 4) autodecremental burst in which the coupling interval of the first stimulus is determined as a certain percentage of the tachycardia cycle length, while the cycle length of the burst is similarly proportional to the tachycardia rate; 5) overdrive burst with extrastimuli that incorporates a combination of a rapid pacing burst with subsequent insertion of one or more premature extrastimuli at the end; and 6) ultrarapid pacing in which a short burst of extremely rapid pacing (3,000 to 5,000 per minute) permits sufficient capture of the reentry circuit to terminate the arrhythmia. The latter technique is yet to be used in an implantable device.

In all patients in whom antitachycardia device therapy is contemplated, careful electrophysiologic assessment is essential in order to establish an appropriate stimulation treatment protocol. As is the case with tiered-therapy devices for treatment of ventricular tachyarrhythmias, several backup therapeutic options may need to be programmed. Additionally, periodic testing is crucial in order to confirm that treatment efficacy is maintained.

The principal factors determining efficacy of pacing treatment include size of the reentry circuit, duration of the excitable gap, and the physical proximity of stimulating electrodes to the reentry circuit. When conditions are optimal, even relatively ineffective pacing techniques such as underdrive pacing can be effective. For example, Curry et al.[20] used electrophysiologic testing to determine the optimum pacing site for tachycardia termination, after which they observed the effective use of implantable dual demand pacing systems in six patients. Ultimately, however, device problems or lack of efficacy occurred in 3 of 6 individuals over an 11- to 47-month follow-up.

Automatic antitachycardia devices have been successfully used in small numbers of patients with relatively few adverse reactions. For example, Jung et al.[21] surveyed their experience with treatment of

SVT between 1985 and 1989. Thirty-two (9%) of 353 patients being evaluated for SVT were treated with antitachycardia pacing systems (Intertach models 262–12 and 262–16). Detection criteria were established by using the noninvasive electrophysiologic testing capability of the device. As a result of this approach, the most frequent diagnostic algorithm used a combination of high rate, sudden onset, and rate stability criteria. Treatment usually comprised a primary and a secondary modality, with the former being autodecremental bursts and the latter being an adaptive scanning mode. In 39 ± 117 months of follow-up, tachycardia was controlled by the device alone in 19 of 32 patients. Concomitant antiarrhythmic medication was needed in a further 10 patients to reduce SVT rate and/or prevent atrial fibrillation. In 3 patients device therapy proved inadequate. Complications included early atrial lead dislodgement in 1 patient, lead fracture in 1 patient, and pocket infection necessitating system explantation in 1 patient.

In a recent review of antitachycardia pacing experience from several Italian cardiac centers, Boccadamo and Toscano[22] reported outcomes in 55 patients treated with Symbios 7008 between 1983 and 1989. Among these patients, 26 were treated for AV nodal reentry tachycardia and 21 of 26 (81%) were reported to be entirely controlled during a mean follow-up of approximately 50 months. Similarly 7 of 10 (70%) patients with AV reentry were reported to have had successful outcomes. The response to atrial flutter, however, was quite poor.

An overall sense of the usefulness of modern implantable antitachycardia pacing systems can be derived from the findings of Kappenberger et al.[23] In a multicenter report encompassing 63 patients followed for an average of 30 months, the authors reported adequate arrhythmia control with pacing alone in 44%, and with concomitant antiarrhythmic drug therapy in 49%. Outcomes were less favorable in the remainder.

In conclusion, sophisticated automatic implantable antitachycardia devices offer an effective treatment modality for terminating reentrant SVT. However, set-up is time consuming, attrition of efficacy is common, and clinical acceptance has been substantially eroded by the advances which have occurred with alternative treatments.

Prevention of Tachycardia

There has been relatively little experience with use of pacing techniques for prevention of reentrant SVTs. Coumel et al.[24] demonstrated that simultaneous stimulation of the atria and ventricles was capable of preventing reentrant arrhythmias presumably by depolarizing the AV junction and maintaining a refractory state in a critical element of the reentry circuit. Thus, Fields et al.[25] were able to use an early AV sequential pacemaker for effective tachycardia control in a relatively large group of patients. Similarly, Spurrell and Sowton[26] used a comparable technique in which an atrial synchronous pacemaker with a short AV delay (30 msec) prevented tachycardia by early ventricular capture. The latter forced part of the reentry circuit into refractoriness, thereby blocking reentry. Comparable success was achieved in three patients with drug resistant tachycardia by Levy et al.[27] A similar device was also apparently successful for prevention of tachycardia in the report by Medina-Ravell et al.[28]

Although prevention of reentrant SVT by pacing techniques may have had appeal at one time, it is evident that the vast majority of patients who are not adequately controlled by drugs can now be better treated by ablation techniques. Nevertheless, since these latter methods may not be either immediately available or acceptable to all patients, pacing therapies for prevention of paroxysmal reentrant AV nodal or AV tachyarrhythmias may continue to have a small following. More likely, however, such techniques are likely to find more extensive application in treatment of primary atrial tachyarrhythmias.

Clinical Experience With Pacing Systems for Primary Atrial Tachycardias

Tachycardia Termination

Among the primary atrial tachyarrhythmias, implantable antitachycardia systems have only been applied with any degree of frequency for treatment of atrial flutter of the common type. Although a relatively common arrhythmia, atrial flutter only infrequently proves to be a long-term recurrent problem, and in most instances is managed quite adequately by antiarrhythmic drugs. Additionally, newly developed transcatheter ablation techniques may prove valuable in many cases. However, in those cases in which atrial flutter is recurrent, implantable antitachycardia pacing systems may be appropriate. As summarized by Wettenstein,[18] the use of implanted pulse generators for treatment of atrial flutter follows directly from previous investigative work indicating a relatively high success rate in converting the common form of atrial flutter either directly through entrainment, or secondarily following conversion of the arrhythmia to a brief unstable episode of atrial fibrillation.

The autodecremental or ramp burst technique, under manual control in the electrophysiology laboratory, has been shown to be particularly useful for entraining and subsequently terminating flutter episodes.[29] The burst technique has also been reported to be effective in terminating atrial flutter in both the electrophysiology laboratory and in implantable devices. Olshansky et al.[30] indicates that successful pacing termination of atrial flutter is best achieved by starting the pacing bursts at a rate approximately 10 beats per minute greater than the atrial tachyarrhythmia rate. The burst is maintained for 5–15 seconds. If the initial application is unsuccessful, repeat bursts are applied using cycle lengths progressively shorter by 10-msec decrements. However, cycle lengths < 150 msec have a greater tendency to induce atrial fibrillation than do longer cycle lengths. For example, in a recent study of pacing protocols for atrial flutter, Hii et al.[31] reported an overall 73% success rate but atrial fibrillation was observed in a substantial number of individuals (18 of 30). However, pacing-induced atrial fibrillation was sustained in only three cases. Other investigators report transient atrial fibrillation occurring in this circumstance in 12% to 63% of patients undergoing overdrive atrial pacing for atrial flutter. However, transient atrial fibrillation is not usually a clinically significant complication and in many cases simply marks one mode by which the transition from pacing therapy to resumption of sinus rhythm is achieved.

Several investigators have described the use of implanted antitachycardia systems for atrial flutter control (Figure 6). In one of the few reports providing longer term follow-up, Barold et al.[17] found that patient activated pulse generators in three individuals (Medtronic model 5998) and automatic programmable antitachycardia devices in two individuals (CyberTach model 262–01, and Tachylog™ model P46 [Siemens Pacesetter Inc., Sylamar, CA) were able to terminate paroxsymal atrial flutter safely and reliably during follow-up periods of 24–60 months. In 4 of the 5 patients, however, concomitant drug therapy remained necessary although at a lower level than prior to device implant.

Apart from overdrive bursts and ramps, Hii et al.[31] also examined the use of rapid atrial pacing followed by extrastimuli to convert atrial flutter. Compared to burst pacing technique, the extrastimulus method proved effective far more frequently (extrastimulus method: 62%; short burst: 8%; long burst: 18%). In this methodology, atrial overdrive pacing was initially begun at a pacing cycle length 20 msec shorter than the spontaneous atrial flutter cycle length. The short burst was set at 20 beats. Long bursts were performed for 1 minute. The atrial extrastimulus method incorporated an 18-beat pacing drive followed by two atrial premature extrastimuli. The A_1-A_2 and A_2-A_3 intervals were initially set 10 msec shorter

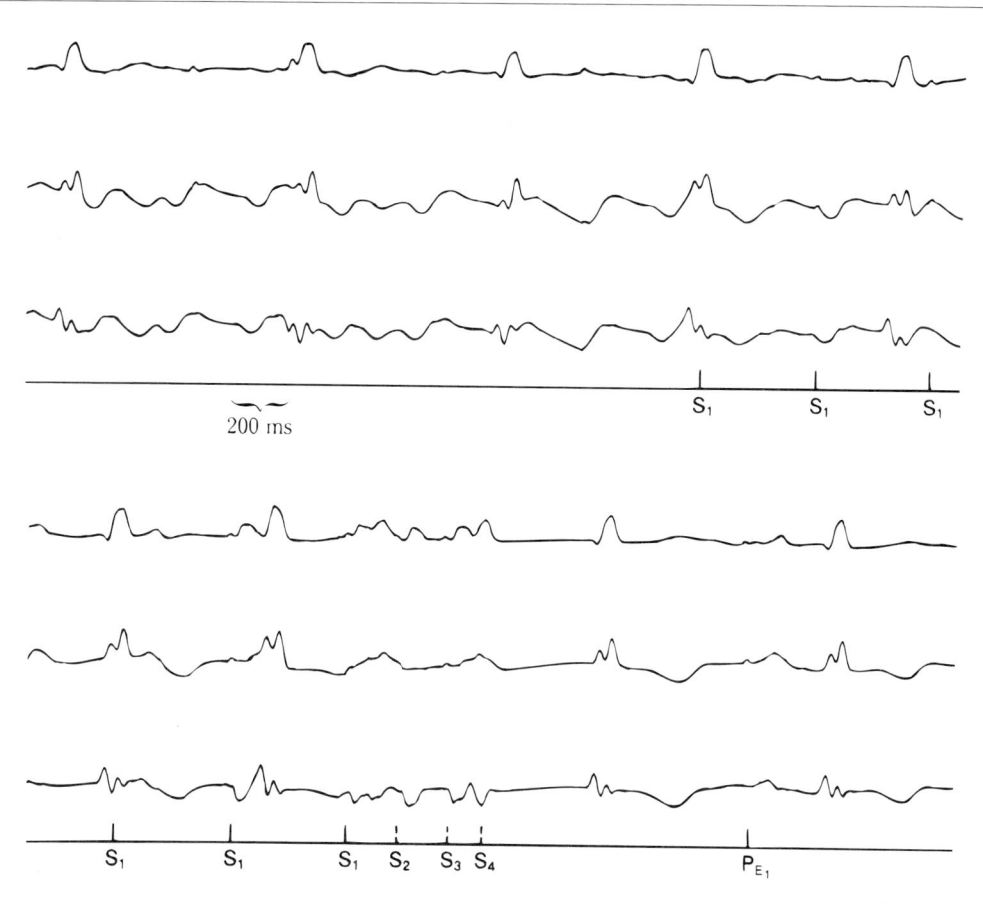

Figure 6. Termination of atrial flutter (cycle length = 280 msec) by atrial pacing (S$_1$) and extrastimulis (S$_2$, S$_3$, S$_4$) using the noninvasive electrophysiologic capabilities of an implanted Synergist II™ (Medtronic Inc., Minneapolis, MN) pulse generator.

than the drive train and progressively decreased by 10 msec until atrial refractoriness was reached. If all three therapies failed, the sequence was repeated after reducing the atrial basic drive train by a further 10 msec.

Unlike atrial flutter, conventional antitachycardia pacing techniques are not suitable for treatment of atrial fibrillation. This is not surprising given current concepts regarding the simultaneous presence of multiple reentry wavelets, and the narrow (or perhaps negligible) excitable gaps associated with each.[32,33] Nonetheless, recent experimental studies leads one to believe that specialized pacing modalities may ultimately prove useful in the treatment of atrial fibrillation patients. Specifically, findings from Allessie et al.[34] suggest that multiple point atrial pacing may prove effective for termination of atrial fibrillation. Using chronically instrumented canines, the authors were able to demonstrate atrial capture within a region of 3-cm radius despite ongoing atrial fibrillation. The findings suggest that within local regions a short excitable gap is present during atrial fibrillation. Ultimately, if similar pacing techniques can be successfully applied at multiple sites, the mass of tissue available for fibrillation may be functionally reduced to the point where fibrillation can no longer be maintained.

Tachycardia Rate Control

In a few patients with refractory atrial flutter, and in many patients with chronic atrial fibrillation, control of the ventricular response is the primary therapeutic objective. As a rule, drugs that directly modify AV nodal conduction (eg, β-adrenergic blockers, calcium channel blockers), and not infrequently Class I and Class III antiarrhythmic medications, are the first options chosen to achieve this end. However, certain pacing techniques have been described that may prove useful on their own or in conjunction with medications, particularly in the case of atrial fibrillation. Wittkampf et al.[35] initially reported substantial regularization of ventricular responses during atrial fibrillation by right ventricular pacing at a rate somewhat faster than the mean ventricular response during the arrhythmia prior to pacing. Subsequently, it was possible to develop a pacing algorithm capable of automatically regularizing ventricular responses in atrial fibrillation patients.[36] As yet, however, this technique has not been applied in an implantable device.

The mechanism by which ventricular pacing regularizes cardiac responses during atrial fibrillation is presumed to be analogous to that proposed for the prolongation of ventricular responses observed when spontaneous ventricular ectopic beats occur in atrial fibrillation patients. In essence, retrograde conduction of ventricular paced or ectopic events are presumed to conceal into the specialized conduction system and AV node.[37] As a consequence, it may be anticipated that a refractory wake prevents or delays antegrade conduction of the next supraventricular impulse. Once established, the regular insertion of retrogradely concealed impulses would be expected to preclude successful transmission of excessively early atrial events and thereby tend to regularize the ventricular response.

The technique proposed by Wittcampf et al.[35,36] could be readily integrated into conventional implantable pulse generators. However, unless the technique proved to be effective at slower pacing cycle lengths, it would have to be considered inefficient from an energy consumption perspective. Further, adverse hemodynamic consequences of rapid pacing may obviate any advantages obtained by regularization of the ventricular response.[38]

An alternative pacing technique for regularization of ventricular response in atrial fibrillation has recently been described.[38] In this method, which appears to avoid the potential adverse consequences of rapid ventricular pacing, ventricular paced complexes were coupled to spontaneously conducted QRS complexes in patients with atrial fibrillation. The coupling interval was chosen in such a manner as to just exceed the effective refractory period of the ventricle during spontaneous rhythm (mean coupling interval 232 ± 28 msec, range 175–290 msec). By this intercalated pacing technique the hemodynamic impact of atrial fibrillation with a rapid ventricular response was substantially diminished, since there was now a single pulse waveform generated by the conducted and pacing impulses (the former probably being more important). In addition, retrograde concealment into the AV nodal region likely proved beneficial by delaying the next conducted impulse. In a series of 10 patents with lone atrial fibrillation, the heart rate was substantially reduced by this technique (from 137 ± 26 to 75 ± 134 beats per minute). Additionally, in five patients with severe mitral stenosis, intercalated pacing appeared to improve cardiac output (3.1 ± 0.2 versus 3.4 ± 0.2 L/min, $P < 0.04$), and reduce transmitral valve gradient (16 ± 8 versus 10 ± 5 mm Hg, $P < 0.02$).

The use of coupled pacing to slow heart rate response during sustained tachycardia was originally proposed in connection with ventricular tachyarrhythmias.[39] In that approach, an extrastimulus was inserted after each tachycardia cycle. This concept permitted resetting the tachycardia circuit, thereby both slowing the effective rate of the tachycardia and improving left ventricular filling time. In terms of atrial fibrillation, the method described by Lau et al.[38] could be applied in conventional implantable pulse generators. It appears to be relatively energy efficient, and unlike rapid ventricular pacing, would probably have negligible adverse impact on myocardial oxygen consumption. Although it is unlikely that pacing techniques will supplant drugs for modification of the ventricular response in atrial fibrillation, it is possible that an automatically responsive pacing algorithm may prove effective for optimizing hemodynamics and at the same time avert the need for exposure of patients to aggressive chronic drug therapy for treatment of intermittent events.

Tachycardia Prevention

To this point, considerable emphasis has been placed on the utility of pacing techniques for termination of spontaneous atrial tachyarrhythmias. However, of comparable practical importance is the potential for prevention of spontaneous tachycardia episodes by appropriate pacemaker selection. In particular, there is growing evidence that even certain currently available antibradycardia pacing modes may reduce the incidence of atrial fibrillation in susceptible individuals.[40-43] Additionally, it appears likely that innovative application of current systems and/or relatively straightforward modifications of such systems could further enhance their prophylactic value.

Currently, sinus node dysfunction is the most common indication for cardiac pacing in western countries, accounting for 40% to 55% of device implants.[43] Among these patients, the development of atrial fibrillation is quite frequent and consequently techniques designed to diminish this susceptibility are welcome. In this regard, retrospective analyses in large numbers of patients suggests that atrial-based pacing techniques (ie, AAI, AAIR, DDD, DDDR, etc.) are superior to ventricular pacing alone with respect to avoiding development of atrial fibrillation. For example, Sutton and Kenny[41] reviewed findings from 18 studies in which the pacing mode could be clearly determined. Among 410 patients treated with atrial-based pacing, 16 developed atrial fibrillation. This represented an incidence of 3.9% during a mean follow-up of approximately 33 months. In contrast, among 145 of 651 patients paced in the VVI mode, developed atrial fibrillation (incidence of 22.3%), a value statistically significantly greater than was observed in the atrial-based pacing patients. In a similar analysis of 12 additional studies using atrial-based pacing, Brandt et al.[44] reported a 4.8% incidence of new atrial fibrillation among 908 patients followed for a mean of 46 months. This implies an approximately 1.3% annual incidence which is almost identical to that calculated by Sutton and Kenny.[41] Finally, one additional report by Brandt[45] reported outcomes in 213 patients receiving atrial-based pacing systems for sinus node dysfunction. Once again, the incidence of new onset atrial fibrillation during follow-up was 7.0%, or 1.4% per year.

Although the studies alluded to are all retrospective in nature, the extensive volume of patient experience strongly suggests that atrial-based pacing is efficacious in markedly reducing susceptibility of sinus node dysfunction patients to develop chronic atrial fibrillation. Additionally, a small body of knowledge suggests that atrial pacing may also reduce the frequency of paroxysmal atrial fibrillation in patients susceptible to such arrhythmias.[46,47] For example, in a preliminary report examining a Mayo Clinic experience comprising follow-up in 649 patients receiving DDD pacemakers between April 1981 and June 1989, Hayes and Neubauer[48] observed a 5% incidence of new onset atrial fibrillation. Importantly, however, among 49 patients who had had paroxsymal atrial fibrillation prior to pacing, 25 (51%) had no apparent documented recurrence of atrial fibrillation after device implantation. Consequently, apart from the incidence of new atrial fibrillation being quite low in patients treated with atrial-based pacing systems, there also appears to be benefit provided in terms of reducing the frequency with which previous paroxysmal atrial fibrillation recurs. A similar outcome has also been reported in a shorter term multicenter follow-up using a DDDR capable pulse generator.[48]

Additional evidence favoring the usefulness of atrial-based pacing for prevention of atrial fibrillation has been provided by Feuer et al.[49] In this study, the effects of dual-chamber cardiac pacing (DDD/DDI) was compared to the effects of fixed rate ventricular pacing (VVI) on long-term development of atrial fibrillation in patients who were in sinus rhythm at the time of pacemaker implantation. This study comprised 110 patients in each of the two groups. Comparison of clinical characteristics revealed the DDD/DDI group to comprise more women and to be somewhat older (71 ± 12 years versus 66 ± 12 years). Hypertension, however, tended to be more common in the VVI paced group (45% versus 29%). In terms of other clinical criteria, such as the incidence of coronary artery disease, congestive heart failure, chronic pulmonary disease, and history of previous supraventricular tachyarrhythmias, the groups were well matched. In follow-up, atrial fibrillation developed more frequently in the VVI paced group than in the dual-chamber paced patients (18% versus 8%, $P < 0.05$). The mean duration of follow-up was 40 ± 80 months in the DDD/DDI group compared to 48 ± 35 months in the VVI paced patients (P = NS). There did seem to be a trend toward a greater frequency of atrial fibrillation development in those patients carrying a diagnosis of sinus node dysfunction than in those who were paced for AV block. Consequently, the study tends to support the notion that physiological atrial-based pacing systems can be helpful in preventing atrial fibrillation and that this benefit appears to be particularly important in patients with sinus node disease. Nonetheless, appropriate pacing selection may be reasonably expected to be comparably beneficial in preventing atrial fibrillation from complicating follow-up in patients being paced for AV block.

A final consideration in the use of atrial-based pacing for prevention of atrial fibrillation is the concept that provision of rate adaptive behavior provides further antiarrhythmic protection. Jordaens et al.[50] provided the first insight into the potential for rate adaptive pacing to suppress exercise-related arrhythmias. In their study, single-chamber rate adaptive pacing was compared with fixed rate ventricular pacing in 8 patients. Among these individuals, 3 of 8 developed exercise-induced arrhythmias while being paced in the fixed rate mode. These arrhythmias were noted to be completely suppressed by rate-adaptive pacing. A similar beneficial effect was subsequently observed during ambulatory electrocardiographic monitoring. It was suggested, that the provision of an appropriate increase in heart rate associated with exercise had a direct effect on suppressing arrhythmia. In part, the relatively physiological rate response provided by rate adaptation may have diminished the magnitude of catecholamine release, and as a consequence reduced susceptibility to arrhythmia.

Recently, Kato et al.[51] suggested that rate adaptive atrial pacing may be more effective than fixed rate atrial pacing for prevention of atrial arrhythmias. In a preliminary report, Bellocci et al.[52] have provided similar observations. Although confirmation of this potential benefit remains to be obtained, it seems clear that the key element is atrial pacing, not merely the presence of rate adaptation. In support of this latter contention, Vanerio et al.[53] examined outcomes in 33 patients with tachycardia-bradycardia syndrome (sinus node dysfunction) who were also treated with either single-chamber (VVIR mode) or dual-chamber (DDIR mode) rate responsive systems. Among the 22 VVIR paced patients (followed for a mean duration of 25 months) chronic atrial fibrillation developed in 54%. By contrast, in the 11 patients paced in the DDIR mode (mean follow-up 18 months) the development of chronic atrial fibrillation was noted in smaller percentage of cases (27%). Although the numbers of patients were small and the differences were not statistically significant, there appeared to be a trend suggesting that atrial-based rate adaptive pacing is superior to ventricular-based rate adaptation for preventing atrial fibrillation in high-risk patients.

A novel and potentially important additional perspective on the use of atrial pacing to prevent primary atrial tachyarrhythmias is based on the concept that prevention of arrhythmogenic intra-atrial conduction delays by pacing at a number of atrial sites in close succession may diminish arrhythmia susceptibility. Recently reported preliminary clinical experience suggests that atrial pacing from two sites reduces the frequency of atrial tachyarrhythmias.[54] By this relatively simple approach, intra-atrial conduction delays are minimized by pacing right atrial and left atrial sites with small programmed interatrial timing delays (programmed in a fashion comparable to AV interval delays). Extension of this concept to multiple sites could conceivably offer additional benefit and will be a technical challenge, but may prove highly effective in both preventing atrial fibrillation and terminating episodes should breakthrough occur.

Low-Energy Cardioversion/Defibrillation Techniques for Treatment of Atrial Tachyarrhythmias

Nomenclature for an Atrial Directed Pacemaker Cardioverter-Defibrillator

In this chapter, a device capable of atrial antitachycardia therapy using pacing techniques, low-energy cardioversion, or relatively high-energy defibrillation (high relative to the atrium but probably still ≤ 5 J) has been termed an atrial directed pacemaker cardioverter-defibrillator. A North American Society of Pacing and Electrophysiology (NASPE)/British Pacing and Electrophysiology Group (BPEG) committee charged with the task of developing an abbreviated code for defibrillator systems has addressed, within their comprehensive examination of this problem, the nomenclature for such systems.[55]

The proposed NASPE/BPEG code uses four positions comparable to the coding system currently in vogue for conventional cardiac pacemakers: Position 1: the chamber receiving a shock (atrium [A] ventricle [V], both [D], none [O]); Position 2: the chamber receiving antitachycardia pacing; Position 3: the manner in which tachycardia detection is achieved (electrogram processing [E], hemodynamic assessment [H]); and Position 4: the chamber in which antibradycardia pacing is provided (atrium, ventricle, both, neither).

The NASPE/BPEG code is designed to modify the device designation defibrillator (or perhaps when appropriate, pacemaker cardioverter-defibrillator. Thus, the NASPE/BPEG code for a pure implantable atrial directed pacemaker/cardioverter-defibrillator with electrogram monitoring for tachycardia detection and backup atrial antibradycardia pacing would read AAEA device. However, were the device to include antibradycardia pacing in the ventricle as part of a dual-chamber pacing system, yet only deliver antitachycardia capability in the atrium, it would be designated as an AAED defibrillator. Other combinations can be easily derived from these examples.[55]

Experimental Studies

The concept that transvenous electrode catheters could be used for cardioversion of atrial tachyarrhythmias is attributed to Mirowski et al.[56] In experimental studies, as described almost 16 years later by Mirowski and Mower,[57] these investigators apparently had used acetylcholine applied topically to the atrial appendage to effect a reproducible model of atrial fibrillation and thereby evaluate the usefulness of transcatheter intraatrial cardioversion. Although the design and surface area of the electrode catheter used for these experiments was not adequately described, the authors claimed 100% success in 125 episodes tested. They

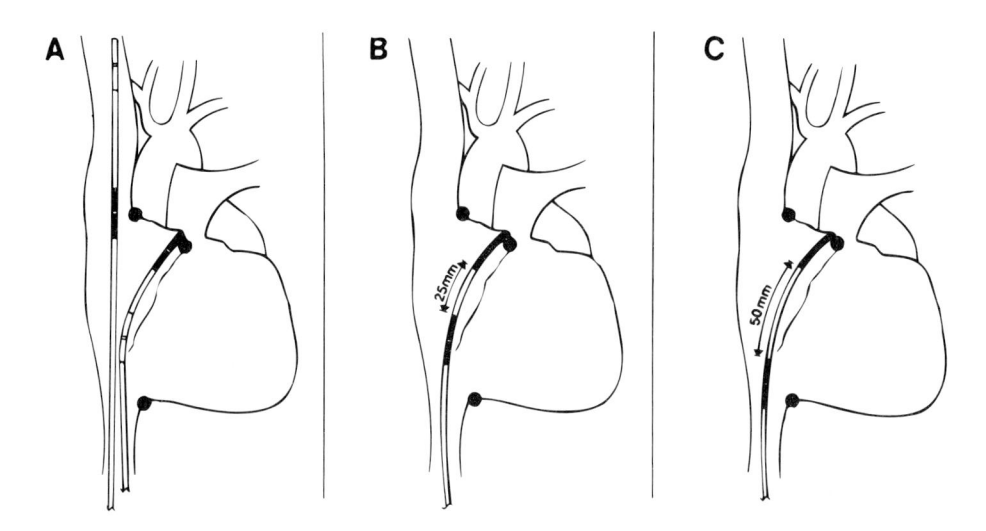

Figure 7. Schematics illustrating catheter positions and interelectrode spacing used in the experimental studies reported by Dunbar et al.[58] The anode positions were in the superior vena cava (panel A), and mid-right atrium (panel B), and the inferior vena cava (panel C). (Reproduced with permission from Reference 58.)

indicated that shocks of 0.05–0.5 J were usually effective and only occasionally were shocks in the 1–3 J range required. In contrast, in this model transthoracic shocks in the range of 40–100 J were necessary in order to achieve cardioversion. Furthermore, as was later observed by others,[58] Mirowski and Mower[57] noted that cardioversion of atrial tachyarrhythmias was not always associated with immediate tachycardia termination, but that not infrequently (approximately one third of episodes) the return to sinus rhythm occurred several seconds after the cardioversion impulse. The possibility was raised that this finding represented only partial defibrillation of the atrial tissue, but that there was insufficient mass of fibrillating tissue remaining to permit persistence of the tachycardia.

Despite these early experiments with transcatheter atrial defibrillation, the idea of an implantable device largely remained latent while the principal focus of attention was directed toward investigation and development of techniques for transcatheter cardioversion of ventricular tachyarrhythmias. During the course of the latter evolution, Jackman and Zipes[59] observed induction of atrial tachyarrhythmias and their subsequent termination by DC shocks in the 1.0-J energy range. About the same time, Benditt et al.[60] reported the results of a preliminary series of studies examining transcatheter termination of atrial tachyarrhythmias in an open chest talc pericarditis canine model (Figure 7). In that study, an existing external defibrillator was modified to provide low stored energy levels (0.16–6.1 J) in calibrated increments of 0.1–0.2 J. The waveform was a rapidly decaying truncated exponential pulse of variable amplitude delivered between a distal electrode (electrically negative) and a proximal electrode pole. The electrode configurations encompassed electrode stimulating areas of 85, 53, 20, and 26 mm^2, respectively. The corresponding interelectrode distances were 16, 16, 22, and 20 mm. The largest surface area electrodes (Medtronic models 5816 and 5818) exhibited better efficacy than was obtained with the smaller stimulating areas (Medtronic model 6904A and USCI [Billerica, MA]) quadripolar catheter with the proximal two terminals paired and the distal two terminals paired). Overall, termination of atrial tachyarrhythmias was successfully achieved in 16 of 70 trials (23%). In seven attempts, energies < 0.3 J were required. In no case did stored energy > 0.6 J succeed when lesser energy levels had failed. It was also observed that extended periods of atrial tachycardia (usually > 5 minutes) was associated with a lower success of cardioversion.

In a subsequent series of studies from our laboratory,[58] a closed chest canine model was used. Specially modified 10F electrode catheters (Medtronic model 6880) were introduced via the femoral veins (Figure 8). The catheter had four stainless steel electrodes, each with the surface area of 1.25 cm². The distal pair of electrodes at the catheter tip were separated by 5 mm. There was then either a 25-mm or 50-mm space between the distal electrode pair and proximal electrode pair. The proximal electrode pair was also separated by 5 mm spacing. In these studies, again using talc pericarditis to facilitate atrial tachyarrhythmia induction, the efficacy of cardioversion was compared using the following shock vectors: 1) right atrial appendage to superior vena cava; 2) right atrial appendage to mid-right atrium (25 mm proximal to the distal electrode); and 3) right atrial appendage to low right atrium (50 mm proximal to the distal electrode). In six dogs used for examining the efficacy of the various anode positions, successful cardioversion was achieved at each of the three anode positions with energy levels of 0.75 J or less. Overall, cardioversion

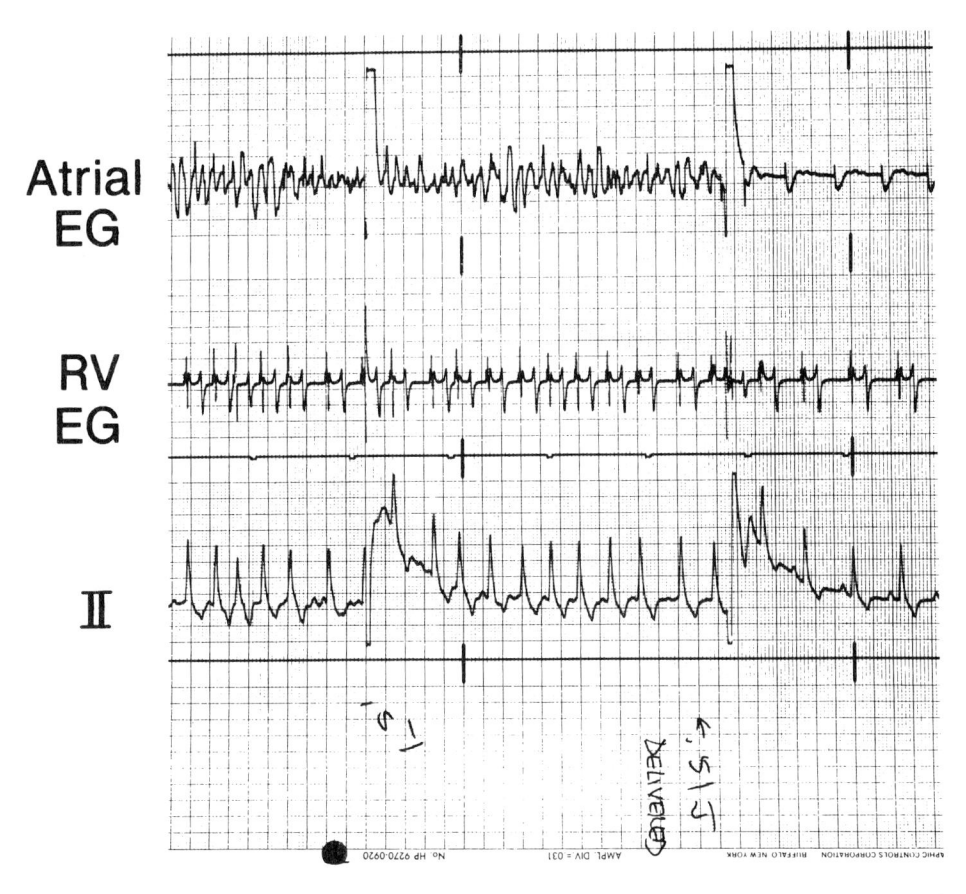

Figure 8. Electrocardiographic recordings and intracardiac tracing illustrating termination of sustained atrial fibrillation induced in a canine talc pericarditis model using low-energy (0.51 J) transvenous catheter technique.

was successful in 18 of 53 attempts (34%). It did not appear that either the frequency of successful cardioversion or the energy threshold for a cardioversion was influenced by either the anode position or the order of testing. On several occasions it was noted that cardioversion delivery was followed by alteration of the atrial tachyarrhythmia characteristics (usually a change in atrial cycle length) with subsequent occasional spontaneous conversions occurring more than 5 seconds after energy delivery. In an additional element of this study, the reproducibility of effective cardioversion energies was examined in dogs subjected to 139 atrial tachyarrhythmia events. Finally, although a wide range of energies were required to achieve cardioversion in each of these animals, a substantial portion of the successful cardioversions were achieved with energy levels of 0.75 J or less (Figure 9).

Recently, Kumagai et al.[61] reexamined the feasibility of low-energy synchronous transcatheter cardioversion of atrial tachyarrhythmias in the dog talc pericarditis model. In these studies a conventional 6F quadripolar catheter was introduced via the femoral vein and positioned at the right atrial appendage. For cardioversion, a single distal electrode pole was used as the anode and a proximal pole floating in the atrial cavity was used as the cathode. A truncated exponential waveform of 6-msec duration was delivered using a variety of energy levels. Atrial tachyarrhythmias were induced by rapid atrial pacing and exhibited an atrial cycle length of 100–180 msec. When the energy was delivered between the two poles of the catheter, successful car-

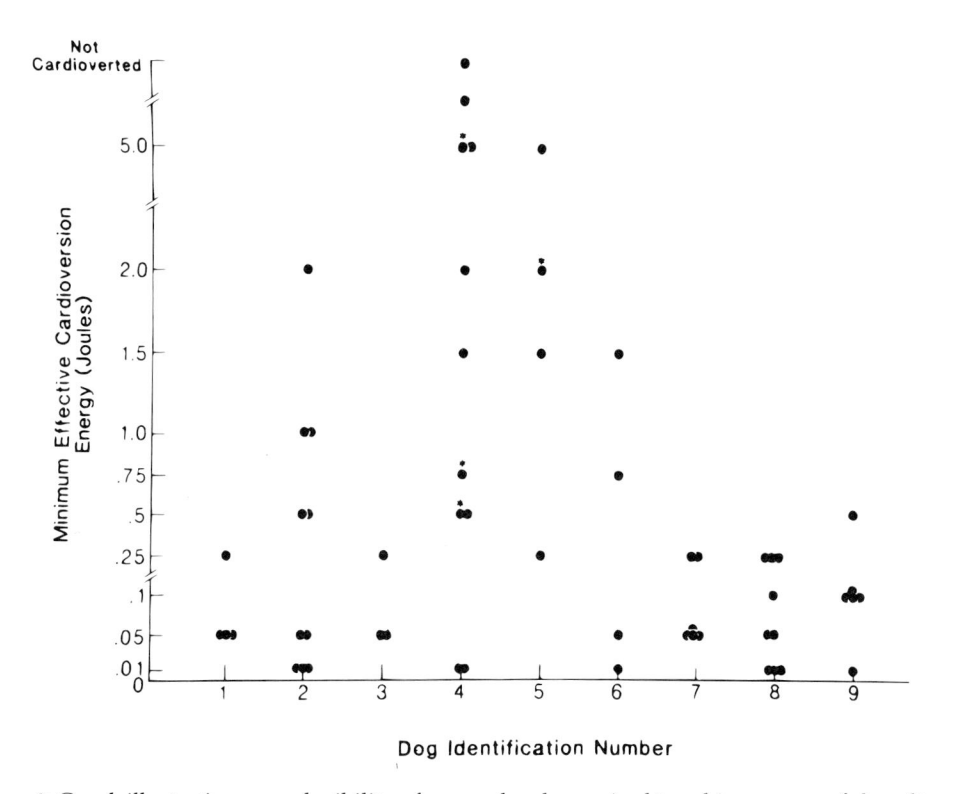

Figure 9. Graph illustrating reproducibility of energy levels required to achieve successful cardioversion of atrial tachyarrhythmias induced in nine dogs using a canine talc pericarditis model. See text for details. A wide range of minimal effective energies was observed rather than a discrete energy threshold. (Reproduced with permission from Reference 58.)

dioversion was achieved in all 68 attempts with shocks ≤ 5 J. Shocks ≤ 1 J were successful in 74% of trials, and shocks ≤ 0.5 J were successful in 47%. These results are quite encouraging and compared well to the outcomes associated with the delivery of shocks between the proximal electrode (cathode) and a backplate (anode).

The most recent experimental report examining efficacy of low-energy cardioversion of atrial fibrillation used an anesthetized sheep model with the chest wall closed by surgical clamps after instrumentation.[62] In this setting, a large surface area stainless steel spring coil electrode (surface area 655 mm^2, CPI, St. Paul, MN) was positioned in the right atrium and used as the cathode. A cutaneous patch electrode with a surface area of 50.3 cm^2 (R2 Medical Systems) was used as the anode and was positioned over the left precordial region. An external programmable defibrillator, delivering biphasic shocks with truncated exponential waveforms and programmable energy levels was used. Atrial fibrillation was induced by rapid atrial pacing, and a total of 768 cardioversions were attempted in 16 animals. Termination of tachycardia was successful in 31% of trials using energy levels of ≤ 0.3 J, 47% at energy levels of ≤ 1 J, and in 83% at energy levels of ≤ 6 J. An energy level in the range of 5 J was uniformly successful except in one animal. Once again, these findings support the feasibility of successful transvenous cardioversion of atrial tachyarrhythmias with relatively low energies.

The appropriate electrode catheter positions and electrode configurations for optimal atrial defibrillation have yet to be resolved. Scott et al.[63] suggest that cardioversion between a right ventricular apex electrode and a right ventricular atrial appendage electrode can be quite effective. However, the methodology and observations of their study are poorly described and consequently difficult to place in context with other reports. More recently, Cooper et al.[64] examined optimal electrode locations for internal cardioversion of atrial fibrillation in sheep. Multiple intracardiac vectors were examined using both a 3-msec monophasic and a 3/3-msec biphasic waveform. In these studies, a biphasic waveform using a right atrial appendage to coronary sinus vector had the lowest successful peak voltage requirement for tachycardia termination (150 ± 22 V) and lowest energy requirement (1.1 ± 0.3 J). Of note, the authors indicated that the superior vena cava to right atrial appendage vector was associated with a higher incidence of postshock sinus arrest, while vectors incorporating the mid-right atrium and low right atrium to coronary sinus tended to exhibit a higher incidence of postshock AV block. In an even more detailed examination of optimum transvenous atrial defibrillation electrode positions, Ayers et al.[65] compared atrial defibrillation thresholds for shocks delivered between a right atrial appendage catheter and catheters located in various aspects of the coronary sinus and great cardiac vein. Findings suggested that a defibrillating vector encompassing the more distal elements of the coronary sinus/great cardiac vein (ie, anterior descending vein, left atrial appendage region) were more effective than vectors in which the more proximal elements of the coronary sinus were tested (obtuse margin, or body of the coronary sinus itself). In the case of the anterior descending vein and left atrial appendage regions, cardioversion thresholds (defined as the energy required to achieve > 10% success) were 0.7 ± 0.4 J and 0.6 ± 0.2 J respectively. These outcomes were not only more than 50% less than the thresholds observed for catheter positions in the more proximal regions of the coronary sinus, but also bring defibrillation energies into a range which may be clinically tolerable.

In conclusion, experimental studies suggest that low-energy transvenous cardioversion of atrial tachyarrhythmias is feasible. It appears that the defibrillation vector should encompass a region from the distal aspects of the coronary sinus to the right atrium. Avoidance of sinus node and AV nodal regions is desirable for prevention of even transient dysfunction in the postshock period. Additionally, biphasic waveforms with large surface area electrodes appear to be critical for both assuring relatively low defibrillation thresholds and optimizing the frequency of successful cardioversion. Finally, synchronization of shocks with the QRS complex is essential for safety.[58]

Clinical Studies of Transvenous Atrial Cardioversion/Defibrillation

Low-Energy Transcatheter Cardioversion

To date, human studies of transcatheter atrial defibrillation have been extremely limited and provide no real insight into the potential value of the technique. Mirowski and Mower[57] indicate that as early as 1972 they undertook attempts at atrial cardioversion using internal electrodes in humans. The outcome was apparently quite disappointing with shocks up to 3 J being described as "not particularly effective." However, the characteristics of the defibrillating electrode system are not described, and given the limited electrode configurations available at the time, it is likely that a suboptimal arrangement was used. The authors concluded that "although an implantable atrial cardioverter was technically feasible, more clinical experience with ventricular arrhythmias was needed before actually undertaking such a project."[57] Nevertheless, they did proceed to obtain patents related to the overall concept.[66,67]

In a more recent small series of patients, Hartzler and Kallock[68] used Medtronic 6880 catheters with 10-cm interelectrode distance to terminate reciprocating tachycardia with 0.5-J shocks in patients with accessory pathways. However, this same technique proved unsuccessful in attempting to cardiovert two episodes of atrial fibrillation and six episodes of atrial flutter using energy levels up to 5.0 J. In these attempts, the cathode was positioned at the right ventricular apex with the anode in the right atrium.

Nathan et al.[69] have also reported results of attempted cardioversion of atrial tachycardias using atrial and ventricular shocks. In the atrial position, Medtronic 6880 catheters with a 10-cm interelectrode separation were positioned with the cathode on the interatrial septum using the subclavian vein or femoral vein approach. The anode position was not specified. Five episodes of reciprocating tachycardia using an accessory pathway were successfully cardioverted with low-energy shocks. However, atrial shocks were unsuccessful in cardioverting atrial flutter (14 shocks at 0.004–1.43 J), or atrial fibrillation (5 shocks, 0.011–5.0 J). Of clinical importance, it was noted that patients felt the atrial shocks to be more painful than ventricular shocks of comparable energy levels.

High-Energy Transcatheter Cardioversion

Recently, the safety of transcatheter intraatrial shocks for treatment of atrial tachyarrhythmias has been evidenced by the successful use of high-energy transvenous shocks for treatment of chronic atrial fibrillation.[70,71]

In an initial series of 10 patients in whom atrial fibrillation had been resistant to external DC cardioversion (300–400 J) as well as pharmacological intervention, Lévy et al.[70] used conventional electrode catheters (6F quadripolar catheters, USCI) to deliver 200–300 J shocks within the right atrial cavity (proximal intracavity electrode as cathode, with backplate as anode). Successful restoration of sinus rhythm was achieved in 9 of 10 cases, although in 2 individuals atrial fibrillation recurred within a few minutes. During longer term, atrial fibrillation recurred in 3 additional patients at 8 days, 2 months, and 4 months, respectively. Nonetheless, despite inevitable recurrences, the safe and effective use of intracavitary shocks was demonstrated.

Further evidence of the potential utility of intracavitary high-energy shock for resistant atrial fibrillation has been provided by

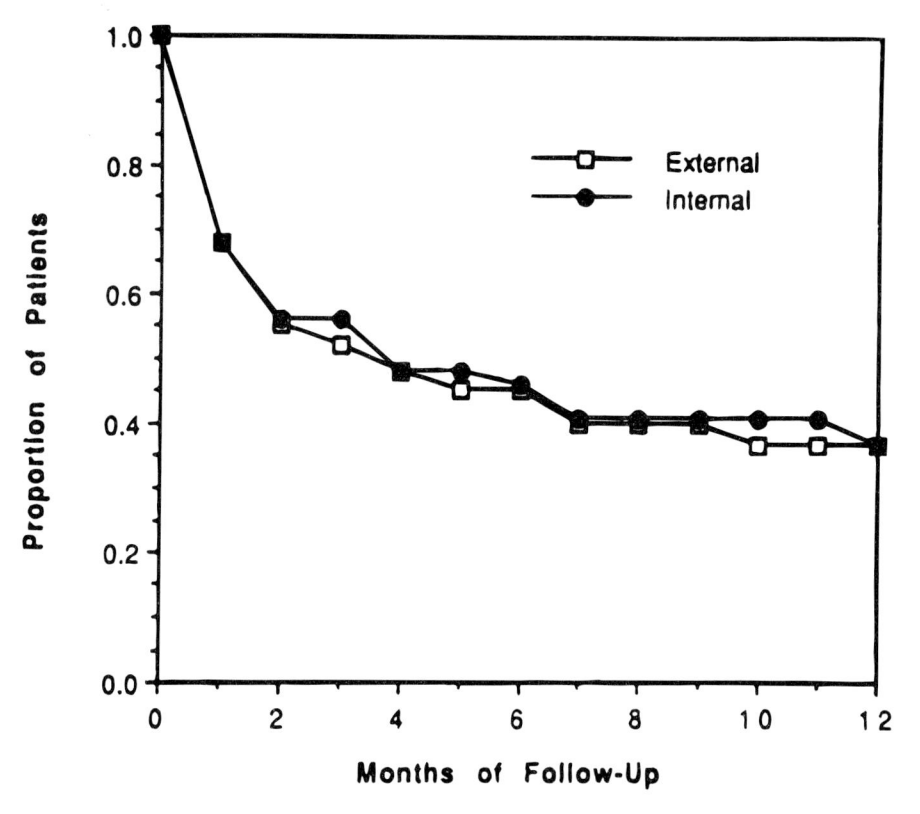

Figure 10. Graph illustrating the proportion of patients remaining in sinus rhythm after successful internal (filled circles) or external cardioversion (open circles). (Reproduced with permission from Reference 73.)

Chauvin et al.[71] Using a technique similar to that described by Lévy et al.,[70] intracavitary shocks of 150–250 J were delivered. The minimum effective energy appeared to be 200 J, with immediate success in 22 of 28 patients (79%) in whom previous external shocks were ineffective. Once again, only transient sinus bradycardia or AV block were the only observed complications.

In one additional uncontrolled trial of intracavitary cardioversion, Kumagai et al.[72] reported success at an initial procedure in 10 of 10 patients (100%). However, early recurrence (≤ 30 days) occurred in 5 patients, in whom a second procedure was successful in 3 of 5 patients. Sinus rhythm was then maintained for follow-up periods of 12–22 months in 8 of the original 10. There were no clinically worrisome complications associated with the procedure.

Recently, Lévy et al.[73] reported results of a randomized comparison of external and internal cardioversion shocks for treatment of atrial fibrillation of 1 month or greater duration. Patients were randomly assigned to external (300–360 J) or internal cardioversion (200–300 J), after a 1-month amiodarone (200 mg/day) pretreatment period. The internal cardioversion used the protocol described by Lévy et al.,[70] while external cardioversion used paddles applied at the ventricular apex and the right infraclavicular region. Although this comparison has been vigorously criticized by Ewy,[74] the findings clearly revealed a substantially greater cardioversion percentage with the internal method (91%) compared to this commonly clinically used external approach (67%). During follow-up of 1 year, 37% of patients remained in sinus rhythm. Not unexpectedly, there was no difference in reversion rate with respect to the type of cardioversion procedure (Figure 10). In terms of complications, the authors noted one thromboembolic event among the externally converted group, and an instance of acute pulmonary edema among the internally cardioverted patients.

In summary, high-energy internal cardioversion appears to be a highly effective and relatively safe technique for termination of resistant atrial fibrillation. It provides a potentially valuable additional technique for selected patients.

Although the utility of high-energy atrial cardioversion using intracavity electrodes is not likely to be appropriate for implantable systems,[70] it is evident that the atrium is well able to sustain intracavitary energies of 200–300 J with apparently little adverse effect. Consequently, it seems likely that synchronized low-energy transvenous cardioversion for treatment of recurring paroxsymal atrial fibrillation can be undertaken safely. Nonetheless, there remains a concern that ventricular fibrillation may be induced in an occasional instance.[58] Additionally, the safety of even low-energy shocks applied to a coronary sinus electrode is unclear. Therefore, considerable additional experimental and clinical experience is required before implanted atrial cardioverter-defibrillator will prove readily accepted by the medical community.

Acknowledgment: The authors are grateful to Edwin Duffin, PhD for providing Figures 1, 2, and 3 and also wish to thank Stephanie Wiebke, Wendy Braatz, and Barry L.S. Detloff for valuable assistance in the preparation of the manuscript.

References

1. Ryan GF, Easly RM, Zanoff LJ, et al: Paradoxical use of a demand pacemaker in treatment of supraventricular tachycardia due to the Wolff-Parkinson-White syndrome. *Circulation* 38:1037, 1968.
2. Krikler DM, Curry PVL, Buffet J: Dual-demand pacing for reciprocating atrioventricular tachycardia. *Br Med J* 1:1114, 1979.
3. Smyth NP, Kesheshian JM, Bacos JM, et al: Permanent pervenous atrial pacing. *J Electrocardiol* 4:299, 1971.
4. Fletcher RD, Cohen AI, DelNegro AA: Noninvasive electrophysiologic studies using implanted pacemakers. In: *Modern Cardiac Pacing*. Edited by S Barold. Mt. Kisco, NY: Futura Publishing Company; 1985, p. 421.
5. Fletcher RD, Wish M, Cohen A: The use of the implanted pacemaker as an in vivo electrophysiology laboratory 1:425, 1987.
6. Goyal SL, Lichstein E, Gupta PK, et al: Refractory reentrant atrial tachycardia: successful treatment with a permanent radiofrequency triggered atrial pacemaker. *Am J Med* 58:586, 1975.
7. Wyndham CR, Wu D, Denes P, et al: Self-initiated conversion of paroxsymal atrial flutter utilizing a radio-frequency pacemaker. *Am J Cardiol* 41:1119, 1978.
8. Peters RW, Scafton E, Frank S, et al: Radiofrequency-triggered pacemakers: uses and limitations. A long-term study. *Ann Intern Med* 88:17, 1978.
9. Den Dulk K, Bertholet M, Brugada P, et al: Clinical experience with implantable devices for control of tachyarrhythmias. *PACE* 7:548, 1984.
10. Spurrell RAJ: Artificial cardiac pacemakers. In: *Cardiac Arrhythmias*. Edited by DM Krikler, JF Goodwin. London: WB Saunders; 1976, p. 238.
11. Bertholet M, Demoulin JC, Waleffe A, et al: Programmable extrastimulus pacing for the long-term management of supraventricular and ventricular tachycardia. Experience of 16 cases. *Am Heart J* 110:582, 1985.
12. Spurrell RAJ, Nathan AW, Camm AJ: Clinical experience with implantable scanning tachycardia reversion pacemakers. *PACE* 7:1296, 1984.
13. Nathan AW, Cochrane T, Bexton RS: Relationship between pacing cycle length and the duration of pacing for the termination of reentrant tachycardias (abstract). *Circulation* 68:313, 1983.
14. Gilli N, Carr S: Two years of clinical experience with a second generation automatic antitachycardia device (abstract). *Clin Prog Physiol Pacing* 4:101, 1987.
15. Zipes DP, Prystowsky EN, Miles WM, et al: Initial experience with Symbios model 7008 pacemaker. *PACE* 7:1301, 1984.
16. Griffin JC, Sweeney M: The management of paroxysmal tachycardia using the Cybertach-60. *PACE* 7:1291, 1984.

17. Barold SS, Wyndham CR, Kappenberger L, et al: Implanted atrial pacemakers for paroxsymal atrial flutter: long term efficacy. *Ann Intern Med* 107:144, 1987.
18. Wettenstein EH: *Automatic Antitachycardia Pacing for the Control of Atrial Flutter: A Review*. Intermedics Inc, June 1992.
19. Fisher JD, Johnston DR, Kim SG, et al: Implantable pacers for tachycardia termination: stimulation techniques and long-term efficacy. *PACE* 9:1325, 1986.
20. Curry PVL, Rowland E, Krikler DM: Dual-demand pacing for refractory atrioventricular re-entry tachycardia. *PACE* 2:137, 1979.
21. Jung W, Mletzko R, Manz M, et al: Clinical results of chronic antitachycardia pacing in supraventircular tachycardia. In: *Interventional Electrophysiology*. Edited by B Luderitz, S Saksena. Mount Kisco, NY: Futura Publishing Company, Inc.; 1991, p. 197.
22. Boccadamo R, Toscano S: Prevention and interruption of supraventricular tachycardia by antitachycardia pacing. In: *Interventional Electrophysiology*. Edited by B Luderitz, S Saksena. Mount Kisco, NY: Futura Publishing Inc.; 1991, p. 213.
23. Kappenberger L, Valin H, Sowton E, et al: Multicenter long-term results of antitachycardia pacing for supraventricular tachycardia. *Am J Cardiol* 64:191, 1989.
24. Coumel P, Cabrol C, Fabiato A, et al: Tachycardia permanente par rythme reciproque. *Arch Mal Coeur* 60:1830, 1967.
25. Fields J, Berkovits BV, Matloff JM: Surgical experience with temporary and permanent A-V sequential demand pacing. *J Thorac Cardiovasc Surg* 66:865, 1973.
26. Spurrell RAJ, Sowton E: Pacing techniques in the management of supraventricular tachycardias: Part II. *J Electrocardiol* 9:89, 1976.
27. Levy S, Berkovits B, Mandel W, et al: Refractory supraventricular tachycardias: successful therapy with double demand sequential pacing (abstract). *Am J Cardiol* 45:457, 1980.
28. Medina-Ravell V, Castellanos A, Portillo-Acosta B, et al: Management of tachyarrhythmias with dual chamber pacemaker. *PACE* 6:333, 1983.
29. Ward DE, Camm AJ, Spurrell RAJ: The response of regular re-entrant supraventricular tachycardia to right heart stimulation. *PACE* 2:586, 1979.
30. Olshansky B, Wilber DJ, Hariman RJ: Atrial flutter: update on the mechanism and treatment. *PACE* 15:2308, 1992.
31. Hii JTY, Mitchell LB, Duff HJ, et al: Comparison of atrial overdrive pacing with and without extrastimuli for termination of atrial flutter. *Am J Cardiol* 70:463, 1992.
32. Moe GK, Abildskov JA: Atrial fibrillation as a self sustaining arrhythmia independent of focal discharge. *Am Heart J* 58:59, 1959.
33. Allessie M, Lammers WJEP, Bonke FI, et al: Experimental evaluation of Moe's multiple wavelet hypothesis of atrial fibrillation. In: *Cardiac Electrophysiology and Arrhythmias*. Edited by DP Zipes, J Jaliffe. New York, NY: Grune & Stratton; 1985, p. 265.
34. Allessie M, Kirchhof C, Scheffer GJ, et al: Regional control of atrial fibrillation by rapid pacing in conscious dogs. *Circulation* 84:1689, 1991.
35. Wittkampf FHM, de Jongste MJL, Lie HI, et al: Effect of right ventricular pacing on ventricular rhythm during atrial fibrillation. *J Am Coll Cardiol* 11:539, 1988.
36. Wittkampf FHM, de Jongste MJL: Rate stabilization by right ventricular on-demand pacing in patients with atrial fibrillation. *PACE* 9:1147, 1986.
37. Langendorf R, Pick A, Katz LN: Ventricular response in atrial fibrillation: role of concealed conduction in the AV junction. *Circulation* 32:69, 1965.
38. Lau C-P, Leung W-H, Wong C-K, et al: A new pacing method for rapid regularization and rate control in atrial fibrillation. *Am J Cardiol* 65:1198, 1990.
39. Fisher JD, Kim SG, Furman S, et al: Role of implantable pacemakers in control of recurrent ventricular tachycardia. *Am J Cardiol* 49:194, 1982.
40. Rosenqvist M, Brandt J, Schuller H: Atrial versus ventricular pacing in sinus node disease: a treatment comparison. *Am Heart J* 111:292, 1986.
41. Sutton R, Kenny R-A: The natural history of sick sinus syndrome. *PACE* 6:1110, 1986.
42. Zanini R, Facchinetti AI, Gallo G, et al: Morbidity and mortality of patients with sinus node disease: comparative effects of atrial and ventricular pacing. *PACE* 13:2076, 1990.
43. Rosenqvist M: Atrial pacing for sick sinus syndrome. *Clin Cardiol* 13:43, 1990.
44. Brandt J, Anderson H, Fahraeus T, et al: Natural history of sinus node disease treated with atrial pacing in 213 patients: implications for stimulation mode selection. In: *Permanent Atrial Pacing. Clinical Studies*. Edited by J Brandt. Lund: Bloms Boktryckeri Ab; 1991.
45. Brandt J: *Permanent Atrial Pacing. Clinical Studies*. Lund: Bloms Boktryckeri Ab; 1991, p. 19.
46. Denjoy I, Leclerq J-F, Druelles P, et al: Comparative efficacy of permanent atrial pacing in vagal atrial arrhythmias and in bradycardia-tachycardia syndrome (abstract). *PACE* 12:1236, 1989.
47. Benditt DG, Wilbert L, Hansen R, et al: Late

follow-up of dual-chamber rate-adaptive pacing. *Am J Cardiol* 71:714, 1993.
48. Hayes DL, Neubauer SA: Incidence of atrial fibrillation after DDD pacing (abstract). *PACE* 13:501, 1990.
49. Feuer JM, Shandling AH, Messenger JC, et al: Influence of cardiac pacing mode on the long-term development of atrial fibrillation. *Am J Cardiol* 64:1376, 1989.
50. Jordaens L, Vandekerckhove Y, Van Wassenhove E, et al: Does rate-responsive pacing suppress exercise-related ventricular arrhythmias? *Stimucoeur* 14:93, 1986.
51. Kato R, Terasawa T, Gotoh T, et al: Antiarrhythmic efficacy of atrial demand (AAI) and rate responsive atrial pacing. In: *Progress in Clinical Pacing*. Edited by M Santini, M Pistolese, A Alliegro. Amsterdam: Excerpta Medica; 1988, p. 15.
52. Bellocci F, Nobile A, Spampinato A, et al: Antiarrhythmic effects of DDD rate responsive pacing (abstract). *PACE* 14:11, 1991.
53. Vanerio G, Maloney JD, Pinski SL, et al: DDIR versus VVIR pacing in patients with paroxsymal atrial tachyarrhythmias. *PACE* 14:1630, 1991.
54. Mabo Ph, Berder V, Ritter Ph, et al: Prevention of atrial tachyarrhythmias related to advanced intra-atrial block by permanent atrial resynchronization (abstract). *PACE* 14:648, 1991.
55. Bernstein AD, Camm AJ, Fisher JD, et al: The NASPE/BPEG defibrillator code. *PACE* (in press).
56. Mirowski M, Mower MM, Langer AA: Low-energy catheter cardioversion of atrial tachyarrhythmia (abstract). *Clin Res* 22:290, 1974.
57. Mirowski M, Mower MM: An automatic implantable defibrillator for recurrent atrial tachyarrhythmias. In: *Atrial Arrhythmias: Current Concepts and Management*. Edited by P Touboul, AL Waldo. St. Louis, MO: Mosby Year Book; 1990, p. 419.
58. Dunbar DN, Tobler HG, Fetter J, et al: Intracavitary electrode catheter cardioversion of atrial tachyarrhythmias in the dog. *J Am Coll Cardiol* 7:1015, 1986.
59. Jackman WM, Zipes DP: Low-energy synchronous cardioversion of ventricular tachycardia using a catheter electrode in a canine model of subacute myocardial infarction. *Circulation* 66:187, 1982.
60. Benditt DG, Kriett JM, Tobler HG, et al: Cardioversion of atrial tachyarrhythmias by low energy transvenous technique. In: *Cardiac Pacing: Proceedings of the VIIth World Symposium on Cardiac Pacing*. Edited by K Steinbach. Darmstadt: Steinkopff; 1982, p. 845.
61. Kumagai K, Yamanouchi Y, Tashiro N, et al: Low energy synchronous transcatheter cardioversion of atrial flutter/fibrillation in the dog. *J Am Coll Cardiol* 16:497, 1990.
62. Powell AC, Garan H, McGovern BA, et al: Low energy conversion of atrial fibrillation in the sheep. *J Am Coll Cardiol* 20:707, 1992.
63. Scott S, Accorti P, Callaghan F, et al: Ventricular and atrial defibrillation using new transvenous tripolar and bipolar leads with 5 French electrodes and 8 French subcutaneous catheters. *PACE* 14:1893, 1991.
64. Cooper RAS, Alferness CA, Wolf PD, et al: Optimal electrode location and waveform for internal cardioversion of atrial fibrillation in sheep (abstract). *Circulation* 86:I-791, 1992.
65. Ayers G, Ilina M, Wagner D, et al: Cardiac vein electrode locations for transvenous atrial defibrillation (abstract). *J Am Coll Cardiol* 21:306A, 1993.
66. Mirowski M, Mower MM, Langer AL: Command atrial cardioverting device. US Patent No. 3,952,750, 1976.
67. Mirowski M, Mower MM, Langer AL: Command atrial cardioverter. US Patent No. 4,572,191, 1986.
68. Hartzler GO, Kallok MJ: Low energy transvenous intracavitary cardioversion of tachycardias. In: *Cardiac Pacing: Proceedings of the VIIth World Symposium on Cardiac Pacing*. Edited by K Steinbach. Darmstadt: Steinkopff; 1982, p. 853.
69. Nathan AW, Bexton RS, Spurrell RA, et al: Internal transvenous low energy cardioversion for the treatment of cardiac arrhythmias. *Br Heart J* 52:377, 1984.
70. Levy S, Lacombe P, Cointe R, et al: High energy transcatheter cardioversion of chronic atrial fibrillation. *J Am Coll Cardiol* 12:514, 1988.
71. Chauvin M, Koenig A, Theolade R, et al: La place du choc electrique interne dans le traitement de la fibrillation auriculaire permanente. *Arch Mal Coeur* 84:377, 1991.
72. Kumagai K, Yamanouchi Y, Hiroki T, et al: Effects of transcatheter cardioversion on chronic lone atrial fibrillation. *PACE* 14:1571, 1991.
73. Lévy S, Lauribe P, Dolla E, et al: A randomized comparison of external and internal cardioversion of chronic atrial fibrillation. *Circulation* 86:1415, 1992.
74. Ewy GA: Optimal technique for electrical cardioversion of atrial fibrillation. *Circulation* 86:1645, 1992.

Chapter 32

Rationale for an Implantable Atrial Defibrillator

Jerry C. Griffin, Gena Sears, Gregory M. Ayers, John Adams, Clif A. Alferness, Ross Infinger, and Kurt Wheeler

Atrial fibrillation has been characterized as "totally disorganized atrial depolarizations without effective atrial contraction."[1] It is a common cardiac disorder resulting in more than twice as many hospitalizations annually as bradyarrhythmias or serious ventricular arrhythmias.[2] A recent editorial raised the question of whether an implanted defibrillator designed for atrial use, might constitute an effective therapy for these patients.[3] This chapter explores this concept and examines the rationale for such a device.

Epidemiology of Atrial Fibrillation

Incidence and Prevalence

Atrial fibrillation is a significant human health problem. By a wide margin, it is the most common cardiac rhythm disorder requiring hospitalization.[2] The most reliable data regarding the incidence of atrial fibrillation comes from the Framingham Study,[4,5] which followed 5,209 men and women for 30 years. They found an overall annual incidence of atrial fibrillation of approximately 0.1% per year among adults aged 25–64 years at the onset of follow-up. This rose rapidly with age from 0.02% in men and women aged 25–34 years at the beginning of the study, to almost 0.4% for men aged 55–64 years at the beginning of the study. Thus, the prevalence in their population, with an initial age range of 25–64 years, was approximately 2%. Other studies, producing similar findings have been reviewed extensively.[6,7] If untreated, paroxysmal atrial fibrillation recurs in most patients. Clair et al.[8] found that over 65% of patients had a second episode within 2 weeks.

Associated Diseases

Atrial fibrillation can occur as an isolated cardiac disease, so-called "lone atrial fibrillation," but most often occurs in association with other forms of cardiac disease. In the Framingham Study,[5] congestive heart failure and rheumatic heart disease carried the highest risk ratios as precursors of atrial fibrillation, but diabetes and left ventricular hypertrophy in both sexes, and hypertensive heart disease in men were also significant. No associated heart disease was present in 30 of the 98 cases of atrial fibrillation

From Singer I, (ed.) Implantable Cardioverter-Defibrillator. Armonk, NY: Futura Publishing Company, Inc.; © 1994.

found during the Framingham Study.[4] In all patients with atrial fibrillation, an important first step is the search for and correction or treatment of any underlying disease processes.

Impact on Prognosis

General

Overall cardiac function is adversely affected by atrial fibrillation in several different ways. The loss of atrial contraction affects ventricular filling and the mean atrial pressure associated with any given ventricular end-diastolic volume. It can affect closure of the atrioventricular (AV) valves, allowing mitral regurgitation. The AV node is bombarded by impulses from adjacent fibrillating atrial myocardium. Too many of these impulses may conduct through the AV node to the ventricles resulting in rapid ventricular rates. This and the irregularity of ventricular contraction may significantly impair ventricular filling on a beat-by-beat basis. Patients may experience marked symptoms including an awareness of heart irregularity, palpitations, fatigue, diminished exercise tolerance, and congestive heart failure. Indeed, in some patients, investigators feel atrial fibrillation may be the causal factor in congestive heart failure rather than a result of it. In some patients, complete or near complete resolution of heart failure occurred after control of the ventricular rate.[9]

Embolic Stroke

The most important recent advance in the understanding of atrial fibrillation is the recognition of the role it plays in the genesis of embolic stroke. Four recent trials have demonstrated the value of anticoagulation in the prevention of cerebral thromboembolic complications associated with atrial fibrillation.[10-13] In all four studies, the annual incidence of stroke in atrial fibrillation patients treated with warfarin was substantially lower (by 37% to 86%) than that observed in the control group (placebo or nothing). Each report recommends that in those patients in whom anticoagulation is not contraindicated, warfarin (and in one study, aspirin) be used to reduce the risk of ischemic stroke and systemic embolism. Furthermore, the studies concluded that warfarin therapy was "quite" or "relatively" safe, with observed increases in minor and major hemorrhage, more than offset by the reduction in ischemic events. The Stroke Prevention in Atrial Fibrillation (SPAF) investigators[12] reported 88% of patients were 80% compliant, and the Boston Area Anticoagulation Trial for Atrial Fibrillation (BAATAF) investigators[11] reported 90% patient compliance.

The BAATAF[11] and SPAF[12] studies stressed that further investigation is needed to try and identify patients at low or high risk for ischemic events so that anticoagulation therapy could be applied selectively. Age and mitral annular calcification appear to be associated with a higher risk of stroke. There is some evidence that patients without other cardiopulmonary disease (lone atrial fibrillation), or those under 60 years of age may constitute low-risk groups.

In all four studies, a sizable population of patients screened were not enrolled—AFASAK[10] reported 30% (505 of 1,711) of willing patients had contraindications to treatment; SPAF[12] excluded 53% (703 of 1,330) of eligible patients from the warfarin study arm, primarily because the patient/physician refused anticoagulation, and the exclusion of patients older than 75 years; the Canadian Atrial Fibrillation Anticoagulation (CAFA) study[13] reported only 13% of all screened patients were study eligible—of those screened, 17% had a medical contraindication to anticoagulation, and most of the balance were excluded for social-psychological reasons. In addition, some portion of enrolled patients had to discontinue warfarin therapy: BAATAF: 10% permanently discontinued[11]; AFASAK: 38% (primarily due to inconvenience of blood draws and side effects)[10]; SPAF: 11% (compared with 5% aspirin and 6.6% placebo groups).[12] Major bleeding complications were not found to be more frequent in those patients treated with warfarin. Minor bleeding, however, was more frequent in warfarin patients, when compared to either placebo or aspirin populations. Thus, it appears that warfarin anticoagulation, although effective, cannot be used in a large subset of patients at risk.

While warfarin substantially reduces the risk of thromboembolism, the case for aspirin is still uncertain. Included in three trials, it had no impact in the AFASAK trial when dosed at 75 mg/day,[10] was not dose controlled or reported separately in the BAATAF trial,[11] and is the focus of an SPAF II study-in-progress to compare the effectiveness of aspirin to warfarin.

In summary, atrial fibrillation is far from a benign problem. In the Framingham study[4,5] the total and cardiovascular mortality rate for individuals developing atrial fibrillation was twice that of patients maintaining sinus rhythm.

Current Therapy

External Direct Current Cardioversion

External DC cardioversion provides an effective means of converting atrial fibrillation to sinus rhythm. In a recent study by Lévy and colleagues,[14] 38 of 57 patients (67%) were converted to sinus rhythm with external cardioversion (a 300-J shock followed by a 360-J shock if unsuccessful). Unfortunately, external cardioversion deals only with the immediate problem and the recurrence rate is high.[8] Lévy et al.[14] also found that only 37% of patients remained in sinus rhythm 1 year after cardioversion despite treatment with amiodarone. Because of the discomfort of shocks of this magnitude either heavy sedation or brief anesthesia must be used at the time of cardioversion. Typically it is performed during an overnight hospital stay or in a hospital outpatient facility. Thus, while external cardioversion is a useful tool in the management of atrial fibrillation, it is rarely useful as a sole method of treatment.

Drugs

Drugs are currently the mainstay in the management of atrial fibrillation.[15] For long-term treatment, a three-pronged strategy is usually required: 1) the AV conduction system is blocked to control the ventricular rate; 2) antiarrhythmic drugs are used to lower the recurrence rate of atrial fibrillation; and 3) warfarin is given to reduce the risk of stroke.

Control of Ventricular Rate

In atrial fibrillation, impulses constantly bombard the AV node for conduction to the ventricles. The number conducted is modulated by the decremental properties of the AV node, which in turn are modulated by the antonomic nervous system, circulating catecholamines, disease of the conduction system, and directly or indirectly by a variety of drugs. The principal drugs used to slow ventricular rate are the β-adrenergic and calcium channel blockers and digoxin. These drugs are effective but their effects are easily reversed by the effects of the sympathetic nervous system or catecholamines. In addition, the calcium channel and β-blocking drugs are negative inotropes and the calcium channel blockers are vasodilators. While these properties do not limit usefulness in some patients, including some with heart failure, others cannot tolerate adequate doses to control the ventricular rate in atrial fibrillation, particularly during exertion. Often a combination of blocking drugs is required. Some of the drugs used for preventing recurrence also have AV nodal blocking properties.[15]

Drugs for Prevention of Atrial Fibrillation

Antiarrhythmic drugs may produce conversion of atrial fibrillation in a fraction of cases, but high doses are required and electrical cardioversion is preferred.[1] Due to the high rate of recurrence, antiarrhythmic drugs are routinely continued after electrical cardioversion. The Class IA drugs (quinidine, procainamide, disopyramide) are all used for prevention of atrial fibrillation.[16] These drugs do not block the AV node, and through their vagolytic effect, some may increase conduction and ventricular rate. The Class IC drugs (flecainide and propafenone) have also been shown to diminish recurrence rate.[17-20] These drugs have some blocking effects on AV conduction. The Class III drugs sotalol[20,21] and amiodarone[22,23] also decrease the recurrence rate and block the AV node. Drugs may be used serially in a staged or step-care approach to take the best advantage of their probabilities of efficacy and safety.[24,25]

Drugs to Reduce the Risk of Embolization

As noted above, warfarin has rather convincingly been shown to reduce the risk of stroke in atrial fibrillation. Unfortunately contraindications, adverse effects and the complexity and cost of follow-up limit its use.

Ablation and Pacing

Ablation of the AV conduction system is an effective form of limiting ventricular rate in patients with atrial fibrillation.[26] A permanent pacemaker is used to control heart rate, usually a VVIR pacemaker, but occasionally a DDD or DDDR device if circumstances warrant.[27] Some patients with paroxysmal atrial fibrillation will benefit significantly from having AV synchrony preserved when they are not in fibrillation.

Surgery

A surgical procedure, the "Maze" operation, has been proposed for preventing atrial fibrillation.[28] With the patient on cardiopulmonary bypass, the surgeon makes linear incisions in the left and right atria. The scars that result form paths for directing the activation wave front down corridors so that the atria activate but reentrant arrhythmias are minimized.

Limitations of Current Therapy

Drugs

In order to be effective drug therapy often requires a complex regimen. All three goals must be achieved: the rate controlled, fibrillation prevented, and the stroke risk lessened. The latter may be achieved indirectly if drug therapy is completely successful in preventing fibrillation episodes. However, as we shall see below this is not often the case, so warfarin anticoagulation is usually needed. To manage this complex regimen frequent patient evaluations and laboratory tests are used to monitor drug effects and screen for organ toxicity. These include ambulatory ECGs (Holter studies), electrocardiograms, treadmill exercise tests, prothrombin times and a variety of hematology, blood chemistry, and other studies depending upon which specific drugs are used.

Despite its complexity, medical therapy generally has limited effectiveness. Although Coplen et al.[16] found quinidine effective compared to placebo, only 58% of patients remained in sinus rhythm after 6 months. In a prospective comparison of quinidine and flecainide only 11% and 22%, respectively remained in sinus rhythm after 2 months.[17] Comparing flecainide and placebo, Anderson et al.[18] found 31% of treated patients without recurrence but only 8% receiving placebo. The median interval between attacks increased to 27 days for treated patients.

Results were similar in a trial of propafenone and sotalol with 41% and 46% without atrial fibrillation at 6 months.[20] Finally, in another trial of sotalol compared to quinidine the results were 52% to 48%, respectively.[21] While these and other studies[29] vary in patient population, methodology, and duration of follow-up, as a group they confirm the low rate of efficacy of individual drugs. Used in series, in a staged care approach, they provide adequate suppression for a bare majority of patients.[24,25] In order to identify those patients for whom drugs will provide adequate suppression, a significantly larger number will have to undergo multiple trials of different agents. All will be exposed to the risk of proarrhythmias, organ toxicity, and side effects. For most of the drugs used to treat atrial fibrillation, this risk may be quite significant.

Falk[30] has summarized the risk of proarrhythmia in patients undergoing therapy for atrial fibrillation. Although difficult to quantify precisely, fatal complications of therapy for atrial fibrillation do occur. Coplen et al.'s meta-analysis,[16] although criticized, showed a higher death rate with quinidine than placebo. Perhaps most impressive are the data of Flacker et al.[31] and the SPAF investigators, who compared atrial fibrillation patients receiving and not receiving antiarrhythmic drugs. Since this trial was primarily to test the hypothesis that anticoagulation lessened stroke risk, randomization failed to prevent differences in the makeup of these two groups. However, analysis of known risk factors failed to identify a predictable bias between the groups. The authors looked at survival as a function of whether the patient was taking antiarrhythmic drugs. The risk of arrhythmia death in patients receiving antiarrhythmic drugs was 2.6 times that of patients not receiving such drugs. This risk was exacerbated in treated patients having a history of congestive heart failure, 3.7 times that of untreated patients. When the data were adjusted to exclude patients with a history of ventricular arrhythmias, the risk in treated patients with congestive heart failure increased to 5.8 times that of untreated patients. Reimold et al.[20] followed 100 patients for 12 months treated with either sotalol or propafenone. Two patients died suddenly, and one death was documented to have resulted from torsade de pointes.

Several other recent studies suggest that therapy with antiarrhythmic drugs may carry significant risk. Although these studies examined outcomes after the treatment of ventricular ectopy[32-35] or after resuscitation from sudden cardiac death[36,37] and not atrial fibrillation, the patients contained in the studies were similar to many with atrial fibrillation. That is, they were of advanced age, had significant underlying (often ischemic) heart disease, and left ventricular dysfunction. While none are conclusive, these studies certainly raise concerns about the use of antiarrhythmic drug therapy in patients with atrial fibrillation.

In addition to life-threatening issues, antiarrhythmic therapy is associated with a high incidence of side effects that are often sufficient to require that the drug be discontinued.[24,29] Finally, a number of potentially dangerous drug-drug pharmacokinetic interactions among the anticoagulants, antiarrhythmics, and AV nodal blocking agents commonly used in the treatment of atrial fibrillation exist.[38]

Ablation and Pacing

Ablation and pacing, while beneficial in the late stages of atrial fibrillation for control of rate, offer little for less refractory cases. Ablation and pacing only offer ventricular rate control, requires permanent destruction of the normal conduction system, and substitutes one abnormal rhythm for another (ventricular pacing for rapid, irregular but normally conducted beats). There is growing evidence that a paced ventricular contraction is less hemodynamically effective and efficient than a normal contraction.[39] Since the atria continue to fibrillate the stroke risk is not lessened. Thus, it is likely that ablation and pacing as a therapy of choice will be limited to those patients who can no longer be cardioverted to sinus rhythm.

Surgery

Surgery for the prevention of atrial fibrillation has been performed in a small group of patients, as yet only followed for a short period of time. Although early success has been reported, little data are available to demonstrate that the atria remain hemodynamically functional. The procedure is also associated with the development of other atrial dysrhythmias such as atrial flutter and sinus node dysfunction. Finally, there are no data on the long-term results of the procedure. Unless overwhelming benefits are demonstrated, it seems likely that cost, risk, and morbidity will limit the application of open heart surgical procedures for the treatment of atrial fibrillation.

Cardioversion Using Transvenous Intracardiac, Catheter Electrodes

Conversion of atrial fibrillation has traditionally been done with drugs or external cardioversion using energy levels from 50 J–300 J. Recently, internal cardioversion using percutaneous transvenous catheter electrodes has been tested in both animals[40-50] and humans.[14,51-58]

Studies in Animal Models

Mirowski and Mower first reported transvenous atrial defibrillation in 1974. Their work in both animals and humans is summarized in a recent article.[40]

Powell et al.[45] evaluated the safety and efficacy of internal atrial defibrillation in a sheep model of atrial fibrillation. They found that low-energy defibrillation (from < 0.3 J to maximum of 5 J) using a right atrium/left chest wall cutaneous patch electrode configuration was effective in converting atrial fibrillation to sinus rhythm. The probability of successful defibrillation depended on the energy used. It ranged from a 31% success rate for energy levels < 0.3 J to a success rate of over 80% for energy levels of 5 to 6 J. In this study, there was a risk of ventricular fibrillation associated with a failure of reliable R wave detection. Eighteen episodes of ventricular fibrillation (VF) occurred during 768 shocks and all were associated with improper R wave synchronization (the mean interval between R wave and shock was 201 ± 38 msec). The probability of VF did not vary with shock intensity.

Kumagai et al.[44] compared two methods of low-energy synchronous catheter cardioversion of atrial flutter and fibrillation in dogs with conventional external cardioversion. Method A delivered shocks between the proximal electrode and the backplate. Method B delivered shocks between the proximal electrode and the distal electrode. In both of these methods, all 149 cardioversion attempts were successful with shocks ≤ 5 J. Shocks of ≤ 1 J were 70% successful using these methods while external cardioversion at the same energy level showed only a 12% success rate. The mean, minimally effective cardioversion energy levels were not significantly different between the two transcatheter methods (0.62 ± 0.67 versus 0.58 ± 0.71 J). No complications of heart block, ventricular fibrillation, or pathological evidence of severe shock-induced atrial injury were noted in this study.

Cooper et al.[46] performed an extensive study of atrial defibrillation using transvenous leads. A variety of electrode positions were tested (Figure 1). Those with left-right shock vectors tended to outperform those with only right-sided electrodes. The best vector was between the right atrium and the great cardiac vein, just beneath the left atrial appendage. Both monophasic and biphasic waveforms were tested and in a variety of durations. Biphasic waveforms performed best with a duration of 3 msec for each phase. Using the best lead location and waveform, the defibrillation thresholds were 1.3 ± 0.4 J. Shocks were delivered synchronously with the R wave and no episodes of ventricular arrhythmia were initiated when that was the case.

We refined the optimal lead location, demonstrating that sites more proximal in the coronary sinus produced less good thresholds.[47] With this knowledge we also demonstrated that both electrodes could be placed on a single lead without compromising thresholds and increasing the ease of lead placement.[48] Electrode lengths be-

RA - CS
1.3±0.4 J.

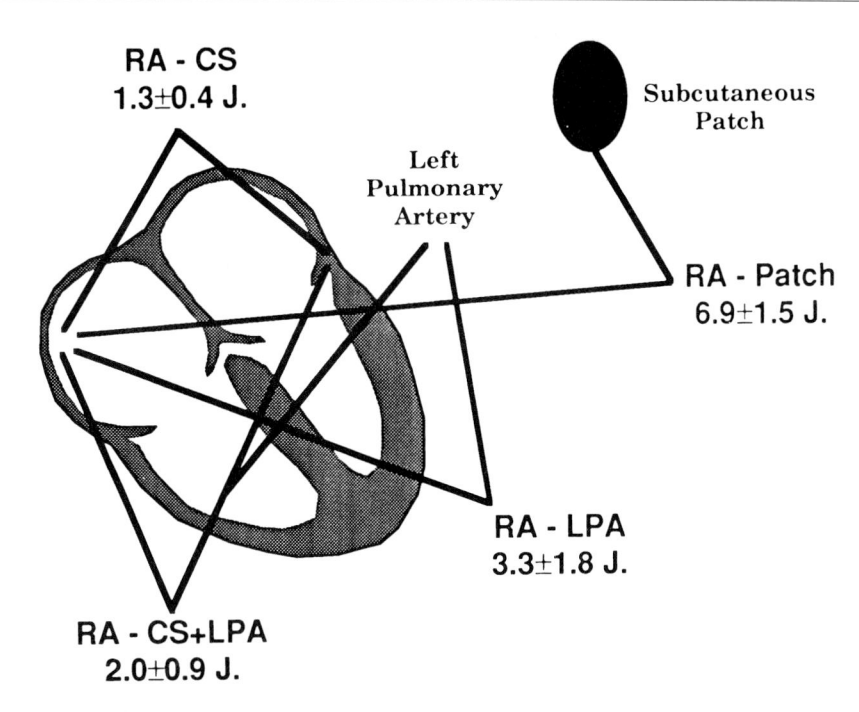

Subcutaneous Patch

Left Pulmonary Artery

RA - Patch
6.9±1.5 J.

RA - LPA
3.3±1.8 J.

RA - CS+LPA
2.0±0.9 J.

Figure 1. Atrial defibrillation varies by shock vector. This diagram shows the mean (± SD) atrial defibrillation threshold associated with various shock vectors. (Data from Cooper, et al. PACE 15: 259, 1992.)

tween 3 and 9 cm provide roughly equivalent values for atrial defibrillation threshold.[49]

We also investigated the issue of ventricular proarrhythmia resulting from shocks delivered to the atrium.[50] Using a right atrial-coronary sinus shock vector, 16 sheep were studied, half (group A) shocked at 80% of atrial defibrillation threshold and half (group B) at twice threshold (Table 1). Shocks were delivered according to four protocols (Figure 2): 1) a shock synchronous with the last paced beat of an eight-beat sequence (S_1); 2) a shock synchronous with a programmed premature stimulus (S_2) after an eight-beat drive (S_1); 3) a shock synchronous with an S_3 following an S_2 delivered at the longest interval not allowing sinus escape after an eight-beat drive (S_1); and 4) in atrial fibrillation during a 50-msec window beginning at some programmed interval following the previous beat. In each case, after delivery of a shock, either the programmed paced beat or the window were moved closer toward refractoriness and the shock repeated. Intravenous epinephrine was used to achieve minimum refractory periods in the ventricle. When the cycle length preceding shock delivery was ≤ 300 msec, a ventricular arrhythmia was induced after 11 of 964 shocks (Table 2). When the preceding cycle length was > 300 msec no ventricular arrhythmias were seen (895 shocks). There was no difference in the likelihood of proarrhythmia between subthreshold and twice threshold shocks.

Table 1
Atrial Defibrillation Threshold Values

	Group A*	Group B*
ADT, V.	128 ± 48	136 ± 37
ADT, J.	0.71 ± 0.6	0.79 ± .4
Shock, V.	107 ± 48	272 ± 74
% Success	52 ± 31	48 ± 29

* Mean ± SD; ADT: atrial defibrillation threshold. V: volts; J: joules.

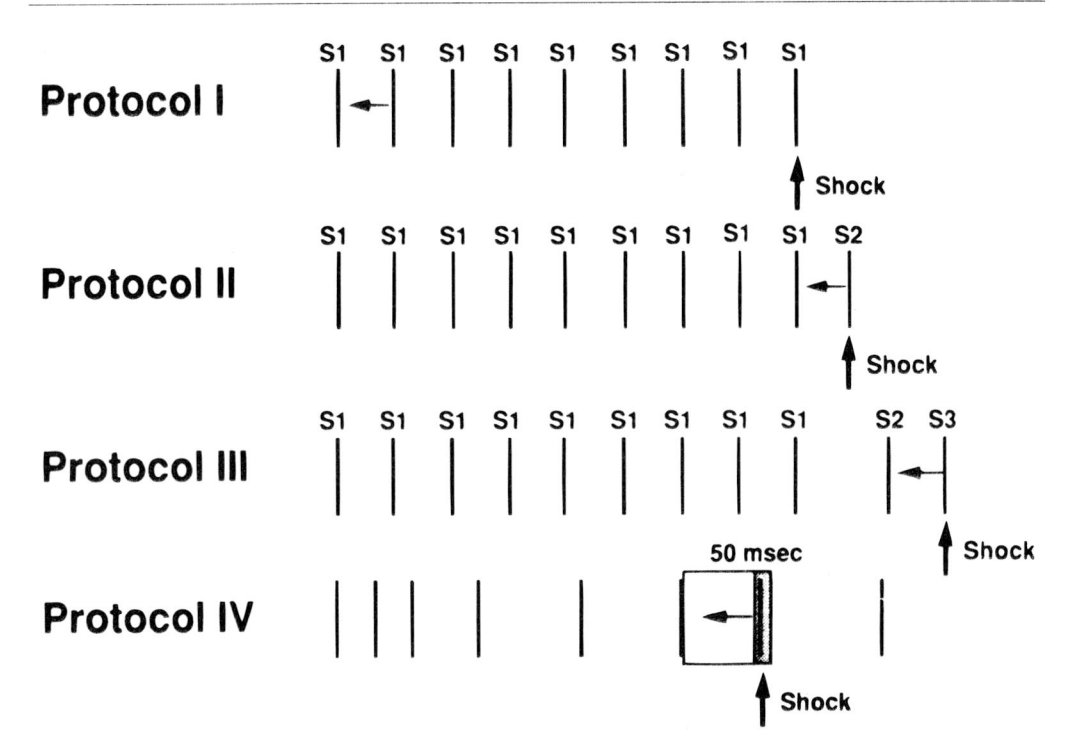

Figure 2. Diagrammatic representation of the four protocols used for testing shock proarrhythmia. For Protocols I–III the shock was delivered synchronous with a paced beat indicated by the vertical arrows. The horizontal arrows in Protocols I-III indicate which pacing cycle lengths were decreased until ventricular refractoriness was encountered. In Protocol IV shocks were delivered on a native beat during atrial fibrillation. The defibrillator scanned R-R intervals until one fell within a 50-msec window coupled to the previous R wave. In Protocol IV the horizontal arrow indicates the reduction in coupling interval of that 50-msec window.

Studies in Humans

Most human studies of atrial defibrillation have used high-energy shocks delivered between an electrode in the right atrium and a skin electrode.[14,53–57] The patients in these studies were generally refractory to external cardioversion. Typically a single shock was delivered to convert fibrillation usually at 200–300 J. Thresholds were not measured. Short-term success rates in these studies ranged from 70% to 100%, but the sample sizes of these studies were small. Transient AV block was reported in two studies. No traumatic complications or ventricular fibrillation were reported.

In humans, early attempts using internal, transvenous, low-energy cardioversion[51,52] had little success, probably due to the suboptimal placement of the electrodes. In Hartzler and Kallok's study,[52] one of the electrodes was positioned in the junction of the right atrium and the superior vena cava while the other electrode was positioned in

Table 2
Cycle Lengths (msec) Preceding Shocks that Resulted in Ventricular Fibrillation

Group / Protocol	I	II	III	IV
Group A 80% ADT		230 240	280	240
Group B twice ADT	250 300	230 230 250	260	198

ADT: atrial defibrillation threshold.

the right ventricular apex. In Nathan et al.'s study,[51] the active electrode was positioned against the right atrial septum causing the indifferent electrode to be positioned in the right atrium, superior vena cava, or inferior vena cava depending on the vein used for cannulation. Neither of these studies incorporated any part of the left atrium in the current path.

Much better results were obtained by Keane et al.[58] who used a right atrial to coronary sinus electrode pair. Patients with recent onset of atrial fibrillation were cardioverted with a mean energy of 3.4 J. This lead field allows more of the atrial mass to be positioned directly between the shocking electrodes. In the ventricle this appears to be the principal determinant of defibrillation threshold.[59]

Safety of Coronary Sinus Leads

Higher energy internal defibrillation (≤ 30 J) with one of the electrodes temporarily or permanently placed in the coronary sinus, has been used safely for the termination of ventricular tachycardia in animals[60] and patients.[61-67] This electrode configuration was found to be effective in terminating ventricular tachycardia and fibrillation using a variety of waveforms and energy levels within the range of existing implantable cardioverter-defibrillators (shocks up to 55 J in pigs and 30 J in patients). In several of the acute studies, the design allowed the investigator to visually inspect the coronary sinus after shocks were delivered. No complications were noted in any of these studies. Similar electrode systems incorporating a coronary sinus lead are now being permanently implanted for use with ventricular defibrillators. Preliminary reports suggest that these leads function well with no long-term complications.[65-67]

Attributes of an Implantable Atrial Defibrillator

A device for the management of paroxysmal atrial fibrillation should have several characteristics: low thresholds using only transvenous electrodes, small size with several years of implant life, and freedom from ventricular proarrhythmia. The small size is necessary to minimize the morbidity of implantation by allowing the devices to be implanted in the infraclavicular area. Low transvenous thresholds will allow cardioversion with a minimum of discomfort, using small capacitors. Shocks in the range of 1–2 J appear to be generally well tolerated in the conscious patient (unpublished data). Finally the device must be safe, at minimum safer than drug therapy to which it will most likely be compared. If such a device could be built, would it be used? An ideal target for the design might be the sophisticated dual-chamber pacemaker. If an effective, safe, atrial defibrillator could be built such that it rivals those devices in size and implantability it will very likely be used because pacemakers combined with ablation are an accepted therapy in selected cases now. Given the frequency of recurrence of atrial fibrillation, and the costs associated with the treatment of arrhythmia recurrence as well as drug induced and other preventable complications such as stroke, devices may be able to provide cost effectiveness and an improved quality of life.

References

1. Zipes DP: Specific arrhythmias: diagnosis and treatment. In: *Heart Disease*. 4th Edition. Edited by E Braunwald. Philadelphia, PA: W.B. Saunders; 1992, p. 682.
2. Bialy D, Lehmann MH, Schumacher DN, et al: Hospitalization or arrhythmias in the United States: importance of atrial fibrillation. *J Am Coll Cardiol* 19:41A, 1992.
3. Lévy S, Camm AJ: An implantable atrial defibrillator: an impossible dream? *Circulation* 87:1769, 1993.
4. Kannel WB, Abbott RD, Savage DD, et al:

Epidemiologic features of chronic atrial fibrillation: the Framingham Study. *N Engl J Med* 306:1018, 1982.
5. Kannel WB, Wolf PA: Epidemiology of atrial fibrillation. In: *Atrial Fibrillation: Mechanisms and Management*. Edited by RH Falk, PJ Podrid. New York, NY: Raven Press, Ltd.; 1992.
6. Cairns JA, Connolly SJ: Nonrheumatic atrial fibrillation: risk of stroke and role of antithromboatic therapy. *Circulation* 84:469, 1991.
7. Kalman JM, Tonkin AM: Atrial fibrillation: epidemiology and the risk and prevention of stroke. *PACE* 15:1332, 1992.
8. Clair WK, Wilkinson WE, McCarthy EA, et al: Spontaneous occurrence of symptomatic paroxysmal atrial fibrillation and paroxysmal supraventricular tachycardia in untreated patients. *Circulation* 87:114, 1993.
9. Grogan M, Smith HC, Gersh BJ, et al: Left ventricular dysfunction due to atrial fibrillation in patients initially believed to have idiopathic dilated cardiomyopathy. *Am J Cardiol* 69:1570, 1992.
10. Petersen P, Boysen G, Godtfredsen J, et al: Placebo-controlled, randomized, trial of warfarin and aspirin for prevention of thromboembolic complications in chronic atrial fibrillation: the Copenhagen study. *Lancet* 1:175, 1989.
11. Boston Area Anticoagulation Trial for Atrial Fibrillation Investigators: The effect of low-dose warfarin on the risk of stroke in patients with nonrheumatic atrial fibrillation. *N Engl J Med* 323:1505, 1990.
12. Stroke Prevention in Atrial Fibrillation Investigators: Stroke prevention atrial fibrillation study. *Circulation* 84:527, 1991.
13. Connolly S, Laupacis A, Gent M, et al: Canadian atrial fibrillation anticoagulation (CAFA) study. *J Am Coll Cardiol* 18:349, 1991.
14. Levy S, Lauribe P, Dolla E, et al: A randomized comparison of external and internal cardioversion of chronic atrial fibrillation. *Circulation* 86:1415, 1992.
15. Podird PJ, Falk RH: Management of atrial fibrillation—an overview. In: *Atrial Fibrillation: Mechanisms and Management*. Edited by RH Falk, PJ Podrid. New York, NY: Raven Press, Ltd.; 1992. p. 389.
16. Coplen SE, Antman EM, Berlin JA, et al: Efficacy and safety of quinidine therapy for maintenance of sinus rhythm after cardioversion. A meta-analysis of randomized control trials. *Circulation* 82:1106, 1990.
17. Lau C, Leung W, Wong CK: A randomized double-blind crossover study comparing the efficacy and tolerability of flecainide and quinidine in the control of patients with symptomatic paroxysmal atrial fibrillation. *Am Heart J* 124:645, 1992.
18. Anderson JL, Gilbert E, Alpert BL, et al: Prevention of symptomatic recurrences of paroxysmal atrial fibrillation in patients initially tolerating antiarrhythmic therapy. *Circulation* 80:1557, 1989.
19. Clementy J, Dulhoste MN, Laiter C, et al: Flecainide acetate in the prevention of paroxysmal atrial fibrillation: a nine-month follow-up of more than 500 patients. *Am J Cardiol* 70:44A, 1992.
20. Reimold SC, Cantillon CO, Friedman PL, et al: Propafenone versus sotalol for suppression of recurrent symptomatic atrial fibrillation. *Am J Cardiol* 71:558, 1993.
21. Juul-Moller S, Edvardsson N, Rehnqvist-Ahlberg N: Sotalol versus quinidine for the maintenance of sinus rhythm after direct current conversion of atrial fibrillation. *Circulation* 82:1932, 1990.
22. Middlekauff HR, Wiener I, Saxon LA, et al: Low dose amiodarone for atrial fibrillation: time for a prospective study? *Ann Intern Med* 116:1017, 1992.
23. Kopelman HA, Horowitz LN: Efficacy and toxicity of amiodarone for the treatment of supraventricular tachyarrhythmias. *Prog Cardiovasc Dis* 31:355, 1989.
24. Crijns HF, Van Gelder IC, Van Gilst WH, et al: Serial antiarrhythmic drug treatment to maintain sinus rhythm after electrical cardioversion for chronic atrial fibrillation or atrial flutter. *Am J Cardiol* 68:335, 1991.
25. Antman EM, Beamer AD, Cantillon C, et al: Therapy of refractory symptomatic atrial fibrillation and atrial flutter: a staged care approach with new antiarrhythmic drugs. *J Am Coll Cardiol* 15:698, 1990.
26. Scheinman MM: Catheter ablation. Present role and projected impact on health care for patients with cardiac arrhythmias. *Circulation* 83:1489, 1991.
27. Sui A, Bradley D, Chazouilleres AF, et al: *J Am Coll Cardiol* 21:95A, 1993.
28. Cox JL, Boineau JP, Schuessler RB, et al: Successful surgical treatment of atrial fibrillation: review and clinical update. *JAMA* 266:1976, 1991.
29. Pritchett ELC: Management of atrial fibrillation. *N Engl J Med* 326:1264, 1992.
30. Falk RH: Proarrhythmia in patients treated for atrial fibrillation or flutter. *Ann Intern Med* 117:??, 1992.
31. Flacker GC, Blackshear JL, McBride R, et al: Antiarrhythmic drug therapy and cardiac mortality in atrial fibrillation. *J Am Coll Cardiol* 20:527, 1992.
32. Echt D, Liebson P, Mitchell LB, et al: Mortality and morbidity in patients receiving encai-

nide, flecainide, or placebo. *N Engl J Med* 324: 781, 1991.
33. Fish FA, Gillette PC, Benson DW for the pediatric electrophysiology group: Proarrhythmia, cardiac arrest and death in young patients receiving encainide and flecainide. *J Am Coll Cardiol* 18:356, 1991.
34. Morganroth J, Goin J: Quinidine-related mortality in the short-to-medium-term treatment of ventricular arrhythmias: a meta-analysis. *Circulation* 84:1977, 1991.
35. Aronow WS, Mercando AD, Epstein S, et al: Effect of quinidine or procainamide versus no antiarrhythmic drug on sudden cardiac death, total cardiac death, and total death in elderly patients with heart disease and complex ventricular arrhythmias. *Am J Cardiol* 66:423, 1990.
36. Moosvi AR, Goldstein S, Medendorp SV, et al: Effect of empiric antiarrhythmic therapy in resuscitated out-of-hospital cardiac arrest victims with coronary artery disease. *Am J Cardiol* 65:1192, 1990.
37. Hallstrom AP, Cobb LA, Yu BH, et al: An antiarrhythmic drug experience in 941 patients resuscitated from an initial cardiac arrest between 1970 and 1985. *Am J Cardiol* 68: 1025, 1991.
38. Jaillon P, Ferry A: How do kinetics relate to toxicity of antiarrhythmic drugs? *Eur Heart J* 9(Suppl B):45, 1988.
39. Rosenqvist M, Isaaz K, Botvinick EH, et al: Relative importance activation sequence compared to atrioventricular synchrony in left ventricular function. *Am J Cardiol* 67:148, 1991.
40. Mirowski M, Mower MM: An automatic implantable defibrillator for recurrent atrial tachyarrhythmias. In: *Atrial Arrhythmias: Current Concepts and Management*. Edited by P Tauboul, AL Waldo. St. Louis, MO: Mosby Yearbook; 1990, p. 419.
41. Jackman WM, Zipes DP: Low-energy synchronous cardioversion of ventricular tachycardia using a catheter electrode in a canine model of subacute myocardial infarction. *Circulation* 66:187, 1982.
42. Dunbar DN, Tobler HG, Fetter J, et al: Intracavitary electrode catheter cardioversion of atrial tachyarrhythmias in the dog. *J Am Coll Cardiol* 7:1015, 1986.
43. Scott S, Accorti P, Callaghan F, et al: Defibrillation of ventricular and atrial fibrillation using new transvenous tripolar leads with 5FR shocking electrodes and 8FR subcutaneous catheters. *PACE* 14:1893, 1991.
44. Kumagai K, Yamanouchi Y, Tashiro N, et al: Low energy synchronous transcatheter cardioversion of atrial flutter/fibrillation in the dog. *J Am Coll Cardiol* 16:497, 1990.
45. Powell A, Garan H, McGovern B, et al: Low energy conversion of atrial fibrillation in the sheep. *J Am Coll Cardiol* 20:707, 1992.
46. Cooper RAS, Alferness CA, Smith WM, et al: Internal cardioversion of atrial fibrillation in sheep. *Circulation* 87:1673, 1993.
47. Ayers G, Ilina M, Wagner D, et al: Cardiac vein electrode locations for transvenous atrial defibrillation. *J Am Coll Cardiol* 21: 306A, 1993.
48. Alferness CA, Ilina MI, Wagner DO, et al: Comparison of a dual to a single lead system for transvenous atrial defibrillation. *PACE* 16:854, 1993.
49. Tacker WA, Schoenlein WE, Janas W, et al: Catheter electrode evaluation for transvenous atrial defibrillation. *PACE* 16:853, 1993.
50. Ayers GM, Alferness CA, Ilina M, et al: Ventricular proarrhythmic effects of ventricular cycle length and shock strength in a sheep model of transvenous atrial defibrillation. *Circulation* 89:413, 1994.
51. Nathan AW, Bexton RS, Spurrell RA, et al: Internal transvenous low energy cardioversion for the treatment of cardiac arrhythmias. *Br Heart J* 52:377, 1984.
52. Hartlzer GO, Kallok MJ: Low energy transvenous intracavitary cardioversion of tachycardias. In: *Cardiac Pacing: Proceedings of the VIIth World Symposium on Cardiac Pacing*. Edited by K Steinbach. Darmstadt: Steinkopff; 1983, p. 853.
53. Lévy S, Lacombe P, Cointe R, et al: High energy transcatheter cardioversion of chronic atrial fibrillation. *J Am Coll Cardiol* 12:514, 1988.
54. Lévy S, Bru P, Cointe R, et al: Cardioversion by internal electric shock of permanent atrial fibrillation. *Arch Mal Coeur* 82:1529, 1989.
55. Germonpre E, Jordaens LJ, Clement DL: Intracardial shock for the conversion of chronic atrial fibrillation. *Nederlands Tijdschrift voor Geneeskunde* 134:1213, 1990.
56. Chauvin M, Koenig A, Brechenmacher C: Internal electroshock in the treatment of chronic atrial fibrillation resistant to external cardioversion. *Ann Cardiol Angiol* 40:47, 1991.
57. Kumagai KM, Yamanouchi Y, Hiroki T, et al: Effects of transcatheter cardioversion on chronic lone atrial fibrillation. *PACE* 14:1571, 1991.
58. Keane D, Sulke N, Cooke R, et al: Endocardial cardioversion of atrial flutter and fibrillation. *PACE* 16:928, 1993.
59. Oeff M, Abbott JA, Scheinman ED, et al: Determination of patch electrode position for the internal cardioverter-defibrillator by cine computed tomography and its relation to the defibrillation threshold. *J Am Coll Cardiol* 20: 210, 1992.

60. Jones DL, Klein GJ, Rattes MF, et al: Internal cardiac defibrillation: single and sequential pulses and a variety of lead orientations. *PACE* 11:583, 1988.
61. Yee R, Jones DL, Klein GJ, et al: Sequential pulse countershock between two transvenous catheters: feasibility, safety, and efficacy. *PACE* 12:1869, 1989.
62. Bardy GH, Allen MD, Mehra R, et al: An effective and adaptable transvenous defibrillation system using the coronary sinus in humans. *J Am Coll Cardiol* 16:887, 1990.
63. Bardy GH, Allen MD, Mehra R, et al: Transvenous defibrillation in humans via the coronary sinus. *Circulation* 81:1252, 1990.
64. Bardy GH, Troutman C, Johnson G, et al: Electrode system influence on biphasic waveform defibrillation efficacy in humans. *Circulation* 84:665, 1991.
65. Yee R, Klein GJ, Leitch JW, et al: A permanent transvenous lead system for an implantable pacemaker cardioverter-defibrillator. *Circulation* 85:196, 1992.
66. Hwang C, Kass RM, Chen PS, et al: Safety and efficay of coronary sinus electrodes for implanted cardioverter defibrillators. *PACE* 16:896, 1993.
67. Bardy GH, Swerdlow C, Reichenbach DD, et al: Anatomic findings in patients having had a coronary sinus defibrillation lead. *PACE* 16:903, 1993.

Chapter 33

Automated Rhythm Systems

Mark H. Anderson and A. John Camm

Introduction

For centuries man has attempted to exert control over cardiac arrhythmias using antiarrhythmic drugs. The limitations of drug therapy and the narrow therapeutic/toxic dose ratio of drugs have been recognized for over 200 years.[1] The use of electrical devices to control cardiac arrhythmias is < 40 years old, and yet, dramatic technical development has occurred during this period. The initial development of implantable bradycardia support pacemakers was followed by antitachycardia pacemakers and most recently implantable defibrillators. The development of these devices has occurred in parallel with developments in electronics that have resulted in increasing complexity and substantial miniaturization during the development of each device. The implantable cardioverter-defibrillator (ICD) is currently the most complex arrhythmia management device available, yet despite the sophistication of the latest ICDs none can yet be described as an automated rhythm system (ARS). Although the functioning of the device is truly automatic, it requires time-consuming programming at implant and follow-up to optimize its function. The development of a true ARS will require the development of devices capable of some degree of self-programming, based on feedback and learning. Improved diagnostic capabilities using additional sensor technology will be needed to enable highly sensitive and specific identification of ventricular and supraventricular arrhythmias. Detailed data logging of episodes of arrhythmia and on the performance of the device in treating these episodes is required and may enable the recognition of precursors of arrhythmic events with the use of prophylactic therapies such as subthreshold stimulation, pacing, or drug delivery to prevent the occurrence of arrhythmia. Therapy delivery by the device would be extended to enable control of atrial and ventricular arrhythmias. This chapter considers the limitations of current arrhythmia control devices and the potential for development of a true ARS.

History

Although the concept that electrical stimulation of the heart might be useful in patients with bradycardia dates back over 100 years,[2] the first implantable rhythm control system was the bradycardia support pacemaker first described by Elmqvist and Senning[3] in 1959. Since then bradycardia support pacing has undergone dramatic technical evolution with the development of demand pacing,[4] dual-chamber pacing,[5]

From Singer I, (ed.) Implantable Cardioverter-Defibrillator. Armonk, NY: Futura Publishing Company, Inc.; © 1994.

and rate responsive pacing.[6] These developments have all occurred in response to problems noted with earlier generations of simple pacemakers and have served to improve the quality of pacing therapy and to widen its applicability for the treatment of patients with symptomatic bradycardias.

The first pacemakers paced at a fixed rate regardless of the underlying cardiac rhythm. Demand pacing, where the pacemaker regulates its output based on feedback from a ventricular sensing circuit, represented the first attempt at automation within an implantable rhythm control device. Rate responsive pacing, where the pacing rate varies depending on the physical activity of the patient represented an additional level of automation but the early rate responsive pacemakers requires manual "tuning" of the sensitivity of the rate response circuitry in order to obtain an appropriate rate response in each individual. More recently rate responsive pacemakers have been developed that adjust their own rate response depending on the activity levels that they sense over a period of days or weeks.[7] This represents the development of second-level automation where the device is using stored information to adjust its own programmed parameters to achieve an appropriate pacing rate.

The concept of antitachycardia pacing dates from 1963 when Moe et al.[8] described an intranodal tachycardia in canines that could be terminated by single or double extrastimuli. A number of publications on the use of the technique in humans followed[9-11] and enthusiastic development of a number of implantable automatic antitachycardia pacemakers followed. Antitachycardia pacing for supraventricular arrhythmias has been shown to be efficacious[12] and cost effective compared to antiarrhythmic drug therapy.[13] Although this therapy was briefly in vogue in the 1980s it has largely been overshadowed by the development of radiofrequency ablation techniques for supraventricular arrhythmias. The use of simple antitachycardia pacemakers for the treatment of ventricular tachycardias has always been limited by concerns over the incidence of arrhythmia acceleration in response to antitachycardia pacing.[14]

Second-level automation has also been developed in antitachycardia pacemakers with the development of devices such as the Intertach II™ (Intermedics Inc., Freeport, TX) that stores information about which pacing therapy was effective for the last tachycardia treated and uses this therapy as the first choice for the next tachycardia occurrence, reverting to the programmed sequence of therapies if this fails.

The concept of automatic defibrillation dates back to Zacouto's patent of 1953[15] but practical development of an ICD had to wait for medical and technical developments and was pioneered by Mirowski et al.[16] and Schuder et al.[17] in 1970. The first device implanted in a dog weighed over 1 kg and was implanted in a sterile rubber glove. Despite skeptical comment on the potential usefulness of such a device[18] development continued during the 1970s culminating in the first implant in a human in 1980.[19] After early encouraging reports of the potential efficacy of the device in reducing the risk of sudden cardiac death,[20] the number of devices implanted increased dramatically over the decade (Figure 1). This decade also saw a rapid increase in the complexity of the device. The earliest version of the device used a simple probability density function algorithm (Figure 2) to detect the occurrence of ventricular fibrillation and deliver a defibrillating shock. However, it soon became clear that in many patients the occurrence of ventricular fibrillation was preceded by ventricular tachycardia[21] and the probability density function has relatively poor sensitivity for ventricular tachycardia[22] and may occasionally be satisfied by sinus tachycardia.[23] Accordingly, R wave electrogram sensing was added to enable the device to deliver cardioversion therapies for ventricular tachycardia giving rise to the automatic implantable cardioverter-defibrillator (AICD™, [CPI, St. Paul, MN]).[24] Survival with this device was improved compared with the earlier devices, but a number

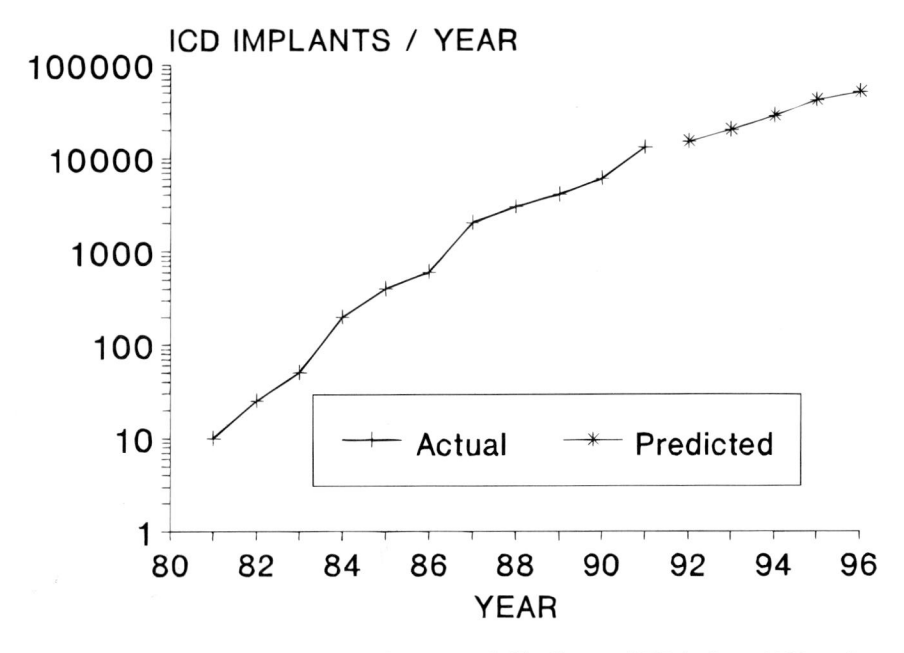

Figure 1. Implant rate of implantable cardioverter-defibrillators (ICDs) since 1981 and predicted implant rates for the 1990s (Data from Cardiac Pacemakers Inc., St. Paul, MN). Implant rates have shown a steady exponential increase since 1981, although the rate of increase is predicted to slow in the future.

of sudden deaths continued to occur, possibly due to asystole that had been observed after delivery of appropriate and effective defibrillating shocks.[25] This observation resulted in the development of the so-called second-generation devices that incorporated bradycardia support pacing in addition to cardioversion/defibrillation functions. The combined use of antitachycardia pacemakers and implantable defibrillators was reported as a means to reduce the incidence of shock therapies in patients with pace-terminable ventricular tachycardias.[26] The complexity of using two separate devices and the potential conflicts in programming led to the development of the so-called third-generation ICD that incorporated an antitachycardia pacing function. First used in 1989 reports of the efficacy in reducing the number of shock therapies first appeared in 1991[27] and have continued. These devices represent the current state of the art in terms of the development of an ARS incorporating as they do the three

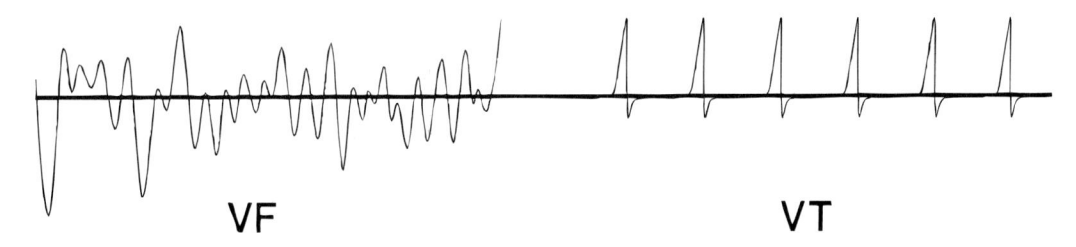

Figure 2. The probability density function measures time spent by the electrogram away from the baseline. In ventricular fibrillation (VF) the electrogram spends more time away from the baseline than during ventricular tachycardia (VT).

main types of device based antiarrhythmic therapy (bradycardia support pacing, antitachycardia pacing, and cardioversion/defibrillation).

Limitations of Currently Available Third-Generation Implantable Cardioverter-Defibrillators

Although third-generation ICDs incorporating bradycardia support and antitachycardia pacing are very sophisticated, there are a number of significant limitations with these devices that must be overcome before a true ARS can be developed.

Arrhythmia Detection

Third-generation ICDs rely entirely on an analysis of ventricular rate, and to a lesser extent ventricular rhythm to classify tachycardia. A few devices still incorporate the probability density function, which behaves as a crude form of electrogram morphology analysis (Figure 2). The high sensitivity of the rate-only detection approach for ventricular fibrillation is reflected in annual sudden death rates of 1% or less in ICD recipients.[28,29] When ventricular rate was used only to identify ventricular fibrillation, the risk of inappropriate therapy delivery as a result of atrial fibrillation or sinus tachycardia satisfying the detection criteria was low. However, as ICDs have increasingly been used to treat slower ventricular tachycardias, the risk of misclassification of supraventricular tachycardias has increased as the difference in heart rate between pathological tachycardias and other rhythms has reduced and may occur in up to 30% of patients.[30] Inappropriate therapy delivery as a result of misclassification of arrhythmias may have serious proarrhythmic consequences[31] and has been reported in between 9%[32] and 16%[33] of third-generation ICD recipients.

To counter this problem manufacturers have included features such as rate stability (Figure 3) and sudden onset detection (Figure 4) to prevent inappropriate detection of atrial fibrillation and sinus tachycardia respectively. Both of these approaches can be effective in reducing inappropriate detec-

Tachycardia detection interval (TDI) = 400ms

Rate stability 60ms

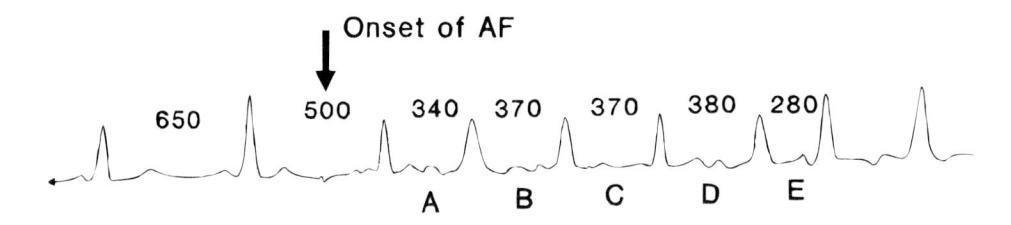

Onset of AF

650 500 340 370 370 380 280

A B C D E

The first four intervals of AF (A,B,C,D) satisfy the TDI

Interval E differs from the mean of B,C & D by more than

60ms and tachycardia detection is reset

Figure 3. The rate stability criterion used to minimize inappropriate therapy delivery due to atrial fibrillation.

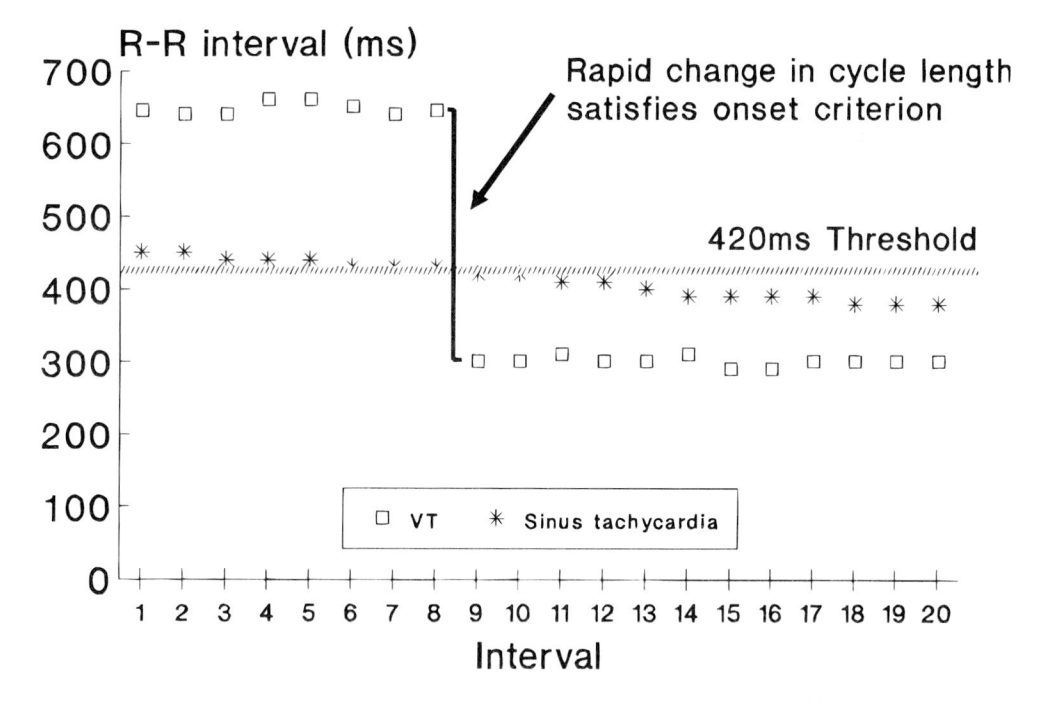

Figure 4. Use of the onset criterion to minimize inappropriate detection caused by sinus tachycardia. The gradual change in sinus rate on exercise fails to satisfy the onset criterion, whereas the sudden change associated with ventricular tachycardia does.

tion, but because of their potential for reducing the sensitivity of tachycardia detection they are used only after the occurrence of inappropriate therapy delivery and require time consuming electrophysiologic study or exercise testing to assess their impact[32,33] on the sensitivity and specificity of arrhythmia detection. Antiarrhythmic drugs are of limited use in modifying the sinus and tachycardia rates to reduce the risk of inappropriate therapy.[30]

Therapy Delivery

Implantable cardioverter-defibrillators currently offer a limited range of therapies. For ventricular fibrillation, they can deliver monophasic or biphasic defibrillation shocks at a programmed energy level. For ventricular tachycardias they can deliver antitachycardia pacing of ramp- or burst-type, and if this fails, can progress to deliver low- or high-energy cardioversion shocks. The therapeutic response to ventricular tachycardias may be further subdivided on the basis of tachycardia rate with faster tachycardias proceeding directly to shock therapy while slower ones receive initial pacing therapy. Heart rate alone governs the delivery of therapy in these devices with up to four heart rate zones programmable on some devices. This approach to tachyarrhythmia termination has become known as tiered-therapy and has the potential to terminate over 99% of episodes of ventricular fibrillation and 85% of episodes of ventricular tachycardia[32] (Figure 5).

However, the range of this therapy is limited to that programmed by the physician. If the device is programmed to deliver antitachycardia pacing prior to a cardioversion shock and this pacing therapy is always ineffective the device will nonetheless continue to deliver the pacing therapy first for each subsequent recurrence of the tachycardia. The therapy delivered takes no account of the hemodynamic effects of the arrhyth-

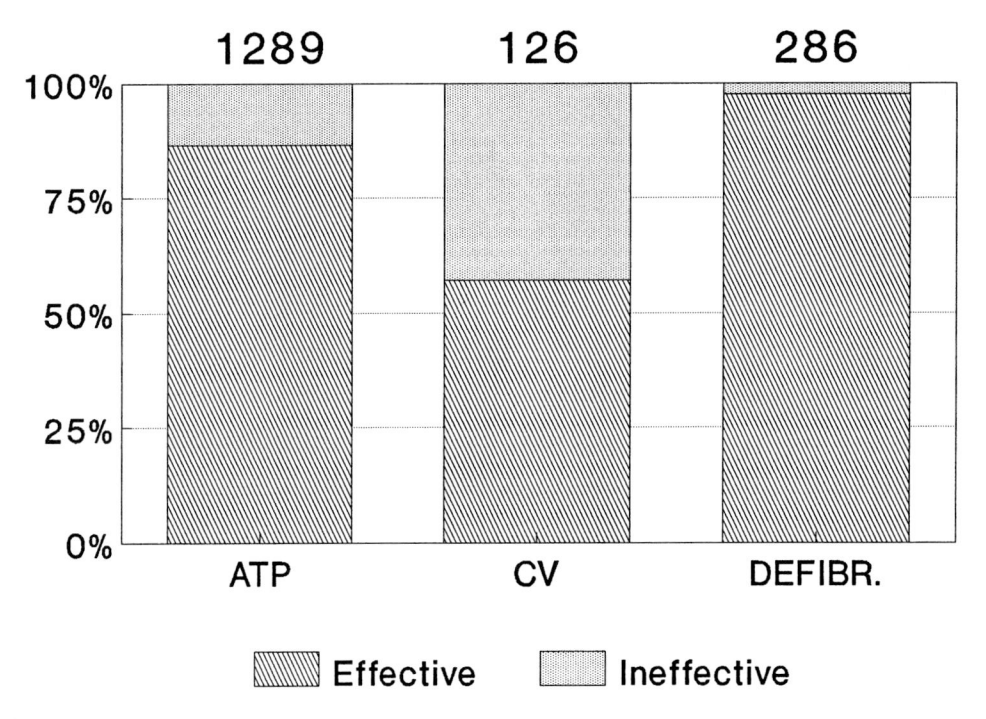

Figure 5. Efficacy of therapies for ventricular arrhythmias (numbers of episodes in brackets) delivered by a tiered-therapy implantable defibrillator in 102 patients. (Reproduced with permission from Reference 32.)

mia so prolonged pacing therapies can be delivered for an arrhythmia that is hemodynamically unstable. Some devices now include a "prolonged high rate" criterion that may be programmed to prevent continued pacing attempts during faster tachycardias but this has to be manually programmed. Although supraventricular arrhythmias are responsible for a significant proportion of inappropriate therapy deliveries no ICD is able to treat these arrhythmias so that their persistence increases the risk of further inappropriate therapy delivery.

Data Logging

The latest ICDs have begun to incorporate data logging of arrhythmia episodes that result in therapy delivery or in aborted therapy delivery. The exact nature of the data stored varies between devices, but most now record the time and date, the cycle lengths of the arrhythmia prior to and after therapy delivery, the number and type of therapies delivered, and in most cases, electrograms recorded from the pace/sense or defibrillation electrodes (Figure 6). Simple data logging of R-R intervals enables the correct classification of the majority of arrhythmia episodes but suffers from the same diagnostic limitations as the ICD itself.[34] A regular supraventricular arrhythmia triggering inappropriate ICD therapy may be impossible to separate from a genuine ventricular tachycardia. Newer devices offer the option of electrogram storage that may facilitate separation of ventricular from supraventricular arrhythmias in two ways. First, it may be possible to identify P wave activity on signals recorded from the defibrillation electrodes (Figure 7).[35] Second, ventricular tachycardia is associated with a change in the morphology of the electrogram recorded from the pace-sense or defibrillation electrodes in over 90% of tachycardia episodes.[36] However, this analysis has to be performed manually, and ad-

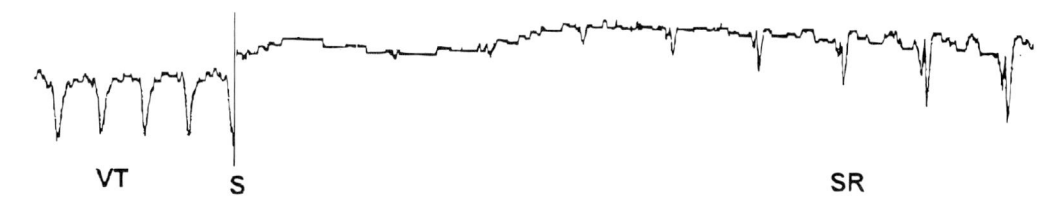

Figure 6. Intracardiac electrogram of the termination of a spontaneous episode of ventricular tachycardia (VT) by a cardioversion therapy (S). The signal is recorded from the defibrillation electrodes. It shows an initial dramatic loss of amplitude before it is clear that sinus rhythm has returned.

ditionally, the ability to differentiate arrhythmias based on the morphology of the ventricular electrogram depends on the site of the sensing electrode.[37] Potentially, storage of electrograms and R-R intervals may also allow recognition of patterns associated with the triggering of ventricular arrhythmias.[38] While the quality of data logging has improved, our ability to correctly identify the sequence of events leading to ICD therapy is limited by the diagnostic limitations of sensing the electrogram from a single intracardiac lead and by the inability of the current devices to use information other than the R-R interval derived from the signals sensed by this lead.

Physical Characteristics, Morbidity, and Mortality of Device Therapy

The original ICD weighed 225 g and had a volume of 250 mL. This bulk made implantation even in the abdomen difficult. A steady reduction in size and weight has occurred with more recent devices (Figure 8) such that prepectoral implantation of the device is possible in some patients in conjunction with transvenous lead systems.[39] Nonetheless even the smallest devices now available are likely to continue to require abdominal implantation and a further reduction in size and weight is desirable.

The earliest implanted defibrillation electrode systems were a combination of epicardial patch and superior vena cava transvenous electrodes, but it was subsequently demonstrated that entirely epicardial patch electrode systems gave lower defibrillation thresholds.[40] However, the desirability of avoiding a thoracotomy in patients who had poor underlying cardiac function, the average implant related mortality in several series of 2.4%[41] and the known poor performance of chronic epicardial pace-sense electrodes[42] led to continued interest in the development of transvenous electrode systems. Early postoperative complications (the majority were of minor significance) occurred in between 6% and 30% of patients with epicardial system. Infection of the ICD system remains the most significant problem and has been reported

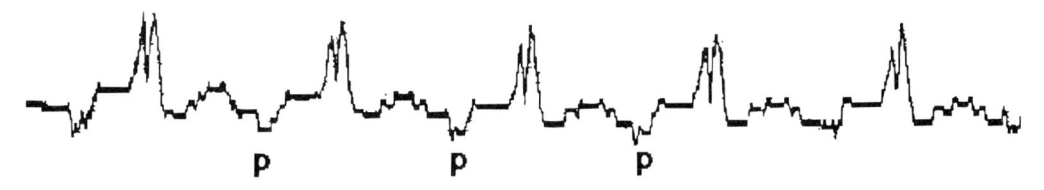

Figure 7. Intracardiac electrogram recorded from the defibrillation electrodes of an implantable defibrillator. Although the recording suffers from some digitization artifact, atrial activity is clearly seen (p).

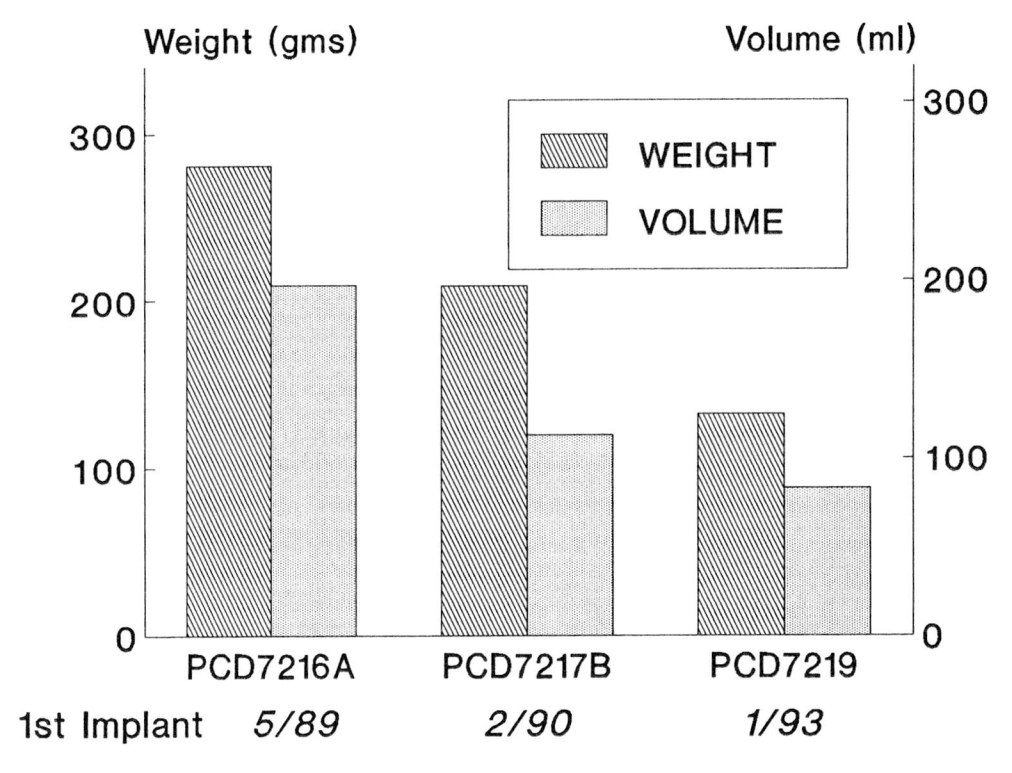

Figure 8. Progressive reduction in volume and weight of third-generation implantable defibrillators. (Data from Medtronic, Minneapolis, MN.)

in between 3% and 7% of patients[43] requiring removal of the system in around 3% of patients. Electrode-related problems due to insulation breakage, electrode fracture, migration, or patch crinkling can occur in 5% to 8% of patients.

Transvenous defibrillation electrode systems have been under evaluation since 1986 and have tended to be associated with lower implantation mortality. The best evidence for this comes from an intention-to-treat analysis of 379 patients that showed an overall mortality for transvenous implantation of 1.6% versus 4.7% for epicardial implantation.[44] However, evidence from two large studies suggests that transvenous lead systems are associated with a higher incidence of lead displacement and lead fracture.[45,46] While the advantage in reduced implant mortality outweighs this problem, it is clear that further work is required to achieve acceptable levels of reliability in chronically implanted transvenous lead systems. There may also be a continuing role for epicardial patches implanted by means that avoid the need for a thoracotomy.[47]

Desirable Features of a True Automated Rhythm System

The features required of a true ARS are summarized in Table 1.

Arrhythmia Detection

The limitations of arrhythmia detection by conventional ICDs using rate sensing signals from a single ventricular sensing electrode have already been described. Analysis of the morphology of the ventricular electrogram may be able to improve the

Table 1
Desirable Features of an Automated Rhythm System

Arrhythmia detection	*Rapid, sensitive and specific diagnosis of:*
	Bradycardias
	Tachycardias—VF
	—VT
	—Atrial Fibrillation
	—Atrial flutter
	—Supraventricular tachycardia
	Recognition of arrhythmia precursors (VPCs, heart rate variability, etc.)
Therapy delivery	Bradycardia support pacing—Atrial/Ventricular
	Antitachycardia pacing—Atrial/Ventricular
	Ventricular cardioversion
	Ventricular defibrillation
	Atrial defibrillation
	Antiarrhythmic drug delivery
Data logging	Arrhythmia episodes
	Heart rates
	Device performance parameters
Arrhythmia suppression	Arrhythmia suppression pacing
	Subthreshold stimulation
	Antiarrhythmic drug delivery
"Intelligent" self-programming	Selection of therapies in the basis of previous success (feedback/learning)
	Use of haemodynamic, activity sensor and electrogram data to decide most appropriate therapy
	Recognition of arrhythmia precursors
Ease of Implantation	Smallest possible device size
	Simple, durable lead system
	Avoidance of need for thoracotomy

VPCs: ventricular premature contractions.

specificity of diagnosis of ventricular arrhythmias, but these techniques have significant limitations and it may not be possible to achieve the high levels of sensitivity and specificity required for a true ARS without the integration of information derived from a secondary sensor or sensors. Additionally, future ARSs should have the capability of treating atrial arrhythmias, and therefore must be able to positively identify supraventricular arrhythmias rather than just classifying them as "not ventricular." The challenge of the next few years will be to identify which secondary sensor or combination of sensors offers the greatest improvement in the sensitivity and specificity of arrhythmia classification and how the information from this sensor can be integrated with that derived from the ventricular sensing lead.

Improving Specificity from a Single Sensor: Ventricular Electrogram Analysis

Diagnosis of ventricular tachycardia from the surface ECG relies on the presence of a broad QRS complex and a number of morphological criteria, which when combined, can enable the diagnosis to be made with a sensitivity of 100% and specificity of over 85%.[48] Therefore, it is not surprising that attempts should be made to improve the specificity of ventricular arrhythmia detection by morphology analysis of the electrogram derived from the ventricular sensing electrode.

The simple measurement of the width of the QRS complex is not of use because of the local nature of the bipolar electrogram. A variety of alternative techniques have been used to examine the morphology of

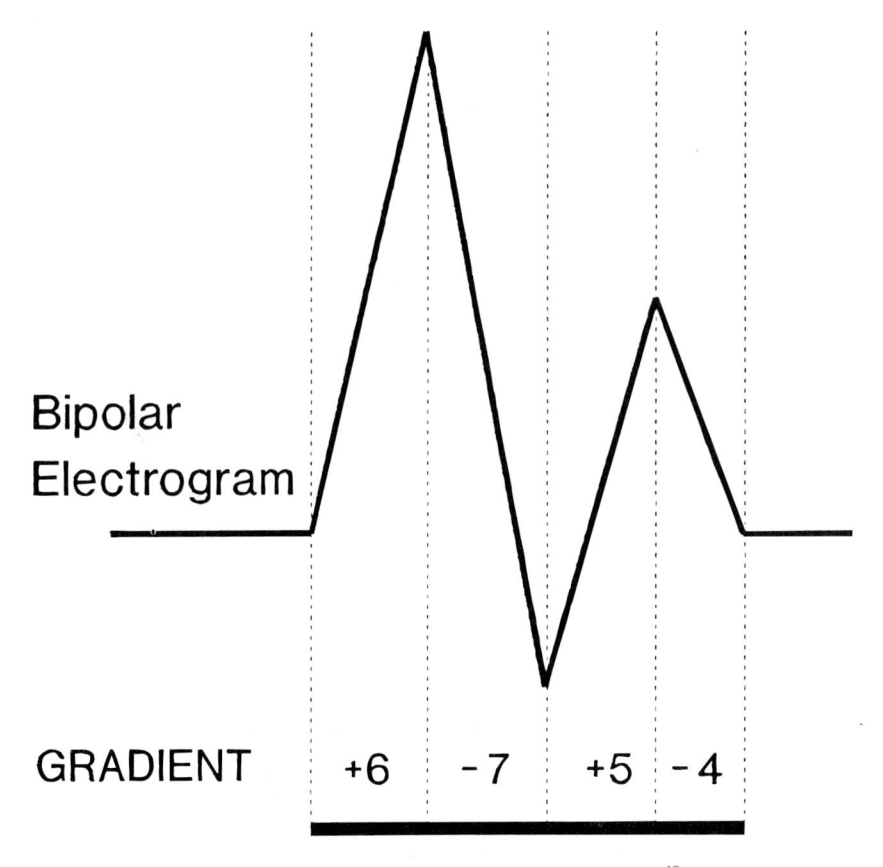

Figure 9. Ventricular electrogram analysis by gradient pattern detection.[49] The electrogram is characterized by a series of alternating gradients that may be used to compare it with other electrograms.

the electrogram. Gradient pattern detection was used by Tooley and colleagues[49] to distinguish between ventricular and supraventricular electrograms (Figure 9). This system characterizes the electrogram as a series of segments with differing gradients. This system was capable of categorizing electrograms with a high degree of accuracy, but required previous exposure to these electrograms during a learning phase. It requires relatively little computing power and could easily be incorporated in an implantable device.

Temporal electrogram analysis[50] is another relatively simple approach to morphology analysis (Figure 10). In this system the time that the electrogram spends outside a threshold value (defined by upper and lower rails) away from the baseline and the order (positive/negative) in which the rails are crossed is used. However, a marked deterioration in performance occurs when a temporal electrogram analysis algorithm is used to analyze recordings made during sinus tachycardia. With manual rail adjustment, ventricular tachycardia could be correctly identified in 26 of 27 patients (96% sensitivity). However, during exercise, 6 of 15 patients were incorrectly labeled as having ventricular tachycardia by the same algorithm (60% specificity). In addition, when a simple automated threshold setting for the rail positions was adopted, the sensitivity of the system for ventricular tachycardia was reduced to 81%. These problems result from the variability of the intracardiac electrogram that can occur during exercise and alterations of autonomic tone.[51]

Template analysis represents a third

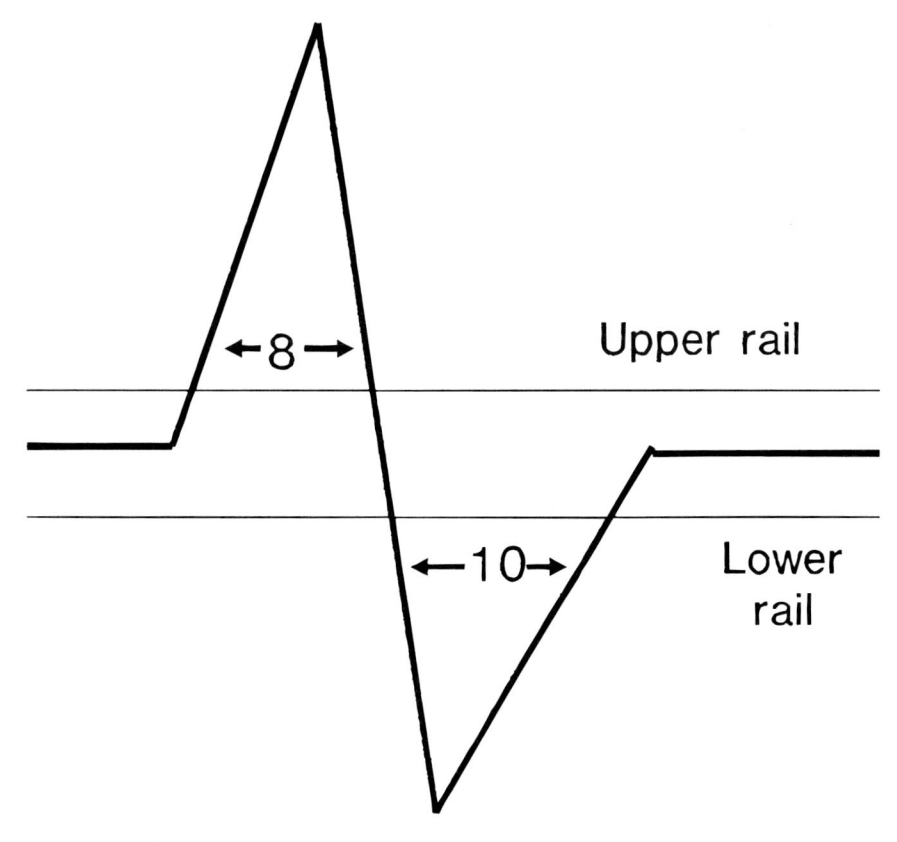

Figure 10. Temporal electrogram analysis.[50] The electrogram is characterized by the order and time at which rails on either side of the baseline are crossed.

approach to electrogram analysis. Each electrogram is compared with a template stored during known sinus rhythm.[52,53] A variety of computational techniques have been used to compare the shapes including the normalized area of difference method (Figure 11) and the less computationally demanding correlation analysis method (Figure 12).

Recognizing the complexity of the mental processing used by humans in their analysis of the differences between two shapes, computer models of neural networks have recently been applied to electrogram morphology analysis. These models mimic the synaptic connections within the brain and the complex interaction between multiple neurons. Before use they are exposed to a large number of electrograms that have already been classified. After this exposure they are able to correctly classify electrograms that differ from any of those to which they have been exposed during the training process.[54]

All techniques based on analysis of the ventricular electrogram are limited by the site of the recording electrode, which may affect the ability to separate ventricular tachycardia from sinus rhythm,[37] by the potential computing power required, and by the need with some types of analysis for prior exposure to arrhythmias to enable correct identification. The ability of these techniques to perform satisfactorily in a clinical environment has still to be shown. While electrogram analysis techniques may have a role to play in improving the specificity of arrhythmia detection the use of secondary sensors may enable diagnosis of a wider range of arrhythmias

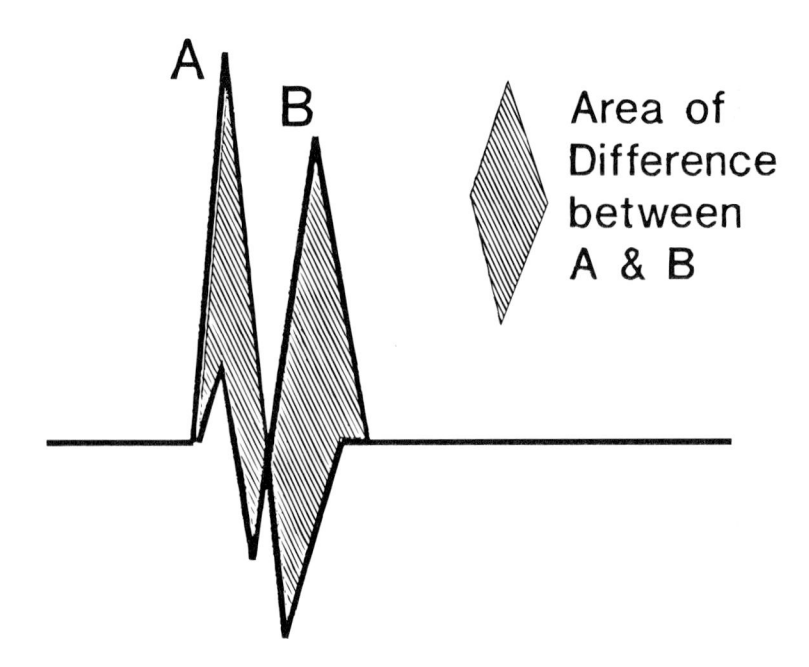

Figure 11. Electrogram analysis by the area of difference method. The area of difference between the sensed electrogram and a stored electrogram template is measured. A large area of difference suggests a significant change in electrogram morphology.

and require less sophisticated computing power.

Secondary Sensors

Atrial Electrogram Sensing

The ability to reliably sense the atrial electrogram using a dedicated atrial electrode over a period of many years has been demonstrated in the context of dual-chamber pacing.[55] Most of the research using atrial electrogram sensing has concentrated on its ability to improve the specificity of detection of ventricular arrhythmias, but in the context of a true ARS the ability to classify supraventricular arrhythmias on the basis of the atrial rate would also be useful.

Schuger et al.[56] used a simple algorithm that for ventricular tachycardia the ventricular cycle length be shorter than the atrial cycle length. In their study of 25 patients, this criteria was consistently met in 83% of patients. In a further 14% this criteria was met for at least 14 seconds at the onset of tachycardia (by which time the ARS should have classified the arrhythmias) before the onset of 1:1 ventriculoatrial conduction. Thus, 97% of ventricular tachycardia episodes would have been correctly classified by this algorithm. The incorporation of waveform analysis and atrioventricular interval analysis may further improve specificity,[57,58] although it may be beyond the computing power currently available in an implantable device.

The development of atrial sensing from floating dipole electrodes on the body of a right ventricular electrode may enable reliable atrial sensing in some patients without the addition of an atrial lead,[59,60] but this technology has yet to be assessed in defibrillator recipients whose underlying cardiac disease may make such indirect atrial sensing more difficult.

As yet, there has been little work looking at the classification of atrial arrhythmias using signals derived from atrial electrodes, but the separation of atrial fibrillation from

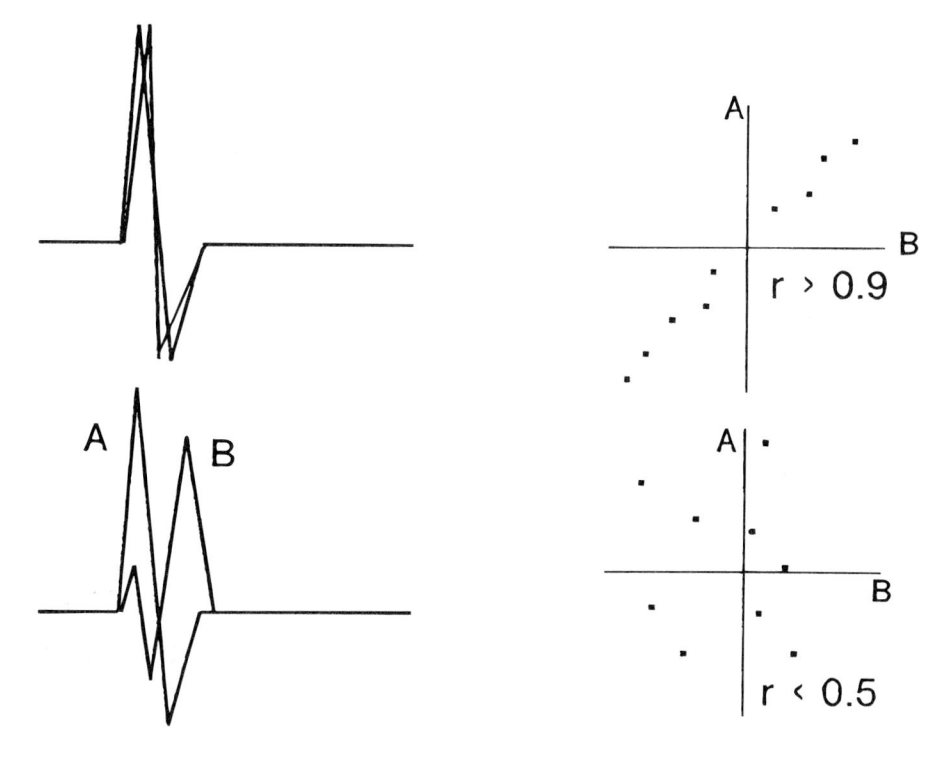

Figure 12. Electrogram analysis by correlation. The sensed electrogram is compared with a template by examining the correlation of voltage at selected time intervals. During sinus rhythm (top) the electrogram is similar to the template and the correlation is good, during ventricular tachycardia the electrogram is different and the correlation is poor.

other supraventricular arrhythmias should be straightforward based on rate and rate stability alone.

Hemodynamic Sensors

Hemodynamic sensors are designed to measure the effect of the tachyarrhythmia on the circulation. The feasibility of such sensing from pressure transducers mounted on electrode bodies is well established. A number of approaches to using hemodynamic data derived from these catheters have been evaluated.

One approach involves the examination of the right ventricular pressure alone. A variety of algorithms have been used. Erickson and colleagues[61] used a threshold of 30% change in either the rectified waveform area of the right ventricular pressure or the right ventricular pressure area (1/2 × pulse pressure × cycle length) and demonstrated that sensitivities of up to 84% and specificities of 100% could be achieved in the separation of stable and unstable ventricular tachycardias. In contrast, right ventricular dP/dt_{max} has been shown to correlate poorly with tachycardia cycle length, mean arterial pressure, and systolic blood pressure.[62]

Atrial pressure analysis may prove a useful alternative. Kaye and colleagues[63] have demonstrated the characteristic atrial pressure patterns that occur with atrial flutter and fibrillation, atrioventricular nodal reentrant tachycardia, atrioventricular reentrant tachycardia, and ventricular tachycardia with or without ventriculoatrial conduction. Beauregard et al.[64] demonstrated a significant rise in right atrial pressure associated with ventricular pacing at cycle lengths between 600 and 333 msec. No significant rise occurred during atrial pacing at the same cycle lengths and there was no significant change in mean right ventricular pressure during either atrial or ventricular pacing.

A combination of heart rate, and atrial and ventricular pressure analysis has been used in an algorithm by Cohen and colleague.[65] They defined unstable tachyarrhythmias as producing a fall of ≥ 25 mm Hg in mean arterial pressure during the first 15 seconds. They compared a simple algorithm of heart rate > 150 beats per minute to one combining heart rate > 150 beats per minute, ≥ 4 mm Hg rise in mean right atrial pressure, and ≥ 5 mm Hg fall in right ventricular systolic pressure over a 15-second interval. The algorithms were compared in a prospective study. The conventional (rate-only) algorithm gave a sensitivity of 100% but specificity of only 68%, whereas the combined rate and pressure algorithm had 100% sensitivity and 100% specificity. As an alternative to intracavity pressure sensing, intramyocardial pressure sensing may provide a means to detect changes in ventricular wall loading associated with arrhythmias and the use of such a system has been described in dogs.[66]

Oxygen Saturation Sensors

An alternative approach to assessing the hemodynamic impact of tachyarrhythmias uses measurement of mixed venous oxygen saturation. Cohen et al.[67] recorded mixed venous oxygen saturations using a fiber-optic catheter positioned in the pulmonary artery during atrial and ventricular pacing at a variety of cycle lengths between 600 and 250 msec. For any given cycle length rapid ventricular pacing tended to cause a bigger fall in mixed venous oxygen saturation than did atrial pacing. However, ventricular fibrillation and ventricular pacing at cycle lengths < 230 msec produced no effect on mixed venous oxygen saturation until after the termination of the arrhythmia (presumably due to complete circulatory stasis during the episode). Clearly such a sensor would be inadequate when used alone, and so on the basis of these findings, a mixed venous oxygen tiered-therapy algorithm was developed (cycle length ≤ 230 msec = unstable; cycle length > 230 msec and fall in mixed venous oxygen of ≥ 6% over 30 seconds = unstable). This was compared with a rate-only algorithm (rate ≥ 170 beats per minute = unstable) and a combined rate and right atrial pressure algorithm (rate ≥ 170 beats per minute and increase in mean right atrial pressure of ≥ 5 mm Hg over 15 seconds). These three algorithms were tested retrospectively in 113 paced and induced tachyarrhythmias in 10 patients and the results are summarized in Table 2. The combined algorithm using either mixed venous oxygen saturation or right atrial pressure appears to improve the specificity of detection of unstable arrhythmias, and the mixed venous oxygen saturation algorithm does so without loss of specificity.

Table 2

Algorithm	Sensitivity (%)	Specificity (%)
Rate—only	93	71
Rate—mean right atrial pressure	85	98
Rate—MVO$_2$	93	96

Activity/Posture Sensors

Activity sensors of various types have been widely used in rate responsive sensing.[68] In addition to their obvious role in the provision of rate responsive pacing, in a future ARS they may also have a secondary role in the diagnosis of arrhythmias. A sudden onset tachycardia occurring in the absence of physical activity is likely to be pathological. Posture sensors might also provide useful information on patient position at the time of onset of arrhythmia, although the implanted device position would have to be stable for these to be of use.

In summary, a wide range of arrhythmia detection methods are already available for inclusion in a future ARS. More specific classification of arrhythmias is likely to require analysis or rate and morphology of atrial and ventricular electrograms. Hemodynamic and metabolic sensors provide important information on the impact of the arrhythmias and may enable the ARS to select the aggressiveness of the therapy delivered. By incorporating atrial and ventricular sensing together with an activity sensor the ARS would also be able to provide full function DDDR pacing for bradycardias.

Therapy Delivery

The aim of an ARS should be to terminate any arrhythmia as quickly as possible using the least aggressive therapy so as to result in the minimum of symptoms (related to the arrhythmia or therapy) to the patient. An ARS would base its decision on which therapy to use on four factors: 1) site of arrhythmia (ventricular/supraventricular); 2) rate of arrhythmia; 3) hemodynamic effect of arrhythmia; and 4) previous experience of this arrhythmia. It could then select from one of the following therapies:

- Atrial or ventricular bradycardia support pacing
- Atrial antitachycardia pacing (for flutter or AVNRT)
- Atrial cardioversion (for persistent atrial flutter)
- Atrial defibrillation (for atrial fibrillation)
- Ventricular antitachycardia pacing (for ventricular tachycardia)
- Subthreshold ventricular pacing (for ventricular tachycardia)
- Ventricular cardioversion (for ventricular tachycardia)
- Ventricular defibrillation (for ventricular fibrillation)
- Antiarrhythmic drug delivery

Its choice of therapy might also be altered by information about the patient provided by the programming physician or at pre- or postimplantation electrophysiologic study. For example, if the patient is prone to infrequent attacks of atrial fibrillation with a slow ventricular response that are usually self-terminating after a few minutes no therapy need be delivered unless the arrhythmia persists or has an adverse hemodynamic effect.

The use of an atrial pace-sense electrode facilitates the delivery of bradycardia support and antitachycardia atrial pacing without additional implanted hardware. Atrial cardioversion or atrial defibrillation will, however, require the use of additional electrodes. The practicalities of atrial defibrillation via implanted electrodes is only just beginning to be explored in humans, but recent work in sheep has shown the practicality of atrial defibrillation using transvenous electrodes positioned in the right atrial appendage and coronary sinus with low-energy (< 5 J) biphasic shocks.[69] Although an additional electrode would be needed in the coronary sinus for this technique to be used with an ARS, it might be possible to use an existing superior vena cava/right atrium electrode as the second atrial defibrillation electrode.

Interest in the impact of subthreshold stimuli on cardiac conduction dates back to the observation of Weidmann in 1951[70] that the application of a subthreshold pulse to a sheep Purkinje fiber in the early part of the pacemaker cycle can increase the duration of diastole. Termination of ventricular tachycardia by subthreshold stimulation was first reported by Ruffy et al. in 1983[71] and has been demonstrated in 8 of 15 patients with inducible sustained ventricular tachycardia by Shenasa et al.[72] This phenomenon is thought to be caused by capture of tissue in an excitable gap within the reentry circuit and for this reason appears to require close proximity of the pacing electrode site to the reentry circuit. This may limit its application in an implantable ARS using transvenous electrodes. However, subthreshold stimulation has been shown to be effective when delivered via epicardial defibrillation patches, which because of their large surface area may well be in close proximity to the reentry circuit.[73]

Drug delivery systems have had limited application in cardiology probably because of the generally large quantities of most antiarrhythmic drugs required to achieve a therapeutic effect. However, using epicardial defibrillation patches modified to contain a 3.6-mL drug reservoir, Avitall et al.[74] demonstrated the feasibility of iontophoresing procainamide into infarcted myocardium in dogs. Therapeutic levels of procainamide were achieved even in the endocardium and ventricular tachycardia was terminated after between 20 seconds and 7 minutes in all 20 dogs in which this arrhythmia could be induced. Clearly a future ARS could incorporate drug delivery systems of this type or alternatively a separately implanted drug delivery unit could be remotely controlled by signals from the ARS.

Arrhythmia Suppression/Prevention

The concept of using pacing to suppress arrhythmias is not new. Zoll et al.[75] first described the use of transthoracic pacing to prevent the occurrence of ventricular arrhythmias in patients with atrioventricular block. The technique was developed using transvenous pacing electrodes and subsequently extended to use in patients without atrioventricular block.[76] In a proportion of patients with atrial fibrillation, atrial bradycardia is the triggering factor for the onset of the arrhythmia and it is known that the use of AAI pacing instead of VVI pacing in patients with sick sinus syndrome is associated with a lower incidence of chronic atrial fibrillation.[77] Therefore, the potential exists to prevent some ventricular and supraventricular arrhythmias purely by preventing the bradycardias that may precipitate them. More sophisticated arrhythmia suppression may be possible in an ARS by its recognition of changes in heart rate variability[78] or short-term variations in R-R interval[79,80] that are known to occur immediately prior to the occurrence of arrhythmia. By virtue of its data storage capability, the ARS may be able to recognize patient-specific precursors of arrhythmia and avert the onset by pacing in the relevant chamber. Subthreshold stimulation may also have a role to play in the prevention of ventricular fibrillation[81] as there is a period of 60 msec after the vulnerable period of the ventricles during which an apparently nonpropagated stimulus or train of stimuli could abort the arrhythmia that would normally be induced by an extrastimulus delivered in the vulnerable period.[82]

Potential warning of imminent arrhythmias may also involve the use of information from sensors other than the pace-sense electrodes. Intracavity pressure monitoring could be used to assess rise in cavity wall tension, which can be associated with arrhythmias.[83–85] Intravascular ultrasound has been demonstrated to be a practical way of examining wall motion[86] and such a transducer could be incorporated in the defibrillating electrode to detect wall motion abnormalities associated with ischemia, which may be precursors of arrhythmia. Implantable electromagnetic wall motion sensors are also being developed.[87] Substantial technical developments would be required to develop such a device that could operate over a long period of time without causing rapid depletion of the ARS battery. Monitoring of coronary sinus oxygen tension by fiber-optic catheter is also feasible[88] and might provide advance warning of ischemia. Ion electrodes incorporated into the defibrillator leads could enable the monitoring of the concentrations of critical ions such as potassium and magnesium[89] and possibly even antiarrhythmic drug concentrations.

Data Logging

Despite the relatively sophisticated data logging available on current ICDs there are many potential improvements that could be incorporated in future ARSs. Presently, those devices that store electrograms and R-R intervals do so for only a short period immediately adjacent to the arrhythmia episode. With the availability of data from additional sensors and more detailed arrhythmia analysis this could be improved so that several minutes of ECG were available, together with patterns of ectopic beat frequency, heart rate variability, and other factors such as serum potassium levels at the time of the event. The practicality of recording a surface ECG from a small implanted device has already been demonstrated[90] and the storage of such an ECG would further facilitate the analysis of arrhythmic episodes and their comparison with arrhythmias induced at electrophysiology study.

Data storage need no longer be linked specifically to arrhythmia episodes. The device should be able to analyze and store data from any of its sensors at a predetermined interval over a period of days or weeks. In addition to the purely practical applications of such data it would also be immensely useful for research purposes.

The storage of the large volume of data generated by such techniques is a considerable challenge, especially at a time when there is a great desire to reduce the size of the device. Additionally, information stored within the device is only of use to the physician once it has been extracted. Although the practicality of transtelephonic data transmission from the data logs of an ICD to the implanting center has been demonstrated with prototypic devices[91] no system of this type is commercially available at present. Several ICD manufacturers are working on the development of these systems and this may enable the retrieval of large volumes of data from the ARS without the need for unnecessarily frequent review at the implanting center. The development of telemetry with a range of several feet raises the possibility of automatic retrieval of data from the device on a daily basis. While the patient is asleep at night, data could be transmitted to a bedside receiver unit that could automatically transmit the data retrieved to the implanting center. Any electrophysiologic or biochemical abnormalities could then be rapidly acted on. The technology to make such a system feasible already exists[92] and the rate limiting step in its development remains whether the need for such a device is perceived by ICD manufacturers. As the number of ICD recipients increases steadily the economics of such devices become increasingly attractive.

Intelligent Self-Programming

The complexity of ICDs already renders their programming difficult and time consuming and the technical developments outlined above in the fields of arrhythmia detection, therapy delivery, and data logging are likely to increase this problem. The introduction of automation in the programming of an ARS is likely to be necessary if its use is not to be confined to a few specialist centers. Limited automation has already been applied to bradycardia support[7] and antitachycardia pacing.

Automation may take the form of relatively simple second-level automation where the device assesses its own performance and modifies its programmed parameters accordingly, or it may develop into a more advanced form where clinical information on the patient and their arrhythmias is fed into the programmer and appropriate parameters programmed accordingly, with the physician having an advisory and monitoring capacity and with the ability to override device choices as necessary (Table 3).

Ease of Implantation and Long-Term Reliability

The problems associated with the current generation of implantable defibrillators and their lead systems have already been discussed. A continued reduction in the size of the ARS is desirable to allow simple subcutaneous insertion. Dramatic miniaturiza-

Table 3
Implantation and Follow-Up of an Automated Rhythm System (ARS)

Pre-implant	Important clinical data input into ARS:
	  Age
	  Underlying disease
	  Left ventricular function
	  Previous tachycardias (rate & type)

Implant	Defibrillation testing— Device optimises pacing, sensing and defibrillation performance
Predischarge	Maximal exercise test—device assesses sensor inputs, electrogram morphology, etc. Electrophysiologic testing—device optimises therapies for induced arrhythmias

Postdischarge	Device monitors arrhythmias
	  Identifies precipitants
	  Evaluates arrhythmia suppression therapies
	  Adjusts arrhythmia termination therapies

Follow-up	Device reports on performance and programmed therapies

tion of the electronic components has meant that the battery and storage capacitors are the major occupiers of space within the device. Steady development in battery technology means that a further gradual reduction in battery size for a given capacity will occur. A similar gradual reduction in capacitor size is also likely, mainly as a result of improvements in terminal design as current capacitor technology appear to have reached a threshold of energy density requiring a major technological breakthrough to achieve substantial gains. The use of higher shock voltages with smaller capacitors may allow for some further reduction in capacitor size.[93]

Potentially the best way to achieve a reduction in device size is to reduce its energy output, as this enables the use of smaller capacitors and batteries. The use of biphasic defibrillation shocks has been associated with lower ventricular defibrillation thresholds,[94] but this improvement has been used to enable the more widespread application of pure transvenous electrode systems (without the use of a subcutaneous patch), rather than any reduction in device energy output.[95] Further research into shock waveforms is likely to allow the use of devices with reduced maximum energy outputs, at least in selected patients.

The majority of ARSs are likely to use transvenous leads because of the lower mortality associated with their use and relative ease of implantation. Prepectoral implantation may allow the use of the casing of the device as an active electrode.[96] Lead systems are likely to become more complex as the functions of the ARS expand to include treatment of supraventricular arrhythmias and additional sensors are incorporated. It is important that this additional functionality is not gained at the expense of poor chronic performance with high revision rates.

Practical Automated Rhythm System Devices and Their Potential Uses

It is almost impossible to predict the exact design of future ARSs but nonetheless it is feasible to speculate on the type of devices that may be required.

Multifunction Automated Rhythm Systems

This device would be a full-function arrhythmia control and management system

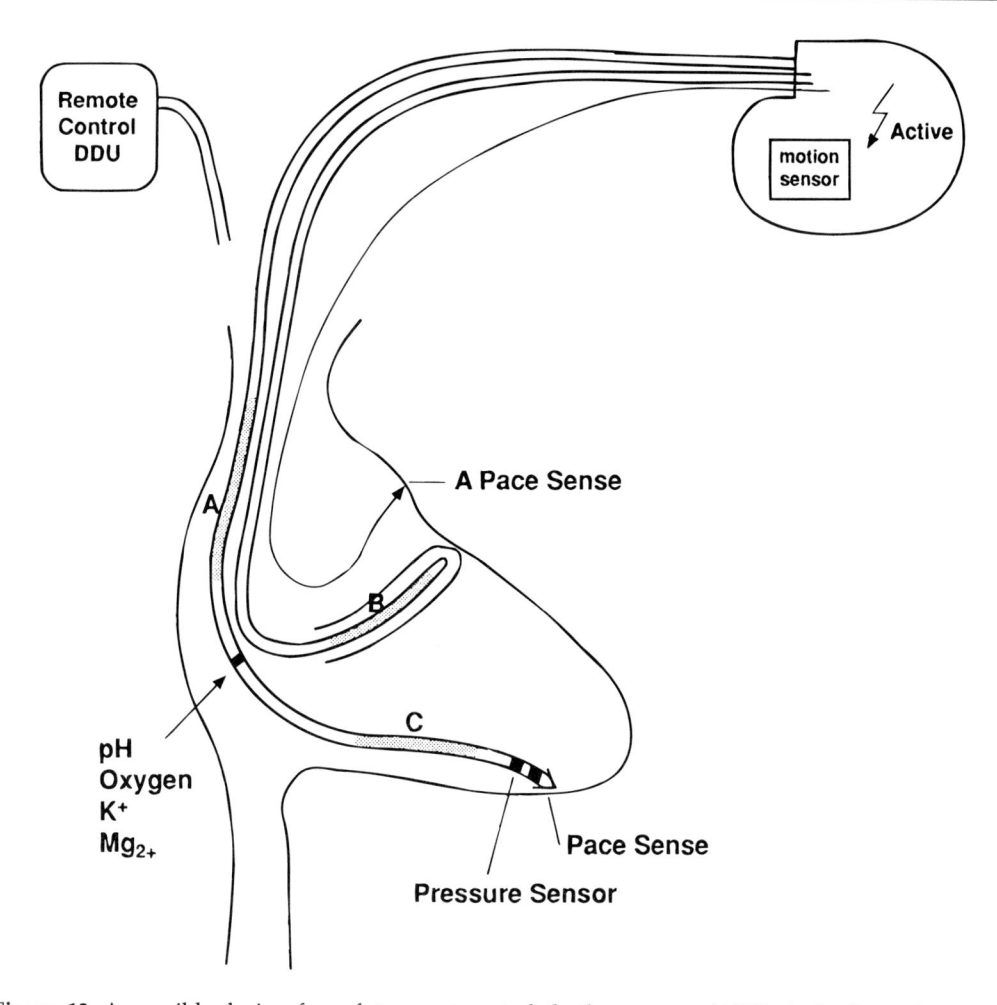

Figure 13. A possible design for a future automated rhythm system (ARS). Arrhythmia diagnosis would be achieved by a combination of ventricular and atrial sensing. Additional information on the hemodynamic impact of the arrhythmia would be obtained from the multifunctional ion electrode in the atrial body and/or from the motion sensor in the device Can. Atrial defibrillation could be achieved using electrodes A (in the atrium) and B (in the coronary sinus) while ventricular defibrillation could use a combination of electrodes A, B, and C with the addition of a far-field electrode in the form of the device Can if necessary to achieve satisfactory defibrillation thresholds. In addition to delivering defibrillation, cardioversion and antitachycardia pacing therapies, the device could trigger antiarrhythmic drug delivery via telemetry to a remotely sited drug delivery unit (DDU).

capable of diagnosis and treatment of atrial and ventricular tachyarrhythmias, arrhythmia suppression (with pacing or via drug delivery), and bradycardia support pacing. A possible design for such a device using three transvenous electrodes is shown in Figure 13.

The range of applications for such a device could be wide. In addition to the accepted indications for ICD therapy[97–99] and the indications proposed by the current series of controlled trials[100,101] the inclusion of arrhythmia suppression therapies might enable the prophylactic use of the device in place of antiarrhythmic drugs, with their potential proarrhythmic side effects.[102] In addition to its purely clinical applications such a device would be a tremendously effective research tool.

Atrial Automated Rhythm Systems

For patients with atrial and supraventricular arrhythmias a more limited device with atrial pacing and defibrillation capacity, but without a ventricular defibrillation electrode might be useful. The low-energy requirement identified in the preliminary studies of atrial defibrillation would enable this device to be a little bigger than a conventional pacemaker and implanted prepectorally.

Conclusions

The last 40 years have seen rapid developments in the concept of the ARS. Evolution from a fixed rate bradycardia support pacemaker to the third-generation implantable defibrillator has occurred in < 30 years. Conceptually there is now no cardiac arrhythmia that could not be treated by some form of implantable device although the realization of some of these concepts is in its earliest stages.

Despite the sophistication of currently available ARSs, there is potential for considerable improvement in all areas of their performance. Reductions in device size, improved reliability and ease of use of lead systems, and the addition of improved data logging are all required. The complexity of these devices already places a strain on the technical and personnel resources even of large electrophysiologic centers. If the use of these devices is to continue to increase they must become more "user friendly" both for the patient and the physician. This aim can best be realized by increasing automation of the functions of the device, paralleling developments in many other fields of technology where despite the increasing complexity of machines automation has been used to improve their simplicity of operation.

While the use of increasing automation could improve the performance of an ARS similar in concept to currently available implantable defibrillators, automation becomes critical in the development of ARS devices whose prime role is arrhythmia suppression rather than treatment. The recognition of arrhythmia precursors and the delivery of therapy to prevent arrhythmias requires the processing and analysis of data from chronic observation that can only be collected by the device itself, rendering the human programmer to a subsidiary monitoring role. It is perhaps in such arrhythmia suppression devices that the future of ARSs lie, as such devices would challenge the current role of antiarrhythmic drugs with their unpredictable side effects. The next decade is likely to see rapid development toward the realization of a true ARS.

References

1. Withering W: An account of the foxglove and some of its medical uses, with practical remarks on dropsy and other diseases. In: *Classics of Cardiology*. Edited by FA Willis, TE Keys. New York, NY: Henry Schuman Inc.; 1941, p. 231.
2. McWilliam JA: Electrical stimulation of the heart in man. *Br Med J* 1:348, 1889.
3. Elmqvist R, Senning A: An implantable pacemaker for the heart. *Proceedings of the Second International Conference on Medical Electronics*. Edited by CN Smyth. London, England: Iliffe; 1959, p. 253.
4. Goetz RH, Dormandy JA, Berkovits B: Pacing on demand in the treatment of atrioventricular conduction disturbances of the heart. *Lancet* 2:599, 1966.
5. Smyth NPD: Atrial programmed pacing. *PACE* 1:104, 1978.
6. Rickards AF, Norman J: Relation between QT interval and heart rate: new design of physiologically adaptive cardiac pacemaker. *Br Heart J* 45:56, 1981.
7. Baig MW, Boute W, Begemann M, et al: One-year follow-up of automatic adaption of the rate response algorithm of the QT sensing, rate adaptive pacemaker. *PACE* 14:1598, 1991.

8. Moe GK, Cohen W, Vick RL: Experimentally induced paroxysmal AV nodal tachycardia in the dog. Am Heart J 65:87, 1963.
9. Massumi RA, Kistin AD, Tawakkol AA: Termination of reciprocating tachycardia by atrial stimulation. Circulation 36:637, 1967.
10. Durrer D, Schoo L, Schuilenburg R, et al: The role of premature beats in the initiation and termination of supraventricular tachycardia in the Wolff-Parkinson-White syndrome. Circulation 336:644, 1967.
11. Haft JI, Kosowsky BD, Lau SH, et al: Termination of atrial flutter by rapid electrical pacing of the atrium. Am J Cardiol 20:239, 1967.
12. Jung W, Mietzko R, Manz M, et al: Long-term therapy of antitachycardia pacing for supraventricular tachycardia. PACE 15:179, 1992.
13. Griffith MJ, Bexton RS, McComb J: Financial audit of antitachycardia pacing for the control of recurrent supraventricular tachycardia. Br Heart J 69:250, 1993.
14. Holley LK, Cooper M, Uther JB, et al: Safety and efficacy of pacing for ventricular tachycardia. PACE 9:1316, 1986.
15. Zacouto F: French patent number. 1,237,702. 1953.
16. Mirowski M, Mower MM, Staewen WS, et al: Standby automatic defibrillator. An approach to the prevention of sudden coronary death. Arch Intern Med 126:158, 1970.
17. Schuder JC, Stoeckle H, Gold JH, et al: Experimental ventricular defibrillation with an automatic and completely implanted system. Trans Am Soc Artif Intern Organs 16:207, 1970.
18. Lown B, Axelrod P: Implanted standby defibrillators. Circulation 46:637, 1972.
19. Mirowski M, Reid PR, Mower MM, et al: Termination of malignant ventricular arrhythmias with an implanted automatic defibrillator in human beings. N Engl J Med 303:322, 1980.
20. Mirowski M, Reid PR, Winkle RA, et al: Mortality in patients with implanted automatic defibrillators. Ann Intern Med 98:585, 1983.
21. Reid PR, Mirowski M, Mower MM, et al: Clinical evaluation of the internal automatic cardioverter-defibrillator in survivors of sudden cardiac death. Am J Cardiol 51:1608, 1983.
22. Lin D, DiCarlo LA, Jenkins JM: Identification of ventricular tachycardia using intracavity ventricular electrograms: analysis of time and frequency domain patterns. PACE 11:1592, 1988.
23. Toivonen L, Viitasalo M, Järvinen A: The performance of the probability density function in differentiating supraventricular from ventricular rhythms. PACE 15:726, 1992.
24. Reid PR, Mirowski M, Mower M, et al: Clinical evaluation of the internal automatic cardioverter-defibrillator in survivors of sudden cardiac death. Am J Cardiol 51:1608, 1983.
25. Thurer RJ, Luceri RM, Bolooki H: Automatic implantable cardioverter-defibrillator: techniques of implantation and results. Ann Thorac Surg 42:143, 1986.
26. Lüderitz B, Manz M: Role of antitachycardia devices in the treatment of ventricular arrhythmias. Am J Cardiol 64:75J, 1989.
27. Almendral J, Arenal A, Villacastin JP, et al: The importance of antitachycardia pacing for patients presenting with ventricular tachycardia. PACE 16:535, 1993.
28. Nisam S, Mower M, Moser S: ICD clinical update: first decade, initial 10,000 patients. PACE 14:255, 1991.
29. Winkle RA, Mead RH, Ruder MA, et al: Long-term outcome with the automatic implantable cardioverter-defibrillator. J Am Coll Cardiol 13:1353, 1989.
30. Paul V, Bashir Y, Anderson M, et al: Antitachycardia pacing and antiarrhythmics combined: a recipe for misdiagnosis (abstract)? PACE 14:722, 1991.
31. Johnson NJ, Marchlinski FE: Arrhythmias induced by device antitachycardia therapy due to diagnostic nonspecificity. J Am Coll Cardiol 18:1418, 1991.
32. Fromer M, Brachman J, Block M, et al: Efficacy of automatic multimodal device therapy for ventricular tachyarrhythmias as delivered by a new implantable pacing cardioverter-defibrillator. Circulation 86:363, 1992.
33. Wietholt D, Block M, Isbruch F, et al: Clinical experience with antitachycardia pacing and improved detection algorithms in a new implantable cardioverter defibrillator. J Am Coll Cardiol 21:885, 1993.
34. Wang PJ, Manadalakas N, Clynce C, et al: Accuracy of rhythm classification using a data log system in implantable cardioverter defibrillators. PACE 14:1911, 1991.
35. Block M, Böcker D, Hammel D, et al: Should implantable cardioverter defibrillators store electrograms from sensing or defibrillation leads (abstract). PACE 16:858, 1993.
36. Callans DJ, Hook BG, Marchlinski FE: Use of bipolar recordings from patch-patch and rate sensing leads to distinguish ventricular tachycardia from supraventricular rhythms in patients with implantable cardioverter defibrillators. PACE 14:1917, 1991.
37. DiCarlo LA, Jenkins JM, Chih-ming C, et al:

Bipolar intraventricular electrogram analysis for ventricular tachycardia detection is site-specific (abstract). *Eur JCPE* 2:A109, 1992.
38. Marchlinski FE, Gottlieb CD, Sarter B, et al: ICD data storage: value in arrhythmia management. *PACE* 1 6:527, 1993.
39. Hammel D, Block M, Borggrefe M, et al: Implantation of a cardioverter/defibrillator in the subpectoral region combined with a nonthoracotomy lead system. *PACE* 15:367, 1992.
40. Troup PJ, Chapman PD, Olinger GN, et al: The implanted defibrillator: relation of defibrillation lead configuration and clinical variables to defibrillation threshold. *J Am Coll Cardiol* 6:1315, 1985.
41. Nisam S, Mower MM, Thomas A, et al: Patient survival comparison in three generations of automatic implantable cardioverter defibrillators: review of 12 years, 25,000 patients. *PACE* 16(1):174, 1993.
42. Oldershaw PJ, Sutton MG, Ward D, et al: Ten-year experience of 359 epicardial pacemaker systems: complications and results. *Clin Cardiol* 5:515, 1982.
43. Bakker PFA, Hauer RNW, Wever EFD: Infections involving implanted cardioverter defibrillator devices. *PACE* 15:654, 1992.
44. Lehmann MH, Mitchell LB, Saksena S, et al: Operative (30-day) mortality with transvenous vs. epicardial ICD implantation: an intention-to-treat analysis (abstract). *Circulation* 86:I-656, 1992.
45. Powers MT, Schwartzman D, Flores BT, et al: Lead-related morbidity in patients with ICDs utilizing non-thoracotomy lead systems (abstract). *PACE* 16:951, 1993.
46. Saksena S, Sakun V, Mitchell B, et al: Complications of third-generation defibrillators using endocardial or epicardial leads: a multicenter study (abstract). *J Am Coll Cardiol* 21:170A, 1993.
47. Goodman GR, Frumin H, Pleatman MA: Implantation of automatic cardioverter defibrillator using thorascopic techniques (abstract). *Eur JCPE* 2:A108, 1992.
48. Kindwall KE, Brown J, Josephson ME: Electrocardiographic criteria for ventricular tachycardia in wide complex left bundle branch block morphology tachycardias. *Am J Cardiol* 61:1279, 1988.
49. Tooley MA, Davies DW, Nathan AW, et al: Recognition of multiple tachyarrhythmias by rate-independent means using a small microcomputer. *PACE* 14:337, 1991.
50. Paul VE, O'Nunain S, Malik M, et al: Temporal electrogram analysis: algorithm development. *PACE* 13:1943, 1990.
51. Paul VE, Bashir Y, Malik M, et al: Variability of the intracardiac electrogram: effect on specificity of tachycardia detection. *PACE* 13:1925, 1991.
52. Greenhut S, Deering TF, Steinhaus B, et al: Separation of ventricular tachycardia from sinus rhythm using a practical real-time template matching system (abstract). *Eur JCPE* 2:A108, 1992.
53. Steinhaus BM, Wells RT, Greenhut SE, et al: Detection of ventricular tachycardia using scanning correlation analysis. *PACE* 13; 1920, 1990.
54. Farugia S, Yee H, Nickolls P: Neural network classification of intracardiac electrograms (abstract). *Eur JCPE* 2:A109, 1992.
55. Parsonnet V, Hesselson AB, Harari DC: Long-term functional integrity of atrial leads. *PACE* 14:517, 1991.
56. Schuger CD, Jackson K, Steinman RT, et al: Atrial sensing to augment ventricular tachycardia detection by the automatic implantable cardioverter defibrillator: a utility study. *PACE* 11:1456, 1988.
57. Jenkins JM, Chiang CJ, DiCarlo LA, et al: Real-time arrhythmia identification from automated analysis of intra-atrial and intra-ventricular electrograms (abstract). *Eur JCPE* 2:A110, 1992.
58. Stability of the atrioventricular relationship during sustained ventricular tachycardias: a clue for an automatic atrial arrhythmias recognition algorithm (abstract). *Circulation* 86:I-58, 1992.
59. Crick JC: European multicenter prospective follow-up study of 1,002 implants of a single lead VDD pacing system. The European multicenter study group. *PACE* 14:1642, 1991.
60. Gross JN, Andrews C, Uri M, et al: VDD pacing: chronic efficacy, incidence of atrial fibrillation and evolution of sinoatrial dysfunction (abstract). *PACE* 16:881, 1993.
61. Erickson MK, Bennet TD, Sharma AD, et al: Detection of hemodynamically stable and unstable VT using right ventricular pressure area (abstract). *PACE* 15:531, 1992.
62. Kapadia KA, Wood MA, Lu B, et al: A prospective study of changes in right ventricular dP/dt during ventricular tachycardia. *PACE* 14:1098, 1991.
63. Kaye GC, Astridge P, Perrins J: Tachycardia recognition and diagnosis from changes in right atrial pressure waveform—a feasibility study. *PACE* 14:1384, 1991.
64. Beauregard LM, Volosin KJ, Waxman HL: Differentiation of arrhythmias by measurement of intracardiac pressures in man. *PACE* 14:161, 1991.
65. Cohen TJ, Bing Liem L: A hemodynamically responsive antitachycardia system. *Circulation* 82:394, 1990.

66. Aubert AE, Denys BG, Ector H, et al: Detection of ventricular tachycardia and fibrillation using ECG processing and intramyocardial pressure gradients. *PACE* 9:1084, 1986.
67. Cohen TJ, Bing Liem L: Mixed venous oxygen saturation for differentiating stable from unstable tachycardias. *Am Heart J* 122:733, 1991.
68. Tyers GF: Current status of sensor-modulated rate-adaptive cardiac pacing. *J Am Coll Cardiol* 15:412, 1990.
69. Cooper RAS, Alferness CA, Smith WM, et al: Internal cardioversion of atrial fibrillation in sheep. *Circulation* 87:1673, 1993.
70. Weidmann S: Effect of current flow in the membrane potential of cardiac muscle. *J Physiol* 115:227, 1951.
71. Ruffy R, Friday KJ, Southworth WF: Termination of ventricular tachycardia by single extrastimulation during the ventricular effective refractory period. *Circulation* 67:457, 1983.
72. Shenasa M, Cardinal R, Kus T, et al: Termination of sustained ventricular tachycardia by ultrarapid subthreshold stimulation in humans. *Circulation* 78:1135, 1988.
73. Termination of sustained ventricular tachycardia by subthreshold electrical stimulation via epicardial patch electrodes (abstract). *Circulation* 84:II-427, 1991.
74. Avitall B, Hare J, Lessila C, et al: Implantable epicardial drug delivery system. *Circulation* 84:125, 1991.
75. Zoll PM, Linenthal AJ, Zarsky LRN: Ventricular fibrillation. Treatment and prevention by external electric currents. *N Engl J Med* 262:105, 1960.
76. Sowton E, Leatham A, Carson P: The suppression of arrhythmias by artificial pacemaking. *Lancet* 2:1098, 1964.
77. Sutton RS, Kenny RA: The natural history of sick sinus syndrome. *PACE* 9:1110, 1986.
78. Coumel P: Modifications of heart rate variability preceding the onset of tachyarrhythmias. *Cardiologica* 35(Suppl 1):7, 1990.
79. Leclercq JF, Maisonblanche P, Cauchemez B, et al: Respective role of sympathetic tone and of cardiac pauses in the genesis of 62 cases of ventricular fibrillation recorded during Holter monitoring. *Eur Heart J* 9:1276, 1988.
80. The role of silent ischemia, the arrhythmic substrate and the short-long sequence in the genesis of sudden cardiac death. *J Am Coll Cardiol* 14:1618, 1989.
81. Verrier RL, Lown B: Prevention of ventricular fibrillation by use of low-intensity electrical stimuli. *Ann NY Acad Sci* 382:355, 1982.
82. Wold M, Seroppian E, Lown B, et al: Protective zone for ventricular fibrillation (abstract). *Am J Cardiol* 29:298, 1972.
83. Franz MR, Burkhoff D, Yue DT, et al: Mechanically induced action potential changes and arrhythmias in isolated and in situ canine hearts. *Cardiovasc Res* 23:213, 1989.
84. Cohn JN, Vheft II study group: A comparison of enalapril with hydralazine-isosorbide dinitrate in the treatment of chronic congestive heart failure. *N Engl J Med* 325:293, 1991.
85. Pye MP, Cobbe SM: Mechanisms of ventricular arrhythmias in cardiac failure and hypertrophy. *Cardiovasc Res* 26:740, 1992.
86. Schwartz SL, Gillam LD, Weintraub AR, et al: Intracardiac echocardiography in humans using a small-sized (6F) low frequency (12.5MHz) ultrasound catheter. *J Am Coll Cardiol* 21:189, 1993.
87. Mueller J, Warnecke H, Grauhan O, et al: An implantable wall motion sensor for rejection monitoring after heart transplantation (abstract). *PACE* 16:895, 1993.
88. DeRossi D, Benassi A, L'Abbate A, et al: A new fiber-optic liquid crystal catheter for oxygen saturation and blood flow measurements in the coronary sinus. *J Biomed Eng* 2:257, 1980.
89. Altura BT, Shirey TL, Young CC, et al: A new method for the rapid determination of ionized Mg^{2+} in whole blood, serum and plasma. *Methods Find Exp Clin Pharmacol* 14:297, 1992.
90. Leitch JW, Klein GJ, Yee R, et al: Feasibility of an implantable arrhythmia monitor (abstract). *PACE* 14:677, 1991.
91. Anderson MH, Paul VE, Jones S, et al: Transtelephonic interrogation of the implantable cardioverter defibrillator. *PACE* 15:1144, 1992.
92. Feldman C, Olson W, Hubelbank M, et al: Improved follow-up of tiered therapy implantable defibrillators with continuous telemetry to a new Holter system (abstract). *PACE* 16:929, 1993.
93. Rist K, Kroll M, Mowrey K, et al: Comparison of epicardial defibrillation energy requirement using 140 and 85 microfarad capacitors (abstract). *PACE* 16:914, 1993.
94. Fain ES, Sweeney MB, Franz MR: Improved internal defibrillation efficacy with a biphasic waveform. *Am Heart J* 117:358, 1989.
95. Block M and the European P2 investigators: Combination of endocardial leads with a new ICD capable of biphasic shocks—first results of a multicenter study (abstract). *PACE* 16:874, 1993.
96. Bardy GH, Johnson G, Poole JE, et al: A sim-

plified single lead unipolar transvenous cardioverter defibrillator (abstract). *Circulation* 86:I-792, 1992.
97. Lehman MH, Saksena S: Implantable cardioverter defibrillators in cardiovascular practice: report of the policy conference of the North American Society of Pacing and Electrophysiology. *PACE* 14:969, 1991.
98. Task Force of the Working Groups on Cardiac Arrhythmias and Cardiac Pacing of the European Society of Cardiology: Guidelines for the use of implantable cardioverter defibrillators. *Eur Heart J* 13:1304, 1992.
99. Dreifus LS, Gillette PC, Fisch C, et al: Guidelines for implantation of cardiac pacemakers and antiarrhythmia devices. *J Am Coll Cardiol* 18:1, 1991.
100. Bigger JT: Future studies with the implantable cardioverter-defibrillator. *PACE* 14:883, 1991.
101. Nisam S, Thomas A, Mower M, et al: Identifying patients for prophylactic implantable cardioverter defibrillator therapy: status of prospective studies. *Am Heart J* 122:607, 1991.
102. The Cardiac Arrhythmia Suppression Trial (CAST) Investigators: Preliminary report: effect of encainide and flecainide on mortality in a randomized trial of arrhythmia suppression after myocardial infarction. *N Engl J Med* 321:406, 1989.

Chapter 34

Dual-Chamber Defibrillator: From Theoretical Concepts to Implementation

Tibor Nappholz

Introduction

Today, implantable cardioverter-defibrillators (ICDs) are an established part of therapy for ventricular tachyarrhythmias. They do, however, have shortcomings, some of which are discussed further in Chapter 36. This chapter addresses some of these deficiencies, and suggests possible solutions using conventional state-of-the art pacing concepts. These concepts are concentrated in the area of sensing, defibrillation, and pacing. Sensors will only be addressed to the extent that they are absolutely essential and are in use in present day dual chamber devices. It should be understood at the outset that a viable DDD based ICD is not yet commercially available and none are in clinical evaluation at the time of this writing. It is hoped that this, perhaps premature discussion, will highlight some of the key relevant considerations for development of such devices in the future.

Benefits of DDD Pacing for Implantable Cardioverter-Defibrillators

The ICD was introduced to clinical practice to treat lethal ventricular arrhythmias and it accomplished this task extremely well.[1] However, the cardiovascular system is not a bistable system, perfectly healthy one minute and in a state of life-threatening arrhythmia the next. Although some patients, especially those with long QT syndrome, may fit this model, they remain in the minority. The majority of patients suffer from a variety of cardiac pathologies that involve the atria and the ventricles. Diverse pathologies may give rise to a variety of conduction and hemodynamic abnormalities and may precipitate lethal arrhythmias that must be controlled by the ICD. These abnormalities in many cases require conventional bradycardia therapy for atrioventricular (AV) block, sinus node disease, sinus bradycardia, and so on.

If the patient requires conventional bradycardia therapy in addition to the tachyarrhythmia control, then it is reasonable to assume that the most effective therapy, in the presence of sinus rhythm, would be an ICD with DDD pacing capabilities. The currently available ICDs are capable of VVI pacing. However, they have limited therapy options and are limited in the amount and type of electrical information that they can gather in order to make the crucial decisions required for the sophisticated multitiered therapy devices. The enhancements that are

From Singer I, (ed.) Implantable Cardioverter-Defibrillator. Armonk, NY: Futura Publishing Company, Inc.; © 1994.

possible with an ICD device backed up by dual-chamber functionality are examined. In this discussion only nonthoracotomy lead (NTL) implants will be considered because there is sufficient evidence to indicate that NTL systems will be used almost exclusively in the future with few exceptions.

Electrical activation sequence ensures optimal function of the heart as a pump. In the case of manifest pathology the pump action may be disturbed in one of several ways: 1) loss of AV synchrony due to AV block, abnormal sinus automaticity resulting in pathological sinus bradycardia or conduction disturbances including bundle branch block, requiring atrial and ventricular pacing; 2) valvular pathologies resulting in a systolic gradient, hypertrophy, and secondary valvular regurgitation; and 3) cardiomyopathy or ischemia leading to contraction abnormalities and impaired left ventricular (LV) relaxation.

Atrioventricular Block, Sinus Bradycardia, and Conduction Disturbances

The benefits of AV synchrony have been extensively discussed.[2-5] Unfortunately, the benefits of "correct" AV delay are still much in question, with some investigators showing a clear benefit to optimizing AV delay to patients' needs,[6,7] and others showing that the precise value is irrelevant.[8,9] The picture becomes even more confusing when it is realized that the correct activation sequence of the left ventricle plays an important role in the optimization of cardiac output.[10-12] This is best summarized in Figure 1, where the penalty of inappropriate sequencing of activation in a group of 12 patients with intact AV delays and without ventricular impairment, is demonstrated. In fact, the gain derived from optimization of the AV delay could, to a certain extent, be counterbalanced by the incorrect activation sequencing due to ventricular pacing at the end of the AV delay. Even patients with left bundle branch block derive benefit from long AV delays that per-

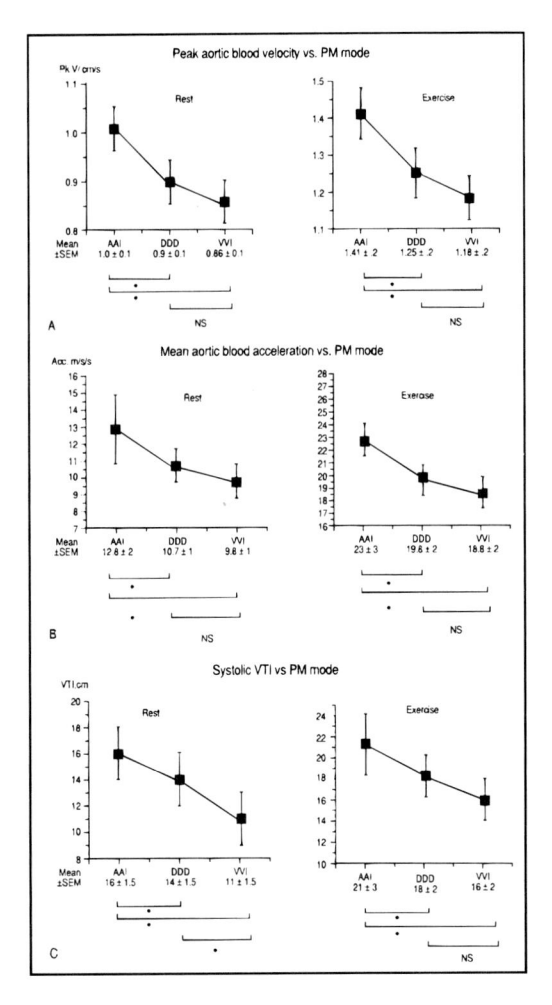

Figure 1. Hemodynamic changes versus pacing mode during rest and exercise evaluated by Doppler echocardiography. **A**: peak aortic blood velocity (PKV, cm/s); **B**: mean aortic blood acceleration (Acc. m/ss); **C**: systolic ventricular time integral (VTI, cm). *$P < 0.05$; AAI: atrial demand pacing; DDD: sequential atrioventricular sensing pacing; NS: not significant; PM: pacing mode; SEM: standard error of the mean; VVI: ventricular demand pacing. (Reproduced with permission from Reference 10.)

mit a more normal conduction.[10] These observations suggest that pacing electrodes should be placed high on the septal wall whenever possible to allow pacing to mimic normal conduction sequence.[12] However, a recent study of 19 patients with congestive heart failure contradicted these concepts and suggested that neither exact AV delay nor correct activation sequence were relevant for optimizing cardiac output.[13] Thus, the controversy regarding AV delay and sequence of activation are still unresolved.

In spite of these conflicting results, AV synchrony results in improved contractility, decreased relaxation time, minimization of cannon waves, and decreased tendency to develop atrial fibrillation.[14-17] During exercise, the presence of an adaptive AV delay may also improve cardiac output.[18] Furthermore, it is now recognized that patients with sinus bradycardia may also benefit from DDDR pacing, where an artificial sensor controls the rate adaptation.[19] This is particularly true for patients with impaired ventricular function where an increase in the contractile reserve is not readily available, hence cardiac output can only be augmented by increasing the paced heart rate during exercise (Figure 2). This particular need for higher paced rates is effectively met by a minute volume ventilation device, since patients with heart failure also happen to have a more rapid increase in minute volume ventilation in response to increased metabolic demand (Figure 3).

Valvular Pathologies and Ischemia

Hypertrophic cardiomyopathy may be due to longstanding systemic hypertension or result from anatomical abnormalities that may cause impedance to blood flow in systole. Patients with hypertropic cardiomyopathy frequently die suddenly. While the

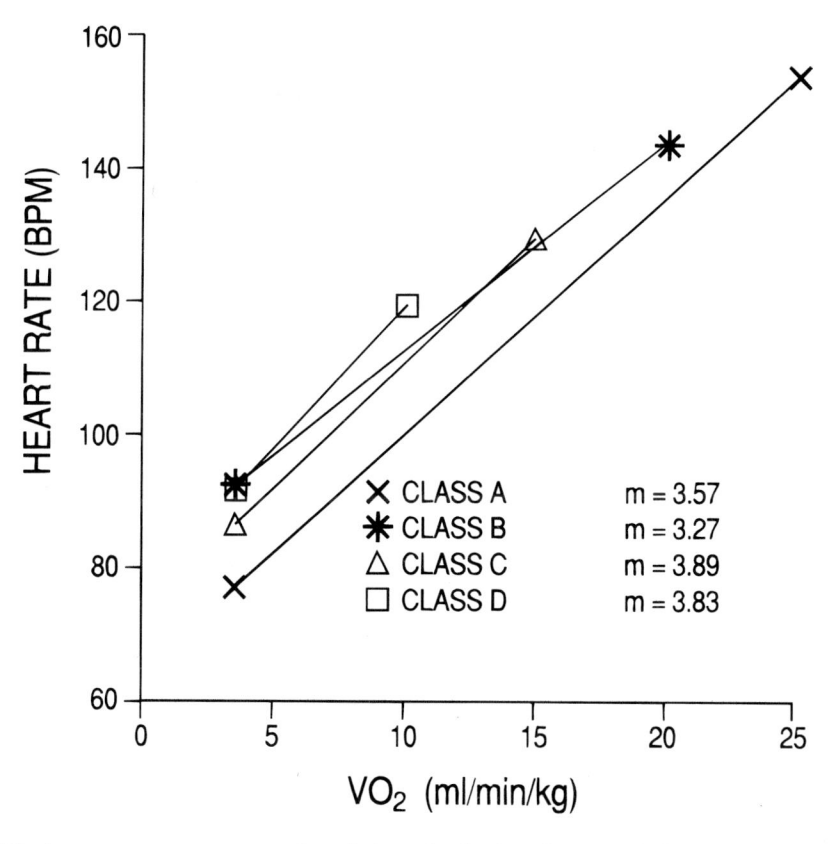

Figure 2. The heart rate to oxygen uptake relations for the four functional classes and their respective slopes (beats per minute per milliliter per minute per kilogram). See text for discussion. (Reproduced with permission from Weber KT: *Cardiopulmonary Exercise Testing*. Philadelphia, PA: W.B. Saunders; 1986.)

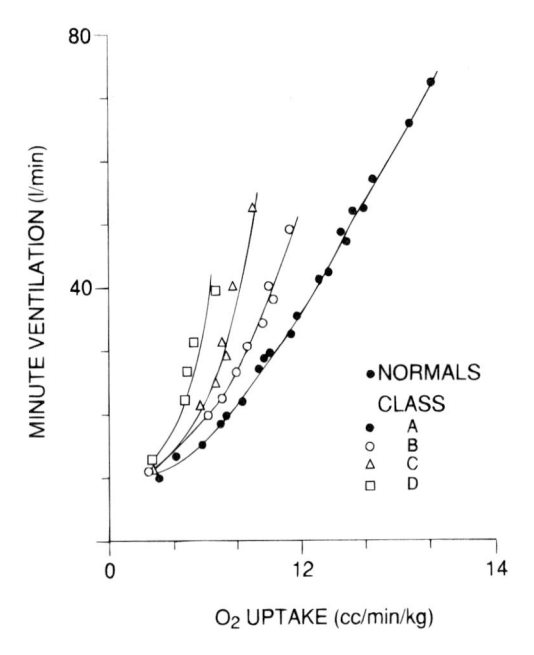

Figure 3. Relationship between oxygen uptake (cc per minute per kilogram) and minute ventilation, demonstrating minute ventilation response during exercise of various functional class patients. (Reproduced with permission from Weber KT: *Cardiopulmonary Exercise Testing*. Philadelphia, PA: W.B. Saunders; 1986.)

mechanisms ultimately culminating in sudden cardiac death are poorly understood, it is currently theorized that the predominant mechanism is "electrical."[20] About 25% of patients with hypertrophic cardiomyopathy also have dynamic obstruction of the LV outflow tract.[21]

In hypertrophic obstructive cardiomyopathy (HOCM) paradoxical motion of the right ventricular (RV) septum is exploited to enhance the flow through a partially blocked LV outflow tract. The reason for this seeming contradiction is illustrated in Figure 4. Due to congenital abnormality or one that is induced pathologically, the mitral valve is sufficiently deformed to allow it to be pulled up against the LV septum by the blood flow through the aortic valve. This force is due to the Venturi effect, enhanced by the constriction between the valve and the septum.[22] The outward motion of the LV septum at the later stage of the contraction cycle allows for the systolic gradient across the aortic valve to decrease, which results in greater blood flow into the aorta and less mitral regurgitation. Atrioventricular delay is a critical factor in determining the degree of mitral regurgitation. This relationship is shown in Figure 5. Advantages accrued due to AV pacing in patients with HOCM are maintained over time as shown in Figure 6, and in fact may lead to a decrease in the severity of hypertrophy.[23]

In patients with dilated cardiomyopathy (DCM) the advantages of DDD pacing with intact AV conduction are equivocal at best.[13] This is because disadvantages of incorrect activation sequence can negate any potential advantage of fine tuning the AV delay. There is little concrete data on what exactly happens to the valvular regurgitation as the AV delay is adjusted.

It has been documented that preexcitation can lead to a decrease in the level of regurgitation with an increase in the stroke index. In one particular study this was achieved in 5 of 8 patients.[24] Minimization of regurgitation does not necessarily lead to improved cardiac output, however, since it is accompanied by a decrease in the stroke index. Since pressure differential between the ventricle and the atrium determines the timing and the rate of closure of the mitral valve, with lower pressures in the atrium the magnitude of regurgitation can increase if the mitral valve cannot close effectively. If the valve can close, lower pressure results in the atrium during ventricular systole. This means that in some cases shorter AV delay is also desirable. The complexity of these relationships is further confounded by the observation that longer AV delays lead to higher diastolic volumes and hence a decrease in myocardial reserve. There is a consensus that with poor inelastic ventricles, often there is a need for an atrial "kick" that may be lost due to poor relaxation. In fact, patients with diastolic dysfunction and prolonged isovolumic relaxation show the greatest improvement when AV delay is optimized.[6]

Patients with distended atria often have excessive delays in the atrial conduc-

![Obstructive HCM and Cavity Obliteration diagrams]

OBSTRUCTIVE HCM   **CAVITY OBLITERATION**

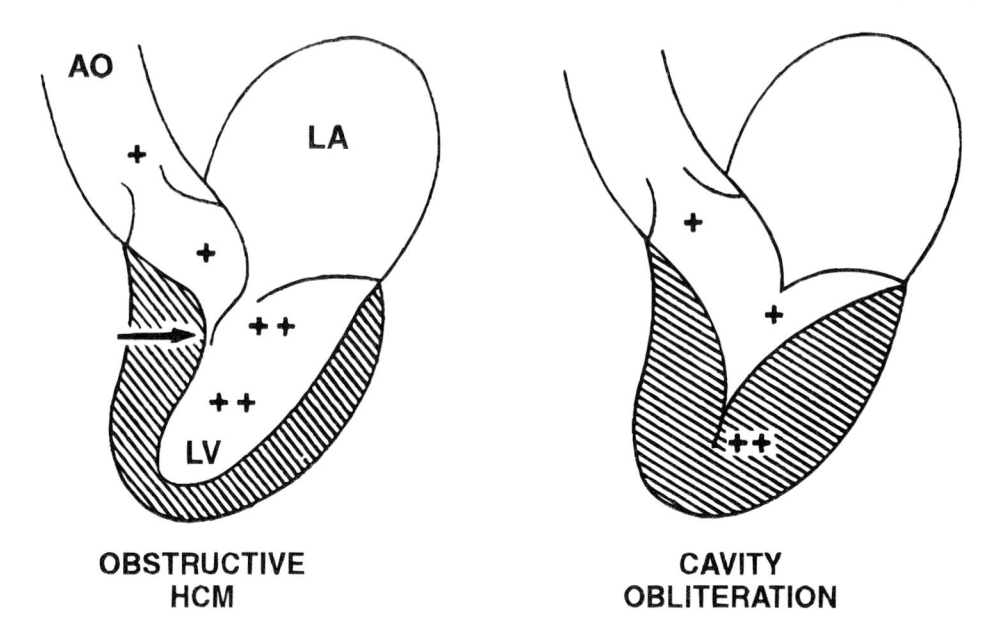

Figure 4. The left ventricular (LV) inflow tract pressure concept. **Left:** In obstructive hypertrophic cardiomyopathy (OHCM), because the obstruction to LV outflow (arrow) is caused by anterior mitral leaflet-ventricular septal contact, the intraventricular pressure distal to the stenosis (and proximal to the aortic valve) is low (+), whereas all ventricular pressures proximal to the stenosis, including the one just inside the mitral valve (the inflow tract pressure), are elevated (++). **Right:** When an intraventricular pressure difference is recorded because of catheter entrapment by the myocardium in an area of cavity obliteration, the elevated ventricular pressure is recorded only in the area of cavity obliteration (++). The intraventricular systolic pressure in all other areas of the LV cavity, including that in the inflow tract just inside the mitral valve, is low (+) and equal to the aortic systolic pressure. Thus the inflow tract pressure is elevated in obstructive HCM but not in cavity obliteration. There are now more than 20 characteristic differences between these two types of intraventricular pressure difference. The three areas of the left ventricle represented by the + signs in each of these diagrams are, from above downward, the outflow tract just below the aortic valve (subaortic region), the inflow tract just inside the mitral valve, and the left ventricular apex. AO: aorta; LA: left atrium. (Reproduced with permission from Reference 22.)

tion times. Maximum AV delay should be allowed after atrial pacing to optimize diastolic ventricular filling for such patients.

From the above discussion then, the advantages of DDD pacing can be identified for patients with AV conduction disorders and especially those with impaired ventricular function. In addition, definite advantages can be obtained in HOCM and in certain patients with DCM and diastolic dysfunction even when their AV conduction is intact. In patients with chronotropic incompetence adaptive pacing may also be beneficial, particularly for patients who suffer from concomitant heart failure with decrease in ventricular contractility. In conclusion, certain percentage of recipients of implanted defibrillators would benefit from DDDR pacing devices. At the present time about 10% of the implants are for patients who also need pacing. In addition, a certain number of patients with HOCM and DCM may also benefit from DDDR pacing. Additional patients may benefit from rate adaptive pacing particularly patients with chronotropic incompetence and sinus node dysfunction.

DDD Pacing for Rhythm Classification

Before discussing signal detection for DDD-based ICDs, a review of some of the

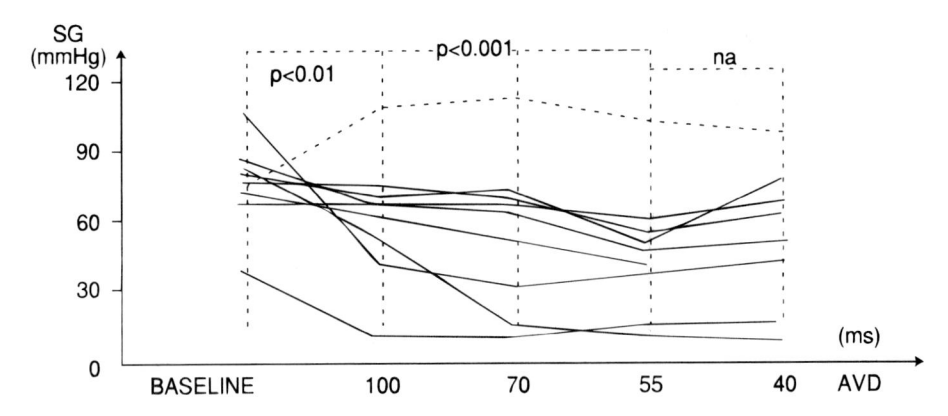

Figure 5. In patients with drug resistant obstructive hypertrophic cardiomyopathy (OHCM), temporary dual-chamber pacing, with measurement of systolic gradient at various sensed atrioventricular (AV) delays, selects patients who will benefit from a pacemaker implantation. (Reproduced with permission from Sadoul N, Simon J-P, De Chillou C, et al: Usefulness of temporary dual chamber pacing to determine indications in patients with drug resistant hypertrophic cardiomyopathy. *PACE* 16:1120, 1993.)

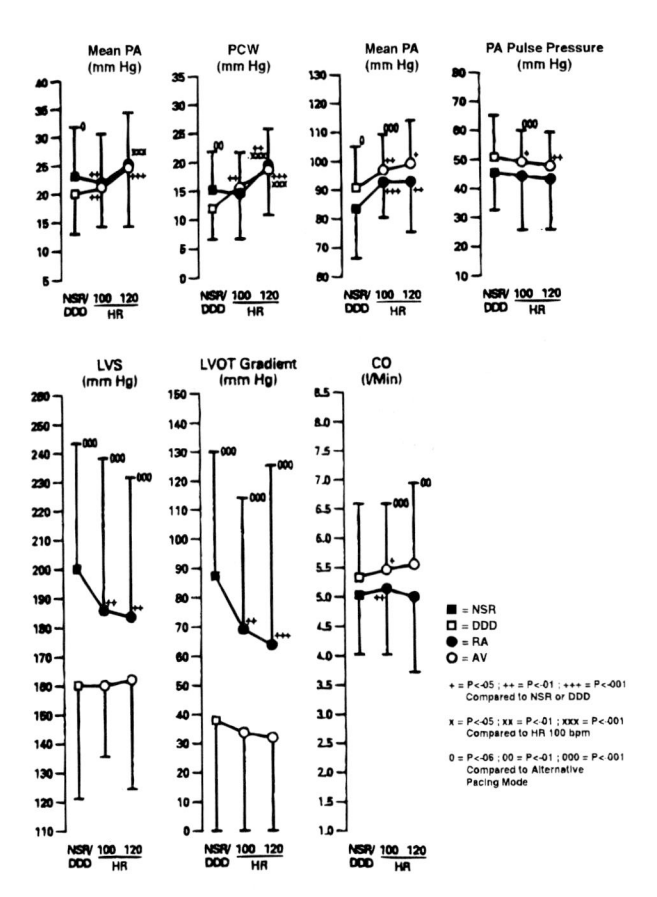

Figure 6. Graphs show comparison of hemodynamic indexes recorded during the baseline study (closed circles and squares) with hemodynamic indexes recorded during the follow-up evaluation (open circles and squares). PA: pulmonary artery; PCW: pulmonary arterial capillary wedge pressure; LVS: left ventricular systolic pressure; LVOT: left ventricular outflow tract; CO: cardiac output; NSR: normal sinus rhythm; RA: right arterial pacing; HR: 100 and 120 paced heart rates (bpm: beats per minute). Mean sinus rate at the baseline study was 79 ± 17 beats per minute; mean sinus rate at the follow-up evaluation was 79 ± 12 beats per minute. (Reproduced with permission from Reference 23.)

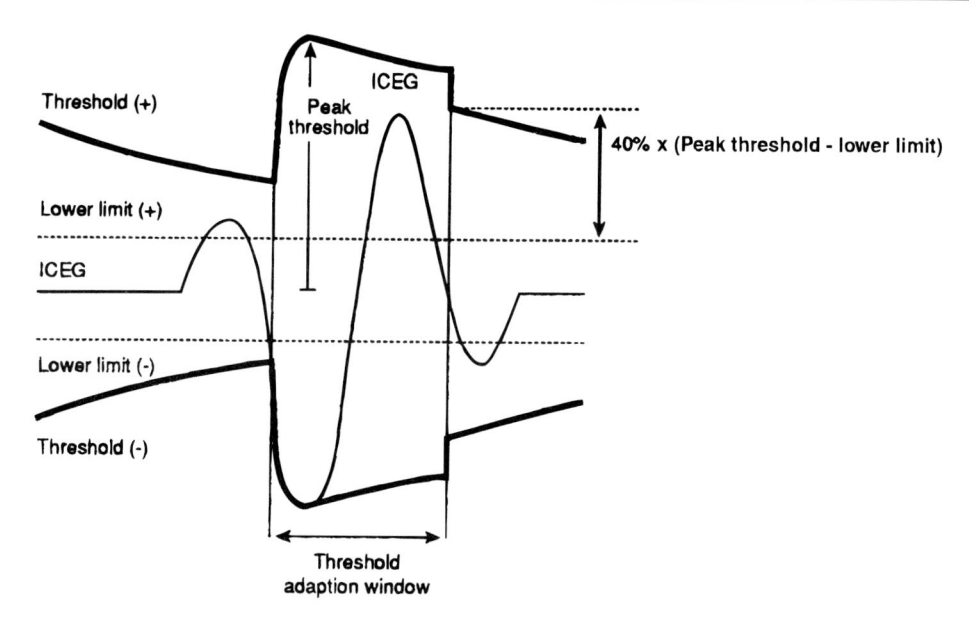

Figure 7. Automatic gain in a present day defibrillator. Threshold is referenced to peak amplitude (positive or negative) and declines through cycle to no less than a preset minimum.

basic approaches used in the present day single-chamber devices is suggested. Currently, sensing is standardized to automatic gain adjustment after filtering. Signals are then counted and checked for rate and suddenness of onset. These concepts are illustrated in Figure 7 and 8. We can see that the automatic gain is adjusted by the signal size and that a gradual decay in threshold is used to eliminate oversensing of extraneous signals, particularly T waves. To meet the rate criteria, an X-of-Y detection, eg, 12 events out of 14, have to be above the programmed rate. For reconfirmation, this criterion will usually change to a lesser number, eg, 6 out of 10 sensed events. The onset

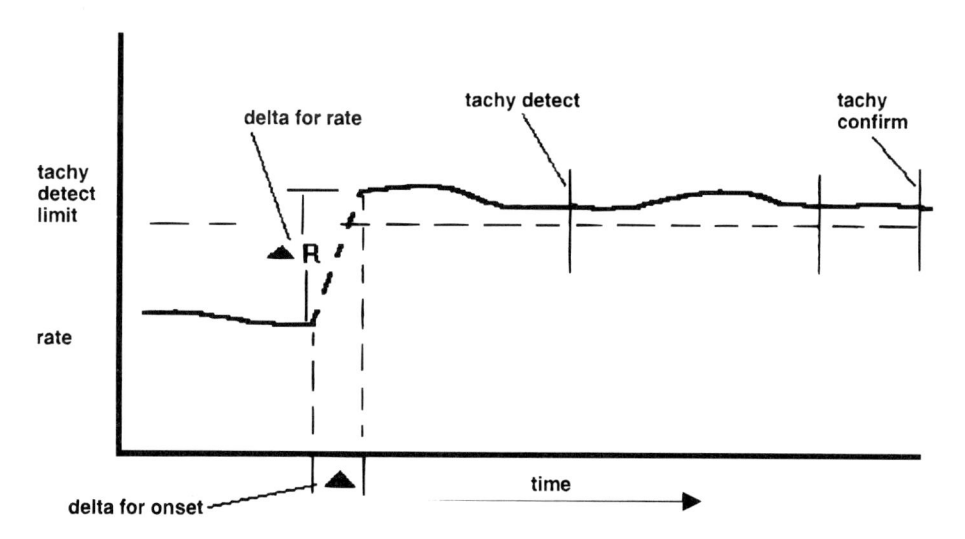

Figure 8. The standard detection routines of present day defibrillators operating from rate alone.

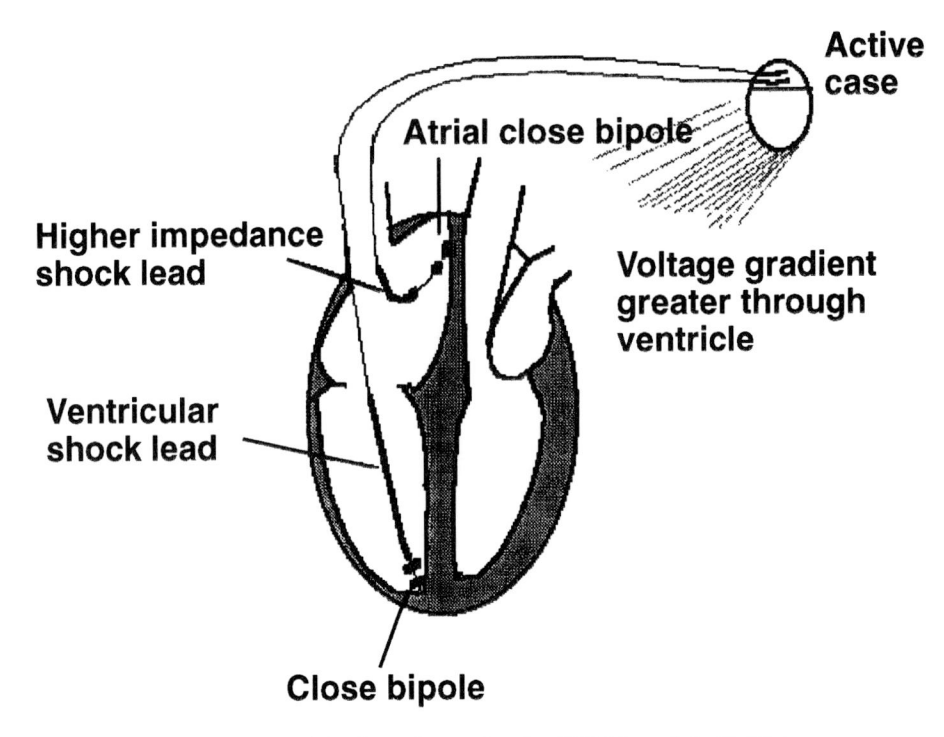

Figure 9. Special lead configuration for DDD based defibrillator.

detection criteria are met when there is greater than a specified decrease in intervals between two sequential sensed events. For each device there are some variations to the above theme, but the concepts are, at the present time, more or less standardized (Figure 9).

The ability of an ICD to deliver correct therapy depends on the correct diagnosis. Third-generation ICDs still misdiagnose supraventricular arrhythmias,[25] with a potential danger of delivering therapy to the ventricle, when in fact the arrhythmia is located in the atrium.

Table 1 summarizes therapies that may be available with a DDD device. "Shock" refers to the conventional high-voltage shock in the present day defibrillator. The shock "U-CON" designates a hypothetical option for the future NTL devices. The design of the defibrillator lead would be such as to allow termination of either atrial or

Table 1
Relationship Between Arrhythmia Type and Therapy

Rhythm/Therapy	VF	VT	Sinus Tachy	A. FIB	A. FLUT	SVT
Shock	X	X				
C'Vert		X				
V PACE		X				X
A PACE					X	X
Shock (U-CON)	X	X		X	X	X

VF: Ventricular fibrillation; VT: ventricular tachycardia; A. FIB: atrial fibrillation; A. FLUT: atrial flutter; SVT: supraventricular tachycardia; C'VERT: cardioversion; A: atrial; V: ventricular.

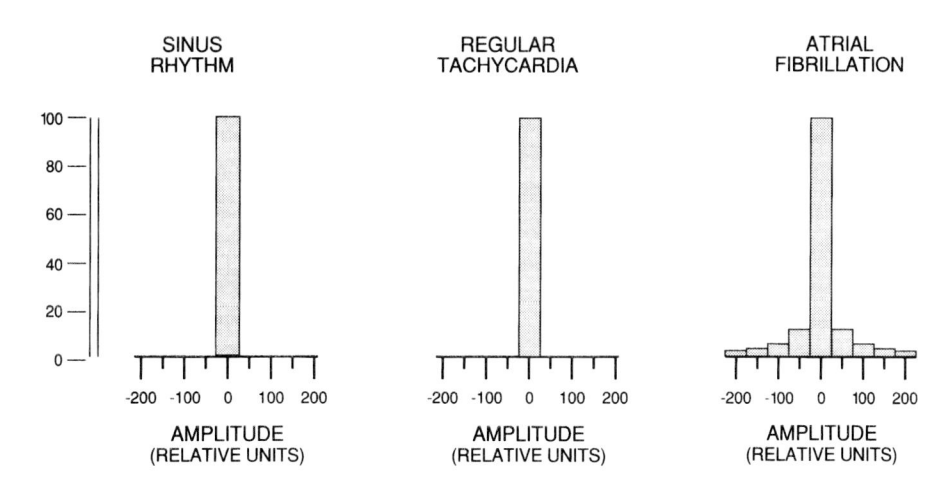

Figure 10. Amplitude probability density function generation. Shown are three examples of amplitude probability density functions from the filtered data segments. Note that the amplitude probability density function for sinus rhythm and regular tachycardia have a large peak around an amplitude of zero while the function for atrial fibrillation is spread out over a wider range of amplitudes. (Reproduced with permission from Reference 27.)

ventricular arrhythmias. A proposed configuration is shown in Figure 10. This design supposes that the component of the lead in the atrium has a higher impedance, so that it generates a lower voltage gradient in the atrium and does not "steal" the current from the ventricle. Nevertheless, it provides enough voltage gradient to terminate an atrial arrhythmia.

Although the U-CON configuration could be effective for termination of atrial or ventricular tachyarrhythmias, pacing is still preferred for arrhythmia termination wherever possible. Pacing termination of reentrant ventricular tachyardias (VTs) and supraventricular tachycardias (SVTs) is a proven therapy with high (> 90%) success rate, and virtually no discomfort to the patient. But what the U-CON can provide is a "safety net" approach to ensure that when an error in the classification is made, it would not result in repeated shocks.

Rhythm Classifier

To allow proper classification of arrhythmias identified in Table 1 we should define the parameters (ie, characteristics) that can be used for the rhythm classification. Currently, tachycardia rate is the most frequently used criterion for the clinically available ICDs.

Table 2 lists the rates (left column) used for rhythm classification. Detection of rate alone is successful for ventricular fibrillation (VF) detection. However, it lacks specificity. Hence, atrial fibrillation and other SVTs may be misclassified as VT or VF. With a DDD system atrial fibrillation may be diagnosed correctly. From previous studies[26,27] we know that the amplitude variability during atrial fibrillation is greater than that recorded during sinus rhythm (Figure 11). This is intuitively correct, except with fine atrial fibrillation. Signal amplitudes, particularly when filtered in the region of 6–36 Hz, can separate atrial fibrillation from sinus rhythm. Figure 11 summarizes the data from an animal study where atrial electrograms were recorded from chronically implanted electrodes.[20] Amplitudes of signals were unfiltered. When signals were filtered in the bandwidth mentioned, the separation was optimal. Peak amplitudes were chosen for the separation of the rhythms because peak amplitude measurements are easiest to obtain

Table 2
Arrhythmia Parameters Used for Classification

Rhythm/Rates	VF	VT	Sinus Rhythm	A. FIB	A. FLUT	SVT
220-Age (AFA)	No	Yes*	Yes*	Yes*	Yes*	Yes*
ARFA-240	No	Yes*	No	Yes*	Yes*	Yes*
>240	Yes	No	No	Yes*	No	No

ARFA: appropriate rate for age, this is conventionally (220-age) beats per minute.
* denotes possibilities for misdiagnosis by presently available ICDs.
VF: ventricular fibrillation; VT: ventricular tachycardia; A. FIB: atrial fibrillation; A. FLUT: atrial flutter; SVT: supraventricular tachycardia.

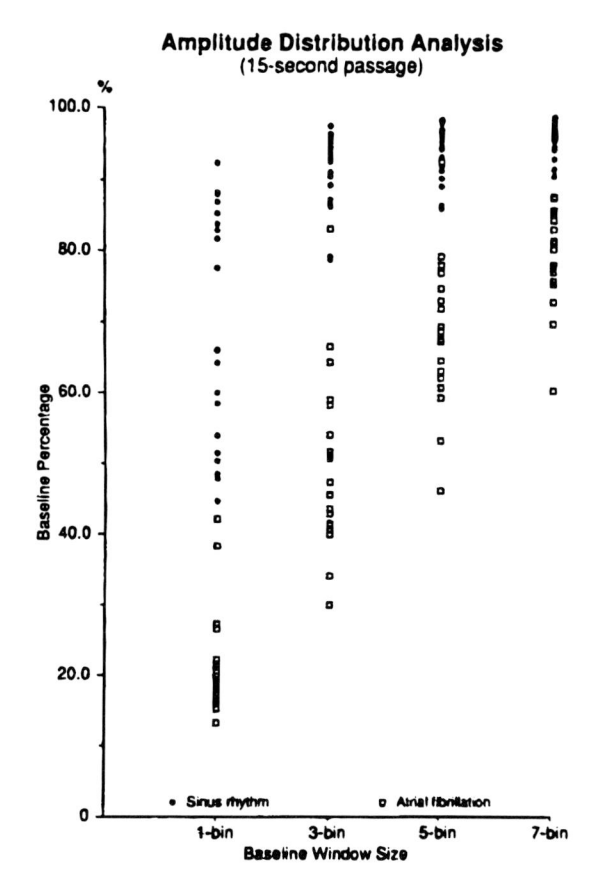

Figure 11. Percentage of signal values falling within a baseline window described on a 32-bin histogram. Each bin represents 1/32 of the maximum peak-to-peak amplitude of the signal in a 15-second passage. During atrial fibrillation, the signal was within the 1-bin baseline window < 43%, and sinus rhythm ≥ 43% of time. Perfect separation was possible with a 43% decision boundary. Decision boundaries for a 3-bin window achieve sensitivities and specificities of 90% or greater. For 5- or 7-bin windows 95% sensitivity and 100% specificity is possible. (Reproduced with permission from Reference 26.)

requiring minimum processing. All that is needed is a resettable peak detector. In fact, the peak value of the signal is needed for the automatic gain adjustment. If the signal during atrial fibrillation is so small that it cannot be separated from asystole, it is possible to measure evoked signals.[28] The evoked signal is the signal obtained immediately after pacing, signifying capture or noncapture, as in the case of fine atrial fibrillation. With the measurement of peak amplitudes as low as 0.15 mV (usually 10% of peak amplitude is a better threshold), the separation by rates may also be possible, since atrial fibrillation rate is usually above 240 beats per minute with few exceptions.[26] The advantage of looking at the peak amplitude of the signal is that it is an integral part of sensing and opens the door to examination of retrogradely conducted signals.

Rhythm Stability Criteria

In atria and ventricles, stability of the rate and amplitude are important to consider. For example, polymorphic tachycardias are frequently associated with hemodynamic instability. For the sake of a consistent framework, the "rate stability criteria" will be regarded as a subset of the "rate criteria" and the amplitude stability will be considered a subset of the wave shape criteria.

Atrium:Ventricle Event Ratios

The ratio of events counted in the atrium to those in the ventricle may be used to indicate location of the arrhythmia.[29,30] This ratio can be used to classify VT and some atrial flutters (Table 3).

Table 3
Atrioventricular Event Ratios Used for Arrhythmia Classification

A/V > 1	A FLUT, A FIB, SVT, S TACH
A/V < 1	V TACH (Oversensing)
A/V = 1	S TACHY, V TACHY, SVT

The A:V ratio is valuable in identifying VTs that do not have 1:1 conduction. It can be of considerable help if the relative instability is a measure of percentage change of rate (or interval) of one chamber compared to the other, but still preserving a unity relationship. If the two are stable, A:V is unity. If A changes more than V, then the ratio is 1+ and conversely if V changes were more than A, then it is 1−.

The use of exact A:V timing has been suggested as an option,[31] but has limited applications. For example, when A:V > 1, the rhythm could be sinus tachycardia with Wenckebach block. Such a situation could be difficult to differentiate from an atrial flutter with AV block. Exact timing considerations are likely to produce problems with rhythm classification.

Onset Criteria and Active Pacing Criteria

The onset criterion has been used extensively in the past for separation of sinus from pathological reentry tachycardias and is a feature of all third-generation defibrillators. The effectiveness of this criterion for rhythm differentiation is equivocal at best.[32-35] Problems of differentiating sinus tachycardia from an arrhythmia is still common. A potentially more dangerous situation could be the reverse, where a pathological tachycardia is misclassified. The main reason for the failure of onset criteria is a rapid onset of sinus tachycardias in younger patients and a slow onset of some pathological arrhythmias. The limitations have been sufficient to recognize the need for improvements.

Atrial prematures were shown to be useful for differentiating sinus tachycardia from pathological rhythms.[33] In a study of 13 patients, application of atrial prematures at 100 msec differentiated a variety of atrial arrhythmias, AV nodal and orthodromic tachycardia from sinus tachycardias. In the case of sinus tachycardia, the delay induced by the atrial premature in the resultant ventricular beat was in excess of 20 msec, com-

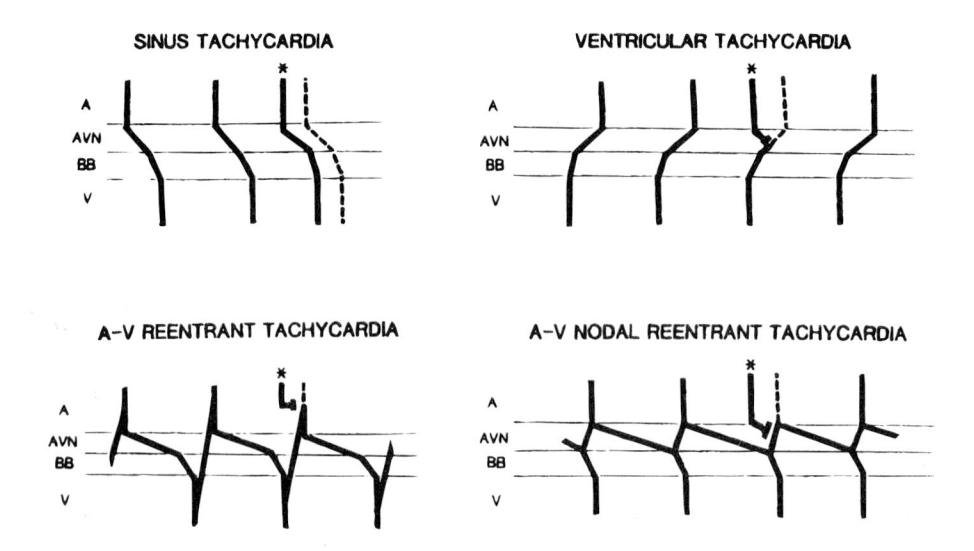

Figure 12. Lattice diagram showing the way atrial extrastimulus can help to identify a fast rhythm as sinus tachycardia. (Reproduced with permission from Reference 33.)

pared to < 10 msec for all other arrhythmias. These concepts are shown in Figure 12. The plot of AV delay response for various prematures is shown in Figure 13. This plot indicates that the delivery of three differently timed premature atrial beats could allow shorter delays to give sufficient definition.

The utility of the method that uses atrial prematures is limited to patients with intact AV delay. In the case of a rhythm where Wenckebach phenomenon is taking place, this method could not be applied. Also, in the case of atrial arrhythmias where the reentrant path is not close to the AV node this approach would not work. It is also inapplicable for VTs.

Metabolic Indicator Criteria

As discussed, there are definite advantages in combining a metabolic indicator with DDDR function. A possible sensor could be minute volume ventilation. It is important to note that with minute volume ventilation some compromising arrhythmias could initiate respiratory response. This response will tend to occur with a delay after the onset of the high heart rate.

Therefore, it would be advantageous to look at the relationship between the heart rate, minute volume ventilation, and the absolute value of minute volume ventilation. It is most likely that this criteria could be used when all the other criteria have established the relative safety of the rhythm for the patient. By definition this test will only be relevant for the appropriate rate for age.

Wave Shape Criteria

Surface ECG analysis of arrhythmias uses timing and wave shapes for rhythm classification. Extensive work has been done with endocardial signals to elucidate the significance of morphology (wave shape) for ventricular arrhythmia discrimination[34,35] and for recognition of retrograde atrial conduction.[36,37] In the atrium, the emphasis has been on recognition of retrograde conduction for the identification of pacer-mediated tachycardias. It is also true to assume because of the nature of propagation of sinus node beats in the atrium with respect to a sensing electrode in the atrial appendage, that all slower SVTs and atrial tachycardias would generate wave fronts emanating from a different directions,

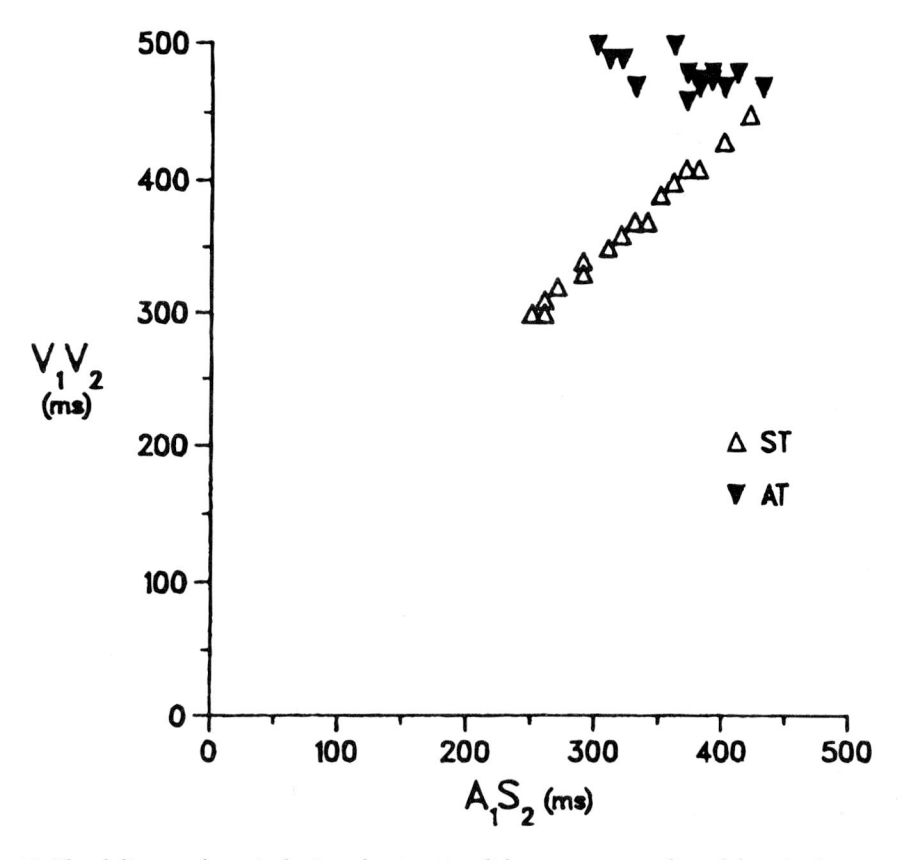

Figure 13. The delivery of precisely timed extrastimuli have corresponding delays in the ventricular cycle, with sinus tachycardia. This is not the case with most supraventricular tachycardias. (Reproduced with permission from Reference 33.)

hence changing the morphology of the detected signals.

From the previous work on the ability to identify VT by template matching to sinus rhythm, the results have shown a near 100% success rates.[34,35] With sampling of the signal at slower rates (< 250 samples per second) the success rates were lower regardless of the type of processing. This means that a simple metrics test or wave shape criteria (amplitude with sign and/or width) was as good as a more complex cross-correlation test. In the case of retrograde atrial signals the initial study[37] indicated 100% successful separation using amplitude alone. It is important to note that with intermittent bundle branch block at higher rates, VT will always be wrongly identified with template matching criteria.

With the use of morphology the diagnostic capability may be improved, noting that during VT with 1:1 conduction atrial and ventricular electrograms will indicate shape changes, since the atrial signal will be retrograde and the ventricular signal will be modified. During SVT the atrial signal will be modified and the ventricular signal will not be. In a recent study using AV relationships and morphology 100% success rate for identifying atrial flutter, fibrillation, VT or ventricular flutter, and fibrillation was documented. Problem remains during intermittent bundle branch block. The only test that is presently viable is to evaluate the ventricular evoked potential. From previous studies[38] we know that the evoked potential does change with VT but not with sinus tachycardia and SVT. Bundle branch block does not change the size of the signal. The reason for not using only the evoked signal for arrhythmia discrimination is that its resolution is poor for slower VTs (< 150 beats per minute). In conclusion then, it seems that morphology can provide a more unified approach than A:V timing alone.

The Final DDD Classifier

In the final summary we have somehow to bring the various criteria together into a single decision making matrix. It is important to understand that apart from "rate" most of the indicators bring additional evidence but cannot be definitive. As an example, "onset criteria" may not discriminate appropriately in younger patients between physiological and pathological tachycardias. In a younger patient, sudden metabolic demand or shock may confuse this criterion, due to a rapid change in sinus rate. To overcome this "fuzzy" logic decision making process may be set up where each of the indicators are weighted and their scores then added. The total score is used to make the final decision on which therapy is based, and in which cardiac chamber it is to be delivered. To allow us to set up the table used for this approach, we will now list the relevant criteria (Table 4).

Table 4 summarizes possible weights for each indicator. The weights are summed for each chamber independently and the chamber with the higher score is the chamber of origin of the arrhythmia. The ratio of atrial to ventricular events contributes more heavily to the decision as to the chamber of origin of the arrhythmia and heavily biases against therapy in the ventricle if the atrium is likely to be the source of the arrhythmia. The relative stability is only a sign saying which chamber is likely the source. Hence a " + " will indicate that it is most likely the source from the atrium. It is important to understand that the weighting is used only to demonstrate the concepts and not an iron-clad proposal for application. A sample of how a decision making may proceed is presented in Table 5.

From Table 5 we can see how the desired therapies could be derived. For the above selected weights pacing therapy

Table 4
Weighting of Scores for use in "Fuzzy" Logic for Arrhythmia Discrimination

Criteria	Description	Score
RC (A or V)	Rate above pedefined limit and its stability	< ARFA = 10 > ARFA and < 240 = 20 > 240 = 50 RATE UNSTABLE = 20
OC (A or V)	Onset of high rate	Maximum score = 20
AVER	Ratio of atrial to ventricular events and relative stability	A/V > 1 = −20 (A = 10) A/V < 1 = 10 (for V) A/V = 1 = 0 = 1+ = −20, − + 10
WSC (A or V)	Wave shape and ampl stablity	Changed = 20 Unchanged = 0 Unstable = 20
MIC	Metabolic indicator criteria	Tracs RC = −20 Not tracs = 20
ACPC	Actively pacing to elicit indication of arrhythmia	Not being weighted at the present

RC: rate criteria; OC: onset criteria; AVER: atrioventricular effective ratio; WSC: wave shape criteria; MIC: metabolic indicator criteria; ACPC: active pacing criteria.

Table 5
An Example of "Fuzzy" Logic Used for Arrhythmia Classification

RC	OC	AVER	WSC	MIC	Score & T'rapy
< ARFA A = 10 V = 10	A = 2 V = 2	A/V = 1 A = 0 V = 0	No change A = 0 V = 0	TRACS A = −20 V = −20	No therapy
< ARFA A = 10 V = 10	Signif. A = 15 V = 10	A/V = 1+ A = 0 V = 0	Change A = 10 V = 0	No trac A = 20 V = 20	A = 55 V = 40 A PACE
> ARFA < 240 A = 20 V = 20	Signif. A = 12 V = 20	A/V < 1 A = 0 V = 10	Change A = 0 V = 20	No trac A = 20 V = 20	A = 52 V = 90 V PACE
> 240 (V) A = 10 V = 100 + 20	A = 2 V = 3	A/V < 1 A = 0 V = 10	Change A = 0 V = 20 + 20	No trac A = 20 V = 20	A = 32 V = 193 V DEFIB
> 240 (A) A = 100 + 20 V = 10 + 20	A = 2 V = 3	A/V > 1 A = 10 V = −20	Change A = 20 + 20 V = 0	No trac A = 20 V = 20	A = 192 V = 33 A DEFIB
< ARFA A = 10 V = 10	A = 2 V = 0	A/V > 1 A = 0 V = 10	No change A = 0 V = 0	TRAC A = −20 V = −20	No therapy

ARFA: appropriate rate for age

would be applied at a threshold of 30 and defibrillation at a threshold of 120. There are a number of other conditions that may have to be applied and the actual weights adjusted in order not to run the risk of not supplying the needed therapy. The general rule is that the application of therapy in one chamber excludes the need for therapy in another. In the last case there is AV block indicated by the need to pace and the rule that the A:V ratio only applies for intrinsic beats. If, however, there were also no "trac" and the wave shape criteria indicated a change in the atrium, pacer-mediated tachycardia would be present. In this case, termination would be achieved by delivering of atrial prematures correctly timed to block the retrograde conduction.

Therapeutic Benefits of DDD Devices

Availability of pacing in the atrium affords additional advantages for treatment of arrhythmias, eg, pace termination of atrial flutter and AV nodal tachycardias. In addition, atrial pacing may stabilize the atria and delay precipitation of atrial fibrillation in patients with frequent atrial ectopy. This benefit has been extensively discussed by Lamas et al.[39] However, no prophylactic benefit was demonstrated for pacing the atrium at higher standby rates.[40,41] There also appears to be some prophylactic benefit in pacing patients with short AV delays, albeit with a considerable hemodynamic penalty.

Pacing Reversion for Supraventricular Tachycardia

This topic has been explored extensively during electrophysiologic studies and with implantable devices from a variety of manufacturers. The majority of patients reported from one study[42] had leads implanted in the right atrium. In 10 patients arrhythmias were terminated from the right

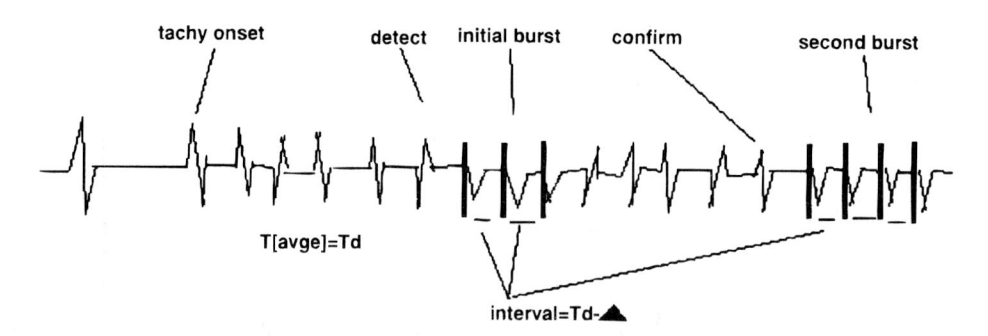

Figure 14. An adaptive scanning burst where the delay of the extrastimuli are timed from the arrhythmia and the number of extrastimuli control the level of "aggressiveness." Autodecremental approach decrements the interpulse interval, starting at Td-▲.

ventricle and in only 5 patients from the coronary sinus. From a recent study[43] more information has been obtained on the rate of success for pace termination of atrial flutter. Permanent atrial fibrillation developed in 27% of patients. This clearly points out the hazards of treating this rhythm with pacing alone. This potential hazard may be minimized by using minimum pacing amplitude possible, keeping the cycle length of the extrastimuli as long as possible, and keeping the number of pulses to a minimum.

The most successful reversion regimes

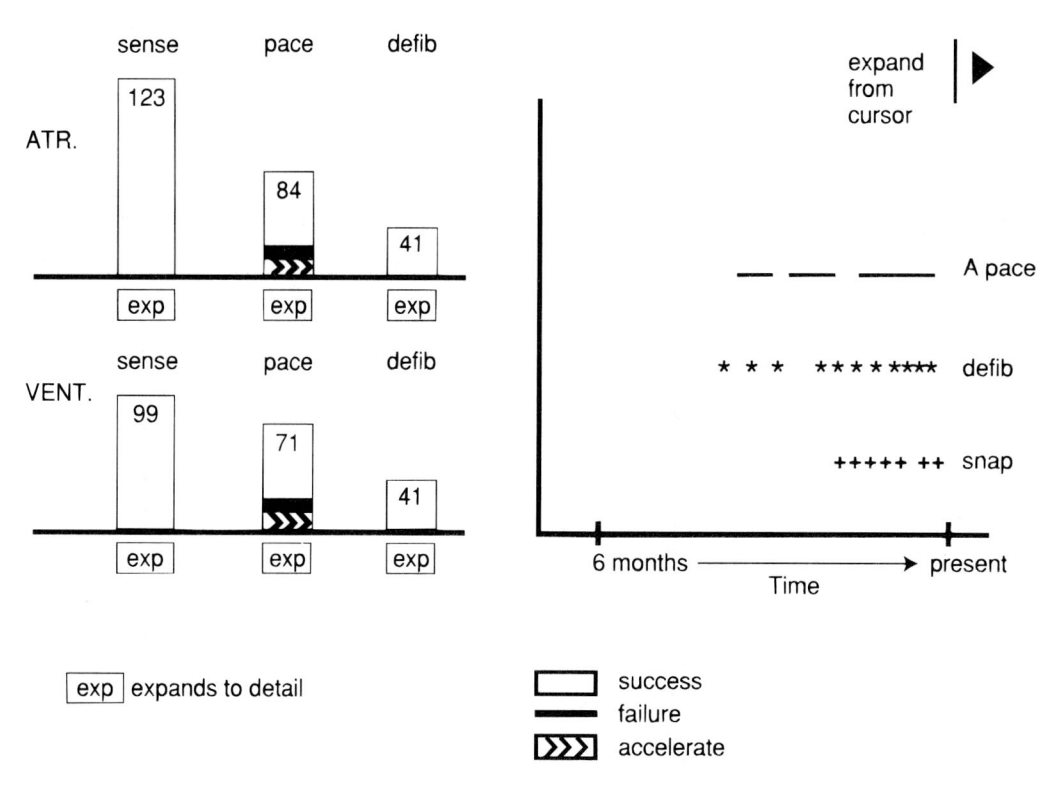

Figure 15. Overview of therapy delivered in the past 6 months by DDD based defibrillator. Expansion (EXP) gives greater definition of data; SNAP: snapshot of arrhythmia.

were demonstrated to be orthorhythmic adaptive bursts, delivering < 16 extrastimuli. The orthorhythmic function allowed the burst to start timing just inside the cycle time of the arrhythmias in question. The success of the autodecremental concept (from Cordis Corp., Miami, FL) and the scanning burst concept (Telectronics Inc., Englewood, CO) (Figure 14), have led to their incorporation into the present day ICDs (Guardian™ ATP 4211, Telectronics, Englewood, CO), and to their general acceptance in the industry.

The use of AV sequential pacing with short AV delays does not generally bring any added benefit for the control of SVTs. As there has been little difference in the efficacy between the scanning and autodecremental algorithms it would be perhaps optimal to standardize and adapt "therapy aggressiveness" so that it could automatically provide the balance between success of termination and frequency of acceleration in the ventricles or in the atria (Figure 14).

Data Logging

Data logging has been accepted as an important diagnostic capability for implanted defibrillators. With the existing ICDs it is in fact a vital link in the programming of the device and understanding relevance of detection criteria.[44] With a DDD-based ICD all of these considerations become even more relevant. However, because of the large quantity of data the pre-

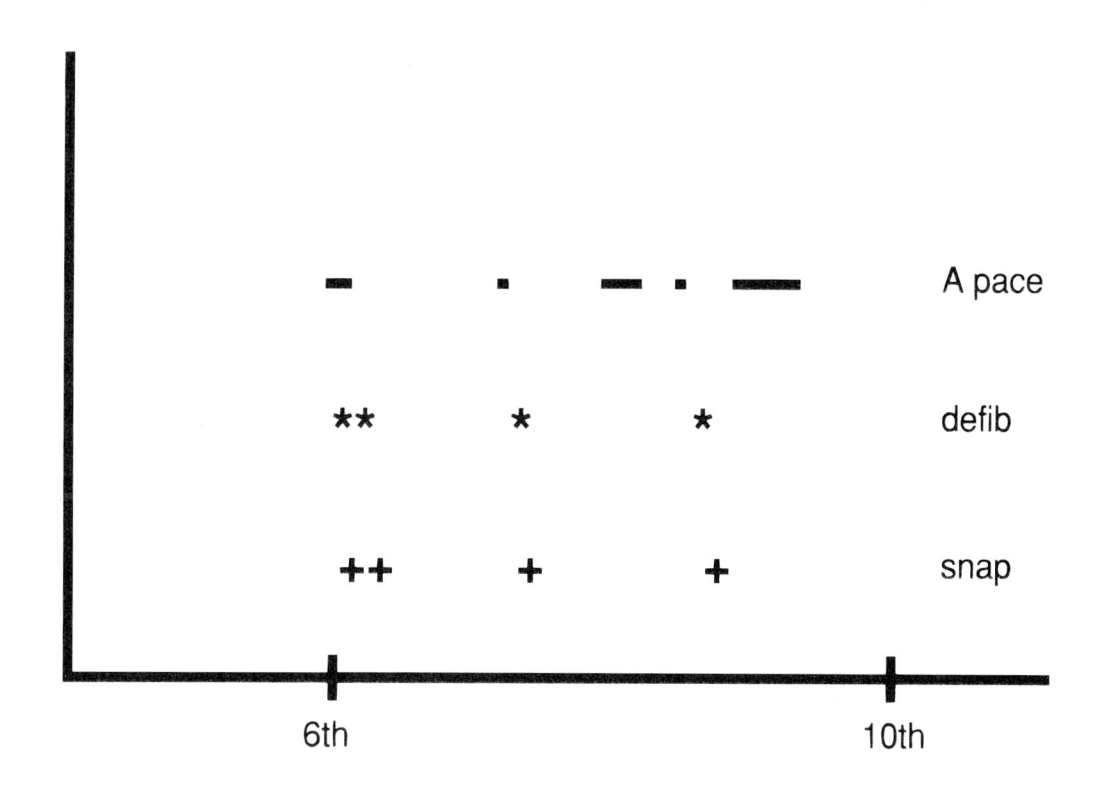

Figure 16. Expansion of the "temporal" display giving more detail of events. Further expansion will allow inspection of precise time of events. A pace: atrial pacing; defib: defibrillation; snap: snapshot.

trocardiographically documented unnecessary spontaneous shocks in 241 patients with implantable cardioverter defibrillators. *PACE* 15:1667, 1992.
26. Jenkins J, Noh KH, Guezennec A, et al: Diagnosis of atrial fibrillation using electrograms from chronic leads: evaluation of computer algorithms. *PACE* 11:622, 1988.
27. Slocum J, Sahakian A, Swiryn S: Computer discrimination of atrial fibrillation and regular atrial rhythms from intra-atrial electrograms. *PACE* 11:610, 1988.
28. Ruetz L, Yee R, Bardy G, et al: Reliable sensing of human atrial fibrillation (abstract). *PACE* 16:902, 1993.
29. Wang PJ, Lu RM, Rastager H, et al: Using the pacing integral to improve ventricular fibrillation detection (abstract). *Circulation* 84(4):I-442, 1992.
30. Jenkins J, Bump T, Munkenbeck F, et al: Tachycardia detection in implantable antitachycardia devices. *PACE* 7:1273, 1984.
31. Schuger CD, Jackson KJ, Steinman RT, et al: Atrial sensing to augment ventricular tachycardia detection by the automatic implantable cardioverter defibrillator: a utility study. *PACE* 11:1456, 1988.
32. Volosin KJ, Beuregard LM, Fabiszewski R, et al: Spontaneous changes in ventricular tachycardia cycle length. *J Am Coll Cardiol* 17: 409, 1991.
33. Munkenbeck FC, Bump TE, Arzbaecher RC: Differentiation of sinus tachycardia from paroxysmal 1:1 tachycardias using single late diastolic atrial extrastimuli. *PACE* 9:53, 1986.
34. Greenhut SG, Deering TF, Steinhaus BM, et al: Separation of ventricular tachycardia from sinus rhythm using a practical real-time template matching computer system. *PACE* 15:2146, 1992.
35. Thorne RD, DiCarlo LA, Jenkins JM, et al: Paroxysmal bundle branch block of supraventricular origin: a possible source of misdiagnosis in detecting ventricular tachycardia using time domain analysis of intraventricular electrograms. *PACE* 13:453, 1990.
36. Thorne RD, Jenkins JM, DiCarlo LA: The bin area method: a computationally efficient technique for the analysis of ventricular and atrial intracardiac electrogram. *PACE* 13: 1286, 1990.
37. Wainwright R, Davies W, Tooley M: Ideal atrial lead position to detect retrograde atrial depolarization by digitization and slope analysis of atrial electrogram. *PACE* 7:1152, 1984.
38. Beltz KM, Ellenbogen KA, Camm AJ, et al: Differentiation between monomorphic ventricular tachycardia and sinus tachycardia based on the right ventricular evoked potential. *PACE* 15:1661, 1992.
39. Lamas GA, Ester NM, Schneller S, et al: Does dual chamber or atrial pacing prevent atrial fibrillation? The need for a randomized controlled trial. *PACE* 15:1109, 1992.
40. Murphy P, O'Keeffe DB: Effect of atrial pacing on the frequency of tachycardia in patients with recurrent junctional tachycardia. *PACE* 14:404, 1993.
41. Chiang C, Jenkins J, DiCarlo L: Real time automatic detection of complex cardiac arrhythmias using rate augmented by intraatrial and intraventricular electrogram analysis. *PACE* 15:529, 1992.
42. Dulk KD, Brugada P, Smeets JL, et al: Long-term antitachycardia pacing experience for supraventricular tachycardia. *PACE* 13:1020, 1990.
43. Jung J, Heisel M, Stopp R, et al: Factors influencing the success of rapid atrial pacing for the termination of atrial flutter. *PACE* 16: 1115, 1993.
44. Marchlinski FE, Gottlieb CD, Sarter B, et al: ICD storage: value in arrhythmia management. *PACE* 16:527, 1993.
45. Block M, Bocker D, Hammel D, et al: Should implantable cardioverter defibrillators store electrograms from sensing or defibrillation leads? *PACE* 16:858, 1993.

Chapter 35

Combination of Drug Delivery Systems and Implantable Cardioverter-Defibrillators: Is There a Possible Future Marriage?

Tibor Nappholz

Introduction

Implantable cardioverter-defibrillators (ICDs) are an accepted reality in the field of cardiac rhythm management. Implantable cardioverter-defibrillators address the most dangerous manifestation of cardiac disease, ie, ventricular tachycardia (VT) and ventricular fibrillation (VF). These arrhythmias account for an estimated 400,000 deaths in the United States alone,[1-3] which represents approximately 50% of all cardiovascular deaths. Although ICDs have fulfilled their stated objective at preventing sudden cardiac death, the overall impact on long-term survival has been questioned by some investigators. It is possible that in a specific subset of patients, sudden death has been replaced by nonsudden cardiac death[4-6] resulting from left ventricular failure (Figure 1). This may be due to the competing concurrent risks of heart failure and ventricular dysrhythmias. This chapter addresses the most difficult problem, that is how to augment the functionality of the ICD, and also addresses other issues contributing to overall mortality.[4]

Implantable Cardioverter-Defibrillator and Infusion

The infusion of cardiac drugs in an acute setting is not a new concept. There are many cardiac drugs that may be infused on a continuous basis using an external pump. The concept of an implanted pump for drug infusion is also not new, and has been in clinical use for a number of years for infusion of insulin,[7,8] administration of chemotherapy, and continuous infusion of analgesics for control of intractable pain,[9,10] but what has not been done is the use of a fully implantable pump for the delivery of cardiac drugs in humans. The main reason for this has been the lack of a demonstrable advantage of this approach over orally administered drugs. Even when it is possible to administer some drugs intravenously (eg, dopamine, lidocaine, bretylium, etc.), the move to an implanted system has not occurred. Again, the explanation may reside in the availability of alternative approaches to achieve the stated goal.

The practical utility of a combined ICD and an infusion pump is the extension of therapy to the congestive heart failure patient. It is estimated that in the United States

From Singer I, (ed.) Implantable Cardioverter-Defibrillator. Armonk, NY: Futura Publishing Company, Inc.; © 1994.

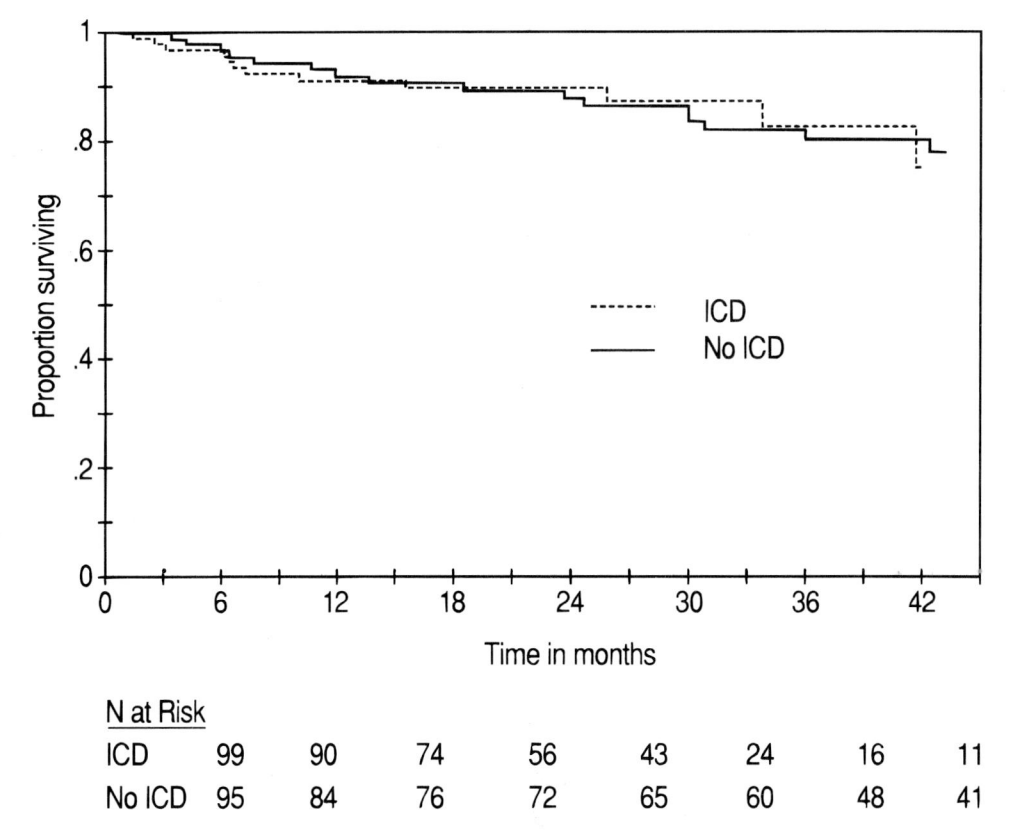

	0	6	12	18	24	30	36	42
N at Risk								
ICD	99	90	74	56	43	24	16	11
No ICD	95	84	76	72	65	60	48	41

Figure 1. Overall survival comparing the groups treated with and without an implantable cardioverter-defibrillator (ICD) ($P = 0.95$). N = number of patients. (Reproduced with permission from Crandall BB, et al: Implantable cardioverter-defibrillator therapy survivors of out-of-hospital sudden cardiac death without inducible arrhythmias. *J Am Coll Cardiol* 21(3):1186, 1993.)

alone over 200,000 patients die annually from congestive heart failure. This figure is continuously increasing.[21] It is one area of endeavor where the most promising therapies of tomorrow may have to be applied.

In broad terms there are two groups of patients at risk of sudden cardiac death. The first group is comprised of patients with no structural cardiac disease (eg, long QT syndrome). The second group is comprised of patients with identifiable cardiac pathology, eg, coronary artery disease. While this classification is broad and controversial, it serves the purpose of emphasizing that there is one group of patients who can be treated for electrically instigated sudden cardiac death and the other, where treating the electrical manifestations of cardiac disease may only be a part of therapy.

Cardioactive Drugs

The quest to discover a "perfect" antiarrhythmic drug probably began with the discovery of quinine. The elusive goal of discovering the perfect antiarrhythmic drug, one with no side effects but one that suppresses all spontaneous ventricular arrhythmias and prevents VF, has been pursued by investigators ever since. The enthusiasm for this quest has been tempered by the realization of the enormity and the complexity of this task.[8] Class I drugs could not be shown to reduce mortality postmyocardial infarction. Modest benefits were demonstrated with β blockers and amiodarone.[12,13] The Cardiac Arrhythmia Suppression Trial (CAST) has demonstrated an increase in mortality with Class IC drugs compared to placebo.[14,15] Failure of the electropharmacological interventions to produce clinically meaningful benefits is due to a multiplicity of causes.

Complex ventricular ectopy is predictive of cardiac arrhythmic mortality.[13] The frequency and the complexity of rhythm disturbances reflects the severity of the underlying disease process, and may represent an epiphenomenon rather than the proximal cause. Suppression of complex ventricular ectopy may not prevent sudden cardiac death due to VF.

Sudden cardiac death in patients with chronic heart failure may result from ischemic and hemodynamic events rather than the progression of nonsustained to sustained ventricular arrhythmia. In patients with chronic heart failure and underlying coronary disease, sudden death is commonly precipitated by an acute ischemic event[17] and in the case of idiopathic dilated cardiomyopathy, sudden death is frequently triggered by hemodynamic events culminating in bradycardia or electromechanical dissociation. In a study of patients with idiopathic dilated cardiomyopathies at the University of California Transplantation Program, 100% of the patients who died suddenly did so from bradycardia and electromechanical dissociation.[17]

Antiarrhythmic drugs have potentially serious side effects, some which may exacerbate underlying ventricular arrhythmia. Antiarrhythmic drugs modify the electrical-characteristics of the depolarization/repolarization sequence. This modification may be proarrhythmic, particularly if the therapeutic level of the drug is not tightly controlled. Antiarrhythmic drugs may exert potent negative inotropic effects.[18,19]

In spite of these shortcomings β blockers and Class III drugs (amiodarone, sotalol) can serve a valuable purpose in suppressing ectopy and frequent tachycardia episodes, thus decreasing overall mortality. A decrease in mortality observed with β blockers is most likely related to antiadrenergic effects (Figure 2).

Electrical Therapy

Electrical reversion of arrhythmias by pacing or defibrillation treats manifestations of the underlying disease process, but does not alter the underlying condition. The advantage of electrical over drug therapy is its specificity. This means that patients treated by "electrical means" do not suffer from drug toxicity, proarrhythmias or the negative inotropic effects of therapy. The disadvantage of electrical therapy is an inability to suppress ectopic ventricular beats and salvos, which may lead to sustained ventricular arrhythmias or VF.

Drugs, Electricity, or Both?

From the preliminary discussion it is obvious that electrical and drug therapy for treatment of arrhythmias address the same issue: control of symptoms of cardiac disease. With the well-recognized side effects of drugs, electrical therapy is likely to be favored in the future. The potential for electrically triggered fatal arrhythmias will always exist in the complex milieu of a diseased heart.

Consequently, to exploit the benefits of concomitant drug therapy we have to use it to stabilize the hemodynamics as much as possible, optimize cardiac pumping function, and try to recover some of the cardiac reserve to prevent the collapse that so often precedes a "not so sudden death." There is some room for the use of antiarrhythmic drugs as concomitant therapy with an implantable defibrillator, and in fact, presently a number of patients are concurrently treated with both.

Purpose and Function of Implantable Cardioverter-Defibrillator Infusion

It is appropriate at this juncture to define the purpose for such a hypothetical device and then follow it logically to its imple-

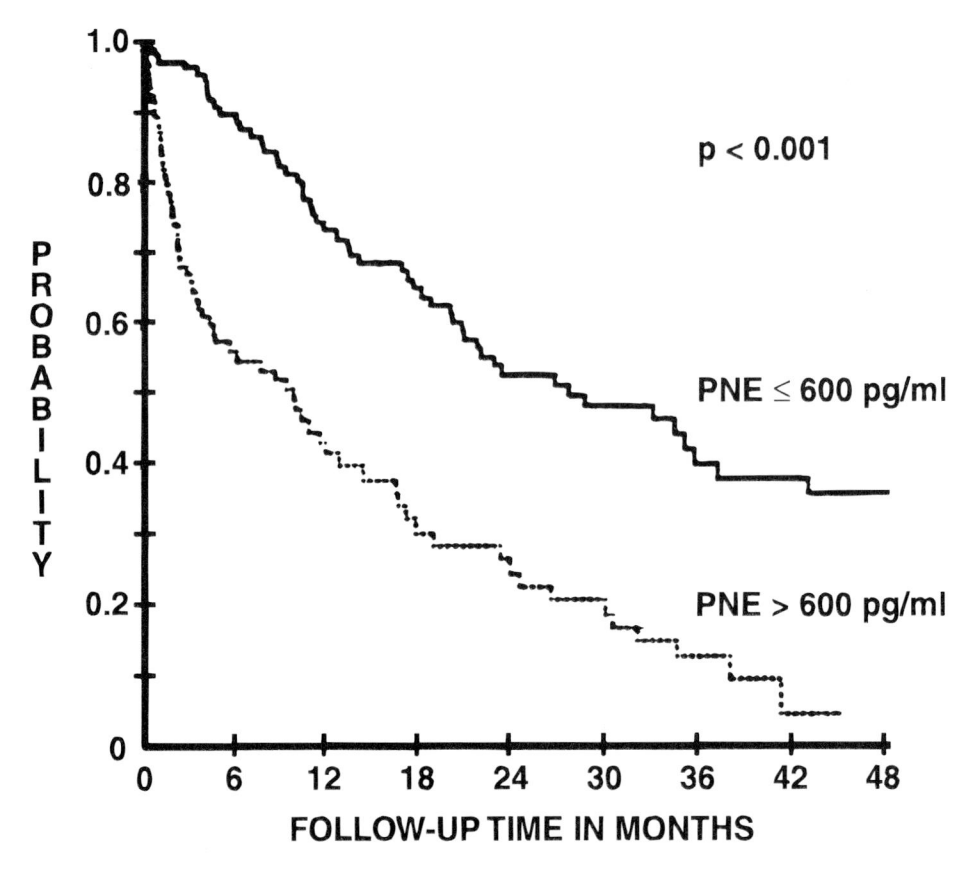

Figure 2. Probability of survival in patients with heart failure whose baseline plasma norepinephrine (PNE) is below or above 600 pg/mL. (Reproduced with permission from Cohn JN: Abnormalities of peripheral sympathetic nervous system control in congestive heart failure. *Circulation* 82(Suppl I):I-59, 1990.)

mentation. For the sake of this analysis the function of electrical therapy and drug therapy will be separated, but in the final device the two functions would be integrated into a single system with the main control center of the device calling for either pacing, cardioversion, defibrillation, or infusion. This discussion begins with the established electrical therapy.

Electrical Intervention

Presently, in third-generation tiered-therapy devices the rate of the electrical depolarizations of the heart is monitored, serving to distinguish sinus rhythm from pathological tachycardias. The change in rate (Figure 3A and 3B) initiates and determines the type of therapy to be delivered (antitachycardia pacing [ATP], cardioversion, or defibrillation). The suddenness or onset of change in rate (Figure 3C), helps discriminate between physiologically appropriate and pathological rate changes (arrhythmias). Stratification of therapies based on the rate detection is shown in Figure 4.

Recognized limitations of the presently available third generation devices include: 1) discrimination of supraventricular from ventricular tachyarrhythmias[20]; and 2) inability to detect small amplitude "fine" VF. Previous studies attempted to better define and differentiate sinus from ventricular and

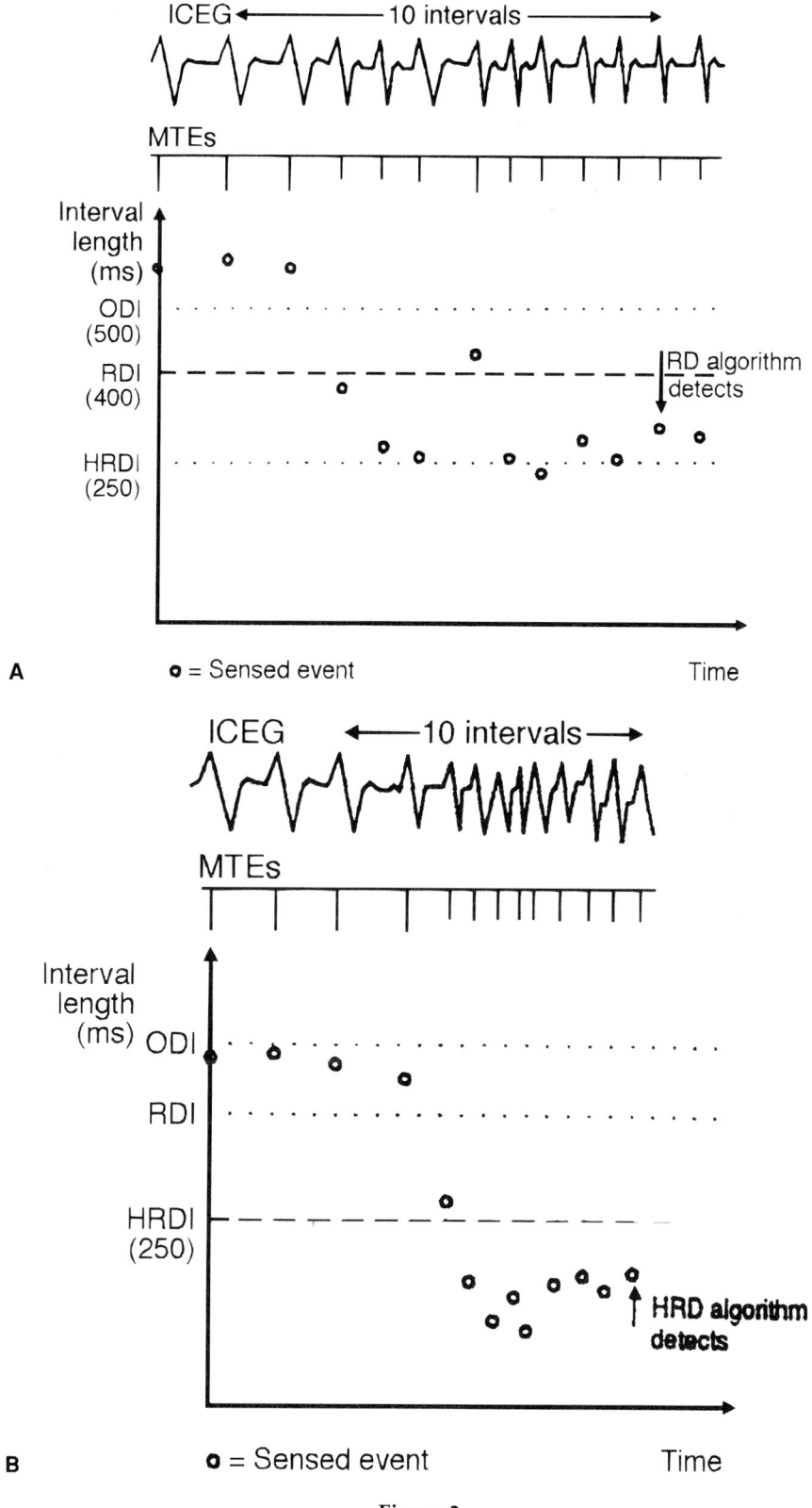

Figure 3.

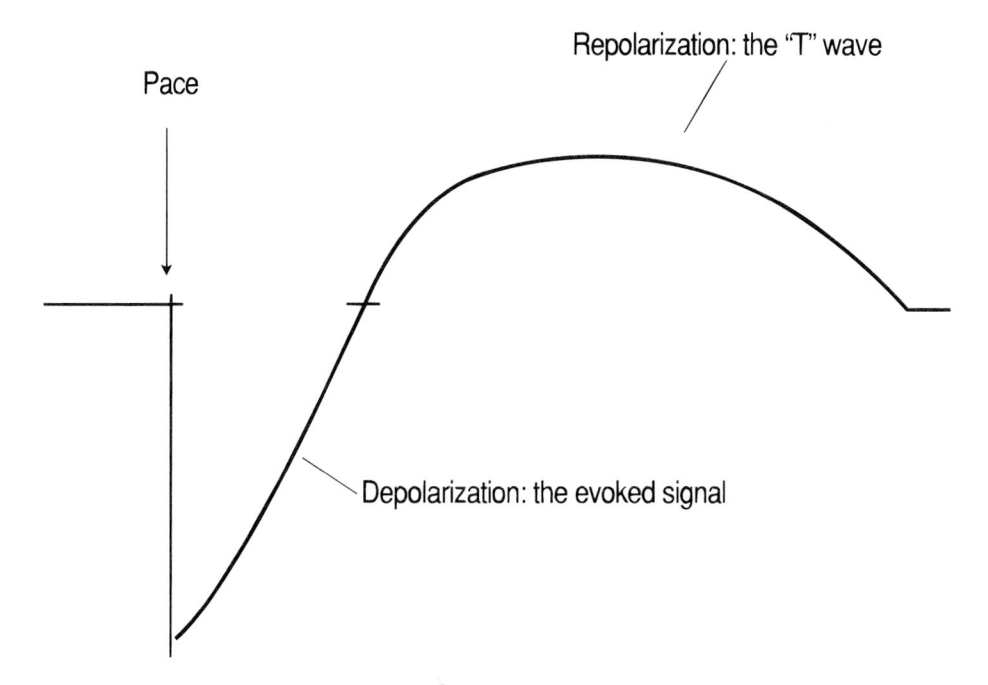

Figure 5. The ventricular response to local (pacing electrode) capture.

aortic root in the animal model.[26] The aortic route was successful in all animals in 2–4 seconds. The CS route was only successful in 7 out of 13 animals. This approach (aortic root infusion) is not acceptable for use in humans and the CS would not be sufficiently reliable.

4) Chemical control of atrial defibrillation. Paroxysmal atrial fibrillation is a frequent arrhythmia. A number of Class I drugs are known to be effective for atrial fibrillation. With ICD drug infusion there would be an option for control of atrial fibrillation or therapy for ventricular tachyarrthymias, with additional availability of atrial defibrillation.[27]

5) Control of contractility. Inotropic drugs (eg, dobutamine, dopamine) activate β_1-receptors in the heart. Continuous infusion of β_1-agonist drugs is hampered by gradual desensitizing effect on the receptors over time. Intermittent infusion of these drugs based on hemodynamic requirements, however, may be feasible.

6) Control of vasodilation of large arteries and coronary arteries. This is another potentially attractive option. This option opens the doors for better control of angina. A relatively new agent, adenosine, is a possible candidate for this application. It is fast acting, potent coronary vasodilator and also a potent vasodilator of large vessels. Unfortunately, it may intensify angina and increase defibrillation thresholds.[28] A comparison of the effect of an inotrope and a vasodilator drug is shown in Figure 6.

From this discussion it seems that at the present time the most obvious application of combined ICDs and infusion devices would be to optimize hemodynamics and decrease arrhythmia frequency.

Mechanics of Infusion Pumps

The most practical approach for an implanted system that incorporates pacing and defibrillation functions would be to infuse cardioactive drugs in the right heart chambers. In this configuration the drug behaves as if there were two or more compartments that it infuses into. For the purpose

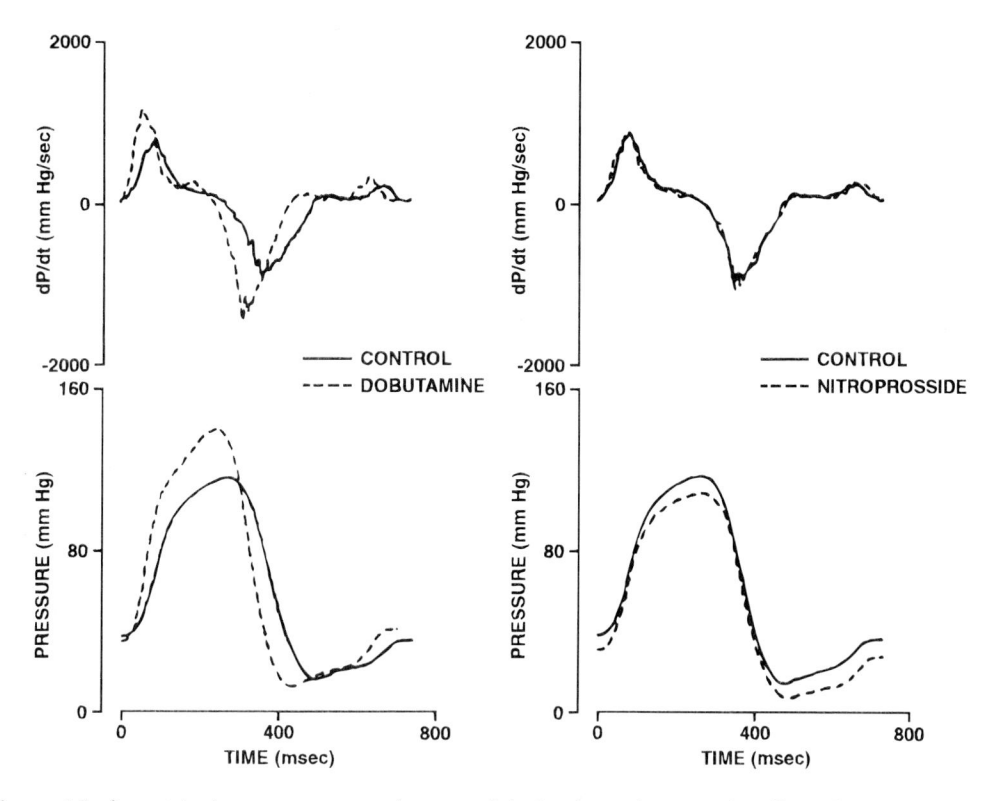

Figure 6. Left ventricular pressure waveforms and derivatives, showing the effect of inotrope (dobutamine) and vasodilator (nitroprusside). Note the influence on end-diastolic pressure. (Reproduced with permission from Walsh RA: Sympathetic control of diastolic function in congestive heart failure. *Circulation* 82(Suppl I):I-52, 1990.)

of this analysis a good approximation is to use a two-compartment model. The first compartment consists of a rapidly equilibrating volume, circulating blood, and highly perfused organs. With a bolus, the time it takes to get 50% of the drug distributed in this initial compartment is the alpha half-life as shown in Figure 7. The second compartment equilibrates with the drug in the first compartment over a longer time and is shown as the beta. Another important pharmacokinetic parameter is clearance. In the case of a bolus, the beta is the result of equilibration in the second compartment and the clearance process. To maintain a steady-state concentration the rate of infusion of a drug has to be equal to the rate of clearance and the actual serum drug concentration is related to the rate of throughput. Figure 7 shows how to achieve a desired level of serum drug concentration.[29] This applies even for fast acting drugs where the equilibration and clearance could be in the order of seconds.

The goal with most cardioactive drugs in a chronically implanted system would be to have fast acting drugs and to avoid the side effects. By definition, fast acting drugs will be influenced less by the second compartment kinetics than the slow acting ones.

With the infusion pump as part of the implantable defibrillator it is most practical to place the infusion catheter into the same vein as the electrodes, ie, the subclavian or cephalic veins. The drug will then enter the heart readily from the right ventricular location, which would be important for rapid mixing and dispersion.

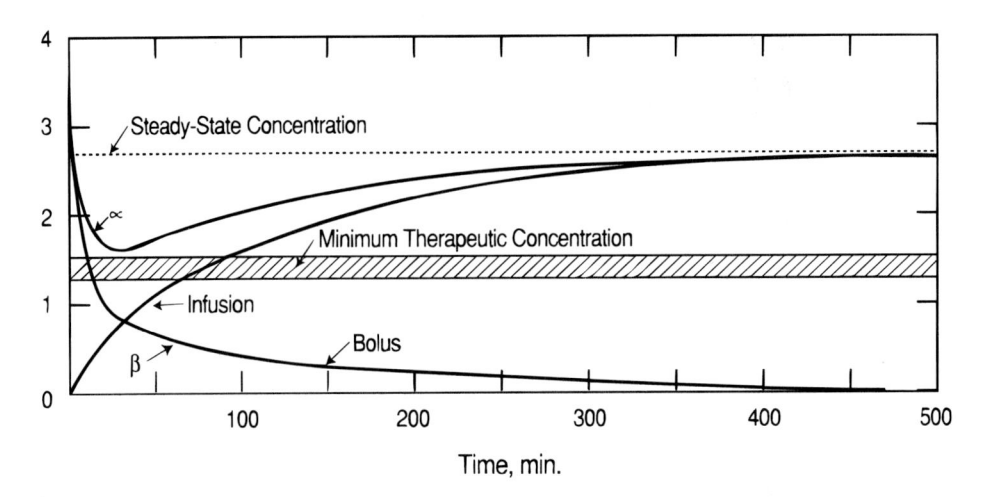

Figure 7. Lidocaine blood levels achieved optimally by a bolus (B), followed by the predefined "infusion" level to give the desired outcome (DO). The objective is to exceed the minimum therapeutic concentration "followed by infusion."

Drugs for Chronic Infusion

As discussed previously one of the drawbacks of cardiac drugs available today are undesirable side effects. The most potent drugs may also be toxic if continuous serum levels are not maintained.

From the previous discussion, there are a number of potential applications that we have targeted for drug use. They are: 1) manipulation of the β-adrenergic receptors of the heart; and 2) dilatation of coronary vessels and peripheral arteries to decrease the wall tension (afterload), and to improve coronary blood flow.

To make the selected drugs acceptable for long-term infusion they need to be infused at an acceptable rate, and require infrequent refilling of the drug reservoir. In addition, the drug has to be stable over time at body temperature for at least several months. As an example, esmolol a fast acting β-blocker would have to be dispensed at about 1 gram per month. This is quite acceptable, for an implantable pump with a 20-mL reservoir. Another potential candidate, nitroprusside is stable for long periods of time provided it is not exposed to light. Adenosine requires similar infusion levels to esmolol (50 ug/kg per minute compared to 300 ug/kg per minute).

Dopamine and dobutamine have been the two most frequently used drugs to enhance contractility.[30,31] However, both drugs result in desensitization of β receptors with continuous infusion. Intermittent infusion could yield better results.

Control Parameters for Infusion

The control parameters are the information that the algorithms use to control the infusion rate of a particular drug. We will address each, ie, type of drug and the sensors that could be useful for regulation of drug infusion.

Control of Adrenergic Stimulation

Esmolol is a potential candidate for this application because of its short half-life. The algorithm would track heart rate. As the heart rate increases the infusion rate would also increase. If supraventricular tachycardia is diagnosed, a bolus of β blocker would

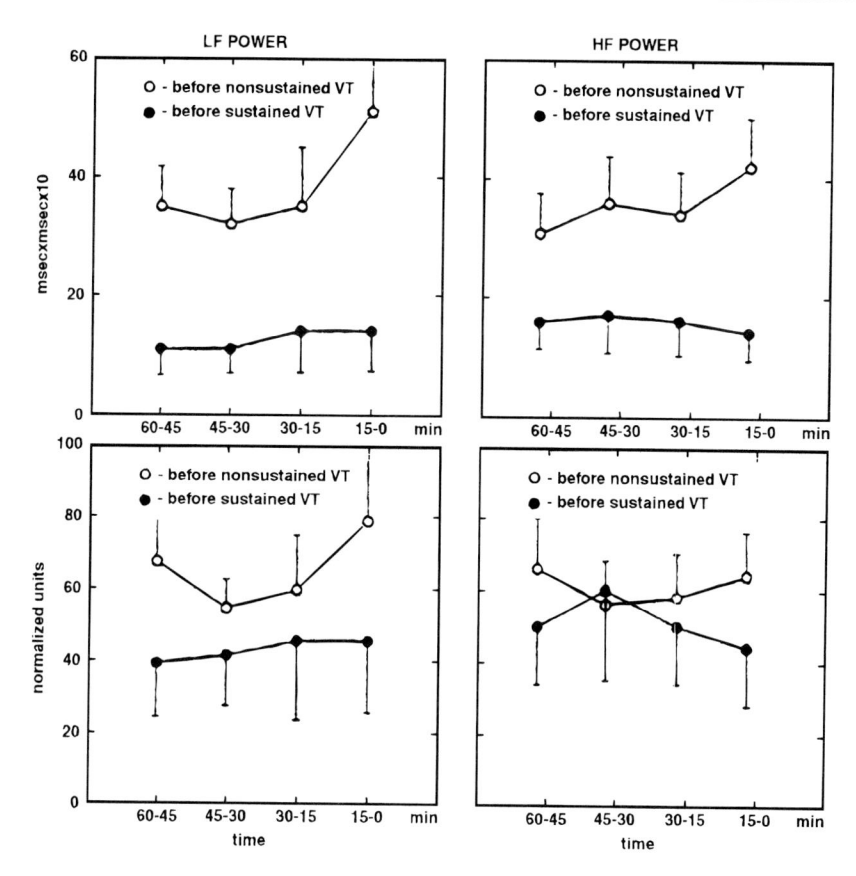

Figure 8. Graphs showing low-frequency (LF) and high-frequency (HF) powers of heart rate variability in absolute units (upper curves) and normalized units (lower curves) before the onset of ventricular tachycardias (VTs). The LF component increased significantly before the onset of nonsustained VT ($P < 0.05$). (Reproduced with permission from Reference 32.)

be delivered in an attempt to slow the ventricular rate or to abort the tachycardia. There is a suggestion from recent work[35] that the total power of the heart rate variability and particularly the low-frequency (LF) component can predict VT up to 15 minutes prior to the episode (Figure 8). If this is so, a bolus of β blocker might be used to prevent the arrhythmia.

There is also an indication that QT dispersion in patients with long QT syndrome could signal excessive sympathetic tone and foreshadow an arrhythmic event.[33] Infusion of a drug bolus could be used to prevent the arrhythmic event. If adenosine was available, it too could be used to terminate reentrant supraventricular tachyarrhythmias almost instantly.

Control of Ischemia

Monitoring of ECG between the shocking electrode and a subcutaneous lead or between the subcutaneous lead and the device case may be used to detect ischemia. When detected a rapid acting vasodilator such as nitroglycerin or equivalent could be infused to minimize or abolish ischemia. Ischemia may also occur during exercise. The availability of a metabolic sensor may be used to assist in the decision to increase the rate of vasodilator infusion.

Modulation of End-Diastolic and End-Systolic Pressures

The ability to minimize end-diastolic pressure and enhance left ventricular relaxation is the primary objective in heart failure patients. This may be accomplished more effectively with an infusion system with a powerful vasodilator drug. This in turn could enhance coronary blood flow and increase myocardial oxygen availability. The relevance of end-diastolic pressure is shown in Figures 9–12. With impaired relaxation, a paradoxical increase in diastolic pressure occurs during tachycardia. Figure 9 illustrates the penalty of high-diastolic pressure on cardiac performance. Increase in diastolic pressure at higher rates increases myocardial oxygen consumption and this is where a vasodilator would be most crucial. Monitoring of pressure generated in the left ventricle would be perhaps most optimal with a pressure sensor inserted into the septal wall, as shown in Figure 13. The sensor would be inserted just far enough to monitor left ventricular pressure but would stay just beneath the endocardial surface so as to minimize a potential for thrombus formation in the left ventricle. The sensor could be either a small piezoresistive diaphragm surrounded with a silicone bubble or an optical sensor also surrounded in a silicone bubble. In this way the peak systolic and diastolic pressures could be monitored. It is preferable to monitor the left ventricular chamber pressures rather than the intra-

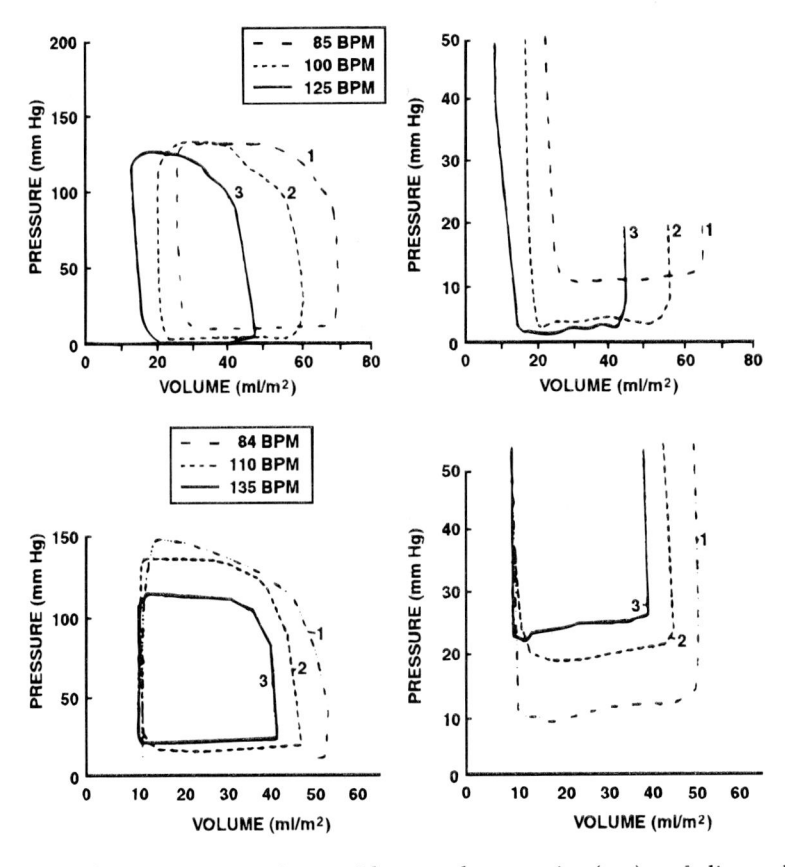

Figure 9. Effect of fast pacing on patients with normal coronaries (top) and diseased coronaries (bottom). Note dramatic upward shift in diastolic pressure in patient with coronary disease. (Reproduced with permission from Grossman W: Diastolic dysfunction and congestive heart failure. *Circulation* 82(Suppl III):III-1, 1990.)

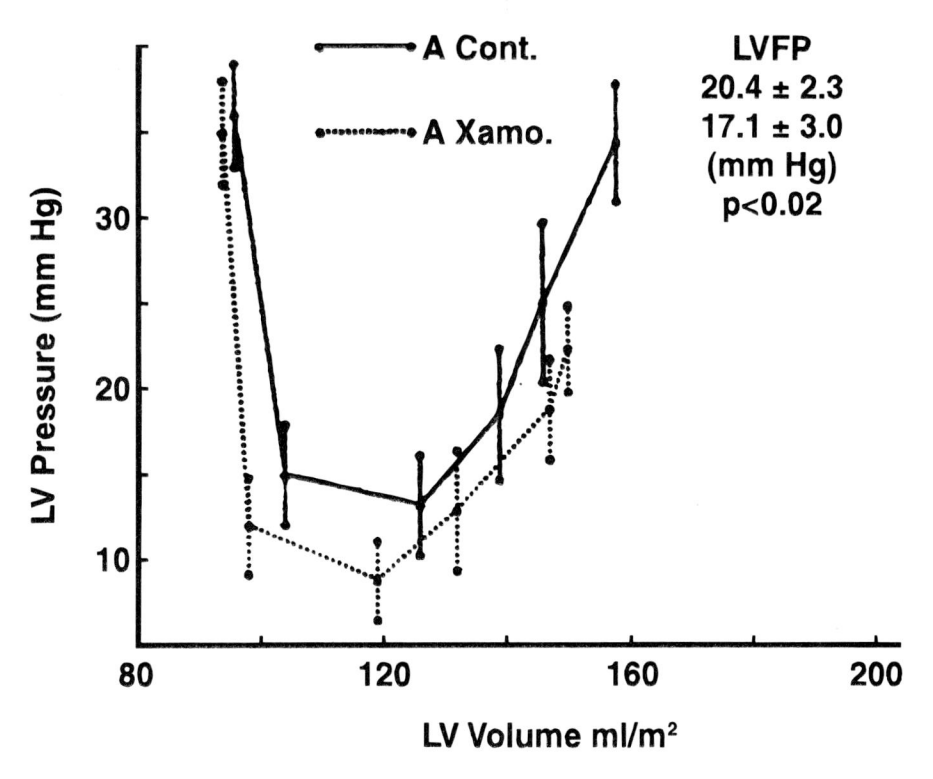

Figure 10. Average left ventricular (LV) pressure-volume relation during diastolic filling in 12 patients of group A before and during xamoterol therapy. LVFP: left ventricular filling pressure. Data are mean ± SEM. (Reproduced with permission from Pouler H, et al: Relationship of diastolic function and exercise capacity in ischemic left ventricular dysfunction. *Circulation* 82(Suppl I):I-89, 1990.)

mural pressures as the former would provide global information identical to the peak arterial pressure.

Enhancement of Cardiac Output

This is a controversial issue. Unloading the heart with vasodilators may be the soundest approach. It is desirable in a system such as the one discussed to measure true cardiac output. This could be done by the use of an ultrasonic Doppler system[34] similar to the conventional esophageal ultrasonic measurements. The sensor would be mounted in the supraventricular vena cava (SVC), the right atrial appendage, or in the pulmonary artery (Figure 13). One of the most difficult questions in such a system would be to know when the cardiac output was appropriate for the patient's needs. With the availability of a pressure-volume loop assessment derived from a sensor that could monitor left ventricular pressure and volume relationships, the objective could be to shift the loop to the left as much as possible. The less effect the inotrope has the more likely it is that the receptors are maximally saturated. A continuous monitoring of the pressure-volume loops may be used to predict deterioration to electromechanical dissociation.

Control of systolic pressure and cardiac output is a complex process.[31,35] Nitroprusside, for example, has a time constant of about 5 minutes and dopamine in excess of 10 minutes. For infusion of nitroprusside the controlling factors are the patient sensitivity to the drug, the initial transport delay, recirculating fraction of the drug, the recir-

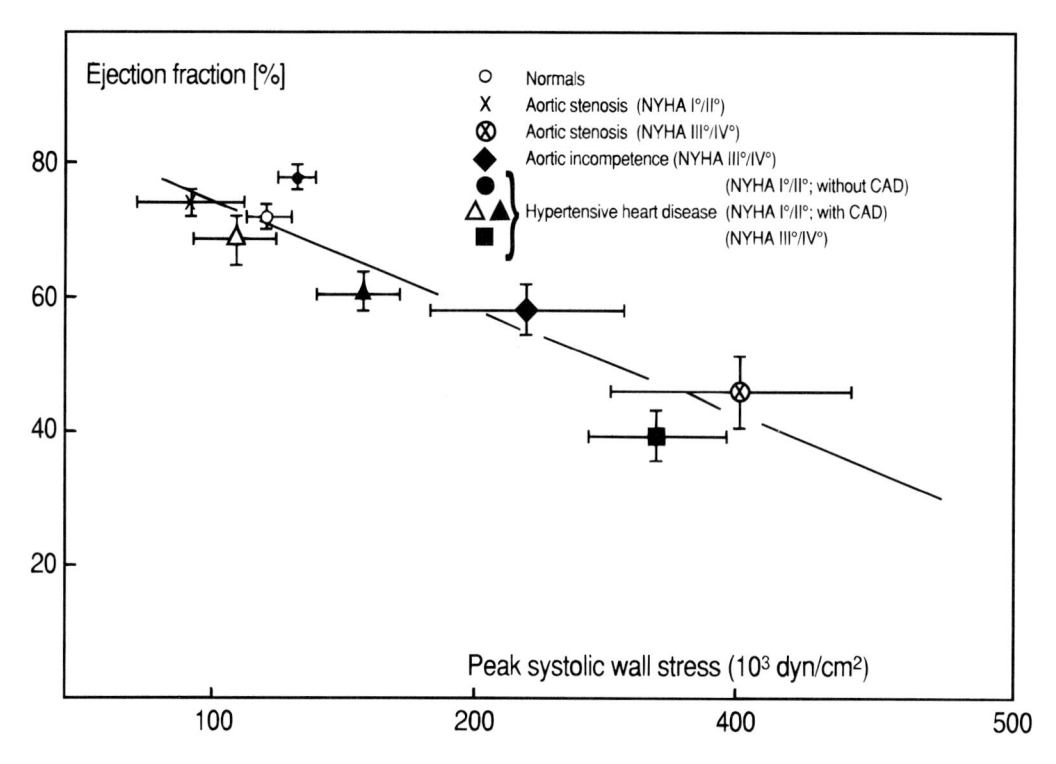

Figure 11. Scatterplot of correlation between systolic wall stress, reflecting left ventricular afterload, and ejection fraction of the left ventricle. There is a reduction of ejection fraction with increasing systolic wall stress that is valid for different forms of the pressure-overloaded left ventricle. NYHA: New York Heart Association. (Reproduced with permission from Schwartzkopff B, et al: Heart failure on the basis of hypertension. *Circulation* 87(Suppl IV):IV-66, 1993.)

culation time, and the response time. Most of these parameters would change in patients undergoing exercise. This is why it would be desirable to use fast acting drugs to minimize long delays and only stimulate and dilate the vessels when needed. This is particularly relevant in situations where the patient has adequate cardiac output at rest and only needs augmentation during exercise. To enable such control a fast acting drug is required with a metabolic indicator, eg, minute ventilation.

Dobutamine could be used with an implanted device, ($t_{1/2}$ 2 minutes) to augument contractility. Dobutamine and esmolol have opposing actions, and could potentially be used in a same patient to achieve opposite effects.

Complex, changing parameters related to drug transport, metabolism, and excretion, will need special attention with a chronic infusion system. One approach[36] is to use a limit cycle method. This is a technique where small pulses of the drug are infused at regular intervals and the response of the system is monitored. The response would enable continuous characterization of the system and checks of the drug infusion process.

Hardware Configuration

The implantable hardware to allow accurate infusion of drugs has been available for about 20 years. The first single rate infusion pump from Infusaid was followed by the development of programmable pumps by Medtronic, Pacesetter Systems, and Siemens.

The main driving force for the develop-

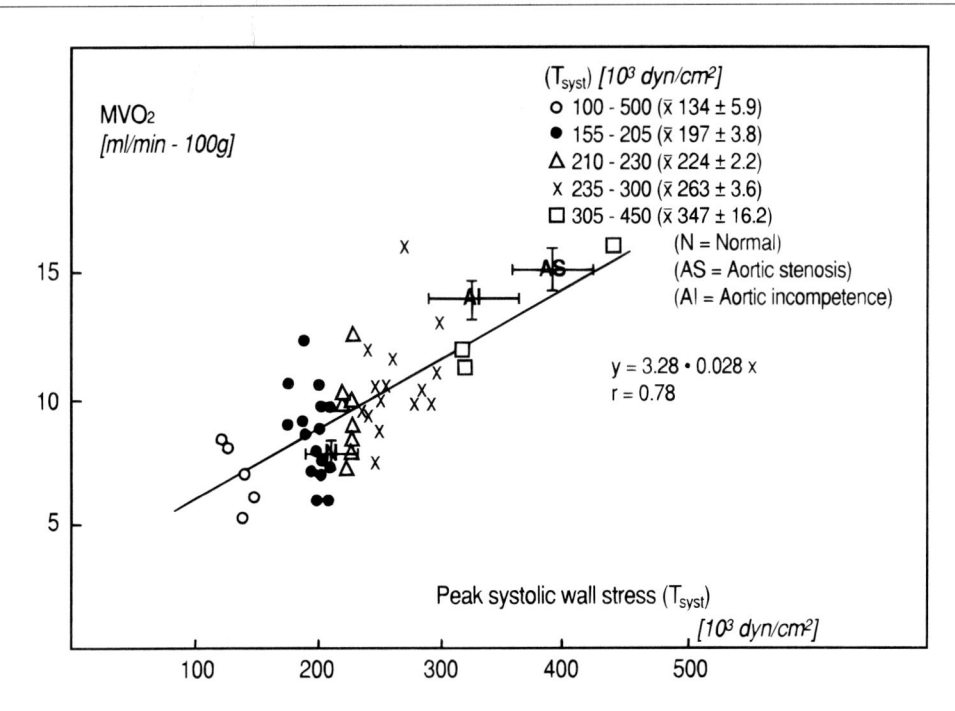

Figure 12. Scatterplot of correlation between systolic wall stress and myocardial oxygen comsumption (MVO$_2$) per 100 g myocardium. There is an increase in MVO$_2$ with increasing wall stress. (Reproduced with permission from Schwartzkopff B, et al: Heart failure on the basis of hypertension. *Circulation* 87(Suppl IV):IV-66, 1993.)

ment of implantable pumps has been for dispensing insulin in patients with diabetes. MiniMed implantable pump, MIP-2001™ (MiniMed Technologies, Sylmar, CA) is an excellent example of the sophistication achieved by these pumps. It is a totally self-contained system (Figure 14) with its own telemetry, electronic controls, and power source. The resolution of drug infusion is down to 0.5 μL per stroke and uses an electrically driven pulsatile delivery system. In addition, it has multiple safety features like an audible alarm and negative pressure in the reservoir to allow injection of insulin into the reservoir. This system has been undergoing intensive clinical trials under the auspices of the United States Food and Drug Administration. It is important to note that insulin, originally too unstable for use in an implantable pump, has now been stabilized effectively for this application.

The pumps currently in use utilize vapor pressure power, peristalsis, or reciprocation accumulator delivery modalities singly or in combination. The most common implementation is the vapor pressure pump where the drug is contained in a bellows-type reservoir surrounded by a chamber containing volatile liquid (charging fluid). Vapor pressure from the enclosed volatile liquid expels the drug into a reciprocating chamber that fills and is emptied by a solenoid into the outlet port and catheter.[37] The drug is dispensed into the reservoir via a special self-sealing port percutaneously. With many of the new pumps a special port exists, flushing the catheter with an appropriate biocompatible fluid. A pump that embodies the simplicity of such devices was developed at the University of Minnesota, and is shown in Figure 15. The driving power for the drug is the elastomeric spring and the drug is delivered via the reciprocating chambers by a solenoid.

The combination of defibrillator and infusion pump could take the form shown in

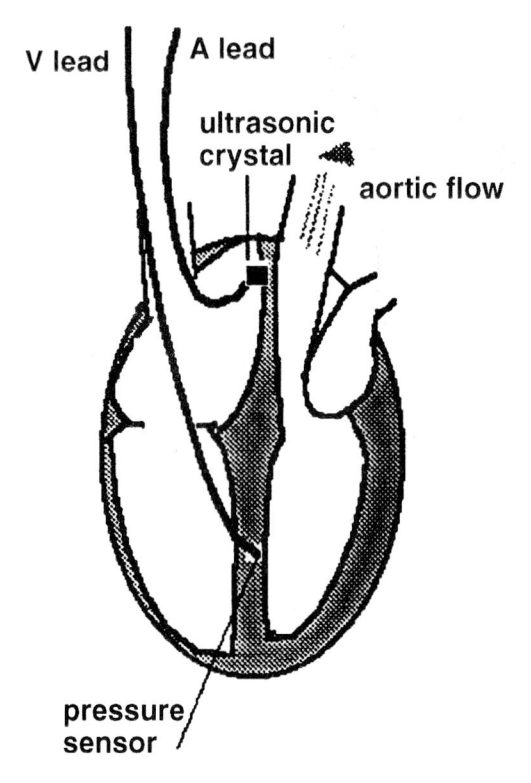

Figure 13. Sensors on conventional leads for measuring aortic flow and left ventricular (LV) pressure.

Figure 16. The control of the infusion pump would be via a single control line from the defibrillator, to drive the solenoid. This control line would be a port on the implanted microprocessor giving the defibrillator a total control of the infusion rate. As the device can keep track of the amount of drug dispensed, in most cases it will be able to warn the patient when it is running low. However, in the long run some indicator of the actual amount of drug in the reservoir remaining would be needed. This could be accomplished with a sensor on the wall of the reservoir that could be sensed by the defibrillator without adding any more ports, or a flow sensor which indicates that drug is being pumped out. Probably both would be needed. When two drug reservoirs are required, as with a β blocker and a vasodilator, additional control circuitry would be added for the pump to direct control, and to perform certain checks, eg, correct filling, level of the reservoir, etc. An alternative would be to keep the pumps electrically simple and to connect sensors back to the main cardioverter-defibrillator controller.

With the availability of left ventricular

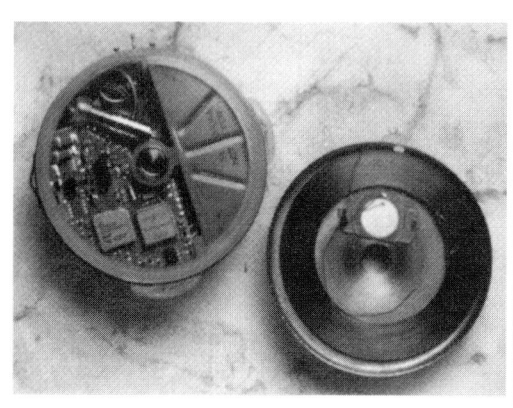

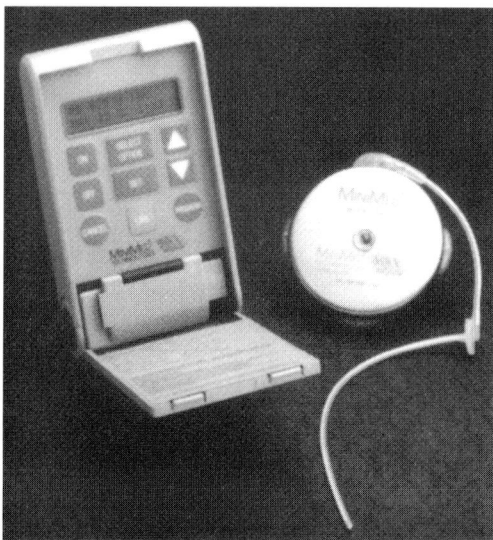

Figure 14. The MiniMed implantable pump and external programmer. The implanted controls, telemetry, and pump make this as sophisticated as an implantable defibrillator. (Photographs courtesy of MiniMed Technologies, Sylmar, CA).

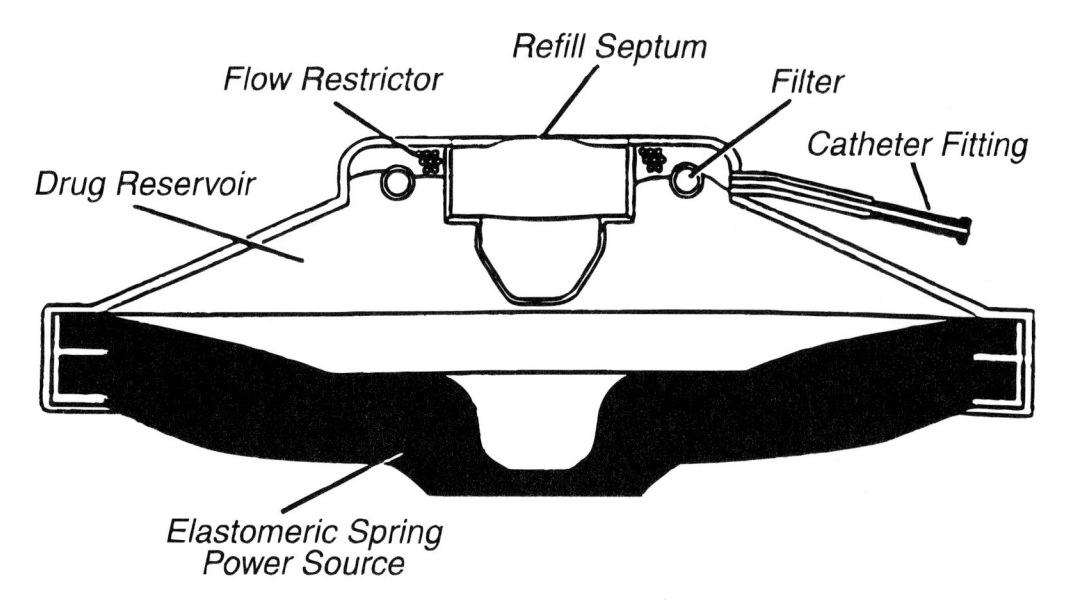

Combination of Drug Delivery Systems and ICDs • 747

Figure 15. Cross-sectional view of a spring-driven implantable pump. (Reproduced with permission from Buchwald H, Rhode TD: Implantable pumps: recent progress and anticipated future. *ASAIO J* p. 772, 1992.)

DEFIBRILLATION AND INFUSION PUMP

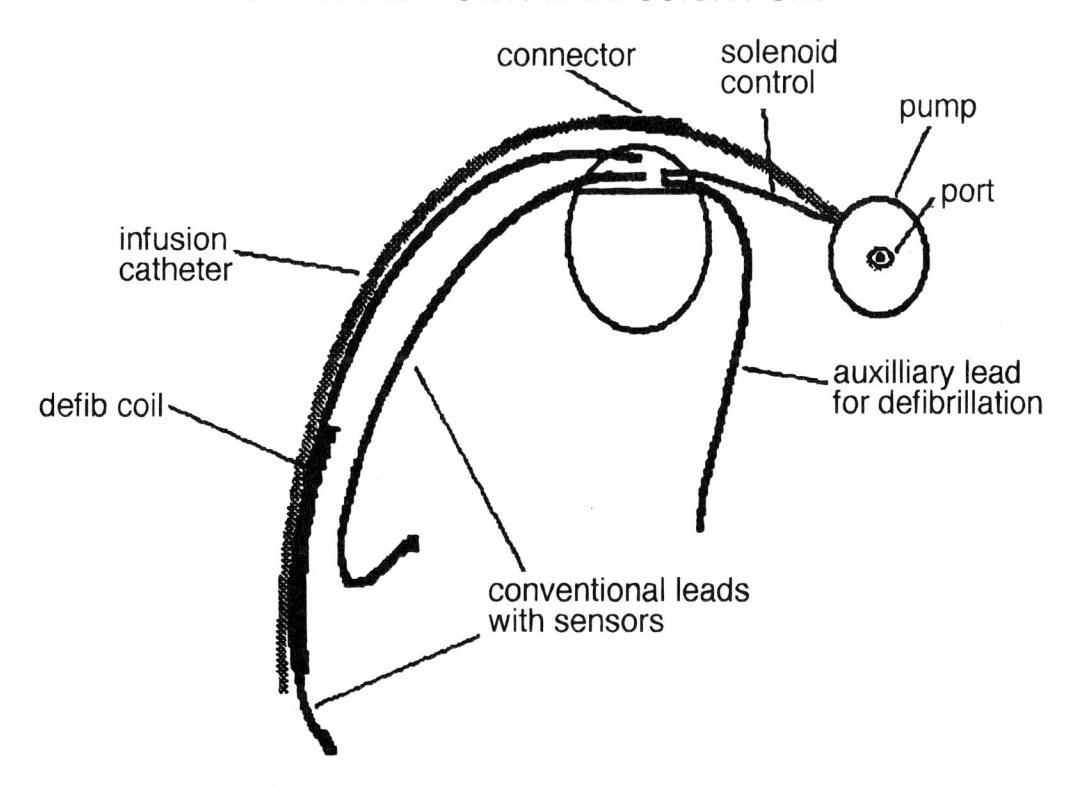

Figure 16. A schematic of an implantable system with sensors and infusion pump.

pressure and stroke volume sensors the system could keep track of the power generated by the heart and cardiac output. This capability would make the function of the defibrillators totally automatic, since the system could determine with precision the consequences of arrhythmias and "decide" which therapy to use (ATP, defibrillation, or infusion).

Summary

The realization of a combined defibrillation and infusion pump is contingent on the establishment of a specific medical rationale critical for its use. In this chapter the emphasis was placed on what this need may be. At the present time, a large number of patients suffering from congestive heart failure and frequent arrhythmias have poor prognosis. Perhaps the ability to intervene on a continuous basis electrically and chemically will benefit these patients. But before we can implement this concept, we have a ways to go with our understanding of the pharmacology of fast acting drugs and to perfect sophisticated implantable sensors. Complex feedback loops would have to be developed to automatically control and adjudicate between various sensors, a task which may require increased computational powers and additional electrical power to provide sufficient energy to drive the system with reasonable battery longevity. Nevertheless, the concept is intellectually intriguing and presents a formidable engineering challenge to implement.

References

1. Myerburg RJ, Castellanos A: Cardiac arrest and sudden cardiac death. In: *Heart Disease. A Textbook of Cardiovascular Medicine*. Edited by E Braunwald. Philadelphia, PA: WB Saunders, 1988, p. 742.
2. Myerburg RJ, Kessler KM, Bassett AL, et al: A biological approach to sudden cardiac death: structure, function and cause. *Am J Cardiol* 63:1512, 1989.
3. Wolf F, Akhtar M: Sudden cardiac death. In: *Heart Disease and Rehabilitation*. Edited by ML Pollock, DH Schmidt. Houghton Mifflin; 1979, p. 12.
4. Kim SG, Fisher JD, Furman S, et al: Benefits of implantable defibrillators are overestimated by sudden death rate and better represented by total arrhythmic death rate. *J Am Coll Cardiol* 17:1587, 1991.
5. Guarnieri T, Levine JH, Griffith LFC, et al: When "sudden cardiac death" is not so sudden; lessons learned from the automatic implantable defibrillator. *Am J Cardiol* 62:803, 1988.
6. Kuck KH, Siebels J, Schneider M, et al: Preliminary results of a randomized trial, AICD vs drugs (abstract). *Rev Eur Technol Biomed* 12:110, 1990.
7. Spenser WJ: A review of programmed insulin delivery systems. *IEEE Trans Biomed Eng* 28:237, 1981.
8. Rupp WM, Barbosa RJ, Blackshear TD, et al: Continuous infusion of insulin in 5 adult onset diabetic patients with an implantable insulin pump (abstract). *Circulation* 64:IV, 1981.
9. Leavens ME, Hill CJ, Cech DA, et al: Intrathecal and intraventricular morphine for pain in cancer patients: initial study. *J Neurosurg* 56:241, 1982.
10. Naofrio BM, Yakesh TL, Arnold PG: Continuous low dose intrathecal morphine administration in the treatment of chronic pain of malignant origin. *Mayo Clin Proc* 56:516, 1981.
11. Packer M: Prolonging life in patients with congestive heart failure: the next frontier. *Circulation* 75(Suppl IV):IV-1, 1987.
12. Yusuf S, Teo KK: Approaches to prevention of sudden death: need for fundamental re-evaluation. *J Cardiovasc Electrophysiol* 2(Suppl):S223, 1991.
13. Pitt B: Role of β adrenergic blocking agents in prevention sudden cardiac death. *Circulation* 85(Suppl):I-107, 1992.
14. The Cardiac Arrhythmia Suppression Trial (CAST) investigators: Preliminary report: effect of encainide and flecainide on mortality in a randomized trial of arrhythmia suppression after myocardial infarction. *N Engl J Med* 321:406, 1989.
15. Akhtar M, Breithardt G, Camm AJ, et al: CAST and beyond: implications of the Cardiac Arrhythmia Suppression Trial. *Circulation* 81:1123, 1990.
16. Wilson JR, Schwartz JS, St. John Sutton M, et al: Prognosis in severe heart failure: rela-

tion to hemodynamic measurements and ventricular ectopic activity. *J Am Coll Cardiol* 2:403, 1983.
17. Lu M, Stevenson WG, Stevenson LW, et al: Diverse mechanisms of unexpected cardiac arrest in advanced heart failure. *Circulation* 80:1675, 1989.
18. Velebit V, Podrid P, Lown B, et al: Aggravation and provocation of ventricular arrhythmias by antiarrhythmic drugs. *Circulation* 67:886, 1982.
19. Gottlieb SS, Kikin ML, Medina N, et al: Comparative hemodynamic effects of procainamide, tocainide and encainide in chronic heart failure. *Circulation* 81:860, 1990.
20. Grimm W, Flores BF, Marchlinski FE: Electrocardiographically documented unnecessary spontaneous shocks in 241 patients with implantable cardioverter defibrillators. *PACE* 15:11:1667, 1992.
21. Thorne RD, Jenkins JM, DiCarlo LA: A comparison of four new time domain techniques for discriminating monomorphic ventricular tachycardia from sinus rhythm using ventricular waveform morphology. *IEEE Trans Biomed Eng* 38:561, 1991.
22. Greenhut SE, Deering TF, Steinhaus B, et al: Separation of ventricular tachycardia from sinus rhythm using a practical real time template matching computer system. *PACE* 15:2146, 1992.
23. Jung W, Manz M, Tebbenjohanns J, et al: Incidence of atrial fibrillation following shock delivery of an implantable defibrillator. Comparison of two lead systems (abstract). *PACE* 15:567, 1992.
24. Wang PJ, Lu RM, Rastager H, et al: Using the pacing integral to improve ventricular fibrillation detection (abstract). *Circulation* 86(Suppl I):I-442, 1992.
25. Langberg JT, Underwood T, Gallagher M, et al: The effect of Ibutilide applied to the epicardium on defibrillation threshold (abstract). *J Am Coll Cardiol* 21:244A, 1993.
26. Cammilli L, Musante R, Perna AM, et al: Immediate pharmacological defibrillation in swine: a new algorithm for a device performed to suppress ventricular fibrillation by drug injection in coronary bed (abstract). *PACE* 16:1119, 1993.
27. Arzbaecher R, Bump TE: Development of an automatic implanted drug infusion system for the management of cardiac arrhythmias. *Proc IEEE* 76(9):1204, 1988.
28. Egelstein D, Bruce BL: Adenosine mediated increase in transmyocardial defibrillation threshold is attenuated by heptanal. *J Am Coll Cardiol* 21(2):305A, 1993.
29. Krugger-Theimer E: Continuous intravenous infusion and multicompartment accumulation. *Eur J Pharmacol* 4:317, 1968.
30. Miller RR, Awan NA, Joye JA, et al: Combined dopamine and nitroprusside therapy in congestive heart failure. *Circulation* 55:88, 1977.
31. Yu C, Roy RJ, Kaufman H, et al: Multiple-model adaptive predictive control of mean arterial pressure and cardiac output. *IEEE Trans Biomed Eng* 39(8):765, 1992.
32. Heikki V, Volkama JO, Airaksinen KEJ, et al: Frequency domain measurement of heart rate variability before the onset of nonsustained and sustained ventricular tachycardia in patients with coronary artery disease. *Circulation* 87(4):1220, 1993.
33. Priori SG, Napolitano C, Diehl L, et al: Dispersion of repolarization as a marker to predict efficacy of antiadrenergic therapy (abstract). *J Am Coll Cardiol* 21(Suppl A):94A, 1993.
34. Valenta HL, Wrigley RH, Ellenbogen KA: A new hemodynamic sensor for pacemakers and defibrillators (abstract) 14:659, 1991.
35. Behbehani K, Cross RR: A controller for regulation of mean arterial blood pressure using optimum nitroprusside infusion rate. *IEEE Trans Bioeng* 38:513, 1991.
36. Mandel JE, et al: Characterization of blood pressure response to sodium nitroprusside by limit cycle behavior. In: *Proceedings of the Ninth Annual Conference of IEEE*. EMBS 1987.
37. Buchwald H, Rohde TD: Implantable pumps: recent progress and anticipated future. *ASAIO J* p. 772, 1992.

Chapter 36

Implantable Cardioverter-Defibrillators: An Overview and Future Directions

Edwin G. Duffin and S. Serge Barold

Introduction

The demonstrated efficacy of the automatic implantable defibrillator has allowed it to become a mainstream therapy for the prevention of sudden arrhythmic cardiac death.[1-3] Although the defibrillator has been greatly refined since its first appearance[4] in 1980 there is room for improvement.[5] Pulse generators are generally too large for pectoral implantation. Simpler, more effective transvenous lead systems are needed to provide rapid, minimally invasive implants with high assurance of success, and with greater patient comfort. Detection algorithms need greater specificity without any sacrifice of sensitivity.[6] More extensive monitoring is needed to document performance and to facilitate appropriate programming. Dual-chamber antibradycardia pacing is needed to provide hemodynamic support and, perhaps, to minimize the progression of heart failure and reduce the occurrence of atrial fibrillation.[7-10] Generator longevity is limited, particularly for use in pacing-dependent patients, and the therapy remains costly. These issues are being addressed by medical researchers and the various manufacturers, and progress should mirror that seen with the implantable pacemaker.

Transvenous Leads

Lead placement requiring entry through the chest has been a major encumbrance to the use of the implantable defibrillator. It is associated with approximately 3% to 4% perioperative mortality,[11-13] significant hospitalization time (mean stay of 28 days in one study)[14] and complications,[15] patient discomfort, and high costs. The mortality and complication rates may be dependent on the inclusion of additional surgical procedures at the time of defibrillator implantation. Watkins and Taylor[16] reported 2% mortality with combined surgery versus 3.2% with defibrillator implantation alone. Gartman et al.[15] noted that defibrillator implantation with concomitant surgery requiring cardiopulmonary bypass was associated with a 4.9% mortality rate and an incidence of 19.5% postoperative complications whereas isolated defibrillator implantation was associated with a mortality of 3.3% and a postoperative complication incidence of 11.6%. Although several approaches have been proffered to minimize the surgical procedure, including subcostal, subxiphoid,[16,17] and thoracoscopic,[18,19] the ultimate solution is the development of fully transvenous lead

---

From Singer I, (ed.) Implantable Cardioverter-Defibrillator. Armonk, NY: Futura Publishing Company, Inc.; © 1994.

systems with acceptable defibrillation thresholds.

Early transvenous leads had unacceptable dislodgment rates,[20] fractures,[21] and sensing problems.[22] More recent versions of these systems offer significant performance improvements while achieving acceptable thresholds in 67% to 95% of patients attempted. Mean defibrillation thresholds range from 10.9–18.1 J,[13,23–26] significantly higher than the thresholds obtained with epicardial lead systems,[13] and these minimally invasive systems require extensive testing of multiple right ventricular (RV), superior vena cava (SVC), coronary sinus (CS), right atrium (RA), right atrial appendage, and subcutaneous lead configurations and electrode spacings.[23,27,28] Nonthoracotomy lead systems have been reported to require nearly twice as much defibrillation test time (57 minutes versus 32 minutes) than is required for epicardial systems.[26] Moreover, patients object to the discomfort caused by the subcutaneous electrodes that are frequently required to obtain suitable thresholds. Long-term reliability data are still evolving for these systems, and they do not offer low enough defibrillation thresholds to allow reductions in generator output energy, and as a consequence, size. Despite the need for improvement, nonthoracotomy leads already offer advantages beyond the avoidance of major surgery. They are easier to remove should there be infections or a need for lead system revision. Although it has been claimed that the pacing thresholds of current transvenous defibrillation electrodes are superior to those of epicardial systems,[23] the reported values were identical to those reported by others for epicardial systems (0.96 ± 0.39 V versus 0.96 ± 0.5 V).[23,29]. The transvenous lead electrogram amplitudes (16.4 ± 6.4 mV) were somewhat larger than the epicardial lead electrograms (13.7 ± 5.9 mV). The eventual application of steroid technology should provide increased pacing efficiency with transvenous lead systems.

Recently, a simple approach that makes defibrillator implantation parallel that for a unipolar pacemaker has been reported. A single RV lead having bipolar pace/sense electrodes and one RV high-voltage electrode is used in conjunction with a defibrillator housing that serves as the second high-voltage electrode (Figure 1). With the generator electrode placed in the patient's left pectoral region biphasic pulse defibrillation thresholds for 37 patients averaged 9.4 ± 5.9 J.[30] This technique appears to be practicable only with generators suitable for pectoral placement, but such devices will become increasingly available.

It is hoped that further refinement of transvenous lead systems will yield simpler systems that require minimal time and effort to place while achieving defibrillation thresholds below 5 J.

Generator Size

Size reduction is a major imperative for defibrillator improvement. Although there have been limited reports of totally pectoral implantation of defibrillators,[31,32] this approach is not the norm given the size of currently available defibrillators. A transvenous defibrillator small enough for implantation in the pectoral region would: shorten implantation procedures; eliminate the need for an operating room; obviate the need for lead tunneling; minimize the number of incisions; reduce the likelihood of infections; simplify lead repositioning or replacement when necessary; reduce lead length and resistance thereby increasing electrical efficiency; and reduce implantation costs.

Defibrillators must convert battery voltages of 2.8–6.5 V to the 600–750 V needed to defibrillate the heart. The voltage conversion process cannot supply this high voltage at current strengths needed for defibrillation, so the defibrillator circuits accumulate the high-voltage charge in electrical components called capacitors that account for 20% to 30% of the volume of a typical defibrillator. The capacitors are large because they need to operate at high voltages.

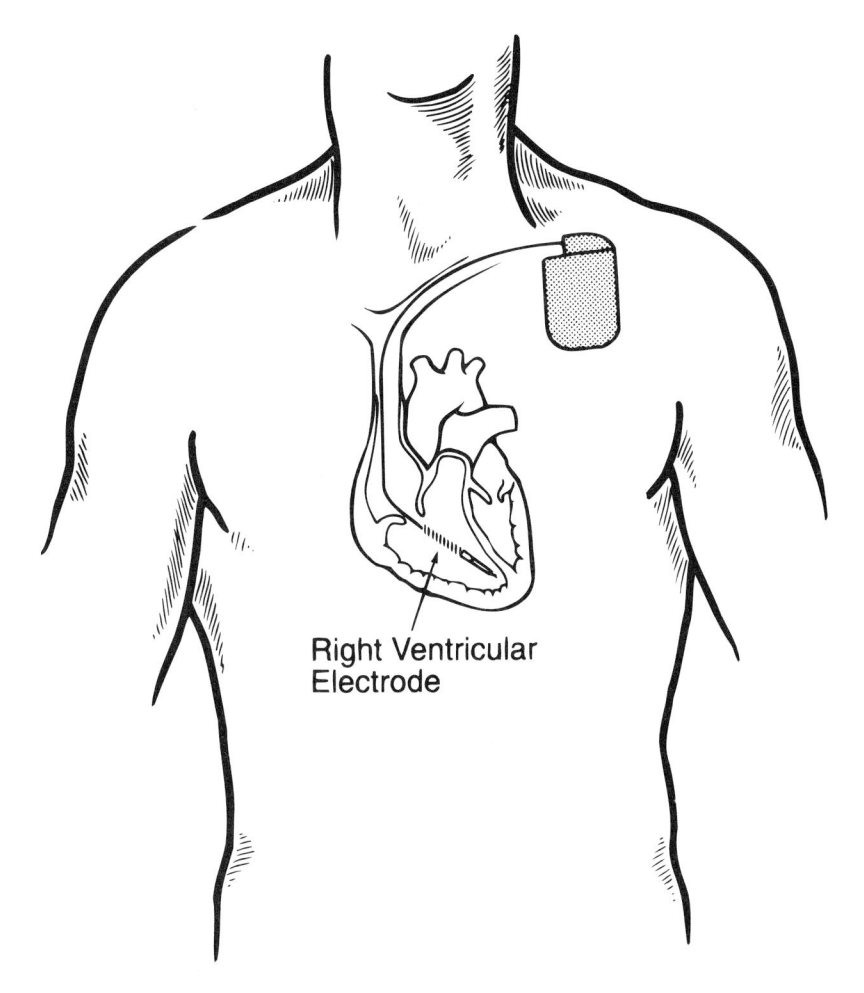

Figure 1. Schematic representation of an implantable defibrillator in which the pulse generator housing provides one of the high-voltage defibrillation electrodes. This generator is used in conjunction with a single transvenous lead system having one high-voltage electrode in the right ventricular cavity and a bipolar electrode pair in the right ventricular apex for pacing and sensing. This system provides thresholds of 9–10 J with pectoral placement of the generator.

Capacitors are, in essence, a series of electrically conductive plates separated by an insulating material, the dielectric, that must not allow charge to pass from plate to plate. High operating voltages require relatively thick insulating layers that, in turn, result in physically large capacitors. Unfortunately, the thick insulating layers reduce the effective storage capacity of the devices making it necessary to increase the surface area of the conductive plates. This exacerbates the size problem. Currently available capacitors suitable for defibrillator use are formed electrolytically and the insulating dielectric will degrade and become leaky if the capacitors are not charged regularly. Defibrillators must have their capacitors charged periodically for this reason. The process is commonly referred to as "reforming the capacitors." If this is not done, the charge time prior to defibrillation can become excessively long because some of the charge that is placed on the plates leaks off before charging is complete. Early defibrillators require that the patient periodically return to the clinic to have the capacitors reformed, while newer devices automatically reform the capacitors at preset or programmable times. Eventually, it is anticipated that new capacitor technology, perhaps ceramic or thin film, will offer higher storage densities, greater shape variability for denser component packaging, and freedom from the need to waste battery capacity performing periodic reforming charges. Packaging density has already improved from 0.03 J/cc for devices such as the early cardioverter, to 0.43 J/cc with some investigational implantable cardioverter-defibrillators (ICDs). Capacitors that allow conformal shaping could readily increase this density to more than 0.6 J/cc.

Commercially available implantable defibrillators weigh between 197 and 237 g, and have volumes ranging from 113–145 cc. Clinical trials are in progress on devices having volumes ranging from 178 cc to 78 cc, and weights between 275 and 132 g. Smaller devices are on the drawing boards, and size reductions will be dramatic with the introduction of improved capacitor and integrated circuit technologies, and lead systems offering lower pacing and defibrillation thresholds. Progress should parallel that made with antibradycardia pacemakers that have evolved from 250 g, nonprogrammable, VOO units with 600 μJ pacing outputs to 26 g, multiprogrammable, DDDR units with dual 25 μJ outputs (Figure 2).

Detection

Defibrillator designs have been intentionally biased to overtreat in preference to the dire consequences associated with failure to treat. It is not surprising, then, that there is a significant incidence of inappropriate therapy delivery. Most commonly these unwarranted therapies are triggered by supraventricular tachyarrhythmias, especially atrial fibrillation, or sinus tachycardia associated with rates faster than the ventricular tachycardia (VT) detection point.[6,33] Additional causes include nonsustained VTs[6,33]; oversensing of T waves[33,34]; double counting of R waves; and pacing stimuli

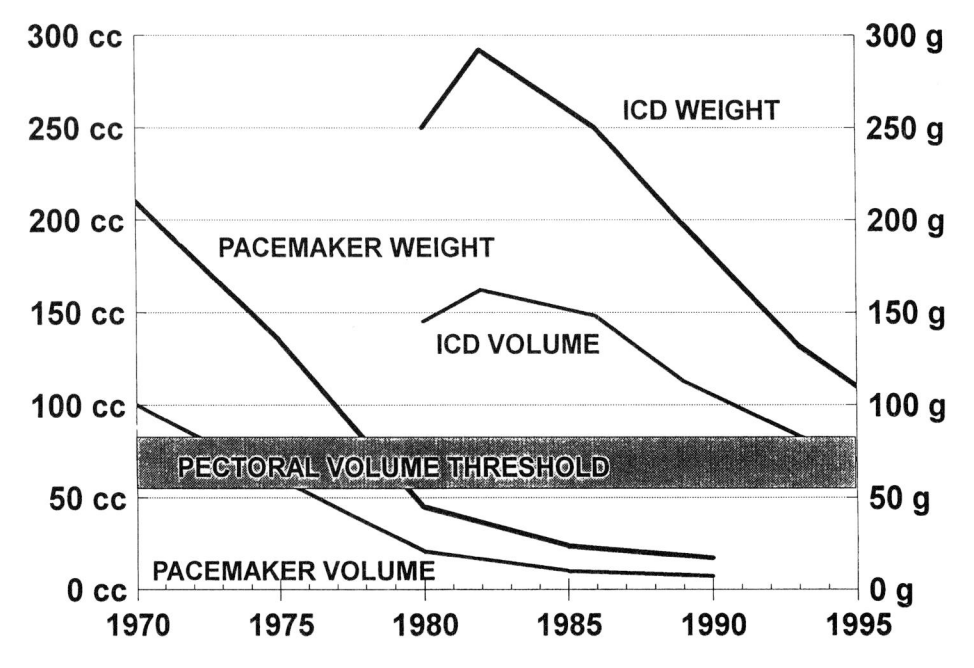

Figure 2. Evolution of implantable defibrillator weights and volumes contrasted with similar data for implantable antibradycardia pacemakers.

from brady pacemakers,[35] and technical faults such as loose lead-generator connections or lead fractures.[33,36,37]

Most defibrillator detection algorithms rely primarily on heart rate to indicate the presence of a treatable rhythm. Additional refinements sometimes include: simple morphology assessments, as with the probability density function, and analysis of rhythm stability and rate of change in rate.[38,39] These additions can increase algorithm specificity, making them useful in carefully selected patients, but they also reduce detection algorithm sensitivity and must be used with care.

The probability density function evaluates the percentage of time that the filtered electrogram spends in a window centered on the baseline. It has been received with some reservation because there appear to be no reliable clinical guidelines for use of the algorithm in individual patients, it may result in nondetection of narrow complex tachycardias, and, in most patients, it adds nothing to the detection of tachycardia.[40,41] Moreover, it has been reported that at elevated rates the probability density function rarely determines a normal complex rhythm to be nonventricular in origin.[42]

The rate of change in rate or onset evaluation discriminates sinus tachycardia from VT on the basis of the typically gradual acceleration of sinus rhythms versus the relatively abrupt acceleration of many pathological tachycardias.[43] This technique also suffers from lack of clinical guides for application in specific patients, and even when programmed optimally it will prevent detection of VTs that evolve during sinus tachycardia.[44] It can also be fooled by premature ventricular contractions that occur while sinus rhythm accelerates through the detection rate threshold.[45]

The rate stability function is designed to bar detection of tachyarrhythmias as long as the rate variability exceeds a physician programmed tolerance, thereby reducing the likelihood of inappropriate therapy delivery in response to atrial fibrillation. This concept appears to be one of the more successful detection algorithm enhancements.[46] It must also be used with caution, however, as it can prevent detection of polymorphic tachycardias with irregular cycle lengths.

Because these additions reduce sensitivity, some defibrillator designs offer a supplementary algorithm that will trigger therapy in response to an elevated rate with prolonged duration. These extended high-rate algorithms bypass all or portions of the normal detection screening, resulting in low specificity for rhythms with prolonged elevated rates such as exercise-induced sinus tachycardia. Consequently, use of this algorithm generally increases the incidence of inappropriate therapies.

Improvements in arrhythmia detection specificity would be welcome, but they must not decrease the excellent sensitivity offered by current algorithms. It would be desirable to configure algorithms that go beyond simple detection of elevated rates. They should classify the rhythms in order to elicit the most appropriate therapeutic responses. The inevitable introduction of defibrillators incorporating dual-chamber pacemaker capability will certainly help in this quest, since it will then be possible to obtain an atrial electrogram to assist the classification process. It would also be desirable to have a means of evaluating the patient's hemodynamic tolerance of the rhythm, so that the more comfortable pacing sequences could be used as long as the patient was not syncopal, yet branch quickly to a definitive shock should the patient begin to lose consciousness.

Although various detection processes have been proposed,[47,48] many have not been tested clinically, in some cases because the requisite processing power was not available in implantable systems, and in some cases because sensor technology was not yet ready for long-term implantation. These barriers are constantly being lowered, offering hope that eventually some of these elegant proposals may prove practicable. Examples of the myriad of proposed detection enhancements are as follows.

Enhanced Analyses of Cardiac Event Timing

- Evaluation of PR and RR stability to distinguish VT and supraventricular tachycardia (SVT)[49]
- Analysis of atrioventricular (AV) interval variation to distinguish VT with 1:1 ventriculoatrial (VA) conduction from sinus tachycardia[50]
- Analysis of the temporal distribution of atrial electrogram intervals and of ventricular electrogram intervals[51]
- Analysis of the timing differences and/or coherency of multiple ventricular electrograms[52,53]
- Analysis of the ventricular response to a provocative atrial extrastimulus to distinguish sinus tachycardia from 1:1 paroxysmal tachycardia[54,55]

Electrogram Analyses

- Evaluation of the paced depolarization integral to distinguish VT from various supraventricular rhythms[56,57]
- Various morphology analyses of RV electrograms to distinguish VT from supraventricular rhythms[58–65]
- Morphology analysis of atrial electrograms to distinguish retrograde from antegrade atrial activity[66]
- Combined analysis of atrial and ventricular electrograms[41,67–69]

Hemodynamic Parameters

- Right ventricular pulsatile pressure for VT[70,71]
- Mean right atrial and mean RV pressures to detect hemodynamically unstable rhythms[72]
- Wedge CS pressure to indicate systemic pressure[73]
- Static RV pressure, right atrial pressure, RV stroke volume, mixed venous oxygen saturation, and mixed venous blood temperature for hemodynamic tachycardia detection[74]
- Measurement of left ventricular impedance or intramyocardial pressure gradient for the detection of pace terminable tachyarrhythmias and malignant VT[75]
- Evaluation of changes in transcardiac impedance to detect ventricular fibrillation (VF)[76,77]
- Measurement of aortic and pulmonary artery flow using ultrasonic sensors[78]

Physical Motion Detection

- Motion sensors to distinguish nonexercise-related tachycardias[79]

The continuing evolution of implantable sensors for antibradycardia pacing and implantable monitoring purposes will complement similar activities in defibrillator development. The rapid improvement in microprocessor speed, memory capabilities, and energy efficiencies will also contribute to making these advanced arrhythmia classification and detection schemes practicable. Perhaps the day will come when it is no longer necessary to prescribe drugs to adjust rhythms to fit defibrillator detection requirements.

Although defibrillators are biased for high detection sensitivity, undersensing does occur. Documentation of such behavior is not easily had, even with expanded memories and recording systems, since devices rarely record events that they do not detect, but undersensing has been shown to result from: inappropriate detection algorithm programming, such as an excessively high tachycardia detection rate; inappropriate amplifier gain characteristics[80]; and electrode designs that place the sensing terminals too close to the high-voltage electrodes with a consequent reduction in electrogram amplitude following shocks.[22] Undersensing can also result in the induction of tachycardia should the amplifier gain control algorithm result in undersensing of sinus rhythms.[81]

Therapy

Pioneering implantable defibrillators were capable only of defibrillation shocks. Subsequently, synchronized cardioversion was added to the therapeutic repertoire. When needed, antibradycardia pacing had to be provided by implantation of a standard pacemaker in addition to the defibrillator and, if antitachycardia pacing was prescribed, it was necessary to use an antitachycardia pacemaker. In 1993 the FDA approved commercial distribution of implantable defibrillators offering integrated ventricular demand pacemaker function and tiered antiarrhythmia therapy pacing cardioversion/defibrillation. Various antitachycardia pacing algorithms are offered and they all seem to offer comparably high success rates.[82,83] These expanded therapeutic capabilities improve patient comfort by reducing the incidence of shocks in conscious patients,[84,85] eliminate the problems and discomfort associated with implantation of multiple devices, and contribute to a greater degree of success since the prescribed regimens can be carefully tailored to specific patient needs. Availability of devices with antitachycardia pacing capability significantly increases the acceptability of the implantable defibrillator for patients with VT.[86-88] The high efficacy that antitachycardia pacing achieved in the various clinical studies was obtained in private practice centers as readily as it was in academic centers, suggesting that the use of these less traumatic therapies will be widespread.

Despite the tremendous progress of the past decade, there is room for improvement in the high-energy therapeutic options offered by implantable defibrillators. Patch sizing and positioning can be manipulated to obtain decent thresholds in the majority of cases,[89] but there are patients who present with high defibrillation thresholds despite efforts to optimize electrode placement. In one study, 18% of a series of 125 patients had epicardial thresholds > 25 J, and 6% had thresholds exceeding 30 J using two patch electrodes and monophasic waveforms.[90] In this study, the high-threshold patients had lower ejection fractions and a higher incidence of previous heart surgery, but were otherwise unremarkable in comparison to patients with normal thresholds. These patients were managed by using high-output defibrillators, a spring vena cava lead plus patch configuration, or alternative medical therapy. In another series of 236 patients, 5% had two-patch monophasic thresholds exceeding 30 J.[91] These patients were managed by using three or four patch electrodes. Newer generators ameliorate this problem by offering biphasic waveforms[92] or sequential pulse delivery options.[93] Moreover, as electrode designs continue to evolve, the overall system efficiency appears to be improving.[94]

Threshold issues are even more pressing with nonthoracotomy lead approaches. Typical defibrillation energies of 18 J for transvenous lead systems make it difficult to consider reducing the output energy and, thus, the size of implantable generators. Lower shock energies would allow the use of physically smaller capacitors with lower voltage ratings, smaller electronic circuit components, and physically smaller batteries.

The incorporation of biphasic waveforms, proven more effective than monophasic waveforms in human clinical trials,[95,96] is a significant therapeutic advance. Although the reason for this improved performance is unknown,[97] speculative mechanisms include the large voltage change that occurs at the transition from the first to the second phase[98] or hyperpolarization of tissue and reactivation of sodium channels during the initial phase, with resultant tissue conditioning that allows the second phase to more readily excite the myocardium.[99] Investigation of the influence that wave shape plays on defibrillation efficiency continues, and there appears to be opportunity for further gains if the mechanisms can be established.[100,101]

Some defibrillators are designed to deliver a therapeutic shock once the output capacitors are charged no matter what the patient's rhythm. This committed mode of operation avoids the risk of undersensing with consequent failure to confirm tachycardia should the fibrillatory electrogram amplitude diminish in amplitude during capacitor charging. The disadvantage is that nonsustained rhythms or electrical noise can trigger delivery of unnecessary shocks. Other designs reconfirm the presence of tachycardia before delivering antitachycardia shocks, but retain the committed behavior for defibrillation shocks, while still others reconfirm all arrhythmias before delivering any shocks.[102,103] No approach is ideal for every patient, so future systems may allow the physician to program committed or noncommitted behavior on a patient by patient basis.

Antitachycardia pacing and cardioversion are not uniformly successful. There is some incidence of ventricular arrhythmia acceleration with antitachycardia pacing and cardioversion, and it is also not unusual for cardioversion to induce atrial fibrillation that in turn triggers unwarranted therapies. Research continues in an attempt to define pacing, cardioversion, or hybrid approaches that will have a higher success rate and/or a lower risk of acceleration. So far, none have been notably better than current offerings. An ideal therapeutic solution would be capable of preventing the occurrence of tachycardia altogether. Prevention techniques have been investigated, among them the use of precisely timed subthreshold stimuli,[104] simultaneous stimulation at multiple sites,[105] and pacing with elevated energies at the site of the tachycardia,[106] but they generally require a degree of prescience on the part of the device in order to deliver the appropriate preventative measures, use of a more complex lead system, or they are not efficient in terms of energy consumption.

The VVI antibradycardia pacing of current defibrillators is rudimentary, lacking rate responsiveness or dual-chamber pacing capability. Consequently, some defibrillator patients require implantation of a separate dual-chamber pacemaker for adequate hemodynamic support.[107,108] Given the incidence of congestive heart failure in defibrillator patients and the evolving evidence that atrial-based pacing significantly reduces the progression of heart failure, the incidence of atrial fibrillation, and even mortality,[8,10] it is inevitable that future generations of defibrillators will offer dual-chamber pacing capabilities. This will also contribute to better arrhythmia detection algorithms.

Atrial fibrillation that occurs either as a consequence of defibrillator operation or as a natural progression in many defibrillator patients is a major therapeutic challenge. It is certainly possible to adapt implantable defibrillator technology to treat atrial fibrillation, but the challenge is to do so without causing the patient undue discomfort. Studies in sheep demonstrated atrial defibrillation thresholds as low as 1.3 J (50% success rate) using biphasic waveforms applied to electrodes in the CS and right atrial appendage.[109] Canine studies have demonstrated successful defibrillation with internal electrodes having thresholds of 495 V (80% success rate).[110] Biphasic waveform defibrillation of acutely induced atrial fibrillation has been demonstrated in humans with an 80% success rate at 0.4 J using epicardial electrodes.[111] Stand-alone atrial defibrillators are in development and, if they are successful, it is likely that this capability would be integrated into the mainstream ventricular defibrillators as well. However, most conscious patients find shocks above 0.5 J to be unpleasant,[112] and it remains to be demonstrated that a clinically acceptable energy level will be efficacious when applied with transvenous electrode systems to spontaneously occurring atrial fibrillation.[113] Moreover, a stand-alone atrial defibrillator must either deliver an atrial shock with complete assurance of appropriate synchronization to ventricular activity,[109] or it must restrict the therapeutic energy delivery to atrial structures in order to prevent inadvertent induction of a malignant ventricular arrhythmia.

Safety/Ease of Use

Defibrillator implantation and follow-up are complex propositions. Until 1993, all FDA approved implantable defibrillators used epicardial patch electrodes, requiring major surgery.[17] Perioperative complications with such systems are not insignificant,[17] and are exacerbated when the implantation is combined with concomitant surgery.[11] One series of 101 implants reported a morbidity of 15%, perioperative mortality of 4%, and an 11% incidence of VT postoperatively.[15] Various centers have reported perioperative mortality rates ranging from a low of 0% to as much as 9%, with arrhythmia being cited as the most frequent cause of mortality.[11,17] Infection rates as high as 7% have been reported for generator replacement procedures at a major center.[114]

Epicardial systems are used infrequently in centers with access to transvenous electrodes because the physician and patient benefits of the transvenous approach are substantial. Perioperative mortality statistics for implantable defibrillator patients receiving nonthoracotomy leads are typically in the range of 0.7% to 2.2%, lower than is common with epicardial systems,[115–117] while morbidity is typically in the range of 18% to 21%, primarily because of lead dislodgments.[23,118] Hospitalization times are dramatically shortened with current transvenous systems,[23,119] and newer designs promise to decrease this time even further. Dislodgment problems with early transvenous lead systems seem to have been resolved with newer designs and lead anchoring techniques.[23] Early transvenous lead systems were less efficient than epicardial systems, but the newest approaches combined with biphasic defibrillation waveforms are yielding thresholds below 10 J without the time consuming need to evaluate multiple configurations.[30] Moreover, these systems eliminate the use of subcutaneous patch electrodes that cause some patient discomfort and add to the cost of the system. It appears that the certainty of obtaining a successful defibrillator implantation will soon approximate the success rate seen with conventional pacemaker implantation.

The large size of implantable defibrillators has contributed to the complexity of implantation. Abdominal generator placement requires tunneling of leads to the upper chest, taking time, causing trauma, and necessitating the use of long wires with energy wasting internal resistance. As generators become small enough for pectoral implantation these problems will disappear. Pulse generator volume has already decreased to 83 cc,[120] and it is clear that further size reductions are on the drawing boards. Defibrillator implantation may soon be comparable in complexity to the implantation of a unipolar pacemaker, although patient selection and evaluation will continue to be complex.

Noninvasive Electrophysiologic Capabilities

Virtually all implantable defibrillators offer provocative stimulation capability to allow intentional initiation of arrhythmias to study or reconfirm the efficacy of antiarrhythmia therapies and to test the performance of the automatic arrhythmia detection algorithms.[121] These capabilities typically include multiple manually initiated premature stimuli, manually initiated rescue shocks, and a range of manually or automatically initiated antitachycardia pacing and shock therapies.

For testing of defibrillation efficacy the devices frequently supplement the premature stimuli with rapid fixed frequency or accelerating pulse trains that, unfortunately, are not always successful in inducing true fibrillation. One suggested invasive solution has been the application of DC from a 9-V battery using a bipolar catheter.[122] A promising technique for noninvasive induction of fibrillation with an implantable defibrillator is the delivery of a modest 50- to 100-V shock into the T wave.[123] This appears to be highly effective at inducing true fibrillation without the preceding overture of erratic hemodynamics that is common with rapid pulse trains or alternating current techniques.[124]

Implantable Monitoring

Until recently, available defibrillators had limited monitoring capabilities, making it difficult to ensure that the detection and therapy programs were selected appropriately. Many rhythms are treated so rapidly that the patient may believe that a delivered shock was uncalled for when it was, in fact, appropriate. At other times atrial fibrillation, sinus tachycardia, or lead and connection faults may trigger totally unwarranted therapies. With limited monitoring the physician is hard pressed to ensure that detection programming offers sufficiently sensitive yet specific behavior. It is equally difficult to be certain that therapies are not ineffective or, worse, proarrhythmic. The latest devices offer recordings of electrograms and diagnostic channel data showing device behavior during one or more tachyarrhythmia episodes. These devices also offer various counters that present a broad, though less specific, overview of device behavior. Monitoring capability in some of the newest devices appears to be the equivalent of about 32,000 bytes of random access memory, allowing electrogram waveform records of approximately 2-minutes duration, with some opportunity for later expansion by judicious selection of sampling rates and data compression techniques. Electrogram storage has proven useful for: documenting false therapy delivery due to atrial fibrillation, lead fractures, and sinus tachycardia; determining the triggers of arrhythmias; documenting rhythm accelerations in response to therapies; and demonstrating appropriate device behavior when treating asymptomatic rhythms.[6,33,125–128]

Electrograms recorded from bipolar ventricular electrodes and processed through the heavily filtered and blanked sense amplifiers of a typical defibrillator are somewhat difficult to interpret. Future designs could allow recording of high-fidelity electrograms from a programmable choice of electrodes using amplifiers designed specifically to preserve the morphology of the cardiac waveforms. As an example, pectorally placed devices with generator housings that serve as a high-voltage electrode could provide an electrogram recorded between the Can and the RV high-voltage electrode so that atrial activity could be visualized.

Electrograms provide useful information by themselves, but they cannot indicate how the device interpreted the cardiac activity. Increasingly, electrogram records will be supplemented with event markers that indicate how the device is responding on a beat-by-beat basis. These records can include measurements of the sensed and paced intervals, indication as to the specific detection zone an event falls in, indication of charge initiation, and other device performance data.

Defibrillator memory is currently quite limited in comparison with the 1–8 million bytes of memory common in virtually all personal computers. Future implantable devices will incorporate larger memories to improve the physician's ability to make well informed decisions regarding necessary programming changes. Indeed, with increased memory recording times could be extended to between 8–16 hours, giving the defibrillator the qualities of implantable ambulatory monitors, and allowing documentation not only of device detections and interventions, but nonsustained arrhythmic events as well. With additional logic, these jumbo memories could make it possible for the implantable generators to fine-tune detection and therapy settings automatically in response to recorded data. A challenge to designers of these large-memory devices will be the telemetry bottleneck that currently slows data retrieval. Larger memories will need accompanying improvements in the accessing, processing, and management of these data.

Follow-Up

Defibrillator patients and their devices require careful follow-up to ensure that the potential benefits of these devices are realized. One major study that involved primarily epicardial systems reported that 53% of 241 defibrillator patients experienced one or more complications during an average exposure of 24 months. These complications included infection requiring device removal in 5%, postoperative respiratory complications in 11%, postoperative bleeding and/or thrombosis in 4%, lead system migration or disruption in 8%, and documented inappropriate therapy delivery, most commonly due to atrial fibrillation, in 22%.[5] A shorter study of 80 patients with transvenous defibrillator systems reported no postoperative pulmonary complications, transient nerve injury (1%), asymptomatic subclavian vein occlusion (2.5%), pericardial effusion (1%), subcutaneous patch pocket hematoma (5%), pulse generator pocket infection (1%), lead fracture (1%), and lead system dislodgment (10%). During a mean follow-up period of 11 months, 7.5% of the patients in this series experienced inappropriate therapy delivery, half for atrial fibrillation and the rest for sinus tachycardia.[23]

Although routine follow-up can be accomplished in the clinic, detection and analysis of transient events depends on the recording capabilities available in the devices or on the use of various external monitoring equipment.[36] Examination of the collected information generally requires that the patient present at the clinic to provide access to the data. With one recent system, transtelephonic monitoring capability has been used to read out and transmit the complete set of stored data and program settings, thereby reducing the need for clinic visits.[129] The technology required to accomplish this is relatively expensive, and it is not clear that the current medical economic climate will support widespread usage, but the concept is feasible, and, in principle, could provide transtelephonic programming to correct problems on the spot. To address the cost issue, a simpler system has been implemented using a conventional pacemaker transtelephonic ECG monitor to send limited data encoded as a series of single and double pacing stimuli. The data rates with this approach are low, but the system is relatively inexpensive.

Economics

The annual cost of ICD therapy is dropping as a consequence of better device longevity and simpler implantation techniques. Early generators that lacked programmability, antibradycardia pacing capability, and event recording had 62% survival at 18 months and 2% at 30 months.[130] Some recent programmable designs that include VVI pacing capability and considerable event storage exhibit 95% survival at 42 months.[131] It has been estimated that an increase in generator longevity from 2–5 years would lower the cost per life-year saved by 55% in a hypothetical patient population with a 3-year sudden mortality of 28%.[132] More efficient energy conversion circuits, and finer line-width integrated circuit technology with smaller, more highly integrated circuits and reduced current drains, will yield longer lasting defibrillators while continuing the evolution to smaller volumes.

Cost of the implantation procedure is clearly declining as transvenous lead systems become commonplace. Total hospitalization duration, complication rates, and use of costly hospital operating rooms and intensive care facilities all are reduced, providing significant financial benefits. One study reported requiring half the intensive care unit time and a reduction in total hospitalization from 26 to 15 days when comparing transvenous to epicardial approaches.[119] Another center reported a mean hospitalization stay of 6 days[23] for patients receiving transvenous defibrillation systems.

Increasing sophistication of the implantable defibrillators paradoxically contributes to cost efficacy. Incorporation of single-chamber brady pacing capability eliminates the cost of a separate pacemaker and lead for those patients who need one. Eventually even dual-chamber pacing capability will be available. Programmable detection and therapy features obviate the need for device replacement that was required when fixed parameter devices proved to be inappropriately specified or too inflexible to adapt to a patient's physiological changes.[133]

Follow-up frequency, and thus costs, will be reduced with devices that do not require capacitor forming in the follow-up clinic every 2–3 months. Some devices will use timed capacitor charging to accomplish this function automatically while others may use capacitor technology that avoids the need for reformation altogether.

Significant cost savings may be obtained by better patient selection criteria and processes, obviating the need for extensive hospitalization and costly electrophysiologic studies prior to device implantation in some patient groups. One frequently discussed issue is the prophylactic role that implantable defibrillators will or should play.[134–136] To date, no studies have established the means for selecting appropriate patients for a prophylactic device, but, if this issue is successfully resolved, economic factors will be the ultimate arbiter. Simply reducing total shock capacity or eliminating antitachycardia pacing will not significantly reduce the overall cost of providing each patient with an implantable defibrillator. Unless a means is found to build far less expensive devices that can be placed with minimal time and facilities, the lifesaving yield for prophylactic defibrillators will have to be high if they are to be cost effective. This remains an open issue.

Conclusion

The implantable defibrillator has been a remarkable success story, flying in the face of early opposition from powerful and knowledgeable experts. Along the way it has engendered acrimonious legal battles. Nevertheless, it is now an established and powerful therapeutic tool. The impending transition to pectoral implants with biphasic waveforms and efficient yet simple transvenous lead systems will streamline the implant procedure and drastically curtail the need for the sweaty-palms process of inducing and terminating fibrillation to demonstrate adequate system performance. These embodiments will make the implantable defibrillator easier to use, more cost effective, and more palatable to patients and their physicians.

References

1. Dreifus L, Fisch C, Griffin J, et al: ACC/AHA task force report. Guidelines for implantation of cardiac pacemakers and arrhythmia devices. *J Am Coll Cardiol* 18:1, 1991.
2. Flowers N, Armstrong W, Curtis A, et al: Indications for implantation of the automatic implanted cardioverter defibrillator. *Cardiology* 19:6, 1990.
3. Lehmann M, Saksena S: NASPE policy statement. Implantable cardioverter defibrillators in cardiovascular practice: report of the policy conference of the North American Society of Pacing and Electrophysiology. *PACE* 14:969, 1991.
4. Mirowski M, Reid P, Mower M, et al: Termination of malignant ventricular arrhythmias with an implanted automatic defibrillator in human beings. *N Engl J Med* 303:322, 1980.
5. Grimm W, Flores B, Marchlinski F: Complications of implantable cardioverter defibrillator therapy: follow-up of 241 patients. *PACE* 16:218, 1993.
6. Grimm W, Flores B, Marchlinski F: Symptoms and electrocardiographically documented rhythm preceding spontaneous shocks in patients with implantable cardioverter-defibrillator. *Am J Cardiol* 71:1415, 1993.

7. Firstenberg M, Moore S, Ching E, et al: Prognosis following treatment with a pacemaker and an implantable cardioverter defibrillator. *PACE* 15:509, 1992.
8. Rosenqvist M, Brandt J, Schuller H: Long term pacing in sinus node disease: effects of stimulation mode on cardiovascular morbidity and mortality. *Am Heart J* 116:16, 1988.
9. Hochleitner M, Hortnagl H, Hortnagl H, et al: Long-term efficacy of physiologic dual chamber pacing in the treatment of end-stage idiopathic dilated cardiomyopathy. *Am J Cardiol* 70:1320, 1992.
10. Alpert M, Curtis J, Sanfelippo J, et al: Comparative survival following permanent ventricular and dual-chamber pacing for patients with chronic symptomatic sinus node dysfunction with and without heart failure. *Am Heart J* 113:958, 1987.
11. Meesman M: Factors associated with implantation-related complications. *PACE* 15:649, 1992.
12. Mosteller R, Lehmann M, Thomas A, et al: Operative mortality with implantation of the automatic cardioverter-defibrillator. *Am J Cardiol* 68:1340, 1991.
13. Saksena S, and the PCD Investigators and participating institutions: Defibrillation thresholds and perioperative mortality associated with endocardial and epicardial defibrillation lead systems. *PACE* 16:202, 1993.
14. Larsen G, Manolis A, Sonnenberg F, et al: Cost-effectiveness of the implantable cardioverter-defibrillator: effect of improved battery life and comparison with amiodarone therapy. *J Am Coll Cardiol* 19:1323, 1992.
15. Gartman D, Bardy G, Allen M, et al: Short-term morbidity and mortality of implantation of automatic implantable cardioverter-defibrillator. *J Thorac Cardiovasc Surg* 100:353, 1990.
16. Watkins L, Taylor E: The surgical aspects of automatic implantable cardioverter-defibrillator implantation. *PACE* 14:953, 1991.
17. Shepard R, Goldin M, Lawrie G, et al: Automatic implantable cardioverter defibrillator: surgical approaches for implantation. *J Cardiovasc Surg* 7:208, 1992.
18. Frumin H, Goodman G, Jarandilla R: Feasibility of thoracoscopically guided defibrillation patch and sensing lead implantation via "mini" thoracotomy. *PACE* 16:895, 1993.
19. Schaerf R, Biderman P, Weigel R: Thoracoscopic implantation of ICD epicardial patches and myocardial pacing leads: potential alternative to major thoracic procedures. *Medtr News* 21:46, 1993.
20. Brooks R, McGovern B, Garan H, et al: Comparison of two different nonthoracotomy cardioverter-defibrillator systems: analysis of 74 patients at one center. *J Am Coll Cardiol* 21:883, 1993.
21. Tullo N, Saksena S, Krol R, et al: Management of complications associated with a first-generation endocardial defibrillation lead system for implantable cardioverter-defibrillators. *Am J Cardiol* 66:411, 1990.
22. Jung W, Manz M, Shah Y, et al: Failure of an implantable cardioverter defibrillator to redetect ventricular fibrillation in patients with a nonthoracotomy lead system. *Circulation* 86:1217, 1992.
23. Bardy G, Hofer B, Johnson G, et al: Implantable transvenous cardioverter-defibrillators. *Circulation* 87:1152, 1993.
24. Block M, Hammel D, Isbruch F, et al: Results and realistic expectations with transvenous lead systems. *PACE* 15:665, 1992.
25. Brooks R, McGovern B, Garan H, et al: Comparison of two different nonthoracotomy cardioverter-defibrillator systems: analysis of 74 patients at one center. *J Am Coll Cardiol* 21:155A, 1993.
26. Frame R, Brodman R, Gross J, et al: Initial experience with transvenous implantable cardioverter defibrillator lead systems: operative morbidity and mortality. *PACE* 16:149, 1993.
27. Saksena S, Tullo N, Krol R, et al: Initial clinical experience with endocardial defibrillation using an implantable cardioverter/defibrillator with a triple-electrode system. *Arch Intern Med* 149:2333, 1989.
28. Jordaens L, Vertongen P, van Belleghem Y: A subcutaneous lead array for implantable cardioverter defibrillators. *PACE* 16:1429, 1993.
29. Lindemans F, van Berlo A, Bourgeois I: Summary of PCD clinical study results. In: *Practical Aspects of Staged Therapy Defibrillators*. Edited by L Kappenberger, F Lindemans. Mount Kisco, NY: Futura Publishing Company, Inc.; 1992, p. 103.
30. Bardy G, Johnson G, Poole J, et al: Simplicity and efficacy of a single incision pectoral implant unipolar defibrillation system. *J Am Coll Cardiol* 21:66A, 1993.
31. Camunas J, Mehta D, Ip J, et al: Total pectoral implantation: a new technique for implantation of transvenous defibrillator lead systems and implantable cardioverter defibrillator. *PACE* 16:1380, 1993.
32. Hammel D, Block M, Borggrefe M, et al: Implantation of a cardioverter defibrillator in the subpectoral region combined with a

nonthoracotomy lead system. *PACE* 15:367, 1992.
33. Hook B, Callans D, Kleiman R, et al: Implantable cardioverter-defibrillator therapy in the absence of significant symptoms. Rhythm diagnosis and management aided by stored electrogram analysis. *Circulation* 87:1897, 1993.
34. Singer I, de Borde R, Veltri E, et al: The automatic implantable cardioverter defibrillator: T wave sensing in the newest generation. *PACE* 11:1584, 1988.
35. Cohen A, Wish M, Fletcher R, et al: The use and interaction of permanent pacemakers and the automatic implantable cardioverter defibrillator. *PACE* 11:704, 1988.
36. Feldman C, Olson W, Hubbelbank M, et al: Identification of an implantable defibrillator lead fracture with a new Holter system. *PACE* 16:1342, 1993.
37. Tullo N, Saksena S, Krol R, et al: Management of complications associated with a first-generation endocardial defibrillation lead system for implantable cardioverter-defibrillators. *Am J Cardiol* 66:411, 1990.
38. Olson W, Bardy G, Mehra R, et al: Onset and stability for ventricular tachyarrhythmia detection in an implantable pacer-cardioverter-defibrillator. *Comp Cardiol* 167, 1986.
39. Geibel A, Zehender M, Brugada P: Changes in cycle length at the onset of sustained tachycardias—importance for antitachycardia pacing. *Am Heart J* 115:588, 1988.
40. Martin D, Venditti F: Use of event markers during exercise testing to optimize morphology criterion programming of implantable defibrillator. *PACE* 15:1025, 1992.
41. Schuger C, Jackson K, Steinman R, et al: Atrial sensing to augment ventricular tachycardia detection by the automatic implantable cardioverter defibrillator: a utility study. *PACE* 11:1456, 1988.
42. Viitasalo M, Toivonen L, Jarvinen A: The performance of the probability density function in differentiating supraventricular from ventricular rhythms. In: *Proceedings of the 10th Asian-Pacific Congress of Cardiology*, OC 36–1, Seoul, Korea, October 6–11, 1991.
43. Fisher J, Goldstein M, Ostrow E, et al: Maximal rate of tachycardia development: sinus tachycardia with sudden exercise vs. spontaneous ventricular tachycardia. *PACE* 6:221, 1983.
44. Model 7217B and 7217D Technical Manual, UC9203800aEN, p. 13. Minneapolis, MN: Medtronic, Inc.; December, 1992.
45. Swerdlow C, Luckett C: Abrupt-onset algorithm enhances discrimination of sinus tachycardia from ventricular tachycardia by tiered-therapy antiarrhythmic devices. *J Am Coll Cardiol* 21:734, 1993.
46. Swerdlow C, Luckett C: Interval-stability criteria enhance discrimination of atrial fibrillation from ventricular tachycardia by tiered-therapy antiarrhythmic devices. *J Am Coll Cardiol* 21:742, 1993.
47. Cohen T, Liem L: Biosensor applications to antitachycardia devices. *PACE* 14:322, 1991.
48. Pannizzo F, Mercando A, Fisher J, et al: Automatic methods for detection of tachyarrhythmias by antitachycardia devices. *J Am Coll Cardiol* 11:308, 1988.
49. Brugada P, Saoudi N, Barnay C, et al: Optimal methods to assess PR and RR stability for automatic recognition of ventricular and supraventricular tachycardia. *PACE* 15:514, 1992.
50. Lehmann M: Tachycardia detection for automatic implantable cardioverter/defibrillator with atrial and ventricular sensing capability. U.S. Patent 4,860,749, Jan 6, 1988.
51. Thakor N, Pan K: Tachycardia and fibrillation detection by automatic implantable cardioverter-defibrillators: sequential testing in time domain. *IEEE Eng Med Biol* March, 21, 1990.
52. DuFault R, Wilcox A: Dual lead fibrillation detection for implantable defibrillators via LMS algorithm. In: *Proceedings of the IEEE 8th Annual Conference on Engineering in Medicine and Biological Science*. 1986, p. 235.
53. Mercando A, Furman S: Measurement of differences in timing and sequence between two ventricular electrodes as a means of tachycardia differentiation. *PACE* 9:1069, 1986.
54. Jenkins J, Bump T, Munkenbeck F, et al: Tachycardia detection in implantable antitachycardia devices. *PACE* 7:1273, 1984.
55. Jenkins J, Noh K, Bump T, et al: A single atrial extrastimulus can distinguish sinus tachycardia from 1:1 paroxysmal tachycardia. *PACE* 9:1063, 1986.
56. Belz M, Ellenbogen K, Camm J, et al: Differentiation between monomorphic ventricular tachycardia and sinus tachycardia based on the right ventricular evoked potential. *PACE* 15:1661, 1992.
57. Nademanee K, Lu R, Bailey W, et al: A new sensor for tachyarrhythmia differentiation—the paced depolarization integral? *J Am Coll Cardiol* 19:288A, 1992.
58. DiCarlo L, Jenkins J, Chiang C, et al: Ventricular tachycardia detection using bipolar electrogram analysis is site specific. *PACE* 15:2154, 1992.
59. Greenhut S, Deering T, Steinhaus B, et al: Separation of ventricular tachycardia from sinus rhythm using a practical, real-time

template matching computer system. *PACE* 15:2146, 1992.
60. Tooley M, Davies D, Nathan A, et al: Recognition of multiple tachyarrhythmias by rate-independent means using a small microcomputer. *PACE* 14:337, 1991.
61. Santel D, Mehra R, Olson W, et al: Integrative algorithm for detection of ventricular tachyarrhythmias from the intracardiac electrogram. *Comp Cardiol* 175, 1986.
62. Lin D, Jenkins J, Wiesmeyer M, et al: Analysis of time and frequency domain patterns of endocardial electrograms to distinguish ventricular tachycardia from sinus rhythm. *Comp Cardiol* 171, 1986.
63. DiCarlo L, Throne R, Jenkins J: A time-domain analysis of intracardiac electrograms for arrhythmia detection. *PACE* 14:329, 1991.
64. Ripley K, Bump T, Arzbaecher R: Evaluation of techniques for recognition of ventricular arrhythmias by implanted devices. *IEEE Trans Biomed Eng* 36:618, 1989.
65. Hartlaub J: Waveform morphology discriminator and method. U.S. Patent 4,552,154, March 12, 1984.
66. Pannizzo F, Amikam S, Bagwell P, et al: Discrimination of antegrade and retrograde atrial depolarization by electrogram analysis. *Am Heart J* 112:780, 1986.
67. Arzbaecher R, Bump T, Jenkins J, et al: Automatic tachycardia recognition. *PACE* 7:541, 1984.
68. Mears D, Pan K, Xin-rong G, et al: Sequential discrimination of atrial and ventricular tachyarrhythmias. *Comp Cardiol* 107, 1990.
69. Duffin E: Method and apparatus for discriminating among normal and pathological tachyarrhythmias. U.S. Patent 5,193,550.March 16, 1993.
70. Sharma A, Bennett T, Erickson M, et al: Right ventricular pressure during ventricular arrhythmias in humans: potential implications for implantable antitachycardia devices. *J Am Coll Cardiol* 15:648, 1990.
71. Ellenbogen K, Wood M, Kapadia K, et al: Short-term reproducibility over time of right ventricular pulse pressure as a potential hemodynamic sensor for ventricular tachyarrhythmias. *PACE* 15:971, 1992.
72. Cohen T, Veltri E, Mower M: A hemodynamically responsive antitachycardia system: theoretical bases for design. *J Electrophysiol* 2:352, 1988.
73. McLellan D, Yee R, Cade D, et al: Wedge coronary sinus pressure during ventricular fibrillation reflects left heart hemodynamics. *J Am Coll Cardiol* 19:287A, 1992.
74. Stangl K, Laule M, Heinze R, et al: Hemodynamic tachycardia detection: what parameters can be used? *PACE* 13:1212, 1990.
75. Verrydt W, Bossche J, Van de Voorde P, et al: Automatic defibrillator, antitachy pacemaker and cardioverter. *Comp Cardiol* 45, 1986.
76. Weiss S, Einstein R, McCulloch R: Can changes in transcardiac impedance appropriately detect ventricular fibrillation? *PACE* 14:352, 1991.
77. Weiss S, Einstein R, McCulloch R: Does transcardiac impedance reflect haemodynamic status in the canine model with twelve-month chronically implanted defibrillation patches? *Eur PACE* 1:50, 1993.
78. Stangl K, Laule M, Heinze R, et al: Aortic and pulmonary ultrasound blood flow measurements for continuous cardiac output determination in implantable defibrillators. *PACE* 13:1212, 1990.
79. Matula M, Mestre E, Alt E, et al: A new approach towards detection of hemodynamic consequences of ventricular tachycardia. *PACE* 13:1203, 1990.
80. Singer I, Adams L, Austin E: Potential hazards of fixed gain sensing and arrhythmia reconfirmation for implantable cardioverter defibrillators. *PACE* 16:1070, 1993.
81. Callans D, Hook B, Marchlinski F: Paced beats following single nonsensed complexes in a "codependent" cardioverter defibrillator and bradycardia pacing system: potential for ventricular tachycardia induction. *PACE* 14:1281, 1991.
82. Newman D, Dorian P, Hardy J: Randomized controlled comparison of antitachycardia pacing algorithms for termination of ventricular tachycardia. *J Am Coll Cardiol* 21:1413, 1993.
83. Calkins H, el-Atassi R, Kalbfleisch S, et al: Comparison of fixed burst versus decremental burst pacing for termination of ventricular tachycardia. *PACE* 16:26, 1993.
84. Leitch J, Gillis A, Wyse G, et al: Reduction in defibrillator shocks with an implantable device combing antitachycardia pacing and shock therapy. *J Am Coll Cardiol* 18:145, 1991.
85. Porterfield J, Porterfield L, Bray L: Ninety-six episodes of spontaneous ventricular tachycardia in 1 week: success of ramp pacing by a pacer-cardioverter-defibrillator. *PACE* 14:1440, 1991.
86. Gross J, Sackstein R, Song S, et al: The antitachycardia pacing ICD: impact on patient selection and outcome. *PACE* 16:165, 1993.
87. Luceri R, Habal R, David I, et al: Changing trends in therapy delivery with a third generation noncommitted implantable defibril-

lator: results of a large single center clinical trial. *PACE* 16:159, 1993.
88. Trappe H, Klein H, Fieguth H, et al: Clinical efficacy and safety of the new cardioverter defibrillator systems. *PACE* 16:153, 1993.
89. Tedder M, Wharton M, Anstadt M, et al: Optimal defibrillator patch configurations include the right side of the heart and left ventricle. *Am J Cardiol* 71:349, 1993.
90. Pinski L, Vanerio G, Castle L, et al: Patients with a high defibrillation threshold: clinical characteristics, management, and outcome. *Am Heart J* 122:89, 1991.
91. Baerman J, Blakeman B, Olshansky B, et al: Use of multiple patches during implantation of epicardial defibrillator systems. *Am J Cardiol* 71:68, 1993.
92. Fain E, Winkle R: Implantable cardioverter defibrillator: Ventritex Cadence. *J Cardiovasc Electrophysiol* 4:211, 1993.
93. Leitch J, Yee R, and the Multicenter Pacemaker-Cardioverter-Defibrillator (PCD) Investigators Group: Predictors of defibrillation efficacy in patients undergoing epicardial defibrillator implantation. *J Am Coll Cardiol* 21:1632, 1993.
94. Kroll M, Anderson K, Supino C, et al: Decline in defibrillation thresholds. *PACE* 16:213, 1993.
95. Wyse G, Kavanagh K, Gillis A, et al: Comparison of biphasic and monophasic shocks for defibrillation using a nonthoracotomy system. *Am J Cardiol* 71:197, 1993.
96. Saksena S, An H, Mehra R, et al: Prospective comparison of biphasic and monophasic shocks for implantable cardioverter-defibrillators using endocardial leads. *Am J Cardiol* 70:304, 1992.
97. Cooper R, Wallenius S, Smith W, et al: The effect of phase separation on biphasic waveform defibrillation. *PACE* 16:471, 1993.
98. Tchou P, Krum D, Akhtar M, et al: Reduction of defibrillation energy requirements with a new biphasic waveform. *PACE* 13:506, 1990.
99. Jones J, Jones R, Balasky G: Improved cardiac cell excitation with symmetrical biphasic defibrillator waveforms. *Am J Physiol* 253:1418, 1987.
100. Hillsley R, Walker R, Swanson D, et al: Is the second phase of a biphasic defibrillation waveform the defibrillating phase? *PACE* 16:1401, 1993.
101. Schuder J: The role of an engineering oriented medical research group in developing improved methods and devices for achieving ventricular defibrillation: the University of Missouri experience. *PACE* 16:95, 1993.
102. Klein L, Miles W, Zipes D: Antitachycardia devices: realities and promises. *J Am Coll Cardiol* 18:1349, 1991.
103. Hurwitz J, Hook B, Flores B, et al: Importance of abortive shock capability with electrogram storage in cardioverter-defibrillator devices. *J Am Coll Cardiol* 21:895, 1993.
104. Prystowski E, Zipes D: Inhibition in the human heart. *Circulation* 68:707, 1983.
105. Mehra R, Gough W, Zeiler R, et al: Dual ventricular stimulation for prevention of reentrant ventricular arrhythmias. *J Am Coll Cardiol* 3:472, 1984.
106. Marchlinski F, Buxton A, Miller J, et al: Prevention of ventricular tachycardia induction during right ventricular programmed stimulation by high current strength pacing at the site of origin. *Circulation* 76:332, 1987.
107. Spotnitz H, Ott G, Bigger J, et al: Methods of implantable cardioverter-defibrillator-pacemaker insertion to avoid interactions. *Ann Thorac Surg* 53:253, 1992.
108. Cohen A, Wish M, Fletcher R, et al: The use and interaction of permanent pacemakers and the automatic implantable cardioverter defibrillator. *PACE* 11:704, 1988.
109. Cooper R, Alferness C, Smith W, et al: Internal cardioversion of atrial fibrillation in sheep. *Circulation* 87:1673, 1993.
110. Scott S, Accorti P, Callaghan F, et al: Ventricular and atrial defibrillation using new transvenous tripolar and bipolar leads with 5 French subcutaneous catheters. *PACE* 14:1893, 1991.
111. Keane D, Boyd E, Robles A, et al: Biphasic versus monophasic waveform in epicardial atrial defibrillation. *PACE* 15:570, 1992.
112. Ciccone J, Saksena S, Shah Y, et al: A prospective randomized study of the clinical efficacy and safety of transvenous cardioversion for termination of ventricular tachycardia. *Circulation* 71:571, 1985.
113. Lévy S, Camm K: An implantable atrial defibrillator. An impossible dream? *Circulation* 87:1769, 1993.
114. Wunderly D, Maloney J, Edel T, et al: Infections in implantable cardioverter defibrillator patients. *PACE* 13:1360, 1990.
115. Norenberg M, Sakun V, Roberts D, et al: Long-term clinical experience with PCD Transvene system: worldwide experience. *PACE* 16:874, 1993.
116. Block M, the European P2 Investigators: Combination of endocardial leads with a new ICD capable of biphasic shocks—first results of a multicenter study. *PACE* 16:874, 1993.
117. Kleman J, Pinski S, Helguera M, et al: An intention to treat analysis of transvenous

and epicardial ICD system implantation. *PACE* 16:874, 1993.
118. Powers M, Schwartzman D, Flores B, et al: Lead-related morbidity in patients with ICDs utilizing non-thoracotomy lead systems. *PACE* 16:951, 1993.
119. Saggau W, Sack F, Lange R, et al: Superiority of endocardial versus epicardial implantation of the implantable cardioverter defibrillator (ICD). *Eur J Cardiothorac Surg* 6:195, 1992.
120. PCD Jewel Technical Manual, UC9300726EN, p. S12, Minneapolis, MN: Medtronic, Inc.; February, 1993.
121. Klein L, Miles W, Zipes D: Antitachycardia devices: realities and promises. *J Am Coll Cardiol* 18:1349, 1991.
122. Weismuller P, Richter P, Binner L, et al: Direct current application: easy induction of ventricular fibrillation for the determination of the defibrillation threshold in patients with implantable cardioverter defibrillators. *PACE* 15:1137, 1992.
123. PCD Jewel Technical Manual, UC9300726EN, p. 7–5. Minneapolis, MN: Medtronic, Inc.; February, 1993.
124. Bardy G, Mehra R, Johnson G, et al: Low energy pulsing on the T-wave: a new programming method for intentional, device mediated induction of ventricular fibrillation for defibrillation testing. *PACE* 15:562, 1992.
125. Marchlinski F, Gottlieb C, Sarter B, et al: ICD data storage: value in arrhythmia management. *PACE* 16:527, 1993.
126. Newman D, Dorian P, Downar E, et al: Use of telemetry functions in the assessment of implanted antitachycardia device efficacy. *Am J Cardiol* 70:616, 1992.
127. Luceri R, Puchferran R, Brownstein S, et al: Improved patient surveillance and data acquisition with a third generation implantable cardioverter defibrillator. *PACE* 14:1870, 1991.
128. Almeida H, Buckingham T: Inappropriate implantable cardioverter defibrillator shocks secondary to sensing lead failure: utility of stored electrograms. *PACE* 16:407, 1993.
129. Anderson M, Paul V, Jones S, et al: Transtelephonic interrogation of the implantable cardioverter defibrillator. *PACE* 15:1144, 1992.
130. Song S: The Bilitch Report: Part B. Performance of implantable cardiac rhythm management devices. *PACE* 14:589, 1991.
131. Song S: The Bilitch Report: Part B. Performance of implantable cardiac rhythm management devices. *PACE* 16:1485, 1993.
132. Anderson M, Camm A: Implications for present and future applications of the implantable cardioverter-defibrillator resulting from the use of a simple model of cost efficacy. *Br Heart J* 69:83, 1993.
133. Winkle R: State-of-the-art AICD. *PACE* 14:961, 1991.
134. Brugada P, Andries E: The rationale for prophylactic implantation of a defibrillator in "high risk" patients. *PACE* 16:547, 1993.
135. Hauser R: Attributes of a prophylactic implantable cardioverter defibrillator: how close are we? *PACE* 16:582, 1993.
136. Bigger T: Prophylactic use of implantable cardioverter defibrillators: medical, technical, economic considerations. *PACE* 14:376, 1991.

Index

Ablative therapy, 31–32, 677, 679
  catheter, 31–32, 308, 633–646
  cryoablation, 31, 617, 623–628
Acceleration, 460, 501
Action potentials, 51–53, 58–59, 64, 161–163
Activity sensors, 700, 756
Adapters of lead systems, 201
Adenosine, 738, 740, 741
β-Adrenergic blocking agents, 516–517, 580, 594–598, 733
AFASAK study, 676, 677
Afterdepolarization, 15
Age in ICD therapy, 310
AICD device, 207, 223, 226, 227, 280, 282
  clinical results with, 477, 483
  development of, 688–689
  sensing system of, 96–97, 98, 382
  testing of, 403, 404
  Ventak ECD for, 229–231
AID device, 471, 520
Air embolism, 425
Alternative therapies, 308, 575–646
Amiodarone therapy, 417, 517–518, 530, 580, 591–596, 733
  CASCADE study on, 600–603
  clinical results in, 475, 511
  compared to ICD therapy, 308–309, 519–520, 523, 524, 551
  compared to other drugs, 598, 600–603
  cost-benefit analysis of, 551
  defibrillation threshold in, 321, 378, 379, 389
Amplifiers, sensing, 75, 76, 125, 197–198
Anesthesia, 358–359
Animal studies, 62–63, 667–669, 680–681
  historical, 3–4, 6–7
  species differences in, 55–56
  on talc pericarditis, 666, 668
  on vulnerable period, 45–46
Antiarrhythmic drug therapy, 30–31, 579–604, 732–733
  β-adrenergic blocking agents in, 516–517, 580, 594–598, 733
  amiodarone in. *See* Amiodarone therapy
  in atrial fibrillation, 677, 678–679
  in automated rhythm system, 702
  clinical results in, 475–476, 511, 519–524, 530
  compared to ICD therapy, 519–524, 551, 733
  defibrillation threshold in, 321, 378–380, 737

  detection of arrhythmias in, 380
  empiric standard, 579–581
  history of, 318
  and indications for ICD therapy, 304, 308–309
  individualized, 581–591, 598, 600
  infusion of, 731–748
  interactions with ICD therapy, 377–383, 445, 448
  limitations of, 678–679, 732, 733
  postoperative, 391
  in primary prevention of sudden death, 516–518
Antibiotic therapy, 344–345, 360, 391, 419
Anticoagulant therapy in atrial fibrillation, 676–677, 678, 679
Antitachycardia pacing, 271–296, 391, 393, 399–400, 651–665
  atrial, 660–665, 701
  clinical results in, 292–295, 496–498, 500–501
  combined with ICD therapy, 280–284, 291–292, 384–385, 757, 758
  complications of, 295–296
  efficacy of, 288–292
  failure of, 441–446
  historical, 651–657, 688–689
  inappropriate, 434–440
  mechanisms of, 271–288
  poor tolerance of, 467
  preventive, 656–657, 659, 663–665
  for rate control, 661–663
  for termination of tachycardia, 651–656, 657–659, 660–661
  testing of, 353
  in tiered therapy, 464–465
Anxiety of patients, 406–411
Arrhythmogenic right ventricular dysplasia, 21, 33, 306, 307–308, 645
Arrhythmogenic substrate, anatomical, 616, 618–619
Arteriography, coronary, 320–321, 492–493
Aspirin, 517
Atrial directed pacemaker cardioverter-defibrillator, 651, 665
Atrial fibrillation, 204, 248, 651–683, 758
  ablation and pacing in, 678, 679
  automated system in, 701, 702
  classification of, 719, 720, 721

Atrial fibrillation (*continued*)
   drug therapy in, 676, 677–679, 738
   dual chamber pacing in, 90–91, 718, 725, 726
   external direct current in, 677
   implantable defibrillator in, 675–683
   multiple point pacing in, 661
   paroxysmal, 466–467, 663, 683, 738
   postoperative, 391, 416
   prevention of, 663–665, 702
   surgery in, 678, 679–680
   transvenous systems in, 665–672, 680–683
   ventricular rate control in, 662–663, 677
Atrial flutter, 248, 670, 720, 721
   antitachycardia pacing in, 651, 660–661
   dual chamber pacing in, 718, 725, 726
Atrial pacing, 661, 758
Atrial sensing, 90–92, 203–204, 698–699
Atrial tachycardia, primary, 660–665
Atrioventricular delay, 712–713, 714–715
Atrioventricular event ratio, 91, 721, 724
Atrioventricular reentrant tachycardia, 657–659
Automated rhythm systems, 687–706
Automatic adjusting thresholds, 75, 76, 77–78, 79
Automatic gain control, 75, 76, 77–78, 79, 266, 438, 717
Automatic ICDs, 224, 226–227
Autonomic nervous system, 48–49
AVID study, 309, 521–523, 524
Axillary vein thrombosis, 428–429

BAATAF study, 676, 677
BASIS study, 517
Batteries, 125, 126–127, 253, 403, 453
Beep-o-grams, 438, 439, 440, 442
Biases in ICD studies, 518–519
Biocompatibility, 183–184
Biphasic waveform, 135, 144, 150, 154, 757
   in atrial cardioversion-defibrillation, 669, 670, 680
   in automatic ICDs, 227
   defibrillation threshold for, 166–174, 350
   duration of, 154, 167, 168, 172–173
   truncated exponential, 166–174
Bipolar lead system, 196–197, 198, 347
Bleeding complications, 425–426
Brachial plexus injury, 426
Bradycardia, 215–216
   sinus, 713
Bundle branch reentrant tachycardia, 636–639, 644
Burst pacing, 46, 285, 286–287, 399, 512
   adaptive, 286, 726, 727
   in atrial tachycardia, 660
   fixed mode, 289–291

CABG Patch trials, 10, 310, 528, 534–540, 563
Cadence device, 8, 253, 254, 255, 424, 440, 453
   antitachycardia pacing, 283, 393, 464, 471
   data log of, 405

   deactivation of, 450
   lead system of, 254
   sensing system of, 74, 82–84, 86, 87, 88, 97, 267, 380
      multiple zones in, 399
      reconfirmation in, 398
   support device for, 232–234
   testing of, 351, 403, 404
Capacitors of ICDs, 125, 127–129, 255–256, 403, 752–754
Cardiac arrest, 304–306, 310, 466
   CASCADE study on, 10, 600–603
   CASH study on, 11, 309, 520–521, 524, 603–604
   cost of ICD therapy in, 556–559, 564
Cardiac output, 712, 713, 743–744
Cardiac Pacemaker, Inc. (CPI) devices, 76, 79, 184, 253, 283, 328
   AICD. *See* AICD device
   deactivation of, 450–452
   ECD, 227, 229–231
   Endotak. *See* Endotak device
   epicardial, 329
   SQ Array, 342, 361, 430
   transvenous, 340, 360
   troubleshooting of, 438, 439, 440, 450
   Ventak. *See* Ventak devices
CASCADE, 10, 600–603
CASH, 11, 309, 520–521, 524, 603–604
CAST, 10, 517, 732–733
Catheter ablation, 31–32, 308, 633–646
Cerebrovascular disorders, 419, 676–677
Chemical ablation, 635
Chronaxie, 137, 138, 144
CIDS, 11, 309, 519–520, 524
Circuitry of ICDs, 75, 76, 125, 129–131
   high and low power, 217, 218–219
   protection of, 219, 383
   switching system of, 129–131
Clinical results of ICD therapy, 7–8, 10–11, 471–513
   compared to drug therapy, 519–524, 551
   cost-benefit analysis of, 548–564
   in randomized trials, 524–543
   with third-generation devices, 496–498, 500–501
   with thoracotomy, 472–476
   with transvenous lead systems, 476–483, 494–496, 498, 500, 501
   in Europe, 507–513
   review of literature on, 511–512
Coagulation, 323
   and anticoagulant therapy, 676–677, 678, 679
Committed devices, 213–214, 398, 406, 758
Complications of ICD therapy, 415–430, 498–500, 751, 761
   infections in. *See* Infections
   lead-related, 422, 426–430, 499, 513, 752, 759
      troubleshooting of, 439, 442, 448
   prevention of, 433–434

Conductors in ICD system, 184, 190–194, 427
Confirmation of arrhythmias, 72, 87, 461
  and reconfirmation, 213–214, 380, 381, 758
Constant energy concept, 135, 143, 149
Contraindications to ICD therapy, 305–306
Converters, DC-DC, 125, 129
Converting enzyme inhibitors, 517
Coping mechanisms, 411
Coronary arteriography, 320–321, 492–493
Coronary artery bypass surgery, 10, 616, 621–622, 626
  annual rate of, 565
  CABG Patch trials on, 10, 310, 528, 534–540, 563
  implantation of ICD after, 321
Coronary artery disease, 18, 20–21, 491, 493, 615–629
  CABG Patch trials on, 10, 310, 528, 534–540, 563
  catheter ablation in, 644, 645
  clinical results in, 494, 510, 527–534
  indications for ICD therapy in, 306–307, 308
Coronary sinus electrodes, 120, 121, 122, 124, 511, 680, 683
Correlation analysis, 88–89, 697, 699
Cost of ICD therapy, 409, 547–571, 761–762
  in unipolar system, 374–375
Coupled pacing, 662
Critical mass mechanism, 156, 157
Cryoablation, 31, 617, 623–628
Current, 24, 109, 131
  shunting of, 198, 199, 200
Cybertach device, 653, 655, 660
Cycle length, 23–24, 50–55, 71, 80

Data log, 404–405, 692–693, 702–703
  in dual chamber pacing, 727–728
  memory capabilities for, 760–761
Deactivation of ICD, 450–453
Death
  nonsudden and noncardiac, 568
  sudden. *See* Sudden cardiac death
Decremental burst pacing, 287, 289–291, 660
DEFIBRILAT study, 10, 540, 542–543, 563
Defibrillation, 153–174
  as bridge to transplantation, 10, 540, 542–543, 563–564
  chemical, 737–738
  duration of fibrillation affecting, 56–58
  theory in, 135–151, 208
Defibrillation threshold, 43, 46, 757
  in anesthesia, 358–359
  atrial, 669, 680, 681
  for biphasic waveforms, 166–174, 350
  in drug therapy, 321, 378–380, 737
  duration of fibrillation affecting, 56, 57
  and energy margins, 240–245, 446–447
  for monophasic waveforms, 165, 167, 168, 171, 172
  testing of, 234–240, 323, 477, 480
    future trends in, 246–247
    intraoperative, 348–350, 361
    for triphasic waveform, 174
    in unipolar system, 365, 367, 370
Demand pacing, 688
Diaphragmatic stimulation, 426–427
Dilated cardiomyopathy, 21, 33, 306, 307, 491, 733
  catheter ablation in, 644
  clinical trials on, 10, 540–542
  device discharges in, 494, 541
  dual chamber pacing in, 714, 715
Direct current
  in atrial fibrillation, 677
  in catheter ablation, 633–634
  DC-DC converters, 125, 129
Dislocation of lead system, 422, 426, 439, 442, 499, 513, 759
Dobutamine, 390, 738, 740, 744
Dopamine, 390, 738, 740
Dose, defibrillation, 135, 145–146
  and response curve, 234, 235, 240–241, 348, 349
Drug therapy, 577–604
  antiarrhythmic. *See* Antiarrhythmic drug therapy
  antibiotic, 344–345, 360, 391, 419
  anticoagulant, 676–677, 678, 679
Dual chamber pacing, 654, 657, 664, 711–729, 758
  rhythm classification in, 90–92, 715–725
Dysplasia of right ventricle, 21, 33, 306, 307–308, 645

Echocardiography, 320
Efficacy margins, 240–245
Effusions, pleural, 416, 417
Ejection fraction, 563
Electric field strength, 138–1143
Electrical stimulation, 135–151
  programmed. *See* Programmed electrical stimulation
Electrocardiography, 19, 29, 318–319, 616
  in antiarrhythmic drug therapy, 563, 582, 583, 584, 600
Electrodes, 110, 186–190, 202
  in atrial cardioversion-defibrillation, 665, 666, 667, 669, 670, 680–683
  cost of, 555–556
  in epicardial systems, 112–119
  fatigue of, 189–190, 202
  materials in, 184, 187–188
  three electrode systems, 110, 117–119, 122–124, 131–132
  in transvenous systems, 119–124, 179, 186–187, 365–375
  two electrode systems, 110, 111–112, 119–122

Electrograms, 20, 73–78, 99, 194–198, 394, 756, 760
  atrial, 698–699
  in automated system, 694, 695–699
  bipolar, 73, 74, 75, 196–197, 685
  endocardial, 73, 74
  epicardial, 73, 74, 194–196
  in lead fracture, 262
  morphology of, 88–90, 100, 695–698
  shunt current in, 198, 199, 200
  in troubleshooting, 440–441
Electromagnetic interference, 95, 440, 445, 452
Electrophysiologic studies, 21–27
  cost of, 556, 558
  in drug therapy, 321, 585–591, 592–593, 598, 600, 603
  limitations of, 400–401
  noninvasive, 759–760
  postoperative, 392–394
  preoperative, 321–322, 493
Electrophysiology
  of fibrillation, 58–62
  of tachycardia, 18–19, 21–27
Electrophysiology laboratory, 23
  device implantation in, 357–362, 375, 512
Embolism, 429–430, 676–677, 678
  air, 425
  pulmonary, 417–418
Encainide, 378, 517
Encircling endocardial cryoablation, 623–628
Endocardial cryoablation, 623–628
Endocardial resection, 617, 622, 628
Endocarditis, postoperative, 419
Endotak device, 9, 74, 189, 192, 329
  clinical results with, 476–481, 496, 499, 511, 512
  complications in, 392, 422
  fixation of, 201
  history of, 8, 181–182, 471, 507
  lead system of, 181–182, 183, 338, 478–479, 508
  materials in, 185, 188, 192
  operative technique in, 337, 339, 342, 343, 392
  sensing system of, 74
Energy margins, 240–245, 348–350, 446–447
EnGuard device, 183, 189, 424, 508, 510
  complications in, 422
  fixation of, 201
  materials in, 192
  operative technique in, 339
Entrainment, 14, 15, 289, 644
Epicardial lead systems, 111–119, 693, 759
  clinical results in, 494, 496, 498
  development of, 179–181
  operative technique in, 327–336, 487–489
  sensing function of, 194–196
Epinephrine, 62–64
Episode termination, 72, 73, 88, 213–214
Erosion of generator, 419–420

ETCD, 227, 229, 231–232
Exit block, 427, 450
External cardioverter defibrillators, 227, 229–231
Extinction mechanism, 156
Extrastimulation, 14–15, 23, 285, 660
  atrial, 91, 92, 722

Family of patient, 410
Fatigue of materials, 189–190, 191, 193
Fears of patients, 406–411
Figure-of-eight reentry, 618, 620
Fixation of lead, 201–202, 203, 422
Flecainide, 378, 379, 517, 678
Fluids, postoperative, 390
Follow-up period, 262, 402–411, 494, 627, 761
Fracture of leads, 191, 202, 262, 263–266, 373–374, 427

Gradient pattern detection, 89, 696
Guardian device, 253, 254, 255, 264
  antitachycardia pacing, 283, 285, 448, 449
  data log of, 405, 407
  programming of, 459
  sensing system of, 79, 85, 86, 87, 88, 380, 381
    dual chamber, 92
    multiple zones in, 399
    reconfirmation in, 398
    undersensing in, 401
  testing of, 351, 352, 403, 404

Hardware of ICDs, 125–132, 217–219
  assessment of, 253–256, 262–268, 346–353
  in automated system, 703–704
  batteries, 125, 126–127, 253, 403, 453
  capacitors, 125, 127–129, 255–256, 403, 752–754
  circuitry. *See* Circuitry of ICDs
  cost of, 548, 555–556
  DC-DC converters, 125, 129
  with drug infusion pump, 744–748
  size of, 693, 694, 703–704, 752–754, 759
Heart rate, 274–280, 719, 720, 724
  in atrial fibrillation, 662–663, 677
  zones of, 80–85, 208–211, 459, 463–465
Heart transplantation, 10, 540, 542–543, 563–564, 565
Hematoma, 420–421, 430
Hemodynamic sensors, 92–95, 400, 699–700, 756
Hemoptysis, 426
Hemothorax, 425
High Voltage Stimulator, 227, 229, 232–234
Historical aspects of ICD therapy, 3–11, 223, 303–304, 471, 487, 687–690
  first implantation in, 7–8, 303, 487, 491
  lead systems in, 179–183
  supraventricular, 651–657
  tiered, 207–208
History of patient, 315, 316

Holter recording, 319–320
Hypertrophic cardiomyopathy, 21, 33, 306, 307, 491
   catheter ablation in, 644
   dual chamber pacing in, 713–714, 715

Impedance, 224–226, 254, 447–448
   measurement of, 347, 348, 397–398, 404, 427–428
Implant support devices, 223–248
Implantation of cardioverter-defibrillator, 327–354, 487–491
   annual rate of, 688, 689
   in automated system, 703–704
   clinical results of, 471–513
   compared to pacemaker implantation, 357–358
   complications of, 415–430, 751
   cost of, 556, 761–762
   endocardial approach in, 337–344
   epicardial approach in, 327–336
   equipment and personnel in, 345–346, 357, 359–360
   indications for, 303–310, 491–493
   in laboratory, 357–362, 375, 512
   operative technique in, 327–354, 361–362, 487–491
   postoperative procedures in, 362, 389–411
   preoperative procedures in, 315–324, 344–345, 360
   troubleshooting in, 353–354
   in unipolar system, 365, 367–370, 374–375
Inappropriate shocks, 354, 378, 405–406, 499–500, 690–691, 754
   troubleshooting in, 434–441
Indications for ICD therapy, 303–310, 472, 491–493
   with pacemaker, 386–387
   programmable, 457–458
   unipolar, 375
Ineffective shocks, 354, 436, 446–450
Infections, 309, 390, 418–419, 512–513
   device-related, 391, 418, 419
   incidence of, 498, 693–694
   prevention of, 344–345, 391, 419
   removal of system in, 498, 694
   source of, 345, 419
Infusion system, 731–748
Inotropic drugs, 738
Insulation
   of lead systems, 184–186, 203, 427–428
   of set screws, 424
Intec devices, 181, 227, 403, 404, 471
Interference problems, 95–96, 361, 440, 445
   in charging cycle, 213
   in circuitry, 218–219
   device deactivation in, 452
   device-device, 361, 438–439
Intermedics devices, 8, 183, 184, 188, 202, 331
   blanking period in, 76
   Cybertach, 653, 655, 660
   Intertach, 655, 656, 688
   Res-Q. *See* Res-Q device
   transvenous, 360
Intertach device, 655, 656, 688
Ionic channels, 58–60
Ischemia, 18–19, 47–49, 617, 741
Isoproterenol, 24, 380, 586

Lead systems, 109–125, 179–204, 651
   complications in, 422, 426–430, 499, 513, 752, 759
      troubleshooting of, 439, 442, 448
   cost of, 548, 555–556
   in dual chamber pacing, 712, 718
   electrograms from, 73–75
   epicardial. *See* Epicardial lead systems
   historical, 179–183
   insulation of, 184–186, 203, 427–428
   low-polarization, 199–200, 203
   migration of, 202, 203, 268, 422
   pacing function of, 347–348, 394–398
   sensing function of, 71–101, 194–200, 203, 346–347, 394–398, 442
   testing of, 254–255, 346–348, 394–397, 404
   transvenous. *See* Transvenous systems
Left ventricle, 320–321
   function of, 309, 476
   tachycardia origin in, 32, 639, 641
Left ventriculography, 320–321
Lidocaine, 378, 379
Lifestyle issues, 409, 410, 411, 548–549, 550
Localization of tachycardia, 27–29
Long QT syndrome, 307, 318, 596, 711, 741

MADIT, 10, 310, 524, 528, 531–534, 561–562
Manual ICDs, 224–226, 227
Mapping, 27–29, 619, 620–621, 624–625
Margin verification, 236–237
Maze operation, 678
Medtronic devices, 184, 283, 471, 652, 653, 654
   blanking period in, 76
   electrodes in, 181, 341, 360, 666, 670
   epicardial, 181, 328, 330
   ETCD, 227, 229, 231–232
   materials in, 179, 186
   patient activated, 655, 660
   PCD. *See* PCD device
   results of, 343
   sensing errors of, 79
   steroid eluting, 200
   Transvene. *See* Transvene device
Memory of ICD systems, 125, 219, 258, 760–761
Metabolic indicators, 722, 724
Metoprolol, 520, 597, 599, 603
Microprocessors in ICDs, 125, 219, 258, 760–761
Migration of lead system, 202, 203, 268, 422
MiniMed implantable pump, 745, 746
Mitral valve prolapse, 21, 33–34, 306, 307, 596

Monomorphic ventricular tachycardia, 19, 53, 54, 639–640, 642
    sustained, 25–27
Monophasic waveform, 135, 144, 150
    in automatic ICDs, 226–227
    compared to biphasic waveform, 166–174
    duration of, 154, 166, 167, 168
    truncated exponential, 153–154, 164–166
        defibrillation thresholds for, 165, 167, 168, 171, 172
Motion sensors, 700, 756
MUSTT, 10, 310, 524, 526–531, 561
Myocardial infarction, 18–19, 562–563, 617–618
    drug therapy in, 518, 596
    history of, 316
    multicenter trial on, 531–534
    postoperative, 416

Nitroprusside, 740, 742
Noncommitted devices, 213–214, 398, 406, 460–461
Nonsustained ventricular tachycardia, 438, 466, 524–531, 561–562, 565
    trial on, 10, 310, 524, 526–531, 561

Onset of arrhythmias, 86, 690, 691, 717–718, 755
    criteria on, 91, 459, 462, 721–722
    in dual chamber pacing, 91, 721–722, 724
Overdrive pacing, 273, 652
Oversensing, 79, 266–268, 354, 403–404, 438, 755, 756
Oxygen saturation sensors, 700

P waves, oversensing of, 438
Pacemakers
    antitachycardia, 271–296, 384–385
    implantation of, 357–358
    interaction with ICD therapy, 96, 361, 383–387, 438–439, 444
Pacing
    antitachycardia. See Antitachycardia pacing
    atrial, 661, 758
    dual chamber, 711–729
Pacing threshold, 199, 216, 254, 347–348, 394–397, 404
Pain, postoperative, 390
Paralysis mechanism, 156
PCD device, 8, 253, 254, 255, 405, 459
    antitachycardia pacing, 283, 285, 385, 471
    clinical results in, 482, 483, 511
    ETCD for, 231–232
    lead systems of, 119, 123
    sensing system of, 80–82, 83, 85, 86, 87–88
Pericarditis, 418, 666, 668
Personnel, 345–346, 357, 359, 403
Philadelphia peel, 622
Pleural effusions, 416, 417
Pneumonia, 416, 417, 419
Pneumothorax, 418, 425

Polarization reduction, 199–200, 203
Polymorphic ventricular tachycardia, 19, 24–25, 53, 54, 211
Polyurethane insulation, 184, 185, 186
Postoperative period, 362, 389–411, 494, 626
Postshock period, 80, 198–199, 214–217, 442–444
Posture sensors, 700, 756
Power source of ICDs, 125, 126–127, 253, 403, 453
    and circuitry, 218
Predischarge testing, 392–393
Premature atrial stimulation, 91, 92, 721–722
Premature ventricular complexes, 21
Preoperative period, 344–345, 360
    evaluation in, 315–324, 344, 621
Proarrhythmia, 382–383, 440, 679, 681
Procainamide, 379, 530, 580
Programmed electrical stimulation, 23, 24–27, 585–586
    in antitachycardia pacing, 273–280, 285
    in induction of tachycardia, 24–25, 398, 525–526
    limitations of, 16–18
    responses to, 14–15, 16, 17
Programming of defibrillators, 146–150, 224–226, 234–245, 457–468
    in automated system, 703
    onset criteria in, 86, 459, 462
    telemetered data in, 261–262
    in tiered therapy, 212–213, 463–465
Propafenone, 378, 520, 524, 530, 678
Psychiatric issues, 406–411, 549
Pulse duration, 135, 136, 137, 138, 141, 143, 144
    in automatic ICDs, 224, 226–227
    in biphasic waveform, 154, 167, 168, 172–173
    formulae on, 150–151
    in manual ICDs, 224–226
    in monophasic waveform, 154, 166, 167, 168
    programming of, 147, 148, 149, 150, 224–226
    and strength-duration curve, 137, 138, 144
    and tilt, 144, 149–150
Pulse generators, 331, 651, 653
    cost of, 548, 555, 565
    erosion of, 419–420
    pocket for, 361–362, 420–421
    replacement of, 353
    size of, 752–754
    testing of, 350–353
    in unipolar system, 365, 366
Pulse shape, 135, 143, 145
Pulse width, 224–227, 254

QT interval, long, 307, 318, 596, 711, 741
Quality of life, 411, 548–549, 550
Quinidine, 379, 530, 580, 678

R wave, 346–347, 437
Radiofrequency ablation, 634–635, 640, 642, 646, 688

Ramp pacing, 285–286, 287, 660
Rapid ventricular stimulation, 273, 274
Rate adaptive pacing, 688
  atrial, 664–665
  bursts in, 286, 726, 727
  dual chamber, 713, 715, 722, 728
Rate detection algorithms, 71, 73, 80–87, 100, 755
  dual chamber, 92
  faulty, 440, 444–445
  in tiered therapy, 210, 211
Rate zones, 80–85, 459
  in tiered therapy, 208–211, 463–465
Reconfirmation of arrhythmias, 213–214, 380, 381, 758
Redetection of arrhythmias, 72, 80, 87–88, 758
Reentry, 13–14, 43–44, 271, 272, 616, 618, 620
  in atrioventricular tachycardia, 657–659
  bundle branch, 636–639, 644
  differentiated from triggered activity, 16–18
  in ischemia and infarction, 18, 47
Reformation of capacitors, 255–256, 403, 753–754
Refractory period, 50–51, 54–55, 271–272
  artificial, 76
  extension mechanism, 156–157, 160–161
Reliability of systems, 370–374, 704
Remote follow-up, 262, 761
Reperfusion, 49
Replacement of ICDs, 253, 254
Respiratory function, 323, 359
  postoperative, 416–418, 425, 426
RES-Q device, 253, 254, 255, 510
  antitachycardia pacing, 283, 285
  sensing system of, 85–86, 88, 267, 268
  set screws of, 424
Rheobase, 135, 137, 138, 139
Right ventricle
  arrhythmogenic dysplasia of, 21, 33, 306, 307–308, 645
  electrodes in, 120, 121, 122–124, 511
  tachycardia origin in, 32–33, 639, 640–641
Risk factors, 20–21, 310, 516, 732, 733

Safety of defibrillation, 348, 349, 370–373, 374, 759
  programming for, 240–245, 397
Scanning techniques, 285, 727
  in antitachycardia pacing, 287, 400, 654
Self-programming, 703
Sensing and detection of arrhythmias, 71–101, 194–200, 203, 754–756
  atrial, 90–92, 203–204, 698–699
  in automated system, 694–701
  bipolar, 196–197, 198, 347
  device-device interactions in, 385–386, 438–439, 444
  drugs affecting, 380, 445
  dual chamber, 90–92

electrograms in, 73–78, 88–90, 99, 100, 194–198, 756
  in epicardial leads, 194–196
  episode termination in, 72, 73, 88, 213–214
  evaluation of, 96–99, 442–445
    intraoperative, 346–347
    postoperative, 394–398, 403–404
  in extended high rate, 84, 460, 755
  future developments in, 755–756
  hemodynamic measurements in, 92–95, 400, 699–700, 756
  oversensing in, 79, 266–268, 354, 403–404, 438, 755, 756
  postshock, 80, 198–199, 442–444
    in tiered therapy, 214–217
  problems in, 78–80, 353–354, 442–445, 755
  in programmable device, 458–463
  rate zones in, 80–85, 208–211, 459
  in third-generation systems, 690–691, 734–736
  in tiered therapy, 208–211
  in transvenous leads, 196, 197
  undersensing in, 78, 79, 215, 266–268, 353, 403–404, 756
  troubleshooting in, 444–445
Sequential pulse defibrillation, 110, 117–118, 122, 123, 131–132, 165
Seroma of generator pocket, 421
Set screws, 422, 424
Shunt current, 198, 199, 200
Shut-down mode, 453
Siemens Pacesetter devices, 280, 281, 282, 510, 660
Silicone insulation, 184, 185
Simultaneous pulse defibrillation, 110, 117–118, 122, 123, 131–132
Sinus bradycardia, 713
Sinus node dysfunction, 664
Sinus rhythm, 28–29, 79, 216–217, 720
Sinus tachycardia, 91, 437, 721–722
Slew rate, 347
Social issues, 406–411, 549
Sodium channels, 58–60
Software of ICDs, 219–220
Sotalol, 308, 309, 380, 523, 678, 679, 733
SPAF, 676, 679
Spontaneous defibrillation, 58–60
SQ Array lead system, 342, 361, 430
Stability of arrhythmias, 85, 459–460, 462, 721, 755
Step-down success protocol, 236–237
Sternotomy, 331–333, 487, 488
Steroid elution, 200, 427
Strength-duration curve, 137, 138, 144
Stroke, 419, 676–677
Subclavian artery injury, 425, 426
Subclavian vein
  stick technique, 418, 424–426
  thrombosis of, 428–429

Subcostal approach, 335–336, 389
Subcutaneous electrodes, 361, 430
Submuscular electrodes, 361
Subthreshold stimulation, 287, 701
Subxiphoid approach, 334–335, 389, 417
Sudden cardiac death, 6–7, 8, 10, 303, 751
  aborted, 22, 472
  cost-efficacy of ICD in, 559, 560, 569–570
  in drug therapy, 597–598, 599, 600, 603
    with amiodarone, 593–594, 595
    individualized approach, 584–585, 588–591
  primary prevention of, 310, 472, 501, 515–543
  risk for, 516, 732, 733
  secondary prevention of, 518–523
  in transvenous systems, 477, 511
Support system of patient, 410–411
Supraventricular arrhythmias, 651–683, 688. *See also* Atrial fibrillation; Atrial flutter
  classification of, 720, 721, 722, 723
  dual chamber pacing in, 718, 719, 725–727
  sinus, 91, 437, 721–722
  troubleshooting in, 437–438
Surgery, 29–30, 31, 308, 615–629
  in atrial fibrillation, 677, 679–680
  coronary artery bypass in. *See* Coronary artery bypass surgery
  for device implantation. *See* Implantation of cardioverter-defibrillator
  endocardial resection in, 617, 622, 628
  mapping in, 619, 620–621, 624–625
Sustained ventricular tachycardia, 19, 25–27, 304, 310, 467–468
Synchronization process, 72, 73, 87

T waves, oversensing of, 438
Tachylog device, 280, 281, 282, 660
Telectronics devices, 76, 79, 253, 254, 255
  antitachycardia pacing, 283, 285, 448, 449, 654
  development of, 8, 179, 181, 183
  EnGuard. *See* EnGuard device
  Guardian. *See* Guardian device
  lead systems of, 179, 184, 200, 201
    fracture in, 264, 265
    materials in, 184, 188, 189
Telemetry, 75, 253–268, 351–353
  in automated rhythm system, 703
  in system evaluation, 253–256, 262–268, 351–353
  in treatment evaluation, 256–258, 435, 437
Template analysis, 89, 696–697, 723
Temporal analysis, 89, 696, 697
Termination of leads, 200–201
Testing of ICD system, 223–248
  energy margins in, 240–245, 348–350
  in follow-up period, 403–406
  future trends in, 245–248, 759–760
  intraoperative, 344, 346–353

  lead assessment in, 254–255, 346–348, 394–398
  margin verification in, 236–237
  noninvasive, 759–760
  postoperative, 392–402
  predischarge, 392–393
  and programming, 234–240, 261–262
  telemetry in, 253–268, 351–353
  threshold assessment in, 237–240, 249
Third-generation devices, 283, 292, 510, 690–694, 718
  clinical results in, 496–498, 500–501
  sensing system of, 690–691, 734–736
Thoracic electrode systems, 120, 122–124
Thoracoscopy, 336, 417
Thoracotomy, 333–334, 472–476, 487
  complications in, 415, 416, 419
  postoperative care in, 389, 390
Thrombosis, venous, 428–429
Tiered therapy, 97, 207–220, 232–234, 734
  antiarrhythmic drugs in, 377
  clinical results in, 496–498
  rate zones in, 208–211, 463–465
Tilt, 135, 143, 151
  calculation of, 148, 149, 154–155
  and pulse duration, 144, 149–150
Tilt table test, 322
Train stimulation, ultrarapid, 285
Transplantation of heart, 10, 540, 542–543, 563–564, 565
Transvene device, 74, 182–183, 189, 471, 507–509
  clinical results in, 481–482, 483, 511
  complications in, 422
  fixation of, 202
  materials in, 188–189, 192, 193
  operative technique in, 339, 391–392
Transvenous systems, 119–124, 489, 751–752
  advantages of, 512, 693, 694, 752, 759
  in atrial cardioversion-defibrillation, 665–672, 680–683
  automated, 704
  clinical results in, 476–483, 494–496, 498, 500, 501
    in Europe, 507–513
    review of literature on, 511–512
  complications in, 389, 422, 752
  cost of, 565–567
  defibrillation energy in, 757
  in dual chamber pacing, 712
  efficacy of, 512, 567
  future of, 512–513, 565–567, 752, 757
  history of, 5, 8, 179, 182–183, 471
  implantation of, 337–344, 365, 490–491
    in laboratory, 357, 358, 360–361
  postoperative care in, 391–392
  preoperative assessment in, 323
  sensing function of, 196, 197
  single electrode, 365–375
  three electrode, 122–124
  two electrode, 119–122

Triggered activity, 14, 15–18, 271
Triphasic waveform, 154, 174
Troubleshooting, 353–354, 433–453
  telemetry in, 253–268, 435, 437
Truncation, 135, 149, 153–154
  of biphasic waveform, 166–174
  of monophasic waveform, 153–154, 164–166
  theory of, 138–144
  of triphasic waveform, 174

Underdrive pacing, 284–285, 651–652
Undersensing, 78, 79, 266–268, 353, 403–404, 756
  postshock, 215
  troubleshooting in, 444–445
Unipolar systems, 365–375
Upper limit of vulnerability, 46, 156, 157–159, 163, 246–247

Vasodilator drugs, 738, 741, 742, 743
Vena cava electrodes, 120, 121, 122–124, 179, 422, 511
Ventak devices, 253, 254, 255, 283
  clinical results in, 477, 481, 482, 483, 496, 511
    compared to drug therapy, 520
  data log of, 405
  ECD, 227, 229–231
  interaction with pacemaker, 386
  programming of, 457, 471
  sensing system of, 84–85, 86, 88, 386, 398
  support systems for, 227
  telemetered data from, 256, 257
  testing of, 351, 403, 404, 497
  troubleshooting of, 450
Ventricular fibrillation, 43–64
  automated rhythm system in, 702
  classification of, 719, 720
  contraindications to ICD therapy in, 306
  dual chamber pacing in, 718
  duration of, 58–61
    and defibrillation success, 56–58, 240, 350
  indications for ICD therapy in, 304, 305, 308
  induction of, 44–46, 49–50, 401–402, 585
  misdiagnosis of, 736
  natural history of, 577–579
  prevention of, 702
  sensing and detection of, 71–101
  testing of, with support device, 223–248
Ventricular tachycardia, 13–34
  antitachycardia pacing in, 271–296
  automated rhythm system in, 701
  catheter ablation in, 633–646
  chronic recurrent, 618

classification of, 719, 720, 721, 722, 723
clinical features of, 19, 616
contraindications to ICD therapy in, 305–306
and coronary artery disease, 615–629, 644, 645
drug therapy in, 30–31, 577–604
dual chamber pacing in, 718, 719
duration of, 460
history of, 317–318
indications for ICD therapy in, 304, 305, 308
induction of, 24–25, 398–401, 525–526, 616
mechanisms in, 13–16, 18, 616–617
morphology of, 19, 53–54, 460, 462–463
multiple, 467
natural history of, 577–579
noninducible, 616
nonsustained, 438, 466, 524–531, 561–562, 565
  trial on, 10, 310, 524, 526–531, 561
pathophysiology of, 617–619
programmed electrical stimulation in, 14–15, 16–18, 23, 24–27
  for induction, 24–25, 398, 525–526
sensing and detection of, 71–101
in structurally normal heart, 21, 32–33, 306, 639–644
surgery in, 29–30, 615–629
Ventriculotomy, 625
  encircling endocardial, 617, 622
Ventritex devices, 8, 254, 255, 328, 360
  antitachycardia pacing, 283, 393, 464, 471
  Cadence. See Cadence device
  High Voltage Stimulator, 227, 229, 232–234
  lead systems of, 179–181, 184, 330
  sensing systems of, 76, 79
Verapamil, 639, 643
Voltage gradient, 109, 131
Vulnerable period, 44–46, 246–247
  and upper limit of vulnerability, 46, 156, 157–159, 163, 246–247

Warfarin, 676–677, 678
Wave shape, 88–90, 153–174
  biphasic. See Biphasic waveform
  correlation analysis of, 88–89, 697, 699
  in dual chamber pacing, 722–724
  monophasic. See Monophasic waveform
  template analysis of, 89, 696–697
  triphasic, 154, 174
Wide QRS tachycardia, 21–22
Wound care, postoperative, 390–391